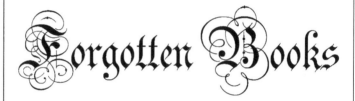

ISBN 978-0-266-99753-5
PIBN 11028599

1 MONTH OF
FREE
READING

at

www.ForgottenBooks.com

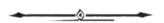

By purchasing this book you are eligible for one month membership to ForgottenBooks.com, giving you unlimited access to our entire collection of over 1,000,000 titles via our web site and mobile apps.

To claim your free month visit:
www.forgottenbooks.com/free1028599

English
Français
Deutsche
Italiano
Español
Português

www.forgottenbooks.com

Mythology Photography **Fiction**
Fishing Christianity **Art** Cooking
Essays Buddhism Freemasonry
Medicine **Biology** Music **Ancient**
Egypt Evolution Carpentry Physics
Dance Geology **Mathematics** Fitness
Shakespeare **Folklore** Yoga Marketing
Confidence Immortality Biographies
Poetry **Psychology** Witchcraft
Electronics Chemistry History **Law**
Accounting **Philosophy** Anthropology
Alchemy Drama Quantum Mechanics
Atheism Sexual Health **Ancient History**
Entrepreneurship Languages Sport
Paleontology Needlework Islam
Metaphysics Investment Archaeology
Parenting Statistics Criminology
Motivational

NEW ORLEANS

MEDICAL AND SURGICAL

JOURNAL.

VOLUME XVII.

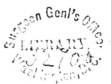

NEW ORLEANS:

PRINTED AT THE BULLETIN BOOK AND JOB OFFICE.

1860.

INDEX TO VOLUME XVII.

THE

NEW ORLEANS
MEDICAL AND SURGICAL JOURNAL.

JANUARY, 1860.

✓ ORIGINAL COMMUNICATIONS.

ART. I.—*On Inflammation:* By WARREN STONE, M. D., Professor of Surgery in the University of Louisiana. (Continued from the November number.)

In a former paper I attempted briefly to give a general idea of my views of inflammation embracing a range of conditions, from the highest degree of excitement, to the lowest degree of depression of the vital forces ; from a condition requiring depressing agents, to lower the excitement, to the condition requiring exciting ones to increase the vital forces.

In this paper I will endeavor to give my views of the action of therapeutic agents and of their adaptation to the various morbid conditions. The most distinct form of active inflammation in which active depressing treatment produces the most decided and unmistakeable good effect, is what is technically called orchitis, or inflammation of the testicle, simply because this inflammation takes place under circumstances favorable to the greatest excitement with the least modifying influences. This inflammation is seated in one of the most vital and highly organized organs ; it is most commonly the result of gonorrhœal inflammation of the urethra, and the fact that the subject has gonorrhœa, is pretty sure proof that his system is in a vigorous state. It is evident that the nature of the cause has nothing to do in giving character to the inflammation, for mechanical irritation, with consequent inflammation, produces the same effect, and it is transmitted through the course of the excretory duct to the testicle, showing itself first in the epididymis and from thence to the body of the testicle. It is fair to infer that even in this case, there is some predisposition in the system, some inappreciable state of the nervous system, which allows an irritation to result in inflammation, that otherwise would have caused some increased sensibility only. This disease is a painful one, and involves an important organ, and it becomes our duty to bring to bear the most effective agents for its cure, although there is very little doubt, but that, a large majority of these cases, if left to nature, would run their course, and finally terminate favorably. But the system would suffer more by the suffering and long confinement, independent of the risk of the permanent loss of the organ or its functions, than by the most active treatment. Bloodletting may not be absolutely necessary in this case (I am supposing one of the acutest forms), but it is a rule, that several agents, all having the same general tendency, but operating differently, will effect the end, with more certainty and with less violence than either one employed alone. Bloodletting to the proper extent relaxes the system, and mitigates all the symptoms, with the least possible injury, and followed with antimony tart., from an eighth to a quarter of a grain—according to the size and vigor of the patient—combined with half the quantity of morphia or an equivalent of opium every one, two or three hours, or so as to produce slight nausea, effects a cure in a few days with great certainty, and furnishes a beautiful illustration of the decided and unmistakeable good effects of these antiphlogistics. The pain ceases first, leaving only soreness, which in recent cases soon subsides, and the swelling gradually subsides. In some cases however, where the disease has had some days the start of the treatment, or from greater constitutional defect, the sensibility of the nerves of the part become more seriously disturbed, and when the acute excitement is subdued as far as the use of the above means can effect it, there still remains some degree of disease, as is shown by the continued soreness, and some degree of pains and the continuance, or perhaps the slow increase of the swelling, and this is usually termed chronic inflammation. In this condition the treatment should be changed to mercury, combined with opium, with a view to its specific effect, unless the diseased action is subdued before this effect is produced. I should remark that ptyalism is not the object, for the effect is just as certain without this effect, often· But we should watch for this effect, for it is evidence that the medicine has been pushed as far as it can be useful, and it is desirable to avoid disturbing the natural functions as much as possible. I should have mentioned that in the acute stage, if a purgative is admissible, a purgative or sedative dose of calomel is highly useful ; and for this purpose from ten to twenty grains are a proper dose. For the constitutional effect one grain of calomel combined with the fourth or a half a grain of opium three or four times a day will be proper. This quantity may be increased or diminished according to circumstances, or if it is desirable to obtain the speedy effect of mercury, it may be obtained by dropping half a grain of calomel in powder on the tongue every half hour or hour—or oftener if the urgency is great—and the effect will soon be obtained.

There is a difference of opinion as to the value of the different salts of mercury. Deference for the authority of Ricord, has brought into general use the iodides, but I prefer the old form, calomel or mild chloride as being more uniform in effect and less liable to lead to mistake. The prompt and almost certain effect which mercury has, when given in the manner and under the circumstances stated above, affords convincing proof of its great value in similar conditions whenever found.

We cannot study pathology, and therapeutics separately, with practical benefit. In our scientific pursuits it is proper that we should push our pathological investigations to the utmost minuteness in pursuit of new light, but practically we must take a less minute view, and confine ourselves to the conditions that can be described so as to be uniformly recognized and appreciated. Therapeutics can be studied in a general way, but we have no knowledge of their precise action upon the minute pathological conditions, and we must confine our investigations to the action of therapeutic agents to precise pathological conditions, or rather to conditions that can be recognized and described. When we learn what will cure one of these conditions, we have the knowledge of a law that we can apply to all similar conditions, wherever and under whatever name found.

The fact that mercury cures indurated chancres and indurated buboes, is proof that it will cure all other indurations that result from chronic or subacute inflammation. If it cures the syphilitic inflammation with the most certainty, it is not because it has any specific effect, but because the syphilitic induration is usually more simple and less likely to be modified by constitutional defects than those inflammations that arise spontaneously. In the case cited of the indurated testicle, and many others of as distinct a character, the effect is as prompt and certain, as in the case of chancre and bubo. Who will undertake to say what the precise action of mercury is in these cases? and yet it cannot be denied, but that we have obtained a law as valuable in practice as if we could explain the whole process.

There is some difference of opinion with regard to the local applications in the variety of inflammation under consideration. Local bleeding is in favor with many, who have discarded general bleeding. Local bleeding in the acute stage of inflammation does but little good unless it is made so free as to produce a general effect, which in children can be easily done. When the active state has been subdued and there is left passive engorgement, or in a case of what Andral would call passive hyperæmia, leeches or scarifications will do some good by way of disgorging and relieving the tension, but in the case in question, the testicle, there is no effect beyond the general one, for the organ, from its anatomical arrangement cannot be affected by it. There ought to be no difference of opinion with regard to the effect of warm and cold applications. In very acute cases, if cold can be steadily applied the sedative effect is highly favorable ; it diminishes pain and heat, leaves contraction of the vessels, etc., but the difficulty of proper application, the bad effect of frequent reactions, and the frequency of rigors, followed by feverish reaction, in our climate, make tepid applications, as a rule, preferable, and in the case mentioned above, I always use a soft cataplasm. Tepid applications relax the parts, favor transpiration, and generally soothe the irritated nerves of the part. This latter effect may be much improved by the addition of laudanum to the local application. Whatever calms the irritated nerves of an inflamed part without doing harm in other respects, does material good, and when we cannot use any powerful controling means we must be content to use anything that will assist nature if it is ever so little, and in truth, the small means should not be neglected in any case. We should bear in mind that a large majority of the cases, we are called upon to treat, would get well without treatment, and many more come so near it, that by a little assistance on our part, quite a number will terminate favorably ; so that while it becomes our duty, in some urgent and active cases, to use prompt and active measures, it behooves us to be on our guard, and limit our remedies to the requirements of the case.

There is a condition quite different from the one just described, for which a different treatment is called for ; and, perhaps, as a specimen, for the purpose of description, with which all are familiar, I will select diffuse cellular inflammation. This form of inflammation occurs occasionally in those of depraved habits ; but its character seems to me to be more generally determined by some epidemic influence, which operates either upon the fluids or solids, or both ; for, when it is prevalent, injuries or wounds upon those, with all the appearance of being in a vigorous, healthy state, will take on this form of inflammation. When it arises spontaneously, it is most likely to take place on the lower extremities, where the circulation is the most languid, and is opposed by the laws of gravitation. It is generally ushered in by rigors or a sense of chilliness ; the seat of the local determination is generally determined by an ulcer or some slight injury, and instead of being circumscribed, as in the case of sthenic or phlegmonous inflammation, it becomes diffused, and instead of the exudation of plastic lymph, it is followed by what Rokitansky calls croupus lymph, which, instead of organizing, it tends to break down and disintegrate the tissues in which it is exuded; or it may be of a more favorable character, and degenerate into impure pus, which, instead of being circumscribed, as in acute inflammation, is diffused in the tissues, or if it is on the surface, ulceration and phagedæna may be the result. In this condition we may find much perturbation of the system, but none of the conditions that would admit of treatment calculated to lower the vital forces permanently. However, on the principle laid down in a former paper, tartar emetic may be given in the early period of the attack, while the rigors are still present, or in the first period of excitement, before exudation has taken place. It may be given with opium, with a view of reducing the pulse, promoting perspiration, and obtaining the peculiar effect of the antimony on the capillary circulation; or it may be given with a view of obtaining its more active effect, that of emesis. Emetics, I am fully aware, should be given with care in such critical conditions, where their action may be good or bad, according as they are properly timed or otherwise, but in certain conditions offending matter may be dislodged, and the circulation of the important abdominal viscera is aroused, and their functions rendered more active and healthy. But antimony, however given, should not be used to produce permanent depression. After the use of the antimony, and free perspiration and relaxation are produced, a full dose of quinine will generally produce a fine effect by promoting or prolonging the sweating, and by the peculiar stimulant effect which quinine has upon the capillaries, tending to prevent or counteract stasis or congestion. Calomel, although its constitutional action is always bad in inflammations that tend to the exudation of croupus or aplastic lymph, may often be given for its local effect on the stomach and digestive organs. It is important in most of these cases to be able to supply the blood with fresh and healthy nutrient matter; but it is frequently, and in fact most commouly in those cases, that the stomach is in no condition to receive nutriment, there being generally engorgement of the mucous membrane and perverted function, which calomel is well calculated to relieve. It is not unfrequent that we find the patient occasionally vomiting a dark green or some unnatural secretion—not constantly, as if there was irritation or inflammation, but occasionally, as if the stomach was secreting its own emetic; for when the fluid is discharged by emesis there is entire relief until the morbid secretion accumulates again. In this condition small and frequently repeated doses of calomel will soon change this morbid secretion, as will be shown by the arrest of the vomiting and by the general relief, as will be shown by the lowering of the pulse in frequency, and an increase in volume. It is at least useless to throw stimulants and nutriment into a stomach in this condition, and it may be injurious. The prostration that is often manifested under these circumstances is more apparent than real, and the system usually rallies under the treatment that is calculated to relieve it.

I will relate a case to illustrate my views. In May last I amputated the thigh of a negro man, for a chronic disease of his knee joint. He had been confined for a long time, but had not suffered severely, and although he had not the normal supply of blood, he was not much reduced in flesh. The double flap operation was made. Chloroform was used, but it produced considerable nausea; and although the stump seemed unusually sensitive, the patient preferred suffering pain during the dressing to breathing chloroform. The small vessels were very much enlarged, requiring an unusual number of ligatures, and there was a hæmorrhagic tendency. The vessels were finally all secured; and after waiting until all oozing had ceased, the flaps were brought together. There was considerable perturbation of the system; pulse 120, and there were unusual pain and a tendency to vomit. Two grains of solid opium were ordered, half a grain of morphia having been given before the dressings were applied, and stimulants, if they could be borne. The patient thought he could relish champagne wine, and it was given. I left him in charge of Dr. Morrison, the house surgeon of my infirmary; and on returning, in about three hours, I found that hæmorrhage had taken place, the dressings of the stump were filled to their utmost with coägulated blood, and there was a considerable loss in the bed. The patient was suffering severely; his pulse was 160 in the minute, and there were frequent and copious vomitings of a dark secretion. The dressings were removed, and it was found that the blood came from the surface of the wound generally. Ice was applied to the stump, and soon arrested the flow; but the condition of the patient appeared extremely unpromising. The patient being reduced in the beginning, and having lost a large amount of blood, both as the immediate consequence of the amputation and subsequently, was in great need of nutriment, but nothing that had been administered rested on his stomach. I ordered two grains of calomel to be placed on his tongue every hour (and at first oftener, until two or three doses were given), until twelve grains were given. The stump was dressed, after having been exposed to the air about four hours. Before all the calomel had been given, the vomiting had ceased, and the pulse had subsided thirty beats. After the calomel was all taken I ordered sulph. magnesia $\mathfrak{z}$i, spts. mindereri $\mathfrak{z}$iv, water $\mathfrak{z}$iv, in a mixture; an ounce to be given every half hour until the bowels were acted upon, which required nearly the whole. A large quantity of dark, tarry secretion was discharged. The perturbation subsided, and the pulse was reduced to 100. Lime water and milk was ordered, which was relished very much; and in a few hours he called for food, and would have relished anything that might have been given him. He continued to nourish finely, and the flaps united so completely by the first intention that the first dressings were not removed until the tenth day.

Those who saw this patient at the worst, thought him hopeless, and so he would have been if his stomach had not been relieved, so that nourishment and stimulants could be received. The excitability of this patient, the disagreement of the chloroform, and I believe the opium, together with great pain and loss of blood, all contributed to produce the great engorgement of the mucous surface of the stomach and bowels, which produced the apparent exhaustion.

The shock of the first onset of an extensive inflammation often produces similar results; and if it does not disappear with the reäction, it ought to be treated as above, that we may have the full use of the assimilating organs, by which we can introduce the proper supports to the system. In an inflammation, when we can afford to pull down, no great skill is required in the management; but when we are required to build up and lend force to the vital actions, much delicacy is required in the management. Having done what we can in the onset to overcome the morbid process, or rather to give it a fovorable start, and prepared the system to receive our assistance, we can properly begin with such means as will best sustain the vital forces, and thereby prevent disorganization.

As a tonic, the muriated tincture of iron is favorable in this condition, as well as in the more specific form of inflammation—erysipelas. It not only acts as a tonic, but it probably has a favorable effect upon the blood, and it certainly has a marked influence on the capillary circulation, when there is passive engorgement, and I am convinced that it tends to lessen the exudation. When the general condition requires stimulants, in the earlier stage at least, carb. ammoniæ is far preferable to alcoholic stimulants. It appears to act upon the mucous system in a peculiar way, and does not much excite the heart's action, while it improves the capillary circulation. Alcoholic stimulants may be admissible in a later stage, when a more potent action is required, or when, what is frequently the case, the patient prefers it from previous habit. I think it is a law of the animal economy, that whatever the general condition of the system requires will be proper for any local condition, and that whenever the alcoholic stimulant is grateful to the senses of the patient, the local derangement will be benefited by it.

Local stimulants, where they can be applied, are often very useful in this form of inflammation; and of this class of remedies I prefer the tinct. of iodine, which can be easily applied and graduated, and when it can be brought to act near the parts involved, it gives a healthier action and a more favorable termination. This form of inflammation may be taken as the type of what may be termed the active form of the asthenic kind; and for the chronic or subacute kind, syphilitic inflammation presents a fair type. We have shown that the indurated variety presents a type of the chronic or subacute variety of asthenic inflammation, and the ulcerative the corroding or phagedenic varieties form a fair type of the asthenic variety. We are in the habit of considering these cases as mere ulcers, but they are the effect of a poison, and the reaction from any cause, whether mechanical or chemical, or an unknown poison, is an inflammation, provided it is so great as to produce exudation. In the indurated variety the exuded lymph is plastic and organizes, while in the phagedenic variety the exuded lymph is of the aplastic or croupus variety, and instead of being organized, it serves only to disintegrate and break down the tissue, producing ulceration, or this process may be more rapid and extensive, and produce sloughing. We also see an intermediate condition, in which the first effect of the poison is to produce a more or less destruction of tissue, but it neither takes on induration nor ulceration, and the recuperative process goes on much better if it is left to nature, or with only such dressings as protect it from mechanical disturbance, than if subjected to the treatment appropriate to either of the extremes. This is a type of many cases of inflammation which we meet with, to which the dietetic system of treatment is properly adapted.

I will not attempt to determine whether these different syphilitic ulcers are the result of different poisons, or different constitutions to which the poison is applied. We certainly see effects quite as different when produced by mechanical causes, when it is very certain that the difference is determined by the temperament. Practically we have to deal with conditions, and even in syphilis, in our treatment we have to keep in view the condition, and guard against being influenced by the name or cause. The treatment in this subacute variety of asthenic inflammation is as plain in its general nature as in the sthenic, although the result is not so marked and certain. In general we have to support the vital forces, allay irritation, and improve the condition of the blood, although we occasionally see a condition of phagedæna bordering on the character of the more acute form, in which antimony combined with opium may be proper. Charmichael, who gave the best classification and treatment of venereal up to his time, speaks of the great good effects in acute phagedæna of tart.

antim., and it will be found that the principle holds good in the same
condition from other causes. I do not mean that it can be given at
random or carelessly in all cases of phagedæna, but when there is
great morbid sensibility in the part, with a marked border of redness
and heat, tart. antimony combined with opium quiet nervous irritation
and the pulse, and diminish local excitement, and consequently the
phagedænic process. The effect, of course, must be watched, and care
taken not to continue so as to disturb permanently the stomach, or
to depress the vital forces. In the use of tart. antimony it is always
safe, so long as we produce no effects that will not subside in the
usual time after omitting its use.

But in general we have only to support and assist nature by the
judicious use of tonics, narcotics, and nutriment. To nourish properly it is not only necessary to furnish healthy and appropriate nutriment, but to see if the digestive apparatus is in condition to furnish
healthy blood out of it. The source must be pure if we would have
the fountain clear. This is not sufficiently kept in view in the treatment of chronic diseases, and more particularly of the class where
the impurity of the blood is one of the causes. A remedy that may
be very good in itself had better be omitted if it disturbs the stomach;
and, as a rule, the use of medicine should not be allowed to interfere
with the nutrition, as the most wholesome, sure, and permanent tonic
is pure and natural nutritive matter.

In many of these conditions we would not purge for the purpose
of depletion, or give mercury for its constitutional effects, and yet we
may use the remedies for the purpose of disembarrassing the digestive apparatus, and enabling it to perform its functions more perfectly.
We may sometimes administer remedies that either improve the blood
by a direct chemical action, or by acting upon the excretory functions,
and thereby depurating it. The iodide of potass. is by many used in
this condition, but I am perfectly satisfied that this valuable medicine
is appropriate to the same sthenic condition as mercury; and although
it may be tolerated in other cases, yet in distinct phagedæna its
effects are injurious. The chlorate of potass. has a different and, in
some cases, a very remarkable good effect, improving the hue of the
skin and the organic actions in the most marked manner. I do not
pretend to say how it acts, and I do not know that I can point out
distinctly the condition in which its action is required, or is the most
appropriate. There is a dirty yellowness of the skin, and a state of

the system bordering on the scorbutic, but not it, and if there is not phagedæna, the lymph that is exuded falls stillborn and does not organize, and, in fact, there is not action enough, good or bad, to entitle it to the appellation of inflammation. The effect is seen very soon, and in three or four days the change in hue is marked, the patient brightens up, and the ulcer assumes a healthy appearance. In all cases of phagedæna I think the effect of this salt is good ; but in the kind I have alluded to, it is the most marked. The truth is, where the natural condition is so much at fault, we cannot expect to do so much as when the disease is more simple in character, as in sthenic disease. This salt, as a medicine, was first brought into special notice in the treatment of cancrum oris, a peculiar inflammation in which the exudation of croupous lymph is abundant, which seems to act like a poison, corroding the parts, and it is found valuable in diphtheritic inflammation.

It is reasonable to suppose—indeed, it is quite certain—that these blood-poisons vary in character, and that the same remedy is not equally effective in all, and a wide field for observation is open to us. We should furnish reasons for what we do in medicine, as far as possible, and apply our remedies according to known laws ; but after all our research, we must yield something to empiricism, and use some remedies, simply because we know them to be good in certain conditions, without knowing why.

Opium may be made use of in this form of inflammation in some cases, but I think it will be found that it is more adapted to the more sthenic form, where the solids are the most affected, than in the lower grades, where the blood is so often at fault, and where the nerve force is lessened. In some conditions the action of opium favors congestion, and it is undoubtedly unfavorable to the elimination of the blood by excretion. Its local action, however, is always good when there is increased sensibility.

These may be considered the extremes of the two forms of sthenic and asthenic inflammation; and as there is nothing specific in their characters, we may expect to find all the intermediate grades, which often make so near an approach in character as to leave the practitioner in doubt whether he had not better look on and watch the progress, rather than risk interference. Some of the most formidable inflammations mankind is afflicted with no doubt derive their character from some epidemic or atmospheric influence. Either extreme of heat or cold, long continued, predisposes the system, so that sudden changes will readily excite inflammatory action, and when thus induced, it mostly falls upon those organs that sympathize with the external surface, the lungs or stomach and bowels. Dr. James Johnson, whose "zeal evidently was not according to knowledge," did much harm by inculcating the doctrine of cutaneo-hepatic sympathy, in his work on Tropical Climates. However, it does not need argument at this time to prove that the internal or mucous surface is the tissue that sympathizes with the external surface naturally, and that among the other organs that under strong predisposition may be excited to inflammation by sudden depression of temperature, the liver is the last. The disturbances that are attributed to the liver under these circumstances belong to the mucous membrane of the stomach and upper portion of the small intestines ; but I may speak of this in another place.

It is well known that long-continued exposure to a low temperature alters the blood, and brings about a scorbutic condition. After a winter of unusually steady cold weather in the North, pneumonia usually prevails when spring begins to open and sudden changes begin to take place. It is a fact that I believe is not generally observed, that in the South, after a long and steadily hot summer, the same scorbutic condition is found, and pneumonia is often prevalent, more particularly among the slave population on plantations, where the sameness of habit and diet are likely to give greater effect to the influence of climate. This is no theory, but a fixed fact, which I have long pointed out to the students at the Charity Hospital. On resuming my service in the hospital, in the fall, I always find more or less scurvy in my wards, and I have observed that the amount depends upon the heat of the previous summer, and if any other element acts as a cause, I have not been able to discover it. The scurvy is not confined to patients who have been in the hospital through the summer, but they are often brought in with it ; and in many cases, where the condition is not very apparent, it may be observed that the color is not healthy, and on examining the lower extremities petechial spots will be found. Nothing can be done with local disease without first attending to this general state. Dysenteries occasionally occur with this class, and will recover under the use of malt liquor, potash salts, fresh vegetable diet, salads with mustard and vinegar, when they would continue to run down under the best regulated medication. This effect of climate may be counteracted in a great measure by regulating the diet and drinks. Subacid fruit of all kinds is of the utmost importance in the South in the summer season ; and if our population would abridge their injurious luxuries, and devote the sum thus saved to the purchase of fruits and the encouragement of their cultivation, they would lose nothing in the enjoyment of luxuries, and contribute very much to health and comfort.

The greatest blessing that can happen to this country would be the introduction of grape culture to the extent that would supply the demand for light subacid wines. It would not only drive alcoholic drinks mainly out of use, but supply a healthful and invigorating beverage, and no doubt, when once established, it would furnish the cultivator a proper remuneration at a reasonable price for the wine.

The pneumonias of the South no doubt derive characteristics from epidemics that precede them, at least when this disease assumes the form of an epidemic. I do not know how it is at the North, but it is beginning to attract attention ; and Dr. Stokes, in a discourse on Clinical Medicine, published in the Dublin Hospital Gazette of December last, refers to it. He says : "Under the action of epidemic and endemic influences, the purely local and accidental diseases take on some, at least, of the character of the essential conditions ; and I believe it will yet be found that a large number of cases of disease hitherto classed as purely local affections—simple inflammations, if you will—not supposed to have relation to fever, or any other essential condition, will turn out to be, in reality, only examples of diseases secondary to a fever, arising, as it were, unconformably—that is, at a period much earlier than is the rule, and by the operation of some law still obscure to us, causing or followed by the disappearance of the general malady. This I offer with diffidence ; but every day increases my belief that many cases of apparently local and accidental diseases are but examples of aborted fevers, and that they are endued with more or less of the character of the parent or antecedent affection, which has disappeared so mysteriously." The connection of the local diseases of winter, with the general diseases of summer and fall, has long been understood in the South and West, but it has, perhaps, attracted too little attention in a practical point of view. Those who depend upon observation, without research into the true nature of these forms of pneumonia, are too much inclined to generalize, and to consider that when they have succeeded in treating one epidemic with success, that they have no more to learn,

when it is probable that the next epidemic will present modifications
so material that the same treatment will be attended with quite different results ; but those who have examined well into the true nature
and character of the different forms, and the various causes that tend
to modify them, and who have studied well the language and signs
of diseased conditions, will be prepared to treat rationally any new
form of disease, and in a short experience will be able to direct their
remedies with comparative accuracy.

A friend, who has a large plantation, and who has, as a near neighbor, a good physician, whom he pays liberally by the year, told me
the other day that he had had pneumonia prevailing on his place, as
a winter disease, for a year or two, but that he managed it himself
by the Thompsonian system and quinine. He at first gave an emetic
of lobelia, and then composition tea, which threw the sick into a copious
perspiration, after which a dose or two of quinine, which prevented
the return of fever. This gentleman, like many more learned in the
prefession, no doubt found pneumonia where it did not exist, very
often, and took credit for curing what would have done quite as well
without treatment in some cases, but no doubt many of his cases
would have resulted in serious pneumonia, and that his treatment
answered well ; but I do not think it adapted to all forms and varieties, any more than the active antiphlogistic or the stimulating treatment, or the let-alone method, all of which may be appropriate in
turn. The above treatment answered well where the disease was
ushered in with a chill, of the character of an intermittent, and where
the local disease is secondary, as is generally the case under like circumstances. The uniform success was due, no doubt, in a great
measure to the fact, that the cases were all considered pneumonia,
and the proper care and protection against exposure for a proper
time were afforded. The local disease is too often overlooked on
plantations until it is so far advanced that the best directed treatment
is not of much service. It is in the early stage of pneumonia that
active means can be used, and it is only in the sthenic form that it
can be continued into the second stage.

Whatever may be said of the asthenic character of spontaneous
inflammation, we do meet with pneumonia and pleuro-pneumonia of
an active character in which plastic lymph is exuded, and which
require active treatment ; and these cases are becoming more common than they were ten or twelve years ago, which is due no

doubt to the change in the general character of inflammation. When we see disease only in an isolated manner and occasionally, changes are not so perceptible, and we find, after a term of years, that our treatment is quite different in many respects from what it was formerly, and we are in doubt whether the change is from the gradual requirements of disease under the principles in which we were educated, or whether we have changed our principles of treatment.

When seen on a large scale, disease can be more correctly compared at different periods. We have always had a large number of cases of penetrating and gunshot wounds in the Charity Hospital, implicating the great cavities of the trunk, and where the result often depends upon the character of the inflammation that follows. In wounds of hollow organs the safety depends upon healthy adhesive inflammation, or the exudation of plastic lymph which will organize and cause an adhesion of the wounded organ to the surface it may be in contact with, and in this manner prevent the escape of any of its contents into the serous cavity. Ten years ago almost every case of penetrating wound of the abdomen involving the intestines was fatal, from inflammation; and post mortem examinations showed the exudation of croupous lymph, soft, and loosely attached to the serous surfaces, or floating in the whey-like effusion—the wound in the intestine being open and free and more or less of the contents of the bowels found in the peritoneal cavity, rendering recovery impossible.

Within the last four or five years a change for the better has taken place; and, for the last two or three years, it is rare to see a fatal case for the want of adhesive inflammation to agglutinate the wounded organ to its opposing surface, and thus preventing the escape of its contents. This change, I believe, will soon be recognized in spontaneous or idiopathic inflammations, and more active treatment will be found proper.

I have before remarked that tart. antimony is proper in all the forms of pneumonia, but that it must be given with care in the asthenic form, and that it is more important in the sthenic form, in which it may be given through the first stage. Bloodletting, also, can be resorted to with advantage in many cases, and in some cases where the symptoms are not very active. I do not urge it, however, as a means that is often imperiously called for, but as one often useful, and that can be used with safety even to relieve plethory and the duty of the lungs. If the inflammation runs into the second stage or that of hepatization, mercury becomes useful on the same principle that it is useful in other inflammations that result in induration or the exudation of plastic lymph. More care and judgment, however, are necessary in the use of mercury in the second stage than in the use of tart. antimony in the first. The effect of the latter is immediate; we can readily tell by the pulse and general condition when we should stop its use ; and, when discontinued, the effect soon disappears ; but in the use of mercury it is important that we should be quite certain of the condition before resorting to its use—for the effect is slow and gradual, and if it should prove injurious the effect does not cease with its omission.

It is quite certain, however, that it is quite proper and useful in cases of red hepatization and injurious in the gray. I will not undertake to point out the precise symptoms by which the appropriate condition for mercury can be distinguished, but the activity of the general symptoms in distinct cases will leave but little doubt. I have said, elsewhere, that where there is doubt it is better to withhold it.

There is no disease, I believe, in which a fixed routine treatment operates so badly as in pneumonia; and those who have continued the old plan of bleeding, when thought admissible, and giving tart. antimony in the first stage, and calomel in the second stage, have been the most dangerous routinists. The prevalent form undoubtedly has been asthenic, and some years ago death often took place from engorgement and effusion before exudation had taken place. I have seen, however, many cases within the last few years, more generally among the slave population, who are in tolerably vigorous health and have had the disease forced upon them by great and careless exposure, in which active treatment became necessary.

It is not my purpose, however, to write a treatise on pneumonia. every one has to acquire whatever is practical himself, and I have aimed to give a few facts and hints in the hope that they may assist some one in his observations.

There are some other special inflammations, however, that I will refer to. Endo-carditis and peri-carditis, as they appear so often in children, accompanied or preceded by the peculiar muscular rheumatism, can generally, if seen, be detected early. There seems to be no fixed plan of treatment adopted by the profession. Some rely upon the saline or alkaline treatment, and others rely upon calomel and opium, local bleeding, blisters, etc. The attention is usually called early to this disease by the accompanying rheumatism, which is generally attended with excruciating pain although with but little swelling. When this is accompanied with great perturbation of the heart and a very frequent pulse, this organ is very certainly implicated, and it would be an unpardonable fault to wait for the usual physical signs (which only appear when the mischief is done) before resorting to active means. There can be no doubt of the great value of mercury in checking the exudation of lymph which nearly always takes place, and even in favoring its absorption, but it has been found difficult to obtain its effect. Within the last few years I have had a number of these cases, some early and some after exudation, and murmurs and friction sound were present, and I have commenced with both mercury and salines, usually the acetate of potass. as it can be given more freely. To allay pain and control excitement I have uniformly given tart. antimony and morphine in equal parts, in doses adapted to the age of the patient, and repeated as often as required to control the pain and procure rest. With this treatment, I have generally obtained the mercurial effect very soon. The effect of the mercury is probably much assisted by the relaxing effect of the antimony, and it may be assisted by the saline. In many cases, where the exudation of lymph is recent, I am sure that these prompt measures cause its absorption, and obviate in a great measure the evil that would otherwise be entailed.

In the case of a young friend, last year, who was most violently attacked with this species of rheumatism, with great perturbation of the heart, the pulse being 150 per minute, this treatment, actively pursued, gave entire relief in about sixty hours. Slight mercurial action was produced, and all the symptoms had vanished.

In a case two years ago, where the disease had some days' start (exudation and pericardial effusion had taken place), the effect of this treatment was striking. The little patient could not bear to have his limbs moved ; breathing became difficult ; the heart's action was obstructed by the effusion, until it was thought death was inevitable ; but this treatment soon brought about slight mercurial action, when the symptoms began to subside, and in a few days loud friction sound was heard over the whole cardiac region. But the circulation was very good, and I found that she did not apparently suffer any inconvenience after she recovered her strength.

The uterus is another organ that deserves special notice, on account of the importance of the organ, the frequency with which it is subject to inflammation, and the improper treatment it is subjected to by the specialists. Notwithstanding the numerous volumes that have been written, to magnify, multiply and mystify the diseases of this organ, and to establish the most barbarous and unscientific modes of treatment, the diseases of the uterus will be found very simple, and nearly all embraced in the term, inflammation. The uterus, like the male organs of generation, rarely takes a diseased action spontaneously, but from its great and frequent exposure to mechanical irritation and other abuses it is far more liable to inflammation. The acute form of inflammation is the least common and is generally understood, but the chronic and subacute forms are usually taken for some undefinable diseased condition, and the whole catalogue of caustics, from the mild to the potential, is arrayed against it. The truth is, that subacute inflammation of the uterus results in the same changes that are produced in other organs of analogous structure, and is modified in like manner, by constitutional peculiarities. In one diathesis it results in induration, and in another in engorgement, as it is usually called. But it is attended by the exudation of lymph, and a kind of hypertrophy. These two conditions are very well represented by the indurated and what is termed the sympathetic bubo. The lymphatic ganglia are subject to inflammation from other causes than venereal poison, and, when persisted in, results in the above conditions. The difference evidently is determined by the diathesis. What is termed the sympathetic bubo presents a spongy, engorged condition, with more or less exudation, which organizes imperfectly, and sometimes disentegrates the tissues, and is properly treated by local stimulants and constitutional treatment that is calculated to increase the nerve force and improve the function of nutrition, while the induration may be treated with mercury and iodide of potass.

We find in the uterus, as we do in subacute inflammation of other tissues, occasionally the extreme conditions, but more frequently the intermediate shades. In the strongly marked indurated condition a gentle mercurial course followed by the iodide of potass. relieves with as much certainty as in any other inflammatory induration. Tepid local applications, in form of half bath, or injections, are far better than cold, although I find that the latter is generally ordered. The cold is followed by reäction and an unpleasant sense of heat, while the warm gives a sense of comfort at the time, promotes secretion, and is not followed by reäction.

It is a subject of astonishment to me that, in this age, it should be thought proper to apply the actual cautery—caustic potass. etc.—to this condition of the uterus. There is as much propriety in applying a caustic to the testicle to cure the result of inflammation. In the other extreme, when the organ is enlarged, more or less tender and soft, and spongy to the touch, the local applications are more appropriate, but not of the potent character mentioned above. The comp. tinct. of iodine is adapted to more cases than any one other stimulant, 'even the universal nitrate of silver. If there are any superficial ulcerations, or others (which I insist are rare), and there seems to be inflammation of the mucous covering particularly, the nitrate of silver may be preferable ; but, in my experience, it is best to make the application of less strength than is usual. Many apply it in substance, others in strong solution, but I am sure it is best of the strength of from ten to twenty grains to the ounce, as a proper wash for the surface, and for more potent applications to effect the deeper parts, the iodine is preferable, because greater effect is produced upon the capillaries of the deep parts with less irritatien of the surface. In some spongy conditions, with less tenderness, a strong solution of the salt alum, ammonia and iron or the perchloride of iron, does well.

Something may be done by constitutional treatment. The muriated tinct. of iron, by some, is as universally given in chronic uterine affections as mercury used to be in supposed affections of the liver, and with as little regard to the nature of the affection. It is, however, often of much service in this condition, by its action on the capillary circulation, and by its general effects as a tonic. Whatever improves the nutritive process and furnishes the system with a proper supply of healthy blood, does more to allay irritability and irritation than all the nicely concocted nervines in use.

In some cases that approach in character the sthenic form, the iodide of potass. is useful, and it may be that mercury may be given, at least for the benefit of the general condition. Ulceration by some is always found, or nearly so, in these cases—but it.is a deception ; and similar conditions of the mucous surface may be seen far more frequently by looking in the throat of patients complaining of these parts. It has so happened that I have seen a large number of chronic cases of disease, both from the city and surrounding country, and it is probable that I have seen a due proportion of chronic affections of the uterus, and I do not recollect that I ever treated a patient especially for an ulcer upon the uterus, except to palliate in malignant disease.

It is not uncommon for a patient to state that she had been treated for several months for an ulcer on her uterus, and that the doctor pronounced her cured, but her feelings continued the same. Seeing so many who have been treated in various parts of the country, I have been surprised at the uniform and prevailing system practised, of looking for ulcers, finding them invariably, and treating them with caustic. The term of treatment, too, is unusual for the cure of ordinary sized ulcers : it usually lasts until the patient or the doctor gets tired ; and then, if the symptoms do not disappear, some other cause is found for them, and a change of air or some watering-place is advised.

A well-marked case of indurated uterus was presented to me last year, in a middle-aged lady, who had given birth to four children in rather rapid succession, but had not been pregnant for six years, on account of uterine disease. The last treatment was for ulcers, and she submitted to the stereotyped course for several months, when the ulcers were pronounced cured ; but feeling no better, she concluded that she had cancer of the womb. I found a plain induration, considerable enlargement, and tenderness. I ordered a grain of calomel three times a day at first, but after a few days gave it only twice a day ; and as she was somewhat anæmic from causes that it is not necessary to enumerate here, I ordered the potassio-tart. of iron. In due time the slight effect of mercury was perceived, when it was discontinued, and eight grains of the iodide of potass. were ordered three times a day. The condition of the uterus was improving, diminishing in size, and becoming softer, when, about six weeks from the commencement of the treatment, other and unusual symptoms for her complaint manifested themselves, which I decided to be signs of pregnancy. The lady would not believe it, partly because she did not wish to, and partly because she thought it impossible ; but time proved that I was correct.

Another case of the opposite condition came under my advice. The lady had a delicate constitution, and though not decidedly scrofulous, she was subject to an affection of the throat, hoarseness, etc., and although not very thin of flesh, there was poverty of blood. She had been married several years, but had never been pregnant, and since her marriage had been mostly under treatment. When I saw her first she had been deprived of exercise for two years, as it was thought to be injurious to her, and she said that she could not take exercise on account of the pain and fatigue. I found the uterus enlarged, and rather soft to the touch, but not much tender, and I could not find in the uterus sufficient reason for her confinement, more particularly as her general condition required exercise so much. I advised her to begin exercise in the open air, according to her strength, and ordered cod liver oil in porter, to furnish more and better blood. She complained at first of the exercise, and said that it increased her pain, but I was satisfied that the uterus had but little to do with it, and on questioning she acknowledged that she often suffered as much when she had been entirely at rest. She continued and increased her exercise, improved in health and strength, and in proportion her uterine symptoms subsided. She took some tincture of iron, and as she suffered some from dysmenorrhœa, which I took to be of a rheumatic character, I gave some guaiac with benefit. The main treatment, however, was simply calculated to establish a healthy supply of blood, and it succeeded so well that she became pregnant in the course of six or eight months. This case, perhaps, ought not properly to be called inflammatory, but the importance of attention to the general health is well illustrated by it, and it is equally important in most of the inflammations of a low grade, and it also shows the value of giving nature full scope, and limiting our treatment to giving aid to her resources over arbitrary interference.

ART. II.—*Diphtheria :** By S. L. BIGELOW, M. D., of Paris ; communicated in a Letter to Professor WARREN STONE, M. D., of the University of Louisiana.

MY DEAR DOCTOR : I have committed myself in a recent letter to you, in answer to your kind favor of August 26th, in which you asked me

* DR. DOWLER : *Dear Sir*—The accompanying communication, on the subject of Diphtheria, from Dr. Bigelow, of Paris, was kindly furnished at my request. When in Paris a year ago, I had some conversation with the doctor on the subject, and finding the disease in our city on my return, I to give you my views upon Diphtheria, membranous sore throat, or angine couenneuse, by promising to do so when circumstances would permit.

I assure you that I feel great diffidence in commencing this task at this epoch, when since two years this is the subject which has held, perhaps, the first place in medical discussion and observation among the highest medical intelligences in the world. What I have to say will be strictly confined to my own personal views upon the subject. This may seem to you presumptuous on my part, and following too closely the letter of your request, ignoring the spirit of it ; but, on the other hand, it would be equally absurd for me to compile a natural history of the disease from documents written by able men during the past two years, which have been accessible to yourself and to other members of the medical profession in America and elsewhere.

So you will understand, my dear doctor, that I have no idea of giving a history of the disease to a novice in medicine, but my own views upon certain capital points in the disease *per se*, and in its relation to membranous croup, to a veteran in the corps (of which I am but a recruit), who knows both diseases better than myself, and will understand those views without description of the diseases in question. I have, then, but ideas to offer in outline, and will be brief.

In the first place I will tell you, as well as I can in words, some of the differences which exist, in my opinion, between the two diseases, membranous croup and angine couenneuse, but some of them are only to be seized by the high faculties of the mind—words can only hint at those points which the reason alone can feel. In one word, it can be felt, but not expressed in its essence.

Firstly, Do you understand what I mean when I say that for me the same relative position exists between these two diseases as exists between the intermittent fevers with which you are so conversant in your part of the country and throughout the United States, and the Syrian or Roman forms of intermittent fevers ? A difference in the intensity of the poison or ferment certainly, and most probably also in its nature, between the croup and diphtheria, and your congestive fever and intermittent, would be an exaggeration.

---

wrote to Dr. Bigelow, and requested as a favor his experience in this destructive malady. No better authority could be appealed to ; for he is an American, and received an American practical education, and then resorted to Paris, to perfect himself, where he has settled in full practice and intimate relation with the leading members of the profession. I trust you will find it a valuable contribution.   Yours, very truly,

                                              WARREN STONE, M. D.

In the second place—and this is less transcendental, if you will pass me the word, than my first proposition—the croup, uncomplicated, kills the patient in but one way—by suffocation. The angine couenneuse, uncomplicated, may produce death in three ways : first, during the acute period of the disease, by suffocation ; and after the disappearance of all membranous exudation in the larynx, even months after, by the effects of the poison or fermènt exhibited in the progressive paralysis which almost always follows the recovery from the acute period of the disease, or by asthenia during an intermediate period. Of this peculiar difference between the two diseases, the consecutive progress in paralysis, I will write more at length later, for to my mind it constitutes an essential point.

In the third place, the croup is a disease which is almost exclusively confined to children, whereas the angine couenneuse attacks indiscriminately children, adolescents, and adults. You may say that this is a loose proposition. True, it cannot be proved by words to difference the natures of the two diseases, but it seems to me that mental discrimination must give the fact an important place in instituting a parallel between them.

I am about touching upon a ground, in my fourth proposition, which is so covered with eggs that I hardly dare try to cross it on tiptoe ! You will appreciate my hesitation if you remember certain of our conversations together while you were in Paris, when I whisper in your ear that word which is to my mind what *bile* is to the mind of the community at large, a scapegoat for the generality of Nature's medical mysteries, contagion. Knowing my sentiments fully upon this subject, you may be disposed to regard the few words I have to offer upon this point as more serious than you would if they came from a contagious sectarian; for you know that I don't believe that a medical *sectarian* can be a sound man, any more than I do that a *religious* sectarian can be a religious man. The croup occurs frequently sporadically, more frequently as an epidemic, but I think few are disposed seriously to consider that it is ever propagated by mediate contagion. Diphtheria *rarely* occurs as a sporadic disease, almost invariably as an epidemic, and now, my dear Doctor, I shut my eyes and make my profession of belief, if there exists a mediately *contagious* disease on earth it is the angine couenneuse, and that the epidemics of this disease are, or may be contagious epidemics. I admit this belief by no means losing sight of atmospheric influences,

which are greater, in my opinion, than all others in the development
and propagation of the disease, but simply to acknowledge that I
believe it to be endowed with a highly contagious element. This is
an opinion founded upon the fairest observation of which I am capable, and by no means a theoretical convenience.

My fifth proposition regards the mode of invasion of the two diseases. Membranous croup commences insidiously, and ordinarily
several days elapse before the symptoms awaken serious apprehensions in the minds of those who surround the patient. The angine
couenneuse, on the other hand, enters upon the field with a certain
conquering magistry, as a general rule, which leaves no time for
parley. The first symptoms are ordinarily, with the exception of the
soreness of the throat, those which announce an invasion of typhoid
fever, general lassitude (the patient expresses it better than I can in
classical professional language by informing you that he feels sick all
over), to which are added pains in the head, back, and limbs, accompanied by a febrile movement for the most part quite intense. The disease
carries the typhoid type with it, if you will permit me the expression,
throughout its entire course, and, if possible, this element is more
marked during the convalescence, which is always an affair of several
months, than during the acute period of the disease. In your letter
to me, announcing your sad affliction for the death of your dear
boy from this disease, you made a remark which proved to me again
your high medical sagacity, for you had seen but two or three cases
as yet in New Orleans from which to form your opinion. It was
that you considered it to be "evidently as general and as much a
blood poison as the New England typhus." It is most certainly all
that and it is *more*—it is deeper and more deadly.

With regard to the treatment of this terrible malady, my views are
to a certain extent in accordance with those generally professed to-
day. It is of an absolute necessity, in my opinion, to apply a mixed
treatment, general and local, from the commencement. I would
much sooner abandon the latter, surgical treatment, as a means of
prolonging life and giving a larger trial of general treatment excepted
than the former. It is evidently a typhoid disease, and as such must
be treated from the start—it is a septic disease, and as such must
be combatted at the earliest moment; it is accompanied by local
accidents, and they must be treated as they present themselves.
First, then, I advise at my first visit an insufflation of about a drachm

of very dry powdered burnt alum, whether I find a commencement of the plastic deposit on the tonsils or in the pharynx or not—you will always find the fauces and tonsils inflamed, and ordinarily a commencement of the deposit in some locality in the throat. Even if I find it already considerable my treatment is the same. At the same visit I also advise a tepid bath of an hour's duration at least, and more frequently of two hours, and a purge of citrate of magnesia (purgative lemonade) six or eight drachms in solution, and dose to be repeated every two hours until it operates. This is to prepare the patient for what is to follow by cleaning the intestines of whatever load of matter they may contain, activating the secretions of the entire canal and irritating the absorbents, if I may so speak, to a more rapid action upon the general medication to follow. The bath is of eminent service in revivifying the powers of that immense organ, the skin, and activating its functions. I can't pretend to explain how, but you will see and feel it as clearly as myself. I prefer the alum as a topic most decidedly to nitrate of silver, as it forms no eschar to blind you at your next visit with regard to the exact state of things in the throat, and also because I have found it really more potent in its good influence as a local application. The tongue is to be held down with a large spoon, and the alum blown in through a single glass tube, six or eight inches long, and one-fourth of an inch in diameter, at the moment when the presence of the spoon in the fauces causes the involuntary act of gagging on the part of the patient. This insufflation I order to be continued every hour until my return. Its frequency must always be determined, however, by the sagacity of the physician, the gravity of appearances taken into consideration. I rarely order it less often than once in two hours. Having thus prepared my patient, I commence immediately upon my general treatment, which consists in the administration, every three hours, of ten grains of the chlorate of potash, and ten grains of the bichlorate dissolved in some convenint vehicle, with the administration ordinarily of one-tenth of a grain of calomel in sugar, dry, upon the tongue, every hour or every two hours, stopping and recommencing its administration according to circumstances which can only be explained or appreciated by the physician at the bedside. This is a proper moment to lay before your consideration a question which has been recently agitated in the medical world, viz: if in the simultaneous administration of calomel and the chlorate of potash, the effects

4

of the latter do not counteract in a measure, or destroy entirely the
specific effects of the former. For my own part, I am prepared to
say that although it may retard or prevent, for aught I know, the
specific effect on the salivary glands, I do not believe that it modifies,
in any way, its effects upon the secretions. This opinion is based
upon many and some very recent observations. However, as we
know nothing positively about the matter, I generally suspend the
one and the other alternately for twenty-four or thirty-six hours at a
time during the course of the disease, in order to profit, if possible,
by the doubt. I always remove with long forceps, or by scraping, or
by any other means, violent or gentle, all accessible portions of the
pseudo-membranous deposit in order to allow the topics to act as
directly as possible upon the secretory surfaces, and also to prevent
as much as may be, the accumulation of a thick, hard deposit which
would act as a serious mechanical obstruction.

In addition to the above, I commence immediately with the use of
tonics, stimulants, and the most nourishing possible fluid animal food.
Quinine every three hours in as large doses as can be borne, without
producing severe cerebral perturbation; bitters composed of cinchona,
gentian, columbo, camomile, quassia, bitter orange peel, etc, formed
into a strong infusion, to which I add brandy and a little syrup. The
following is my ordinary formula :

R   Cort. cinchona flav. cont...ʒij ;
        Rad. gentian, cont...ʒij ;
        Rad. columbo, cont..ʒss ;
        Cort. aurant., flor. anthemis, quassia amara.................aa ʒij ;
        Aq. bulliens...Oij ;
M.   Ft. infus. et add spts. vini gallic...................................ʒvj ;
        Syr. cort. aurant..ʒiv.

Of this I give ordinarily to an adult from half to two-thirds of an
ounce five or six times in twenty-four hours. Strong *bouillon* of beef
mutton, and chicken, cooked together until it forms a jelly on cooling,
from which may be made tapioca or vermicelli soup as a change, a
teacupful every three or four hours, with occasionally a soft-boiled
egg instead. Ale, porter, sherry, brandy and water, from time to
time, in such quantities as may be borne. Of course no fixed laws
can be given for the administration of these various things, but the
sagacity of the physician is always with him to act as his mentor
and guide. If the necessity occurs, I administer, from time to time,

a purge of the citrate of magnesia, *always* in divided doses, repeated at intervals, if necessary, in order not to produce mischief by an intemperative dose. I always repeat, every two or three days, my tepid bath, of an hour. The patient ought always to be visited from three to six times daily, and the first visit should be always very early, and the last one very late. The topical applications should be made as frequently as possible by the physician himself, as his experience and ¡knowledge enables him to perform them with much greater effect than the nurse or member of the family can attain. The insufflations are to be continued day and night so long as a tendency to the formation of the false membrane continues, and I am in the habit of alternating between the powdered alum and tannin at each hour—more to take the benefit of the chances than because I am convinced that I obtain better results. I find that under the above course of treatment promptly applied and vigorously continued, the larynx is in the majority of cases spared from the membranous exudation, but still it too frequently becomes invaded in spite of all we can do to permit me to pass over this terrible accident in silence. And now comes a solemn moment for solemn remarks. Many authors of high merit have counselled and still advise the use of emetic in high doses, to produce the expulsion of the false membrane from the larynx or trachea. I have never yet prescribed a single grain of emetic in a case of angine couenneuse, and I hope that it may never be given me so to do. I protest in the most serious manner against this advice, which may, no doubt, be good at times in membranous croup, for at all hazards, and at all costs, we must maintain the integrity of the stomach and sustain the forces of the patient, not only for the duration of the disease, but for the convalescence, fearful at best. The presence of the spoon in the throat gives rise to efforts of coughing sufficiently powerful to answer all the ends of an emetic in the expulsion of the membranes, and it deteriorates in no wise the integrity of the action of the stomach, and let the stomach fail and I give all up as lost. There are those in authority who counsel bloodletting under certain conditions of pulse in this disease. I would as soon put my lancet into the vein of a moribund typhique, as to take an ounce of blood from a patient with membranous sore throat under any circumstauces of the disease which I have ever witnessed or can imagine. Your baths, which are in no wise debilitating, and your intestinal evacuations by means of gentle aperients, are sufficiently sharp-pointed lancets.

One word more and I am done, my dear doctor and master, with
what I have to offer in regard to the treatment of this formidable and
fearful disease. We have arrived now at the most terrible episode of
the disease which we can encounter—imminence of death by suffocation from the accumulation of plastic lymph in the larynx. The only aim
then left is to still prolong the life of the patient, and then the chances
of aid from general treatment—the only means is *tracheotomy*, and I
know that the word will pale on your ear. I know that you have
said, and under circumstances of the most appalling nature, that you
would never open another trachea in a case of croup. I know, too,
that you have since been guided by the high star of your intelligence
to do it more than once. Do it, dear doctor, and *always* do it, but do
not do it too late. It is impossible to perceive the moment away
from the bed-side of the patient, but to the sagacious physician shall
it be given *to do*, when the time comes. I think that Dr. Gay, of Boston, has *said* the best and *done* the best of any living man, not even
excepting Trousseau, in regard to the question of the proper time to
operate and the proper treatment to pursue after performing tracheotomy in membranous croup—he operates early—and let me assure
you that my profound belief is that you must operate even *earlier* in a
case of angine couenneuse than in a case of croup—for you doom
your patient to a certain death if you allow his vital powers, his powers of assimilation, to arrive at an ebb when ingestion becomes null
before you operate. Operate while he can still assimilate—it is *not* as
Malgaigne would have it in his arbitrary contempt for *medical* surgery,
an operation a thousand times fraught with peril in itself ; it is simply a flea bite in comparison with the sure results of a tardy operation.

And now I advise what I have never seen advised or know to be
put into practice, except by myself, after the operation—not only to
continue the insufflations of alum into the pharynx, but to practise
them immediately, constantly, and vigorously into the trachea through
the tube inserted in the ordinary manner into the trachea, and to perform them also with the same vigor and as well as you can into the
larynx by turning the tracheal tube in the opposite sense and blowing it the most effectively possible upward into the larynx. I need
hardly add that the same general treatment is to be continued constantly the same as before the operation, which only constitutes an
episode.

I find that the " few words " which were to form my letter to you have procreated already to an alarming extent, and as yet I have not said one word in regard to the convalescence from the disease and the accidents which the most frequently accompany it as sad satellites. I promised early in my letter also to speak specially upon the sequent progressive paralysis. If you will still bear with me, I will continue this hasty and wholly unpremeditated document. Convalescence arrives, and we naturally add to our already nourishing fluid diet, solids, such as beef steaks *underdone,* roast beef *underdone,* mutton chops, poultry, game, vegetables, etc. I forgot in my hurried ramble to say that throughout the whole course of the disease I gave an abundance of such fruits as peaches, grapes, apricots, cherries, currants, raspberries, and strawberries, each or all in season, with lemonade and morsels of ice as a beverage, also soda water and syrup of raspberries, currants, or gooseberries as beverage. All this may be continued during the convalescence, accidents to be met as the discretion and judgment of the physician may dictate.

I forgot also to state that I prefer my patient in angine couenneuse to change his chamber daily, or more frequently even as in typhoid fever, and to have free and constant access to fresh air from without.

It is generally two or three weeks after the disappearance of all traces of false membranes from the pharynx that the symptoms of paralysis commence. The muscles of the soft palate are the first to indicate the invasion of this new series of accidents—it is indicated by the nasal sound of the voice, and by the regurgitation by the nose in the act of swallowing of liquids taken in by the mouth. During this period of convalescence, patients, instead of gaining strength, activity, and flesh, lose in each particular respect. Pains in the back and joints supervene, numbness and prickly sensations in the feet and legs manifest themselves, insensibility and partial or complete loss of the power of locomotion. The fæces and urine are evacuated involuntarily, the tongue trembles, and articulation becomes imperfect and sometimes impossible. The appetite generally remains good, the intelligence is preserved, but there is a tendency to indolence. The parts paralyzed become less sensible to the touch, or in some cases entirely senseless to tactile excitation, but the electric sensibility is never destroyed. The superior members are also subjected to the same paralytic phenomena as the inferior, and paraplegia even sometimes occurs in a marked degree. The muscles of the face and eyes even become involved also in their turn in certain cases. There is evidently no coïncidence in this condition of progressive paralytic phenomena with the disease in question, as all known observations show that the accidents commence in the same manner and arrive at the same or similar results. The ordinary termination of these paralytic accidents is recovery. For their cure, iron tonics, generous diet, cold effusions, warm clothing, and exercise in the open air are the best. Strychnine, nux vomica, and electricity have seemed to me to exert no favorable influence in their cure—on the contrary, sometimes the patient dies under this state of things, but no pathological phenomena are left to indicate the material lesion or cause of death. Diphtheretic paralysis is probably the effect of the toxic poison of the disease—but nobody knows. All we can say at present is that it is a disease which leaves no palpable traces in the nervous centres, that it is certainly caused by diphtheria, and that we cannot trace the cause to the effect.

I have said all I have for the moment to say, dear doctor, and I trust in you to excuse my apparent or real egotism in giving you only my own personal views upon a subject which is deeply agitating the entire medical world. You asked it of me, and I have *literally* given what you asked. Let me hear from you again soon, and believe me,

Yours truly,   S. L. BIGELOW.

ART. III.—*A Few Thoughts on the Use and Abuse of the Uterine Speculum, with some Remarks on Uterine Polypus:* By W. .H GANTT, Union Hill, Texas.

THERE seems to have ever been on the part of some members of the medical profession a disposition to have a hobby; and also to hide behind the mystifications of some diseased action of some organ of the body, which, by general agreement, seems more prone to take upon itself a greater amount of obscure morbidity than others; let this peculiarity be either real or in the imagination of the doctor, to hide too often, sorry, am I to say, his entire ignorance of the diseased action in question. I do not wish for one moment to infer that our profession, in my eyes, is more blamable in this respect than others. No l I well know that it is a very hard matter, indeed, for one to say, " I don't know," when it is supposed from his position he knows or should know all about it ; too few men are to be found with the requisite amount of moral courage to act thus ; often, sorry am I to say, the more honest ones are kept from it by the knowledge of the fact, a lamentable one indeed, that some Æsculapian of great and wonderful powers sits watching ready to pounce upon the case, crying aloud his ability in the cure of such cases.

A few years since, in our Southern States, in the days of *Cookism*, the liver was the scape-goat, and had not only to bear its own sins, but likewise the sins of most of the " ills flesh is heir to." Malaria, indigestion, inflammations, heat, cold, wet and dry, it matters not which ; nor was it of much importance whether the disease was in the head or in the foot, whether internal or external, the liver was torpid or the liver was inactive, and on the same principle of the toper's logic, whisky is good to heat and good to cool, calomel ! calomel l was the cry ; and by its abuse this inestimable medicinal agent was cried down, and mineral doctors set aside, and " root and herb " ones taken in their stead. Though this state of affairs, with the advancing of our profession towards a brighter and better day, is yielding, we yet find the fault existing. It is also a pleasing fact to learn, that the liver has of late days improved very much in its actions, as it does not now occupy the place of great fault doer.

The womb, in the female, like the liver in general, has ever been the scape-goat for diseases in a class of our patients, and of late days seems to be growing worse. I am willing to admit that we more frequently of late days find uterine affections among our patients than existed a few years back, owing to a greater amount of luxurious and sedentary living, the peculiar mode of dressing, and other causes, no doubt ; but yet this does not prevent the fact from obtaining, that it is abused, and that this organ has often to bear sins not of its own commission or omission. This, of late days, has with many of our medical profession, both in the cities and in the country, given another hobby for them to ride, and they ride it like a borrowed horse—rather too free.

Ulceration of the os uteri and also of the cervix of this organ,

seems to have sprung into existence, as if by magic. Indeed, I have
known some places where you could scarcely find a woman whose
os uteri was not as well known to the eye of the medical man of the
neighborhood as her face ; or, in the words of a patient of a medical
friend of mine who had this mania, "Dr., you will surely know by
sight the mouth of my womb as well as you know your own child."
The Doctor had *speculumed* her too often for the good of the cause of
medical science, bringing it into disrepute in the community in which
he lived, causing those who really needed it to resist its use. We all
remember the story, current a few years since, of the English doctor
who had become deeply infected with the speculum mania, who,
when an enraged father hastened down to Bath as fast as steam
could carry him, for the purpose of chastising him for *speculuming* his
young daughter, not only by the honeyed words of this medical Nestor,
became satisfied of the need of it in his daughter's case, but likewise
convinced that he needed it, and forthwith was *speculated* on by the doctor
for ulcers of the rectum. So goes the world.

It would seem that some Nemesis had determined in the distribut-
ing of her punishments to the daughters of Eve, to select the os and
cervix and body of the womb, yea, the entire concern, to be their
terror, whose diseases, like the fabled Tityus, grew as fast as consumed ; and the dread of their medical attendant, if he be a conscientious man—for we all know of the difficulty of the cure of many
uterine diseases—and the very fact of these organs being diseased,
bring also a moral shock to the mind of the timid and modest woman ;
and, as her medical advisers, we dread to have to resort to the examination of those parts, and it should never be done for slight and
trivial causes. Now, I don't for one moment wish to be considered
an old fogy in our profession—far from it. I use the speculum, and
when needed, its services are invaluable ; in fact, not to be done away
with in a scientific and thorough investigation and treatment of the
vaginal tract, the cervix and os uteri. I only oppose the indiscriminate use of it, nay, I should say, abuse of it. Nor is it alone the
fact of its free and uncalled-for use, but it becomes the means of ir-
rational and improper treatment.

When the speculum is used, and the mouth of the womb exposed,
too often it is the case, the porte-caustic is too freely handled, armed
with the nit. argent., and where no inflammation did previously exist,
it is now brought about. Every medical gentleman well posted up

and conversant with the appearance of the os uteri in women who have frequently borne children, knows, that very often on the inner face of the ring or rim of the os, there are to be found slight enlargement and hardening of the mucous membrane of that part, sometimes only one, at others several of the little points may be seen, the result, no doubt in my mind, of the tearing and cicatrizing of the mucous membrane during and after labor.* The speculum reveals these, and to one not conversant with them, when it has been used in a case where the urgency of the symptoms did not call for an investigation, the nit. argent. is used time and again, and in a few days we have inflammation of these parts. I have seen such cases more than once. This, with many other equally urgent reasons, has led me often to wish that there was some restriction placed upon its use. But why so, if man must have a hobby?

The womb cannot, like Achilles, claim to be vulnerable at only one point, and greater the pity. While one has ulceration of the mouth and neck, another has prolapsus uteri. Let a woman complain of a pain in the lumbar region, with a sense of weight in the hypogastric region, any part of it, and too often she is doomed by her medical adviser to a disagreeable and unnecessary course of treatment. The doctor seemily has forgotten, that uterine engorgement may exist producing these symptoms, that a rheumatic condition of the womb may produce them, and that, that protean disease hysteria, may also do it, and yet the uterine globe remain *in situ.* This is too often the case, and though the maladies of this organ are better understood by the profession generally than they were a few years ago, yet grave errors do yet exist. The anatomical situation of the womb is known to all, but its relative position with other organs is not as well understood by many as it should be. If this was studied more, a correct knowledge of many cases of supposed prolapsus would be obtained, and a few doses of colchicum and iodide of potassium would relieve the uterine rheumatism, or leeching the cervix uteri, with a well directed general treatment, proper regimen and exercise would overcome the engorgement of this organ.

Hysteria has been called the protean disease; and it most assuredly richly deserves the appellation, for there seems scarcely a disease to which human flesh is heir to, that it may not and does so closely

---

* Not to be mistaken for enlarged glands of Nabothi.

imitate, that the best of our profession are sometimes forced to bear the mortification of a false diagnosis and misdirected treatment. The study of this disease is a field richly abounding in the wonders and mysteries of the nervous action direct and reflexed; and will amply pay the student for his time and his study. Here, again, we have opened for us an avenue for the abuse of the speculum, and it is too often taken advantage of. There being many of the members of our profession who look upon hysteria as the direct consequences of an ulcerative process going on in some portion of the uterine neck, in at least the large majority of cases of hysteria. The speculum is used, and the glands of Nabothi being enlarged, are instantly cauterized or creosotized. Let those thus viewing and treating this disease, read that very readable book, Meigs's "Woman and her Disease," and learn from it. It certainly contains many facts of vital interest to the physician who expects to practise his profession among women ; and in the treatment of hysteria he will learn from it to use the speculum less, to be not over anxious to say ulceration is the great cause of uterine action ; but to direct a general treatment to a neuralgic or rheumatic diathesis, uterine engorgement, and general depravity of the assimilating function more.

I now come to make a few remarks upon uterine polypus; knowing that this disease is often mistaken for other diseases, especially for prolapsus uteri, and likewise knowing that it exists much oftener than many seem disposed to think, I, therefore, am led to pen the following lines.

The symptoms marking uterine polypus, are, in its earliest stages, very obscure; and although we may have no certain symptoms to base a positive diagnosis upon, we have yet many symptoms that may, by proper investigation lead us with very tolerable correctness to the opinion that our patient is laboring under uterine polypus. There is no part of mucous membrane but what is, to a certain extent, prone to the lesions necessary to form an extraneous growth, and it seems to me that there is no part of it that should be deemed more liable to this abnormal condition than that of the uterine cavity. For years subject to regular periods of a congested condition, a hyperæmia, so to speak, of all its vessels, and a super-excited condition of its nervous filaments, lasting for a greater or shorter length of time, is certainly prone, or rather more liable to an irregular action, and to the effects resulting from exposure and various other causes than any other portion of this tissue. Then, again, for months its vessels growing from the smallest to the greatest caliber, subject to frequent congestions and depletions, we may ask, is it not wonderful that lesions of secretion and nutrition, ending in hypertrophy or tumors, are not more frequently met with upon its surface ? But Nature usually saves the parts called upon to undergo frequent and great changes, by her peculiarly wise and well adapted laws, though she sometimes fails, and then we have the various tumors, hypertrophies, etc.

As above said, the symptoms marking this peculiar diseased action of the lining membrane of the womb (for I hold that it is here that it springs into existence), the nervous filament that fails to supply the proper nerve force, and the improper quantity of blood sent there, not called for, it cannot be healthily consumed, or given out to surrounding parts, a tumor or hypertrophy results, and of a hidden character, and requires perhaps more tact to arrive at a fair starting point in its description than one would at the first blush presume. In the early stages of polypus of the womb, the tumor occupies the cavity of this organ, and is alone to be known by general symptoms. A woman complains of pains in the uterine regions, not very severe nor very frequent ; but as the tumor grows, their frequency and force increase, becoming now the cause of distention of the muscular walls of this organ. Many writers upon this subject tell us that the disease is early accompanied by a glairy discharge. This I believe doubtful, for I have seen several cases where it never presented itself. The symptoms of pain and weight go on increasing, and soon the patient becomes satisfied that she is laboring under an attack of prolapsus uteri. An examination per vaginam is made with the finger, and if the physician who makes it be not thoroughly conversant with the peculiar and relative position of this organ when *in situ,* and its varied position in different women, he becomes satisfied that prolapsus exists, and forthwith the woman is subjected to a treatment for this disease ; if upon examination the patient complains of some tenderness upon pressure to the os and cervix uteri, the speculum is used, and bad is made worse by cauterizing an uninflamed womb until there is lit up an active inflammatory condition. In a short time after the first sensation of disturbance or pain has been felt, the next and by far the most important symptom presents itself. I allude to the flow of blood. It is perhaps an improper step to try to specify the period at which we may look for this symptom ; but from a number of cases that I have been called upon to treat, I believe we may say it scarcely appears prior to six weeks after the first disturbance ; generally about the second month we may feel certain that the hæmorrhage discharged proceeds from a tumor of this age, or that our patient has been laboring under it this long. I, as before said, have found that the patient would put the time of this discharge at about this period from the first symptoms of pain and weight. It is, however, true, that sometimes it is longer ; as it is equally true that all tumors do not grow at equal speed.

This hæmorrhagic tendency varies in different individuals ; in some it is profuse from the onset—in others slight at first, grows in quantity, with the growth of the tumor. This symptom most usually is sudden in its appearance, the blood gushing from the patient in rapid and profuse discharge, without any exertion on her part that might give it force. This symptom is not only irregular in the quantity discharged, but likewise varies much in its times of appearance ; in some cases it is daily, in others it is not to be seen more than once in every three or four weeks. There is no such thing as placing any definite time for its appearance, the patient being liable to these hæmorrhages at any time and at any place, rendering her miserable and uncomfortable. Another symptom to be well noted is, the condition of the bladder. When the tumor has passed from the uterine cavity, and occupies the upper portion of the vaginal tract, its pressure upon the bladder gives inconvenience. This inconvenience is, at first, a frequent desire to urinate, the bladder seeming to fill more rapidly than formerly, and requiring more frequent evacuation. At first the pressure of the tumor producing this symptom, does not interfere with the contractile powers of the neck of the bladder ; but as it grows in size, and the general emaciation and enervation of the general powers of life and body goes on, we have incontinency of urine ; the urine escaping with a gush, more especially when the woman rises suddenly from a reclining or sitting posture.

The debility and emaciation that ensue, result necessarily from the frequent and profuse loss of blood, sooner or later brings about hectic diseases. The patient suffers from pulmonary affections oftener than any other form of disease. If the patient is not seen until the tumor has left the uterine cavity, and is occupying the vagina, the touch reveals its presence, usually as a rounded and smooth body of different sizes. Sometimes, however, it is rough to the sense of touch,

being covered with elevations and depressions upon its external surface. If the finger is passed up along the side of the tumor, we most
generally can find the os uteri, and feel likewise the footstalk upon
which the tumor grows ; sometimes, however, the os uteri grasps the
tumor around its body, and may give some trouble in our diagnosis :
but of this, more hereafter.

The symptoms above enumerated, with the exception of those from
taxis, *may* exist without uterine polypus being the producing cause.
They may last for years, and still remain obscure. The polypus may
be for years retained in the uterine cavity, and the sense of touch be
of no avail ; nor can we now do much towards the permanent relief
of our patient. But if I am called to see a woman, who tells me that
for a longer or shorter period she has suffered from hæmorrhage from
the vaginal outlet ; that it is irregular in quantity and time of appearance ; that it is pure blood coagulating and not dependent upon her
monthly courses, and unlike it, as she will very soon learn ; that she
has a sense of weight in the region of the womb, with fleeting pains
there, and pains in her lumbar region ; and that these symptoms preceded the hæmorrhagic discharge, I feel sure of uterine tumor being
in existence in her case. If, upon farther inquiry, I find that there
exists a disposition to frequently evacuate the bladder, this organ
seeming to fill more rapidly than formerly, and upon placing the hand
upon the lower part of the hypogastric region, I feel the womb above
the symphysis pubis ; if upon examination per vaginam with the
speculum, I find no ulceration of great size and depth ; if upon *ballottement* the womb feels heavier and larger than it would in a perfectly
normal condition ; if upon introducing a catheter into the bladder
and a finger into the rectum, I find a large body between the point
of the instrument and the point of the finger, I feel doubly sure of it
—I *know* that a uterine polypus is here. I have diagnosticated thus
several times, and I feel confident of diagnosticating correctly in all
such cases.

If, however, upon introducing the finger into the vagina, I find it
filled with a body, and passing my finger up and around this body, I
find the neck of the womb, with its os grasping either the footstalk
or body of the tumor ; if upon repeating the examination with the
catheter and finger before alluded to, I feel the womb *in situ ;* if my
patient tells me that when she sits down and suddenly rises to her
feet, her urine gushes from her, and she cannot control it, I have now

no doubt, if any before existed in my mind, as to this being a case of uterine polypus. Now, though the symptoms are rather indefinite in the early stages, yet, I think, if the course above laid down be pursued, we may arrive at a very correct diagnosis.

There are some other diseases with which we may place this one, as liable to give us trouble in our diagnosis in its early stages. The sense of weight and pain in the lumbar and hypogastric region, and weight on *ballottement,* may arise, to our mind, as existing in uterine engorgement, or hypertrophy of the entire organ. But when these symptoms are taken in conjunction with the hæmorrhagic condition above alluded to, and the bulk as revealed to the finger introduced into the rectum, we may come to a very correct conclusion.

The next malady that may complicate our diagnosis, is prolapsus uteri. It is only when the tumor has left the uterine cavity, and occupies the vaginal canal, that this fact is obtained. Here the sense of touch, the feeling of the cervix above the body of the tumor, with its os grasping some portion of it. The speculum reveals the condition of the os uteri ; though I knew a case in which a depression in a polypus occupying the vaginal canal so closely resembled the os uteri as to deceive several medical gentlemen of skill and ability. The sense of touch and the eye were both in fault in this case. There is no disease that is so often mistaken for uterine polypus as prolapsus uteri ; and I wish to direct the attention more directly to this fact than a mere general mention of it would do. Having had sent to my care no less than five patients that had been treated for months, and in some cases years, for prolapsus uteri, and from whom I took tumors weighing from three to fourteen ounces, I know that a correct knowledge of the disease in question, is, in many cases, wanting.

If a medical man is called in to see a case of prolapsus uteri, as he has been told, let him inquire into the monthly sickness of the woman, and if she tells him that her menses are irregular in quantity and time, let him ask if they ever come away with a sudden gush, and coagulate sometimes, and if he is answered in the affirmative, let him be very cautious about his diagnosis. He had better search long and carefully for the cervix and os uteri, and find if they are not above the body supposed to be the prolapsed womb ; let him make the rectal examination with the finger, the catheter being in the bladder, and find if the womb is not *in situ ;* let him, I say, be doubly careful, for he will be placed in an awkward position if he treats his case for some time for prolapsus, and then another physician is called in and diagnosticates the case to be a polypus, and removing it, cures the woman. Let him remember that prolapsus uteri seldom if ever is accompanied by hæmorrhage, and though the womb may be the point from which the blood flows, the tumor being of a fibrous character, yet this hæmorrhagic nisus is the direct result of the uterine cavity being occupied by, I may say, a foreign body, or at least an irritating one, and though the fibrous tumor rarely of itself bleeds, yet great caution is required in diagnosticating, and if any of the above described symptoms are obtained, still greater caution is required not to make a mistake in your diagnosis.

In speaking of the treatment of this disease, there may be said to be but one ; that is, extirpation. It is not always our good fortune to find the tumor without the uterine cavity. Growing by a footstalk in some cases, it may readily pass from the uterine cavity to the vaginal strait. In other cases growing from the mucous membrane in a bulky or large space, it is slow, if it ever leaves the womb, and may waste our patient to death either by general depletion, or, as is the case oftener, by bringing on cachectic diseases. The treatment called for then in those cases where the polypus is still within the womb, has, with me, been as follows. I will give a short history of a case of this kind that I was called upon to treat. The patient, a woman aged thirty-six, the mother of four children, the youngest of which was now four years old, was pale and emaciated in body ; supposed to be laboring under prolapsus uteri, with pulmonary tuberculosis. From her I learned that some three years previous, she felt some pain in the region of the womb, with some sense of weight or bearing down. Some four weeks after the first evidences of these symptoms, she had a gush of blood from the vagina, while sitting at her work table ; that this weight and pain with hæmorrhage had increased in quantity and force ; that the flooding was irregular in its time of appearance as well as to its quantity, sometimes being profuse, at others small, and usually every week or ten days at farthest. I examined as directed above, and felt satisfied that she was laboring under uterine polypus. I ordered a generous diet, the metallic iron, and exercise in a carriage over smooth roads for a few days. As soon as she had recovered some little from the flooding that had occurred, just previous to my seeing her, I gave her a strong decoction of the Galega Virginiana in table-spoonful doses every hour until four or

five had been administered. I have found the decoction of the fresh
root of the Devil's shoe-string to produce free contractile action on
the part of the womb ; I have known it three times to produce miscarriage. I did not on the first day succeed with this remedy in
bringing about the desired effect. I continued the general treatment,
and in a few days' time tried the galega decoction again. This produced very fair labor pains which lasted for some three or four hours,
at the expiration of which time, upon examination, I found the uterine os opening, and the tumor seeming to occupy the neck. In three
days' time, the womb having now and then suffered from contraction
of its muscular tissue, the tumor descended into the vagina, when I
threw a ligature around it, and in three days more I withdrew a tumor
weighing six ounces.

This general treatment is certainly called for, and it does seem to
me that mildly moving the muscular structure of the womb promises
some good result. I have ever used this method, and I never have
had cause to regret my so doing. I prefer this article in such cases
to the secale curnutum, being more controlable, and though acting
well as a parturient in most cases, its action, unlike the secale, is
regular, and wanting in that wild and erratic action so often observed
in the ergot, and is a more regular agent in its action in the non-
graved womb than the latter. It is not generally known to the profession that this agent possesses any such powers, the books calling
it an anthelmintic, and giving it but a slight notice.

When we are called to see a patient, and upon examination being
made by the introduction of the finger into the vaginal tract we there
find the canal occupied by some body ; a careful examination made
by passing the finger above it, if possible, feeling the uterine neck
and os ; if we cannot reach this point, the introduction of the finger
of the right hand into the rectum and the catheter into the bladder,
bringing its point so as to be felt by the point of the finger
through the intervening tissues, we can satisfy ourself that the body,
which was felt in the vaginal strait, is not an inverted womb, but the
womb being felt *in situ*, resting between the point of the finger and
catheter, we are satisfied that there is a tumor ; and that it grows
from the mucous membrane of the womb, or upper part of the vagina.
We here proceed to throw a ligature around it. This is best done
with Gooch's double canula. It is unnecessary for me to enter into
anything like a description of the mode of procedure in this opera-

tion with this instrument, as it has been laid down by various authors upon the subject. But sometimes we have not accessible to us Gooch's canula, and have to depend upon other means. I was once called to see a lady supposed to be laboring under prolapsus uteri, but upon my instituting a close and well directed search, I discovered it was not the prolapsed womb that filled the vagina to almost procidentia, but a uterine tumor, and that not all of the tumor was yet delivered from the uterine mouth. I attempted to withdraw by gentle tension upon it with the forceps (a small pair made for this purpose), but it would not yield, so I was forced to desist. I felt satisfied that by ligaturing it at the point nearest the os uteri, that death of the part contained within the womb would likewise occur. Her father, an old and distinguished medical gentleman, assured of this point, agreed to the procedure ; but we had with us no canula. What were we to do without it, was the question. I procured two female catheters, and taking off the upper joints, I proceeded to arm them with a stout silk ligature, confining the ligature to the rings of one of the catheters, I passed it up through the instrument, then down through the other. Finding the one to be held by the assistant, too short, I prepared a piece of wood nicely, and introducing it in the catheter serving as a handle, I could, without much difficulty, manage the other one. Placed side by side, the left hand, or three fingers of it, being introduced into the vagina, served as a guide, along which the instruments were passed until the ends had reached sufficiently far into the vagina ; the handled catheter was now held firmly *in situ* by the assistant, while I slid the other one around the tumor until it had reached exactly the opposite from which it departed, the ligature encircling the tumor nicely. I now withdrew the wooden handle, and tightening the string, found the instruments to fit and the ligature to hold well. The adroitness and tact of my medical friend (the father) was of great service in the easy accomplishment of the operation. The string was confined to the rings of the two catheters, thus holding them together. I tightened it twice a day for four days, when it cut through, and I extracted the portion that rested in the vagina, which weighed three ounces. In forty-eight hours after, the part remaining in the uterine cavity passed down into the vagina, and being extracted, was found to weigh two ounces. The disease had lasted so long, and our patient was so wasted, that she died some weeks after from inflammation of the lungs.

6

Here we will close our remarks upon this disease. We again say that, believing it is a disease more frequently existing than seems to be generally believed by the profession, and so often mistaken and treated as another disease, we have been led to the penning of the foregoing thoughts. We cast them upon the sea of medical literature ; they are our candid and matured opinions, and as such we trust them to the profession.

The remarks upon the hobbyism and the abuse of those hobbies that are found in the first of our article, we are sorry to say have been brought about by actual observation and experience. We have found that often the man styling himself doctor, and trying to ride into practice on his hobby, like Perillus falls by this very work of his own hand ; and a pity it is that it ever fails to be so.

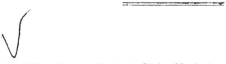

Art. IV.—*Urethro-Vaginal, Vesico-Vaginal and Recto-Vaginal Fistules ; General Remarks ; Report of Cases Successfully Treated with the Button-Suture:* By Nathan Bozeman, M. D., of New Orleans (late of Montgomery, Alabama).

Something more than two years have now elapsed since my last paper upon the subject of *Urethro-Vaginal* and *Vesico-Vaginal Fistules* appeared in the *North American Medico-Chirurgical Review.* I then gave the profession the result of my experience, based upon the report of nineteen cases successfully treated by our new mode of suture. Since that time I have been steadily engaged in prosecuting my labors in this department of surgery, not only in this country, but Great Britain and France, where I was invited to operate in some of the hospitals while on a visit there. Some of my operations in Europe have already been reported ; but having been published in foreign journals, but few of my readers in this country, I presume, have seen the account. For this reason, and the fact that the circumstances under which they were performed have not as yet been fully stated, I must be excused for introducing these cases here in their regular order.

In presenting now another article to the notice of the profession it is my purpose only to preface with a few remarks the report of cases, the only sure way by which the merits of any plan of treatment can be correctly judged of. The point which I would first touch upon, then, is *metallic sutures*, and the best mode of using them in the management of the class of diseases to which our attention is at present directed. The notice which has been given this subject, both in Europe and America, within the last year or two, has had the effect of arousing the entire profession to a sense of its importance. This is unquestionably due to the great success claimed by American surgeons in the treatment of the injuries of which we are speaking. The advantages of metallic sutures over all others as thus shown, had, it is true, been known to us for more than a quarter of a century before, still but litttle had been said or written upon the subject. The fact was familiar to us, and the question that occupied our minds was as to the best mode of employing them. The various plans proposed are familiar to every surgeon, and consequently need not occupy our time here. Suffice it to say the results produced from them in the aggregate far exceeded what had been furnished by the whole of Europe together. At the late period referred to, Great Britain was aroused, as if from a slumber, to the great importance of metallic sutures, as being something new. Prof. Simpson, so distinguished for his zeal in the cause of science, took hold of the subject at once, and we absolutely find him, by experiments on a pig, arriving at results precisely the same as were presented to the profession more than thirty years ago by our countryman, Dr. Levert. His conclusions as to the non-irritating effect of metallic sutures as compared to that of organic, were certainly most satisfactory, and he proved beyond doubt that they were of ancient origin in the treatment of ordinary wounds. What I object to, however, is the preference which he gives to iron-wire sutures over silver, and his manner of using them. Let us see, then, what he predicates this preference upon. It is that iron-wire " is stronger, cheaper, and altogether more easily worked with than silver wire."* Now, that iron-wire is a little stronger and cheaper than silver, does not perhaps admit of a doubt, but in affirming that it is more easily worked with than the latter, he certainly labors under a wide mistake, if the experience of others amounts to

---

* London Medical Times and Gazette.

anything. The result of my own, is that there is no comparison between the two. I have tried the best quality of iron-wire, that manufactured for Prof. Simpson's own use by the firm of Cockers Brothers,
of Sheffield, and even this is greatly wanting in the softness and flexi-
bility characterizing silver. Admitting, however, all he says of what
may be called the working qualities of iron-wire, what are we next to
infer of its effects on the animal tissues as compared to silver? He
here tells us that he has employed "iron-wire coated with tin, silver,
etc., as well as wires of platinum and other metals, but not one of
them fulfills any indication better than the simple annealed iron-wire,"
which, he says, remains "passive" in the tissues, and "not at all liable
to become changed and oxidated."* Now, this does not accord with
my experience. I have never yet seen iron-wire remain in the tissues
even a few days without being turned black. Not only this; I have
always observed where there was much dragging upon the sutures
of this metal, they would cause ulceration and frequently cut out.
This is almost certain to occur in cases of fistule requiring more than
four sutures. I have not the slightest doubt that the failure of Prof.
Simpson's first operation with the button and iron-wire sutures, which
he attributes to awkwardness in adjustment, is to be ascribed to this
cause alone. He tells us that in that operation he employed five
iron-wire sutures, and that the edges of the fistule "united opposite
four of these sutures, but gave way early opposite the middle suture
of the five." Upon this middle suture was the greatest strain, and
for the reason of its irritating effect, it cut out early, thus causing a
partial failure of the operation. Had the same strain been upon the
other four sutures, they would have also cut out and caused a complete failure. This, however, did not exist in the nature of things.
In a line caused by the approximation of the two sides of any incised
wound, the force required to hold them together, whatever may be the
means employed, will be found to diminish as you go from the center
to either angle, and *vice versa*. This same general law obtains when
the edges of a fistulous opening are brought together by sutures;
and here, I may say, if the chasm is of considerable size, it is more
marked than almost anywhere else in the body, as will be indicated
by the intolerance of the tissues to the amount of pressure exerted at
the several points of suture. Every surgeon, I suppose, has observed

* *Op. Cit.*

the above results to a greater or lesser extent in the employment of silk sutures in ordinary wounds. I have myself repeatedly observed the fact. During the whole course of my practice in vesico-vaginal fistule, however, I never saw a more beautiful illustration of it than was presented to my notice about a year ago in London. The case was one which had been operated upon at the "London House" by my highly esteemed friend Mr. Isaac Baker Brown. Mr. B., although he had had unprecedented success in his operations with the button suture, yet was induced, by way of trial in this instance, to substitute Prof. Simpson's iron-wire sutures for silver. The fistule required five of these sutures, which he secured on the ordinary button principle. The ninth day he removed the apparatus, and to his astonishment found all the sutures nearly cut out, the middle one quite so, and a fistulous opening remaining in its tract. Four or five days afterwards he requested that I should see the case with him, but did not tell me anything about his having employed iron-wire sutures. No sooner, however, had he introduced his speculum through the parts into view, than I remarked to him that silver sutures had not been used in the operation, and if so, there was an effect from them I had never before observed. He then stated that he had employed iron-wire in the case, as an experiment, and that the partial failure of his operation, he believed, was to be ascribed to this circumstance alone. Such was the opinion of all who witnessed the result, there being five or six other physicians present. There were red lines on either side of the cicatrix, caused by the healing up of the ulcerated points of the sutures. These lines varied in length, increasing from the first, near the original angles of the fistule, to the center one, in whose tract was situated the remaining fistule, caused doubtless by the suture here cutting out and destroying the cicatrix.

Now, the indications which I have just pointed out that led me to the detection of the use of iron-wire sutures in a case of which I knew nothing, certainly should be regarded as one of the most convincing arguments that could be adduced in favor of silver sutures if such was necessary. Believing, however, as I have before said, that sutures of these two metals admit of no comparison, I deem it a waste of time here to discuss farther the superior claims of the latter. That iron-wire, excepting for hydrocele or other diseases treated upon the same principle, is to take the place of silver sutures, it is a manifest absurdity. But few operators in Europe, and I venture to say, none,

in this country, will be found to follow the example of Prof. Simpson
in his use of it.

It was my intention in the outset to notice Prof. Simpson's proposal
to modify 'our button principle, by what he terms an "iron-wire
splint," but as the results of his own practice with it do not even
warrant the claims set up to improvement, as I have been informed,
I shall pass it over. Whatever success he may have had with this
contrivance, is to be attributed to the principle of our button, differing widely, however, from the latter as to the combination of advantages. It could lay claim to but one, namely, steadiness and support
to the approximated edges of the fistulous opening. This now brings
us to a consideration of our button and the ends we attain by its use.
I here propose a short notice of the principle of its action, for the
reason that it is not generally understood by physicians, as I have
been induced to believe from the many questions asked me about it.
If it can be employed for no other purpose than simply the name of
the thing, why let it be dispensed with. What, then, are the advantages of the button as employed by us ? The conclusions I have long
since arrived at, and which long days' experience serves to strengthen
my conviction as to their correctness, may be thus briefly stated :

1. That our button in conjunction with the sutures comprising the
apparatus, in the treatment of the class of diseases under consideration, does exert a powerful controlling influence in directing and
forcing the edges of the fistulous opening in perfect apposition ; that
is to say, it is the level to which they are applied, and in nowise can
their inversion or eversion take place in being thus secured.

2. That it does give steadiness and support to the edges of the
fistule when adjusted, on the same principle, excepting that it is more
efficient, as the adhesive strips, compress and roller, when applied to
incised wounds generally.

3. That it does protect the denuded edges of the fistule from all
extraneous influences, such as vaginal and uterine secretions and the
urine in cases of double and triple fistules when it is desirable to
close up but one at a time.

Now, that all these points are attained by the employment of the
button as a part of our suture apparatus admits of the clearest demonstration, which any one can test by applying the principle to two
pieces of softened sole-leather with their edges slightly beveled off.
As to the greatest proof I can offer of the efficiency of the contri-

vance, I appeal to the report of my cases, embracing as it does the largest collection on record by any one surgeon, either in this country or Europe, now amounting to nearly fifty. My success in the management of these cases has been such, I conceive, as to justify all that I have claimed for the button suture. So far as I am informed, there is not another method from which such results have been produced, a majority of my cases having been cured by the first operation ; almost every shade of difference, ranging from the simplest to the worst form of the disease, has been met with. Only one case out of the number has been rejected as not admitting of operative procedure. One only, operated upon and afterwards discharged incurable. One terminated fatally from pyæmia. The operation in this case was performed in the Royal Infirmary, at Edinburgh, and as regarded closure of the fistulous opening, it was found, after death, to be complete. This case has been reported by my friend Dr. Keiller, in the Edinburgh *Medical Journal.* But from its general interest, I propose introducing it here among my other cases. Several of the cases that I am now about to report, are of unusual interest ; one, perhaps, the most remarkable on record. This was a case of both vesico-vaginal and recto-vaginal fistulés, and from its peculiarities occasioned the inauguration of a new and successful plan of treatment never before adopted, that I am aware of, and one to be regarded of the greatest practical utility. The vesical opening was of enormous dimensions, involving nearly the whole of the vesico-vaginal septum, together with half an inch of the root of the urethra, and a large part of the cervix uteri. Through it the fundus of the bladder protruded externally in the form of a large red tumor. The recto-vaginal opening, situated about two and a half inches from the anus, was associated with a broad, hard, and unyielding band below it, which prevented any movement of the septum, and consequently any depression of the uteris, which is usually made subservient to the closure of openings in the bladder, attended with such extensive loss of substance. This unyielding nature of the posterior septum could not be overcome by any plan of treatment. This, therefore, left us with no other alternative than the obturation of the vagina at the vulva, according to the method of Vidal (de Casis). In addition, now, to the ordinary objections to the above procedure, there was one in the present instance, that at first appeared insurmountable, namely, the existence of the recto-vaginal fistule. With this remaining, not only the urine and catamenia, but the fæces would have been turned into one common receptacle with no other outlet than the urethra. For the latter to become dissolved in the other two excretions, and be discharged with them, would have been next to impossible. M. Vidal's operation, therefore, was out of the question, unless the recto-vaginal opening could first be closed, and to the success of this there appeared one very great obstacle, namely, the uncontroled urine. This in almost any position of the patient would necessarily come more or less in contact with the raw edges of the fistule when brought together, and by its irritating effect have prevented their union. Relying, however, upon the protective power of our button, as shown on former occasions in the management of double and triple vesico-vaginal fistules, I resolved to hazard an attempt at least to place our patient in a condition for obturation of the vagina, which, however partial the relief promised, seemed to be called for under the circumstances. I say partial relief, because it is well known that closure of the vagina, as directed by M. Vidal, leaves the patient with no control over the urine, to say nothing of the ill consequences arising from the more or less stagnation of this fluid, and the catamenia at the lower part of the vagina. To prevent the latter result, therefore, it required that these excretions should always be freely and completely discharged, whether involuntarily or not. This, in my judgment, could be effected in no other way than by attaching the posterior to the anterior wall of the vagina just below the vesical extremity of the urethra, thus placing our line of cicatrization horizontally and far above the perpendicular one of M. Vidal, just within the meatus urinarius. Therefore, after closing the recto-vaginal opening, if possible, I determined to put into practice this new procedure. Accordingly, I went to work, and to my great astonishment the rectal opening was closed at our first trial. It remained now for me to see what could be realized by the procedure above proposed. The mode of performing this, however, we must defer until the case is introduced in its appropriate place. Suffice it to say, our first operation was attended with entire success, and our patient, contrary to the most sanguine hope, had almost complete control over her urine. I say almost complete, because she retains and passes it at will, dribbling only taking place from the urethra occasionally when she goes too long without emptying the bladder. She keeps perfectly dry at night, not requiring to get up at all, and during the day, when walking about, she can sometimes go three or four hours without any dribbling.

When I performed this operation, I did not for a moment suppose that our patient would regain, to any extent, the power of controlling her urine, if ever so successful. The most that I hoped for was a mechanical obstruction to its flow while the patient was in the recumbent posture, thus enabling her to lie dry at night. The result, however, has proven most conclusively that the vagina, thus occluded, secures to the patient the power of retaining and passing her urine at will, as though the fistulous opening itself were closed up.

This operation, therefore, cannot be regarded otherwise than as a great triumph. It enables us now to manage a class of cases, if not as satisfactorily as we could desire, certainly upon scientific principles, and with results never heretofore attained, as far as my information extends. Vidal's operation, however successfully performed, must, from the very nature of things, always be attended with an involuntary flow of urine upon leaving the recumbent posture, and therewith a downward pressure or unpleasant feeling at the lower extremity of the vagina, caused by the accumulation of urine constantly going on there.

A word now as to the classification of fistules, and I will then be ready to enter upon the report of cases. The rules for classifying all urinary fistules belonging to the female, are laid down in the paper referred to in the outset of these remarks, and consequently need not be repeated here. The object of classifying is to facilitate a correct understanding of the peculiarities of fistules, as well as the various modifications of treatment required for their successful management. Experience led me to the adoption of this course, and I see no reason for departing from it. The many advantages of such an arrangement, it is not my purpose here to enlarge upon; this I have already sufficiently done elsewhere. Suffice it to say, I shall adhere to the same general plan in the following report of cases.

(To be continued.)

7

ART. V.—*Tobacco an Antidote for the Poison of the Rattle Snake:* By HUMPHREY PEAKE, M. D., of Yazoo City, Mississippi.

WHILE Bibron's antidote for the poison of the rattle snake is exciting considerable interest, I deem it proper to call the attention of the profession to an article which I believe exercises some peculiar influ- ence over the poison of this reptile, and the ordinary effects of which are counteracted by it in return. I do not remember to have seen any mention of this in any of the books or journals, and, if the opin- ion be correct, the facility with which the remedy may at almost all times be procured, adds greatly to its importance. The article in question is tobacco, and my opinion of its efficacy is derived from two sources. Among many negroes, and white people of the lower class, it is considered an effectual antidote for the venom of the rat- tle, as well as that of other poisonous snakes. I got this idea from them when a boy. In Arkansas, where I was raised, there is a region of country known as the " Rich Woods," in which the crotalus con- fluentus, or rattle snake, is found in fearful abundance. It is a sin- gular fact that the common hog is a dangerous enemy of this serpent. He attacks him without scruple, and is apparently utterly regardless of the venom of his bite ; when he has slain him, he straightway de- vours him—nay, he sometimes literally eats him up alive. At least this is so in the " Rich Woods," where there are also great numbers of hogs. The result of these circumstances is that a great many of these snakes take refuge in the fields. The negroes there are not unfre- quently bitten by them. Tobacco is their remedy, which they chew and swallow freely on being bitten, and always with success. I know an intelligent man in that region of country who keeps his ne- groes constantly provided with tobacco in the warm season for the especial purpose of an antidote. He is satisfied from actual observa- tion of its power of completely counteracting the poisons of the rat- tle and moccasin snakes—trigonocephalus piscivorus.

The following occurred under my own observation : While en- gaged as a land surveyor, one of my chain-bearers was bitten on the dorsum of the foot by a rattle snake of the largest kind. It was in the month of August, when the poison of this snake is supposed to be more deadly than at any other time. In less than five minutes I had made him chew and swallow near two ounces of common chew- ing tobacco. It did not cause him to vomit ; indeed, so far was this from being the case, that he was not even nauseated by it. His limb swelled but very little, and he was up and about the next day, well. This happened before I had studied medicine, or I should not, perhaps, have been so liberal in supplying him with what certainly acted as an effectual remedy. I have had no opportunity of using it since.

Another domestic remedy, and in my opinion a very good one, is whisky or brandy. I have never seen it used, yet I am fully satisfied of its usefulness. The common people, from whom I have it, give it by pints as soon as it can be procured after the bite has been inflicted. The patient is made to drink almost as much as he can hold. I have talked with many persons who had seen it used, and with some who had thus used it, and they told me that it did not make them drunk, notwithstanding some had drank over a quart. This may have been owing in some degree to the strong mental impression present, but certainly not wholly so. Still another, but a vulgar remedy, is the tearing open of a living chicken, and binding it quivering to the wound.

OCTOBER 23, 1859.

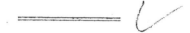

ART. VI.—*On Granulations of the Lining Membrane of the Uterine Cavity:* By JAMES TRUDEAU, M.D., of New Orleans.

THIS affection, which I have often met with here, is of comparatively rare occurrence in the Eastern States, and in the temperate or cool climates of middle Europe—described for the first time by Récamier,* and afterwards mentioned by his pupils, Nélaton and Chassaignac— it has become of late better known to the profession. Last year, several good monographs were published in Paris, on this subject. The most complete is the thesis of Dr. Rouger (*Etudes Cliniques sur les Fongosités Utérines,* Paris, 1858, No. 253).

Uterine fungosities (a new term proposed by Récamier, and a good one, to designate that peculiar state of the mucous membrane of the

---

* RÉCAMIER. Des Granulations dans la cavité Utérine; Annales de Thérapeutique, Août, 1846.

NÉLATON. Des Fongosités Utérines, Gaz. des Hôp., 1853.

CHASSAIGNAC. Sur le Traitement des Granulations Utérines par le Cautérization. Bulletin de Thérapeutique, Déc., 1848.

uterine cavity), do not certainly deserve in the nosological frame, a distant place from small vesicular polypi developed within the cavity of the uterus and non-malignant epithelioma (cancroïd or cauliflower excresences). They are true fibro-plasms located in the cavity of the uterus and that of its neck, and affecting two very distinct forms.

A. Small tumors, with a wide base, originating directly from the mucous membrane. Their size varies from that of a pin's head to that of a strawberry. The larger tumors are often pediculated. Their surface is rough and irregular ; their consistency soft ; they can be easily detached by scraping them gently with the nails, or a scoop. Their color varies from pale pink to red. They are generally found on the mucous membrane of the uterus, at its posterior face, and near the implantation of the fallopian tubes. This variety is seldom found on the mucous membraue of the neck. We designate these small tumors by the name of *cellulo-vascular vegetations.*

B. Pediculated vegetations, smaller in size than the preceding; of a grayish color, of a greater density, elastic and smooth. Their place of election is in the inferior segment of the uterine cavity, and in that of the neck. It is almost impossible to separate their pedicles from the mucous membrane. Those are the *cellulo-fibrous vegetations.*

According to the researches of M. Charles Robin, these vegetations consist of a hypertrophy of the mucous membrane, with numerous cells, fibro-plastic elements, and an increased vascularity for the variety A (see this interesting paper, Archives Générales de Médecine, 4éme série, tom. xviii). The variety B has the same histological structure with fewer vessels, and is protected by a layer of epithelium, like that of the uterus. Those two varieties are sometimes found together, in the same uterus, with small follicular cysts. It is especially the case with elderly multiparous women. Sometimes they are observed at the orifice of the os tincæ, forming small vascular tumors bulging out of the canal. Récamier and Nélatou relate several cases of that kind, which were mistaken for encephaloid cancer. We have observed a very interesting case of the same kind, which will be reported subsequently.

The symptoms of internal uterine vegetations consist, at first, in an increase of the menstrual flow, which soon degenerates into profuse hæmorrhage. These are succeeded by watery leucorrhœal discharges, often tinged with blood, and of greater or lesser abundance, according to the degree of the disease. Sometimes the leucorrhœa is very pain-- ful, causing a sensation of burning, which extends to the neck of the bladder, and even to the rectum. Dysmenorrhœa soon joins that train of symptoms at every menstrual period. It is certainly caused by the presence of a large quantity of blood in the cavity of the uterus, and the subsequent expelling pains to rid the organ of the accumulation. After some time, the menstrual periods become, as it were, subintrant, each one encroaching upon the other, causing the unfortunate patients to be constantly flooding. The loss of blood is not always considerable between the interval of the menstrua ; it amounts, sometimes, to mere oozing, but at the regular turns it is always large, and often alarming. Soon after the first appearance of menorrhagia, the digestive functions are apt to be disturbed. The patients complain of painful sensations toward the epigastric region. At times the craving for food is incessant, but that deceptive appetite disappears after swallowing a few mouthfuls. Oftener they loathe the sight of their once favorite dainties. Digestion, too, becomes difficult ; in one word, all the confirmed symptoms of dyspepsia set in. With these spmptoms, the patients complain of sharp pains at the lumbar, sacral and hypogastric regions. These last are some- times of such a degree of severity as to cause faintness. Not un- frequently, there is a painful spot in one of the iliac regions, extend- ing to the corresponding limb. This last symptom, I look upon as one of great value.

Together with the above mentioned phenomena, the patients lose flesh rapidly. Their features assume that peculiar cast of counte- nance observed in many uterine disorders (facies uterino) ; the skin loses its softness and brilliancy ; the eyes are set deeper in the orbit, and surrounded with a bluish circle ; the extremities are always cold, even during the warmest weather. Anæmia makes its appearance as soon as the loss of blood becomes profuse. With it we have its well known train, palpitation of the heart, difficulty in breathing, etc., and a series of hysterical symptoms of proportionate severity to the nervous irritability of the patients.

The affective faculties experience also great perturbatious. But they are of the same character as those observed in most uterine affections : dejection of mind, peevishness, irritability of temper, and unusual restlessness.

The examination by touch, shows an enlargement of the body of the uterus, with tenderness of the organ, and greater softness of its parietes. The vaginal portion of the neck is often hypertrophied, softer than usual ; the canal dilated so as to admit easily the finger. The speculum discloses a patulous condition of the os, through which a thick, transparent, tenacious, yellowish white mucous is seen to exude. The neck is generally congested and dotted with minute superficial excoriations. With the aid of a peculiar speculum, granulations resting on an inflamed and excoriated membrane can be sometimes traced in its cavity. Occasionally, as I have before mentioned, small fungous masses, project from the orifice of the neck, establishing at once the true character of the disease.

The introduction of the uterine sound is easy, owing to the great softness of the tissues, when the disease invades both the uterine cavity and that of the neck. But when it is limited to the uterine cavity alone, some difficulty is experienced in passing it through the cervical canal. Once introduced, it can be moved in any direction into the cavity of the body of the uterus, showing its increased capacity, and greater thinness. In some cases, even it is carried far enough to allow the instrument to be felt through the abdominal parietes. The introduction of the sound causes often some hæmorrhage.

As it may be seen by the preceding, the existence of uterine vegetations has no pathognomonic symptoms distinguishing it in a positive manner from several other uterine disorders ; yet with a little care the differential diagnosis can always be established, in a satisfactory manner. Uterine polypi of small size may simulate this affection, but, unless enclosed within the uterine cavity, the touch or the speculum will disclose at once the mistake. If small polypi were contained in the cavity of the neck or of the uterus, the treatment being the same in both affections, an error would be of no importance whatever.

In a case of simple menorrhagia, the hæmorrhages, patulous condition of the os, and softness of the vaginal portion of the neck, may induce the belief that these accidents are caused by uterine fungosities. However, let us remember that in uterine fungosities, as well as dysuria, there are always present severe lumbar and hypogastric pains; the hæmorrhages in metrorrhagia take place during the menstrual period ; in uterine fungosities, they become subintrant. The leucorrhœal disharge is generally confined, in metrorrhagia, to a few days before and after the periods; it is constant in the case of uterine fungosities. In metror-rhagia, the*cervical cavity is pale, and as it were, bloodless ; it is red, congested, and often the seat of granulations, in the other disease. With cancer, and especially epithelioma, it may be more readily confounded. In fact, we have in common, profuse hæmorrhages at all periods, discharges, pains, cachectic appearance. A proper examination by the touch and the speculum, cannot fail to establish the true nature of the disease we have to deal with.

This affection progresses, in the greater majority of cases, but slowly ; the general health of the patient is but little affected at first; but when the long train of accidents we have mentioned begin to unroll themselves, the most robust constitution is soon undermined. Yet, the prognosis is seldom unfavorable, and becomes so, chiefly from complications arising either from peri-uterine irritation, or retro-uterine hæmorrhage.

M. Nélaton says that this affection is observed on females who have passed the prime of youth. Seldom had he met it before twenty-five years of age, and oftener at thirty-two and thirty-five. M. Richet confirms this statement (which is in perfect concurrence with our own observations), and remarks farther that it can always be traced to a confinement or miscarriage. There is but little doubt, but that to the puerperal state and to uterine hypersecretions, which are liable to follow the lochia, we can ascribe the true ætiology of uterine fungosities.

The majority of French, German, and English authors, among whom we may mention Aran (1), Scanzoni (2), H. Bennet (3), and Tyler Smith (4), include the description and history of this disease, under the head of chronic metritis. There is no doubt that in sound pathology, their position is perfectly correct ; but on the practical point of view, it is quite different. The treatment required in order to destroy internal vegetations, affecting often a polypoïd character, perhaps even a cancroïd development, is wholly different from that calculated to remedy chronic inflammation, affecting either the uterine mucous membrane or its parenchyma.

The conclusion of this paper, together with the cases related, will, we trust, sustain us in the position we have taken.

(1) Leçons cliniques sur les maladies de l'utérus et ses annexes. (Paris, 1858.)
(2) Traité pratique des maladies des organes sexuels de la femme. (Paris, 1859.)
(3) A practical treatise on inflammation of the uterus, etc. (Philadelphia, 1853.)
(4) The pathology and treatment of leucorrhœa. (Philadelphia, 1855.)

ART. VII.—*Speculative and Practical Remarks on Absorption, the Enepidermic, Iatraleptic, Endermic, and Hypodermic Methods of Medication :* By BENNET DOWLER, M. D.

THE great centre to which all the lines of medical investigation should be converged, is therapeutics, or the prevention and cure of disease. If the whole circle of the medical and auxiliary sciences is occupied by the physician, if he observes and thinks, and thinks and observes again ; if he seeks new routes of experimentation, new interpretations of phenomena, all gravitate towards this centre. Hence every new remedy, or new application of an old one, stimulates hope and excites enthusiasm. Here enthusiasm is meritorious. Although exaggerated expectations are, and have been, doomed to disappointment, yet the human mind never has, nor perhaps will it ever, abandon the cherished hope (illusory it may be) of discovering panaceas and specifics, or at least, remedies which shall possess great certainty and uniformity, if not obsolute universality, for the cure of nearly all diseases, except accidental injuries, the decays of age, and the ravages of a few malignant maladies. This bias of the mind in favor of panaceas or universal remedies, is the great lever by which charlatans move the world of humanity.

If a specific for any disease shall ever be discovered, the remedy will probably cure or alleviate all analogous diseases. As yet, it can hardly be said that a single specific is known for any disease, not even for the itch. Notwithstanding the great advancements recently made in diagnosis, that branch of science is imperfect, especially in diseases considered curable. In a few incurable diseases, as cancer, consumption, etc., diagnosis approximates certainty. If in a single case of disease, a cure can be effected by any remedy, all other cases precisely homological or identical would be cured by the same remedy. This, though an ideal or transcendental axiom, is a necessary truth in therapeutics as well as in physics ; for, the same causes, conditions, or antecedents, must produce the same effects invariably. To suppose that identical antecedents may give rise to contradictory or different sequences, is to renounce the sciences altogether. The application of this rule or axiom is attended with uncertainty in therapeutics. No intellect, however gigantic, has as yet been able to ap-

---

* One object in offering these remarks, is to show the will, if not the ability, to fulfill the requests of some correspondents whose letters of inquiry on these topics remain unanswered.

preciate all of the antecedents of a single malady; that is, the nature of the vital forces, the morbid elements, and essential conditions. Enough, however, is known, to show that in the same malady, as it appears to the senses, each case differs more or less, though the causes and nature of this difference often eludes the keenest research. Hence diagnosis, which is never absolutely perfect and exhaustive, especially in the initial stages of disease, degenerates into probability. Hence, also, the remedy which cures one case will fail to cure another apparently, though not really, identical case. Diagnosis is a barren science without therapeutics. Therapeutics is the science of blunders without diagnosis.

What remedy so ever is beneficial in one disease will be beneficial in analogous even though not identical diseases ; but in the application of this rule, there is, as already stated, great difficulty. This luminous principle of therapeutics irradiates the pages of Professor Stone's papers in the present and preceding number of this journal.

If therapeutics were denied all claim to pure rationalism, it might on the principle of enlightened empiricism, that is, mere experience alone, sustain itself. Having made a reliable diagnosis, it might affirm that the remedy which cured one will cure another, although no reason, physiological or pathological, other than the simple fact, would be assigned in explanation. The significant question put by Bichât, applies to experience or empiricism as well as to rationalism, namely, " Qu'est l'observation si l'on ignore là où siège le mal ? "

With an absolutely perfect diagnosis, experience would enable a physician to decide that a disease, though its cause might be unknown, would or would not terminate fatally if left to nature, and in the same way, the effects of medicines for good or evil, might be known, though their *modus operandi* might not. Although curative agents possessing undeviating certainty and universality in therapy should not be attainable, yet persevering efforts for their attainment will tend to approximate, if they do not fully realize these ends. Disappointment is not necessarily eternal. Scientific optimists hope on and hope ever that certainty, if not universality, will be attained in therapeutics.

Medicine has already, and of late, achieved triumphs little short of mathematical certainty, both in the prevention and cure of disease, which a century ago would have been pronounced utopian. Vaccination is an almost perfect example of a limited panacea (excuse the

8

verbal contradiction), so far as small pox (once the destroyer of millions) is concerned. Scurvy, once the destroyer of unnumbered thousands, has been nearly extinguished by preventive means. Prophylaxis or sanitary measures for the preservation of health, and the adoption of means to prevent diseases which have been developed chiefly in recent times, ennoble medicine, and should convince right-thinking persons that its progress is onward. These, rather than drugs, are the approximate panaceas now the most prevalent in the medical profession.

Anæsthesia, formerly an ideal conception seemingly baseless as a vision of the night, has been of late approximated, if not fully realized. The diagnostic uses and values of percussion and auscultation, by some overrated, by others underrated, have approximate certainty and universality in their appropriate spheres. Practical surgery and physic afford many similar illustrations.

If medicine be viewed from a therapeutical stand-point—if the recent prevalence of the gastric pathology and the consequent fears of exciting or increasing already existing inflammations by drugs introduced into the stomach be considered—if the researches of Dutrochet* and many others on endosmosis and absorption be duly estimated—if the researches of MM. Lembert and Lesieur (made more than thirty years ago), on the endermic method of medication (not to name later writers), be appreciated, it is truly surprising that this and some other forms of the external application of medical agents have been, and continue to be, almost universally neglected. Had these principles been thoroughly tested during the last three decennia, an applied science of external therapy might probably have been founded. But as this matter now stands, who knows the particular articles of materia medica available for this purpose? their number? their best mode of preparation? their precise doses? their physiological, curative, dangerous or toxic effects or symptoms? the celerity or tardiness with which each medicinal agent is absorbed through either the denuded or the sound skin? or the cellular tissues?

---

* *Memoires pour servir a l'histoire anatomique et physiologique des vegetaux et des animaux; avec un atlas. T.* 11. Paris, 1837. This work, published ten years before the author's death, is one of great value, and well deserves to be translated into English; or, if so translated, its republication in the United States would prove very acceptable to thinkers and workers who prefer the physics of physiology to either the incomprehensibilities of neuro-reflex physiology, or the theory of a pure neuro-dynamical pathology. These abstractions may, in many cases, be known by two characteristics, namely, they cannot be proved—they cannot be disproved. Such speculations seldom live more than one generation. Truth, though often neglected for a time, is immortal; if temporarily lost, it will be, almost always, re-discovered.

The masters of the profession in their prelections and writings, on external medication, when they casually allude to it, require as an essential preliminary, the removal of the scarf skin, which is a painful and repulsive procedure for the patient, and a tedious, or at least a troublesome one for the medical attendant. Hear what these masters say : In his article on the endermic method, (Dict. de Méd.), M. Bouillaud lays down as a fundamental preliminary, in this mode of medication, that the epidermis must be removed by a blister or by other means. The late Anthony Todd Thompson, M. D., professor of materia medica in the University of London, in the first volume (pp. 7, 11) of his elaborate work on materia medica (Lond. 1832), says of the mode of medicinal action, that it " can only be referred to nervous sympathy ; we are unable to prove that any chemical change is effected in the circulating mass ; if we admit the principle that medicines can only affect the body through the medium of the nerves, there is no difficulty in understanding it, etc. No medicinal agents applied to the surface of the .body, *when the cuticle is entire*, except to a small portion of the skin, are absorbed, but they exert their influence altogether through the medium of the nerves." Although this author quotes opinions on both sides of this question, he seems, with rare exceptions, to reject the doctrine of absorption through the sound skin. He says : " The opinions respecting cutaneous absorption are very unsettled. The observations and experiments of many celebrated physiologists, tend to disprove the existence of *cutaneous absorption whilst the cuticle remains entire.*"

I will here stop to remark, that those who declaim against physiologico-pathological :vivisections and experiments upon the inferior animals, have only to consider this neurological explanation of the *modus operandi* of medicines, taught by Professor Thomson in the University of London, about a quarter of a century ago, and they will see—thanks to the experiments of Magendie and his successors— how completely this nervous theory is exploded by demonstrative evidence, showing that medicines are absorbed into the blood-vessels, and traverse the entire circulation with a celerity scarcely credible, that is, in a few seconds, even from and through parts, the nerves of which had been severed; while, on the other hand, the arrest of the circulation, the nerves remaining intact, prevented the action of medicinal and toxic agents. These failed to act though applied directly to the nerves.

Professor Wood, one of the latest and most reliable authorities on the Materia Medica, says : " In this (the endermic) mode of employing medicines, the epidermis is first removed, and the medicines then applied to the denuded surface." Dr. Wood says, however, that "medicines are probably absorbed from any part of the body. There can be no doubt that the epidermis opposes a great impediment to absorption. Deprived of the epidermis, the skin admits the entrance of medicines with great facility, though even in this state, somewhat less readily than the gastric mucous membrane, probably because it is less vascular."

Christison, in his work on Poisons, says: " Cutaneous absorbtion is slow, on account of the obstacle presented by the cuticle and by the intricate capillaries of the true skin."

Notwithstanding the experimental evidence extant concerning the advantages of external modification, the principle has hitherto remained a barren rather than a fruitful one in pharmacy, posology and therapeutics.

If a dose exhibited ependermically, endermically or hypodermically, act with more or less celerity and energy than a similar dose given internally, the pharmacopœia should present corresponding formulæ for the preparation and doses of medicines.

Endermic (with analogous modes of) medication, though by no means a novelty, is now rising in importance among therapeutists. The pathological condition of the stomach *per se*, seldom requires, on its own account, the topical application of medicaments. On the contrary, such agents are usually intended to act, not topically, but on the general system, and often secondarily through it on remote special organs. It is reasonable to suppose, that for the most part neither functional nor structural derangements of the stomach and bowels will be so likely to occur from external as from direct stomachic or intestinal applications of certain medicines. If effective medication can be attained by the inoculation, endermic, or ependermic method, with less local or irritating effect either primarily or secondarily upon the stomach, a great good will be achieved and serious dangers will be often prevented. If external medication can be intelligently and effectually accomplished so as to arrest or control morbid action not only without involving the stomach injuriously, but to a great extent leaving its functions intact, a great advantage, present and prospective, will be gained, especially in certain cases in which the sick require considerable nutriment as one of the indications of cure. Moreover, the battle between disease and drugs often reduces the vital forces to the lowest ebb, and a complete victory can be achieved only by bringing up, in good time, those reliable reserves, the nutritive powers of the stomach, thereby reïnstating health.

The paramount importance now attributed to a rich nutritive diet, by many practitioners, affords a striking contrast with the opinions, in that behalf, which prevailed but a few years ago. Broussais regarded what is called good living, " black meats, game, oils, pungent articles,"* as predisposing, and purgatives, emetics, and the like, as exciting causes of gastritis ; and, according to him, gastritis is the primary pathological condition of almost all diseases, especially the pyrexiæ and phlegmasiæ. To the disciples of this school, who hold that there is any virtue in medicinal agents beyond those of gumwater, acidulated slops, and lancets, endermic or analogous medication, ought to be peculiarly acceptable, although their prophet does not mention it, unless cataplasms, baths, etc., be so considered.

All careful observers will admit that the stomach is either primarily or secondarily affected, at least functionally, in most diseases. To say nothing of its anatomical lesions, its digestive and absorptive powers sometimes become weak or paralyzed, so that neither ingesta nor medicine is assimilated or taken into the economy. In some cases, for example, in cholera, medicinal agents, as well as diet, may remain in the stomach unchanged, unabsorbed, not only useless, for the purposes of cure, but irritants, foreign bodies. Here endermic, and still more hypodermic medication inspires hope founded on reported cases and experiments already extant.

Moreover, insane persons, young, obstinate children, and persons during convulsions, coma, epilepsy, hysteria, etc., often will not and sometimes cannot swallow. Upon forcibly pouring medicines into the throat in cases of insensibility, or when there is spasm, or paralysis of the glottis, there is danger that suffocation may occur from the entrance of these into the wind-pipe. Of this there is great danger in sun-stroke in the first degree.

Vomiting, one of the most general symptoms in disease, frequently expels medicine in whole or in part at once and persistently, and it is usuallly difficult to estimate how much is expelled, how much retained,

* "Punch and burnt brandy ought to be regarded as true poisons." *Chron. Phleg. ii*, 137.

and whether a dangerous cumulative effect, or no effect will follow under such dubious circumstances. Thus, on the one hand, there is danger from over-medication, and on the other, from the uncontrolled force of the malady. To wait, in order to decide from the physiological effects, whether the medicine is or is not retained in the economy in cases of cholera, congestive intermittent, and the like, is neither safe for the patient nor pleasant for his attendant.

On the other hand, the alleged danger of causing, or of increasing an already existing gastric inflammation, by the introduction into the stomach of active medicinal agents, has doubtlessly been greatly exaggerated even in cases where the primary disease or lesion is seated in that organ. Calomel, for example, has been charged by its enemies with causing inflammation of this organ as its general natural effect. Not only so : a distinguished teacher and author, who contributed the second article to the first volume of this journal (1844), gave it this alarming title, namely, "*calomel considered as a poison.*" The writer begins by asking and answering the following question : "*What! calomel a poison? It is even so.*"

It would seem that calomel and some other medicines, if not poisonous to, have never agreed so well with French, as with English and American stomachs. The *Medical Times and Gazette* (Oct. 22, 1859), has the following passage upon this subject :

" Our French brethren can't understand the English method of using opium, calomel, and antimony. Mercury as an *alterative* (let the term signify what it may) is with them a medicament unknown. They are astonished at the skill and audacity which we employ in giving large doses of opium. 'If,' says one public writer, 'we were to take from the English physicians their opium and their calomel, they would have to renounce the practice of medicine.' M. Girard Teulon exclaims at the incomprehensible fact of English surgeons attacking stricture of the urethra by opium, *i. e.*, their commencing with the opium instead of the bougie. However, as he very sensibly remarks, when a whole nation systematically carry on the same sort of practice in dealing with opium, calomel, and antimony, it is worth while that we should consider whether it may not have some goodness in it. In compliment to our neighbors, we beg to rejoin that on similar principle, we on this side the channel, seeing that they systematically cure or treat their patients without the continual and daily application of these articles, and we must suppose satisfactorily treat them, ought reasonably to consider whether it be not possible that we use them more frequently and more extensively than is good for the patient who is subjected to their action."

In no department of science is charity more commendable than in therapeutics—charity, not towards the evidently false and absurd, but charity for the earnest inquirers after truth who may differ honestly concerning the efficacy of therapeutic agents. Mathematicians, physicists, and astronomers agree, because the fundamental laws of terrestial and celestial mechanics are fixed, known, demonstrable. But the changeful conditions of morbidity, and the apparently variable actions of medicinal agents, certain enough in themselves, exist in relation to the human understanding as probabilities of varying intensities which cannot be defined and reduced to axioms "having neither variableness nor shadow of turning." The extreme oscillations and revolutions in medical treatment are not generally the results of culpable ignorance, but arise from the real or supposed inefficacy of old measures, or from an enthusiastic expectation that new ones are better. The new remedies soon prove to be neither specifics nor panaceas ; perhaps, they are found to be inferior to the old. In their turn they usually fall. The excessive and unwarrantable use or rather abuse of a valuable remedy, often causes a reaction, whereupon it falls into oblivion, or its real efficacy is underrated ; nay, worse—it may be denounced as a poison. Such has been the fortune af calomel, etc.

The late Dr. Beaumont,* of the United States Army, in his remarkable and prolonged experiments on St. Martin, who had, and still has, a traumatic opening two and a half inches in diameter, into his stomach, resulting from a gun-shot wound in 1822, found, when St. Martin was sick from disorder of this organ, attended with lassitude, debility, fever, dry skin, headache, coated tongue, aphthous and erythematous inflammation, bloody grumous exudations, offensive and vitiated secretions, with muco-purulent matter, and " numerous pustules resembling coagulated lymph spread over the mucous coat of the stomach," with suspended digestive power, and arrested, diminished, or altered states of the gastric juice, that, "on dropping through the aperture half a dozen of calomel pills, four or five grains

* Born 1796 ; spent $3,500 in his experiments ; applied to Congress for a reimbursement of his expenses, in thus promoting scientific discovery ; got nothing ; and died at St. Louis in 1853, deserving a national monument to his memory.

each, the foregoing symptoms and appearances were removed, sometimes in three hours." However, in some instances, longer periods were
required before a cure was effected.

Dr. Beaumont, during eight years' experimentation (1825—1833),
mentions several attacks of gastric disease from which St. Martin
suffered, though in general a very vigorous and healthy man. Some
of these attacks originated spontaneously, some from intemperance,
others from repeated mechanical irritations with cords, muslin bags,
thermometers, and the like, used in experimentation. These attacks
yielded with remarkable celerity and uniformity to pills of calomel
and blue mass dropped into the stomachical opening. Thus all the
phenomena of the diseased appearances, and of the rehabilitation of
the tissues, secretions, and normal functions, were open to ocular
demonstration. Dr. Beaumont's researches in this most extraordinary
case were directed chiefly to the physiology of digestion, but their
pathological import is valuable.

Dr. Beaumont makes the following general statement concerning
the pathological conditions of the stomach, founded on ocular demonstration :

"It is interesting to observe to what extent the stomach may
become diseased, without manifesting any external symptoms of
such disease, or any evident signs of functional aberration. Vitiated
secretions may also take place, and continue for some time, without
affecting the health in any *sensible* degree. In the case of the subject
of these experiments, inflammation certainly does exist, to a considerable extent, even in *apparent health*—greater than could have been
believed to comport with the due operations of the gastric functions."
(P. 252-3 Edin. edit.)

Endermic medication, following as it does a blister or other means
by which the epidermis has been removed, is generally painful in a high
degree, and may occasion local inflammation—inconveniences and
dangers from which the enepidermic mode is free. Even the preliminary blister in the former, may itself cause gangrene in the advanced
stage of some diseases, as scarlatina, etc.

Experiments appear to show that minute division, or best of all,
complete solution (which is virtually a ready mode for dividing most
completely), favors absorption. Hence medicines which are soluble
should if possible be given in that form, when speedy action is
required. And, inasmuch as endosmosis or imbibition is an auxiliary

if not a fundamental physical condition of absorption, in the living organism, each medicinal agent might as far as possible be thus tested by dead membranes or septa, in order to gain all possible information concerning this property, particularly in reference to the external modes of medication. There are probably many medicaments, particularly those of easy solution and of wetting properties, which possess a direct affinity, yet in different ratios of intensity, for the skin (and the subcutaneous tissues and fluids), being adapted to permeate and pass through that porous membrane, and its epidermis into the capillary and general circulation. There is reason to believe that different portions of the skin have, in this respect, different degrees of susceptibility, different times and velocities. Disallowing (what many physiologists might not be willing to concede), the claims of the skin to vital action *sui generis,* or selecting endowment, this tissue as a merely physical medium, is, upon the principle of endosmosis, well adapted for the imbibition of medicaments with great force. From the simplest primordial cell floating in the blood plasma to the solid skeleton, porosity and permeability everywhere exist, and are apparently available for medication, as well as nutrition. Porous membranes, according to Dutrochet, exert a force for the transmission or interchange of liquids of different densities and composition, equal to a pressure of four and a half atmospheres.

The physiological physicists who seem to think themselves freer from prejudice and ignorance than others who think that absorption is not wholly physical, and that the vital economy in both health and disease presents phenomena peculiar to itself over and above physical endosmosis and exosmosis, take a great deal for granted which they do not demonstrate by physics. When cholera develops itself, the absorbent action is greatly if not entirely suspended in the mucous membrane, its glands and vessels, where, an hour or two before, it had been active. It sometimes happens after one or two fæcal evacuations that the digested, scentless, milky chyle is discharged from the upper portion of the bowels. Here the disease surprises the digestive and absorbent functions. The apparatus, membranes, septa, liquids, and general arrangements of the experimenters, have no known existence or peculiar arrangement to explain such a case.

It is necessary to go with the physicist as far as his art and science will explain or aid in explaining the phenomena and functions of the

9

living economy. The physiologist will, however, find thus far parallelism rather than identity; but even parallelism will fail, and he must pass beyond brute matter and occupy other and peculiar grounds in the broad domains of the science of life, and should no more than the psychologist himself "seek the living among the dead." The entire animal kingdom—vertebrata, mollusca, radiata, articulata, present fundamental antitheses to the natural history of inert matter.

The late M. Magendie, a hardened physicist in physiology and an infidel in therapeutics, affirmed that absorption is wholly physical, being sometimes from without, inwardly; from within, outwardly; that is, by imbibition, which is therefore in contrary directions, and is a duality; the one is imbibition proper—the other exbibition; in other words, absorption and exhalation are identical; or, as Dutrochet would say, there is "*un courant d'endosmose—un courant d'exosmose.*" Honor to these illustrious masters for their researches! Their theories are to a certain extent true, homologically, or at least analogically, in their application to science of the living economy, but do not cover the entire field, nor upon mechanical principles account for the phenomena of the latter, in absorption, selection, assimilation, secretion, excretion, and elimination, waste and repair, sensation, passion, intellection, voluntary and involuntary motion, reproduction, calorification, growth, disease, decay, life, death, not to mention the irrepressible expectation of a future.

Magendie regarded the epidermis as a great barrier to imbibition, which, however true, seems to have been exaggerated, and hence little has been done to test the availability of enepidermic medication.

The iatraleptic method, or the therapeutical application of medicaments by inunction, is as ancient as medical history itself. In the first sentence of the first book of Celsus, he mentions this class of doctors in connection with physicians. Of the iatraleiptes or iatralipta, *medicus unguentarius*, or unction doctor, Pliny says that it was an order founded by Prodicus, at Selymbria. Hippocrates used iatraleptic medication, as ointments and fats applied to the skin, sometimes aided by friction. This is only a branch of the enepidermic treatment.

The small esteem in which the enepidermic method is held, is indicated by many writers. Mr. Wilson, in his recent work on the skin, says, that even when aided by friction, "some few substances only can be transmitted through the skin ; and excepting in the single instance of a medicine, the practice is discarded." This exception probably is mercurial ointment.

Without offering at present any direct opinion upon the efficacy of this mode, it may be proper to state, that from recent researches into external medication, this practice is gaining advocates whose experiments and opinions deserve consideration. M. Jeannel, one of the editors of the *Journal de Médecine de Bordeaux* (in his *Mémoires sur les corps gras**), maintains that the metallic oxydes chemically combining with fatty bodies, are absorbed through the skin and are assimilated by the economy. He recommends, in the October (1859) number of the journal above mentioned, oil baths ; or in their stead, as being more convenient, emulsified baths, for which he gives a formula. During immersion in emulsified baths, the fatty matters are deposited upon the surface of the skin, and after thus bathing, the epidermis, notwithstanding repeated frictions, and after having been made dry, remains *lubrified* to a degree altogether remarkable. Such a bath repeated several times daily, has, with him, been found to impart a comfortable feeling, as well as vigor, etc.

The enepidermic and iatraleptic treatment have been very successfully employed by M. J. B. Thompson, who, in a paper published in the *Bulletin Général de Thérapeutique* (Sept., 1859), gives the results of his personal observation and experience in the external application of medicinal agents during the last seventeen years—a condensed translation of which will be given in the course of the present article.

Contrary to the opinion of M. Deschamps, M. Thompson maintains from personal observation, that applications of medicated oils and fats to the sound skin, possess great curative efficacy. Not only so. He has found that grease, *per se*, applied externally is highly medicinal. This is the iatraleptic treatment in the most literal sense.

Dr. Thompson has observed during seventeen years, in a population principally employed in the manufactures of wool, that feeble, puny children in a few weeks after their entrance into the wool-spinning factories, present a striking improvement in their physical appearance ; that the oil (always that of the olive) with which they

---

* See vol. XVI, p. 390, *New Orleans Med. and Surg. Jour.* : *Researches into the influence of Fatty bodies in the Absorption and Assimilation of Metallic Oxydes* ; by Prof. Jeannel, Translated by Dr. Barbot.

work, penetrates into their systems through the skin, in considerable
quantities, influencing, in an advantageous manner, scrofulous affections, and also improving the constitutions of the operatives. This
was proved furthermore, by the increased weight of operatives whose
work brought them thus in contact with great quantities of fatty
matters. This increase was further proven by comparison with
youths employed in cotton and other manufactures, and also with
others not so employed, living in the same locality. Even in the
same factory, those who ceased to work in the grease, lost weight, as
compared with those who continued so to work.

M. Thompson finds, in agreement with these facts, that medicated
ointments, plasters, etc., as of mercury, iodine, belladonna, opium, tinc-
tures, chloric and sulphuric æther, etc., enter the economy, when
rubbed on the forehead, backhead, palms, soles of the feet, and epigastrium, and produce in moderate doses the most favorable effects,
that is, their appropriate actions ; cases of which he details ; from
which it appears, that the external administration proved effectual,
after the internal had utterly failed. Thus in a case of *delirium tremens*, the patient had taken every three hours, for two successive
nights, forty drops *de liqueur de morphine*, without obtaining sleep, who,
on the third night, became quite tranquil from the use of thirty drops
of the tincture of opium, rubbed upon the epigastrium.

I may here stop to remark, that while translating this last passage,
I determined to try the external application of laudanum in an obstinate case of delirium tremens then under my care, in which enormous
doses of morphia and laudanum given internally had wholly failed to
procure sleep, after a continuous wakefulness for a week. The patient, a middle aged gentleman of family, of means, and of general
sobriety (having used neither spirits nor wines for seventeen years),
had more than a week before I saw him, drank a secret alcoholic preparation called bitters, which produced severe sickness, violent tre-
mors, mental agitation, etc. During four days before I saw him, he
had not, as he and others affirmed, slept any. He had been treated
unsuccessfully, with small portions of brandy ; had vomited several times—was constipated ; had taken a purgative of castor
oil, which acted well. I found him bathed in sweat ; thirsty ;
tongue ·tremulous, coated with a brownish fur, but moist ; pulse
soft and full ; restless ; trembling of the arms, hands, and body ;
features expressive of fright ; answers quickly, but with intelligence.

Morphia was substituted for the brandy. Of the former he took about three or four grains daily for nearly three days, which neither brought sleep nor removed the muscular agitations. During this time, however, he took, without advice, another dose of oil which operated, after which his pulse became quick and feeble ; his strength diminished ; he was worse. At night laudanum was freely used internally several times, commencing with a large teaspoonful dose, which produced nausea, but no sleep or relief whatever. Next morning a drachm of laudanum was rubbed on the epigastrium, and the same quantity three hours afterward. Unexpectedly soon after the last application, he fell into a good sleep. In two days after, he left his bed.

In this, as in most other cases where internal medication had preceded the external, I have not been able to draw satisfactory conclusions as to the part taken by the latter. In the epidemic yellow fever of 1839, I practised to some extent endermic medication on the denuded skin, in that disease, chiefly with preparations of quinine, but not having felt justified, in most cases, in omitting the simultaneous stomachical and rectal medications, the curative action, if any, of the former could not be appreciated, because it could not be separately considered.

Dr. Thompson, however, adopted a far more satisfactory mode of experimentation. In order to test in an unequivocal manner, the reality of endermic or rather enepidermic medication, he made numerous experiments upon himself : Thus he used friction with half a spoonful of *café de laudanum*—this experiment he repeated from fifty to sixty times, which produced elevation of the pulse, an increased activity of ideas, followed by confusion and incoherency of mind, with a sensation of fulness in the head ; perspiration ; and at the end of twenty or twenty-five minutes after the application above mentioned, sleep came on insensibly. Chloric and sulphuric æther, in like manner, caused a rise and fulness of the pulse, perspiration, incoherency of ideas, and sleep. In some cases, chloric æther, sulphuric æther, laudanum, or the tincture of hyosciamus, produced no complete sleep, but excitement, revery, and a drowsy feeling for twelve hours.

The condition of the organism, and especially that of the stomach, require to be taken into consideration. If endermic or enepidermic medication be practised when the functions of the stomach are disordered—when it is loaded with food and engaged in digestion—the disturbances of the system are increased, and sleep is accompanied with dreams and agitations. These narcotics, even in small doses applied externally, will in three or four hours, slowly but surely produce soporific effects. In the case of a soldier who was ordered a flax-seed poultice with fifteen drops of laudanum on it, next morning he was found comatose, had spasms and convulsions, and died. It was discovered, that owing to a mistake, an ounce of laudanum had been used in the cataplasm, instead of fifteen drops.

From a very extended course of experimentation both upon himself and his patients for many years, M. Thompson is led to the conclusion that the endermic and iatraleptic medications deserve greater attention on the part of the practitioner, than has yet been accorded to this method—a method which seems to be almost completely ignored among physicians, who appear to regard with almost absolute scepticism, the possibility of introducing through the intact or sound skin, medicinal agents. When he was a student, professors taught that the epidermis should be removed, and the medicine reduced to powder and put on the denuded parts, in order to insure its absorption.

Many physiologists have demonstrated, that water at eighty-two degrees Fahrenheit, passes through the skin and augments the weight of the body. Many alkaline substances, also, rhubarb, certain coloring matters, dissolved in baths, have been refound in the urine. The vaccine vesicle has been produced by placing the lymph in contact with the sound skin.

M. Thompson says that another lesson is taught by the facts which he has witnessed, namely, the bad effects of opiates introduced by the mouth, which may and ought to be prevented by the adoption of the iatraleptic method. The internal administration of narcotics are often injurious in biliary disorder as well as in bowel affections, by lowering the tone of the intestinal canal; and when it or the stomach is inflamed, these agents produce constipation, and not only diminish the vital energy of the canal, but that also of the *vis medicatrix* in her efforts to arrest the disease and repair its disorganization. Narcotics absorbed from the surface, enter the circulation, acting on the general system, as well as locally on the organism.

The reader will bear in mind, that in M. Thompson's cases and experiments, the epidermis was not in any case removed. It is probable, though he does not affirm it, that in all cases more or less friction was used.

M. L. Gosselin, in a communication in the *Gaz. Hebdom.* (Nov. 30, 1855), maintains that liquids, both medicinal and deleterious, are absorbed from the surface of the eyes. Even when the eye is closed, an infusion of Jamestown weed (datura strammonium) applied over the lids and contiguous parts, speedily acts on the iris, as I have repeatedly witnessed before operating for cataract, having used no other preparation either to produce irian dialatation before the operation, or to break up recent adhesions of the iris in both truamatic and idiopathic inflammations.

According to several observers, the lingual mode of medication is, for some medicinal agents, superior to any other. M. C. Hunter, who has taken an active and praise-worthy part in the experimental investigation of the hypodermic treatment, as will be seen in this journal, quotes and adopts Dr. Wardrop's statement, namely, " that there is a remarkable difference in point of time when medicines are absorbed from the stomach or from the mouth, absorption being most rapid from the latter, and the effect is more regular and more equable. Nor is it difficult to see why—the medicine absorbed from the mouth is taken directly into the general circulation, but when absorbed from the stomach, it has *en route* to pass through the portal system ; absorbed from the tongue, the effect is more regular, because the medicine is more certainly absorbed *en masse.* There is, then, much similarity between the hypodermic and the lingual modes. Rapidity of absorption is the great point in the *modus operandi* of each; and with regard to the effect they both have the advantages of rapidity, greater efficacy, regularity, and equability. Can the one method, then, replace the other ? Are they applicable for the same cases and medicines ? No ; they both have their advantages. Dr. Wardrop's plan is best for the administration of *tasteless* medicines, for calomel, *et hoc genus omne,* but it cannot be used for those medicines which are nauseating and bitter, not, in fact, for narcotics generally, not for cases of delirium, patients refusing medicine, etc., which are the cases where the other plan is most desirable." (*Med. Times and Gaz.,* Oct. 8, 1859.)

The reader will have seen in the papers on inflammation, in this journal, that the lingual method is used by Dr. Stone, of the University of Louisiana.

Vesical medication, though scarcely recognized, is not without claims to attention as an avenue to the general system in cases of

emergency when other routes are obstructed or defective, especially
in diseases in which a two-fold treatment, that is to say, a local
and general treatment simultaneously applied, seem to be indicated.
In the following case (a free translation of which is subjoined), the
remedy used in the stomachic method failed, while the vesical application was completely successful. Dr. Lecluyse reports in *L'Union
Médicale* (April 30, 1850), a very interesting case of palsy of the
bladder, which was cured by injecting strychnine into the cavity of
that organ. The history of the case is circumstantially given at
length, from which it appears that the patient, P. D., aged sixty-
eight, of average constitution, having one day been betrayed into a
drunken debauch, contrary to his habits, on returning home, through
the cold, at an advanced hour of the night, experienced a pressing
desire to urinate, but found, to his astonishment, that he could not
discharge a single drop. Dismayed by this untoward incident, he
resumed his bottle ; but his sufferings from the retention of urine
increased and caused him to send for the doctor, who, after drawing
off the urine, directed leeches to be applied to the perinæum, cataplasms, baths, diet, sudorific drinks, etc. From day to day the doctor
was required to draw off the urine. The doctor searched for stone,
but found none ; there was neither urethral stricture, nor spasm, and
the conclusion forced upon him was, that the bladder was totally paralyzed. He had previously recommended oily frictions with camphor,
opium, and belladonna, without any beneficial effect ; but now viewing the case as a paralytic affection of the bladder, he determined to
use stimulating diuretics, such as copaiva, turpentine, uva ursi, cantharides, ergot, and strychnine. The latter he gradually increased to
one grain daily, which caused spasmodic contractions of the muscles
of the trunk and limbs, but no relief to the palsied bladder and retention.

Dr. Lecluyse having continued this internal medication for fifteen
days, at length resolved to make a final effort before abandoning the
case as utterly hopeless, namely, he determined to apply strychnine
directly to the bladder by injection. Accordingly, six grains of
strychnine were dissolved in a little alcohol, which was diluted with
one pound of water, two ounces of which were daily used for an injection, immediately after having drawn off the urine. At first, the
bladder appeared wholly insensible to the contact of the injection.
But on the fourth or fifth day after the commencement of this vesical

medication and after the last injection, the patient had the sensation of water passing (*chose étonnante*), and was able to discharge his
urine. His cure was perfect, as he was observed by the doctor for
months afterwards.

The hypodermic or subcutaneous injection of medicaments, a mode
of treatment which is attracting considerable attention at present,
as the reader will see in another part of this journal, is scarcely ripe
enough for satisfactory deductions or speculation. Dr. Dechambre,
the learned editor of the *Gazette Hebdomadaire* (Oct. 21, 1859), gives
a very brief summary of Prof. Courty's cases of hypodermic medication (from the *Montpellier Médical* of October, 1859). A part of M.
Courty's experiments were, however, no more than repetitions of those
performed by M. Béhier. M. C.'s cases, eleven in number, were
rheumatisms or neuralgias. The principal medicament injected under
the skin, was hydrochlorate of morphia, fifty centigr. of which were
dissolved in ten grammes of water ; from six to thirty drops were
used for an injection. These cases which required thirty-four punctures and as many injections, were either cured or relieved with two
exceptions. These injections produced their medicinal effects rapidly,
and without narcotism or other serious accidents. M. Dechambre
regards the papers of MM. Béhier and Courty as highly interesting
contributions to the hypodermic treatment of neuralgic diseases.

M. Hiffelsheim, in a communication in the *Gazette Médicale de Paris*
(27th Dec., 1851), upon the hypodermic medication with tartar emetic
—termed by him la médication stibio-dermique—says, Orfila killed a
small dog in from thirty to forty seconds by 0.1 gr. of the powdered
emetic introduced into the subcutaneous tissue of the thigh.

The hypodermic or subcutaneous medication is probably liable to
some dangers, which not being well ascertained by sufficient experience, are for that reason likely to render this practice unacceptable
to the cautious practitioner. The advocates of this treatment admit
that there is danger of abscesses, especially if the injection should be
repeated in the same locality. The requisite doses, though small as
compared with either stomachical or rectal doses, have not been ascertained. The rapid and energetic effects from minute doses, which
though constituting the great merits of this method for some purposes, nevertheless foreshodow danger, the prevention of which may
not be possible until farther progress shall have been made. Moreover, this method requires a little surgery, which though a simple
puncture, will ever be repulsive to most patients.

10

ART. VIII.—*Medical Museums and Schools, with remarks on the Radical cure of Hernia :* By J. C. NOTT, M. D., Professor of Surgery of the Medical College of Alabama.

LONDON, 27th Sept., 1859.

MESSRS. EDITORS :—Before leaving for my tour through Europe, I promised, with the best possible intentions, to give you some "pencillings by the way," of such things as might interest the readers of a medical journal, and am now on the eve of turning my steps homeward, without having given you a line in redemption of my pledge. I feel ashamed to leave this continent, without at least making you an apology, and have now time left for little more.

You are aware that we are about starting a medical college in Mobile, and that my main object in visiting Europe, was to purchase the complicated apparatus necessary to put such an institution in motion. Our profession is made up of such an assemblage of sciences, and the material required is so varied, that a mission of this kind must necessarily bring with it a great deal of hard work. I have in the space of about three months, visited every town in England, France, Italy, northern and southern Germany, where I had reason to suppose that anything was to be obtained useful to our enterprise. When you reflect on all this, I am sure you will pardon me for breach of promise. Moreover, the cliniques in Paris, Florence, Vienna, Munich, Berlin, and other cities, were mostly closed for the summer, and it is very difficult in those cities to pick up much about professional matters, except when the public teaching is going on.

It has occurred to me, nevertheless, that I might still say something that would interest a large portion of your readers. Medical schools are springing up in every part of our country—those already established are desirous of improving their condition, and there are many members of the profession who would be glad to have the very kind of information I have been in search of ; and I therefore propose to give you some items of my experience about the collection of materials for a museum—the sources from whence they are to be obtained, etc. I may commence by stating, that circumstances had probably prepared me better for a mission of this kind, than most of those who cross the Atlantic on a similar errand. In the first place, I was attached to the University of Louisiana for a season, as Professor of Anatomy, where there is the most extensive collection of models ever brought to the United States, and where, with the addition of the private collection of Professor Richardson, they have one of the best, if not the very best museum in our country. Having to work through this collection, it gave me an opportunity of knowing the wants of a medical college, the kind of material to be had in Europe, and to a certain extent, the sources from which such articles are to be had. When I state that Professors Wedderburn and Cenas, expended about thirty thousand dollars on this museum in Europe, the reader may form some idea of its extent.

I have been very much surprised at the poverty of the collection of models in Europe generally. You may be astonished to learn, that after the collections in Florence, Vienna, and perhaps Bologna, the one in New Orleans is the most extensive in the world, and does great cridit to the enlightened liberality of our sister State. Before leaving the United States, I had, through foreign correspondence, collected catalogues of preparations, models, chemical apparatus, etc., with the prices of articles, and other information of this kind, which was exceedingly useful in enabling me to form some estimate of the probable expense of each department, and to economize time.

I arrived in Liverpool about the middle of June, and went immediately to London, where I knew exactly what to expect and what to do. My information had led me to the conclusion that I should find little else for sale in London than the beautiful wax models of Mr. Joseph Towne, at Guy's Hospital. I take much pleasure in stating that Mr. Towne is a gentleman in every sense of the word, and that my intercourse with him has been exceedingly agreeable. He is straight forward in his dealing, and perfectly reliable. The models for which he has gained his greatest celebrity, are those of skin diseases, and I do not hesitate to say that they are incomparably superior to any made in Europe—in fact, after seeing these, they are the only models of this class I would think of carrying home. I have seen no others at all true to nature, and from which a teacher could instruct pupils with any exactness. Mr. Towne has been for thirty years living in Guy's Hospital, studying skin diseases at the bed-side, and has worked from nature alone. His models of skin diseases cover the whole range, and besides these, he makes others of pathological specimens, and a few admirable ones of normal anatomy. One of the latter, representing the anatomy of the head and neck, and which I bought at a pretty high figure, I do not hesitate to say has not its equal in Florence, Paris, Vienna, or any where else, for amount of labor, and truthfulness of anatomical detail.

· The models of Mr. Towne, are very expensive, compared with those found on the continent, but it is better to pay any price that can be afforded for models true to nature, than to take as a gift those which are untrue, and can only give false notions to pupils. I have paid four thousand five hundred dollars for about one hundred of his models, nearly all of skin diseases and surgical pathology, and I am sure that no one, able to judge, will look at them without regarding the investment as a good one. You hear much of the famous Dupuytren Museum of morbid anatomy in Paris, and I assure you I would not give the collection I have from Mr. Towne, for the whole collection of models in this museum. I forgot to allude to Mr. Towne's series of models of the brain, in wax, life size—they are perfect, but the series cost about seven hundred dollars—and are included in the collection I procured.

After these models of Mr. Towne, there is not much else to be had in London. There are no depôts of dried or wet preparations, though there are industrious and skillful young anatomists about the schools, who would make such things to order. Microscopic preparations can be very well procured in London, and information on this point may be had from Mr. Carpenter, Mr. Queckett, Mr. Sharpey, Mr. Paget, or any of those gentlemen working in this department. I have found them all obliging in giving me advice and assistance.

From London I went to Edinburgh, and finding nothing there on sale, shaped my course to Paris, which after all, is *the* place where the greatest *assortment* of articles is to be found, and all the models, preparations, etc., which are made there, are much cheaper than in England—I may say in general terms, that almost everything which could be desired, to make up a museum, *except wax models*, can be best procured in Paris, both as to quality and price ; but the wax models are usually very inferior—some of those of normal anatomy may do to make a display on shelve-cases, but are rarely reliable for practical demonstration ; and the *pathological* models here are too inaccurate to be of much use.

The most important establishment in Paris, is that of Vasseur, very near the Ecole de Médecine. Here will be found a superb osteological collection both human and comparative. You have skeletons, both natural and artificial, in every stage of development, from the fœtus of three months, up to adult age, as well as those of extreme old age. Also, a rich collection of diseased bones, illustrating their pathology very fully. M. Vasseur's collection of skeletons, illustrative of comparative anatomy, is very complete, and enables one to select a very full series of types of the different divisions of the animal kingdom. His collection of deformed pelves is very complete, and he has a considerable number of wax and other models, some of which are useful, though this is not a speciality with him. All his articles may be had at fair prices, and I found him obliging and reliable.

With regard to preparations of parts of the human subject, both wet and dry, some difficulty exists in Paris—I found no regular depôts for them. They can be made to order, but this is always an unsatisfactory way of doing business, as I know from experience. In Paris, however, there are always preparations of this kind to be had, if you can find them out, and by inquiring about the dissecting rooms and hospitals, you can hear of some private collection that may be bought. This occurred to me—I found out a gentleman now holding one of the highest positions in Paris, who had on hand a number of superb preparations of the vascular and lymphatic systems, on which he had been at work for years, with an eye to a concour, in which he was finally successful; and having reason to believe that he might be disposed to sell them, I called on him and sounded him at once. He allowed me to make a selection of such as I desired, and I have not seen anything superior to them in any museum in Europe. Some of the same series, are the best of the kind now seen in the museum at the École de Médecine.

There are two other establishments in Paris, devoted almost exclusively to the manufacture of models in *papier maché*. They represent normal, human, comparative, and pathological anatomy. The first is that of Legèr, No. 126 rue d'Enfer, formerly known as the establishment of Thibert, many of whose models are seen in the museums of our country. The models of Legèr represent a very extensive series, and the whole collection would cost some three or four thousand dollars, but there is not more than one-fourth of these worthy of transportation. Wherever they attempt to represent normal, even coarser surgical anatomy with any minuteness, or the delicate shades of pathological anatomy, they are utter failures. The representations, for example, of eye, skin, and syphilitic diseases, of which there is an extensive series, are coarse, untrue, and worthless. On the other hand, there are others, which attempt little more than the portraying of *form* and *size*, that are extremely valuable. For example, the gravid uterus in various stages of development, the displacements of the uterus ; tumors of every kind ; the operations for tying the larger arteries ; a capital series of greatly magnified models of microscopic anatomy ; placentas of every variety ; monstrosities, and many other things, which, with proper caution, may be selected to great advantage.

The other establishment alluded to, is that of Auzoux, where is manufactured what he calls *anatomie clastique,* in some kind of compositiou material. These models are devoted almost exclusively to normal anatomy, human and comparative, and here the purchaser is again cautioned to select with great caution. Where minute anatomy is attempted, they will be found very coarse and untrue to nature. The most valuable are those which are greatly magnified above life-size. These models, are, many of them, so large, that [the members of a class in a lecture room, can see at a distance the structure of those parts which could not be seen at all on the natural subject, and the teacher may thus give a clear and coarse outline to the beginner, of what is afterward to be studied in greater detail. All the parts of the horse are here made with sufficient correctness ; but the most valuable part of this whole collection, I think, is that of comparative anatomy ; there is a series of models representing the structure of those organs which perform the principal vital functions, in the four divisions of the animal kingdom. The types are very well selected, and are of great use to the lecturer on physiology. There are many useful little " odds and ends," both in this establishment and that of Legèr and Vasseur, which I have not time to enumerate.

In speaking of Legèr's enlarged models, I might have instanced, those of the capillary circulation, the minute distribution of nerves, the structure of glands, muscles, nerves, hair, all the tissues, etc. ; these are large enough to be seen across a large room, and are excellent.

One may be well served in Paris, also, in the materia medica and chemical departments. Mènier & Co., for about eight hundred dollars, furnished a very complete selection of those articles necessary to illustrate a course of lectures on materia medica ; they are put up in uniform, handsome bottles, very neatly labelled, and make a very ornamental display in a museum. They have, also, on reasonable terms, every variety of chemical material and apparatus, and the extent of purchases for this department, are without limits. For chemicals, I found M. Deroche, No. 19, rue de l'Ancienne Commedie, very reliable and obliging.

With regard to surgical instruments, I say most decidedly, that if I had my work to do over again, I would supply myself in this department in the United States. Our instruments are quite as good, there is no material difference in the prices, and then I have found Tiemann, in New York, and several makers in Philadelphia, much more punctual and reliable than those of Paris. In London, everything is enormously dear, though the cutting instruments are excellent. A general order for instruments suitable for a college, might be ordered in the United States, and then the purchaser could amuse himself picking up novelties in London and Paris. One intending to come to Europe on a mission of this kind, would do well to procure the catalogues of Vasseur, Auzoux, Legèr, and Chaurière, the instrument maker; they give a full list of all the articles they have for sale, with the prices, which enables you to form an approximative estimate of the amount of money required in each department. The catalogues, also, of Mènièr, and Weiss, of London, will be very useful.

About two thousand dollars with Vasseur, one thousand with Legèr, one thousand with Auzoux, and about the same in the materia medica department, will get a large and very useful assortment of things. Chemicals, books, instruments, may be taken without limit.

Having used up Paris, and being disappointed in the collection of wax models, I determined to continue my march through the other principal cities of Europe. My information had led me to expect the best supply of these in Florence, which has long been celebrated, there being nothing in the world comparable to the collection in the museum of the Grand Duke of Tuscany; but the weather being hot, I determined to take the cooler latitudes first, and accordingly started for Munich, where I had reason to expect some good things. I here was recommended by Professor Bichoff to a gentleman named Paul Zeiller, who is a thorough anatomist and most ingenious modeler. He uses a composition of wax, cotton, and lime, which gives great solidity to his models, and they stand handling as freely as the common *papier maché* ones. I procured from him a series of ten, of normal anatomy, life size, for about one thousand dollars, which I regard as one of the most valuable parts of my collection. This gentleman is talking of moving to London, but I think would be much better paid in New York or Philadelphia. The number of schools growing up in our country, makes it the best market for things of this kind.

From Munich I went to Vienna, which, after Paris, is the most important point of medical education, and I was much disappointed in finding nothing whatever for sale in my line. There are no modelers at all, and although preparations wet or dry might be ordered, there is nothing that I could hear of on sale. The museum of the University is a superb one, and the collection of wax models stands next to that of Florence, but were all made in the latter city.

Leaving Vienna, I went to Berlin and the other principal cities of Germany, and although I saw many handsome museums, I met with nothing for sale.

I next determined to go to Florence, which has always been regarded as the head quarters of wax models. The museum in this department is extensive and gorgeous almost beyond description, and a superficial observer would think here that is collected a full series of models, representing every organ and part of the human frame, with such fidelity as to enable the student to learn minutely the structure of every part, and almost to do away with the necessity of dissections. At first glance, the muscles, brain, blood-vessels, nerves, in short, all the tissues strike you as being wonderful and truthful counterfeits of nature ; but on minute examination, the anatomist detects errors at every step—the muscles want precision in origin and insertion ; the blood-vessels and nerves often branch at the wrong point and run out of their proper course ; the ligaments of joints are generally very incorrect ; and so on with the whole anatomy of the system. I would therefore advise any one who goes to Florence in search of wax models, to purchase nothing but what he can inspect, or if he leaves orders behind him, to employ some competent anatomist to examine critically every model before it is paid for.

I took time to go very deliberately through the extensive collections both in Florence and Vienna, and I did not find a single specimen, where there was much complicated anatomy, that was really true to nature and reliable for purposes of *practical demonstration.* There is moreover a difficulty in procuring these models at present in Florence. Fontana, the great man in this department, is dead, and two others were absent from Florence during my visit. One, I was told, had gone to the United States with some idea of settling there, and another was somewhere in Germany, setting up models for a school. I found very few things there on sale. There are men there who could and would make them to order, but they must be closely watched.

There is a pretty large collection of wax models at the school of Bologna, and from what I have learned, I would rather take my chance there of filling an order, than in Florence. I did not see the man who makes them (he being absent a few days), but he was well spoken of.

As for the cost of fine wax models, they are very expensive—there is in fact no limit. The collection of wax models, alone, alluded to, in the University of Louisiana, must have cost at least fifteen thousand dollars, and the series in Florence or Vienna museums would cost probably five times that amount. So much for museums.

The operation for radical cure of hernia was attracting a good deal of attention in our journals before my departure for Europe, and it being one of very great interest, I determined to make some inquiry as to what was doing in this line among the surgeons here, and was surprised to learn how little favor it has met with among the more sober-minded surgeons.

In Paris I talked with Velpeau, the Nestor of French surgeons, with Nélaton, and others, and they all say that Wutzer's operation, or any other on similar principles, cannot be relied on, the disease returning in the great majority of instances. In fact, the operation is scarcely performed at all now in Paris ; a great many experiments have been made on this principle, since the one of Gerdy ; and all having proven unsatisfactory, the operation is now nearly abandoned in Paris. I had a long conversation with Mons. Charrière, who has been the leading surgical instrument maker there for some thirty years, and he told me that he had no call at all at present for Wutzer's instrument, and kept none for sale in his shop. He told me, moreover, that he had some years ago taken the trouble to go to Bonn, in Germany, where Wutzer resided, to get information on the subject, and that after investigating the matter fully, came back to Paris satisfied that the operation would not do—the rupture soon or late returns, according to his information.

In London, I went round to the hospitals, and talked with several leading surgeons and instrument makers, and I found that the operation was here decidedly losing ground, although it is still performed

11

to some extent. Spencer Wells seems to have gone more deeply into it than any one else in London, from what we see in the journals; and when I alluded to his experience, as published in the journals, to one of the most distinguished surgeons of London, he shrugged his shoulders and said he did not know much about Mr. Wells, and did not think his experience was great.

That the hernial ring may be closed, by this operation, for a time, is certain; that in a very large proportion of the cases the rupture works its way out again, sooner or later, is no less certain; and the points to get at now, are what proportion is really successful, what are the proper cases for the operation, and whether the proportion of successful cases justifies the operation at all. I have performed a few of these operations, but my experience is too limited, and the time since the operation too short, to justify me in forming an opinion, though I am inclined still to think that a judicious selection of cases for operation might be made, and the operation to a certain extent employed.

I shall conclude with a few words about our *rival* medical schools. It is often said that we in our country make schools too fast, and too many. I do not think so. The system of medical education is everywhere imperfect, and the only means I see at present of improving it, is *competition*. You cannot have a good hotel, livery stable, or even bar-room, without opposition, and the professors of our schools are always made to do their work more faithfully by neighboring opposition. It is true that medical schools now are too much the offspring of private speculation and interest, and I am satisfied that there never will be any great improvement in our system until the *State governments* take up medical education and treat it as they do other parts of education. The professors should be paid out of the public purse, put beyond the reach of temptation, and there should be a regular gradation of studies, extending through several years.

But our country is not yet ripe for this, and we must make the best of a bad system. I therefore say to our old friends in New Orleans, devil take the hindmost, we are in for a wattle race, and let us whip and spur each other's donkeys to the utmost. There is plenty of room for us all, and I most heartily wish *them*, as well as ourselves, success.

In haste, very truly yours, etc.,

J. C. NOTT.

Art. IX.—*Historical and Critical Researches into the origin of large doses of the Sulphate of Qninine :* By Bennet Dowler, M. D.

" Amicus Plato, amicus Socrates, sed magis amica veritas."

Within a few years there has been, and there continues to be, much controversy as to individual, sectional, and national priority or originality in the administration of large doses of quinia for the cure of several diseases. Neither the blandisments of friendship nor the biases of country, should sway the inquirer into the history of science, which, without favor or fear, recites truths and facts only.

The eighteenth volume of the *Dictionnaire de Médecine,** which was published May, 1827, at Paris, in referring to the intermitting fevers of Italy, quotes Martinet, Drossi, and Mathœis to show that it was then the established practice in that country to give thirty-five, forty, and even seventy-two grains of the sulphate of quinine for a dose, and arely to give less than from eighteen to twenty-four grains (see M. Guersent's article, *Quinquina,* p. 131, *et. seq*). M. Guersent having alluded to doses ranging from eight to sixteen grains, adds : "Mais il parait constant, d'après les observations de MM. Martinet, Drossi, et M. le professeur Mathœis, qu'il est nécessaire de porter beaucoup plus haut la dose de sulfate de quinine en Italie qu'en France, car ces trois observateurs ont été obligés de donner dans ce pays rarement moins de dixhuit à vingt-quatre grains de sulfate de quinine dans l'intervalle d'un paroxysme à l'autre, pour maitriser une fièvre ordinaire, et quelquefois il était nécessaire de porter la dose beaucoup plus haut, jusqu'a trente-cinq, quarante, et même soixante-douze grains, ce qui est énorme, puisque quarante grains de sulfate de quinine équivalent presque à une livre et demie de quinquina. Il est impossible, quant à présent, d'expliquer la cause de cette différence, si elle est constante."

It will be observed, that Pelletier, who, with Caventou, discovered the preparation of quinia, is one of the editors of this dictionary, as will be seen in a foot note.

The following communication, with the comments upon the same, appeared in the *Æsculapian Register* (July 22, 1824), and may serve

---

* This volume of five hundred and sixty-one octavo pages, has the following title, which will be copied entire : " Dictonnaire de Médecine, par MM. Adelon, Andral, Béclard, Biett, Breschet, Chomel, H. Cloquet, J. Cloquet, Coutanceau, Desormeaux, Ferrus, Georget, Guersent, Lagneau, Landré-Beauvais, Marc, Marjolin, Murat, Ollivier, Orfila, Pelletier, Raige-Delorme, Rayer, Richard, Rochoux, Rostan, Roux et Rullier. Tome dix-huitième. Pse—Rut. A Paris, Chez Béchet Jeune, Libraire, Place de l'École de Médecine, No. 4. Mai, 1827."

to show what were considered large doses of quinine in the United States more than thirty-six years ago.

It will probably be found, upon a thorough investigation, or even upon a hasty superficial one, such as this paper is, that the French and Italian physicians are entitled to the credit or the blame of administering large doses of quinia, sooner than others, after its discovery by Pelletier and Caventou.

Before proceeding farther, the following documents will be submitted to the reader:

"Communication.—*Mr. Editor*—In Dr. Eberle's New Medical Journal, notice is given of the use of sulphate of quinine in large doses, by a foreign practitioner, in such a way as to induce the belief that such doses were novel. I am able, however, to state, that quite as large portions have been frequently exhibited in the vicinity of Philadelphia, and with the happiest results. I have in a number of instances, where I had but little time for the favorable exhibition of the remedy, given ten grains in the course of three hours. To a delicate little girl of about ten years of age I recently gave six grains in the course of one hour, and with the best success, no untoward symptom supervening.

" Two reasons have operated to elicit these remarks—first, a desire that medical men may be assured of the safety of the remedy in large doses ; and, secondly, that we may enjoy the credit, if any there be, of being as enterprising in the use of the sulphate, as any of our distant medical brethren.

"I am, with respect,   Thos. D. Mitchell.
" *Frankford, July* 14, 1824."

" We publish the preceding communication from Dr. T. D. Mitchell, from a wish, as much as in us lies, to extend the knowledge of the perfect safety of so valuable a remedy as the sulphate of quinine. We cannot, however, doubt the fact to have been long familiar to our medical brethren, since scarcely a journal of England or France appeared without a reference to it. So far back as July, 1821, it had been given in doses of six to eight grains repeatedly through the day ; and, since that period, many other instances are recorded. Yet, although safe, such doses, it is to be remembered, are not often necessary ; and personal experience must probably decide the relative doses that individual cases may require."

In the *Medical Review*, edited by Drs. Eberle and McClellan, (vol. 1, Philadelphia, 1824), T. D. Mitchell, M. D., of Frankfort (already quoted), communicated a paper of nine pages on " the merits of the sulphate of quinine," in which he says, that this article " came into use in this region of country, in the first instance, as a remedy for intermittents ; " he refers to certain illusions concerning it, of which he says, " they have *long since* passed away ; " he gave eight grains in less than an hour, ten grains in two hours, and eight grains previously to the hour of bed-time." He says further : "but however successful the sulphate of quinine may have been in the cure of ague and fever, it has appeared to me to be much more triumphant in the *bilious remittents* which we have had so frequently to encounter. The old methods of treating remittents, generally protracted their cure to five or six weeks. Indeed, it was common with some practitioners to affirm that it was impossible, by any means, to prevent those fevers from running their course ; and it appeared to me, that, according to their scheme, the bark answered no other end than to keep up the energies of the system, while nature conducted the patient through, what was supposed to be, the unalterable course of his disease. The sulphate of quinine has taught me (if I had not learned before) the fallacy of such pathological views ; and from the experience I have already had, I feel as confident of being able to cut short the course of a remittent, as I am that I can relieve the pain of toothache, by extracting the offending cause." (612–13.) Dr. Mitchell speaks of " the [then] general use of quinine," and refers to its previous use in France. Thus, in four years after its discovery, large doses of quinine was considered a practice comparatively old upon the banks of the Kentucky river, and, of course, still older upon the banks of the Seine, where it originated. Thanks to medical journals, and rapid international intercourse.

On large doses of Quinine in Atmospheric Fevers. By H. PERRINE, M. D. (Extracted from a letter to William P. Dewees, M. D.)—Laboring under the symptoms of *cholorine* on the eve of my expected return to Campeachy, I cannot depart from this *stage* or *state* without renewing my testimony of the virtues of the sulphate of quinine. I commenced the practice of medicine in Illinois, in the fall of 1819, continued it in that State until the spring of 1824, and in the State of Mississippi until the spring of 1826, when I embarked at New Orleans on account of my health for Cuba, and thence proceeded through Boston to Canada during the summer. The following winter was passed in this city. In May, 1826, I sailed for Tobasco, in Mexico, where I remained during the rainy season, and arrived at my consulate in Campeachy of Yucatan, in November. I returned to Tobasco in July, 1830, and sailed from that port for this city in June, 1831, and in September last was again at Great Sodus Bay, in this State, where I had been a short time in 1826. You will hence perceive that I have had opportunities for medical observation in various degrees of latitude and longitude between the southern shores of our great lakes and the northern base of our Guatemalian mountains.

During the first six years of my practice I used and recommended with gradually increasing boldness, *large doses* of the Peruvian bark, *frequently repeated* during the *paroxysms of fevers.* My communication in your Journal of November, 1827, contains my first essays with *large doses of the sulphate of quinine.* I have since had abundant opportunities of witnessing their effects in the hands of myself, of other physicians, and of *the people.* In 1827, quinine was first known in Tobasco and Yucatan, and was bought by *physicians* at two shillings a *grain.* I introduced its use in large doses, during the febrile paroxysms. In 1831, it was bought by *families* at five dollars an *ounce.* Every person that adopted my practice, has never, I believe, abandoned it. I therefore merely claim common capacity for observation and common veracity for report in submitting very briefly a few general results of my experience :

1. The medium dose of the sulphate of quinine at any period of fever from its incipient to its terminating symptoms is *ten grains* to be repeated every *two hours,* whatever be the state of the pulse and skin.

2. It may be given without interfering with simultaneous, antiphlogistic, stimulant, or other auxiliary measures according to symptoms, any more than an equal quantity of James' powder. Indeed if the quinine be slily substituted in the paper, the physician would express his surprise at the immense sudorific and sedative powers of this new pulvis antimonialis.

3. The retreat of fever under the power of quinine as under the power of nature, is indicated by changes of the hot or the cold skin, and of the strong or the feeble pulse towards their natural condition; and most generally by secretion from the skin, often from the kidneys, occasionally from the bowels, and sometimes from all three in succession.

4. The *general* disturbance of the nervous and vascular systems, called febrile, whether cold and depression or heat and excitement be the alarming traits, may be counteracted on the first day by at most six doses, or on the second, by a dozen ; and thus will be prevented that gastro-enteritis, a *consequence* of endemic or epidemic fever, which Brouissais has mistaken for the *cause.*

I have hence reason to believe that all malignant fevers (even if called the *cholera,* when their force is attracted to previously disordered bowels) may be cut short at their commencement by large doses of sulphate of quinine ; and that local disorder may at the same time or afterwards be corrected by the same means that were effectual for the same symptoms before the attack.

I am happy to see in Magendie's Formulæ, that large doses of quinine are administered by highly reputable physicians of Europe. —*New York June* 26, 1832—*Transylvania Jour. Med.,* vi. 302-3. Lexington, 1833.

Dr. Porter, surgeon U. S. A., in the September issue of this journal, has in unequivocal terms claimed for the late Dr. Harney, surgeon U. S. A., originality in giving, recommending and establishing large doses of quinine in army practice, in 1840-1 ; previous to which he had used large doses, having learned the practice from an older physiclau, whose name he had forgotten. Neither dates nor documents, however, are mentioned, beyond the year 1840. The emphatical manner in which Dr. Porter speaks of one beyond the reach of praise or censure, may be expressive of the general opinion among the intelligent surgeons of the United States Army, upon this topic. " Dr. Harney spoke with indignation of the attempts of some few persons to appropriate the honors to themselves, without giving the least credit to those who introduced this practice into the Florida Army in 1840. The doses he advised were 10, 15, 20 and 25 grains, and even more."

It will be seen in the Medical Statistics of the United States Army (a voluminous work), that a copious appendix, entitled " *Reports on the administration of quinine in large doses*," has been published, founded on fifty-seven special reports from medical officers. These reports were in response to an official circular from the Surgeon-General (Dr. Lawson), in which the following question, among others, was propounded : " In how large doses have you administered it [quinine], both as it regards the *extreme* and the *average* quantity ?" The object of this circular was not, however, to ascertain the *originality* of this practice. The general result, observes Brevet-Brig.-Gen. Lawson, Surgeon General, and assistant surgeon R. H. Coolidge, M.D., who compiled these documents, is, " that to the medical staff of the army belongs the credit of having demonstrated, on an extensive scale, the safety and efficacy of quinine in large doses, and of having thereby largely contributed to revolutionize the treatment of fevers in this country. It has not been found practicable to ascertain from the official records, the *precise* time of the introduction into the army of the practice of giving quinine in large doses. The earliest reports of sick, in which that practice is alluded to, refer to the treatment as having been adopted some time previously. The reports of assistant surgeon (now surgeon) J. J. B. Wright, for the quarter ending June 30, 1841, and of assistant surgeon (now surgeon) Charles McCormick, for the quarter ending September 39, 1841, *are the first which are accompanied with any special or detailed account of this treatment.*"

This statement which claims for the army the credit of having demonstrated the safety and efficacy of quinine in large doses for fever within the last decennium, and made known only in 1856, can-not be accepted by civilians as consistent with the therapeutic history of that medicinal agent for nearly forty years. The army practice, at the utmost, only contributed additional evidence in favor of the pre-existent treatment, but did not "contribute largely to revolutionize the treatment of fever in this country." Anterior to the period above mentioned in the army statistics, quinine in large doses had passed the boundaries of intermittents and remittents, and had been freely given in other fevers, not excepting the yellow fever, and had given rise to the questions of priority. The question of originality in the administration of very large doses of quinine (from twenty to sixty grains, and in some cases even more), in yellow fever of New Orleans, in the epidemic of 1339, was much discussed in private, and also in the public journals at that period, but is foreign to the present inquiry. It deserves a special report and faithful record in this journal, while the facts, so creditable to several physicians of this city, are fresh in the memory of living witnesses.

In fact, the influence of the army practice, restricted as it is to a class, soldiers, could scarcely have been appreciable in civil practice before the official reports of the medical officers appeared in the large quarto published by the Government in 1856. It may be doubted, whether, as yet, one physician in fifty has either seen or read this work, valuable as it is.

The statement, therefore, though an official one, " that to the medical staff of the army belongs the credit of having demonstrated the safety and efficacy of quinine in large doses, and of having thereby largely contributed to revolutionize the treatment of fever in this country," might be altogether reversed, without damage to historical verity. The quinine *regime* had already passed its culminating point and was declining to its proper level, before the army report twinkled above the horizon. Enormous doses, sometimes called "the abortive treatment," had been tried and nearly abandoned, or held in reserve for extraordinary emergencies ; at least, they were no longer prescribed as the ordinary treatment. Scruples replaced drachms, grains scruples. Quinine was not abandoned, but restricted. The revolution had gone backward. New enemies consequent upon this reäction, threatened medicine, namely, scepticism, non-medication, homœopathy, and popular distrust.

A little army of ten thousand men, two-thirds of whom are foreigners, scattered over a territory nearly seven hundred times larger than England, must afford but a limited field of practice for even ten doctors, if all were resident in one locality. The practice of the army surgeons in remote posts and barracks, thousands of miles apart from each other, and often the same distance from civilization, cannot, from the nature of the case, "largely" influence civil practice, much less "revolutionize the treatment of fever in this country," especially before the revolutionary treatment was even made known, that is, before 1856.

The following communication copied from the October number (1859) of the *Medical Journal of North Carolina*, sets forth Dr. Cartwright's claims of priority in the case of large doses of quinine to the exclusion of all others, not only in the South, but in the entire world :

"*Interesting letter from the distinguished veteran*, DR. SAMUEL A. CARTWRIGHT, *of New Orleans, on the Southern form of Pneumonia, and the history of the introduction of large doses of Quinine in Fever :* Published by request of the Granville (N. C.) Medical Society.*

NEW ORLEANS, MAY 7TH, 1859.

DR. MANSON—*Dear Sir :* Yours of the 25th ult. has just come to hand, but not the Virginia Medical Journal containing your article on pneumonia, which I have not had the pleasure of seeing or reading. It is very flattering to an author to have his writings favorably noticed, which have been recently published, but it is doubly so to have them favorably noticed by a new generation, after a third of a century has passed away. My monograph on pneumonia biliosa, published in the *Medical Recorder*, of Philadelphia, bears on its face that it was written in April, 1826, very nearly a third of a century ago. You are pleased to say that you "think it contains the best description of the cold stage in pneumonia which has ever been written," but you desire me to inform you more particularly, "whether the cold stage in this disease, as you (I) observed it, returned periodically or not ? " At page 65† you will see it stated that a "remission of the symptoms generally happens in the morning, or in some other part of the twenty-four hours : it is more favorable when it occurs in the morning." In Natchez, as in New Orleans, Philadelphia, and, I believe, in all of our cities, the remittent fevers and pneumonias are not so decidedly paroxysmal as in the vicinity of water courses, marshes, etc., at some distance from the blocks of the cities. The pneumonia in the vicinity of Natchez partook of the type of the prevailing intermittent and remittent fevers. In the city, the periodical cold stage was less evident, or scarcely perceptible, amounting to nothing more than a coldness of the tips of the fingers, ears and toes, as you describe. You were pleased to ask me "who first used large doses of quinine in the febrile exacerbation in the South ? " Put

---

" * The President (Dr. O. F. Manson) read a lengthy, interesting, and very able letter from the distinguished Dr. Cartwright, of New Orleans, on the treatment of Pneumonia, and giving a minute and circumstantial history of the introduction of quinine as a sedative febrifuge in fever, which, on motion of Dr. P. P. Peace, he was requested to submit for publication in the *North Carolina Medical Journal*. *Extract from the Minutes of the Granville Medical Society.*"

" †Medical Recorder, vol. x. Philadelphia, 1826. "

world for *South*, and I answer, that the records of medicine do not furnish any example of quinine having been used in large doses anything like as far back as April, 1826, when I wrote the article on pneumonia biliosa, strongly recommending the sulphate of quinine in large doses in that disease, with the single exception of a paper published by Dr. Perrine near about the same time, in Chapman's Journal. I may here observe, that Dr. Perrine was a *protégé* of mine, who came from Illinois to Natchez. Dr. James A. McPheeters and myself indoctrinated him into the mysteries of treating fevers and pneumonia with quinine. He settled in the country about twelve miles from Natchez, where the quinine practice in his hands was so successful, that Dr. James Metcalf, in the same neighborhood, was compelled, in self-defence, to adopt it to retain his business. Dr. James Metcalf had a brother a student of medicine in Paris at the time, to whom he communicated the wonderful virtues of the sulphate of quinine in six-grain doses during the paroxysm of certain fevers, attended with very frequent pulse and great determination of blood to the head, snd also as very valuable in pnenmonia biliosa. It was through that brother, Dr. Volney Metcalf, that the French were induced to try the article in large doses. It was more than ten years after the introduction of the quinine practice in certain forms of remittent fever and pneumonia, before the physicians of New Orleans, or anywhere else, adopted the practice, with the exception of Dr. Thomas Fearn, of Huntsville, Ala., who began its use in 1833 or 1834. For a number of years the quinine practice was confined almost entirely to Drs. McPheeters, Perrine, Metcalf and myself, and a .ew young men who learned the practice from us, and adopted it in order to succeed in business. Dr. Bouldin was one of these. Not succeeding in Natchez, he settled in Claiborne county, Mississippi, where his great success with the quinine introduced him to a large and lucrative practice. He mixed prussiate of iron with it—his usual dose being six grains of each. In scorbutic and hemorrhagic conditions of the system, the prussiate of iron was found to be a valuable adjuvant.

"Subsequent experience has convinced me that six grains do better than larger or smaller doses, and that the remedy should never be pushed after it begins to produce its peculiar effects upon the ears. Patients were found to bear it better when given in combination with morphine, Dover's powder, aconite, valerian, extract canabis indica, etc.,—one or more of these articles with warm drinks to determine to the surface, and in pneumonia, with some expectorant. We preferred giving the quinine in solution to pill.

Very respectfully your obedient servant,
SAMUEL A. CARTWRIGHT."

"It is a source of pride and pleasure to the undersigned to have it in his power to present the above letter from a gentleman who has even distinction, not only among his brethren at the South, for his useful contributions to practical medicine, but who has obtained honorable recognition from Northern umpires."

"To those unacquainted with Dr. Cartwright, I may state, that in his younger days, he attained considerable reputation for essays published in this country. In my researches among these neglected and forgotten works, I find it noticed that he received two gold medals from the Harvard University, being the Boylston premiums for dissertations ; on another occasion a silver pitcher was awarded to him by the Medico-Chirurgical Faculty of Maryland, besides other prizes in Philadelphia. Later, however, the Doctor received a present (which he doubtless values most highly) of a magnificent gold vase, valued at above $1000, from the citizens of a settlement near Natchez, for his success in the treatment of an epidemic in 1833. The Doctor's highest claims to distinction, however, rest, I conceive, for the conspicuous part which he has enacted in the introduction of quinine as a sedative in fevers, etc.,—*the great medical fact of the nineteenth century.* —*Medical Journal, North Carolina, Oct.* 1859. O. F. MANSON.

The exact claims of Dr. Cartwright, as set forth in the essay in the *Medical Recorder,* to which he alludes as above mentioned, were duly marked and kindly left at the office of the *New Orleans Medical and Surgical Journal,* and will be found below, in quotation marks, preceded by a few of the principal data in the treatment, abridged from case 6, occupying seven printed pages ; as this is the only case in the essay, in which the large doses of quinine were given, the preliminary treatment, before that of the quinine ought to be indicated, so that the reader may judge the better of the merits of both or either.

This patient affected with pneumonia biliosa, was a delicate lady, aged 20, in the sixth month of pregnancy, whose treatment, for three days before taking quinine, is indicated by the following measures adopted in 'succession : she was bled 1½ ℔s ; bled again more than 1½ ℔s ; had a dose of 20 grains of pulvis antimonialis ; 10 grs. cal., 5 grains pulv. antim., and 5 grains Dover's powder ; bled ½ ℔, blistered 8 by 10 inches ; "her excited mind appeared alone to live, the body seemed already dead ;" 3 grs. of tart. emet. and 5 drops of laudanum every hour ;* took 26 grs. of tartar emetic. "After the tartar was discontinued the sulphate of quinine was given. At the first dose 8 grains were given. Shortly after this dose of quinine the patient fell into a sleep, for the first time since her attack (except a little doze a few hours before, while taking the tartrite of antimony) She slept half an hour, during which time the pulse diminished fifteen beats, but rose to one hundred and ten after she awoke. The sulphate of quinine was continued in four-grain doses every two hours

---

* Her " pulse not easy to count ;" sight began to fail ; could not distinguish the features of those around her. * * * I hoped that tartar emetic would here display its stimulating powers ; that it would awaken the dormant energies of the system, restore sensibility to the surface, which now neither felt blisters nor the hottest applications."

until noon, after which time, a dose of quinine and a purgative powder (composed of 12 grains calomel, 8 grains of aloes, and 8 grains
of scammony every two hours.") These and other measures were put
into operation during the first three days."

The treatment is detailed at length for three days afterward, but
the amount of quinine given is not mentioned. "The patient in
course of a few weeks regained her health and strength."

A few other passages occur in this essay in which Dr. Cartwright
gives a summary of his views of quinine and its doses, namely :

"As some of the most prominent rules of practice in the administration of tartar emetic have already been considered, and the effects
which it produces stated, it will be necessary now to mention some
of the most evident effects of the sulphate of quinine. In the state
of the system which has been under review, after the partial reäction
has been somewhat subdued by tartar emetic, the sulphate of quinine,
in four grain doses every one or two hours, appears to subdue the
existing febrile irritation, and to produce perspiration or expectoration. It sometimes, however, brings on a general and equable
excitement of the arterial system. In either case, it prepares the
system to be properly acted on by other agents, particularly purgatives, does away the disposition to watery evacuations, and equalizes
the excitement. * * * In the event that the tartar emetic only
subdues the partial reäction and diminishes the local determinations
of blood, but does not bring about a general reäction, the sulphate of
quinine, in doses of four grains every one or two hours, I have lately
found to be a valuable remedy in such states of the system. After
the quinine has been used through the day, a purgative given at night
will frequently produce dark bilious evacuations, which will remove
the hepatic or other abdominal congestions, reduce the inflammations,
and strengthen the patient. I have used the quinine in pneumonia
biliosa, not only without *lessening* the expectoration, but have evidently thereby *promoted* that important evacuation. To do this, it
should be given in doses *sufficient* to subdue the violence of the local
excitement, to restore the loss of balance, and to produce secretion ;
or *sufficient* to produce that pathological state of the system which
consists in a general reäction, and thereby to determine to distant
parts a portion of those fluids which, during the previous pathological state of the system, being hemmed in about the inflamed organ,
had aggravated the inflammation and prevented expectoration from
taking place."

It appears that M. Maillot, in 1834, used large doses of quinine
in the treatment of intermittents in the military hospital of Bon, in
Africa. In the same year Dr. Roots treated neuralgia in St. Thomas'
Hospital, with large doses, the details of which appear in the *Medico-
Chirurgical Review* (Jan., 1835) ; upon which the astonished editor
remarks :

" In the foregoing case there was exhibited *bold practice*, in respect to doses.   We know Dr. Roots well, and believe him to be a very judicious physician.   We'should have great confidence in his prescriptions, because we are satisfied that he acts under the guidance of observation and reflection.   Eighty grains of sulphate of quinine, added to a quarter of a pound of carbonate of iron, with a strong dose of morphine, in the twenty-four hours, make, altogether, a *"quantum suff."* that would astonish a Bonhommie, a Quinn, a Hahnemann—or, indeed, any man who had not studied in St. Thomas's Hospital.   We remember, full well, the sensations which we ourselves experienced, some years ago, when taking twenty grains of sulphate of quinine for an intermittent."

In 1832, Dr. Cerioli, an Italian physician, found in numerous cases of intermittent which quinine had failed to cure, that the ferro-cyanate of quinine, in doses ranging up to, and above, eight grains, was effectual.

Dr. David Hosack, whose Lectures on the Practice of Physic were published after his death, which occurred in 1835, says of quinine: " Generally, the best way is to begin with large doses, so as to produce a strong impression at once.   Even eight or ten grains have been given at a dose, and the Italian physicians give even more." (324.)

The North American Medical and Surgical Journal (April, 1828), has among the floating articles of its excerpta, the following statement, which not only shows that *large doses of quinine* had been adopted in Paris, but indicates the doctrine of *its sedative action*, which has been so often claimed, directly or virtually, as more or less original with later writers : " M. Bally, at the *Hôpital de la Pitié*, contends that small doses of the sulphate of quinine—two grains, for example— have very uncertain therapeutical effects, at the same time they are apt to produce syncope, vomiting, and other nervous symptoms referable to *cerebral exaltation*.   He asserts that if this medicine be administered *in large doses, such as twenty or thirty grains* in the day, it will, so far from producing the accidents attributed to it by practitioners, cause the redness and suburral state of the tongue to disappear, and *act as a sedative on the nervous and circulatory systems*. Nay, still farther, M. Bally is induced to believe that in the engorgements of the spleen, the sulphate of quinine acts as a *deobstruent*, by promptly removing all symptoms of enlargement." (450.)

M. Boisseau's " Physiological Pyretology, or a Treatise on Fevers," which first appeared in 1823, at Paris, and which in seven years passed through four editions, was republished in English at Philadelphia by Carey & Hart, in 1832.

M. Boisseau, though a devoted disciple of Broussais, gave quinine, but seldom more than twelve grains for a dose. This must have been previous to the publication of his book in 1823, or at the latest before the edition of 1830, here quoted.

M. Boisseau mentions a case of intermittent pneumonia treated by decoction of bark, to which ten grains of quinine were added, for an enema. The doses were repeated, and the patient recovered. The date of this case is given—namely, November, 1828. M. Boisseau details two fatal cases of pernicious fever, reported at length from M. Gassand (1828), in which quinine, together with decoction of bark, was repeatedly given "in high doses," sometimes designated at 10, 12, 30 grains, etc. (443:4-5.)

Although these cases, and others which might be quoted from this voluminous writer, are probably but representative cases of a pre-existing practice; and, although they represent the large doses of quinine as being three or four times greater than Dr. Cartwright's, the actual dates are two years later than his. But M. Boisseau has given other evidence, as will be seen below.

There can be no doubt that large doses of quinine were administered in both France and Italy anterior to either 1828, or 1826, or 1822. If the evidence already adduced from the 18th volume of the Dictionary of Medicine, published in May, 1827, be not absolutely conclusive, the following evidence is; and, what is remarkable, the case is very nearly a parallel one with that above mentioned in Dr. Cartwright's report:

M. Boisseau says: "Laënnec observed an existence of pernicious peripneumonic fever. A third paroxysm occurred. The chest having been explored, about the middle of the next paroxysm, the respiratory murmur was found unaltered except at the root of the lungs, where it was marked by a *râle crepitant* well characterized, principally on the right side. Laënnec without hesitation, declared the disease a double pneumonia in its initial stage: tartar emetic, six grains, sulphate of quinine, eighteen grains, to be taken in three doses. But as the *râle cripitant* had not entirely disappeared with the cessation of the febrile paroxysm, the two prescriptions were continued. * * * The tartar emetic was discontinued on the fifth day. The sulphate of quinine was continued for some days." (Pp. 433-4.) The patient got well. The exact date in this case is not given, but as Laënnec died in 1822, the quinine must have been given previously to 1822; and, à fortiori, before 1826.

Laënnec (born 1781—died 1822), who gave the world (in 1819) his discoveries, in a work on ausculation, the greatest gift to the science of diagnosis of which the nineteenth century can boast, died of the disease which he had so fully illustrated, namely, consumption. It is probable that he was not engaged in practice for some months before death, which, in this disease, is lingering. Hence it is probable that the large doses of quinine and tartar-emetic for "pernicious peripneumonic fever," which the illustrious Frenchman prescribed in this and probably many other cases, may bo dated within twelve or eighteen months after Pelletier and Caventou's discovery.

In the *Dictionnaire de Médecine* above mentioned (May, 1827), M. Guersent alludes to the experiments which had been already made in order to ascertain the physiological effects of seven or eight grain doses of the sulphate of cinchonine, and the same doses of the sulphate of quinine. Not only so. These experimental doses were increased in a few hours to thirty and forty grains, which, in some cases, produced no appreciable effect on the health, while in other cases the individuals were painfully affected from even three or four grains. Caventou, who, with Pelletier, had the great honor of being the discoverer of the mode of preparing quinia, took his own medicine, in order to ascertain its effects in his own person.

Pelletier and Caventou (names of which every Frenchman should be proud), made known this unequaled preparation in 1820. They received for the same from the Academy of Sciences, the Monthyon prize of ten thousand francs.

It appears from a volume of the Medico-Chirurgical Transactions, published in London, in 1827, and reviewed and quoted in the *Medical Recorder* of 1828 (p. 383), that ten grain doses of quinine were commonly given in London, in periodical fevers.

So great was the demand for quinine, that four chemists of Paris manufactured ninety thousand ounces of this article in the year 1826!

Art. X.—*Remarks and Translations illustrative of the Physiognomy of the Battle field, and the Attitudes of the Dead :* By Bennet Dowler, M.D.

> Like so many Alexanders,
> Have, in these parts, from morn till even fought,
> And sheathed their swords for lack of argument.
>   Shakspeare.

The poet, in every age, has labored to veil the hideousness of the battle-field, the aceldama where victory and glory are won. Here, scattering the flowers of song to the memory of the fallen, he invokes the noblest, mightiest, yet too often the most selfish passion, the love of country, right or wrong, as not only justifying carnage, but requiring unnumbered victims. It is sweet, it is honorable, says the Roman poet, to die for one's country :

> *Dulce et decorum est pro patria mori.*

> " How sleep the brave, who sink to rest
>   By all their country's wishes blest."

But neither the masters of the world nor the poets, can look the grim statistics of the killed and wounded in the face, without comprehending their sad import, the unutterable anguish and bereavement of the families and friends of the slain and mutilated, and sympathising with the living and the dead.

The position of the medical man in the army, and particularly in the field of battle, though he is a non-combatant, is often one of danger, always one of usefulness, but never one of glory, in the military sense of that word. Amid dense smoke, the clangor of arms, the thunderings of artillery, and the rattlings of shot, the surgeon, in modern wars, operates, often immediately on the battle ground, where many of the wounded may be thus saved, who would otherwise perish in a few moments from hæmorrhage, etc. And when the battle is ended, his work in the hospital or ambulance still goes on—as amputations, disarticulations, trephinings, extracting bullets and other projectiles, dressing wounds, fractures, etc. ; while the victorious combatants are partaking of the loud acclaims and blandishments of the public, enjoying festivities and amusements, honors, promotions, and repose. The surgeon in the meanwhile hears, instead of the pæans of triumph, the groans of the mutilated and the last sighs of the dying.

It appears that during the recent battles in Italy, some of the French physicians were directed by their superior medical officers, in addition to their more immediate duties to the living, to study the physiological mechanism, if one may so speak, of death itself, as it occurred in the battle-field; that is to say, the physiognomy, positions and attitudes incidental to death from the arms of war, during, or as soon as possible after, the conflict. Thus the surgeon passed from his operating ambulance to view the fallen. Is not this an intensification of the moral sublime? an unique study? original? French? more than tragedians ever conceived?

Thus Dr. Armand, physician-major of the first class, chief of the ambulance of the head quarters of the fourth corps of the French army of Italy, relates from personal observation some interesting particulars concerning the aspects and attitudes of the slain in the battle-fields of the Crimea, and of Italy—a condensed translation, or sketch, of which (from the. *Gaz. Hebdom. de Méd.* Sept. 16, 1859) will be subjoined, as worthy of consideration, psychically, physiologically, and traumatically.

During the day of the battle of Magenta, including the night, 800 wounded Frenchmen and Austrians underwent capital or minor operations and dressings at the ambulance of Dr. Armand. With his two assistants he had completed his work by the dawn of the following day, when he proceeded to inspect the bloody field of Magenta, and the attitudes of the slain. A melancholy, not a useless study.

Dr. Armand observed that a great number of the dead preserved, as nearly as may be, the same attitudes in which they had been when the messengers of death struck them—a proof that they had passed from life to death without agony, without convulsions. Those struck in the head generally lay with the face and abdomen flat upon the ground, a position which the death-stiffness had not changed, holding, for the most part, their weapons still grasped in their hands.

Dr, Armand mentions a peculiarity often attendant upon wounds of the head, in which the patient thinks himself by no means dangerously hurt, although sometimes he dies, one might say, spontaneously, or by surprise. During the battle of Solferino, a soldier wounded in the head by a ball, entered the ambulance and was dressed by Dr. Lambert The ball had perforated the skull and lodged in the cerebral mass; nevertheless, the patient's intelligence was perfect; he made light of his wound; lay down, having his lighted pipe in his mouth, with his head raised upon his knapsack against the wall, where he was found afterwards, with his pipe still in his mouth. He had expired without movement or noise. Dr. Armand details a similar case, that of a sergeant-major, whom Dr. Lambert (Dr. A's assistant) dressed in the Crimean war. The soldier smoked on for a dozen of days after having been wounded; and, having lighted his pipe for the last time, died suddenly, keeping it still in his mouth. These cases are, therefore, attested by at least two medical witnesses.

Dr. Armand says that soldiers who receive their death-wounds in the heart, fall and rest in the same manner as those do who are killed by injury of the brain, though the death is not so instantaneous but that it may allow an attitude, which, so to speak, is active. We have seen, among others, a Zouave struck fairly in the chest, who was brought together, or doubled upon his musket as if taking a position to charge bayonet, his face full of energy, as if advancing, with an attitude more menacing than that of a lion. It is reported that His Majesty had observed a similar case at Palestro.

On the other hand, an Austrian, who had died by hæmorrhage from a ball which had divided the crural vessels, whose agony had been of some duration, as proven by the blood in which he was bathed, presented the attitude of supplication ; he lay on his back, a little bent to the right, his face and eyes turned towards the heavens, both hands joined together, with the fingers interlaced and contracted. This man died in the attitude of prayer. In fact, religious ideas appeared to have prevailed quite extensively among the Austrian soldiers, as well as among the Russians in the campaign in the Crimea.

In wounds of the abdomen, as the agony was more or less prolonged, the pains were intolerable, attended with vomiting and hiccough ; the face of the corpse was generally found contracted, the hands and forearms crossed and closed upon the abdomen, the body doubled upon itself, and resting on the side.

At Ponte Vecchio di Magenta, a Hungarian hussar, killed (as was his horse), remained nearly in the saddle lying upon the right side, having the point of his sabre in advance, in the position of a horseman when charging. He had roses still fresh in his tolpak, his forehead pierced with a ball ; his horse was riddled with shot in the head, and both had died simultaneously. This case was witnessed by Dr. A. Renard. Dr. Armand relates a parallel case which occurred to an Austrian artilleryman.

At Melegano, several French solders while charging bayonet fell, mortally wounded with grape-shot ; their faces rested on the ground and their bayonets pointed in advance.

At Magenta, among the slain strewed upon the battle-ground, several Austrian officers were recognized of distinguished physiognomy, dressed with the utmost care and propriety in glossy gloves—one might say that they had affectedly made their toilette in anticipation of death. Their fine blond heads of hair and regular features, for the most part different from the common soldiers, had the expression of bravery and resignation.

Next to such a vast panorama of death, the dead-house of the Charity Hospital of New Orleans during a great epidemic of yellow fever, may claim a place. The physiognomy of the yellow fever corpse is usually sad, sullen, and perturbed; the countenance dark, mottled, yellow, livid, stained with blood and black vomit, and swollen; the eyes prominent and blood shotten, and yellow. The veins of the face and of the whole body often become distended; the whole expression is less calm and placid than in most other corpses especially such as have died of hæmorrhages.

The following tableau of the dead body of Goëthe, is by the masterly hand of Eckermann.

" The morning after Goëthe's death, a deep longing seized me to look yet once again upon his earthy garment. His faithful servant, Frederic, opened for me the chamber in which he was laid out. Stretched upon his back, he reposed as if in sleep ; profound peace and serenity reigned in the features of his noble, dignified countenance; the mighty brow seemed yet the dwelling place of thought. I wished for a lock of his hair, but reverence prevented me from cutting it off. The body lay naked, only wrapped in a white sheet; large pieces of ice had been placed around, to keep it fresh as long as possible. Frederic drew aside the sheet, and I was astonished at the divine magnificence of the form. The breast was so powerful, broad, and arched; the limbs full, and softly muscular; the feet elegant, and of the most perfect shape ; nowhere on the whole body a trace either of fat or of leanness and decay; a perfect man lay in great beauty before me; and the rapture which the sight caused made me forget for a moment, that the immortal spirit had left such an abode. I laid my hand on his heart—there was a deep silence—and I turned away to give free vent to my tears."

Independent of experience, the physiologist cognizes no inherent necessity in life itself, nor in any of its organized forms of manifestation, nor in any of its structural adaptations and finalities, for a catastrophe so melancholy—so repugnant to the instincts of humanity, as death. Indeed, the analogies of the material universe wherein stability reigns, or varies only in constantly recurring cycles, seems to teach that man, for whom all things appear to exist, is, what his irrepressible instincts claim, immortal—exempt from death! The stars rise undiminished as on the morning of the creation, and "pursue the even tenor of their way" through infinite space. The earth, a little scarred on its face by volcanic eruptions and accidents, undecayed by age, "spins silently onward with spheres which never sleep; her unwithered countenance being as bright as at creations' day." Trees live thousands of years, and some fishes for centuries. The inferior animals neither foreknow, nor apprehend impending death at every step in life. This unpleasant secret is made known to man alone. A current, he can no more resist than the unfortunate boatman caught by the descending rapids of Niagara, hurries him over a precipice into a realm as tenebrious (after all the researches of mere physical science), as that into which the fabled Styx debouched in the days of antiquity.

Poets and philosophers have sought to bring out in the foreground, pictures more cheering, so as to veil the sombre tableau of death in the distance. Bryant's picture is one of the most pleasing:

> "So live, that, when thy summons comes to join
> The innumerable caravan, that moves
> To the pale realms of shade, where each shall take
> His chamber in the silent halls of death,
> Thou go not like the quarry slave at night,
> Scourged to his dungeon ; but sustained and soothed
> By an unfaltering trust, approach thy grave
> Like one who wraps the drapery of his couch
> About him, and lies down to pleasant dreams."

With unsurpassed beauty, La Fontaine calls death the evening of a fine day:

> "*La mort est le soir d'un beau jour.*"

PROGRESS OF MEDICINE.

ART. I.—*Hypodermic and Enepidermic Medication and Experiments.*

i.—*The Hypodermic Treatment :* By CHARLES HUNTER, late House Surgeon at St. George's Hospital.

[MR. HUNTER, in terminating his papers on hypodermic medication *(Medical Times and Gazette,* July 11, 1859), gives a summary of his conclusions, which will be found below. In the preceding volume of the *New-Orleans Medical and Surgical Journal* (p. 558), the reader will have seen a paragraph giving a brief view of his researches upon this subject as far as then published. It appears from his cases and experiments published some months later, that this mode of medication, though highly efficacious generally, is sometimes the cause of very serious effects which take place " at once," as " severe and distressing sickness."]

1. That certain medicines may be introduced into the cellular tissue beneath the skin with safety and with advantage. 2. That medicines so introduced have a *general* as well as a local effect. 3. That the general effect of medicine so introduced is exceedingly rapid. 4. That this mode of administration is *more certain in its action* than stomachic doses are, for the *exact* amount introduced is known, and the whole of it takes effect, which *may* or *may not* be the case with stomachic doses. 5. Medicines are *more purely received* into the system by this method than when given by the stomach, in which organ they may become contaminated or decomposed. 6. A given amount of a medicine employed hypodermically has a greater effect than the *same* amount administered by the stomach ; *it also acts more quickly.* 7. A given amount of a medicine employed hypodermically has a greater and more rapid effect than when employed *endermically.* 8. That the medicines for which this mode of introduction is especially applicable are the various *narcotics* and *sedatives.* 9. That the *diseases* for which this plan of treatment is especially indicated are for the most part *affections of the nervous system :*—1stly. Where the immediate and decided effect of a narcotic is required. 2ndly. Where narcotics administered by the usual methods fail to do good, and yet are indicated. 3rdly. Where the effect of a narcotic is required, and the patient *refuses to swallow.* 4thly. Where from irritability of the stomach or other cause (such as idiosyncracy, etc.) the patient cannot take the medicine by the stomach (case 2). 10. That to produce a general effect it does not signify whether the remedy be injected into the cellular tissue of the body or of an extremity. 11. That to relieve or cure a local neuralgic affection, there is no ne-

cessity to localize the injection. 12. That whether the object be to treat a local or general affection, it seems advisable each time to change the site for injection, should it be more than once required.

Mr. Hunter, in the *Medical Times and Gazette* (Oct. 8, 1859), gives some further details concerning the mode of employing the hypodermic treatment, a portion of which is subjoined :

The Syringe for Injection.—The little instrument I use is made by Messrs. Whicker & Blaise. It is of the same make (but a little larger as regards the barrel) as their original *caustic syringe.* The barrel is of glass, with silver fittings, and contains a piston which works by a screw-rod, each half-turn of which expels half-a-minim, as a fine drop from the end of the pipe.

Two pipes belong to each syringe, the one larger and stronger than the other.

No Incision is required with lancet, or other instrument, when this syringe is used, for the point of the pipe being very sharp and fine, is readily passed, with proper precaution, beneath the skin ; no blood is shed, and the operation is no more than the prick of a needle.

The Employment of the Syringe.—Having charged the syringe with the narcotic fluid, hold it in the right hand at the junction of the barrel with the pipe, and with the left hand take up, between the finger and thumb, a fold of the skin of the patient, so as to make tense the part beyond your thumb, then the right hand being gently steadied, but not heavily pressed on the patient, let the point of the syringe, which is held at a right angle to the skin, touch the part which is tense, and, with a *quick but steady movement,* be passed through it ; the point being well *through the skin,* the direction of the pipe may be altered so that it may run along in the loose cellular tissue beneath ;* all this is the work of a moment ; the pre-arranged number of drops are then introduced by so many turns of the piston, the pipe is then withdrawn, a finger making slight pressure as near as possible on the punctured spot, the object being both to steady the skin and prevent any drop of liquid escaping ; and lastly, a narrow strip of plaster, cut beforehand and warmed, is placed on the spot.

The strip of plaster is generally a precautionary measure, but it becomes a necessity when the quantity injected is large, say twenty minims ; but it is always useful to prevent the spot from being chafed. A broad piece of plaster is worse than none at all ; it presses on the "little lump," which is caused for a few minutes by the presence of the injected fluid beneath the skin, and not at all perhaps on the punctured spot, and so it does more to press the fluid out than keep it in (I have seen a first injection in a case of delirium tremens fail for this very reason); *but a narrow strip just covers the punctured spot.*

These directions may appear unnecessary, but the operation may fail, as just shown, for want of attention to these little points. If

---

* In the majority of cases the plan above described is best, especially with thin people ; if, however, the patient is very fat, it is better to perforate vertically a portion of skin and subjacent fat, pinched up, and so made tense between the finger and thumb.

the introduction of the syringe be attempted, the skin of the patient being loose, or the syringe held at the farther end, and consequently unsteadily, the patient may by these means be put to a great deal of pain, and the pipe of the syringe may be bent or broken from the socket ; but when it is introduced with a quick steady movement, the skin being tense, the patient does frequently not even know when the point is introduced.

The Tissue to Inject.—The tissue injected is the cellular or areölar tissue of the body ; it may not matter *much* whether the cellulo-adipose tissue, the panniculus adiposus, or the reticular tissue beneath it (not containing fat) be injected, but the latter is to be preferred ; it is the looser of the two, fluid injected into it meets with no obstruction, and cannot easily escape from it ; but if injected into the skin itself as some think it is, or the conjoined cellulo-adipose tissue, it is apt to cause pain, it enters less readily, and is more apt to escape ; nor does it seem to act quite so rapidly as when injected into the loose cellular tissue from which most probably absorption is the more rapid.

The Part of the Body to Inject.—When the object is to quiet the brain, or to produce a general effect, is it material whether·the fluid be injected into the cellular tissue of the body or of an extremity? *No ;* the non-necessity of localision is the basis of this plan of treatment, and is the reason of its applicability in cerebro-spinal affections and general diseases. I need only refer to the various cases detailed in corroboration of this. The site which I, however, most commonly inject, is *the inner part of the arm.* The skin is here thin, easily made tense, and easily perforated ; the cellular tissue beneath is loose, and readily receives the fluid ; there are perhaps more veins here than in some other parts, but they are easily avoided.

The Quantity of Fluid to Inject.—It is as well to have the fluid of that strength that three or four turns of the piston shall be an ordinary injecting dose. Two or three turns can be made in a moment of time, and it is no small relief or surprise to the patient, who has been expecting, perhaps dreading, an operation, to find all over *in less than h lf-a-minute.*

The Dose—Too much caution cannot be employed with regard to the *amount of the narcotic* injected. Two half turns, if your solution is strong, may double the dose, and the life of the patient, for want of due care, be placed in jeopardy ; I would, therefore, urge attention to these points :

1. Be certain of the exact strength of the fluid employed, and the exact value of each turn of the piston.

2. Concerning first injections, never use more than half the ordinary stomachic dose for males, nor more than a third for females.

3. Should a second injection be necessary, let it not be used too soon ; nor in a full dose when the patient is partially under the influence of the narcotic.

These points are of practical importance ; a *certain degree* of narcotism has to be reached for benefit to accrue, and by the injection it can be reached in many cases by a very small quantity of the narcotic, because of the rapidity with which the effect is produced ; what we have to avoid is *too great* an effect ; what we try to produce is a *certain effect* with as *small a quantity* as possible. This leads me to remark that men *bear narcotics much better than women.*

I was not aware to what extent this was the case until I had employed this treatment some little while ; but I now think it may be looked on as a rule, that men in general will bear with no ill effects, but be benefited by, injected doses of narcotics, which doses would very strongly, if not seriously, affect women ; in fact, *this treatment is a test of the exact amount* of a narcotic necessary to produce a desired effect, when taken by direct means into the general circulation. For instance, you introduce beneath the skin the one-eighth of a grain of morphia, the effect which follows is the whole effect of the whole one-eighth ; but you cannot be certain that the effect which follows the administration of one-eighth of a grain, firstly, by the skin, secondly, by the stomach, or, thirdly, by the rectum, is the effect of the whole one-eighth ; but it is the whole effect of the quantity absorbed.

As by this method we get the *whole effect of the known quantity introduced,* which we are not sure of getting by the other modes, we have now a method as accurate as that of venous injection (without its dangers) for testing the precise effect of little-known medicines on animals, and the exact doses and effects of well-known medicines on man, of seeing the difference which the sex requires in the dose, and of ascertaining the minimum amount required to produce a desired effect.

It is impossible to say "what amount is to be injected," without knowing the particulars of the case, as well as the sex and age ; but taking the acetate of morphia for an example, I think that first injections for adult females should vary from the one-eighth to a quarter or one-third of a grain ; for adult males, from the one-sixth to half or three-quarters of a grain.

First injections should be small rather than large, and are good indicators of the amount necessary, should repetition be required. It is true that I have seen used, and employed myself, much larger quantities than those I have mentioned, for first injections ; but the cases have been exceptional, and under close observation.

In the preceding papers on this subject, I have shown the advantages of this mode of treatment over the endermic, enepidermic, and stomachic methods, which, requiring longer to act, are less certain, and apt to fail completely.

ii.—*Hypodermic Injection of Medicines.*— By ROBERT WHITE, M. D., Boston.

So far as I have been able to investigate the matter, I am of opinion that this new method will supersede many of the older and slower modes of procedure in therapeutics. I am sanguine enough to believe, and to predict, that it will produce as great a revolution in the healing art as the electric telegraph has done in the slow-coach system of our ancestors.   *   *   *   *   *

On the 3rd, —— sent for his family physician, who prescribed tincture of opium and fluid extract of valerian. Half an ounce of the former and two ounces of the latter were given in twenty-four hours, without producing quiet, but rather the reverse. Chloric ether was also tried, from the effects of which he would sleep a few minutes, then wake up as bad as ever. Strong hop tea was then administered freely, with an occasional dose of McMunn's elixir, and a bladder of ice kept constantly applied to the head.

When I visited him on the morning of the 5th he was talking incessantly, making frequent attempts to get out of bed, fidgeting and pulling at the bedclothes, with subsultus tendinum, pulse 104, pupils contracted, head very hot, skin dry, tongue moist and coated with a white fur. He complained of dryness of the throat. Bowels regular. Knew all his attendants, and could with difficulty be kept in bed. I advised a suspension of the opium, and to continue the hop tea and valerian, and ordered a solution of bicarb. potass., to relieve an occasional attack of vomiting. Leeches to the temples. Ice to be continued to the head, and plenty of diluent drinks.

The patient continued in nearly the same condition, and under the same treatment, only varied according to circumstances, until the morning of the 8th, when he appeared evidently sinking : pulse very weak and slow, extremities cold, cold clammy perspiration exuding all over him, vocalization constant, muttering and indistinct. He did not recognize his attendants. As a last resource, I ordered a glass of hot brandy punch, and determined to try the effects of injecting morphia into the cellular tissue. I desired his family physician to procure a small glass syringe and a little morphia, which he immediately did. When he returned, he administered the punch to the patient, which was slowly but eagerly swallowed. In the mean time I dissolved a grain of the morphia (muriate) in about half a teaspoonful of cold water, then made a puncture with a lancet into the cellular tissue of the left arm, and injected as much of the solution as I could with my very imperfect apparatus. Yet, notwithstanding all disadvantages, the experiment was perfectly successful. Some said it was the punch that made him sleep ; at any rate, in twenty minutes afterward he was calm, his eyes closed, something was evidently composing him ; and I was well pleased to learn, when I visited him at 2, P. M., that he had slept soundly for two hours and a half. He had evidently rallied, but the delirious symptoms continued, though much abated. I had determined to repeat the injection, should the first have no effect ; but he was so much better that I hoped he would sleep more, and I deferred it until the evening. I then left him, but in an hour after was sent for. The messenger said he had grown violent, and could not be kept in bed. I visited him directly ; he was out of bed, partly dressed, poking about the room, tossing everything upside down. I dissolved one grain of sulphate of morphia, which I had brought with me, in about the same quantity of water as before, and repeated the punch, which was vomited immediately. Now, said I, there will be no blame to the punch. I then requested him to sit down on the bedside, and made a puncture in the other arm, large enough to admit the point of the syringe, and with the small blade of a penknife extended the puncture beneath the skin, about three-eighths of an inch, without enlarging the orifice. I then introduced the syringe as far as I could, elevated

14

the skin, and withdrew the syringe a little, so as to free the point from the cellular tissue, then pushed the piston home. The solution whizzed in, forming an areöla around the puncture, about the size of half a dollar; withdrawing the syringe, I pressed a moment on the puncture, and then applied a little adhesive plaster, to prevent the solution oozing out.

In a few minutes afterward, he started off round the room again, tossing over and examining everything, then went to the window and looked out, making remarks on the weather. The morphia was evidently operating. In a short time his eyelids began to close, and his head to grow heavy. I suggested the propriety of his going to bed, to which he immediately assented, and sat down on the bed-side, put off his pantaloons with a little assistance, lay down as docile as a child, and in ten minutes was sound asleep. I saw him again at 11, P. M. He was awake, but had slept upward of five hours. Subsultus tendinum much abated. He felt comfortable, but drowsy and thirsty, and when left alone would go right off to sleep. When I visited him again, next morning, he was wide awake, after sleeping nearly the whole night, perfectly sensible, the subsultus tendinum completely gone, he had no headache, bowels had been open during the night, no unnatural thirst, and he was completely convalescent. He dozed a good deal during the day, and slept naturally the succeeding night. He continued to improve rapidly, and in three days he was up and dressed, arranging his affairs.

I have injected since in three other cases, and have used a vaccinating lancet and a small glass syringe, with the piston well packed, and have found them to answer admirably every desired object in the operation.—*Boston Medical and Surgical Journal, December* 1, 1859.

iii—*Experiments on some of the various circumstances influencing cutaneous absorption :* By AUGUSTUS WALLER, M. D., F. R. S., Professor of Physiology, Queen's College, Birmingham.*

In some former experiments† I endeavored to elucidate the phenomena of cutaneous absorption on the lower animals (batrachia), by immersing the hinder extremities in various solutions, and afterwards watching the period at which the absorbed substances reached the tongue, where their presence was detected by means of some reagent applied to its surface; as, for instance, a salt of iron, when the legs were immersed in a solution of yellow ferro-cyanide of potassium ; Prussian blue was then formed as soon as the ferro-cyanide was brought to the tongue.

Furthermore, I was able to detect, by the aid of the microscope, the " lieux d'élection," or preference spots, where the cyanide escaped from the vessels.

On the present occasion I shall endeavor to elucidate cutaneous absorption on the higher animals, and, if possible, to give a more

* In the November number of the *New Orleans Medical and Surgical Journal, p.* 875, a brief extract is given from Dr. Waller's previous papers on cutaneous absorption.

† Waller "Absorption of various substances through the skin of the frog."—*Frorieps Tagesberichte,* 1851.

definite view of this function, by determining, by accurate measurement, the degree of rapidity, the peculiarities, etc., which it may offer in various conditions.

A very simple mode of demonstrating the existence of cutaneous absorption is by immersing the leg of a young guinea pig, not more than half-grown, into a mixture of equal parts of chloroform and tincture of aconite. After fifteen minute's immersion, the part will be found insensible at the surface and extremities, and, after a short time, symptoms of poisoning by aconite will supervene, viz : nausea, efforts at vomiting, sometimes vomiting of bile, coldness of the surface and extremities, circulation very weak, laborious respiration, slight convulsive symptoms, and death.

The influence of age, or of thickening of the cuticle, is easily seen in the same way ; for, if instead of a young animal we take an adult one, we obtain no poisoning, but merely local insensibility and slight disturbance of respiration, etc.

Another not less instructive experiment consists in replacing the mixture of chloroform and tincture of aconite by simple tincture of aconite. In this case, the limb may be indefinitely immersed without our obtaining either local insensibility or death, or indeed any symptom whatever of the presence of aconite in the system.

A fourth experiment, which consists in dividing the sciatic nerve, shows the influence of innervation on the function of absorption ; for if performed on an adult animal, and consequently one incapable of absorbing aconite in quantity sufficient to cause death, the powers of absorption will be generally found so much augmented, that the animal will be poisoned by immersion of the limb in simple tincture of aconite.

In this experiment I attribute the acceleration in the cutaneous absorption to the paralysis of the blood vessels, as in my experiments on the sympathetic nerve, where I showed that in blood vessels the passage of the blood is completely regulated by nerves springing from the spinal cord. When the vascular nerves are paralysed, the artery becomes greatly distended, and the blood flows faster within it. The foot, after the section of the sciatic, is on this account more hot and red ; and for the same reasons it is easy to account for the more rapid absorption of medicinal agents.

A fifth experiment consists in placing a ligature on the limb, in order to impede the powers of absorption of the animal. Although the ligature does produce this result, I was rather surprised to find how much less efficient it was than is generally represented ; for, whenever the least symptoms of a toxic influence made their appearance, a ligature placed over the limb rarely succeeded in saving the animal.

In order to obtain results more susceptible of measurement, I proceeded to substitute atropia for aconite, and to make use of the albino rat in lieu of the guinea pig. By this means, I possessed an agent whose intervention was immediately detected by its action on the iris. My choice of the albino rat was for the like reason, i. e. the facility which it offered for exact and easy measurement, in which respect this animal is far preferable to any other with which I am acquainted, unless we except the white mouse, which, however, is so liable to die from slight causes, that it is little adapted for most physiological experiments.

The *modus operandi* which I generally adopt is to immerse the limb into a small two-drachm bottle containing sufficient of the mixture to cover the foot and part of the leg. The strength of the solution of atropia being generally that from half a grain to one drachm of some menstruum, such as chloroform, alchohol, etc., I generally prefer simply to hold the animal during the experiment to any other mode of restraint. By these means I am able to guard against several causes of error, such as the direct contact of the solution with the eye or mouth, and, at the same time, avoid any unnecessary discomfort to the animal.

Chloroform and Atropia.—A solution of atropia in chloroform will generally be found to cause dilatation of the pupil after the foot has been immersed from two to five minutes. The dilatation, having once commenced, is usually very rapid, and the pupil very soon attains double or triple its normal diameter, which is about $\frac{1}{4}$ to $\frac{1}{2}$ a millimetre during day-time. It is easy to recognize that this dilatation is not in very simple ratio to the time occupied in its expansion, the expansion of the pupil being more nearly in proportion to the square of the time occupied than in a simple arithmetical ratio. Immersion of one limb causes both pupils to dilate equally, except in some few instances, where one pupil expands much more than the other, from some constitutional peculiarity, which remains the same whichever foot be immersed.

Although I have never failed to obtain dilatation of the pupils by the immersion of the foot in this solution of atropia, yet, in some cases, it takes more slowly than in others. The age of the animal has, in this respect, a most marked retarding influence. On animals only about a third grown, it will often occur at about $2\frac{1}{2}$ minutes after immersion, while in the adult it generally requires five minutes and upwards.

The local effects of immersion are redness, heat, and swelling of the foot, accompanied sometimes with extravasation from some smaller vessels, when the immersion has been prolonged for ten minutes and upward. The sensibility of the part is likewise diminished, but in no case so as to produce insensibility. The amount of irritation is of course variable, according to the duration of the immersion. It is, however, important to remark that full dilatation of the pupils may be obtained without any symptoms beyond those of a temporary active vascularization of the part, which quickly disappears when the irritating cause is removed, and which presents no more active symptoms than those produced by neuro-paralysis of the vessels after section of the sciatic nerve.

If instead of immersing the limb as above, we merely plunge it for a moment in the solution, we likewise may have dilatation of the pupil, but more slowly.

The same effects are obtained even although the limb be washed on its withdrawal from the solution, which would lead to the inference that the effect in that case is owing to the absorption of the atropia, at all events beneath the cuticle.

In the case of a solution of atropia in turpentine, a still more curious effect is observed, viz : that during immersion in the liquid the pupil scarcely, if at all, dilates ; whereas, immediately after the removal of the limb, the dilatation commences. Dilatation of the pupils will generally persist from twenty-four to thirty-six hours, and the return to the normal size is very gradual. In some cases the pupil may be affected after an immersion of nine minutes, the dilatation reaching three millimetres ; while in others. only a very slight influence is obtained on the pupil after an immersion of from twelve to fifteen minutes. If the limb is then removed from the solution, the pupil dilates to its maximum in a few minutes. After two or three minutes' immersion, the animal shows signs of considerable pain. Much inflammation of the part follows the action of this solution, which is followed by œdema.

When we immerse the tail of the animal instead of its foot, absorption takes place much more slowly, dilatation of the pupil being produced only after the lapse of about twenty minutes.

Atropia and Alcohol.—If we substitute alcohol instead of chloroform as a solvent, we find that absorption is extremely slow. Instead of obtaining dilatation of the pupils in two or three minutes, we find that an immersion of twenty to thirty minutes in the alcoholic solution will only produce very slight effects. At the same time the local irritation is much less than that caused by chloroform. Alcohol of various strength, from proof spirit upwards, had the same result as a solvent.

Atropia in water, with the addition of sufficient acetic acid for its solution. —The absorption of atropia in this state is very slow, thirty minutes' immersion frequently producing no dilatation of the pupils. Dilatation is then promoted by the removal of the limb from the solution.

Watery Extract of Belladonna.—When rubbed over the leg and tail, this substance was not found, after the lapse of an hour, to produce any dilatation of the pupil.

Tincture of belladonna, with half its quantity of chloroform. produced dilatation at the end of fifteen minutes. The part was found on removal to be completely insensible, and considerably swollen from œdema, which lasted for several days.

Atropia with strong alcohol and ammonia produced dilatation of the pupil, after twenty-five minutes' immersion. In this case the ammonia was added for the purpose of ascertaining how far irritation of the part was conducive to absorption. Slight vesication was the consequence of the presence of ammonia. The acceleration of the absorption was very slight, as the solution produced no dilatation until after twenty-four minutes' immersion.

Absorption of Morphia.—The foot of a young rat, at one-third of its growth, was immersed in a solution of half a grain of acetate of morphia in twenty drops of alcohol and one drachm of chloroform. In five minutes the pupils gradually dilated to the maximum ; the limb was then withdrawn ; foot hot, red, and rather swollen. Irritation of the skin caused no cry, the animal merely withdrawing the part. Somnolency existed, from which any noise aroused it, but only for a moment. When placed on its back, the animal remained in that

position. Respiration accelerated. Vision, when roused, very imperfect, as was shown by its falling off the table. The pupils continued fully dilated, the iris being reduced to an almost imperceptible
circle, the dilatation exceeding that which I have been able to attain
even with atropia. I will not dwell more fully at present on this last
interesting fact, which is opposed to what we generally meet with in
the administration of morphia. Twelve hours after, pupils normal,
animal quite well.

Strychnia and Chloroform.—After three minutes' immersion of foot
dilatation of pupils ensued. After five minutes the immersed limb
was very sensitive, apparently more so than normal. Limb removed
from solution ; spasms about the throat now appeared, which were
rapidly succeeded by stiffness of the trunk, increasing into tetanic
spasms. Death two minutes after removal.

Strychnia and Alcohol.—Foot immersed in a solution of alcohol and
strychnia for upwards of thirty-five minutes ; no symptoms of strychnine poisoning. Removed from solution and washed. Twelve hours
later, no dilatation nor contraction of pupils.

The above observations evidently show that medicinal substances
may be very rapidly absorbed into the circulation under certain circumstances, among which, the most important is the choice of the
menstruum in which they are dissolved.

It remains for us to examine into the effect of temperature, inflammation, neuro-vascular paralysis, etc., on absorption. But, what is
of still more importance, we have to see how far these facts are
applicable to man in health and disease.

Meanwhile I take this opportunity to state that a remarkable uniformity exists between cutaneous absorption in man and in the lower
animals ; and I believe that the application of these facts to practical
medicine promises to be very important and extensive.—*Journal of
the Royal Society.—Dublin Hospital Gaz., Oct.,* 1859.

On the Endermic application of Iodide of Glycerine—By Dr. FERDI-
NAND SZUKITS.—The author of this paper, after enumerating the several
forms in which iodine has hitherto been endermically applied, proceeds to remark, that all the solvents in ordinary use take up only a
small quantity, with the exception of alcohol. It was therefore
desirable to discover a solvent which, without affecting the skin like
the alcoholic tincture, should take up as large a quantity as possible
of the iodine. This solvent was found in 1854, by Cap, in glycerine.
Cap attributed to glycerine the part of a simple solvent, and he proposed it, among others, for the solution of bromine, iodine, oxide of
lead, strychnia, veratria, atropia, morphia, etc. To Dr. Richter belongs
the credit of having first introduced into practice the solution of iodine
in glycerine. He combined the iodine with iodide of potassium, in
order to facilitate the solution of the former : combined with this, it
may be dissolved in any quantity up to the proportion of almost
three to five. But in this concentrated state it is a caustic solution,
and too strong for common endermic use ; and the author has proposed a solution of one part of iodine and five parts of glycerine, as
a solution which may be applied for a long time to the parts about
the neck and to the female breast, without any inconvenience except

a slight burning. In the neck and the female breast, the application, after two or three paintings, causes smart burning, and after four or five it produces more or less large excoriations, which require the discontinuance of the remedy and the application of cold fomentations. On the abdomen and in other parts, these symptoms occur much later. After a longer application of the iodide of glycerine, the epidermis peels off on the painted parts. The paintings were performed once a day in the author's cases, and paper of gutta percha was laid over the painted places, to prevent evaporation. The paintings may be continued for a month without producing *iodism*, and without causing the slightest disturbance in the well-being of the patient. According to the experiments of Bonnet, the absorption and elimination of iodine may take place to the amount of a gramme of iodine (15.4 grains) per diem for several weeks, without any injury to the general health. The number of the cases in which Dr. Szukits has employed the iodide of glycerine was twenty-four, in some of which the most satisfactory results were obtained.—*Brit. and For. Med.-Chir. Review.*

iv.—*Poisoning from Belladonna Plaster.*

[THE following extract from the *Boston Med. and Surg. Journal*, is suggestive of the existing uncertainty which hangs over external medication, though practised by skillful physicians :]

Poisoning from Belladonna Plaster.—Dr. Lyman reported the case. The patient was a woman aged twenty-nine, of a highly nervous temperament, and for several years had been in feeble health with pulmonary symptoms, and had suffered much of late with palpitation, for which, on Sunday, Nov. 6th, was ordered a belladonna plaster, two by four inches. She was cautioned against wearing it too long at a time. It was applied Sunday evening and removed on Monday morning, the palpitation being quieted. It was applied again on Tuesday, and worn all day. Tuesday evening, when she retired, she was advised by her husband to remove it ; but deriving comfort from it, she delayed so doing, and fell asleep with it on. At two o'clock the following morning, Wednesday, 19th, she awoke with severe pain in the top of the head, vomiting, dryness of the fauces, spasmodic action of the muscles of the throat and chest, and an indescribable sensation of sinking. Dr. L. saw her at six o'clock. The above symptoms continued, with the exception of vomiting, which had ceased. Her pulse was *quick* and thready ; the irides were very much dilated, though contractile; there was no disturbance of vision; the face and eyes were suffused ; the extremities cold, the tongue moist, and the skin dry. Spasmodic action and faintness returned every few minutes. There was no exanthematous eruption or disturbance of the bowels or kidneys. Seidlitz powders, sinapisms to the feet and epigastrium, were ordered, together with brandy and strong coffee. At half-past nine, the symptoms were about the same, with the exception that the headache was less. At noon, free perspiration occurred, followed by very marked relief. At five, P. M., the spasmodic action still occurred at intervals, causing much distress; the patient was otherwise better. The pulse was full and tolerably forcible, but ranging as low as from twenty-eight to thirty-two! Skin moist, respiration normal. Neither the bowels nor kidneys having acted, liquid acetate of ammonia was ordered, also an enema and continuance of the stimulus of which she had partaken during the afternoon very moderately. The enema caused a free evacuation of the bowels and bladder. During the night, she complained of numbness of the face and inability to raise the lids. She urinated several times, with severe scalding and irritation of the bladder; and slept a little at intervals after midnight, the pulse ranging from twenty-eight to forty-two. During Thursday, the symptoms all disappeared, with the exception of the dilated pupils and slow pulse. On Friday morning the irides had recovered their natural appearance; but the pulse, though more full, was still at twenty-eight, and intermitting every one, two, or three beats. On Saturday evening, the pulse was fifty-two, though quite feeble. She was in good spirits, and sailed with her husband, Sunday morning, for Port au Prince, where they had previously made arrangements for passing the winter.

Dr. Lyman remarked that he was much in the habit of using this plaster, but he recollected only one instance in which the slightest unpleasant cerebral effect was produced, and that hardly appreciable. He had been since informed, by a very intelligent gentleman, that a precisely similar train of symptoms occurred in the case of his own wife, from the application of a poultice of the leaves to her abdomen, the pulse remaining in this depressed condition for many weeks.

Dr. Bethune said that he had known *atropine* to be absorbed through the skin, and produce its characteristic effects.

Dr. Williams mentioned a patient under his care with cataract, who, whenever a solution of atropine, in the proportion of five grains to the ounce, was applied to the conjunctiva, had dryness of the fauces and nausea.

ART. II.—*On the Internal Employment of Medicines in Vapor:** By J. BIRKBECK NEVINS, M. D., *London, Lecturer on Materia Medica in the Liverpool Royal Infirmary School of Medicine.*

THE subject of the present paper is one which I had the honor of bringing before the Medical Society of this town (Liverpool) some time since ; and to the members of that Society who then heard it, I must offer an apology for something so like a twice-told tale; but the favorable manner in which it was then received encourages me to hope

----

* Read at the Twenty-seventh Annual Meeting of the British Medical Association, held in Liverpool July 27th, 28th, and 29th, 1859.

that they will pardon some inevitable degree of repetition, whilst I trust that the addition of extended experience, and also some variety in the mode of applying remedies in this manner, will be accepted by them as my excuse.

There are several diseases which are constitutional in their commencement, and are at first most suitably treated by constitutional remedies, but which become chiefly local in their latter stages, and would at this time be most effectually relieved by topical remedies. Such a case is acute bronchitis—which at first affects the constitution generally, whilst in its latter stages, we have often few constitutional symptoms, and the chief complaint of the patient arises from the copious secretion from the bronchial membrane, and the cough which is excited by the effort to get rid of it. In this chronic stage of bronchitis, then, we have chiefly a local disorder, yet it is one which we are generally obliged to treat by constitutional remedies only, from the difficulty of applying topical agents to the lining membrane of the air passages. The profession has long been familiar with the change of treatment adopted when acute inflammation of the bladder subsides into the state of chronic catarrh of the organ. In the first instance, antiphlogistics, opium and diluents, are used; but when the disease has become chronic, injections of alum or other astringents into the bladder are employed with the greatest benefit. Upon the same principle, I lately made a patient inhale an impalpably fine powder of alum, gum, and morphia, in the manner brought before the Liverpool Medical Society by Mr. Bickerton, and in four and twenty hours the expectoration was reduced from above a pint and a half daily to nearly half the amount, with corresponding benefit to the patient.

Again, there is a class of diseases situated in organs so difficult of access, that we are frequently obliged to resort to counter irritation in the neighborhood, or to other methods of cure more or less inefficient, from our inability to apply our remedies to the affected surface itself. Such are chronic affections of the chordæ vocales, the Eustachian tubes, the frontal sinuses, and the passages in the nose. In these cases, we are generally unable to apply our remedies locally, and we therefore resort to blistering in the neighborhood, injections which we have but little hope of directing with accuracy to the part affected, and other means which we feel to be more or less unsatisfactory.

It is to meet such cases as these that the method I propose to lay before you offers considerable advantages; for if we can obtain our curative agent in the state of vapor, it may then be applied topically to every part which is traversed by the air we breathe; and may, therefore, be made to pass over a diseased laryngeal surface, by every effort of inspiration and subsequent expiration; or it may be passed through the nose by expiration through that organ; or driven into the Eustachian tubes or the frontal sinuses by forced efforts at expiration when the mouth and nostrils are closed, so as to prevent the actual escape of the air.

I propose now to mention a few cases illustrative of the general principle here laid down.

A patient had suffered from complete loss of voice for above a

15

year, not being able to speak above a whisper; the affection was evidently purely local, probably dependent upon a thickened condition of the chordæ vocales. She had no pain or any constitutional symptoms, and had long since given up treatment. She used the mercurial cigarette, to be described hereafter, for a month, and perfectly recovered.

A patient in the last stage of phthisis suffered from pain in the larynx, and utter inability to sleep for days and nights together, from the incessant cough and expectoration. Other treatment had been without avail; and I then made him inhale the vapor of strong nitric acid poured into a saucer, and placed near his mouth. He soon experienced relief from it; the pain abated, and the cough ceased to such an extent that he obtained some hours of refreshing sleep. He continued to adopt this means of relief at intervals until his death.

The trouble and annoyance of strong nitric acid in the neighborhood of a sick bed are, however, so great, that the inhalation of the nitrous acid fumes obtained by the combustion of nitrite of potash, is far preferable, and is easily accomplished. A young lady, who suffered much distress from the cough in a rather advanced stage of phthisis, and could only lie on one side, found far more relief from the inhalation of the fumes arising from brown touch paper burning in the bottom of a breakfast cup, and held near to her mouth or far from it as her own comfort dictated, than she did from the employment of cough medicines, the local application of the solution of nitrate of silver, or any other means which she had employed.

In a very chronic case of offensive discharge from the nostrils, with a sense of uneasiness in the frontal sinuses, the patient was quite cured in about a month by the use of the mercurial cigarettes. He held his nose after taking a mouthful of the smoke into his mouth, and then forced it into his nostrils, in the manner sometimes practised by accomplished smokers.

Another patient, who suffered from polypus in the nose, and had been operated upon in London by Mr. Fergusson, and subsequently in this town by myself, is now able to keep the disposition to form fresh polypi in check, by smoking the cigarette, and expelling the smoke through his nose, when he feels uneasiness, which warns him that he has to fear a recurrence of the disease.

In the treatment of the form of deafness which is dependent upon an obstructed Eustachian tube, I have increasingly numerous cases in which the smoke forced into the tympanum from the throat, gradually restores the sense of hearing. The circumstance which first led me to adopt this method, was hearing a deaf patient on one occasion remark that, when he was sneezing the day before, he heard perfectly; the violent effort appeared for the moment to have dilated the Eustachian tube, and hearing was the result. I have at present under my care a patient who has been deaf for seven years, and he has benefited more by this method of treatment than by any other. In this case, however, simple brown touch paper made into cigars, appears to be of more service than the mercurial cigarettes.

Such is an outline of the cases likely to be benefited by this mode of treatment, and the various methods in which it may be employed.

It offers a reasonable appearance of advantage in what are often very intractable diseases; and in bringing it more prominently before the profession, it is with the hope that it may prove a useful addition, in however small a degree, to the remedial agents at present in our possession. Modifications of the method itself, and the employment of other agents capable of being converted into the form of vapor, will, no doubt, suggest themselves to the experienced practitioner,.if he is satisfied by the results of trial that the principle itself is a beneficial one.

I use, for making the mercurial cigarettes, fifteen grains of nitrate of mercury, fifteen minims of strong nitric acid, and six drachms, or as much as may be sufficient, of water. Dissolve the nitrate in the nitric acid diluted with the water, and aided by a gentle heat (such as the top of an oven), and soak in the solution thick white blotting paper (eight by six inches.) Divide it into eight slips, which are to be rolled round a quill or pencil into cigarettes before they are quite dry, and gummed along the edge. If the paper is quite dry before it is rolled, it becomes brittle, and breaks in the folding.

There are various modifications of this mode of employing medicines mentioned in *L'Art de Formuler*, by MM. Trousseau and Reveil, from which work I obtained the suggestion in the first instance.—*British Med. Jour., Sept.* 24, 1859.

ART. III.—*Quinine in large doses in the Phlegmasiæ—Rheumatism and Heart Diseases.*

PARIS, October 24, 1859.

IN a recent number of the *Medical Times and Gazette* one of your distinguished correspondents expresses some doubts as to the efficacy of the sulphate of quinine in large doses in the treatment of some of the phlegmasiæ, and more especially in acute rheumatism and peritonitis; and, as he stated at the same time, that he would be glad to have some details as to the treatment of these affections by the above mentioned agents, I have much pleasure in placing before him three cases selected from many others which have come under my notice. They will be found to exhibit in a pretty strong light the connection existing between deafness and other symptoms resulting from quinic intoxication and its therapeutical action. These three cases were treated at La Charité, by M. Beau, of whose practice I have already spoken pretty fully on more than one occasion. The notes were carefully taken at the bedside of the patient, and all the details may, consequently, be strictly relied on.

Case 1.—C. R. aged thirty; employed at the Paris Telegraph Office, admitted into the Salle St. Felix, January 23, 1859. This patient is of middling stature and thin, with blue eyes, fair complexion, and lymphatic temperament ; has inhabited Paris since the age of eighteen, and has generally enjoyed good health. At the age of ten, had a first attack of rheumatism which lasted six weeks, since which he has been subject to cardiac palpitations; had a second attack of the same disease at the age of twenty; he now suffers from a third attack, induced by exposure to cold about a fortnight ago. On the present occasion the knees were first affected, but other parts of the body soon became involved. No active treatment hitherto had recourse to. The patient is lying on his right side, and is quite unable to assume any other posture; the left knee is the seat of considerable tumefaction, attended with heat, redness, and intense pain; it remains half bent, and all movement is impossible. Although not so seriously affected, the right knee also is swollen, red, and painful; no fluid is perceptible in either of the two articulations; the left shoulder and elbow are also the seat of very considerable pain, and all the metacarpo-phalangeal articulations of the left hand are red, swollen, and painful. On auscultation, a rough murmur is found to accompany the second sound of the heart; it extends over a large space, but its maximum is observable at the base of the organ; there is considerable dulness over the precordial region; the pulse is strong, full and jerking, eighty; skin hot, and covered with profuse perspiration; tongue furred, thirst, and loss of appetite; bowels regular. Diagnosis pronounced by M. Beau, "Acute rheumatism, with insufficiency of the semilunar valves." January 24.—Two grains of tart. antimon. are prescribed, which induce copious evacuations both from stomach snd bowels. January 25.—The pulse remains at eighty, though the patient is in other respects very feverish. M. Beau supposes that, in a state of health, this individual's pulse is naturally slow; the joints are swollen, painful, and stiff. Ordered sulph. quinæ, twenty-seven grains, in a potion, to be given in three doses—at midday, eight in the evening, and four in the morning. January 26.—No marked effect produced by the quinine, the patient having been deaf only about half-an-hour; the articulations as painful as they were yesterday; pulse eighty. Ordered quinæ sulph., thirty-six grains. January 27.—Marked symptoms of quinic intoxication from noon until eight in the evening, the patient having been deaf all the time; the joints are much better; pulse eighty. January 28.—The deafness is increased; pain and swelling of the joints diminished; pulse seventy-two. January 29.—The pain, redness, and swelling of the joints have disappeared; pulse sixty-four; the appetite is returning; ordered two soups. January 30.—Pulse sixty; the patient doing well. February 3.—Pulse fifty-six; patient continues in a very satisfactory state; the sulphate of quinine is reduced to twenty-seven grains. February 5.—Pulse fifty-two; patient no longer deaf ; joints continue quite free from pain; the quinine is reduced to eighteen grains, and the patient is allowed one portion of solid food. February 6.—The quinine is now entirely discontinued. February 7.—Has been up all day, and feels remarkably well; appetite good. February 12.—Was to-day discharged cured.

Case 2.—P. M., married, aged forty-three, private coachman, admitted into the Salle St. Felix, January 28, 1859. This patient is stout, short, and thick-set, with dark eyes and black hair; face very pale; has lived in Paris for the last twenty years. Had a first attack of rheumatism about eleven years ago, which was slight, but which made a permanent impression on his heart, as evinced by palpitations to which he has been subject ever since; in other respects has enjoyed good health. His present attack of rheumatism commenced six weeks ago. The left knee was first affected; but after a short time the right also became implicated. The patient lies on his back, and can with difficulty move; the palpitations are stronger than usual, accompauied with a little dyspnœa. The left knee is red, swollen, painful, and stiff; the right knee, the ancles, and the left shoulder are also much affected; the passage of the extensors under the annular ligament of the tarsus is peculiarly painful; all extension of the feet or movement of the toes is impossible. Auscultation reveals a rough murmur, accompanying the first sound of the heart, which extends over the entire precordial region, but has its maximum of intensity at the apex; a soft murmur attends the second sound, exclusively at the base of the organ; considerable dulness exists over the cardiac region, aud the heart's pulsations are excessively strong. Pulse, ninety-two; full and rebounding; the carotids are also the seat of a rough murmur, which immediately precedes the second sound of the heart. Lungs healthy; tongue furred; loss of appetite, and intense thirst; bowels regular, skin hot, and covered with a profuse perspiration exhaling an acid odor. *Diagnosis of M. Beau is acute rheumatism attended with mitral stricture and insufficiency of the semilunar valves.* January 29.—Two grains of tart. antimon. are prescribed, to be followed as soon as the vomiting shall have ceased, by thirty-six grains of the sulphate of quinine, exhibited as in the preceding case. January 30.—The stomach has been relieved of a large amount of bile, and patient feels more comfortable; he is almost entirely deaf; the joints are less painful; pulse has fallen to seventy-six. January 31.—Continues to do well and remains deaf ; the pulse has, however, risen to eighty-eight. February 1.—The rheumatic pains have returned; he is no longer deaf; pulse, ninety-two; sulphate of quinine increased to fifty-four grains. February 2.—He is quite deaf ; pulse fallen to seventy-six; the joints still a little painful. February 3.— Continues to improve; pulse seventy-two. February 4.—The patient is greatly agitated, having received bad news from home; tongue furred; constipation; pulse eighty-eight; deafness continues; is ordered two grains of tartar emetic, while the quinine is to be continued. At five in the afternoon, the patient had had copious evacuations: pulse, one hundred. February 6.—Feels relieved; deafness continues; pulse, seventy-six; joints free from pain. February 7.— Continues to improve; deafness persists; pulse, seventy-two; appetite returning; sulphate of quinine reduced to forty-five grains; two soups ordered. February 8.—Is much better; the joints are in their natural state; pulse has fallen to sixty-eight; appetite good; deafness continues; quinine reduced to thirty-six grains. February 12.— Quinine is entirely suppressed; ordered one portion of solid food. This patient remained in the ward until March 12, on account of his heart disease; but during the whole of this time he was quite free from rheumatism.

Case 3.—L. F., waiter, aged twenty-three, admitted into the Salle St. Felix, September 18, 1859; small in stature, dark eyes and brown hair, complexion rather pale, and has the look of having been badly fed; has lived in Paris since the age of eighteen. Three years ago had a first attack of rheumatism, which lasted three months; had a second attack in January last, and is now suffering from a third attack, which commenced yesterday. Both knee-joints invaded at once. Patient is sitting up in bed; the lower limbs alone being affected. The knees are red, hot, swollen, and painful, more especially the left one, all movement of which is impossible; both limbs are extended. On auscultation, a very slight murmur is heard to accompany the first sound of the heart, heard only, however, over a very limited space over the apex; skin hot and dry; pulse, one hundred, strong and full; tongue furred; loss of appetite; intense thirst; bowels regular. *Diagnosis: acute rheumatism, attended with very slight mitral stricture.* September 19.—Two grains of the tart. antimon. prescribed, which produced free evacuations. September 20.—Patient feels relieved; pulse, ninety-two; joints still very stiff and painful; ordered twenty-seven grains of sulph. quinæ. September 21.—Is quite deaf; pulse, seventy-six; joints still painful. September 22.—Pulse fallen to sixty; complete deafness; swelling of joints much diminished. September 23.—Pulse, sixty; deafness continues; joints no longer painful; the murmur attending the first sound of the heart is now very faint. September 24.—Pulse, fifty-six; continues to improve. September 26.—Pulse, fifty-two; the joints now in their natural condition; the quinine reduced to eighteen grains per day; two soups ordered. September 27.—Pulse, fifty-two; patient feels a little giddy; deafness continues. September 28.—Pulse, fifty-four; no pains in the joints; deafness persists; quinine is reduced to nine grains daily; one portion of solid food ordered. September 30.—The quinine is entirely suppressed. October 8.—Patient quite free from every symptom of rheumatism, and the sounds of the heart being all but perfectly normal, he is transferred to the Convalescent Asylum.—*Med. Times and Gazette.*

ART. IV.—*Phthisis, Bronchitis, Pneumonia.*

i.—*On the elements of Prognosis in Phthisis: By* DR. POLLOCK.

Dr. Pollock read before the Harveian Society the following paper on the elements of Prognosis in Phthisis, which he illustrated by the exhibition of several photographic portraits of patients in whom the disease had been arrested. The following is an abstract of the paper :

Dr. Pollock began by observing that the subject of phthisis had fallen into disrepute with medical men, who were accustomed to bestow the largest amount of attention only on what is new and striking. The prevalent idea that the disease is incurable, and that its progress is only a continuous declension towards the fatal result, also retarded new researches—the profession conceiving that it was to be palliated, but never eradicated. This condition of the professional mind was most to be deprecated, as from it would spring no progress, and under its influences even an impartial examination of facts became impossible. It were inflicting a mental blindness on ourselves to allow this State of things to continue without a protest occasionally from those who have large opportunities of seeing this disease. For some years the author had enjoyed these opportunities at the Consumption Hospital ; and he proposed, without reference to theories, to offer a few rules for guidance in forming an opinion on the probabilities regarding the future course of any case of phthisis. The value of correct prognosis was very great, involving the personal interests of the patient and his friends, and the character of the physician. The applause and the highest pecuniary rewards of the public also attend on our proficiency in solving these questions ; and the author conceived that he should not exaggerate their importance if he stated that more fortunes had been made by scientific accuracy in prognosis, and more credit lost by mistakes in the same, than by all other incidents of professional life put together. The recent practice of insurance offices to accept diseased lives at an increased premium, also added to the importance of an accurate knowledge of the subject. To the attainment of this careful observation and precise knowledge, must be added individual tact. In speaking of consumption, he must be understood to mean a deposit of tubercle indicated by the known physical signs. The first stage meant a simple deposit ; the second, its softening ; the third, an excavation. Medical language and that of the public greatly confuse one another : the latter desiring to indicate the degree of danger alone. Patients die in all three stages : a fatal result often occurring with extensive deposit only, which had never softened—the sick person being thus in the first stage of tubercle, but in the last of the disease. Let it at once be stated that the degree of disease in the lung and the condition of the patient cannot be expressed by the same formula. Physical signs can never be the measure of the danger, any more than symptoms alone ; both must be studied together. It was first necessary to ascertain the average duration of the disease—all stages and varieties being put together. Here we found great difference of opinions, of which the following is an abstract : Portal says it may last from 1 to 40 years ; Louis and Bayle in 314 cases found the mean to be 23 months—of these more than half (162) terminated in 9 months, and the greatest proportion between the third and ninth month ; the average duration was 18 months. Andral, at La Charité, found the average duration 2 years ; Sir James Clark, in the upper classes "enjoying advantages," 3 years; Dr. Williams, assuming the average duration to be two years, considers (in the last addition of his work) that it has been doubled, or raised to four years, by the introduction of cod-liver oil as a remedy.

Three years would be the medium of these opinions. The author inclined to place the duration at a much higher figure, and was satisfied that if cases were earlier recognized, they would be found to last much longer than now supposed. The method of invasion of the disease, and its progress, were next dwelt on. It was evident from the study of some thousand cases which have been under the author's care, that phthisis proceeds by a succession of attacks, and he doubts if even galloping consumption is ever present without a previous, but perhaps unnoticed attack—an opinion which has been expressed by Louis. The symptoms and physical signs of such an attack of tubercle were then described, the patient presenting with slight dullness of percussion, prolonged expiratory murmurs, roughness of respiration, and slight increase of vocal resonance—the symptoms being fever, more or less severe, of a remittent form, cough, and slight evacuation, with or without an hæmoptysis. From this there is partial recovery, but the patient ever after remains below his normal standard of health. Dr. Pollock has seen perfect recovery occur, though rarely, the physical signs being occasionally quite removed. Now, it is obvious that if the subsidence of the attack were overlooked in prognosis, we might deliver a false opinion as to the danger of our patient. A second invasion of disease invariably occurs at a shorter or longer interval. The circumstances which might be considered favorable as regards duration (or the disease becoming chronic) were then dwelt on. These are the softening being limited in extent; the fresh deposit occurring in the same lung lower down ; and a clear respiratory sound persisting at the base. The limitation of disease to one lung, whatever be its extent or stage, is more favorable for prolongation than if the affection be double, and the stage earlier.

Two varieties of very chronic phthisis were then described. One, a limited excavation, of well defined character, in one apex, the physical signs showing consolidation of the lung tissue below this, and the base being quite free from deposit ; the other consisting in a cessation of all activity on the stage of softening, and a coincident improvement in symptoms. The physical signs evidence a diffused deposit, shown by a crepitation of a dry character, with here and there a bubble, intervals existing in which the respiratory sound is bronchial and dry, and nothing to indicate a cavity in any part. The expectoration is moderate, the cough confined to certain hours of the day, the health tolerable, but on a low par; but there is considerable dyspnœa on exertion. Dr. Pollock has known such cases to last as long as fifteen or twenty years in persons who outlived middle age, and some interesting photographs were handed round, of young girls who had been for some years in this condition, who appeared in tolerable flesh, and were in good general health, the menstrual health becoming established, with improvement of all the symptoms. It would thus appear that there are two kind of tubercle, one prone to rapid softening, the other presenting inert features. Dr. Pollock also cited cases to prove that there occasionally exist cases of strumous deposit in the lungs in young persons, analogous in all respects to that in the cervical glands, and which become slowly absorbed in the same manner. The prognosis in children must therefore be most guarded.

The importance of examining *the whole chest* was then dwelt on in forming an opinion as to the probable duration of a case. The localization of the deposit is worth observing. Softening most frequently begins at the posterior part of the apex, and its signs, when not discoverable under the clavicle, may often be found above the spine of the scapula. In tubercle which assumes a chronic form of diffused deposit, it is not uncommon to find the following order : First, one apex ; next, the opposite apex ; third the base of the side last attacked. The most chronic is, however, often diagonal, as right apex left base, left apex right base successively. A curious result of some thousand observations may be thus stated : When the observed and customary order of physical signs is reversed, or in any important respect anomalous, the chances of prolonged life are greater. For, example, when the base is first attacked and the apex secondarily, the case will be a long one. One anomaly again generally implies several, as when softening began at the base, there was often absence of hæmoptysis or of hereditary taint, etc. In a word, the more each case approaches to the ordinary type of the disease, the more rapidly fatal is it sure to be. The conditions which are either antagonistic to tubercle, or which are rarely found in combination with it, were then noticed, and the rule deduced that where any of these are present the case tends to great prolongation. Tubercle seems to monopolise the system. Skin disease (excepting syphilis and the milder rashes, as acne simplex, urticaria, and herpes), external suppurating scrofulous abscess, cancer, gout, tumors, aneurism, and eminently emphysema of the lung are among these. Acute rheumatism after a deposit of tubercle is rare, but not unfrequently precedes it. Of all these combinations, that with emphysema tends to the greatest longevity. Persons with dark hair and eyes, although prone to phthisis, generally exhibit it in the chronic form. A freckled state of skin is rarely seen in the consumptive, and the influence of solar light as a counteractive agent was hinted at. Simple anæmia is rarely found in the first stages of the disease ; in the latter it occurs as a symptom of blood impoverishment. Of tubercular symptoms it may be remarked that an early profuse hæmoptysis is unfavorable. A single, late, profuse hæmoptysis is often accompanied by relief to the symptoms, and followed by a pause in the progress of the disease. Dry pleurisy (indicated by *frottement*) is theoretically an almost necessary occurrence to insure insulation of diseased parts, and is not unfavorable to prolongation of all favorable symptoms. A quiet pulse and the absence of fever are the most important. Hectic often occurs early before physical signs are present. Its recurrence in advanced cases is invariably associated with either an advance in the stage of existing disease or with a fresh deposit. The wasting of the tissues in consumption has its meaning in keeping the system at a balance with the respiratory power, and a uniform spare habit of body is the most favorable for chronicity. With this is often associated a most,valuable condition, which may be called nervous vitality, conferring on the system great powers·of endurance.

Dr. Pollock next exhibited a table of the particulars of about 190

16

cases of phthisis under his care which had already lasted upwards of four years, each case being noted and examined by himself :

Cases over four years :

Males..111
Females.. 82
Under 20.. 25
Under 30... 71
Under 40.. 60
Over 40... 36
First stage.. 60
Second stage... 56
Third stage... 71
One lung affected... 84
Both lungs affected... 97
Hæmoptysis..124
None 65
Have taken cod-liver oil...144
Have not taken cod-liver oil. 44
Diarrhœa 39
No diarrhœa..151
Larynx affected.. 21
Larynx not affected..170
Hereditary predisposition.. 69
No hereditary predisposition..113
Have taken cod-liver oil three months........................ 82 .
Have taken cod-liver oil six months............................ 87
Have taken cod-liver oil for years................................ 32
Degrees of waste :
   First (slight)... 97
   Second (decidedly thin)... 80
   Third (extreme).. 12
Hectic, marked by sweatings :
   Now 88
   Formerly 30
   Not.. 38

An analysis of the above tables is in favor of males.

Advanced age shows increased toleration of phthisis. An individual is not only less likely to contract consumption after thirty-five; but if he has it the disease inclines to the chronic form. The remarkable number of seventy-one are found with cavities, and the emaciation was not in proportion to the stage, for only twelve were in the extreme of wasting. One half had never spat blood, the ordinary proportion of all cases together being about sixty-three per cent. This illustrates the rule of anomalous occurrences referred to above. The absence of hereditary taint is very remarkable. The secondary affections, diarrhœa and disease of larynx, were exceedingly rare. The presence of hectic was also rare. Finally, the favorable conditions in phthisis may be thus summed up :

From Physical Signs.—1. Limited quiescent deposit in one lung. 2. Limited well-defined cavity in one lung. 3. The sounds denoting softening becoming dryer in a one-sided deposit. 4. The concurrence of emphysema of the lower parts of the lungs with tubercle in the upper. 5. Any unusual localization of physical signs.

From Symptoms.—1. The absence or rarity of fever. 2. The concurrence of skin diseases, external struma, gout, tumors, aneurism, fistula in ano. 3. The lymphatic temperament. 4. A spare habit of body without much variation in the weight.—*Medical Times and Gazette, Sept.* 17, 1859.

ii.—*Alcoholic Liquors in Tubercular Disease.*

Dr. John Bell, of New York, to whom was awarded the Fiske Prize (June 1, 1859), for his essay upon this subject, after much statistical research, arrives at the following conclusions :

1. The opinion so largely prevailing as to the effects of the use of alcoholic liquors, viz : that they have a marked influence in preventing the deposition of tubercle, is destitute of any solid foundation. 2. On the contrary, their use appears rather to predispose to tubercular deposition. 3. Where tubercle already exists alcohol has no obvious effect in modifying the usual course run by that substance. 4. Neither does it mitigate, in any considerable degree, the morbid effects of tubercle upon the system, in any stage of the disease.—*Am. Jour. Med. Science.*

iii.—*On the causes of the Independence of Bronchitis in relation to Pneumonia :* By M. ROBIN.

These M. Robin has never found stated by any author, and that arises, he believes, from the faulty notions which prevail as to the elementary structure of the organ of respiration. It is customary to represent the tissue of the lungs as a mere continuation or expansion of the bronchi, which is as incorrect as it would be to represent the uriniferous tubes of the kidney as a continuation of the urethra, bladder and ureter. As long as he believed in this doctrine, M. Robin never could comprehend why bronchitis should not constantly be passing into pneumonia. Nothing, however, can be more distinct than the pathological anatomy and symptoms of the two affections, which may be sometimes observed co-existing, but never passing from the one into the other.

The differences between the two diseases, marked as they are, must remain incomprehensible to those who consider the entire tube as lined with an uninterrupted mucous membrane from the larynx to the extreme subdivisions into *cul-de-sacs.* The real state of things is, however, as follows : Having passed through a certain number of subdivisions, the bronchi, now no more than one or two millimetres in diameter, lose their portions of the cartilaginous rings, and have no longer transverse muscular fibres, elastic longitudinal fibres, or a mucous membrane separable from the bronchial wall properly so called. They no longer possess a prismatic epithelium with vibratile cilia—losing, in fact, all the characters of bronchi. The pulmonary or respiratory canalicules, erroneously termed ultimate bronchial ramifications, continue to subdivide and terminate in rounded or ovid *cul-de-sacs* (improperly called bronchial or pulmonary cells), which at the period of birth are from five to eight hundredths of a millimetre large, and in the adult atiain the size of one or two tenths. These canals have not the structure of the bronchi, but are characteristic of the pulmonary parenchyma. They are surrounded by intimately interlaced bundles of elastic fibres, mingled with fibres of the laminated tissue, formed of fibro-plastic elements, and of vessels. These vessels form on the interior of the canalicules (which presents slightly projecting folds), a network differing from that of the bronchi. This network consists of large capillaries, which nearly touch each other, so as to leave intervals smaller than the capillaries themselves. It is distributed on the very tissue of the walls of the pulmonary canalicules (there being no mucous membrane separable from the elastic parenchyma), and is only separated from the cavity of these conduits by a layer of pavement epithelium with large nuclei, which commences where the cylindrical epithelium of the bronchi ceases. Thus the pulmonary canals, in which hæmatosis is accomplished, have a different structure to that of the bronchi which convey the air necessary for respiration. It is not possible to detach a mucous membrane distinct from the pulmonary parenchyma and the laminated tissue, in which, or on the surface of which, the capillary network is distributed, as is the case in the bronchi still provided with cartilages. In this way we may explain the rapid absorption which takes place in the lung, as compared with the slower absorbing power of the organs provided with mucous membranes—as also the easier rupture of these capillaries, with discharge of blood, or of substances injected by the air-passages. There is, in fact, as great a difference in texture between the bronchi and the pulmonary parenchyma, as between that of the excretory duct of a gland, and of the gland itself.

It will therefore be seen that affections seated in two portions of the apparatus so different, may well present great distinctions in their course, etc. But a still more important cause also explains the rarity of the extension of inflammation from the bronchi to the pulmonary tissue. Thus, in the case of bronchitis, the portion of the capillary system which is the seat of inflammation belongs to the general capillary system, properly so called, and receives its blood from the aortic or red-blood system; but in the case of pneumonia, the capillaries of the lesser circulation, deriving their supply from the black blood of the pulmonary artery, are in question. It is at the expense of this black blood that the morbid products of pneumonia are formed, as in hepatitis it is at the expense of the black blood of the vena porta that abscess of the liver is produced. We know, in fact, that although the pulmonary artery accompanies the bronchi throughout their entire extent, it gives no branch to them, nor to the interlobular partitions, and that it does not anastomose with the bronchial arteries. The latter entirely cease at the points where, or at a little beyond where, the small cartilaginous nuclei disappear from the bronchi, i. e. where the bronchial canalicules are only one millimetre, or a little more in diameter. This is the exact spot where the capillary distribution of the venous artery begins to take place between the contiguous walls of the pulmonary canalicules, forming on their sub-epithelial surface a net work of quite a special type of mesh-work, which is also found in the lesser circulation of all classes of vertebrate animals, even to the branchial plates of fishes. Beyond the bronchi, the bronchial arteries only furnish *vasa vasorum*, and branches to the interlobular laminated tissue, which extend as far as the pleura.

These circumstances supply not only an answer to the question proposed in this article, but also explain some of the differences which distinguish the nature and progress of inflammation of the lungs from that of other parenchymatous organs.   It explains also the differences of pneumonia, according to age, differences not exhibited so decidedly in the inflammations of any other organ, and which arise, not only because the parenchyma and the respiratory canalicules undergo notable modifications, but also because modifications in its nature and course are produced upon the inflammation by the nature of the circulation.   These are no where so decided as in the lesser circulation, which unites anatomically and physiologically the two sides of the heart, although its disturbances are often only caused indirectly, in consequence of lesions of the left side of the heart, instead of directly by changes on the right side.

Independently of the special type of distribution presented by the pulmonary capillaries, differing from that of the bronchial, their structure also differs in some points from that of the general capillaries. They are, in fact, amongst the largest of the body, and their parietes present smaller, more numerous, and more approximated nuclei than those of the other capillaries.   It is, however, to be observed that the capillaries of the portal system in the liver present the same peculiarities of structure.   These facts are not without their value when we call to mind that inflammation is a disturbance of the capillary circulation.—*Medical Times and Gazette, Oct.* 22, 1859.

ART. V.—*The African Station and Climate — Colonization—Guinea Worm—Vital Statistics.*

i.—George Clymer, M. D., Surgeon of the African Fleet, in a communication to the United States Medical Bureau, giving sundry notices, climatic, statistic and medical, concerning the African station in 1855–6–7 (published in the *Am. Jour. Med. Science*), says : " Freetown, the capital of Sierra Leone, contains a population of 16,000 negroes and 150 whites—the colony itself, 46,000."

A few extracts from Dr. Clymer's discriminating remarks upon the Republic of Liberia will be subjoined, possessing as they do, particularly at present, paramount interest for the Southern portion of the United States, including the Colonization Society.

" Monrovia (Lat. 6° 19′ N.), the capital of Liberia, is a missionary station, colonized by negroes from the United States.   It is planted on a promontory, called Cape Mesurado, washed on two sides by the Atlantic, and on the third by a creek, or inlet of the sea, called Mesurado River ; whilst interiorward stretches an interminable tract of impenetrable mangrove swamp.   This, at all times steaming with miasmata under a burning sun, becomes, in the rainy season, a vast morass, covered with mud and ooze from the overflowing of the St. Paul's River and Stockton's Creek, which wind their sluggish way through this flat and miry region in the neighborhood of the town. It is, in a higher degree than at any other period of the year, after the subsidence of the rains in the autumnal months, and at their commencement in the spring, when the soil is reeking under a torrid sun, and the atmosphere is stagnant, that it becomes loaded with paludal exhalations, which are a fruitful source of endemic sickness, and which but for the frequent tornadoes at those seasons, might render all this portion of the coast uninhabitable to any except the native.   The character of the diseases here, as elsewhere on the coast, is nearly uniform, consisting, as they do, of fevers of the intermittent or remittent type, and of diarrhœas and dysenteries, often causing by the frequency of their recurrence chronic disorders of the viscera, and, in particular, enlargement of the liver and spleen.   More than nine-tenths of the emigrants from the United States suffer from the endemic sickness.   This is miscalled the acclimating or seasoning fever, as an attack is an initiation rather than a prevention ; and the treatment to be effective, must be to anticipate and prevent the attack by *the* remedy, sulphate of quinia.   Whatever acclimation may consist in; whether, as the name implies, it is anything more than a habituation of the system to the climate—that is, to the temperature, the dryness, or moisture, the miasmata, and, indeed, to the condition of the atmosphere in all respects—an attack of fever does not here appear to confer protection or immunity, but rather to predispose to and invite a recurrence or repetition.   These attacks are apt to return at invals during the first two or three years of the emigrant's sojourn on the coast, and, in a measure, to disqualify him for much labor in the meantime.   To provide, in a degree, against this drawback to the well-being of the emigrant, the Colonization Society sent from the United States, last fall, two " receptacle houses," capable each of comfortably accommodating one hundred emigrants.   One of these has been put up at Monrovia, and the other at Cape Mount, forty-two miles northward on the coast.   Here the emigrants who desire it are received on their arrival, and are lodged and fed for six months; after which they are expected to provide for themselves.   Those who are then able to labor, and some who are not, repair to the interior, some twenty or more miles up the St. Paul's River, to cultivate the land, of which the Government gives to each adult five acres ; whilst the poor, the indolent and the sickly are apt, on coming out of the " receptacle," to loiter and lounge about the town, a tax upon its scanty resources and its charities.   A third " receptacle" sent from the United States, has this winter been put up some sixty or seventy miles from the coast, in an elevated and healthy locality.   To this, in consequence of sickliness of the coast, emigrants are to be transferred in boats up the St. Paul's River, immediately from the vessel in which they arrive, without putting foot on the coast.   This, it is hoped, will save the health of the emigrants, and enable them, with comparatively little interruption from sickness, to proceed to support themselves by the cultivation of the soil.

"I have said enough to convey my opinion that Liberia, with its enervating and sickly climate, was unfortunately selected as the locality on which to colonize the emigrant negro from the United States. It stretches some 400 miles through a low tract of variables and calms, which no trade breeze ever refreshes, and which is exceeded by no other, and equalled by few on the coast, in its oppressive heat, its sultriness, and its unhealthfulness, constituting it little better, in its effects on health, than an overheated, ill-ventilated swamp. These are essential drawbacks to its prosperity.

Dr. Clymer says that Liberia contains a population conjecturally estimated at 75,000 natives, and 10,000 emigrants from the United States, 1500 of which latter class constitute, with a few missionary families, the city of Monrovia.   *   *   *

"Leaving Cape Palmas on the day after our arrival, we passed the Ivory Coast, and, on the 16th of December, anchored at Elmina on the Gold Coast, at the distance of 387 miles, and in lat. 5° 5' N., and long. 1° 23' W. The southerly and south-westerly trades, which we struck after leaving Cape Palmas, sweep gently up the entire Gulf of Guinea, and confer upon the coast a climate in every respect more agreeable than that which we had just left. Elmina, the principal Dutch station on the coast, consisting of a native town of stone and mud, with thatched roofs, and containing ten thousand inhabitants, is remarkable for its conspicuous white castle—the largest on the coast, and built by the Portuguese, for the traffic in gold dust and palm oil—and in a hygienic point of view, for the two classes of disease there endemic, viz: dysentery and the Guinea worm. Whilst it was represented to me, by the surgeon of the castle, to enjoy a nearly total exemption from fever, so destructive to the health of the unacclimated on the coast of Liberia, the exhalations from a marshy creek at the edge of the town exposed it to annual autumnal visitations of dysentery, which, though especially fatal to the Dutch officers and other Europeans who led irregular lives, did not wholly spare the natives. The natives, of both sexes, and particularly the women, who appeared especially to abound in the shaded streets of Elmina, were a well-formed and well-developed race. But especially was I interested by the opportunity here presented of seeing specimens of those fortuitous and temporary inmates of the human body, peculiar to some warm climates, and which are popularly known by the name of Guinea worms. The surgeon of the castle, who had always many cases of it on hand, showed me samples of this filiform parasite (the *filaria medinensis* of nosologists) in various stages of its progress, from the earliest perceptible irritation beneath the skin in a single point, to fluctuation and approaching ulceration at that point, with a distinctly felt development of the worm in its waving or serpentine direction in the subcutaneous cellular tissue, and finally to its semi-extraction at the ulcerated point. Its length he stated to average eighteen inches, but to range from one foot to three. These worms he represented to exist sometimes singly, sometimes in succession, and sometimes numbers at a time in different stages of development in the same individual, and sometimes to appear a long time after leaving the coast of Guinea. Though they usually infest the lower extremities, I saw one, of eighteen inches, half extracted from the side of an individual who had two in the lower limbs. The extracted part looked and felt like a string of catgut ; whilst the other could be distinctly traced by the fingers, like a whip-cord, beneath the skin. The sinuous tract in which the worm was lodged was sensitive on pressure, particularly at its orifice ; and traction caused some degree of pain. On this account, as well as to avoid the risks of a rupture of the worm, the traction is not carried beyond a quarter, or at most, a half of an inch at a time, and is renewed daily, or twice a day, until its complete extraction. The protruded portion dangled at the side ; though it is usually recommended, as well to protect it from injury as to prevent retraction, to coil it around a quill of cotton, or other cylindrical substance, and to secure it near the aperture by adhesive plaster or other retentive means. The Guinea worm, as I was assured, requires two or three months to run its course, during which time the patient, though partially disabled, may walk freely about. Whilst it lasts, the soldier at the castle is relieved from duty. An attack secures no exemption for the future, but may be followed by a series of invasions. It has been observed that the officers, and others who are properly clad, are nearly, if not entirely exempt from Guinea worm, which attacks, in great numbers, the natives, whose limbs are exposed with little or no clothing, and who bathe in the stagnant waters near the town. May we not, then, refer the origin of these subcutaneous worms to the penetration (after the reputed manner of the pulex penetrans or Chigoe) of the animalcules, from the waters, in which they may be supposed to abound, through the skin into the cellular tissue, where, finding a nidus adapted to their nourishment and growth, they attain, at length, a development and activity which lead, through the irritation and inflammation which they create, to their expulsion from their human habitation as no longer to be tolerated inmates ? The opinion that they are due to the drinking of water charged with the entozoäl germs, which, traversing the absorbents and the route of the circulation, come to be deposited beneath the skin, there to find a home, and to receive their development, is destitute of the support of physiology and analogy ; though it does not want advocates, among whom is the surgeon of the castle at Elmina. The idea of their spontaneous generation will hardly be maintained in these latter days."

ii.—In an article on Liberia and the Colonization Society, by Mr. E. Ruffin, in *DeBow's Review*, for November, 1859, the writer quotes reliable documents, which show a steady decrease and deterioration of population in that colony :

"Mr. Cowan (who approves the colonization of the negroes and has recently written a book on Liberia) shows the decrease of population to be 3,551 more than all the births which have occurred since the first settlement. On *data* partly official, and all of which he deems reliable, he computes the total population of Liberia, of colonists and their descendents, in 1858, at 7,621, including all living children.

(p. 166.) The American Colonization Society had sent out in all, 9,872 up to January, 1858. This makes the actual decrease of these, 2,261, besides all the births in thirty-eight years. The Maryland Society acting separately at first, had sent out to Cape Palmas 1,300 —by both societies, 11,172. After thirty-eight years, of this number, *with their offspring*, 7,621 are living, the then total colonial population, leaving for deaths 3,551, exceeding births, which is thirty-three per cent. loss by death, and of absolute decrease in thirty-eight years." (p. 166.)

Mr. Ruffin concludes his series of papers with the following summary :

" In short, the colony has been throughout, and the 'independent republic' of Liberia continues to be, a worthless and hopeless pauper community, subsisting, to a great extent, on the alms and care of the misdirected charity of benevolent and deluded contributors in the United States—and without which aid and support being continued, Liberia, as an independent and civilized community, will soon cease to exist, after its long-continued maintenance has already cost the government and the people of the United States many millions of dollars ; of all which expense, much the larger proportion, and especially of the individual and special donations and contributions, has been borne by the people of the slaveholding States, to whose great interests the designs and operations of the Colonization Society have already been greatly injurious, and are tending to produce much more of injury and danger."

Whatever may be the ethical opinions of the reader concerning negro slavery in the United States, there cannot be, for the physiologist and vital statistician, a more luminous, but as yet unexplained fact, than that of the extraordinary vital progression, increase and longevity of the black race as witnessed in the Southern States of this republic, while, everywhere beyond the limits of the latter, that race, especially the free portion of it, is either steadily declining or remains stationary. It is astonishing that vital statisticians ignore instead of making this a point of departure for their investigations. Every hundred thousand slaves originally imported had, long ago, increased to more than a million, and now the original two or three hundred thousand have increased so as as to be very nearly equal in number to that of the pure blooded negroes of the whole western coast of Africa, the land of their ancestors for thousands of years.

ART. VI.—*Official Report of the Last Illness of His Majesty King Oscar the First, of Sweden, and of the Post-Mortem Examination of the Body;* translated from the original, by WILLIAM DANIEL MOORE, M: B , of Trinity College, Dublin ; Honorary Member of the Swedish and Norwegian Medical Societies.

THE examination of the body of the late King of Sweden took place, by command of his present Majesty, Charles the Fifteenth, at the Palace of Stockholm, on the 12th day of July, 1859, at 10 o'clock in the forenoon.   A large number of the great Officers of State, and of members of the medical profession, having assembled in accordance with summonses issued by His Excellency Count Lewenhaupt, Marshal of the Kingdom, and the latter high functionary having given permission for the commencement of the business of the day, P. O. Lilje-walch, First Physician in Ordinary, read the following:

Report of the Last Illness of His late Majesty King Oscar the First.— The late King was, with the exception of the chest, not strongly built; nevertheless, during the greater part of his life, he enjoyed tolerably good health.   Having, as a youth, passed through a severe typhus fever, he was, in full manhood, attacked by rheumatic fever ; both diseases, however, went through their ordinary course without leaving behind them any injurious consequences.   His Majesty was therefore able, on ascending the throne, to devote himself, with indefatigable industry and undisturbed health, to the functions of his high calling, and this he did with a zeal indicative of the keenest sense of duty. In the commencement of each spring, however, a troublesome irregularity in the heart's action not unfrequently occurred.   Still the morbid symptom was generally not of long duration, but yielded in a short time to gentle measures; and as His Majesty almost every year during the milder season made excursions to remote parts of the country, or to the Kingdom of Norway, and most frequently did not return to the capital till late in the autumn, his system regained, through country air and the increased exercise attendant on his excursions, what it lost during the winter by hard work, often continued to a late hour of the night, combined with a more sedentary life.   But in the course of the year 1851, his health became seriously implicated; the heart's action was constantly irregular, digestion was impaired, and the liver increased in size.   The most important central organ of the nervous system, too, showed unmistakable traces of exhaustion, and absolutely required rest.   In consequence of this, His Majesty repaired, in the summer of 1852, to the baths of Kissingen, and at the end of his stay at that watering place made a tour in Switzerland, returning to Sweden in the autumn, cured of his liver complaint, and with his health in other respects also improved.   But now his paternal heart was smitten with the sad loss of a beloved son, and in a short time the Royal parent lay on the sick bed, suffering from the same disease which had opened the grave for his bitterly lamented child.   A particularly tedious typhoid fever now for many weeks threatened His Majesty's life, but finally terminated in convalescence, which, although slow, gave hopes of a future complete restoration to health.   These expectations were, to a certain extent, fulfilled, and would, no doubt, have been completely so, had not the political circumstances of the time laid too strong a claim upon His Majesty's exertions, and determined him to neglect the care of his own person in order to devote himself wholly to the protection of the interests of the two nations, whose welfare constitued the highest object oi his sense of duty. The over-exertion of the mind to which His Majesty consequently subjected himself, the omission or curtailment of his summer tours, and the neglect of a necessary visit to the baths, at last told upon him, and in the beginning of 1857 his health again began to give way in a manner calculated to cause great uneasiness, with evident congestion of blood to the head. The lower extremities, the muscles of which were always weak, began to totter under the weight of the body, and at the same time that the power of combination for the motions of these parts was impaired. His Majesty was troubled with vertigo, particularly accompanying the movements of the head, and with vomiting, which symptoms, in combination with dimunition of strength and the occurrence of involuntary muscular spasms, indicated the existence of a more deeply seated affection, probably a softening in the central nervous system. Incapacity to discharge his Royal functions now brought on a deep melancholy, and His Majesty even in the commencement of his illness expressed his conviction of its incurability. Although this conviction could not, unfortunately, but be participated in by those who were privileged to be His Majesty's Physicians, we did not at that time consider it our duty publicly to express it. The means employed to combat the disease were, moreover, without any essential efficacy ; the paralysis, which commenced in the lower extremities, gradually increased, and after the King, feeling his inability any longer to fill the high position to which Providence had called him, transferred into the hands of his then Royal Highness the Crown Prince, the Government of the United Kingdom, his deep melancholy gave way to a progressive indifference, even for those things which in his health he had regarded with the most lively interest. The disease henceforward progressed slowly towards its end, and the paralysis began so steadily to extend to the other voluntary muscles, that towards the end of last June both lower and upper extremities, and the sphincters of the excretory passages were almost entirely paralyzed, while involuntary spasms from time to time agitated the right leg. The appetite, too, had now disappeared, and, although digestion continued undisturbed, the body had greatly emaciated, while the hitherto superficial bed sores, which had often been nearly healed, and had already existed more than six months without causing any great pain, began to extend and to assume a gangrenous appearance. Under all this the patient's strength gradually sank; the power of speech, previously very limited, latterly was altogether lost ; the lungs filled with mucus, which, in consequence of incipient paralysis of the muscles of respiration, could only with increased difficulty be expectorated ; and on the 8th of July, at eight o'clock in the morning, His Majesty quietly expired, supported in the arms of his Royal consort, who during his more than two years' illness never left his side, and surrounded by all the other members of the

Royal Family, kneeling with her and weeping bitterly around the death bed of the never-to-be-forgotten and long tried head of their illustrious house.

The first trace of the nervous disease, the development of which I have now described, and which brought the late King to the grave, manifested itself long since, although it was not until within the last six or eight years of His Majesty's life, that, as we have seen, it occurred with more definite, and at last with such threatening symptoms. No one who had the good fortune to approach His Majesty's person, and who had an opportunity of observing him during a long period in his daily intercourse, could avoid being amazed at the very extraordinary power His Majesty always exhibited of retaining in his memory the most varied details, or could cease admiring the rapid apprehension, the unerring judgment, and the singular clearness of statement which were exhibited whenever he spoke. But at the same time he would not fail to recollect how His Majesty sometimes in the middle of a conversation to which he was directing all his attention, would of a sudden appear to be abstracted, and would really transfer his thoughts to some other subject on which, unless he might be disturbed, he would allow them to rest, usually only for a few moments, but sometimes for many minutes; after which the conversation would be resumed, as if it had not been interrupted. The peculiar expression of His Majesty's features, particularly his look assumed on such occasions, and the spasmodic state, or the involuntary movements which at the same time took place in one or other part of the muscular system, render it probable that this distraction, which at times was of frequent recurrence, was due to an incipient affection of the central organ of thought. This symptom, referable to the most important organ of the nervous system, was of late years accompanied, as has already been mentioned, with increasing weakness in the muscles of the lower extremities, and with uncertainty in the combination of movement, probably depending on a commencing organic change, either in the organ alone, on which the power of motion depends, or also in that by which the harmonization of movements is effected. The anatomical investigation which is now about to be made will show, whether any discoverable change of structure exists in the central parts of the nervous system, or whether the disturbance of function has taken place, without the naked eye being able to detect the seat or nature of the change, which must be supposed to be present, when the function of the organ is deranged. This examination ought also to demonstrate what morbid change has taken place in the structure of the heart, as a cause of the irregular movements to which this organ was occasionally subject.

Before I close this brief report of the late King's last illness, I ought to observe that Professors Huss and Malmsten took part in the treatment from the commencement of the disease, and that Professors Conradi and Heiberg were called into consultation from the Kingdom of Norway, as Professor Faye, the Norwegian Physician in Ordinary of his late Majesty, was at the time on an extended foreign tour. It should likewise be mentioned, that the treatment of His Majesty's disease was, during two months of last year, intrusted to Dr. Kuylenstjerna, to ascertain whether animal magnetism [!!] might not have some beneficial influence, after the attendant Physicians had stated that the restoration of His Majesty's health lay beyond the power of art.   P. O. LILJEWACH,

First Physician in Ordinary to his late Majesty King Oscar.
STOCKHOLM, July 12, 1859.

As a preparatory step, the Royal remains were, with a view to prevent decomposition, on the 9th of July, at 1 o'clock in the afternoon, injected with an arsenical solution. The following observations were on that occasion made as to the *external appearance of the body*. The Royal corpse, which was at once recognised by all present, and the features of which presented a tranquil expression, was found laid on a table in the late King's bed-chamber. Cadaveric rigidity existed only in the joints of the right knee and foot, and in the under jaw. The whole body was greatly emaciated. The tuberosities of the long bones and ribs, and the spinous processes of the vertebral column were prominent. Over the entire back and the upper part of the posterior surface of the thigh were slightly livid spots. On the left side of the nose, about an inch and a half from its point, and close to its dorsum, was a small abrasion, said to have occurred after death in the removal of a cast of the face. On the front of the legs (*anti-crura*), but chiefly on the left limb, were found some light brown spots, varying from the size of a pin's head to that of a pea. These spots were in some places distinct, in others they were confluent, and were not raised above the surface of the skin. On the right side, over the lower edge of the sacrum, towards the anus, was an oval dark brown spot, an inch in length, and above it and continuous with it was a yellowish, somewhat larger, semilunar, similar spot, both together forming the mark of an imperfectly-healed bed-sore. On the left side, in a spot corresponding to that just described, was a bed-sore three inches in length by two in breadth, on which the slough still remained. Over the right os ilium, about at its junction with the sacrum, was a superficial abrasion, three-quarters of an inch in length, and on the spinous processes of the seven inferior vertebræ (lumbar and dorsal), were similar, but still smaller abrasions.

After the foregoing inspection, the left carotid artery was opened, and into it was injected, towards the heart, about a pound and a-quarter of finely elutriated arsenic, four pounds of distilled water, and five pounds of rectified spirit of turpentine, impregnated with essential oils. The incision made in the skin was then united, and the Royal corpse was replaced in bed.   In fidem protocolli,

DR. A. HILARION WISTRAND.

The foregoing having been read, the post-mortem examination was made on July 12, by Professor Baron von Düben, assisted by Professor Santesson and Prosector Lovén. With respect to external appearances, the following additional observation was made: The Royal corpse has not during the last few days undergone any other change than the formation on the anterior surface of the right shoulder of some reticulated, grayish brown spots (*vibices*). The slough on the bed-sore already referred to, on the left side over the sacrum, is found on incision to extend in the centre to the depth of one and a-half lines, and

at the edges to the depth of one line; while the cutis vera, as well as
the subjacent adipose tissue is, to a certain extent, infiltrated with
blood.

Inspection of the Internal Parts—Head.—The scalp is pale and deficient in blood. The cranium is thin, with very little, almost no
medullary substance; its inner layer exhibits deep impressions left by
the vessels and *glandulæ Pacchioni*, rendering the skull in some places
very transparent. Small, fine osseous granulations are found in the
course of the vessels on the inside of the cranium (*osteophytes*). The
dura mater is strongly adherent to the inside of the skull; it is everywhere thickened, particularly towards the falx cerebri, and is adherent to the arachnoid and pia mater in the course of the longitudinal
sinus. After the separation of the dura mater, the cerebral mass
swells out and exhibits the arachnoid and pia mater tolerably full of
blood and healthy, with the exception of a somewhat thicker edge along
the longitudinal sulcus, whence on both sides proceed numerous Pac-
chionian granulations. The convolutions of the cerebrum are flattened, so that the sulci between them are almost wholly effaced. The
color of the cerebral mass on the surface is pale grey with a slight
tinge of red. On pressure over the lateral ventricles, evident fluctuation is felt. On section the cerebral mass appears of a greyish
white color, and is tolerably copiously studded with sanguinous dots.
The lateral ventricles together contain rather less than three ounces
of somewhat turbid serum; they are considerably dilated, particularly
the posterior cornua. Their inner investment, with two or three lines
of the adjoining cerebral mass, is softened and pale, resembling coagulated milk (*emollitio alba*). In the posterior hemispheres of the cerebrum this white softening extends on the right side nearly an inch,
on the left side nearly an inch-and-a-half, reckoning from the walls of
the ventricles; forming foci of *ramollissement* on the right side of the
size of a small walnut, and on the left of that of a hen's egg. The
septum lucidum is also for the most part softened. The corpus callosum is likewise softened. The choroid plexuses are pale and compressed. The other parts of the cerebrum exhibit no morbid change;
the blood-vessels are healthy and open.

On taking out the cerebellum its right half is found, for the extent
of more than an inch, attached to the dura mater by means of old,
firm adhesions; in this part the mass of the organ is of a reddish-
brown color, and is somewhat swollen, containing a tumor of the
size of a small hen's egg, which is easily distinguishable from the rest
of the cerebellar mass, and on section is seen to contain a round
cavity, half-an-inch in diameter, imperfectly filled with a shrivelled
pale yellow, broken down, fibrinous coagulum; the cavity is surrounded by a fully organized sac of connective tissue. Around this
the cerebellar mass is found, to the extent of fully half-an-inch, softened, infiltrated with blood; and on microscopic examination appears
broken up and mixed with coloring matter, granular cells and corpuscles. The rest of the substance of the cerebellum is healthy.

The pons Varolii and the medulla oblongata exhibit no morbid
change. The inner lamina of the skull is also, at the base, rough
with small osseous granulations. In the right receptaculum cerebelli,

where the adhesion already mentioned existed, the dura mater is easily separable from the bone, which underneath it is found to be rather cribriform and corroded. In the foramen magnum, the odontoid process of the second cervical vertebra is felt to be very prominent.

Chest.—The integuments of the thorax contain a layer of fat about half-an-inch thick. All the cartilages of the ribs, especially of the superior, are ossified. The thoracic viscera retain their normal relative situations. Each pleural sac contains about four ounces of dark red serum. Both lungs are free, distended with air, full and rich in pigment. In the apex of the left lung is a small cicatrix, slightly drawn under the surface. In other respects the lungs are perfectly sound. The pericardium is rather abundantly covered with fat, and contains a couple of spoonfuls of dark red serum. The right side of the heart is also somewhat loaded with fat, and its walls are thin and have undergone some fatty change. The valves and orifices of the right side are healthy; the papillary muscles are particularly small. The left ventricle is somewhat dilated; its walls are of rather less than ordinary thickness; the trabeculæ and papillary muscles are thin and flat, the latter at their apices are changed into connective tissue. By this tissue the efferent tendons are partly united to one another. The mitral valves are somewhat attenuated and short, but are otherwise healthy. The semilunar valves of the aörta have undergone morbid change, the right valve being along the whole of its free margin thickened, and as it were doubled, by an excrescence one line in height, comb-like, filamentous at top, and running along the inner surface of the valve. Farthest to the right is a conical calcareous excrescence, adherent at the base, the base of which extends somewhat into the ventricle. The two other semilunar valves are joined to one another, the septum between them having almost disappeared. These valves are, moreover, considerably thickened, contracted, and somewhat convoluted. The free valve is $1\frac{3}{4}$; those which have grown together are exactly two inches in breadth. The greatest width of the left ventricle is eight inches. The aörta immediately above the valves is $4\frac{1}{2}$ inches in circumference. The walls of the auricles are particularly thin.

• *Cavity of the Abdomen.*—In the abdominal integuments is a considerable layer of fat, one inch in thickness. The peritoneum is healthy, but on each side is an external inguinal rupture, capable of admitting three fingers laid together. The omentum, one-sixth of an inch in thickness, covers the abdominal viscera, which occupy their normal, positions, and do not exhibit any morbid adhesions. The stomach almost empty, is rather thick anteriorly towards the pylorus; the mucous membrane in that part is slightly hypertrophied; the coats of the stomach are otherwise everywhere sound. The intestinal canal contains in its upper part thinner, in the lower part more solid mucus and brownish-green excrementitious matters; the small intestines are healthy; on their mucous membrane at the iliocæcal valve, and about three inches upwards, the mouths of the glands are open, and the membrane itself is there particularly thin and clammy. The large intestine is throughout healthy. The mesentery is rigid, with a layer of fat three-quarters of an inch thick. The pancreas is healthy. The liver is very small, especially its left lobe; its substance is close and hard, but without any trace of cicatrix or cirrhotic change. The liver is 8 inches broad, 7 high, and 3½ thick. The gall bladder contains about a tablespoonful of dark brown grumous bile. The spleen is somewhat turgid, but exhibits no morbid change. The kidneys are imbedded in a layer of fat a couple of inches in thickness, which extends into their pelves; their substance is healthy. The ureters are open and healthy. The renal capsules are also healthy. The urinary bladder contains a couple of tablespoonfuls of turbid urine; its walls and mucous membrane are healthy; the third lobe of the prostate gland is somewhat enlarged.

Cavity of the Spinal Column.—The medulla spinalis is surrounded by a great quantity of fat, its membranes and substance are healthy. Nothing else worthy of note was observed.   Visum, repertum,
Stockholm, July 12, 1859.   GUST. VON DUBEN.

The pathological changes above described, compared with the symptoms detailed in the history of the case and in the published bulletins, lead to the following conclusions as to the connection between them: 1. The irregularity of the heart's action, which for many years was sometimes more, sometimes less troublesome, depended on the existence and growth of the morbid products found in the aortic valves, which, arising in the course of the rheumatic fever mentioned in the report, subsequently continued and increased, causing attenuation of the wall of the left ventricle and dilatation of its cavity. These morbid products, although discoverable by means of the stethoscope, were by the efforts of nature in time smoothed and modified, so that the heart was able to discharge its functions, although less regularly and perfectly. 2. The distraction of mind described in the report, which was observed for many years back and was connected with more serious symptoms, subsequently developed signs of congestion of the head and diminution of strength, finds its explanation in the morbid changes of the dura mater, which, in consequence of an insidious chronic inflammation, extending likewise to the inner table of the skull, was both thickened to an unusual degree, and became adherent on the one side to the skull, and on the other to the arachnoid and pia mater, and through them to the outer surface of the superior convolutions of the brain. 3. The extravasation of blood found in the right half of the cerebellum, which, from its character, as above described, and its effects on the subjacent bone, appears to have been of long standing, probably took place at the same time, or the commencement of the year 1857, betraying its origin by the increase of the before-mentioned cerebral symptoms, and by the supervention of vertigo and vomiting, and manifesting its continued influence in the derangement observed in the muscular movements, particularly of the lower extremities, and in the want of control over these movements. 4. Soon after the softening, found on dissection, began to be developed in the cerebrum, the posterior lobes, the walls of lateral ventricles, the septum and corpus callosum, with consequent effusion into the ventricles and dilatation of the latter, which change was characterised in its commencement by the increasing morbid apathy, and afterwards by the progressive paralysis of the voluntary muscles, and finally of the excretory passages and the muscles of speech and respiration. 5. Lastly, it may probably be inferred that, as no other sign of inflammation was found in the body, the recent inflammatory process, of which the results were observed around the old clot of blood in the right lobe of the cerebellum, was the cause of the feverish symptoms which occurred during the closing period of his Majesty's illness, and which were mentioned in the published bulletins. Consequently these feverish indications and the post-mortem appearances left by the inflammatory process, on which they depended, are to be regarded as the latest symptomatic and anatomical phenomena in the present case.

Verified, ex-officio, GUST. VON DUBEN.
Dr. A. HILARION WISTRAND.
Medical Times and Gazette, Oct. 1, 1859.

REVIEWS.

REV. I.—*A System of Surgery ; Pathological, Diagnostic, Therapeutic, and Operative :* By SAMUEL D. GROSS, M. D., Professor of Surgery in the Jefferson Medical College of Philadelphia, etc., etc. 2 vols. 8vo., pp. 1162 and 1198. Blanchard & Lea: Philadelphia, 1859.

THE long-promised work by the distinguished Professor of Surgery in the Jefferson Medical College, has at length made its appearance, and two portly tomes of nearly twelve hundred pages each are thus added to the literature of surgery. We sincerely congratulate the author upon the termination of his task, which, however, has doubtless been to him a labor of love, and we think we have abundant cause to congratulate the profession upon so valuable an addition to their means of information. We can now point our foreign detractors to a work on this branch of medicine, at least, which will favorably compare with the boasted productions of their most eminent surgeons ; and it may not be amiss here also to remind our own teachers of surgery, that in future they can have no good excuse for ignoring the mention of a single home treatise on this subject in their annual lists of books recommended to students. Indeed, in reference to the former, we may go so far as to state that with the exception of South's translation of Chelius, and Townsend's translation of Velpeau (the latter exclusively a work on operative surgery and not therefore properly belonging to the same category as the former), the work of Professor Gross has no rival in the English language. Great Britain, notwithstanding her great wealth of professional talent, her numerous working societies, and her vast and well-appointed hospitals, has not, strange to say, ever produced a truly great work deserving to be called a " System of Surgery." We would not underrate the partial treatises of Cooper, Liston, Pirrie, Druitt, Paget, Miller, Skey, nor the most excellent text-book of Mr. Erichsen, all of which the profession of this country have shown their high estimate of in a way most flattering to their authors; but what we mean to say is, that no one of these, or others which we need not mention, can be considered a complete exposition of the science and art of surgery. The treatise of Professor Gross is not, therefore, a mere text-book for undergraduates, but a systematic record of more than thirty years' experience, reading and reflection by a man of observation, sound judgment and rare practical tact, and as such deserves to take rank with the renowned productions of a similar character by Vidal and Bozer, of France, or those of Chelius, Blasius and Langenbeck, of Germany. Hence we are disposed to admit the claim which the author sets up (see preface) of having embraced " the whole domain of surgery, allotting to every subject its legitimate claim to notice in the great family of external diseases and accidents," and do not hesitate to express the opinion that it will speedily take the same elevated position in regard to surgery that has been given by common consent to the masterly work of Pereira in Materia Medica, or of Todd and Bowman in Physiology.

To analyze such a book, as it should be done, would require more talent than has fallen to our lot to possess, and more space than the pages of our journal will permit ; but as most of our readers would probably be gratified to know the opinions of the author upon some of those points of doctrine and practice, which are not considered as positively settled, we have selected a few of the more important, and shall limit our notice to a brief statement of the mode in which they are discussed and the conclusions at which he has arrived.

And here, before entering upon our task of picking up curious stones from the vast quarry of massive truth that lies before us, we would commend the judgment of the author concerning the unity of medicine to those in the profession who have fallen in with the popular but derogatory notion that surgery is only a collection of rules for carving the human body with grace and skill.

" Surgery thus improved and perfected can no longer be separated from medicine ; any attempt to produce such a severance must prove abortive. They are, in point of fact, one and the same science, and therefore indivisible. No surgeon can practise his profession with credit to himself, or benefit to his fellow creatures, if he is not an enlightened physician, or deeply grounded in a knowledge of the great doctrines of disease. He may, it is true, be an excellent operator, a good mechanic ; but unless he is an able pathologist and therapeutist, he is unworthy to be intrusted with the health and life of the humblest citizen that may be so unfortunate as to fall into his hands."

The first four chapters of the work, covering nearly two hundred and fifty pages, are devoted to inflammation and its results; the latter including deposition of serum, fibrinous exudation, suppuration, hemorrhage, mortification, hospital gangrene, ulceration, granulation and cicatrization, to the elucidation of which the author brings all his large acquirements in pathology and pathological anatomy, and a mind long trained in logical deductions and skilled in practical application. Recognizing in this subject all the great principles of surgery, he endeavors to impress its paramount importance upon the student, and is evidently unwilling to proceed to the consideration of special diseases until it is thoroughly disposed of. All enlightened surgeons will so far accord to him abundant praise, however much they may differ with him upon certain points of doctrine as well as of practice. But let it not be supposed that he has attempted to settle dogmatically or even to clear up the numerous disputed questions which have vexed the minds of pathologists for so many centuries as to the nature of inflammation, the cause of excessive fibrinous development in the blood, etc., etc. He does no such thing, but upon many of these points, while suggesting explanations, he acknowledges his inability to speak with positiveness. Thus, in regard to the latter of the two questions mentioned, i. e., the cause of the increase of fibrin in the blood as an accompaniment or a result of inflammatory action, he gives as his opinion that "it takes place in the arteries, in consequence of the manner in which the blood is agitated in passing through the different parts of the body, its various ingredients being forcibly pressed and rubbed against each other, and against the sides of the vessels by the increased powers of the heart," producing a kind of disintegration of its own structure; but at the same time he admits that " it is still a mooted question which it will require further observation to solve." Did time and space permit, we ourselves would join issue with him here, and show, as we think has been done by others, that the excess of fibrin is due not to any change in the blood itself, but to a vital disintegration of the tissues through which the fluid passes, the former being consumed, as it were, more rapidly than in health, and thus yielding a corresponding amount of debris or ashes.

Upon the subject of the "Mode of Healing Wounds," our author discusses with marked ability the doctrines concerning the repair of solutions of continuity, and after passing in review the five methods described by modern writers on surgery, he concludes that there are really but two modes, as established long ago by Hunter. We give his own words:

"If what has now been said be correct, it follows, as a necessary corrollary, that there are only two modes in which wounds unite, long recognized by surgeons, easily comprehended, and in perfect harmony with the results of observation and experience. These two modes are, as was previously stated, adhesive inflammation, or union by the first intention, and repair by granulations, or union by the second intention; in other words, there is no form of union without inflammation and lymph; and the only difference in the two processes here mentioned is, that in the one the plastic matter serves as a direct bond of connection between the opposed surfaces, while in the other it is converted into a series of elaborately organized bodies which, by their coalescence, ultimately fill up the gap left by the retracted edges of the wound."

Upon the question concerning the extirpation of malignant tumors, embracing under this head scirrhus, encephaloid, colloid, melanosis and cancroid, Professor Gross holds the following conservative opinions:

"In regard to *extirpation*, all experience has proved that it cannot be relied upon as a means of permanent cure. The only benefit which it can confer is temporary relief for a few months, or, at most, for a year or two; and this is true no matter in how masterly and thorough a manner the operation may be executed. Hence, not a few surgeons of the present day have expressed themselves as averse to such a procedure, believing that it will only serve, in the great majority of instances, to hurry on the case to a fatal crisis. My own conviction is that interference with the knife is, as a general rule, only productive of harm, and that the patient will live quite as long without as with it, and, on the whole, in a state of greater comfort. Nevertheless there are cases, although it is difficult to define their character, where we occasionally see an operation followed by highly beneficial results, not only ameliorating pain, but apparently preventing an extension of the disease, and relieving the mind of that terrible feeling of anxiety which is so sure to attend the more severe forms of carcinoma. The cases which have done best in my own hands, after operation, were females with scirrhus breasts, which, after having been long in a quiescent state, at length assumed a threatening ulcerative tendency, or which had actually, in a slight degree, yielded to this process."

"Epithelial cancer is less liable to recur after extirpation than scirrhus, encephaloid, or melanosis. Removed in its earlier stages, there is occasionally a strong probability that there will be either no relapse at all, or only after a considerable period. One reason probably of this is the fact that the disease is more of a local character than the ordinary forms of carcinoma."

Turning to the chapter on "Syphilis," we find that the author recognizes but two primitive forms of chancre, the soft and indurated. Phagedena and gangrene he considers as accidental occurrences, and likely to manifest themselves in connection with either variety.

In the treatment of the non-indurated or soft variety, after the period for the employment of abortive measures is passed, he relies principally upon local means, conjoined however, with due attention to the state of the patient's system. The internal use of mercury in such cases, he considers not only uncalled for in the majority of instances, but often positively detrimental, and not by any means preventive of constitutional infection. In the indurated form, the true Hunterian chancre, he agrees with every other good surgeon in his high estimate of the value of this remedy. In the treatment of the secondary results he places most reliance upon tartar emetic given in small doses, say from one-eighth to one-sixth of a grain several times in the twenty-four hours. The tertiary form he treats with iodide of potassium conjoined with minute quantities of bi-chloride of mercury, where there is no constitutional contra-indication to the employment of the latter. In infantile syphilis, he bears testimony to the importance of mercurialization.

Although by no means averse to adopt new remedies and new modes of operating, Professor Gross exhibits a laudable disposition to withhold his sanction of such measures until they are fully tested either in his own hands or in those of competent and unbiassed judges. We are not surprised, therefore, that he should place a very low estimate upon the value of the ecraseur, which, notwithstanding the extravagant claims set up for it by Mons. Chassaignac and other equally enthusiastic Frenchmen, is, we are happy to say, rapidly falling into disuse, except for the removal of internal hemorrhoids, vascular tumors of the head and face, and the neck of the uterus. Indeed, it is a matter of astonishment to us that rational, humane men should ever have even contemplated the application of this barbarous instrument to the extirpation of the breast, amputation of the extremities, and such like capital operations.

In the treatment of burns and scalds the author still adheres to the use of white lead, as a local application. Having ourselves had frequent opportunity to witness its beneficial effects, we can bear testimony to its great value.

The diseases of the eye, although frequently omitted in works on general surgery, are here treated of with that fullness of detail which their importance deserves, more than a hundred pages being devoted to their consideration. In looking through this section of the work, we observe that Professor Gross prefers, in operating for cataract, laceration and depression to extraction of the lens. The following is his language upon this point :

"In regard to the relative merits of these operations, we are not in possession of any statistical facts which can aid us in deciding the question. My favorite method, as before intimated, has been for a long time the double operation of laceration and depression ; and such is my confidence in its superiority, that I shall continue to practise it until I have more substantial reasons than I now have for abandoning it. We have already seen that no one procedure is exclusively applicable to all cases, and there can be no question that each is capable of affording excellent results in the hands of a judicious surgeon. Destructive inflammation will occasionally follow, no matter how careful we are ; no honest man will pretend to uniform success ; every thing may go on well for a number of days, and the case may be in every respect most promising, when, all of a sudden, some unfavorable circumstance may arise, and the eye be irretrievably lost. Such a contingency should put us upon our guard, and render us cautious in respect to our prognosis. It is far better, after every operation for cataract, to promise too little than too much."

In bringing this imperfect and hasty notice to a close, we would take occasion to express our admiration of the style in which the work is published, and the liberality of the eminent publishers in consenting to the introduction of such an immense number of original engravings.

To our readers we would say—buy the book, read it, and reflect upon it.

REV. II.—*Review of a Contribution to, and the Editorship of, the New Orleans Medical and Surgical Journal.* By G. W. OUTLER, M. D.

EUTAW, LIMESTONE Co., TEXAS, October 27, 1859.

DR. DOWLER—*Dear Sir :* Your excellent Journal (The N. O. Medical and Surgical) is doubtlessly in the hands of many medical practitioners who take all its teachings as orthodox and good authority in their profession : and it *is* mainly scientific and reliable, but there does occasionally appear articles in its pages calculated to lead such into error, and to cause grave blunders in their practice ; and to counteract, to some extent, the evil they effect in this way, I suggest that you append a brief criticism to all such articles as you do not endorse, and point out what you conceive to be their errors. I do not make this suggestion in a spirit of dictation, nor do I wish to see the Journal a medium of petty controversy ; but the estimation with which I regard your talents and attainments, and the interest I feel for the cause of humanity and the science we pursue, induce me to ask you to add that much more to the already abundant and efficient labor bestowed on that most excellent periodical. I doubt not that all your readers would be pleased to have your views on the treatment of every published case, as well as the principle of every theory mooted in your pages. It is legitimately your province to criticise every thing you publish ; and I am almost sure no author would feel aggrieved by it, unless there should appear something personal in the criticism, manifesting a disposition to gratify some selfish spleen.

In every periodical I read I would be glad to have the views of the editor on every article he publishes, but especially in this, for the reasons already assigned. I could name quite a number of articles that have appeared in this Journal during the last ten years, which I think have had deleterious effects on the practice of many credulous individuals, who are accustomed to let others do their thinking, and always take as authority the last thing they may have read on any subject—articles, I am sure, which neither you nor your predecessor, the lamented Dr. A. Hester, ever would endorse, and which your protest would successfully forestall. But that which has more immediately prompted the writing of this letter, is the seventh article of the fifth number of Vol. XVI, published in the month of September, written by Dr. McPheeters, of Natchez, Mississippi, which gives the practice of Dr. McClintock, "accoucheur" in the Dublin Lying-in Hospital, and that position gives more weight to his testimony, more authority to his example, and will induce some the more readily to adopt his practice as a legitimate precedent, and therefore the more urgent is the call for criticism, as I think the doctor was too hasty in his interference with the *lex naturæ*.

His first case, it seems, was a natural labor ; head presenting, parts dilating well, uterine contractions good ; no malformation, nor any obstruction whatever ; yet in less than twelve hours from the first pain, the forceps were applied, which, after slipping off and being reäpplied, were laid aside without success, and the vectis tried, with the same result. Craniotomy was then resorted to, "with little re-luctance, as the fœtal heart could not *now* be heard." The italics in the quotation are my own ; and I think the word now, intimates that the fœtal heart had been heard before the use of instruments. What was there then to stop the beating of that heart, unless it was those same instruments that so bruised and mangled the head of the child in his fourth case that it was asphyxiated, and probably caused the sloughing of the vagina of the mother, as also the tenderness over hypogastrium, and the puerperal mania, which came so near landing her in eternity ? I think it more likely, however, that the beating of that heart had not then ceased, but that it was probably so enfeebled, by the officiousness of the "accoucheur" that he failed to detect it. I have frequently failed to recognize the sound of the fœtal heart, where it was afterwards proven to have existed by the birth of a living child; and I have seen more practical ears than mine fail similarly. It is a true old maxim that "meddlesome midwifery is bad midwifery." The most use there is for a physician with natural labor is, to prevent ignorant, sympathizing women from being too meddlesome.

Labor is divided by several good writers into three stages; the first including the passage of the head through the os uteri ; the second the birth of the child ; and the third the expulsion of the placenta. I believe that all the best authorities agree that tediousness in the first stage, according to this division, is attended with very little, if any, danger, to either mother or child. Churchill furnishes a table of cases, in which the labor lasted twenty-four hours and upwards, giving the length of the first and of the second stages, and the results to both mother and child; in which nearly five-sixths exceeded thirty, about one-third exceeded forty, and from that on up to one hundred and seventy-seven hours, in the first stage ; and even the second stage frequently exceeded the time of McClintock's first stage. The table contains one hundred and forty-three cases, every mother in which did well, and every child but ten, and one of them was born putrid, in none of which did the attendants think it necessary to resort to *any instrument*, much less "Smellie's scissors," or any other cranial perforator.

The only reason given for this resort to instruments by the Dublin accoucheur is, that the head of the child was "still high up at the superior straight" after the os uteri had been well dilated, the mem-branes ruptured, and the pains strong and frequent for *three* hours. I have frequently witnessed such a state of affairs as that for forty or fifty, and as high up as seventy hours, in cases that finally resulted favorably to both mother and child, simply by waiting on nature, without any artificial help whatever. I think such hasty proceedings as were had in the case under consideration rash, to say the least of them; and that they cannot be too strongly reprobated.

In his second case we are not told when labor commenced. But it was a foot presentation, and a first pregnancy ; and a short time after admittance a quantity of meconium passed, demonstrating the existence of uterine contractions, and progress ; and in one hour a foot protruded through the vulva, which could only just be felt through the membranes at first, which I think indicates as speedy progress, and as efficient pains as were desirable in a primipara of twenty-six years; but at the end of another hour, our hero thinking the contractions rather feeble for his ideas of double quick time, gives half a drachm of ergot, and in one hour more, being satisfied, as he tells us in his fourth case, that a child cannot live in utero two hours after the mother has taken that drug, his assistant (by his orders, I presume) lays violent hands on the feet of that little innocent, and with a hard struggle, as is evinced by pulling off the cuttle of its legs, and tearing open the perinæum of its mother, drags it into the world.

In foot presentations, the great danger is, that the progress of expulsion will be more rapid than the dilatation of the mother ; hence, the indication is more rational to impede than to accelerate that progress, if art *must* be invoked to some interference. Women who have lived twenty-six years without bearing children, very naturally require more time for that dilatation than the mother who has had several children, more than one who has just matured into full womanhood. Hence, I think, the administration of the ergot was unadvisable, and the tearing away the child fully as much so.

As to the child's having had scarlatina, *in utero,* when the mother had not had a symptom of it, as is supposed in a kind of resumé at the close of the history of this case, I think it more likely that the violence used in the extraction caused that "scaling off of cuticle, etc." The mother may have had scarlatina after delivery, as stated, but a "red tongue and fauces" with a "rash on the body," are sometimes seen in puerperal fever, without any scarlatina ; and I cannot resist the conclusion that this woman, and her child, would both have fared better had she been entirely alone until her babe was born.

In the third case, I think it likely, that there was another living child's brains gouged out unnecessarily ; for we are told that they

19

only waited half an hour after the pulsations in the prolapsed portion of the funis ceased, and that there was neither hæmorrhage nor any other " occasion to hasten delivery." The circulation in the funis may, I am sure, be so much obstructed by pressure as to render the pulsations imperceptible for more than half an hour, and yet admit a sufficiency of the vital fluid to sustain fœtal life. Even if the presentation had sacrificed the life of the child, if it was impossible to change it so as to extricate the cord in time to prevent its perishing, there is no complication stated calculated to render evisceration essential to delivery; and I cannot see the necessity for such mutilation.

The other two cases described in the article in question were both primiparæ considerably advanced in age, in which ergot was used, and almost immediately afterwards the forceps ; the first of which was, perhaps, called for, as it is stated that the second stage had lasted sixteen hours ; but in the last case, the first stage had only reached fourteen hours, and there is, to my mind, nothing stated to justify instrumental interference.

Although I cannot endorse all the therapeutical treatment of these cases, I have not reviewed that, because I think it less reprehensible, and less likely to influence the practice of others than the operative, which I have censured.

I have no ambition to flourish in the periodicals of the day, nor any inclination, dear Doctor, to obtrude long articles on your pages; neither do I know anything, either personally, or from character, of the gentleman concerned in the article I have reviewed. The main object of this communication is the suggestion with which it begins, and the article in question is referred to as an illustration of the assertion with which I set out—that you send around occasionally articles that may, if not controverted, influence deleteriously the practice of some of the weak brothers of the medical fraternity.

One more suggestion, Doctor, in a few words, and I am done. Ever since I commenced the reading of physic, and first ascertained that I could not procure a complete standard pronouncing medical dictionary, I have felt the want of such a book to be a desideratum in medical literature, and have been surprised that none of the bookmakers in the profession have seen the necessity for such a work, nor undertaken to supply it. If it be answered that professional men should always be scholars and understand the idiom and orthoëpy of every language of which the technicalities of medical science are made up, I reply that it is *not* the case, if it should be; and that many of our most sensible, and consequently most reliable and skillful physicians, have but little oral teaching from such as are capable of pronouncing correctly all the terms used in our science. Indeed I believe there is no uniformity in the pronunciation of many of our terms among the best informed of the profession; and I think it very desirable there should be some standard of pronunciation by which all physicians who speak the English language, at least, might learn to call things by the same name, as well in spoken as in written language. To start this ball in motion is another task I wish to impose on you. I merely make the suggestion, and ask you to argue the case. Such a work would certainly pay well, if well done, for nearly all the physi- cians, and *every one* who expects to become such, would want the book. I would that every medical journal in the English language were in- duced to importune the scientific world until such a work be pro- duced.

The following critique is from E. McAllister, M. D.:

PORT GIBSON, MISS., Nov. 29th, 1859.

BENNET DOWLER, M. D.—*Dear Sir:* If Dr. McPheeters' exposition of treating lying-in women in the Dublin Hospital, as given in the September number of the *N. O. Med. and Surg. Jour.*, be correct, I am of opinion that I could not make a worse wish on them for this world, than to wish them to become patients in that department of that institution. What say you?

Very respectfully yours,

E. McALLISTER.

[The truth of the facts related and the justness of the opinions expressed by contributors are not necessarily vouched for by the editors of this journal, but must stand upon their own inherent merits and verity. Although an editorial *imprimatur* cannot be inferred from the mere acceptance of an article for publication, yet a journal whose first principle of action is to do no harm, and whose second is to do all possible good in its sphere, should not, when justice demands it, hesitate to sacrifice expediency or the biases of friendship to these fundamental principles. In many speculative and not a few practical matters, an agreement to differ is allowable and even praiseworthy in the absence of positive evidence on either side. Even speculative treason, though a crime, is not, without an overt act, indictable. It is the same in some speculations in obstetrics. If the obstetrician, should upon insufficient grounds, levy war with forceps and cranial perforators against the helpless child, thereby endangering the mother, the speculative gives place to the concrete, that is to say, steel, blood, and brains, and investigation into the good or evil of such procedure concerns the well being of society. A few months ago, Dr. Tyler Smith, of London, publicly advocated *"the abolition of craniotomy from Obstetric Practice,"* which, according to him, sacrifices annually 1,800 children, and from three to four hundred mothers in England and Wales—a proportion more than twice as great as among the French, and four times greater than in Germany. Against the total abolition of craniotomy valid objections may be urged, but none against its restriction and limitation to a few conditions, as deformity, monstrosity, difficult labor, with death of the child, etc. Sometimes, indeed, the accoucheur or midwife begins this operation, and before a particle of the brain can be extracted, the child is expelled by the natural powers, having a cranial wound from which it dies slowly and miserably.

Craniotomy is more frequent in rural than in city practice. In the former medical criticism and opinion have little influence to deter from the performance of an operation which the patient and her friends demand most urgently in some cases wherein there is not the least necessity for instrumental interference, the mother believing that her life is in immediate danger—an opinion in which her friends are apt to coïncide. Usually the operator instead of losing, gains reputation in the vicinity by craniotomies.

In regard to the cases reported by Dr. McPheeters, which have elicited several dissenting criticisms, it must be borne in mind that he relates what he says he observed; what he observed he is not re-sponsible for, not having had any control or power in the premises.

B. D.]

———

REV. III.—*Etudes Chimique sur l'Action Physiologique et Pathologique des Gaz injectés dans les tissus des animaux vivants :* Par C. LECONTE, Pro-fessor *Agrégé à la Faculté de Médecine de Paris,* et J. DEMARQUAY, *Chi-rurgien des hôpitaux. Archives Gén. de Méd.* Oct. et Nov. 1859.
Chemical Investigations into the Physiological and Pathological Action of Gases injected into the tissues of living Animals.

In the last number of the *New Orleans Medical and Surgical Journal* a slight notice was given of the extended, laborious and able researches of MM. Ch. Leconte and J. Demarquay, on the injection of gases into the tissues of living animals, which in part had already appeared in the October number of the *Archives Générales de Médecine,* and which have since been continued in the November issue of that journal.

MM. Leconte and Demarquay commenced a series of experiments illustrative of this problem, in September, 1856, which they continued until May, 1858. The gases with which they experimented by injections into the cellular tissue and the peritoneal cavity, were oxygen, carbonic acid, hydrogen, nitrogen, and also atmospheric air. These authors have studied the isolated, combined and mutual influences, actions and reactions of injected gases in the living economy. The animal which they selected for experimentation was the rabbit.

A description of their modes of operation, experiments, apparatus, analyses, conditions and tables, cannot be reproduced even in a condensed form in the remaining limits of this Journal. They cover nearly fifty pages of the *Archives Gén.* for October and November, and abound with the numerical tables, resembling books of arithmetic, being, like many good things, hard to learn and analyze thoroughly, especially during the holidays.

MM. Leconte and Demarquay give a historical sketch of the erroneous opinion which was universally prevalent in former times, concerning the deleterious effects of atmospheric air upon wounds in general, more particularly such as opened the serous cavities, whether accidentally or during surgical operations. Of this assumed noxious or deadly influence of the air, John Bell spoke doubtingly as early as 1812. Dr. John Davy, in 1824, made certain experimental investigations by injecting gases, but not with the view to ascertain the question of the danger or the innocuousness of air on wounds or in the cavities, but to determine their gaseous relation and composition, as modified in the economy. Sir A. Cooper and others subsequently proved that air injected into the tissues produced no ill effects ; although, when injected in a considerable quantity directly into the blood vessels, it constantly and quickly proved fatal, owing to the mechanical obstacle which it interposes to the circulation.

As already stated, it is intended on this occasion neither to specify the individual experiments with air, oxygen, hydrogen, carbonic acid and their mixtures which were injected into the cellular tissue and serous cavities in animals during fasting and repletion and in varied temperatures, nor to detail the chemical analysis made, it may be proper and altogether sufficient for practical ends to give the general conclusions which have been drawn from the whole experimental series.

1. That air, nitrogen, oxygen, carbonic acid and hydrogen, produce no injurious effects when introduced into the subcutaneous cellular tissue or into the peritoneal or serous cavities.

2. That these gases are resorbed after a period more or less prolonged, and with a rapidity which varies from forty-five minutes (for carbonic acid gas), to several weeks (for nitrogen), the rapidity being always in the order following respectively, namely: carbonic acid, oxygen, hydrogen, air, nitrogen.

3. That any gas whatsoever injected either into the cellular tissue or peritoneum constantly determines or leads to an exhalation of such gas so contained in the tissues and blood.

4. That there is readily produced after the injection of these gases, a mixture in which that gas which is least resorbable is held in check being the last to undergo resorption, and does not, until after having been mixed in certain proportions with these gases, begin to be exhaled with them.

5. That in general, the exhalation of these gases from the blood or from the tissues, in these experiments has been more abundant during digestion than fasting, and more active in the peritoneal cavity than in the cellular tissue.

6. That the rapidity of absorption does not appear to be modified either by fasting or by the process of digestion.

7. That of all the gases thus injected, hydrogen is that which is exhaled the most actively from the gases of the blood, until the hydrogen previously mixed has disappeared, and although the volume of that part of the animal where the injection is made, remains unaltered, so that one might think no absorption of this gas had occurred, if no chemical analysis be made proving the contrary.

8. The rapidity of the absorption of the gases by the blood is not always in the ratio with their solubility in water (as nitrogen and hydrogen).

9. That from the injection of air into the cellular tissue and peritoneal cavity, a constant absorption of oxygen from it and an exhalation of carbonic acid take place, so that these phenomena relatively approximate what occurs in pulmonary respiration, yet these two facts should not be considered indentical with it, for in the case of injections, the ratios or relations between the carbonic acid exhaled and the oxygen absorbed, vary perpetually.

10. The rapidity of absorption and exhalation of these gases injected from without into tissues of living animals is in proportion as the compound is soluble in the blood and in a ratio to the quantity of atmosphéric air introduced with these gases.

11. The exhalation of these gases from the blood thus mixed with the injected gases, is in a ratio with the solubility of the compound in the gases of the blood and existing quanity of atmospheric air in this gaseous mixture.

This experimental memoir, though important as a contribution to physiological chemistry, has not been applied by these authors to therapeutics, with the exception of wounds, in which they seem to show that the gases mentioned above including the atmospheric air in the tissues and great cavities, are not necessarily dangerous. If this fundamental postulate be true—if these gases do no harm—a point of departure is thereby fixed, from which experimenters may hope to find from these gases, in certain morbid states of the economy, positively medicinal virtues to a much greater extent than has hitherto been supposed, not only by the means which they have adopted, but by inhalation and by injections into the natural openings, as the rectal, vaginal, uterine and vesical, the indications for which may possibly be securely founded, in part, at least, upon physiological and pathological chemistry. The unsystematic, fragmentary experience already extant, is sufficient to afford many valuable practical suggestions, as well as to stimulate farther investigations.

How little soever the respiration of pure oxygen may be adapted to the normal condition of the economy, an artificial addition of that gas to the air inspired, might, upon theoretical grounds be supposed beneficial in its action in conceivable conditions of disease attended with a low oxidating power or partial paralysis of the pulmonary organs and functions. Prof. Lehmann in his Physiological Chemistry says: "The latest experiments of Regnault and Reiset, on dogs and rabbits, show that the respiration of air which is richer in oxygen than the atmosphere, does not produce effects differing from those yielded under the normal relations; the animals did not exhibit any distress from the inhalation of air containing two or three times more oxygen than our atmosphere, and the products of respiration were precisely the same as when the animals had breathed the atmospheric air. It is therefore the more striking, that the earlier experimenters on respiration in pure oxygen should have led to tolerably decisive results; among these we must include the observations of Lavoisier and Seguin, as well as those of Allen and Pepys on man, and those of Marchand on frogs. According to these observers, the excretion of carbonic acid was only slightly or not at all increased by breathing in pure oxygen, although *far more oxygen was absorbed than under ordinary conditions.* According to Marchand, for instance, there remained more oxygen in the blood (which was not expended in the formation of carbonic acid) than in the respiration of ordinary air. The experiments of Allen and Pepys, exhibit, moreover, no inconsiderable exhalation of nitrogen. Sir Humphrey Davy's experiments (according to which most of the vital functions are performed with augmented energy after the prolonged inhalation of oxygen) are worthy of being carefully repeated with such improved means as Lespasse has lately employed in his observations." (ii, 440.)

The innocuity (this word if not English, should be,) of carbonic acid gas injected into the tissues and cavities, as also when taken into the stomach in sparkling wines, soda waters, soda powders, effervescent draughts, many mineral springs, etc., while at the same time this gas, even when mixed with a considerable per centage of air, causes immediate death when inhaled in respiration, presents a curious problem, which *à priori* reasoning could not have solved independently of experience. In clinical practice the development of carbonic acid in the stomach (as by a simple soda powder, etc) is not only innocuous but medicinal in many cases of gastric perturbation, nausea, vomiting, etc., being occasionally more efficacious than morphia, or perhaps any other article of the Materia Medica.

In view of the extraordinary known effects, both physiological and psychological, of nitrous oxide, upon being inhaled in suitable quantities, it might be reasonably supposed that its action in certain morbid conditions would be beneficial.

The inhalation of gaseous and vaporiform medicinal agents (to which the recent introduction of anæsthetics have given an impetus), warrants the expectation of therapeutic improvement by this method of medication.   B. Dowler.

Mortality Statistics of New Orleans, from October 2, to December 11, 1859, compiled from the Weekly Reports politely furnished by Dr. Baldwin, Secretary of the Board of Health. Population of New Orleans by the last census, 188,000.

Time.	Total Deaths.	Children under 2 yrs.	Under 20.	U. States
October (4 weeks)	611	194	261	304
November (4 weeks)	663	181	274	332
December (2 weeks)..	248	96	113	146

Principal Diseases.	October (4 weeks.)	November (4 weeks.)	December (2 weeks.)
Still born	35	38	16
Trismus Nascentium	26	18	11
Teething	15	23	5
Cholera Infantum	7	7	0
Infantile Convulsions	37	22	17
Infant. Marasmus	12	17	5
Croup	10	5	3
Diphtheria	13	2	0
Scarlatina	8	6	1
Rubeola	9	0	0
Variola	0	0	0
Tetanus	6	0	0
Diarrhœa and Dysentery	36	71	33
Gastro-Enteritis	5	4	3
Inflammation of Liver	5	6	4
Inflammation of Lungs	5	24	9
Phthisis	76	93	20
Apoplexy	4	8	3
Congestion of Brain	14	22	8
Fever, Typhoid	27	33	7
" Miasmatic	51	20	5
" Yellow	59	28	1

All the deaths from yellow fever reported by the Board of Health have occurred between September 27 and December 11. Total for the year 1859, 89.

S. E. C.

MONTHLY SUMMARY—METEOROLOGICAL REGISTER.—*From the Medical Purveying Office, U. S. Army, N. O.* New Orleans, La., Lat. 29 deg. 57 min. 30 sec. N.; Long. 90 deg. W. Altitude of Barometer above the level of the sea, 35 feet.

1859.	BAROMETER.			THERM. ATTACHED.			THERMOMETER.		
MONTHS.	Max.	Min'm.	Mean.	Max.	Min'm	Mean.	Max.	Min'm	Mean.
October ...	7 A. M. 30th. 30.450	2P. M. 27th. 29.880	30.178	2, P. M. 17th. 83	7 A. M. 30th. 52	71.93	2 P. M. 17th. 83	7 A. M. 30th. 50	70.74
November	7 A. M. 14th. 30.536	2 P. M. 17th 29.898	30.243	2. P. M. 28th. 78	7 A. M. 13th. 46	67.69	2 P. M. 28th. 79	7 A. M. 14th 44	65.67

1859.	HYGROMETER.			PREV'G WINDS.	WEATHER.		RAIN.	
MONTHS.	Max.	Min'm	Mean		Fair.	Cloudy.	Days.	Quantity.*
October ...	2&9 P.M 17th 80	7 P. M. 30th. 46	66.81	N.; N. E. & E.	23	8	3	2.17.
November	2 P. M. 28th. 74	7, A. M. 14th 41	63.97	N.E.; E. & S.E.	21.33	8 66	4	2.79.

* This is the smallest quantity for these months on this record, which was commenced in 1855.

White frost on the mornings of 13th and 14th November, the first this winter.

T. HARRISON, Clerk.

THE

NEW ORLEANS

MEDICAL AND SURGICAL JOURNAL. .

MARCH, 1860.

ORIGINAL COMMUNICATIONS.

ART. I.—*On Union by the First Intention and Purulent Absorption:*
By WARREN STONE, M. D., Professor of Surgery in the University
of Louisiana.

THE tendency of us all is to fall into a routine, and to adopt some
mode of practice, and apply it to all cases and conditions ; and hence
the opposite systems of practice, often seen, not only in different
countries, but in the same country and in the same city, and even in
the same hospital.   This is strikingly illustrated by the exclusive and
opposite methods of dressing wounds adopted by the American and
French surgeons.   The American surgeons dress with the view of
obtaining union by the first intention in all cases, whether it is probable it may be effected or not.   The French surgeons fill their wounds
with lint to prevent union, if there should be a disposition to it.   The
French, however, I believe, are not so exclusive in their mode of
dressing as the Americans, but both are undoubtedly wrong.   It is
undoubtedly true that our mode of dressing is far better adapted to
our country than to France, but it is evident that neither method is
adapted exclusively to either country.   The American surgeon dresses
all cases alike, whether there is a prospect of immediate union or not.

20

The wounded or divided parts are brought in close contact, regardless of the consequence of confining dead animal fluids upon surfaces not protected by the exudation of plastic lymph. The French surgeon, fearing purulent absorption, or the absorption of other impure animal matter, leaves the wound open, or fills it with charpie, to absorb any fluid that may accumulate, and to stimulate the surfaces. It is quite certain that, in the French hospitals, at least, adhesive inflammation does not take place so favorably as it does in ours, and I will not pretend to determine how far they are wrong in their exclusive method of dressing ; but, favorable as our country is, I am sure that we are as much in error in our exclusive method as they are in theirs. We have not attached sufficient importance to the danger of confining by dressings the effused fluids in the depths of wounds that do not take on healthy, adhesive inflammation. Even if absorption does not take place and affect the system generally, the local effect is bad, causing unhealthy action, and in some cases favoring gangrene. This is shown by the unhealthy inflammation that often follows contused and lacerated wounds, where the blood is diffused in the tissues and the air has sufficient access to it to favor decomposition.

Hunter, in his work on the blood, warns us against making an opening to discharge the blood that may be extravasated in the tissues after contused wounds, but without giving any other reason, except the fact that such opening is liable to be followed by an ill-conditioned inflammation. While blood is excluded from the air, it remains harmless, and plastic lymph will be exuded around it ; but if the air has access to it, decomposition may change it to poison, which will change the character of the inflammation entirely, and reduce the blood to the capacity of the absorbents, and it may be absorbed, and produce more or less constitutional disturbance. I am sure this takes place, under certain circumstances, from blood extravasated into the large serous cavities, for I have seen cases of death, with all the symptoms of animal poisoning, shown by the experiments of Magendie, when the consequent inflammation was very little. This should furnish a plain indication in the management of wounds of this kind ; and in the dressing of wounds generally, we should be cautious in confining the animal juices or effusions.

When union by the first intention cannot be expected, it is, at best, useless to bring the surface of wounds closely together, and even if no other serious consequence follows, the wound itself often takes on unhealthy inflammation, and does not granulate as well as if it had been left more open for the ready discharge of any effused fluid, and for the application of stimulants, if necessary.

It is a great object, in many cases, to effect union by the first intention, in large wounds such as are left after amputation, for the diminished irritation and the saving of the drain of suppuration may often be the means of saving the life of the patient. Something may be done before dressing to lessen the effusion that always takes place from exposed surfaces, and to favor healthy reäction. The effusion of serum would cease, of course, if we waited long enough before dressing, but this is not generally done, and, indeed, in many cases it would require many hours' exposure. The application of ice answers the double purpose, that of drying the stump and affording healthy reäction and the adhesive process. This, I believe, is a perfectly safe application (unless rigors are produced by it), and when the capillary circulation is feeble, or when it is feared that too little reäction will take place, there is no other stimulant so wholesome, or that produces so natural and healthy a reäction.

In the French hospitals, purulent absorption is the great dread, and this has led to a more general use of the ecraseur than would otherwise have been given it, for it is asserted (and I believe with truth) that wounds made by this instrument heal more favorably than those made with the knife, and are much less liable to what is termed in Paris purulent absorption. I have reference only to the Paris hospitals, for union by the first intention cannot be contemplated when the ecraseur is used. The favorable result, however, of wounds or operations by this instrument, goes to prove what I have asserted of the bad effects of the effused animal fluids in wounds, either directly on the surface of the wound or by absorption. The ecraseur does not make a rough and ragged wound, as is generally supposed, but the tissues are cut as with scissors, but in such a gradual manner as to give time for the closure of vessels of moderate sizes, and consequently there is no oozing or exuding from its surfaces, and it remains dry, and is followed by no ill-conditioned inflammation. Why is this, when incised wounds are disposed to behave so badly under the same circumstances and in the same hospital? I can see no reason but the effusion of animal juices that takes place in incised wounds, which is prevented by the ecraseur. The incised wound produces less violence, and if everything is favorable, union by the first intention will follow, which cannot be expected of a wound by the ecraseur under the same favorable circumstances. The keen cutting instrument is far preferable in most, if not all cases, and so far as any absorption of impure matter is dangerous, the effect can be entirely obviated by the application of ice in favorable cases, and if necessary, the application of the alum iron or per-chloride of iron, which arrests at once all oozing of the fluids, and produces a wholesome stimulant effect. These last two applications are only recommended when union by the first intention is not expected, and when there is a general disposition to unhealthy inflammation.

I have been surprised at the readiness with which wounds heal when I have found it necessary to apply these potent styptics, and the uniform healthy character of the reaction after their use. The ecraseur is better adapted to the removal of hæmorrhoids than anything else ; but fifteen minutes to a half hour must be taken for each application, or there will be danger of hæmorrhage. I have been in the habit of using scissors, and applying immediately a sponge of suitable size, saturated with a strong solution of alum iron, which arrests the bleeding with certainty, and the parts give very little trouble afterwards. In a pure state, there is not much difference in effect between the per-chloride and the alum iron, but the per-chloride decomposes readily, gives down a sediment, and leaves an excess of acid, while the alum iron is always neutral. Whether the French surgeons mean by purulent absorption the actual absorption into the circulation of pus, or mean to express a pyæmic condition, I am unable to determine, though it is certain that they do not mean that pus, in its natural state, is absorbed, for it is decided that this cannot take place. They apply it to that pyæmic condition which is attended by great depression, and the formation of matter in various parts of the body, which they attribute to the absorption of impure matter from wounds ; it may be disintegrated pus, or other animal fluids. This never takes place in healthy and vigorous subjects, in which healthy exudation of lymph follows wounds, and it is quite plain that its frequency in the Paris hospitals is due, in a great measure, to the want of fresh air and proper nourishment. I speak of the deprivation of fresh air from personal observation, and judge of the diet from the general appearance of the patients. In the London hospitals, surgical patients presenting the appearance of the generality of those in the Paris hospitals, would be ordered beef, mutton, and porter or port wine, etc. This general poverty of the blood prevents adhesive inflammation, and leaves wounds in condition to absorb the unhealthy fluids that form in them, and the general system in a state to be most seriously affected by it.

By proper preparation, by means of tonics, and proper diet, much may be done to prevent this unfavorable result. Several years ago, and for several years, operations were disposed to take on a kind of diffusive, unhealthy, cellular inflammation, and in all cases that admitted of delay, I was in the habit of preparing them, by the use of tonics and attention to the stomach and diet, and by these means I almost always avoided this unhealthy process. The late Professor Wedderburn, who was one of the visiting surgeons of the Charity Hospital during the time referred to, made local applications for the same purposes. His usual application was a strong solution of sulph. quinine, with a slight excess of acid, and he thought it almost a specific. I believe it was of some service, but the more potent applications before mentioned, I am confident, are more sure, if the case should be imminent enough to warrant their use, and I hold that these applications would be warranted in all cases where union by the first intention cannot be expected, and when unhealthy inflammation is probable. These cases, however, are different from the cases of pyæmia in the Paris hospitals, and are probably due more to some epidemic poison and deterioration than to poverty of the blood. Pyæmia has also at times been prevalent, as if some epidemic influence was operating. Tonics, fresh air and proper nutriment constitute the general treatment, and stimulants or potent astringents are proper local applications, and very effective, at least as much so as the ccraseur.

ART. II.—*Dissection Wounds:* By W. C. NICHOLS, M. D.

THE diligent student of anatomy is often troubled with the reflection that the acquisition of knowledge in this department of science is replete with difficulties. Perhaps by stealth, and at midnight, he procures the material suited to his purpose ; and were he not led on by elevated aims, he might abhor this encroachment on the sanctity

of the tomb. Thus it happens that many in passing along the intricate paths of this science, consider the way too toilsome, and deem
the value of the acquisition hardly commensurate with the hazard of
the adventure. Though filled with repugnance at the mutilated body,
the student must reflect that all learning is slow in coming to maturity. Attempts must be made barren of success, experiments without satisfactory results ; and it must be early discovered, that, as
there is a vast difference between the outlines of a shadow and the
life-like picture of the master, so there is a wonderful distinction
between the first rudiments of an art and its extreme perfection—
between cultivated fields and fallow ground.

Being constantly engaged in the study of anatomy, and consequently much exposed to the noxious influence of cadaveric effluvia,
and having also witnessed serious disease from septic inoculation,
I have deemed it appropriate to mention a few peculiarities of this
affection. In this, as in other things, a timely hint may protect the
unwary from danger, and, at the same time, allay the needless alarm
of the timid.

It has been often remarked that those who assiduously prosecute
anatomical dissections, passing each day several hours in the midst
of an unwholesome atmosphere, undergo some depreciation of healthy
vigor. The putrid exhalations from the bodies taken into the system
with every breath, occasionally cause a sallow hue of countenance, and
generate dyspepsias and diarrhœas. In point of fact, with many persons, a flux from the bowels seems to be an initiatory step, an acclimation, as it were, to research in practical anatomy. This opinion is almost
confirmed by the fact equally noticeable, that a temporary withdrawal
from the cause of sickness gives relief, and in the majority of instances,
no recurrence of the disease will take place even during a long continuance in dissections. Putrid effluvia, when concentrated and
inhaled, give rise to constitutional disturbance ; and though the preservative tendency of habit may render some immunity from their
usual influence, adynamic fevers and dysenteries have been generated,
and when decomposing materials, from whatever source derived, are
inserted into wounds, the local mischief and the contamination of
the circulating fluids give origin to serious disease. The cook that
caters for the taste of the epicure receives from high game painful
eruptions and abscesses ; and in thus finding the system infected by
applications of a deleterious nature to the exterior of the body, we

are surprised that lovers of tainted food should so frequently escape sickness ; but such is the protective influence of habit in reconciling the palate to the dainty morsel, that the luxurious liver grows obese and gouty on food that would be insupportable and destructive to those unaccustomed to eat it in this state. Nor is a knowledge of this property of dead matter confined alone to the learned, for the vengeful savage, in deadly hate, hurls against his enemy the dart steeped in the fetid body of his murdered companion. Disastrous consequences have originated from fetid odors, when allowed to escape, either by accident or design, from bodies far advanced in decomposition ; so that from the upheavings of cemeteries sudden and fatal diseases have had their birth.

But it is not the anatomist alone who suffers from putrescent matters ; for it appears that in certain persons a peculiar aptitude to this disease exists. This predisposition, however, does not present itself at all times in the same individual ; for, by some change of constitution, a person may be susceptible to its slightest influence, whilst on another occasion he will resist evident exposures. Concerning this topic, Dr. Gross, in his recent valuable treatise on surgery, holds this language : " There is no question that some persons are peculiarly prone to suffer from this poison. I am acquainted with a physician who was formerly much engaged in pathological researches, who rarely opened a dead body without having a dissecting boil on his hand, thumb, or finger. Occasionally the consequences were more serious, the disease extending up the arm, along the course of the absorbents, as high as the axilla." Furthermore, many persons worn down by the arduous duties of student life, suffer from any slight abrasion. Direct absorption in these instances may not take place, but the local irritation generated by the constant maceration of the hands in putrid matter, may give rise to constitutional fever. This irritation may be thrown along the absorbents, even to the axilla ; yet in such cases we never witness that sudden depression of vital resistance which is so characteristic of the transmission of the virus into the general circulation. In the one case, the local mischief precedes the general disturbance, whilst in the other, the constitutional irritation over proportions the local inflammation ; and, in the language of Mr. Travers : " The local inflammatory action is an unessential and subordinate feature of the disease in its severest form, the disease itself consisting of a direct prostration of the vital forces, marked by a preternatural excitement and rapid exhaustion." Besides, mere local abscesses at the point of contact of the matter, we occasionally find that painful tubercles may arise. Several eminent anatomists of our country have been 'afflicted with this rare form of the disease.

In discussing this question of animal poison, it becomes a subject of some moment to consider the circumstances under which this disease may be produced. The assertion has been made by high authority, that the effects of morbid animal matters could only be generated and made efficient at an early period after the vital powers have 'become extinct. Could such a theory be established, could it be clearly proved that this deadly poison, brought into activity ere vitality was dissipated, is soon to be evolved by putrefactive changes, the practical anatomist would have achieved a great boon. Mr. Travers, in his work on "Constitutional Irritation," confirming the view that the disease arises from the absorption of the fluids of fresh bodies, holds the following language : "Of all the examples of the disease which I have given or selected, it is remarkable that the subjects were recent. Not one had been buried, some were yet warm. Even of those in which, not inspection, but demonstration, was the object, the bodies were in a perfectly fresh state. If, as is probable, at the moment of expiring vital influence, or of deanimalization, new combinations give birth to a specific matter of contagion, it is to be presumed that the ultimate state of dissolution and decay which we term putrefaction, so alters its quality as to neutralize and render it inert. And it is in conformity with observation, that actual putrescency is in some degree a security from the effects of this species of injury." In the paragraph immediately succeeding that above quoted, he attempts to deduce an analogy from comparative pathology. Vegetables, at the expiration of life, are known to undergo such chemical changes that new combinations are generated, which must also disappear previous to' the final decay annihilating the original structure ; and the author concludes with the reflection that "chemical observation and analysis directed to the subject, would, and probably one day will throw light upon the fact that the first changes which take place in the animal body, after the utter extinction of the vital influence, produce a fluid more deleterious in its effects upon the living body than any which succeed it, and will also determine whether the fluids generated by disease, when undergoing these changes, possess more or less of this property."

Though the above opinion in regard to this malady obtains with many, and would be highly satisfactory in the use of prophylactic measures, we yet have reason to believe that fatal effects may result from subjects far advanced in decomposition, and even from the living. Innumerable accidents of this character prove that morbid poison may be induced from specimens long kept ; and, in corroboration of the belief that morbid fluids from the living may produce disastrous consequences, I will offer the following quotation from a letter addressed to me by Dr. J. Roby, the able Professor of Anatomy in the University of Maryland. After making allusion to the general nature of this infection, he remarks : " My brother-in-law, Dr. Sharpe, of Boston, was also very ill for months. His case arose from poison received from a living, not a dead subject. The main points are as follow. A dispensary patient, recently confined, came under his care. He saw her for the first time on Saturday, and was obliged to empty her bladder with the catheter. She evidently had puerperal peritonitis. On Sunday he used the catheter again. On Monday, while riding, he was suddenly attacked with intense headache, pain in the back, and severe rigor. I saw him on his return home, still in the chill, and complaining of great pain in the back. He supposed that he was about to have typhus fever, or small-pox. There being great nausea, I advised an emetic of ipecachuana, which he took. The pain, however, continued, and he was very ill through the night. The next morning, I asked him, ' if he had any patients with erysipelas ?' He then told of the case he was attending. I examined his hands, and found on the end of his left forefinger an almost imperceptible abrasion. The case was clear to me. He was suffering from *morbid poison*. Soon the usual symptoms followed— intense restlessness, headache, pain in the back, delirium and prostration. In truth, his condition was an exact transcript of Morla's. A large abscess formed under his pectoral muscles, and he barely escaped with his life. Morla's case you saw. I had no doubt of its character from the beginning, and if you remember, predicted the course and event."

The case above alluded to as resembling Dr. Sharpe's, was that of a medical student, occurring in the Baltimore Infirmary, in the summer of 1857, during my term of service as house physician to that institution. On a sultry summer evening of that year, a poor sailor died of a cancerous affection of the stomach. He had lingered long,

21

and an autopsy was held about 10 o'clock on the night succeeding his death. The body still retained warmth, and during the examination Mr. Morla received several abrasions on the left forearm, from the cut ends of the ribs. His hands were smeared with the secretions of the body, and at this time the contact of the matter gave no sense of irritation. At noon of the following day, he complained of chilly sensations, the conjunctivæ of his eyes were injected with blood, and his restlessness and jactitation evinced irritation of the nervous system. Not being satisfied with the unfavorable symptoms in this case, I sent a messenger for Dr. Miltenberger, the visiting surgeon of the Infirmary, who, arriving late in the afternoon, found Mr. Morla in an active delirium. He had great heat of skin, and a bounding pulse. At this time, no signs of inflammation were evident about the abrasions. As his cerebral symptoms were untoward, and his pulse justified the procedure, he was bled from the arm. After losing several ounces of blood, he fell asleep, and on the succeeding morning was quite rational.

At this period of the disease, we could approach a correct diagnosis ; for he now complained of irritability and numbness of the · left arm, attended with excessive pain in the axilla and beneath the pectoral muscles. Recurring to the autopsy of the previous night, conjoined with the extreme distress and prostration, we were obviously dealing with poison from animal matter.

Mr. Morla suffered much, and, though carefully attended, many weeks elapsed before recovery took place. His frame, naturally robust, had to contend, not only with the sedative influence of the poison, but large abscesses having speedily formed under the pectoral muscles and down the arm as far as the elbow, the continued suppuration from such an extensive surface almost drained the fountain of life.

Since coming to New Orleans, I have witnessed an instance of septic inoculation similar to the one above detailed. A man suffering from the effects of intemperance, inflicted a mortal wound on his wife, and then attempted suicide. Both man and wife came to the Charity Hospital in a mutilated condition, and the latter, lingering a few days, died. Mr. Shelby, a resident student of the Hospital, having charge of the ward to which she was consigned, assisted at the coroner's inquest. From an abrasion on the right hand, the toxic material was absorbed. The usual phenomena—chill, pain in the

axillæ, and fever—soon supervened ; and abscesses discharging profusely, formed about the axillary glands, and many weeks elapsed
before recovery took place.

In both instances just mentioned, the subjects from which the
malady resulted were recently dead ; and, had we not opposing evidence, I would subscribe to the testimony of some, that the peculiar
poison " produced by the textures before their vital properties and
cohesions are quite extinct," could be only rendered baneful at an
early period after death.

The symptoms attending this malady are generally characterized
by extreme depression of the nervous system. At the point of contact, there is rarely any evidence of inflammation beyond slight redness ; and so agonizing and violent are the effects, that the local
action can only be regarded as a secondary and unimportant feature.
Indeed, the severity of the rigors, the intensity of the pain, the
nausea and delirium, all testify that a blood poison has been absorbed.
In Mr. Morla's case, little irritation was shown about the abrasion
till the more serious trouble in the axilla had declared itself. On the
third or fourth day after the reception of the poison, a small vesicle
appeared on the wrist of the left arm, which eventually desquamated
without attracting further attention.

It has been supposed that the disease was allied to the malady of
which the infected body died. But such a view is erroneous, since it
is well ascertained that similar results have ensued from the examination of bodies dead by accident ; yet it must be admitted that diseases
attacking serous surfaces have manifested the greatest disposition to
cause infection. In truth, in all bodies recently dead, this poison
exists in various grades of activity, irrespective of any form of disease. And furthermore, the symptoms of this disease somewhat
resembling those of pestilential epidemics, can only be understood by
the supposition that the circulating fluids are contaminated, and that
the nervous system is oppressed by a peculiar irritant. In some cases,
this virus must be generated long before vitality is extinct ; for it is
thus only that we can harmonize the above views with the fact that
the living occasionally cause inoculation. And in those isolated
cases where poison has been absorbed from handling pathological
specimens, we must conclude that the preservative fluid, whether
alcohol or other menstrua, in arresting putrefactive alterations,
retained the septic element, to be rendered effective and deadly when
brought in contact with the abrased hand of the curious.

In the majority of the cases on record, the poison was taken from
bodies recently dead, and its virulence manifesting itself within
eighteen hours after reception, the sad story of their issue is told in
speedy death or a tedious convalescence.

It is well worthy of remark, that the axillary glands are the foci
around which inflammation originates destructive action on the tissues. It appears that nature offers in this situation some resistance
to the offending material ; but, so diffusive and blighting is this
subtle agent, so rapidly does it pervade the organism, that the most
robust frame is made to totter under its toxic effect.

In a disease always formidable, and often extremely fatal, it
behooves us to understand the preventive measures placed in our
power. If, as some suppose, the virulence of the poison is proportionate to the freshness of the body dissected, we who study anatomy
in New Orleans should maintain the greatest caution; for none of the
material used in our demonstrations has ever been buried. But,
happily, though the heat of climate and the constitutions of our students, may predispose to disease, I have never known an instance of
poison to occur in the dissecting rooms of the University of Louisiana.

In consequence of the high degree of temperature peculiar to this
latitude, great care is maintained in the ventilation of our rooms, and
in the speedy withdrawal of all offensive matter. Moreover, as every
dead body brought into our dissecting rooms has been preserved with
a solution of the chloride of zinc, the student need not apprehend any
danger from poison, for no other disinfectant creates such alterations
in the tissues of the body; and thus far, the records of medicine furnish no instance of inoculation following the dissection of bodies
injected with this valuable agent. In this respect, New Orleans presents to the student of medicine unsurpassed facilities for the acquisition of knowledge in anatomy. Possessed of ample material, which
can be reclaimed from the destructive tendency of disease and climate,
not only during our short and mild winters, but even during the heat
of midsummer, when epidemics are rife, our dissecting rooms can
satisfy the avidity of every earnest worker in this department of
science. Although persuaded that inoculation can scarcely take place
we recommend to students, in order to allay fear, in case of cuts and
abrasions on their hands, to resort immediately to the use of water
and sucking the wounded part with the lips. We eschew the use of
caustics and other irritants; for, from their free application to simple

injuries, troublesome sores have been produced. Besides, as the action of this poison is almost coïncident with its insertion into the wound, it would be unavailing.

When the specific virus has been absorbed, the disease resembles other affections of this class; and in our efforts to bring about a favorable issue, we should have recourse to such means as may sustain the flagging powers of life. The patient, in point of fact, has his own cure in his capacity of vital resistance. The strong man will quickly divest himself of the deadly poison, whilst the feeble will sink under the depressing cause. Every animal poison, whether originating from venomous reptiles and insects, or from the dead body, engenders a depressing influence on the vital powers; and whatever tends to facilitate the introduction of the virus into the circulation, will add to the dangers of the disease. In all cases of blood poison, the struggle that ensues between the action of the poison and vital resistance so alarms the functions of life, that many of the symptoms of inflammation are simulated. Few persons can undergo depletory measures, which would diminish the vigor of the constitution, and increase the rapidity of absorption; for this disease, like erysipelas, typhus, and similar affections, compels us to do nothing that may weaken the inherent strength of the patient. Rarely would we think of resorting to the lancet in erysipelas; for though its outburst with fever, pain, delirium, and a full pulse, may tempt us to such a procedure, yet in the majority of instances, a short lapse of time will evince the fact, that the calm is approaching when judicious care and every ounce of blood are requisite to carry the patient to a favorable termination. As yet, we are ignorant of any constitutional remedies that can be of positive efficacy when directed against septic poisons. In one of the cases referred to in this paper, that of Mr. Morla, the iodide of potassium was administered, but this agent exerted no antidotal properties. Perhaps further investigation may elicit knowledge corroborative of the information already set before the medical world in reference to the depurative effects of bromine and iodine in cases of animal poison. In the incipiency of this disease, palliative treatment, and the use of such measures as will alleviate pain and prevent suffering, should be the sole aim of the judicious surgeon. Proper vigilance will indicate the time for supporting the patient amid the adverse chances of the disease, which, like kindred ailments, much resembles in its course an oceanic voyage that, barring accidents, will have a happy termination.

ART. III.—*Acquired Occlusion of the Os Uteri in a Lady who had borne five Children; Operation successful for Mother and Child.* By J. T. SUGGS, M. D., of Harrisburg, Pontotoc county, Mississippi.

OCTOBER 11th, 1856, 3 o'clock, evening, called to Mrs. P. C. L., in labor. Pains regular, not severe or very frequent. About 12, at night, the pains becoming more frequent and harder, thought it necessary to proceed to digital examination. Upon making a careful and thorough investigation, could find no os tincæ; was satisfied there was a depression where it seemed to me the os should be. The pains shortly after the examination becoming lighter, the patient went to sleep and rested tolerably well till next morning.

12th, 7, A. M., pains returned. I made another very careful and thorough examination; but with all the caution and nicety of manipulation I could bring to bear, I found it impossible to detect any opening in the uterus, but was more certain of a depression and something of a puckering where the os had been. (She was the mother of five children.) I was brought to a stand, (for I had never met with any thing of the kind before).

I sent home, several miles, and got a case of metroscopes. The pains increasing, I placed the patient so as to get the advantage of a strong light, and with the help of the instrument brought the depression fully into view, the appearance of which was that of a striated cicatrix; the striæ converging to the centre of this depression were the obliterated os uteri; consequently, an operation was indispensable.

Having no cutting instrument, except a thumb lancet, I set my ingenuity to work to make that answer the purpose, and proceeded as follows: I wrapped the lancet to within the eighth of an inch of the point with a strip of fine tough paper, then tied the lancet (with the handles turned back straight with the blade) to a probe of sufficient length (the probe made of a piece of switch); having reinserted the metroscope (and here I would say that owing to the great relaxation of the vagina I had to use trivalve cylinder), and with the lancet tied to the probe I made an opening through the cicatrized os, by cutting very cautiously with the lancet point; the structure was firm, about one-sixth of an inch thick, and difficult to cut.

At this stage of the case, the patient became dreadfully alarmed, in consequence of which the pains left her entirely. Being utterly unable to convince her that the danger was assuredly past, so far as the operation was concerned, and that a return of the pains was all that was required to bring about a safe delivery, I had my friend, Dr. Frazier (now of Arkansas), sent for.

At 3 o'clock, P. M., we gave an opiate, which procured some sleep; after which the pains not returning, and the parts being well relaxed, we gave 20 grs. of ergot, which brought on the requisite action. The case terminated entirely satisfactorily in a short space of time.

Mother and child have both done well, and are at this date alive and well.

December 8, 1859.

ART. IV.—*Retrocedent or Remitting Parturient Labor successfully treated with the Sulphate of Quinine.*

PALESTINE, Anderson county, Texas, Dec. 7th, 1859.

DR. B. DOWLER—*Dear Sir:* Thinking that the relation of a case of retrocession of labor, which fell under my observation, might not be uninteresting to you and some of the numerous readers of your Journal, I submit it to you for publication, if, after perusing it, you deem it worthy.

On Sunday, the 21st of August, at 9 o'clock, A. M., I was called to see Ann, a servant girl of Mrs. B., who had been then an hour in labor. On making an examination, I found the os uteri dilated to the size of an American dollar, and quite patulous. I inquired of her the probable duration of her pregnancy, and was assured that it was about the eighth month; as she had, she said, "kept particular count."

The pains were regular but not of much force, coming on at intervals of twenty minutes. This state of things lasted an hour, at which time the pains began to grow weaker, and had ceased altogether by 3 o'clock, P. M. No advancement of labor, (save a slight protrusion of the bag of membranes, through which could be distinctly felt a head presentation) took place. As she was fatigued, and had some fever, I concluded to give her 10 grs. pulv. Doveri.

On visiting her again on the morning of the 22d, to my surprise I found her up and attending to her regular avocations. I was called hurriedly to her again on the 28th, just a week from my previous call. I found her as at first seen on the 21st, apparently in progressive labor. Pains regular, at intervals of twenty minutes; membranes slightly protruding, with a soft and dilatable os. After remaining an hour, and there being no further advance of labor, and not believing in the speedy termination of the case, I left, and called again at 2 P. M. As I expected, I found the pains diminishing in force and frequency, and by 3 o'clock, an hour from the time I called, she was quiet, having, however, as before, considerable fever. After witnessing these two cessations of labor in the same individual, I was lead to believe that the periodicity manifested in the uterine contractions, had a miasmatic origin. I therefore had quin. sulph. administered to her on the following Saturday night (3d Sept). I called on the morning of the 4th, at 9 o'clock, and found her again suffering some slight pain, which, however, lasted hardly an hour. I ordered her quin. sulph. again on the following Saturday (the 10th Sept.), and called on the morning of the 11th, finding her well. The quinine was kept up for four more Saturday nights, the pains in the meantime not returning. On the morning of the 9th October, at 9 o'clock, I was again called, and this time found it no "fuss and feather" affair, for she was soon delivered of a well-grown male child.

Yours, with the highest regard,

JNO. R. WOODWARD, M. D.

ART. V.—*Cases Treated and Reported :* By Drs. SCALES and GILMAN, of Crawfordsville, Mississippi.

CASE I. *Dislocation of the head of the humerus into the axilla, and fracture of its neck.*—On the 18th July last, we were called to see a negro boy about nine years old, and on examination, found the head of the humeral bone in the axilla, and a fracture of the neck, which we thought was oblique. We seated the patient in a chair, and passed a girth around the chest, and secured it to the bed post, by which we had seated him. We then directed an assistant to take hold of the wrist with one hand, and the humerus, just above the condyles, with the other, and make extension, first outwards and upwards, then downwards and inwards, with directions to let loose his hold with the last extension, we, at the same time, placing our thumbs on the shoulder and the fingers of each hand in the axilla, behind the head of the bone, and drawing it out after the shaft, as the arm was extended. Just as the extension was made downwards and inwards, and the limb let loose, the head of the bone entered the socket with a slight jar. By holding the head of the bone with one hand and rotating the shaft with the other, the crepitus was as distinct as before the reduction. Knowing that such cases sometimes terminate in false joints, we determined to have our partner, Dr. J. T. Gilman, to see the case before dressing. On examination, he pronounced the reduction of the head of the bone and the fractured ends in proper position, but thought it was the anatomical neck fractured. We dressed the part after Boyer's method, and on the 22d of the month again visited our patient. Finding the bandage loose, and not feeling the limb entirely secure with that mode of dressing, we applied the bandage after the method of Prof. Dudley, putting a pad in the axilla, as at first, and passing the roller around the chest and arm, when it had first been carried from the hand to the pit of the shoulder. Then placing the forearm in a sling, we left the patient in charge of his young master, a first course student, with instructions to inform us if the bandage got too loose. We did not repeat our visit, nor was the dressing removed, till the fifth week, after which the boy was put to work. In the latter part of November we paid our patient a visit, and found him in the field, picking cotton. A casual observer would hardly notice any difference in the two joints, but, on close examination, we found slight enlargement at the fractured part of the injured limb, and the motions of the joint not quite so perfect as the other, although the arm could be raised above the head with facility, and the usual motions easily made.

Sir Astley Cooper, in his lectures on surgery by Tyrrell, reports the case of a child ten years old, that met with a fracture of the neck of the humerus, with dislocation in the axilla, the head of the bone remaining in the socket, and says such cases may occur with the young or old, but rarely with the middle-aged.

Mr. Fergusson reports two well-defined cases of fractured neck with dislocation of the head of the bone into the axilla, in his surgery by Norris, and states that a false joint was the result in each.

22

CASE 2. *Operations with the Ecraseur.*—A negro man, laborer on the Mobile and Ohio Railroad, disabled from work by a pile, was sent to us for treatment. For a few days we administered laxatives, and applied cold water, with instructions to push the pile within the sphincter, and, if possible, keep it there. Finding this course availed nothing, we put the patient under the influence of ether, and, with the ecraseur, cut the pile off. There was no pain, and but few drops of blood lost. The balance of the treatment consisted in a few doses of morphia, laxatives and cold water injections, the part incised being as smooth as if cut with a knife, three days after the operation. The boy was able to resume his labor in a few days. Some weeks afterwards we saw him, and learned there had not been the first symptom of a return of the disease. We mention this case merely to show how great suffering may be relieved by an operation so simple, to say nothing of the labor saved.

CASE 3. *Removal of a portion of the Rectum.*—Mr. B. W. W., medical practitioner, sent for us on the 30th June last, about fifteen miles, to cut off his piles. On examination, we found about two-thirds of the circumference of the rectum in a state of prolapse. The distress was so great in riding that he was not able to attend his practice ; and after being informed that a portion of the bowel protruded, instead of hæmorrhoids, and that the protruded portion consisted of the mucous lining, he determined to have it removed. After the administration of chloroform, the ecraseur was applied, and the prolapsed portion cut off. There was but a very small quantity of blood lost, and on the sixth day after the operation, the patient was up, and rode in a buggy some twelve or fifteen miles to his county town. This case shows the great advantage of the ecraseur over the ligature, in such operations.

CASE 4. *Fistula in Ano.*—A Mr. F., about 35 years of age, had been afflicted with fistula *in ano* for many months before his application to us, which was the latter part of May last. On examination, we found the opening in the bowel so high up that we determined to operate with the ecraseur, to avoid hæmorrhage. We fastened one end of the chain of the instrument with a silk ligature, in the eye of a curved needle, about the size of an ordinary speying needle, passed it up the fistula into the bowel, and brought it out through the sphincter, by which means we included all the substance between the fistula and mucous membrane of the bowel. We then applied the ends of the chain to the instrument, and laid open all the parts included, with the loss of very little blood—probably not more than two drachms. Preliminary to the passing of the needle and chain through the fistula and the operation, we administered chloroform, through the assistance of Dr. Fant. The patient made a good recovery, without anything worthy of notice in the after treatment.

CASE 5. *Use of the grooved staff in Strictures of the male Urethra.*—A negro man, 40 years old, was brought to us on the 30th July last, with strictures of the urethra, of nine years' standing. We found two strictures between the glans penis and bulb, as well as one in the membranous portion. At times, before his application to us, the warm hip bath, with diuretics, had to be used to get the urine off at all. The boy could sometimes get a small catheter in the bladder, but frequently failed. After introducing a gum catheter, No. 5, we could not get a gum catheter or bougie of larger size to pass the stricture in the membranous portion of the urethra. At that time we had no metallic catheter or bougie smaller than a No. 8 ; and while reflecting what we should do, as we could not introduce No. 8, it occurred to us to use a small grooved staff, which we did, and followed it by a larger one, which produced the sensation of a tearing or dull cutting instrument, as it passed through the stricture, accompanied with considerable hæmorrhage, and followed by two or three chills. After this, we increased the size of the instruments with facility, till the full size was passed, on the 6th September, there being no symptoms worthy of note further than those mentioned, fourteen catheterisms having been performed in the meantime. The staff used was a French instrument, the groove terminating suddenly one half inch behind the round point.

CASE 6. *Stricture.*—A gentleman, 35 years of age, called on us the 30th August last, stating he had some disease of his urinary organs, and had asked the advice of a number of physicians, some saying it was prostatic enlargement, some irritable bladder, and some inflammation of the urethra, and among them gave him (to use his own terms) his hat full of balsam, with a variety of other remedies of a similar class, without the least permanent relief. We expressed the belief that he was strictured, and proposed an examination, which he readily consented to. We commenced with a No. 10 gum bougie, which we could pass through a stricture in front of the bulb of the urethra, but when we reached the membranous portion we could get it no further. We then reduced the size to the infant bougie before we could possibly pass the last named stricture, after which we were able to increase the size of the gum bougie to a No. 6, and pass it into the bladder. We could not introduce a gum or metallic bougie larger than the No. 6, just mentioned, without using more force than we thought justifiable ; and, as in the previous case, we passed the grooved staff into the bladder, tearing the stricture, which was followed by considerable hæmorrhage, but no chills. On the 26th October, we introduced a full-sized bougie, the patient's symptoms having been greatly relieved, and requiring only an occasional introduction of the bougie since.

CASE 7. *Fracture of the Skull.*—A little son of Mr. D. G. Holbrook, about ten years old, was, on the 6th August last, amusing himself in the performance of what he called " skinning the cat," on the limb of a tree, some twelve or fifteen feet from the ground. While engaged in the performance, he lost his hold, and fell head-foremost, the right side of the frontal bone striking the root of the tree, and producing a large circular fracture, extending from just behind the superciliary ridge, back, near the parietal bone, and down, near the temporal, driving in the circular piece, and producing a longitudinal fracture of it. We saw the patient a few hours after the accident, and found the right eye entirely closed by ecchymosis ; the pulse small ; the pupil of the left eye dilated ; the skin cool, a disposition to sleep, and rather stupid, but able to answer questions intelligibly. After shaving the scalp, we made a circular incision in the line of the fracture, some three inches or more, and commencing above the os temporis, behind, and continuing upwards, having several arteries to tie, there being pretty free hæmorrhage. On raising the flap, we found the bone slightly shivered at the junction of the circular and longitudinal fracture. The longitudinal fracture, we think, extended from the front to the back part of the circular piece, and a little below its centre. Just at their junction behind, we applied the instrument, and trephined, including a very small portion of the edges of the fractured portions in the circle taken out. We raised the fractured portions, and found considerable effusion of blood on the brain, with constant oozing. After closing the incision with a few stitches, we put the patient to bed, and administered a dose of epsom salts, with instructions to repeat, at intervals of a few hours, till the bowels were moved. The salts operated well, and the symptoms continued to improve till about the 15th of August, when headache was complained of, with inability to sit up. There was also a circular prominence just above the superciliary ridge, about the diameter of a silver half dollar, which, on pressure, presented the feel of a depression in the bone. We determined to investigate its nature, and made a circular incision around a portion of its circumference, when a small quantity of blood was discharged, and showed a communication under the scalp with the fluid that was discharged from the first incision. The occipito-frontalis muscle was here fractured the entire round of the circle, and the fractured bone was slightly elevated on the sound bone, instead of being depressed. The flap was dressed after the manner of the first operation, and our patient continued to improve for some three weeks, when vision in the right eye began to fail, objects being seen double, and finally not seen at all ; but, in the course of a few weeks more, vision was gradually restored, and he is now in the enjoyment of good health.

We anticipated necrosis of the circular piece of bone that was depressed, owing to the great injury done in breaking up its connection with the surrounding bone, and that done to the portion of scalp covering it. We think the circular fracture of the muscle, just over the eye, was the part that struck the root in the fall. There were some fungous granulations sprouting up along the line of the first incision, some month or more after the operation, which were removed by the application of caustic. We cannot say why it was that the amaurosis made its appearance at the time it did, but suppose it may have been owing to the pressure of a clot of blood and a restoration of the function of the eye, owing to the absorption of the coagulum.

In both operations, we had the assistance and concurrence of our friend, Dr. Owen, of Choctaw Agency, Mississippi.

CASE 8. *The bandage and adhesive straps in Chronic Ulcers of the Legs.*— Patsy, a negress, about 65 years old, was sent to us on the 5th of August last, suffering from jaundice, dropsy of the lower extremities, and ulceration of the left leg. The ulcer was narrow, and about three inches long, situated on the front central part of the leg. The legs were both much swelled to the knees, with dropsical effusion. We cut the adhesive strips long enough to encircle three-fourths of the leg, and drew them tight over the ulcer. We then applied the common roller, about three inches wide, from the feet to the knees, pretty tight every morning, till the 9th, inclusive. On the 12th, we found the dropsy in the legs removed, the rollers remaining till that date without removal ; the ulcer much improved. The ulcered leg was dressed with the straps, and again bound, on the 12th, with a view of making a final cure of the ulcer. Two days after, the bandage was removed, being wet, and we found the inside of the leg in a solid blister, from the ankle nearly to the knee. Previous to this we had given the patient a dose of calomel and jalap, which produced free purging, and was followed by an opiate to stop it, when free salivation followed. We laid aside the ·dressing to the leg, applied nitro-muriatic acid to the mouth, and gave comp. syrup sarza and iodide potass, internally, alternated with muriated tinc. iron. The jaundice persisting, and the dropsy partially returning, we changed our prescription to iodide potassa grs. v ; nitrous ether ʒi.; given in water, three times daily ; giving the muriatic tinc. iron in 20 drop doses intermediately through the day. By a perseverance in this course for about six weeks, we made a complete cure of all the symptoms, the dropsy disappearing with the jaundice, and neither from the system fully, till the free action produced on the kidneys by the last remedies named. The quantity of urine discharged daily was greatly increased, and we attribute the success to this circumstance. We were not able to account for the blistering of the leg under the use of the bandage, but had another case, in a gentleman about 55 years old, who had a small circular ulcer on the lower front part of his shin, treated with straps and the bandage, as in the preceding case, when, in a few days, the ulcer was almost healed, and a blister made its appearance all around it, involving a circle of some two inches or more in diameter, that was a little discolored from previous inflammation. This case was also cured ; and to support the part from a future return, a silk stocking was worn.

CASE 9. *Ulcer of the Leg.*—Lucinda, a negress, 35 years old, bearing children, was sent to us from Masheclerville, this State, on the 24th of June last, with an ulcer of long standing, about three by two inches deep, and occupying the right leg, just above the internal malleölus. The leg was very large up to the knee ; the edges of the ulcer thick and indurated. This case had baffled all the *Doctors* that chanced to try it, and, finally, amputation was advised as the only hope. We made free incisions around the thickened edges of the ulcer to its bottom ; cut the adhesive straps from three-quarters to one inch in width, and drew them on as tight as we possibly could, and applied the bandage, also, as tight as we could draw it, from the foot to the knee, taking great care to have its pressure uniform. This course of treatment we continued almost daily for four months, when our patient was entirely relieved ; and, to test the result, we put on a silk stocking, and retained the case under our charge a month longer, when, being satisfied, we sent her home. We had two other cases, not mentioned, treated in the same way, with similar results, except the stocking was not required after the cure was completed. When the bandage is applied with as much pressure as we use, its folds should be smooth, and no successive turn should be tighter than the preceding, or great suffering may require its removal and reäpplication.

DECEMBER 9, 1859.

ART. VI.—*The Auricles of the Heart Act by their Elasticity and Contractility, not by Muscles:* By CHARLES SMITH, M. D., New Orleans.

To demonstrate this fact, we shall first expose the heart, and then follow the current of blood.

Tie the pulmonary veins above the auricle ; perforate the mitral valves of the ventricle, and inject through the aörta, and fill the left ventricle and auricle to their fullest capacity, and lay the preparation aside until perfectly dry ; when the auricle will appear transparent as glass, and the ventricle perfectly opaque.

This proof that the auricles have no muscles, or muscular fibres, ought to convince any one who has not committed himself upon the subject. I must confess that I have often admitted to my professor that I could see the muscular fibres in the auricles ; nor could I contradict it, until I had lectured upon anatomy and physiology myself, and given the subject special attention.

We say, then, that the auricles act, upon the principle of ELASTICITY and CONTRACTILITY, dependent upon the ventricles. During the action or contraction of the ventricles, the auricles are distended with blood, and continue so until the reäction of the ventricles, when the blood flows (upon the principle of the laws of fluids) into the ventricle, which again contracts, and propels it into the arteries.

We may simply say here, that, if muscular action were necessary for the purpose of emptying the auricle, the pulmonary veins would have valves, to prevent the regurgitation of blood. But, as yet, none have ever been discovered. In all the course of the circulation, we find valves in proportion to the force applied. Hence we might reasonably infer that the auricles do not really act—only passively.

The idea, then, that muscular fibres could be seen in the auricles, I believe to be an error that ought to be corrected ; and if they can be shown to exist, then it is certain that the circulation of the blood does not obey the laws of force, and motion, and fluids.

If this view, then, be correct, the auricle is a passive, not an active appendage, and the blood would be acted upon the same as it would in the suction pump, where the column of water is subservient to the action of the piston.

So, in the circulation, the blood in the auricles depends upon the action of the ventricles. If passive, the auricles are only RESERVOIRS, and adapt themselves to the amount of blood required for the use of the ventricles.

In the structure of the heart, we see the vast difference between the right and left ventricles, in the comparative thickness of their parietes and the remarkably great strength of valves, to prevent reflux—all adapted to the two circulations, the general system and the pulmonary.

Now, if it is necessary to provide against regurgitation in one part of the circulation, where active force is used, it must be in all ; therefore, if there were any muscular action, or other kind but passive, there would certainly be valves at the auricles, or in the course of the pulmonary veins, otherwise the capillary circulation would be completely arrested, and the grandest object in the circulation defeated.

December 22, 1859.

Art. VII.—*Nature and Art in the Cure of Disease.* By Thomas T. Wall, M. D., of Campte, Natchitoches Parish, Louisiana.

No one man knows all things. Superiority in some degree belongs to every man, and no man is so ignorant but that something can be learned from him. Yet there is nothing new under the sun; but there are a great many things existing which have never been found out, for the want of a persevering investigation and practical observation, to understand the phenomena of nature both in the organic and inorganic world, and to analyse their equivalents and affinities, will show that they are invariably fixed under like circumstances. According to Liebig, no experiment can contradict truths derived from the observation of nature.

But we are not capable of appreciating those truths existing in nature, without a physical or a chemico-physiological investigation of her laws. He who is acquainted with the workings of nature, both in her morbid and healthy action, possesses the best proximate knowledge of what is the cause of her derangement, truth and certainty of action being the foundation of all information. Being well instructed in the functional and organic laws of man, we can see at a glance any deviation from her natural course. Then, by fixing on the memory an extensive collection of facts, derived from experience and observation, from which our conclusions can be drawn, these will direct us in the proper course of procedure. And this can only be accomplished by becoming our own reasoners, thinkers and observers of physical evils and pathological sequences, depending on no man's *ipse dixit*. A mind that is ever credulous and ready to endorse new doctrines, because they emanate from men who want to be the oracles the profession, will be always distracted as to what shall be the proper course to pursue when called to the bedside of the sick, who stand in need of assistance.

Owing to the discordant state of opinions and the misrepresented systems of therapy promulgated at home and across the broad Atlantic, the mind is sometimes left shivering in the gale, tempestuous winds conveying it to an unknown shore, where it will be stranded in mystery without, knowing what to do, if said mind is not freighted with the proper ballast ; and, according to my humble opinion, this ballast consists, first, in common sense; second, an ability to analyze and discriminate between what is, and what is not; third, extensive reading, in order that we may not be led away by the opinions of any one man, but carefully examine the testimony of all, and draw our conclusions therefrom (sometimes flowers grow amongst thorns, and the darkest hour is before the dawn); fourthly, practice or experience, that we may be able to compare events or facts, with each other to know the true and guard against the false.

23

I contend that there is no position on earth so all-important as that of a physician when placed at the bed-side of his patient. Here, indeed, he is autocrat, while the sick and their friends are calling aloud for help. No man stands more in need of judgment, humanity and divine assistance. It is even sometimes allowable and necessary for man to have some doubt of his own learning, that he may become wise and not be possessed of a too daring disposition, when human life is involved.

Is the assistance of art capable to counteract a morbid process? I advocate the affirmative. But there are certain requisites for us to be in possession of that we may be able to assist Nature, and afford her the proper amount thereof. We must know the nature of the disease—and where located—its cause and nature, if benign or malignant, its complications, its relation with other organs, particularly with those organs that are essential to life, and what effect it will have upon the general system, provided its progress is not arrested; the age, race, sex, season, and, from physiology, what kind of a constitution we have to act upon. After making due investigation into all the circumstances with which the case is surrounded, and coming to the conclusion that life is threatened, and that quickly, our treatment must· be active, no matter what kind of a disease it may be. If life is not threatened speedily, the treatment should be less active. Where disease will cure itself, according to Sir John Forbes, M. D., all active remedies should and ought to be abandoned. But in what do the resources of our art consist, if we are to be deprived of active medication? Take away from us wine, brandy, quinine, camphor, opium, etc., etc., and we never want to have to attend on a case of typhoid fever, nor its allied diseases, etc. But are we to consider Sir John Forbes the judge of what kind of remedies we shall administer in our treatment of disease in the State of Louisiana? (a man so remote from us, and, as I might say, ignorant of the nature of disease in this country, and of our soil and climate). He who does take away all active medicines had better quit the practice of medicine, that it may fall into abler hands, and not have the lives of our citizens placed in jeopardy.

Admitting that it is necessary to know all the antecedents above mentioned, and that we are posted therein, before we commence our treatment, we must then ascertain what kind of medicine we must give, the medical property of which is capable of counteracting the morbid phenomena that have so much disturbed the system.

We must also determine how much to give, what effect it will have upon the disease, if any; or, whether we are to increase or diminish the dose; how long to continue; when to quit or alter the prescription, etc. Although man is born to die, yet this fact does not supercede the skill of the physician, nor the good effects of medicine in many maladies. And even though man's hour cometh, his life may be prolonged through the goodness of God and the medical attendant, as it was in the days of Isaiah, when the latter applied a poultice of figs to the king's boil, and his life was prolonged fifteen years. There is a way that appears right to some great minds, yet it leads to the overthrow of science and the destruction of man; and the reason of it must be, too great a strain of the understanding, already biased by passion, to attempt some object before it has been maturely deliberated upon, before truth has been separated from falsehood, and an illusory imagination, a fanciful idea, filling the place of truth.

Sir John Forbes asserts that it is not only useless, but injurious to attempt *to suppress a morbid process by strong remedies.*

If each organ has independent action within itself, a unity of this action in the aggregate constitutes the phenomena of life. We frequently see that in grangrene of a part, a line of demarcation is drawn by the powers of nature between the dead and the living, and this in proportion to the degree of vitality. If the judicious aid of art be timely administered to this veto-physiological action, her efforts will be doubly vigorous, in casting off the morbid process that has revolutionized the healthy status. Life is contrary to death. The shock to this life-force may be too great, and it become asphyxiated. May not resuscitation be established by and through the instrumentality of nature and art combined, and derangement be counteracted in man as well as in other organic bodies? The means that we possess must be equal to the ends, or the indications to be accomplished, let it be strong, stronger or strongest. We have been frequently called to see those that are sick, and after carefully examining into all the circumstances connected with the case, and prescribing according to the conclusions that we had then fixed upon, yet it frequently happened that we had to increase the dose, or shorten the time of its administration, etc. Here, like the united action of the strong men who lifted the burden from off the tender sapling, which was again planted, and it grew, the means applied were equal to the ends in view, and a return to health as a consequence thereof.

I admit that the action of medicine on the system is carried to too great an extent by some professors of the healing art. I entirely oppose the profuse salivations practised by others, as such a change, brought on by mercury, vitiates the fluids, and, as a consequence, the solids, and predisposes the organism of man to gout and rheumatism, and disqualifies him to undergo the vicissitudes of the weather and the changes of the seasons with the same security as he otherwise might have done. Yet I am, in justice, compelled to say that mercury is an excellent remedy, if used with moderation. The abuse of anything does not disqualify its use. The mechanism of man endeavors to relieve herself of her detritus through the medium of the lungs, liver and kidneys. The bowels and the skin may become torpid, or their action suspended, but by giving the proper remedies, the latent vital power that in them lies dormant, may be aroused and brought into efficient action ; but to know what is the matter, what to give, how much, and when to stop, are the great desiderata. And these must be learned, first in the schools adapted for the instruction of medical students; afterwards by experience, observation, and practical analogy.

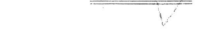

ART. VIII.— *Urethro-Vaginal, Vesico-Vaginal, and Recto-Vaginal Fistules ; General Remarks ; Report of Cases Successfully Treated with the Button Suture:* By NATHAN BOZEMAN, M. D., of New Orleans (late of Montgomery, Alabama).

[Continued from page 49.]

CASE XX.*—*Vesico-Vaginal Fistule of large size, complicated with loss of the Cervix Uteri; two Operations with the Button Suture; Cure.*— Mrs. ——, of Greenville, Alabama, applied to me for treatment of her case, in the month of November, 1857. She is of tall and slender figure, aged about 33, and had always enjoyed pretty good health, until the birth of her last child, five years ago. This was her fifth labor, being tedious, as all previous ones had been. In no instance

---

* It is proper that I should state that the numbering of my cases here is a continuation from the November number of the North American Medico-Chirurgical Review, my report of cases at that time having reached nineteen.

before, however, did instruments require to be used, the efforts of nature being quite sufficient to complete delivery. This time they failed, after continuing uninterruptedly for sixty hours. The phys. icians in attendance applied the usual remedies, but no action of the uterus could be gotten up. A thorough examination now not only showed that the child was unusually large, but that its life was extinct.

With this state of things, it was thought advisable to employ instruments. Craniotomy was accordingly performed, and speedy delivery effected.

Patient states that there was more or less dribbling of her urine all the next day ; the day after there was still some, though not enough to relieve the bladder. Distension of the organ, with no ability to relieve itself, was the consequence. From this there was considerable suffering. An attempt was now made to relieve the bladder by introducing a catheter, but the instrument, it seems, could not be carried far enough to answer the purpose. Relief from this cause, however, soon followed, by a slough of the vesico-vaginal septum—caused, doubtless, by the long pressure of the child's head there. Constant dribbling of the urine now was the result. It was several months before the patient got out of bed, and when she did, her general health was very indifferent. Her menstruation, however, came on at the usual period after delivery, and continued pretty regular up to the present time, which is somewhat remarkable.

In almost all cases, according to my observation, and especially when the injury to the vaginal walls is considerable, as it was in this instance, there is almost a total cessation of the catamenia. There is certainly nothing like regularity in its return.

Examination.—Fistule belonged to my fifth class—second variety. It was somewhat triangular in shape, with its base downwards, and the apex formed by a rent in the anterior part of the cervix uteri. Three fingers could almost be introduced through the opening into the bladder, and owing to this enormous size, the mucous coat of the bladder kept pretty constantly protruded. The extent of the cervix lost was considerable, there being no trace of either lip present. With this there was also very great contraction of its canal, the parts around being very much indurated. The posterior edge of the fistule proper and the uterus, at first allowed of but very little de-pression—nothing like enough to effect apposition with the opposite

side. Here, then, was a very great obstacle in the way of a successful
management of the case. Knowing, however, that closure of the
chasm could be effected in no other way, I set to work to overcome
this difficulty, as a preparatory step. This I did by forcibly drawing
the parts down every day, stretching them, so to speak. The instrument I employed for the purpose was a pair of strong forceps, having
circular blades, with a groove on the face of one and a corresponding
ridge or tongue on the other. With this kind of appliance the upper
edge of the fistule could be seized and drawn down with considerable
force, without danger of being cut or torn. By this procedure I was
enabled, in the course of ten days, to get the two sides of the fistule
together with perfect ease, and to secure such an amount of elasticity
of the parts as to remove all apprehension as to the probable cutting
out of our sutures.

Operation —The patient being placed in the usual position, upon
her knees and elbows, and the speculum introduced and held by an
assistant, I proceeded to pare the edges of the fistule. What was
peculiar in this process, was the free trimming of the corners of the
cleft cervix, together with the adjacent septum, done for the purpose
of reducing this border of the opening to a suitable shape to match
the one of the opposite side. This being done, our sutures, eight in
number, were next introduced. Two of these were carried through
the stump of the cervix, one upon either side of the canal. Upon
being adjusted now, a button, bent upon its convexity and notched
in the upper edge, was slid down upon them, and secured in place by
compressed shot. For a view of the kind of button used in this case,
excepting that it has no curve upon its convexity, see figure 13, in
the *North American Medico-Chirurgical Review* for July, 1859. The line
of perforations in this button, it will be perceived, is straight, and
such was the feature of the button I used in the present instance.
The result, however, proved that I was mistaken as to its adaptation
to the parts. The operation was a partial failure. A small triangular
opening was left, it being the apex of the original fistule. Through
this small opening nearly all the urine passed, after the catheter was
laid aside. The strain, too, upon the newly-formed cicatrix I found
to be very considerable, and after the patient was allowed to get up,
it began to give way at each angle of the fistule, and so continued
until the whole of it had yielded, thus leaving the opening in the
bladder larger than it was in the outset. We had, therefore, to commence our treatment *de novo*.

The mistake I made in the adjustment of the suture apparatus, in this instance, was as to the extent of elasticity belonging to the anterior border of the fistule, and the manner of introducing the central sutures. This border of the opening, in attempting approximation, could not be brought up to the straight line of perforations in our buttons ; and in the upper border we lost all mechanical advantage over the apex of the fistule, by having; our ‘sutures upon either side too far removed from it. The consequence of this was an imperfect coäptation of the two edges of the fistule in the center, and a certain failure to unite to that extent.

In my next operation, therefore, I was prepared to take advantage of these oversights. The difficulty was easily overcome, and a perfect cure of our patient secured. Instead, now, of employing a button with the line of perforations straight, I had it curved to correspond exactly with the anterior border of the opening, and next, instead of having the central sutures in the upper border off to either side of the apex of our triangular opening, I placed them directly over it, so as to secure the greatest possible amount of power here, to force coäptation. The removal of the suture apparatus on the ninth day, showed how perfect its adaptation had been. Complete union throughout was the result. After a few days our patient was allowed to get up. She at first had some incontinence of urine, doubtless the result of weakness. This gradually disappeared, and after a couple of weeks she was going about as well as she ever was, having perfect control over her urine.

Remarks.—I have thus minutely described my operation in the above case, thinking it of such interest as to warrant it. It illustrates, I conceive, several important points in practice, which the surgeon should never lose sight of ; namely, a close inquiry into the nature of the parts before proceeding to operate, and a careful adaptation of the mechanical appliances called for. It was inattention to these that doubtless caused the partial failure of my first operation. I have nothing to say of our ultimate success in the case ; certainly nothing could have been more satisfactory than it was.

CASE xxi.—*Urethro-Vaginal and Vesico-Vaginal Fistules; Partial Obliteration of the Urethra ; all the Result of Lithotomy through the Vesico-Vaginal Septum, and Sloughing Caused by the " Clamp Suture;" Obliteration of the Urethra overcome, and both Fistules closed with the Button Suture; Perfect Control over the Urine afterwards.*—The subject

of this case was a mulatto girl, Louisa, sent to me by Mr. John
Bondurant, of Marion, Alabama, January the 18th, 1858. She is
about 18 years old, of large stature, and apparently in good health.
Upon being interrogated, she stated that, as far back as she
could recollect, there had been great difficulty, at times, in passing
her urine, and now and then it would be mixed with a little blood.
This trouble continued to increase as she grew older; and finally,
when about nine years old, it became so severe that it was thought
advisable to put her under some physician for regular treatment.
Dr. J. M. Sims, then residing in Montgomery, Alabama, was put in
charge of the case, who, upon examination, detected the existence of
a calculus in the bladder. The account of the case, while under the
care of Dr. S., I give from my own recollection, knowing, as I did,
something of its management. Dr. Sims' proposal was to rupture
the hymen, and to dilate the vagina to a sufficient extent to allow of
the stone being removed by an incision through the vesico-vaginal
septum ; afterwards to close the opening with his "clamp suture."
The preparatory treatment, then, having been gone through with,
which required several weeks, Dr. S. proceeded to perform the operation above indicated, in the presence of myself and several other
physicians. The incision was made through the septum longitudinally,
and about an inch in length. Through this opening the stone, about
the size of a partridge egg, was easily extracted. This part of the
operation, as well as the application of the clamp suture afterwards,
was done with the utmost skill and dexterity. The case was now
conducted on general principles ; such as position upon the back,
catheter in the bladder, light diet, opiates to hold the bowels in
check, etc.

After waiting the usual length of time, the suture apparatus was
removed ; but, unfortunately, closure of the wound had not taken place.
A vesico-vaginal fistule, with all the ill consequences of one arising
from tedious and badly managed labor, now remained.

Operation after operation Dr. S. performed, though without success.
The patient says that she was under treatment eighteen months or
two years, and underwent, first and last, about eight or ten operations ; thinks that her suffering was worse after removal of the stone
than before. Menstruation did not take place until the age of seventeen.

Examination.—Upon placing the patient in the usual position, procidentia uteri was found to exist—a very unusual position, certainly, of this organ for a woman who had never borne a child. This " falling of the womb," she said, had existed for two or three years.

I had no difficulty in replacing the organ. This being done, the speculum was next introduced, and the opening in the vesico-vaginal septum brought into view. It was situated in the median line, and about half an inch above the mouth of the urethra ; its size was sufficiently large to admit the point of the index finger. A catheter now introduced into the urethra, and passed on, made its appearance in the vagina, about one inch and a quarter from the meatus and an inch from the opening above described. All my efforts to pass the instrument beyond this point failed. The smallest size probe was then attempted to be passed, but with no better success. Obliteration of the passage above this point was the cause of the trouble. Both fistules were situated pretty much upon the same line, with reference to the longitudinal axis of the vagina.

Operation.—This was performed in the presence of Drs. Fowler, Weatherly, and Gaston, in the following manner : Both openings were converted into one, in the first place, my object being to reëstablish the urethra, and to simplify the main steps of the operation. This was effected by a long and narrow bladed knife, entered in the urethra at the meatus, and brought out at the opening near its root, and then carried through the other one, into the bladder. With its edge then turned towards the symphysis pubis, and by a sawing motion, the parts were easily laid open to a depth sufficient to reach the opposite side of the obliterated portion of the urethra. This being done, I next pared the edges of the two fistules, and introduced my sutures, seven in all, four to the urethra and three to the bladder. The closure of the whole was effected over an elastic catheter. The button employed was of the ordinary shape, and when adjusted, lay longitudinally.

The after treatment was conducted upon general principles. It being desirable not to remove the catheter, choking was prevented by passing through it, as often as necessary, a small wire.

On the eighth day, removed the suture apparatus, and found union of the parts complete, all to a small point corresponding to the original seat of the urethro-vaginal opening. This I had to close at another operation, which left the cure complete, the patient with

24

entire control over her urine. The procidentia uteri gradually disappeared under the free use of astringent injections.

Remarks.—The above case being somewhat out of the ordinary course of things, the few reflections that I may make here will not, I trust, be regarded as foreign to the subject.

The occurrence of the injuries, under the circumstances stated in this case, together with the long suffering of the patient afterwards, and the consequent procidentia uteri, make it rather unique, and certainly not devoid of interest. As to the propriety of the general course of treatment that was adopted in the outset for the removal of the stone in the bladder, it is not my purpose to criticise. Such a procedure as this, I am convinced, should be the established practice in older subjects, especially those who have borne children, now that our method of closing up the wound has become so simple and easy.

The risk of incontinence of urine, and consequent misery, perhaps for life, would be entirely avoided in this way. In such subjects, dilatation of the urethra, with or without incision, is exceedingly liable to be followed by the above result, especially if the calculus to be removed is rough, and of any considerable size. The vagina, in this class of cases, being already sufficiently dilated, we have only to make the required incision through the septum, remove the stone, and apply the button suture for closure of the wound. The whole thing is quickly done, and our patient placed in the very best condition for a permanent cure in a few days, without any risk whatever.

In young subjects, however, as the above case was, when the hymen has to be ruptured, and a long course of dilatation of the vagina—in short, complete defloration has to be instituted as a preliminary treatment only, to say nothing of the removal of the calculus afterwards, then the question as to the best operative procedure becomes a matter of grave consideration. As to the course that should be pursued under such circumstances, there is no doubt in my mind. The procedure ascribed to Paul Dubois is the one I should most certainly adopt ; namely, dilatation of the urethra by incision, to a sufficient extent to allow of the easy removal of the calculus. In giving preference to this method, however, I do it, not because I think that I should not be able to close the wound through the vesico-vaginal septum, as happened to the distinguished surgeon whose name I have mentioned in connection with this case, but that by adopting it time and trouble would be greatly lessened, and the defloration of our patient avoided ; both matters, I conceive, of the very greatest importance, when the result is, perhaps, more satisfactory than could be obtained in any other way. This operation, in very young subjects, is simple and easy to perform, and as a general rule, is attended with the most satisfactory results, as there is abundant testimony to prove. My own experience, though small, fully warrants me in saying what I have.

Not quite two years ago, I had occasion to perform this operation upon a little girl, not quite three years and a half old. The stone was almost as large as the one in the above case, and yet there was no sort of difficulty experienced in its removal through the dilated urethra. Our little patient could scarcely be kept in bed for twenty-four hours after the operation. Not an untoward symptom followed. There was the most perfect control over the urine, and now she is as healthy and sprightly as any child of her age. At some future time, I hope to be able to report the details of this case at length, and some others of a similar nature, in the mode in which I adopted an operative procedure not heretofore practised, that I am aware of, to any extent, in this country. I allude to the operation with the *rectangular staff*, as performed by Professor Buchanan, of Glasgow, Scotland.

CASE xxii.—*Vesico-Vaginal Fistule of large size; Successful application of the Button Suture.*—The subject of this case, Mrs. O., of Conyers, Georgia, was sent to me by my friend Dr. Dean, of the same place, in the month of March, 1858. Her history is as follows : æt. 41, of medium stature, good form, and always enjoyed good health until the birth of her ninth and last child, eight years ago, at which time she became the subject of her present affliction. She says that all previous labors were easy, excepting two, and these were not very tedious. At the time of her injury, labor lasted only twenty-four hours, and terminated naturally. She does not recollect, however, of passing any urine during the time, nor for thirty-six hours afterwards, and then only by the use of a catheter, when a large quantity was drawn off, very much to her relief. Her suffering, for some hours previous to the use of the catheter, was such as she never before experienced, even in her confinements. Very soon after this, dribbling of her urine took place, which has continued ever since, with an almost constant scalding effect.

About six months previous to consulting me, this patient applied to a distinguished surgeon, of Augusta, Georgia, who performed several operations upon her, though without any material benefit. She next consulted a surgeon at Atlanta, who, after putting her upon the table, and giving her chloroform for an operation, declined performing it. Such was the discouraging account given by herself, upon applying to me.

Examination.—This revealed the existence of a fistulous opening, large enough to admit easily two fingers into the bladder. It was oval in shape, with its long axis transverse, and belonging to my fifth class, first variety.

Ten days after my first examination, I proceeded to operate, in the presence of Drs. Gaston and Norton, of Montgomery, and Dr. Johnson, of Notasulga, Alabama. Seven sutures were required to close the opening, these being carried through the anterior lip of the cervix uteri. The usual shaped button for this form of fistule, was used. (See figure 13, *op. cit.*)

Patient got on remarkably well, after the operation. Ninth day removed the suture apparatus, and found union perfect, all to a small point at the right hand angle, which, however, closed up in two or three days, without further trouble.

After getting up, there was a little incontinence of urine, and an inability to go longer than two or three hours without emptying the bladder. In both of these respects, however, there was a constant and rapid improvement.

About a month after the operation, our patient was discharged, with no incontinence of urine, but still an inability to go longer than three or four hours without emptying the bladder. This I was disposed to attribute to long disuse of the organ, and diminution of its cavity.

I very recently received a letter from my friend Dr. Deane, in relation to this case, it having been nearly two years since my operation. He states that the inability to retain the urine any great length of time still continues, and that, upon a thorough examination, he can report a permanent closure of the fistule.

Remarks.—Considering the nature and size of the fistulous opening, and the discouragement the patient had met with before applying to us, the result of our operation cannot be regarded otherwise than of the most satisfactory nature. Her inability to retain the urine as long as formerly, results from an unnatural cause, which is beyond the reach of art (diminution of the capacity of the bladder), and, therefore, should not be considered as lessening the fullest extent of success, to which we might with propriety lay claim.

CASE xxiii.— *Vesico-Vaginal Fistule; First application of the Button Suture successful.*—Mrs. T., of Elkton, Kentucky, consulted me, March the 25th, 1858, in relation to her case : æt. 26, rather large and fleshy, and, to all appearances, in the enjoyment of perfect health; states that she was confined at full term with her first child, February, 1856 ; was in labor only seventeen hours, and delivery natural; does not recollect of passing any urine during the time. After delivery it had to be drawn off with a catheter, which required to be kept up daily, for more than a week. Soon after leaving off the instrument, first noticed dribbling of the urine, which has continued unabated ever since. Three operations, she says, have been performed for closure of the fistule, but without affording her any relief whatever.

Examination.—Fistule was found to belong to my fourth class, first variety ; that is to say, it involved both the trigonus vesicalis and the root of the urethra. It was rather oval in shape, with its long axis corresponding to that of the vagina. Its edges were quite red, and very much thickened ; I suppose, from a quarter to a third of an inch of the urethra had sloughed away.

March 26th, I proceeded to operate in the usual manner (see *op. cit.*). In paring the edges, I took special care to so shape them that the line of approximation should be transverse to the urethra. This is a very important point, and should always be borne in mind in the management of cases belonging to this class. It is only when our sutures are introduced antero-posteriorly, in such cases, that we can produce an easy and natural coäptation of the parts, and, consequently, prevent an undue amount of traction, which would otherwise take place. The reverse of this was the plan followed by the surgeon who preceded me, and to this circumstance, I doubt not, is to be attributed his failures.

Four sutures were called for, two upon either side of the urethra. A button of the usual shape for this class of fistules, was used (see figure 10, *op. cit.*).

In the after treatment there was nothing worthy of note. On the ninth day, removed the suture apparatus, and had the satisfaction of finding perfect union throughout. In a few days, our patient got up and went about, as well as she ever was, having entire control over her urine.

Remarks.—This case, as well as the preceding one, illustrates, in a very striking degree, the fact that tedious and protracted labor is not always essential to the production of such accidents. In one, labor lasted only twenty-four hours, and in the other seventeen. Another fact too, worthy of note is, that in neither case were instruments employed.

CASE xxiv.—*Vesico-Vaginal Fistule of large size, requiring for its closure ten Sutures; First operation with the Button Suture successful.*—This patient, a colored girl, was very kindly sent to me for treatment by my friend Dr. W. P. Reese, of Selma, Alabama, March, 1858. She is about 28 years old, spare built, and rather delicate-looking ; states that the confinement at which she became the subject of the above injury occurred only six or eight weeks before, it being her eighth, and, this time, with twins. All previous labors had been easy. In the present instance, however, it was tedious, lasting about fifty-two hours. The first child was delivered naturally, about twenty-eight hours after the commencement of labor, and the second one by forceps, about twenty-four hours after this. Says that she passed but very little urine until after the birth of the first child, and then no more until after the delivery of the other. Soon after this, noticed that it was dribbling off, without her having any desire to pass it in the natural way.

Examination.—Fistule was found to belong to my fourth class, third variety. It was of enormous dimensions, admitting readily three fingers into the bladder. The fact is, nearly the whole of the septum, with at least a third of an inch of the urethra, had sloughed away. The chasm was almost circular, the transverse diameter being a little the longest.

April the 3d, operated upon the case. After paring the edges in the usual manner, ten sutures were found to be necessary. The uterus, in this instance, had to be pulled down, in order to close the opening, its anterior border being immovable. This step of the operation was easily effected, and perfect coäptation of the two denuded surfaces secured. (For a view of the button here employed, see figure 22, in the number of the Journal previously referred to.) After treatment the same as usual. Ninth day, removed suture apparatus, and found union of the parts throughout.

By way of experiment, I introduced, at my operation, two zinc wire sutures, one at each angle of the fistule. My object was to see what would be the effect of this metal on the tissues, as compared with that of silver. The result was anything but satisfactory. When I came to remove my button, I found both of these sutures so brittle that they could scarcely be withdrawn, and along the track of each there was considerable ulceration—more, indeed, than we would have expected from silk sutures. A small secondary fistule followed the use of each of these sutures, but, being very favorably situated, they both closed without my having to resort to another operation. Our patient was discharged a few weeks afterwards, entirely well, having complete control over her urine.

CASE XXV.—*Two Vesico-Vaginal and one Recto-Vaginal Fistules, complicated with Retroversion of the Uterus; all successfully closed with the Button Suture.*—While on a visit to this city, in January, 1858, I was requested by my distinguished friend Dr. Cartwright, to visit and examine a colored girl, belonging to Mr. Geo. Moore, of St. James parish. He stated that the girl had been under his treatment for a disease known as *Yaws*, of which she was almost, if not entirely relieved, but that there still existed the condition above stated, which he hoped I could do something for. A very accurate and interesting account of the case, and its treatment while under his charge, may be seen by reference to the number of this Journal for July of last year. The history of the case, upon coming under my care, is as follows : Mary, æt. 30, under medium size, and rather delicately formed; states that she has had six children, the first at the age, of fifteen, and the last at twenty-three, when she sustained her present injuries. Labor, this time, lasted forty-eight hours, and during the time she passed but little if any urine. The child's head being unusually large, and the circumstances of the case demanding it, the physician in attendance thought it advisable to resort to instruments. Craniotomy was accordingly performed, and delivery effected in the usual manner. The next day she discovered dribbling of the urine, and very soon after this, its entire passage through the vagina took place; and so it has continued to the present time. Patient is somewhat reduced in flesh, and has the appearance of one who has endured great suffering. Menstruation is scanty, and very irregular.

Examination.—The patient, on being placed in the usual position, upon her knees and elbows, and the speculum introduced into the vagina, my attention was first called to a change in the relationship of the parts ; indeed, so great was this that I could form no conception of the nature of the injury I was in search of. There was the most complete retroversion of the uterus I had ever seen. The fundus rested very low down, between the posterior wall of the vagina and the rectum, with the cervix turned into the bladder through the fistulous opening, and presenting upwards. The organ appeared to me to be almost entirely reversed. To restore the organ, now to its proper position, I found to be highly necessary for a further and satisfactory examination of the parts involved. This end I attained by passing a blunt hook through the fistulous opening and along the cervix, until I could hitch it in the os uteri. This having been accomplished, I then drew the cervix downwards and backwards, at the same time, with a probang resting against the fundus of the organ, I forced this upwards and forwards, thus causing it to assume its normal position. Both the anterior and posterior walls of the vagina could now be clearly seen, in their proper relationship with the apertures in them. The recto-vaginal opening I had not before suspected, my attention not having been called specially to it by the patient. It was situated just below the posterior lip of the cervix uteri, almost circular in shape, and of a size sufficient to admit of a No. 8 bougie. It admitted the passage of a large portion of the fæces into the vagina, when in a fluid state.

On the other side now of the vaginal canal there were to be seen two vesical openings, both quite large. One situated in the *bas fond* of the bladder, and the other, the trigonus vesicalis, and separated from each other by a narrow bridge of the septum, say half an inch wide. Each one measured upwards of an inch in its transverse diameter, and was rather oval in shape. Seeing now that the intervening substance was not of sufficient width to allow of the opposite sides of both openings being attached to it, I concluded to remove it entirely, thus converting both fistules into one which would belong to the third variety of my fourth class. This little operation I easily performed with a pair of curved scissors; there resulted from it considerable hæmorrhage, however, which I had some trouble in arresting. The next thing I did after this was to introduce a large tube into the vagina for the purpose of keeping the uterus in its place, which it did most effectually. This was removed every day, and the vagina syringed out with cold water. Under this preparatory treatment, our patient was soon ready for the operation of closure of the fistulous openings.

March 16th, every thing being in pretty favorable condition, I proceeded to operate upon the vesico-vaginal fistule in the usual manner. After the paring was done, nine sutures were found to be necessary. Upon approximating the two sides of the opening, the line thus formed showed itself to be somewhat semi-circular, its con-cavity presenting upwards and its convexity downwards. In addition to this, the surface on which our button was to stand was undulating. In accordance with these peculiarities of the parts it had to be formed and adjusted. In the first place it was made semi-circular, and then grooved and floored upon its edges in the ordinary manner. The line of perforations was made to correspond to the line of approxi-mation, and thereby binding it upon its convexity and twisting it in several ways, it was made to conform to the inequalities of the parts upon which it was to stand. The whole adjustment was easily and quickly done, and the apparatus when secured in place set most beautifully.

There was nothing which required to be noted in the after treat-ment, excepting a slight leakage, which was noticed after the third day, indicating that a partial failure of the operation, at least, had to be looked for.

On the ninth day I removed the suture apparatus, and sure enough found the line of union incomplete. At the right hand angle there remained an opening not larger than a pin's head. About half an inch from this there was another one of about the same size. Through these little openings, after the button was removed, a considerable quantity of urine escaped.

Another operation therefore was called for, and in planning this, I resolved to attempt closure not only of these fistules, but the recto-vaginal also. Accordingly on the 3d of April, I operated. Two sutures were employed for each of the vesico-vaginal openings, and three for the recto-vaginal.

On the eighth day removed the suture apparatus, but found only one of the vesical openings completely closed; the other, and the rectal opening partially so only. The former failed, I was disposed to think, from imperfect paring, the light having been very bad at the time of our operation. The urine escaping through this, found its way beneath the button on the rectal opening, and thus prevented this from closing. Another operation, therefore, was called for, which I performed after waiting a suitable length of time.

Our patient now was not in a favorable condition for the operation, her general health being somewhat impaired. Both openings, at this sitting, were closed.

Upon removing suture apparatus on the eighth day, I found another failure. The vesical opening was greatly reduced in size, but the other opening was about the same. Our patient after this was sent to the country to recuperate her health. So soon as this took place, strange to say, the small vesical opening closed spontaneously, leaving the patient with entire control over her urine. Only the rectal opening now remained, and at another operation this was closed, and the cure of our patient thereby completed.

Remarks.—I have detailed this case at length, even risking being considered tedious, to state all the circumstances connected with its management. It is, I think, interesting in several respects. The existence of two fistulous openings, involving nearly the whole of the vesico-vaginal septum, and their complication with recto-vaginal fistule and retrocession of the uterus, the difficulty experienced in obtaining a complete result, the final cure after so many years of suffering, are all points of no ordinary interest. Our first operation, considering the size of the fistule and the tendency of the cervix uteri to fall through it into the bladder, was, it must be admitted, attended with a highly satisfactory result. The two small points that remained unclosed were doubtless owing to imperfect paring, not to any cutting out of the sutures or imperfect adaptation of other parts of the apparatus. Our failure, at subsequent operations to close these small openings, as well as the one in the bowel, is such that every surgeon may expect now and then to meet with. One who is constantly operating is liable to become careless in attending to small matters, which frequently leads to unfavorable results when it might not otherwise have happened. I am not exempt from this fault myself, and I think if I had taken a little more pains with my operations in this case, I would not now be under the necessity of recording my two failures.

Case xxvi.—*One Urethra-Vaginal and Two Vesico-Vaginal Fistules, with great Contraction of the Vagina; Failure of the " Clamp Suture;" Case that led to the adoption of the Button Suture; Closure of all the Fistules; Relapse; Case finally discharged uncured.*—Matilda, colored girl, property of Col. M. Stamper, of Early county, Ga., was put under my care February, 1855. Æt. about 21; short, heavy built and stout; was confined with her first child in 1850. Says that she was in labor about two days; child was removed with instruments; does not recollect anything about passing urine during labor; very soon afterwards first noticed it dribbling from her without having any desire or ability to pass it in the natural way; was for several months confined to bed, and during this time had great soreness of the parts. Amenorrhœa now; general health somewhat impaired.

Examination.—Found the vagina very much contracted by indurated bands extending across it. One just below the cervix uteri occasioned such narrowing of the canal that the point of the index finger could scarcely be passed through it. On the posterior side of the organn the induration and contraction were greatest, giving rise here to considerable shortening of the canal and drawing in the labium of one side. Communicating with the urethra very near the meatus, there was a small opening; further back, just across the beginning or root of the urethra was situated another, about three-quarters of an inch in length, and of course communicating with the bladder. About half an inch above this last and to the extreme right was situated still another opening, about the same size. These two last, one having its longest diameter transverse and the other longitudinal, represented two sides of a square.

In attempting now to pass a catheter through the urethra into the bladder, I found great difficulty, owing to distortion at its neck, caused by the anterior border of the fistule situated there being drawn up to the pubic bones.

Having considered now the case in all its bearings, I determined to make an application of Dr. Sims's "clamp suture," this being the suture at that time I was employing. Before proceeding to the operation, however, the question arose in my mind as to the possibility of closing both of the vesical openings at once by two sets of clamps, this appearing to me to be the preferable course. Upon a minute examination now of the parts with reference to the practicability of such a procedure, I was convinced that it could not be done, owing to the narrowness of the intervening tissue upon which both sets of clamps would have to rest. Thus applied, one of each set of clamps would necessarily cross the other. Seeing this difficulty, therefore, I determined upon the only alternative, which was to close one opening at a time. The upper one I selected for my first operation, thinking by this to avoid to some extent the irritating effect of the urine passing through the lower opening. As a preparatory measure now for this operation, I had to make deep incisions in the contracting bands of the vagina, and then dilate the organ by the use of tents. This took up considerable time, and was the cause of much suffering to the patient, owing to the excessive irritability of the parts.

Operation.—March the 23d, 1855, everything being as favorable as we could expect under the circumstances, the operation above indicated was performed. Owing to the great induration and contraction of the parts, I encountered no little difficulty in going through with the different stages. Three sutures were required to close the opening after its edges were thoroughly pared. These being introduced, transversely of course, the clamps were applied and secured as Dr. Sims directs. The edges of the opening came together well enough, but they were not accurately adapted to each other, owing to a greater thickness of one than the other, and the consequent elevation of the corresponding clamp above its fellow.

With this condition of things our patient was put to bed and a catheter introduced into the bladder to convey off as much of the urine as possible. Very little of it, however, passed through the instrument; it continued its old course through the vagina. The clamps were allowed to remain the usual length of time. When I came to remove them I had no need of scissors. The whole concern had sloughed out and lay loose in the fistulous opening, now greatly enlarged.

The result of this operation thoroughly satisfied me that I should never be able to close successively the fistulous openings in this case. The whole failure I, attributed to the poisonous effect of the urine upon the denuded edges of the fistule and the raw surfaces caused by the embedding of the clamps. So well was I convinced of this fact that I should have discharged the patient without ever making another trial, had not the idea fortunately occurred to me of protection to the approximated edges of one fistule from the irritating effect of the urine passing through the other. From this thought, scarcely need I say, the principle of our button suture originated and was put into practice. Although the principle of protection was suggested to me as above stated by the peculiarities of this case, yet the first trial of it was not made here. Having at the time other cases ready for operation, I applied the principle in them. From the great success I had with it in these cases, I was now encouraged to believe that I would soon be able to effect a cure in this one. So accordingly I commenced a course of treatment preparatory to an operation. This consisted in making daily incisions into the indurated bands, and then dilating the vagina as far as was practicable, as I did before my first operation with the clamps. Although, after several months' perseverance I succeeded in dilating the parts pretty well, still there remained great hardness and a disposition of them to return to their former condition. I took advantage of a favorable opportunity, however, and operated, selecting again the upper fistule.

After paring the edges thoroughly, three sutures were called for, and a button of the ordinary shape. Everything did as well as could be expected under the circumstances. On the ninth day, removed the suture apparatus, and was delighted to find union complete. Upon examination of the parts, several days afterwards, however, I discovered that the newly-formed cicatrix, at its lower extremity, had given way—in short, there was a partial re-production of the fistulous opening. This was my twelfth operation with the button suture, and I may add, my first failure with it.

My next operation was to close this small fistule, which had been re-produced, and the one just across the root of the urethra, which I did under one button. Four sutures were required for the lower one and two for the upper. The former were introduced antero-posteriorly, and the latter transversely. A single button, as above stated, was used for both fistules. The case progressed very well to the ninth day, when we removed the suture apparatus. We now found that the upper opening had failed to close, and the lower one had closed only partially, the failure being at the right hand extremity. After this operation, there was considerable irritation, and some ulcerative inflammation of the vaginal mucous membrane, occasioned by a more acrid condition of the urine.

I next concluded to try the urethral opening. This, it will be recollected, was situated very near the meatus urinarius. The narrow bridle separating the one from the other, I laid open as a preliminary step, and then treated it as an ordinary rent, employing my peculiar form of button for this injury. (See figure 9, in the article previously referred to).

Upon removing the suture apparatus on the eighth day, I found union of the parts so near complete that I considered our operation successful. Only the two small vesical openings, both the result of partial failures, now remained. These I worked upon in good earnest, hoping to obtain a complete result in spite of the ulcerative inflammation now and then set up, and the tendency of the vagina to recontract. Operation after operation I performed, with varying success, until finally the last one was closed, and our patient pronounced cured. Our consolation at this gratifying result, however, was of short duration. Four or five days had scarcely elapsed before ulcerative inflammation of the vagina supervened, and partially destroyed the cicatrix of the last fistule closed. By this unfortunate result, urine was again allowed to pass into the vagina, which now appeared more acrid or irritating in its effects than ever. Months were required now to subdue this inflammatory action, and to overcome the contraction of the organ, which followed as a consequence. During this period, the patient's general health suffered very much.

Still not discouraged at the above unfortunate results, I concluded to renew my operations; believing, however, that there was considerable doubt as to my ever being able to effect a permanent cure, owing to this proneness of the parts to take on morbid action. After this, every operation, or even an incision made in the dilating process, would be followed by the peculiar form of inflammation which we have mentioned. Instead now of advancing our patient towards a cure, the reverse was observed. Every effort of ours, seemingly, was attended with a loss of ground, until finally one cicatrix after another yielded to destructive morbid action, and our patient was placed where we started with her. In this condition I discharged her, April, 1858, she having been under treatment something over three years. I performed in all, according to my recollection, ten operations.

Remarks.—This is one of the two cases referred to as being still under treatment, in the concluding remarks of my article, published in the *North American Medico-Chirurgical Review* for July, 1857. The case I have reported here at length, for the reason that I am desirous of recording, in regular order, my unsuccessful as well as my successful operations. The result, as above shown, is, I conceive, by far more interesting, in a practical point of view, than if it had been ever so successful. It certainly illustrates, in the most striking manner, some of the difficulties to be encountered in practice, and the perseverance that is sometimes necessary to overcome them.

Again, I may say, the case is interesting in other respects. First, it was its peculiarity of triple fistules which first caused me to see the imperfection of the so-called clamp suture, and to lead me to the adoption of our protective principle, or button suture. Secondly, the case is interesting as being the first in which the latter form of suture had failed in my hands, this being the twelfth application of it. Thirdly, the case is remarkable as being the only one I ever discharged uncured, when a fair trial of the button suture had been made.

(To be continued.)

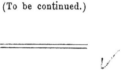

ART. IX.—*Researches into Animal Heat :* By BENNET DOWLER, M. D.

ANIMAL heat possesses paramount interest and significance for the physiologist, the pathologist, and organic chemist. Its physical or chemical exposition upon the Lavoisierian theory of oxygen has long occupied the medical mind as a fundamental study. It is not intended in this paper to examine at length either this or any other theory, but to give a hasty outline, chiefly of a numerical aspect, relating to experiments made more than sixteen years ago, showing the temperature of the human body before and after death from yellow fever. If space, time, and the printer's progress will permit, perhaps, some other data of later date may be referred to in this relation.

These researches during the last sixteen years have been repeated, varied, and greatly extended with unwearied patience and diligence. The special details of later and more complete data (many of which have been published), will on this occasion be omitted. The data now produced were originally transmitted to, not published in, *The Western Journal of Medicine and Surgery* (printed in Louisville), during the winter of 1843–4, but were returned to me, unpublished, with a request that I should make an abstract from the same, as the original documents were alleged to be, and with reason, too voluminous for admission into a monthly Journal. Whatever value they then possessed, they still possess, undiminished by age.

The reader will, therefore, bear in mind that neither the special histories upon which the following tables are founded, nor the tables themselves, were published in the journal referred to, excepting one table of only six lines, which has been extensively copied. I transmitted a short abstract together with some numerical analyses, to that periodical, taken from the returned papers, already mentioned, one of which bears date in March, and the other in July, 1844, both of which appeared in the same year ; the first in the June, and the last in the October number of the journal, and will serve to fix these dates beyond the possibility of dispute. To the same journal, I had fortunately, in a previous year, contributed several papers entitled "Post Mortem Researches," and "Contributions to Morbid Anatomy," including experiments on muscular contractility, the capillary circulation, etc., the dates of which have, since that period, served to settle questions of priority, and have led to honorable retractions and corrections worthy of commendation, especially as experience has often shown, in medical history at least, that abstractions which no one can clearly conceive, nor refute, nor prove, have nevertheless for generations swayed men's minds more than the great land marks of facts, documents, and dates, whenever the latter conflict with a cherished theory.

To give a tabular classification of pathological and biotic data, is peculiarly difficult, owing to the occult nature, apparent variation and instability of the phenomena themselves. Numerical tabulation restricted as it is to a few salient points of observation, excludes continuous details, progressive developments, and the enumeration of the modifying influences incidental to vital and morbid actions, remedial measures, etc. The natural history or course of disease, even where copious details are admissible, is seldom witnessed and studied apart from the complications which the remedial elements, as blood-lettings, cathartics, tonics, stimulants, baths and the like, introduce among those which are strictly pathological. In reporting cases, it is often a matter of difficulty and always one of importance to determine what and how much, may be omitted in detail as being non-essential.

In observing and recording complex facts and data, such as are now under consideration, the most careful and conscientious historian is liable to errors of commission and omission, which, however, are of little importance when the experiments and observations are very numerous.

In some instances in the data which follow, the temperature of the air was not actually taken upon the spot where the experiments upon the living and dead were made ; but was taken from other sources, or estimated at intervals between the known thermometrical data of the day. Many original records concerning age, sex, race, and so forth, have been intentionally omitted, as being not only cumbrous, but of little value for, or rather incompatible with the scope and the purposes of the tables which follow. The methods of procedure, which are of much importance, having been fully explained in former papers in this and other journals, cannot be repeated in this place. Nor is it intended to enunciate at length, formal propositions, arguments, and doctrines which have a bearing either upon the normal · origin, or pathological aberrations of animal heat.

In investigations of this kind there may perhaps be some readers who think life too short, art too long, time too precious, and patience too limited, to study the prolonged and minute history of cases, facts, and processes, being content with the consideration of the conclusions or results of the whole ; while another class, being unwilling to accept conclusions without scrutinizing all of their antecedent data and the routes pursued in an investigation, deem details of fundamental importance in a science which can advance only by experimental progress and cumulative processes. Such is medicine. The ability to observe, compare, classify, and apply medical facts and reasonings exists in various degrees. Even those who possess in the highest degree this knowledge, may find it difficult, perhaps impossible, to impart it to others, particularly by writing. It is often equally difficult to know what to omit as unimportant and non-essential, and what to record as necessary elements of the case—that is to say, significant facts. As a general rule, it is best for the observer in making his original histories to record minutiæ, though they may seem of little value or relevancy. These, at his leisure, and in the further progress of his experience, after having made numerous records, he can revise and eliminate, so as reduce pages to paragraphs without omitting necessary facts pertinent to the history. It is, in truth, often more difficult in this way, to make a short essay or treatise than a long one. At first view it seems to be labor lost to write what only a few will read, whether this be owing to indifferentism on the one hand, or to the author's prolixity on the other. The writer who seeks refuge in the brevity of arithmetical tables can

26

hardly expect to attract readers who wish to trace vital or pathological facts by their peculiar individuality, as well as in their points of contact, parallelism and identity. Numerism, in its practical application to the medical sciences, is liable to errors incidental to the classification of very complex and variable phenomena as analogous or identical. Imperfection clings to all methods. Nevertheless general results of great certainty are often obtained by this method, to which no other can lay claim.

TABLE I.—Showing the temperature* of the primary period of Yellow Fever in persons who recovered.

History. No.	Age.	Hours sick.	Air.	*Hand.	Axilla.	OBSERVATIONS.
69	27	3½	88 °	102°	106 °	V. S., *ad del.*, cured in six days.
71	28	20	84	102	105	V. S., *ad del.*, well in six days.
91	24	8	83	101	103	V. S., *ad del.*, well in seven days.
74	30	9	88	100	106½	Cured in thirty-eight days.
76	...	5	88	102	104	Intermit. type, well in eight d'ys.
77	30	12	86	105	105	Cured in six days, V. S., *ad del.*
80	25	13	86	102	104	Cured in seven days.
86	24	14	89	102	104	Cured in ten days.
92	27	13½	88	102	104	Cured in twenty days.
79	21	16	88	107	107	Cured in seven days.
83	28	19	70	102	104	Cured in three days.
75	29	22	88	102	104	V. S. *deliq.*, well in four days.
87	25	28	88	102	106	Cured nine days after.
90	23	26½	81	102	104	V. S., *ad del.*, cured in 14 days.
95	41	48	82	99	102	
96	30	48	85	98	104	V. S., *deliq.*, conval. in one day.
98	22	48	80	104	106	
100	21	48	91½	.....	102	Next day conval.
103	28	48	85	97	103	Next day conval.
104	26	48	81	105	.....	Cured in ten days.
105	29	48	84	97	102	Cured in six days.
72	23	60	86	.....	103	Cured in seven days.
180	34	24	83	99	102	
84	31	14	70	95	102	Cured in twenty days.
Mean.	25·5	26.81	81·3°	101·22°	104·12°	

* These experiments were made with Réaumer's thermometer, the degrees of which are reduced to those of Fahrenheit, without giving the decimal fractions or minute differences between the degrees of the two scales. The thermometers which I invented and subsequently used, are incomparably better for easy application, rapid movement, and minute division of degrees.

TABLE II.—*Showing the temperature of the middle period of Yellow Fever in those who recovered.*

History. No.	Age.	Days sick.	Air.	Hand.	Axilla.	OBSERVATIONS.
165	30	6	85°	106°	108½°	Third day convalescent.
69	27	2	85	102	105	
74	30	1½	86	99	105	
......	...	2½	86	102	102	
75	29	2	85	100	102	Cured in three days.
94	34	4	86	102	104	Cured in ten days.
......	...	5	86	......	102	
101	21	2	85	97	103	Cured in nine days.
104	26	6	85	97½	100	Cured in five days.
182	24	14	60	100	104	
......	...	16	58	106	106	
106	24	8	86	97	102	Cured iu thirty days.
166	29	5	83	102	109	Cured in twelve days.
107	38	4	87	100	102	Cured in two days.
108	23	4	90	100	104	Cured in fifteen days
156	19	16	88	104	104	Convalescent in five days.
109	38	4	84	102	104	Cured in nine days.
157	38	12	84	95	102	Recovery in fifty days.
111	27	4	80	99	104	Convalescent in four days.
162	22	9	75	103	104	Cured in twenty-eight days.
113	34	5	82	99	100	Cured in six days.
117	20	4	86	97	100	Cured in five days.
174	82	7	75	100	103	Cured in ten days.
118	24	5	85	99	100	Cured in six days.
120	32	6	86	100	102	Conval. in six days.
122	22	3	88	100	108	
126	22	4	75	100	104	Conval. in four days.
127	20	4	80	100	107	Cured in four days.
131	25	6	80	107	107	Cured in eight days.
135	28	6	86	102	.102	Cured in seven days.
138	30	8	88	101	●102	Cured in five days.
139	18	7	86	102	104	
144	21	9	80	101	102	Cured in sixteen days.
147	23	...	80	97	101	Cured in twelve days.
148	27	4	90	104	108	Cured in seven days.
149	85	12	81	91	102	
150	22	7	82	93	100	Cured in six days.
152	18	11	85	102	102	Cured in four days.
155	24	9	80	94	97	Cured in ten days
95	41	2	82	99	102	
Mean.	26·94	5·92	82·52°	100·42°	103·11°	

TABLE III.—*Showing the temperature of the period of convalescence in Yellow Fever patients.*

History. No.	Days sick.	Air.	Hand.	Axilla.
76	2	85 °	100°	99°
69	5	84	96	100
71	3	83	100	102
74	4	85	93	99
...	5	82	91	97
77	4½	86	99	98
79	2½	75	86	97½
80	1½	83	97	100
94	9	86	...	97
104	7	83	97½	83
106	9	91	94	100
134	6	90	95	99
139	8	83	96	99
...	9	85	93	95
148	5	86	...	95
149	16	...	97	98
150	10	83	100	100
162	18	74	95	98
163	8	90½	...	102
164	7	87½	97½	101
167	8	86	99	101
180	1	83	98½	102
183	...	85	100	102
95	2	80	98	100
122	5	72	95	97
Mean.	6.5	82°	96°	98 46°

TABLE IV.—Showing the temperature of the primary period of those who died of Yellow Fever.

History. No.	Hours sick.	Air.	Hand.	Axilla.	OBSERVATIONS.
1	12	86°	102°	105°	
56	12	85	103	107	
70	12½	80	105	105	Died in seven days.
78	24	82	104	107	Died in four days.
85	28	75	107	107	
88	15	89	.....	102	
...	37	90	97	102	
89	26	86	104	109	
93	29	85	107	109	
97	34	74	103	104	
99	42	85	97	102	
73	24	88	99	100	Died in two days.
Mean.	24·62	83·75°	102·54°	104·91°	

TABLE V.—Showing the temperature of Yellow Fever, in the middle period, of those who died.

History. No.	Days sick.	Air.	Hand.	Axilla.	OBSERVATIONS.
88	1	86°	95°	104°	
6	5	88	101	104	
2	5	82	97	102	
1	3½	80	100	105	
97	5¼	74	100	105	Died in three days,
102	2	86	100	102	Died in four days.
110	4	84	104	107	Died in three days.
121	3	85	100	104	Died in three days.
123	4	86	102	105	
.....	5	84	91	102	
130	6	88	100	105	
130	6	80	102	105	A relapse.
132	7	85	98	100	Died in four days.
136	8	89	93	99	Died in three days.
146	5	80	99	104	
178	8	70	102	102	
.....	12	75	106½	105	
73	1	88	99	100	
142	6	81	100	104	Died in two days.
123	7	84	91	102	Died in three days.
175	7	75	101	104	
177	8 ·	70	102	102	
.....	12	75	105	106½	
.....	14	73	101½	103	Died in three days.
99	6	...	99	.....	Died in three days.
Mean.	6·04	81·16°	99·4°	103·89°	

TABLE VI.—Showing the temperature in the fatal stage of Yellow Fever, with some account of the respiratory action.

Hist. No.	Hours bef. d'th.	Air.	Hand.	Axilla	
151	10	81°	101 °	102 °	Resp. quick and uneasy.
2	24	87	95	104	Resp. quick.
153	8	90	...	101	Coma; seven inspirations per minute.
3	1	89	91	100	Resp. loud, heaving.
4	1½	88	94	100	Resp. noisy, quick, laborious,
158	6	85	89	100	Resp. noisy, slow.
5	2¼	77	70	95	
159	9	80	94	100	Resp. imperfect, quick, irregular.
7	21¼	71	95	100	Resp. noisy.
8	21½	79	104	106	Resp. irregular.
161	11½	75	81	90	
113	11	79	88	100	Resp. quick, wheezing; coma.
145	10	75	84	95	Resp. easy.
15	7½	79	86	97	Resp. laborious, irregular.
141	12	85	95	102	Stertor; coma.
33	11	80	89	95	Resp. quick and irregular.
160	12	82	...	99	Resp. noisy, quick, laborious.
35	6	86	83	.....	Resp. imperfect, small, unequal, quiet.
161	7	...	81	90	Resp. extremely laborious, gasping, suf.
41	26½	84	104	105	Coma: stertor.
43	24	90	...	100	Resp. hurried; coma.
45	21½	89	97	104	Coma; stertor.
46	23	89	89	98	Resp. quick.
48	1	82	84	95	Resp. slow, loud, heaving.
178	67½	73	101½	103	Resp. imperfect.
60	5¼	84	100	101	Resp. quick and irregular.
179	12	80	102	102	Resp. quick.
88	40	86	...	97	Resp. quick.
112	24	81	89	100	Resp. loud, laborious, rattling; coma.
181	1	75	...	102	Resp. loud, puffing.
114	2	74	...	100	Resp. loud, quick; coma.
173	48	82	88½	97½	Resp. quick, puerile.
115	2½	74	89	99	Resp. stertorous; coma.
116	24	86	93	97	Resp. hurried, unequal.
119	28	86	102	104	Resp. easy.
123	72	71	88	101	Resp. quick, but easy.
168	5	87	...	95	Resp. rapid, small.
124	9	83	...	98	Resp. hurried, suffocative.
125	4½	71	89	97	Resp. easy.
128	24	80	91	101	Resp. imperfect—thirteen per minute.
170	24	65	88½	102	Resp. wheezing, puffing, rattling, cough.
129	2	89	93	97	Resp. irregular, laborious, quick.
133	24	82	66	95	Resp. quick, puerile.
137	12	70	93	101	Resp. quick, puerile, loud.
140	12	90	...	100	Resp. hurried.
169	30	87	104	106½	Resp. hurried.
.....	4	83	102	104	
171	6	71	...	96	Resp. short, imperfect.
143	12	81	100	101	Resp. 57; coma.
154	24	85	100	103	Resp. stertorous—comatose.
158	5	85	89	100	Resp. noisy, slow.
Mean.	16·01	81·24°	92·25°	99.56°	

POST MORTEM SERIES.

TABLE VII.—Showing the Post Mortem Heat of regions.

History No.	Time Dead when Obs. Began H's.	M.	Time Obs. Lasted H.	M.	Air.	Axilla.	Thigh.	Rectum.	Perineum.	Pelvis and Abdomen.	Liver.	Epigast.	Chest.	Heart.	Brain.
2	...	10	4	8	90½°	109°	113°	.....	......	......	112°	111°	......	109°	....
3	...	5	2	...	89	107	107	105°	......	106°	106	105	106°	104	....
4	...	30	...	33	88	104	.....	102	102	......	......	103	......	......	102
5	...	15	1	5	79	102	102	104	......	......	......	101	100	100	....
6	...	5	...	31	70	106	102	......	......	......	......	106	......	......	101
7	...	10	1	...	71	96	98	......	......	......	......	90	97½	......	93
8	...	•50	1	...	82	103	102	......	......	......	......	104	......	......	100
9	3	•...	2	...	80	101	100	100	......	......	102	101	......	......	95
16	1	...	1	9	82	103	104	......	......	......	108	104	97	......	99
17	...	10	1	51	80	106	108	......	......	......	......	106	......	...	101
19	...	10	2	20	84	106	107	......	......	......	......	109	......	......	....
20	3	...	...	51	85	106	105	......	......	......	......	109	107	......	....
21	2	...	2	...	80	102	103	......	......	......	......	104	103	......	....
22	...	20	1	40	90	106	106½	......	104	......	......	106	105	......	....
23	...	30	...	45	86	108	100	......	......	......	......	105	......	......	....
24	3	...	...	10	82	106	.....	105	......	......	......	......	......	......	....
25	1	...	2	...	84	106	106	......	......	......	......	106	106	......	....
26	...	30	...	33	90	108	.....	......	106	......	......	......	......	......	....
27	2	...	1	41	91	.....	103	102	......	......	......	104	101	......	....
29	...	5	1	8	86	104	108	104	......	......	......	106	103	......	....
30	...	15	1	45	88	104	106	......	......	......	......	109	......	106	....
31	...	15	2	...	89	104	106	109	......	......	......	108	104	103	....
34	1	30	...	20	82	104	......	104	......	......	102	105	......	......	....
36	...	15	1	45	82	102	104	101	......	102	105	104	102	99	....
38	...	20	3	20	83	108	109	......	104	107	104	109	104	......	....
39	2	...	1	30	80	105	......	104	......	......	......	105	......	......	....
40	2	30	3	50	86	109	......	107	109	107	107	105	102	102	....
41	...	30	1	4	83	107	108	......	......	106	......	109	102	102	....
42	...	30	1	40	87	105	......	104	104	107	......	104	104	......	....
43	...	1	4	...	90	103	102	......	102	104	104	104	105	105	....
45	...	30	4	...	90	106½	......	111	109	......	......	......	......	......	....
46	1	...	3	...	89	103	......	102	104	......	......	......	......	......	....
47	...	15	4	45	86	107	109	......	104	106½	109	108	106½	106½	....
48	...	15	1	...	82	102	100	......	......	......	......	102	......	......	....
49	...	15	2	..	84	104	103	107	......	......	......	110	......	......	....
51	...	10	...	...	85	107	107	......	......	......	......	107	104	......	....
52	...	10	...	26	85	103	104	......	......	......	......	......	102	......	....
53	...	5	...	17	75	107	107	......	......	......	......	......	......	......	....
54	...	30	...	20	87	100	100	......	......	100	......	......	102	......	....
55	2	...	...	35	84	100	......	98	......	......	......	......	......	......	....
56	...	25	...	55	85	103	......	102	101	......	......	......	......	......	....
57	...	5	...	12	90	106	......	106	......	......	......	......	......	......	....
58	...	10	...	36	85	103	104	......	......	......	......	102	......	102	....
Mean.	...	58½	1	32	84.4°	104.44°	104.71°	104.05	104.45	105.05	106.33	105.48	102.95	103.5	98

TABLE VIII.—Showing the decline of post mortem heat, the antagonism of the surrounding media or incipient reginal refrigeration the fore-runners of putrefaction.

History No.	Time Dead When Obs. Began. H.	M.	Duration of Experi'nt. H.	M.	Air.	Epigast.	Lungs.	Heart.	Liver.	Rectum and Pelvis.	Thigh.	Axilla.	Brain.	OBSERVATIONS.
38	3	20	...	40	81°	104°	104°	...	...	104°	...	...	...	Buttock a little flattened; cornea opaque.
40	4	50	1	10	86	105	...	102°	107°	102°	99°	...	...	Rigid except the neck; abdomen a little convex.
44	4	...	...	15	82	100	93	...	...	...	92	...	...	Jaws rigid; limbs supple; eyelids non-elastic.
61	10	...	...	9	90	93	...	...	...	...	103	...	...	Cornea brilliant; muscles powerfully contractile; ab-
49	2	...	...	10	84	106	104	...	...	...	88	...	...	Rigid except the neck. [domen depressed; supple.
51	3	...	...	15	85	...	...	...	...	...	...	88¼	86°	Eyes natural; rigid only in the neck; muscular con-
11	5	...	...	28	66	93	...	...	...	...	99	...	...	[tractility; abdomen depressed.
10	4	30	...	30	70	100	97	...	...	...	89	...	98	Cornea and pupils natural; limber; abdomen de- [pressed.
12	12	...	...	55	79	92	91	91	...	91	93	...	84	Rigid except the neck; abdomen concave; putrid odors; [marbled hues.
13	11	...	...	25	80	96	...	93	...	...	93	...	85	Abdomen concave; body rigid except the neck.
28	6	...	...	8	91	102	...	...	...	...	100	...	...	Limbs rigid.
32	3	...	...	20	86	104	...	...	...	...	100	100	...	Rigid; abdomen a little convex; faint putrefactive odor.
33	18	...	...	10	80	95	...	...	...	...	93	100	...	Neck and legs supple; arms rigid; marbled.
89	6	...	...	20	80	103	...	...	...	...	100	...	...	Rigid.
68	15	...	...	30	86	92	91	...	...	...	87	...	84	Rigid except the neck.
14	10	...	...	20	80	91	...	87	...	...	86	...	84	Partly dissected before observation.
18	3	...	1	...	61	84	80	...	86	...	84	...	30	
Mean.	6	48	...	27	86.29	97.5	94.28	93.25	96.5	99	94.26	96.8	85.33	

TABLE IX.—Showing the coincidence of temperature between the dead body and the atmosphere at the period of incipient putrefaction.

Hist. No.	Hours Dead.	Temp. of room.	Epiga-strium.	L'ngs.	Brain.	Axilla.	Thigh.	OBSERVATIONS.
1	16	87°	89°	89°	...	...	89°	Abdomen spotted greenish, distended with gas; cornea glassy, relaxed; neck limber; arms rigid.
8	28	90	92	92	...	...	88	Neck supple; legs rigid; arms becoming limber; foetid gas in the abdomen.
15	14	80	88	84	78	...	81	Neck only limber; marbled; abdomen concave; foetid scent.
29	19	86	89	89	...	...	86	
33	18	88	95	...	...	...	93	
86	27	86	86	...	...	...	82	Cornea depressed; abdomen convex; green discolorations of the groins and neck.
59	20	91	91	...	74	...	91	Arms, neck and spine limber; legs rigid; cornea lustreless; abdomen convex, green.
60	16	71	...	...	...	...	88	Neck limber; abdomen and intestines greenish; four hours after, skin turned green.
61	10	90	93	...	...	...	92	The neck only limber; slight abdominal convexity; in an hour, the arms relaxed.
62	15	90	93	...	...	...	88	Neck limber; abdomen convex; green at the flanks; rigidity soon disappeared.
63	15	86	92	91	...	...	87	Abdomen undistended; universal rigidity.
64	19	88	91	...	...	...	88	Abdomen concave; groins green; rigid.
65	18	88	90	...	...	...	88	Belly green and distended, emitting foetid gas.
66	22	90	90	...	...	...	...	Supple, except the legs; abdominal convexity and greenness; putrefactive odor.
67	12	70	...	...	...	86	...	Skin blue; cuticle everywhere loose; abdomen depressed; neck limber; red stripes.
68	6	91	...	...	...	91	...	
176	24	54½	...	...	83	...	56¾	Abdomen depressed; neck supple; arms a little so; legs rigid.
188	17¾	83	65¾	...	81¼	...	89	
....	...	94	82	...	81¼	82½	79	
Mean.	17·04	84·39°	88·11°	89°	79·12°	86·5°	85·35°	

Complete, or even partial refrigeration of the dead body, with or without congelation, must, upon physical principles (independently of endosmotic action), obliterate or change certain anatomical lesions, especially such as congestion, vascular injection, color, etc. The death-rigidity probably contributes to these conditions. In the living economy, the application of cold, as all know, produces striking changes. Cold air produces contraction, pallor, goose-flesh (cutis anserina), shrivelling of the skin. Cold feet and hands, as well as the whole surface of the body, during the cold stage of an inter-mittent and the collapse of cholera, present marked changes, with appearances of anæmia or bloodlessness; while, on the other hand, the immersion of the feet in a hot foot-bath produces expansion and distension of the bloodvessels, capillary congestion, and rubefacient redness, simulating inflammation. Cold acts on the dead body in an inverse manner. Refrigeration, which proceeds from the surface to the centre, contracts the peripheral vessels, repels the blood towards the warmer, softer, more spongy, more vascular, more dilatable parenchymatous organs, whereby pathological congestions may be obliterated, and post-mortem ones, simulating morbidity, created. Neither the residuary vital actions which persist for a time after death, nor the physical agencies which act upon and modify the cadaver, have obtained, as yet, sufficient appreciation in autopsical reports; and, consequently, pathological anatomy, as to color, vascularity, congestion, softening, and inflammation, is more or less dubious. Thus, in certain states of the weather, the brain, in a few hours, may be softened from causes purely physical.

POST MORTEM SERIES.

TABLE X.—Showing the comparative temperature, taken at variable periods after death, in several regions of five different bodies, amounting to forty maxima.

MAXIMA OF EIGHT REGIONS COMPARED IN FIVE CADAVERA.							
Thigh.	Epig'm.	Axilla.	Chest.	Heart.	Brain.	Rectum.	Liver.
118°	111°	109°	107 °	109°	132°	111°	112°
109	110	109	106½	106	101	109	109
109	109	108	106	105	101	107	108
108	109	108	106	104	100	107	107
108	109	107	105	104	99	106	106
Mean. 109·4°	109·6°	108·2°	106·1°	105·6°	100·6°	108°	108·4°

It will be seen by Table X (*Post Mortem Series*), that the average of five *maxima* of the epigastrium are nearly the same ; but if we select ten *maxima* from each of these regions, the thigh will be found the hotter of the two by 0·3°. This is the more remarkable, as the observations were made (owing to the emergencies incidental to an epidemic) at irregular, sometimes at lengthened periods after death, when, the thigh more especially, from its comparative smallness and greater exposure, had parted with more or less of its morbid caloric, by contact and radiation.

In one series of cases of yellow fever, taken without selection, the following results were obtained : Fifteen patients who recovered, whose temperatures were taken at a period which averaged 15⅓ hours after the invasion, and afforded a mean temperature for the hand of 101·8°, and for the armpit 104·84° ; nine persons who died, gave, at an average of 22⅓ hours after the invasion—for the hand, 103·62° ; for the armpit, 105·44°.

The maxima of these classes coïncided, but not the minima. In those who died, the average was higher ; in the hand, the maximum reached by both was 107°; the minimum in the hand among those who recovered, was 95°, and of those who died, 99°; the maximum of the former, in the axilla, 107°; of the latter, 109°; the minimum of the former, in the same region, 102°, and of the latter 100°, the latter being *in articulo mortis.*

The extraordinary fact, that, in some bodies recently dead the temperature, at various periods thereafter, rises higher than it had risen during any stage of the maladies which preceded—much higher than in their latter stages—has been fully confirmed, as well as another, still more extraordinary; namely—that, at uncertain periods, usually, perhaps less than an hour, though occasionally later, the centre and periphery will attain to, and remain at a stationary, perhaps a high temperature, which, for a considerable time, will neither rise nor fall. But, still further than this, either the centre or circumference, or both together, having reached a certain temperature, will sometimes fall and rise several degrees, repeating these movements several times. These internal and external fluctuations may or may not coïncide in time, degree, and duration. Assuming that these thermal currents originate in different regions, independently of each other, and pursue different, perhaps curved routes, occasionally uniting at certain points or foci, it might be expected that, at these points of contact or convergency the maximum heat would be found. These foci are not found in a marked degree, even in the centre of the brain, far less in the inferior extremity below the knee, where the calorifacient power is most feeble or null in cadavera.

How hot soever the patient may have been during the progress of fever, the heat generally recedes before and at death; and this recession will, upon averaging a great number of cases, approximate natural standards, at least in the armpits and some other accessible regions.

The development of post mortem calorification does not appear to be materially accelerated or retarded by the atmospheric temperature, humidity, or dryness. This heat is not the effect nor the accompaniment of, but antagonistic to, putrefaction. When calorification ceases, physical refrigeration begins; and when the latter is reached, putrefaction is rapidly developed, if the weather be sufficiently warm.

The laws of post mortem calorification are numerous and complex. Its increment, decrement, degree, duration, and repeated ebbings and flowings, differ in different bodies so much that neither physics nor physiology has as yet furnished any satisfactory standard, explanation but a parallelism. Periodical diseases, in which paroxysms of cold and heat alternate, serve to indicate analogy, if not identity, as do the great, but little known, fluctuations of the normal temperature during morning, noon, evening, and night, among persons in health.

I will here stop a moment, in order merely to refer to the experiments concerning these fluctuations, the data of, and the deductions from which appeared *in extenso* in *The Western Journal of Medicine and Surgery*, in the year 1844 ; so that the friends of Dr. John Davy, if they choose, as upon a former occasion, to assert his priority herein may consult documents and dates, as a number of copies of these papers were sent immediately to both insular and continental Europe, and, in some instances, were republished almost entire. (See *Northern Jour. of Medicine*. 1845: Edinburgh.) An abstract from Dr. Davy's researches will also be subjoined, in the second paragraph below.

The horary oscillations of the normal temperature during the day are very considerable : thus, during ten consecutive days in January, the external temperature ranging from $39\frac{1}{2}°$ to $79\frac{1}{2}°$, that of the room where the observations were made being never lower than 61°, nor higher than $73\frac{1}{4}°$; from 7 to 10 A. M., the hand gave an average of 90·15°. At noon, the room ranging from 68° to $74\frac{1}{2}°$, the hand, averaged 97·71°; at 3 P. M., room 67° to $75\frac{1}{2}°$, the hand averaged 97·15°; at 9 P. M., the room ranged from 70° to 77°, the hand averaging 99°. A similar series for nine days gave the same mean result, with the exception of the inconsiderable fraction of $\frac{5}{8}$°. The hand averages, in bed, at 6 A. M., 98·45°, but falls about 9° during the morning hours in winter. In the warm season of the year, the morning declination of temperature is less in the extremities, but is still very considerable. These observations were published in detail, in 1844. There is, therefore, a remarkable parallelism between the normal heat and morbid heat in numerous cases of the latter. In most febrile maladies, there is very marked remission of the temperature in morning, even in fevers called continued. These data will be found *in extenso* in the Western Journal of Medicine and Surgery for the year 1844.

In the Philosophical Transactions, for 1850, quoted in the *Br. and F. Med.-Chir. Rev.*, for July, 1851, is given a summary of Dr. John Davy's observations on the temperature of man within the tropics, chiefly at Barbadoes, during a period of three and a half years, the mean temperature of the Island being 80°, and the range 10° to 18° in the open air : " The observations were made three times a day ; the temperature of the body being noted, with that of the external air, the pulse and the number of respirations per minute : 1. The average temperature of man within the tropics is a little higher— nearly 1°—than in a temperate climate, such as that of England. 2. Within the tropics, as in the cooler regions, the temperature of the body is almost constantly fluctuating. 3. The order of fluctuating is different from that in a cooler climate, the minimum being early in the morning, after a night's rest, and not at night. 4. All exertion of body or mind, except it be very gentle, has a heightening effect on the temperature ; while passive exercise, especially carriage exercise, has a lowering tendency. * * * 7. When laboring under disease, however slight, the temperature is abnormally elevated, its undue degree being some criterion of the intensity of the diseased action. 8. Within the tropics, there is comparatively little difference of temperature of the surface of the body and the internal parts ; the skin is the most active in its functions—the kidneys less active ; the former state being connected, perhaps, with a rapid desquamation of cuticle ; the latter, with an absence of lithic acid. 9. The effect of wine, unless used in great moderation, is commonly lowering as to temperature, whilst it accelerates the heart's action, followed, after a while, by an increase of temperature. 10. The tendency of seasickness, like that of disease, is to elevate temperature. 11. The tendency of a sea voyage, apart from seasickness, is to equalize the temperature, without permanently elevating it."

A sudden breaking out of sweat, either spontaneously or from nausea excited by drugs, venesection, etc., as I have noticed more than once, will be attended with a sudden fall of the mercury, amounting to three degrees more or less ; while, on the other hand, a hot mustard foot bath will cause an elevation.

When, however, post mortem temperature is no longer generated, the calorifacient power being exhausted, the real refrigeration which then sets in proceeds from the surface towards the centre, according to the recognised physical law of all cooling bodies.

Conceding the materiality of caloric, it is not unreasonable to sup-pose that possibly it may consist of several varieties, kinds, or modi-fications—as physical, vital, morbid ; which, however, the mere ex-pansion of the mercury in the thermometer may fail to indicate. Thus, I have found, from a limited number of observations, that blood freshly drawn from the arms of patients parts with its caloric in a ratio slower than that of the same blood after refrigeration, on being reheated artificially to the original point of departure. If physical heat is dissipated from the same body, under identical cir-cumstances, in a different ratio, either slower or faster than animal heat, whether normal or morbid, this would establish an important differentiation which, however, my experiments have been neither sufficiently varied nor numerous enough to demonstrate beyond the possibility of mistake, seeing the difficulty of artificially arranging circumstances precisely identical in the procedure mentioned.

The sense of touch, it is believed, will recognize a difference be-tween the heat of typhus and that of a biscuit or potatoe of equal temperature, as tested by the thermometer.

Where least expected, experimental evidence has been adduced, showing that even physical heat presents marked differentiations or varieties. Thus, " a plate of glass placed before a common fire, will intercept the heat until it becomes itself sufficiently heated to radiate. When, however, the source of heat is more intense, a small portion will be directly transmitted ; while, for the solar rays, we find the heat is transmitted as well as the light." Here domestic heat and solar heat of equal intensities are, in the one case, intercepted by, and in the other, instantly transmitted through, the same medium, apparently under the same conditions. Other differences, relating to both its transmission and radiation, might be indicated, tending to show analogically that animal heat may be of different kinds, especially in diseases.

Assuming that the chemical history of respiration may be interpreted either as a refrigeratory or heat equalizing process, and that while the absorption of oxygen during respiration may generate heat, on the other hand the parting of carbonic acid gas and aqueous vaporization from the lungs, together with the incessant respiration of the air, almost always much cooler than the body, must refrigerate the animal economy; that, for all that has been proved to the contrary, oxidation and deoxidation, repair and waste, composition and decomposition, inhalation and exhalation, are mutually compensating or equiponderant in the regulation of animal heat ; and that, while it may be plausibly assumed that nearly the whole series of organs and organic functions, especially those of nutrition, contribute directly or indirectly to the origin and distribution of animal heat during life, post mortem calorification might to some extent be accounted for by assuming that respiration is not a heating but a refrigerating process, which, ceasing with apparent death, ceases to liberate the free caloric of the economy; whence the calorifacient function, not being in many instances extinguished with the respiration, persists, and for a long time accumulates faster than it can be radiated into the surrounding media. When the respiratory function is impaired or obstructed by direct disease, or indirectly, as in coma, with infrequent breathing (as may be seen in one of the above tables), there is not only no corresponding depression of the temperature, but often a comparatively augmented ratio of calorification before and during the agony.

During hot weather, animals, especially after violent exercise, instinctively accelerate their respiration, as if for the purpose of cooling themselves, although, according to the prevalent theory of pulmonary combustion, increased respiration ought to produce corresponding increase of heat. In diseases which affect the pulmonary organs, and which impede their full and complete action, as pneumonia, consumption, bronchitis, catarrh, pleurisy, croup, fevers, sunstroke, etc., a preternatural heat obtains in a ratio more or less approximating that of the actual embarrassment of the pulmonary apparatus and its consequent failure to render latent the free caloric developed in the general economy. Cholera represses the calorifacient function, either directly or secondarily by the refrigerating processes of exudation, sweating, evaporation, general waste resembling liquefaction, and by the suspension of the nutritive action.   Even the air expelled in breathing in the hottest weather, is in cholera sometimes very sensibly cooled. As soon, however, as breathing ceases, post mortem calorification generally begins, and may mount far above the normal standard, and still farther above that of the antecedent disease in algid cholera.

A curious fact, quite adverse to the theory which makes the lungs the heating furnace of the entire animal economy, has been often tested by the thermometer; namely, that the greatest and most persistent $_h e_{at}$ is not found in these organs however, either soon or late after death.

Tabular views and average numbers, where the principle of selection is excluded, may and ought to be sometimes rejected, and replaced by the selection of cases in which the highest or maximum numbers or phenomena are obtainable. If, for example, two observations be made, in order to decide the pulmonary theory of calorification, one body being 75° and the other 113°, the average would be 94° and would be inconclusive ; whereas a single case in which the temperature increased after death beyond that of the normal or morbid temperature, would invalidate the whole theory, and show that post mortem calorification must have some other than a respiratory origin. The following observations (anno 1860) will forcibly illustrate this proposition.

George Henry Lewes, Esq.,* long distinguished as an elegant author

---

*The Glasgow *Medical Journal* says, that " at the last meeting of the British Association Professor Owen read a paper from the pen of Mr. G. H. Lewes (a gentleman who is earning for himself as high a reputation in physiology as he has already acquired in general literature and as a novelist), on ' *The Spinal Cord, a Sensational* and Volitional Centre.' "

The sensational and volitional functions of the spinal cord were fully established by numerous vivisections and experiments made, and also published in the *New Orleans Medical and Surgical Journal*, many years ago, as the readers of the Alligator papers will testify, as will many witnesses who either assisted or were present at these vivisections.

Mr. Lewes, a few weeks since, in a paper presented to *The British Association*, maintained on " anatomical and experimental evidence, that the supposed essential distinction between sensory and motor nerves did not exist ; but that both, in properties and functions, the two nerves were similar." (See his communication in the *Lancet*, Jan. 1860. Am. Ed.) The readers of the *New Orleans Medical and Surgical Journal* must have seen, more than a decennium ago, numerous reports of experimental researches, together with an extended exposition of the fundamental deductions made from these experiments, among which are the very conclusions at which Mr. Lewes has arrived. The book compilers have been gradually, with the least possible acknowledgment, modifying the existing text books, yet without suddenly drawing out, and thereby weakening the bundle of sticks which they had previously tied together with theoretical cords.

of various literary works, who of late has been equally distinguished for his physiological research, has in a work on physiology now passing through the press of Messrs. Appleton & Co. of New York, adopted the conclusions established by experimental evidence in New Orleans seven years ago.

Mr. Lewes says : " While, therefore, it is still undecided whether carbonic acid and water arise in the organism by a process of direct oxidation, the theory of animal heat, which is based on such an assumption, must necessarily be held questionable.   Meanwhile, we may look a little more closely into the evidence which declares that Animal Heat is the direct product of respiration, rising and falling with it, dependent upon it, as effect upon cause.   That a mass of evidence can be adduced is perfectly true, because, whatever theory we may form, we must still perceive that *an* intimate relation exists between respiration and animal heat ; if only on the ground that all vital processes are intimately related, and in the organism one function is necessarily dependent on another.   The question, however, is not whether *an* intimate relation exists, but whether *the* casual relation exists, whether the two phenomena are in invariable correspondence—the one never feeble when the other is energetic—the one never acting when the other has ceased.

" Disregarding the mass of evidence which may be adduced in favor of the correspondence, let us here fix our attention solely on some striking exceptions.   The cases are by no means very rare in which a corpse has preserved a high temperature for many hours ; and, as respiration must altogether have ceased, these cases have great significance for us.   Dr. Livingstone mentions a case which came under his own eye, of a Portuguese lady, who died of fever at three o'clock in the morning of the 26th of April.   'The heat of the body continued unabated until six o'clock, when I was called in, and found her bosom as warm as ever I did in a living case of fever.   This continued for three hours more.   As I had never seen such a case in which the fever heat had continued so long after death, I delayed the funeral till unmistakable symptoms of dissolution occurred.' Mr. George Bedford informed me of a case which he had under his own eye.   A soldier given to drink died, I forget from what cause, and next day Mr. Bedford was quite startled at finding the body still warm.   Dr. Bennet Dowler, of New Orleans, has likewise observed that, in many cases, the temperature *rises* after death.   *   *   *   Dr. Dowler found that

28

where the highest temperature during life was 104° under the armpit, it rose to 109° in ten minutes after death; fifteen minues afterwards it was 113° in an incision in the thigh; in one hour and fifty minutes it was 109° in the heart.   Three hours after all the viscera had been removed, an incision in the thigh showed the temperature to be 110°. When we remember that, even after death, processes of growth and secretion have been observed to take place, there is nothing incredible in these examples of continued heat after death ; but we cannot see how the advocates of the respiratory theory reconcile such facts as the complete absence of respiration during several hours with no dimunition of animal heat.   According to theory, the two phenomena are in immediate dependence, the intensity of heat corresponding with the energy of respiration; but here there is no respiration, nor has there been any for some hours, yet the heat continues to be produced. *   *   *   There are, moreover, numerous facts which show a similar want of correspondence,"* etc.   (Vol. I. 359–360.)

Whether abnormal animal heat be considered in its ætiological or symptomatic character, it is more intelligible than many assumptions that have been adopted as fundamental principles in ætiology and nosology.   The thermometer indicates a nosological distinction long prevalent, which divides maladies into the pyretic and the apyretic—the febrile and the non-febrile—a distinction which often

---

* Mr. Lewes (pp. 264–5) admits that not only may animal heat be developed after death, but other phenomena which are of a physiological or vital character, as the capillary circulation, etc. Upon the circulation of the blood he discourses as follows: " But the objections to the Harveyan doctrine do not end here. The heart may be removed in cold-blooded animals, and the capillary circulation will continue for some time in spite of that removal. This has been done more than once; and although I had myself observed it some time ago, yet in preparing these pages for publication I again investigated the point ; and for this purpose removed the heart of a Triton, with as much care as possible, and found the circulation going on in the tail for some minutes afterwards, nor did it entirely cease on separating the tail from the body.

"While the fact was thus indubitable, I had many doubts as to the cause. But the fact is enough for our present purpose; and that it is also true of warm-blooded animals may be inferred, since after death various processes of secretion, and some even of growth (as of hair, beard, etc.), are known to take place; and this seems to imply capillary circulation. 'After most kinds of death,' says Dr. Carpenter, the arterial system is found, subsequently to the lapse of a few hours, almost or completely emptied of blood; this is partly, no doubt, the effect of the tonic contraction of the tubes themselves; but the emptying is commonly more complete than could thus be accounted for, and must therefore be partly due to the continuance of capillary circulation. It has been observed by Dr. Bennet Dowler that in the bodies of individuals who have died from yellow fever, the external veins become so distended with blood, within a few minutes after the cessation of the heart's action, that when they are opened the blood flows in a good stream, being sometimes projected to the distance of a foot or more. It is not conceivable that the slowly-acting tonicity of the arteries could have produced such a result as this ; which can scarcely therefore be attributed to anything else than the sustenance of the capillary circulation by forces generated within itself.' "

affords therapeutic indications nearly allied with physical certainty, because cold represses excessive heat, and heat, cold; remedies which in the present state of scepticism and uncertainty in therapeutics, should be neither scorned nor rejected. Here, at least, there is a ray of light to guide to rationalism.

Although the scope of this paper excludes the further considera-tion of free caloric in its varied relations to physiology, ætiology, diagnosis, pathology, morbid anatomy, and therapeutics, it may be allowable to make the general remark, that, if all gaseous, liquid, and solid substances, whether celestial or terrestrial, organic or in-organic, be, as some cosmologists assert, animated, the vitalizing agent which possesses the greatest universality, energy, adaptation and claim to " this high argument" is caloric—an agent which is in-herently dynamical and developmental, at once the means and ends of all movement and organization, or at least, the essential condition, throughout the whole realm of nature. In its absence, universal inertia, torpidity, or hibernation, would reign everlastingly over in-organic matter, and over vegetable and animal organisms. Its derangements and excesses produce disorder and destruction. Its normal distribution holds in equipoise whatsoever is :

> " That, changed through all, and yet in all the same,
> Great in the earth as in the ethereal frame;
> Warms in the sun,
> Glows in the stars, and blossoms in the trees ;
> Lives through all life, extends through all extent,
> Spreads undivided, operates unspent."

Caloric binds and unbinds, unites and separates, creates, develops, changes, and, at first view, seems to destroy; but its decompositions and apparent annihilations are but new compositions, new forms resulting from new affinities, which contribute to the perpetuation of the mighty stream of life. Viewed from this stand-point, death appears but an illusion. The quantity of heat and the quantity of life, if not identical and interchangeable phases of a common principle, present, at least, striking parallelisms. From the polar regions, where dwarfed shrubs will not grow, and where animals are reduced to a few hardy kinds, life is augmented and diversified as the equatorial regions are approached. Before man's advent upon the earth, and the multiplication of the human race, colossal plants and animals, whose fossilized remains are indelibly recorded in the rocks of the earth's crust, prove that in remote geological ages life abounded—was, perhaps, exuberant, corresponding to the then higher temperature which must have reigned in the arctic or cold regions, where the fossilized remains of gigantic floras and faunas of a tropical character, now extinct, have been disinterred. It is easy to offer objections to all speculations which have been broached upon this subject. Neither organization nor life is known to be the necessary effect of caloric or any physical agent.

PROGRESS OF MEDICINE.

ART. I.—*Dr. Brown-Séquard's Physiological Researches.*

[THE following elaborate summary of Dr. Brown-Séquard's experimental researches and discoveries, taken from the July number (1859) of *The Glasgow Medical Journal,* is the latest and appears to be the fullest exposition that has appeared, and will doubtlessly be acceptable to the readers of the *New Orleans Medical and Surgical Journal.* The extensive bibliographical list, in *The Glasgow Journal,* of Dr. Brown-Séquard's papers, which covers a considerable portion of two pages preceding the article, contains erroneous dates not very creditable to to the proof-reader of that excellent journal.

Before proceeding to the paper concerning the distinguished physiologist whose name stands at the head of this article, the reader will excuse a few preliminary remarks.

As the editor of *The Glasgow Medical Journal* quotes, as the sequel shows, from Dr. Brown-Séquard to prove that Walker anticipated Bell in announcing the so-called sensational and volitional nerves, the editor of that journal, as well as all other editors and book builders in both hemispheres, might have read the voluminous works whose entire title pages will be found below in a foot note* ; nevertheless the editor has quoted (*anno*, 1859) from Dr. Brown-Séquard, the evidence of Walker's priority in this respect. Dr. Brown-Séquard had doubtessly seen my papers, which had disinterred the Walkerian documents many years ago—not long after Dr. B.-S. entered the ranks of the profession. Walker, after a long career of authorship, mostly of a semi-popular character, such as books on Beauty, Intermarriage, etc., descended to the tomb within the last year or two. Among other expositions of his theory, the fullest is given, together with numerous quotations, in the *New Orleans Medical and Surgical Journal of* 1847, and subsequently, clearly showing the physiological injustice done him by ascribing to Bell the so-called discovery of two distinct kinds of nerves, the sensory and volitional or motory. While denying the reality of this dogma, the ground taken was, that how true or erroneous soever it might be, in either case, its full announcement should be awarded to Walker.

In 1851, in the seventh volume of this journal (p. 51), Walker's claims are reïterated in the following words : " I have already proved that Mr. Alex. Walker preceded Bell in the so-called double function of the nerves, the unanimity of the British and American writers to the contrary notwithstanding. If any more evidence be wanted to establish this, my protest, against one of the greatest historical falsehoods of the century, I am prepared to give it without delay."

Soon after the appearance of my papers, in which full justice was demanded for Walker, several brief notes, if I recollect rightly, appeared in *The Lancet*, expressive of the fact that a mistake had been

---

*Let the sceptical reader examine the following works, the first two of which have been long in my library, namely: " The Nervous System, Anatomical and Physiological: In which the Functions of the various parts of the Brain are for the first time assigned; and to which is prefixed some account of the author's earliest discoveries, of which the more recent doctrines of Bell, Magendie, etc., are shown to be at once a plagiarism and a blunder associated with useless experiments, which they have neither understood nor explained: Being the first volume of an Original System of Physiology adapted to the advanced state of Anatomy : By ALEXANDER WALKER, author of Physiognomy founded on Physiology. London : Smith, Elder & Co., Cornhill, booksellers to their Majesties. 1834. Pp. 704. 8vo."

" Documents and Dates of Modern Discoveries in the Nervous System. Pp. 172. 8vo. London: John Churchill, Prince street, Soho. MDCCCIX."

" Natural System of Medical Science, 1808."

"Archives of Universal Science," Jan., 1809; April, same year ; July, same year. The *unpublished* work of Bell on the Brain claims to have been dated in 1811—that is two years later.

These works contain the original papers of Walker, with the dates commencing in 1803. The very headings are remarkable: " Discovery of the Functions of the Cerebel in 1803;" " Discovery of the Distinction between the Nerves of Sensation and the Nerves of Volition, in 1809, as explained in earlier works," etc.   B. D.

made in giving Bell the credit due to the former. But a long "flash of silence" for nearly half a generation, ensued. That two continents should have acquiesced and persisted in this error, and made it the chief staple of their courses of medical lectures and elementary books upon the nervous system, is not only a discredit to historical verity, but a psychological curiosity, for which the text books on insanity have no name. Sir Charles Bell's latest and most authoritative statements contain internal evidence that he could have made no physiogical discovery whatever, because he positively rejected experi ment, the only method yet discovered in that behalf.

B. Dowler.]

On a previous occasion we directed the attention of our readers to the labors of Dr. Brown-Séquard as an experimental physiologist, in a notice of the first number of his journal of physiology. Since then the courses of lectures which he has delivered in London, Edinburgh, Glasgow and Dublin, have made his name familiar to the profession in this country, and have widely disseminated a knowledge of the many important discoveries which he has made respecting the physiology and pathology of the nervous system. He has, by his labors and discoveries, entitled himself to be placed in the foremost rank of living physiologists. His powers as an observer and experimentalist are of the highest order; and the extent, variety and importance of his researches may entitle us to place him by the side of such men as Magendie and Claude Bernard. It is not our intention in this review to follow him over the wide field, which a critical analysis of the numerous memoirs placed at the head of this paper would require of us; but we shall confine ourselves to a brief notice of some of the more important observations and discoveries which they contain. Those who wish to become acquainted with the details of the experiments, which are extremely interesting, must study the works themselves, as our limited space will not permit us to enter, however briefly, on this part of the subject. It is the conclusions founded on these experiments which will at present exclusively engage our attention. We may here remark, in reference to all such experiments by vivisection, that the repugnance felt by physiologists in this country to their performance, has been one of the chief causes why the investigation of many physiological questions has been materially interfered with, and many important discoveries, which could not be arrived at in any other way, have not been made. We have given expression in this journal to opinions unfavorable to their prosecution ; but we must admit that since we have witnessed the experiments performed by Dr. Brown-Séquard, our objections to them have been considerably modified, and that, in the hands of so able an experimenter, the apparent cruelty is the less offensive in proportion as the results which they demonstrate are more conspicuous. At the same time we must be permitted to state that we should regard it as a great calamity—as a crime worthy the severest reprobation, if such experiments were indulged in from motives originating in any but the purest scientific aspirations. All that we can say for it is, that the end in view is the only justification which we can offer for the means employed. In France there appears to be less scruple in this matter than has hitherto prevailed in this country; and we could almost go the length of saying that we should feel content that the *status quo* should remain as it is, even though our continental brethren should continue in advance of us in matters pertaining to experimental physiology.

The existence of paralysis of sensation and of voluntary motion, isolated from each other, naturally leads to the question whether those parts of the nervous centres, and those nerves which serve the purposes of sensation are not distinct from those which serve the purposes of voluntary motion. It does not appear, however, that this idea was formally stated till the early part of this century, when Alexander Walker had the merit of enunciating it in the following terms: "As in certain cases sensation exists without volition, and as all the nerves have their origin in distinct filaments, I believe that everywhere, when a part, at one and the same time capable of sensation and voluntary motion, receives a nervous trunk, that trunk contains a nerve of sensation and a nerve of motion;" and "that the action which commences in sensitive organs passes to the cord by the anterior roots of the spinal nerves, which are consequently the nerves of sensation, and ascends the whole length of the anterior columns of the cord;" and, again, "that the voluntary action descends along the posterior columns of the cord, and distributes itself by the posterior roots, which are consequently the nerves of volition."[*]

Sir Charles Bell seems to have adopted the general principle advanced by Walker, but he completely reversed the particular views which he had enunciated respecting the functions of the anterior and posterior roots. He ascribed to the anterior roots the voluntary motor, and to the posterior the sensory function. The demonstration of this important fact constituted the greater part of the discovery of Sir C. Bell. He did not carry his investigations sufficiently far to enable him to make any important discovery respecting the functions of the different *columns* of the spinal cord. He first entertained the view that the posterior columns are the continuation of the posterior roots; but afterwards formed the opinion that the lateral columns are continuous with the posterior roots, on the ground that the posterior columns do not terminate in the cerebrum, but in the cerebellum. His discoveries respecting the functions of the roots of the spinal nerves were fully confirmed by other physiologists, particularly by J. Müller,[†] Valentin and Panizza. The only difficulty started was that raised by Magendie in 1839, respecting the occurrence of sensation in the ante-

---

[*](Archives of Universal Science, July, 1809, quoted by Dr. B.-S.)

[†] When Müller published these experiments, Bell repudiated them, declaring that "he preferred to build on *anatomy* and the *vital powers*, not on the galvanic conducting powers of the nerves. All such experiments are much better omitted; they never can lead to satisfactory conclusions. The nerves dead or alive may convey the galvanic power like a wet cord. Experiments never have been the means of discovery; and a survey of what has been attempted of late years in physiology will prove that the opening of living animals has done more to perpetuate error, etc. I have made few experiments," etc. (See Bell's *New System; passim;* also this journal for Sept., 1847; and numerous other papers. B. D.

rior roots, who afterwards found that it was not directly, but by recurrence only that these roots appeared to be sensitive.

The greatest claim which Dr. Brown-Séquard has upon our admiration as a physiologist, arises from the light which his experiments have thrown upon the most obscure part of the physiology of the nervous system; upon the question, what part of the spinal column transmits the orders of the will to the muscles, and what part of this organ transmits impressions to the sensorium.　It was at this point that the investigations of Bell ceased; and it is here where the investigations of Brown-Séquard begin.　The want of correct and accurate information on this subject has given rise to a great diversity of opinion.

1. It was the opinion of Backer, Kuerschner and Longet, that the posterior columns of the spinal cord are the only channel for the transmission of sensitive impressions.　2. According to Bellingeri, the grey central substance is the only mode of transmission.　3. According to Stilling, the posterior part of the grey substance is the only channel. 4. The lateral columns are alone charged with the transmission of sensitive impressions, according to Ludwig Türck. 5. Eigenbrodt held the view that the posterior columns are the principal vehicle for the transmission of sensitive impressions, but that the grey matter, probably from the white fibres which it contains, is also capable of transmission.　6. According to Schiff, both the posterior columns and the grey substance possess this function, and the one can supplement the other.　7. All parts of the spinal cord, according to Rolando and Calmeil, can transmit sensitive impressions.

Dr. B.-S. accounts for the contradictory nature of these opinions by the ignorance on the part of experimenters of one or more of the following circumstances :　1. The existence of reflex movements.　2. The existence of the cross-transmission of sensitive impressions in the spinal cord.　3. The possibility of the existence of the power of transmitting sensations in a part not itself endowed with sensibility.　4. The possibility of laying bare the spinal cord without producing too great hæmorrhage, or exhausting the sensibility of the animal.

The view advocated by M. Longet, that sensitive impressions are conveyed by the posterior columns of the cord, has been very ably refuted by Dr. B.-S., by arguments drawn from human and comparative anatomy, from the anatomy of structure, and from vivisections.　The experiments on which M. Longet founded his opinion, consisted in making cross-sections of the spinal cord, and applying stimulants, such as galvanism, to the cut surface of the several columns.　He found that the animal gave expression of pain, only when the posterior columns were stimulated.　Dr. B.-S. does not admit the validity of these experiments, till it has been shown that impressions cannot be conveyed except by a part which is itself sensitive.　This objection does not seem to have occurred to M. Longet; and Dr. B.-S. has proved, in opposition to him, that parts, which in themselves are not sensitive, have the power of transmitting sensitive impressions.　Besides experimental proofs, M. Longet rested his opinion upon pathological observations which he made. The most of them, however, were of little or no value, as in some, though the posterior columns were much diseased, there was no loss of sensibility; while in others, the posterior roots of the spinal nerves were also affected, as well as the posterior columns; and, consequently, the loss of sensibility could not be ascribed to the disease ، of the posterior columns. On the other hand, Dr. B.-S. has collected a large number of pathological facts, which prove that sensitive impressions are transmitted, even though the posterior columns are chiefly affected by disease.

Without entering into the arguments derived from other sources which he brings to bear against the views of M. Longet, we shall notice briefly some of the experiments, by which he proves, in opposition to that physiologist, that sensitive impressions are conveyed by the central grey matter of the cord, and that they cross along the whole length of the cord, to the lateral half opposite to the side from which the impressions come—that is, that sensitive impressions coming from the right side of the body, pass to the left lateral half of the cord, and *vice versa.*

1. By the first experiment he proves, that when the posterior columns are cut through, the parts below the section, instead of loss, have an increase of sensibility. 2. By a second experiment, all the posterior columns, the posterior grey cornua, and a part of the lateral columns, were cut through, and still the sensibility of the posterior limbs was greatly exaggerated. This experiment at least proves that the posterior columns are not the only channel for the transmission of sensitive impressions. 3. The third experiment consists in cutting the posterior columns at the last dorsal vertebra, and at the second cervical. It was found that the sensibility was greatly increased in irritating the superior surface of the first section made. 4. The fourth experiment consisted in cutting the posterior columns transversely, on a level with the point of the calamus scriptorius. In this case, when the restiform bodies (the continuation of the posterior columns) were severely irritated, no trace of pain was expressed; while, on the contrary, the irritation of the posterior columns, immediately behind the section, was excessively painful; and it was found that the extremities and surface of the body had become endowed with a remarkable degree of sensibility. 5. In the fifth experiment, the spinal column was laid bare in the whole lumbar region; and a longitudinal section was mode through its whole extent, dividing it into two equal lateral parts; and it was found that sensibility was completely destroyed in the limbs. 6. In the sixth experiment, the whole of the spinal cord was cut through, except the posterior columns on a level with the second dorsal vertebra, and no amount of irritation could produce any symptom of pain. The foregoing experiments lead, by a process of exclusion, to the conviction, that it can only be by the grey substance that sensitive impressions are conveyed. The following experiments also lead to the same conclusion : 7. In this experiment the spinal cord is laid bare in the dorsal region of three animals. In one, the posterior columns and the central grey substances are cut across without injuring the antero-lateral columns. In a second, the lateral column of one side and the central grey substance is cut. In a third, the lateral column of one side, the anterior

columns, and the central grey substance are cut. In all these, sensibility is found to be entirely gone in the posterior extremities. 8. By means of an instrument made for the purpose, the central grey substance is cut through with as little injury as possible to the white substance of the cord; and the result is found to be complete insensibility of the posterior extremities.

The conclusions drawn by Dr. B.-S. from these experiments, are as follow : 1. It is not by the posterior columns, as is generally admitted in France, that sensitive impressions, received from the trunk and limbs, are transmitted to the brain. 2. It is by the grey substance of the cord, more particularly its central part, that this transmission takes place.

It may be objected to this doctrine, that the central grey substance, not being itself sensitive, cannot convey sensitive impressions. But there are numerous facts to prove that the very reverse of this is true, viz : that sensibility cannot exist in parts capable of transmitting sensitive impressions, proceeding from sensitive surfaces. As instances of this, we may adduce the brain proper, and, perhaps, the cerebellum and the fibres of the trifacial nerve, which are not sensitive, but are capable of transmitting sensations. Besides, it has been shown that the nerve trunks, which convey the tactile sensations, are not themselves sensitive.

In further investigating this subject, Dr. B.-S. has made a series of experiments relative to the distribution of the fibres of the posterior roots in the spinal cord, and has found that these fibres decussate, and that the impressions from one side of the body pass to the opposite side of the cord, and reach their ultimate destination by means of the central grey substance. It is abundantly proved by Dr. Brown-Séquard's experiments, that while the motor nerves decussate only in the upper extremity of the spinal cord, and chiefly in the medulla oblongata, the sensitive nerves decussate throughout the whole extent of the cord.

In connection with this subject, it is interesting to remark that, on the 20th of June, two memoirs were presented to the French Academy of Sciences, by M. Flourens, in name of their authors, Professor Paolini, of Bologna, and M. van Kempen, of Louvain, relative to the functions of the spinal cord, which are confirmative of the experiments of Dr. Brown-Séquard. The following are the conclusions arrived at by Professor Paolini : 1. The posterior and lateral columns of the spinal cord are endowed with an exquisite sensibility, 2. The division of these columns does not prevent the transmission of sensitive impressions to the brain. 3. The impressions transmitted by the posterior spinal roots, after a short passage across the medullary fibres of these columns, pass into the grey substance. 4. The grey substance, though insensible itself—that is to say, incapable of receiving immediately impressions which excite sensations—appears to be the indispensable means of transmitting these impressions to the sensorium. 5. The posterior columns alone being cut transversely, the sensibility of the parts of the animal situated below the section is temporarily increased. 6. The posterior columns preserve their own sensibility, even when cut in two or three points at a certain

distance from one another.   7. The anterior columns are insensible
to the immediate application of stimuli.   8. Lastly, the anterior columns are essentially motor, but they do not appear to be totally devoid of the production of feeling.

The following are the conclusions of Professor Van Kempen, of
the University of Louvain :   1. In frogs, the transmission of conscious sensibility is crossed in the whole length of the spinal cord;
that of movement is direct in the lumbo-dorsal region, and crossed in
the cervical portion.   2. In pigeons, the decussation of the conductors
of conscious sensibility occurs through the whole length of the spinal
cord.* The transmission of voluntary movement is direct in the
lumbo-dorsal, and partially crossed in the cervical region.   3. In
mammals, the transmission of conscious sensibility is crossed through
the whole length of the spinal cord.   The transmission of voluntary
movement is direct only in the lumbo-dorsal region; in the cervical
region it is partly crossed, but is for the most part direct.   These conclusions, arrived at independently by eminent physiologists, strongly
conduce to our cordial acceptance of the views of M. Brown Sé-
quard.—*The Glasgow Medical Journal, July,* 1859.

[Experimental physiology should save itself from distrust and contempt, by avoiding the vain and temporary successes attendant upon
the *construction of theories out of mere words, instead of things.
The word-theories of physiology seem for a time captivating, and even
true, from being labelled as experimental; but when another contradictory or variant theory is in like manner inaugurated, scepticism
justifies itself in regard to the whole, not believing that revolutions
so sudden and contradictory can be found in the economy of Nature.
A faithful verification of facts, with a history of their antecedents,
the order, connections, conditions, sequents, uniformity, and universality, will not thus change several times during a single generation.
The law is the thing in a generalized form.   But, if a word is to be
adopted as a thing, experimental physiology had better come to a
standstill, than to accept automatic, sensori-volitional, excito-motory,
excito-secretory, transmitted impressions, reflex actions, etc., all of
which claim to be things which set out, things that travel along
things (roads), things which arrive at places and come back as things,
by crossings, curves, semicircles, circles.   Not one of these things is
either seen in any experiment, or known by intuition or consciousness.   In the living unity, of which all the parts are mutually means
and ends, dependent and depending on each, the whole economy
contributes, more or less, to the functional finality of any one organ,
which latter returns the compliment and the complement.   When the
finger is cut there is a pain in the finger ; all the things that travel

to or from the cerebral sensory spot are unknown and unnecessary to the case. If the nerves be divided, palsy or something else may take place, as the effect of the injury of the particular part, or of the organic unity of the whole. The antecedents of a phenomenon, such as sensation, voluntary motion, etc., may be numerous, and the change in any one of these agents might render the common or compound result an impossibility.

The physiological antecedents, conditions, and agents, of which the writing of this sentence with the right arm is the result, are numerous. Among these may be named, as the simplest, the muscles, nerves, and the circulation. Divide the muscles or the nerves, or cut off the circulation of the blood, and at once the writing is arrested ; divide the nerves, leaving the muscles entire, and the same effect follows; leave the muscles and nerves intact, but cut off the circulation completely, and the result is the same. If these mutilations should be invariably attended by the same or similar morbid phenomenon on the other side, or left arm, it would not necessarily prove *per se* that a *thing*, or even a metaphor, crossed to the other side. It would only prove the fact that, when one part of the living machine is disorganized, another is. The words crossed, reflex, arched, transmitted, as applied to any known *thing* going to the sensorium, spinal roots, columns, etc., are purely hypothetical, and far more unintelligible than the old terms, sympathy, consent of parts, and the like. Even these were used as metaphors, and did not mislead the physiological anatomist by imaginary diagrams of multitudinous routes to and fro. In the last edition of his Anatomy and Physiology, Sir Charles Bell exclaims : " How much vain theory has been suggested from the simple experiment of loss of power in consequence of tying a nerve; and yet it was not the compression of the tubes of the nerve, but the obstruction of bloodvessels, which produced the effect." It is remarkable that, with all the maps extant showing the different kinds of nerves, neither anatomists nor microscopists can distinguish them in the human body. Were they known and fixed, the existing and conflicting theories of their action could not be established without further evidence. The prevalent theory, which assumes that the nerves are wholly insensible conductors to an exclusively sensorial spot in the brain, and that sensation is not immediate, but representative, or through an agent or intermedium—that is to say, transmitted impressions, and not a directly felt relation between the object impressing and the subject impressed, without any known transmitted impression or secondary intervention—can have no existence but in books, being opposed to the highest of all evidence, intuition, and therefore incapable of proof. B. D.]

Art. II.—*Modern Physiology*.

[*The Glasgow Medical Journal*, in an extended article on the progress of modern physiology, maintains that "five-and-twenty years ago, physiology stood on an intelligible and sound footing; it does so no longer; and that it now rests on a footing which is continually shifting," etc. A few extracts will show the scepticism and distrust with which the paper is imbued.]

Alas! how is the gold become dim! how is the most fine gold changed! since the days, not yet thirty years ago, when Alison (psychologist and physiologist both, and of no mean order) gave us an exposition of this department of our science, which, alike in its groundwork and its details, to this day contrasts favorably, we think, with that of those (and these not a few) in this country and on the continent, who have come after him, and have superseded him as a guide and an authority in what he was fond to call the "noble" science of physiology.

As to the causes which have led to this change—to this mutilation of mind by our physiologists, and to its almost complete expurgation by them from their science—they are very various. We will not mention, although we believe it to be the case, that psychology has never acquired its due and rightful ascendancy among our English physiologists, who have of late taken the lead in giving tone and character to physiology. But we will say—and let us say it at once and boldly—that one cause lies in the *undue* prominency which has of late years been given to what is called the "reflex function" of the spinal cord, which, crammed down the throats of our physiologists in the first instance, whether they would or not, gained at length the firm footing in physiology it has *temporarily* got, through the untiring perseverance of the late Dr. Marshall Hall, and which function of "reflex" agency, we (who have strong convictions the other way) regret to say has, under the fostering care of Dr. Laycock and Dr. Carpenter, been extended to the brain. So great is the ascendancy which "unconscious (and purely organic) reflex agency" has acquired in physiology, that we not only breathe by it, and eat and defecate by it, but walk by it, and talk by it. "Automatic agency"—*i. e.*, an agency of or belonging to an automaton, a machine—has supplanted "habit," viewed as mind

become expert in act through use of its own inherent power ; and to
" unconscious cerebration," it is now suggested, we owe even the
highest achievements of human genius.   We will not charge these
physiologists with materialism.   They disavow it themselves, and we
do not think them really chargeable with it, at least in its ordinary
and vulgar sense.   But we will say, that the kind and extent of power
they assign to living nervous matter, in relation to mind, are such
and so great, as, in our judgment, to degrade the mind to the level of
a spiritual puppet—or, in effect, to put the sovereign prerogatives of
mind into commission, or under trust.

We are glad to see that, in his work, Dr. Noble, although to no
small extent imbued with the spirit of this school of physiologists,
discountenances this doctrine of unconscious cerebration:

> " I conceive that the particular facts which seem to countenance the theory of
> unconscious cerebration, will certainly admit of some more obvious and simple in-
> terpretation, than one which renders it necessary to regard nerve-substance as
> elaborating and perfecting thought *without thought*—a process, it appears to my-
> self, which would be not altogether unlike the production of melody by a notori-
> ously unmusical instrument, without the sensible manifestation of sounds."*

And he pays this compliment to Dr. Laycock's arguments in support
of his doctrine of " the reflex function of the brain," that " it is not
very obvious how the evidence of facts can be made to corroborate
them, or otherwise ;"† while, with respect to Dr. Marshall Hall's
theory—premising that we have never yet seen any attempt made
fairly to meet the objections which Dr. Alison, following Whytt (particularly in his " Remarks on the Sympathy of the Nerves"),‡ long
ago urged against it, both in his " Outlines of Physiology,"§ and in
the pages of the *British and Foreign Medical Review*‖—we rejoice to see
indications of renewed opposition to it.   At the last meeting of the
British Association, Professor Owen read a paper from the pen of Mr.
G. H. Lewes (a gentleman who is earning for himself as high a reputation in physiology, as he has already acquired in general literature, and as a novelist), on " The Spinal Cord, a Sensational and Volitional Centre;" and in the *North American Medico-Chirurgical Review*
for May last, we have a paper by Dr. George Paton, of Galt, on " The
Perceptive Power of the Spinal Cord"¶—in both which papers we

---

* Pp. 94-95.

† P. 109.

‡ Edinburgh, 1764.

§ Third edition, pp. 211-12, taken in connection with p. 385, *et seq.* See also his paper on " The Physiological Principle of Sympathy," in Edin. Med. Chir. Trans., vol. ii, p. 174, *et seq.*

‖ Vol. iii, p. 29, *et seq.*

¶ Were it not that the author's meaning sufficiently appears from his paper, this title would be as ex-
ceptionable as the expression, " unconscious cerebration." But with Dr. Patton it is not really the cord
in the spinal column, it is the mind that is conscious of and perceives what is perceived, and is con-
sciously felt in consequence of the impressions made upon the cord. This organized and living structure
furnishes the conditions under which sensations are felt, and it forms the medium through which different mental acts affect various muscles; nay, nor these only, but likewise all the vital organs and their
functions. This has long been acknowledged on all hands; and this being the case, we cannot (with all
due respect for the ingenuity and perseverance of Dr. M. Hall) perceive that any great effort of genius
was required to show that (as in his experiments) all functions of our bodies in which mental acts are, in
the natural state, essentially concerned, must be liable to excitement, and so far (to use an expression
of Dr. Alison's) to be *imitated* by *injuries* of different portions of that part of the nervous system which
—so essentially requisite in order to these acts, and to their agency on the body, and so carefully constructed with that view—is (it is worth while observing) so effectually protected naturally from injury.

have *facts*, bearing out the inferences implied in their respective titles, and which we would commend to the serious attention of the devoted adherents of the late Dr. Marshall Hall.

And to bring to a conclusion this branch of our subject, we will merely express our gratification at the *havoc* which Dr. Brown-Séquard is just now making of long-established notions in neurology, and particularly at his calling in question—what seems to be held as no less than a first principle in the science—the distinction between the grey or vesicular nervous matter, "as the seat of *primary change;*" and the white or fibrous, "as a mere *conductor*, or channel of transmission," of the influence originating in the grey. "There is nothing," says Mr. Lewes, "like the sharp angle of a paradox to prick the reader's attention;"*, and it may, perhaps, aid us in the object we have in view in this article—which is, to assert for mind its own proper rank, as a power in nature of the first magnitude, as well as its proper place in physiology—if, with Mr. Lewes, we go a step further, and confidently affirm, on the ground of *fact*, "that both contractility and sensibility, (sensation, perception, will, mind) are manifested by animals *totally destitute* of either muscles or nerves;"† nay, if we affirm that, in man himself, there is a stage in his history when his mind, latent it may be, exists in his body independently of nervous matter, because prior to the formation or evolution of this matter from the *homogeneous* germinal membrane, of which alone, at this stage, his body consists.

Revolutionary these remarks may seem, and their spirit wanton. But believing the doctrines assailed to be no true doctrines, or, some some of them, at least, to be of that order which can neither be proved nor disproved, and the whole basis of this department of animal physiology, as sometimes treated, to be unsound, we deem it right in the interest of physiology to say what we think without reserve. Our desire is simply to show cause why the existing system of physiology, as it relates to the purely "animal functions," should be reconsidered —to move for a new trial, and to pray the court—shall we say of "*Common Pleas?*"—that mind may again be put in possession of .its lawful rights in relation to the nervous system, as lord paramount therein, and the nervous system denuded of powers and offices which do not of right belong to it, otherwise than as the seat and instrument of the mind. And we trust cur learned brother, Dr. Carpenter, will not consider that, in anything we have said hitherto, we have exceeded the license freely accorded to counsel.

*　*　* If, indeed, the physiologist desire or hope to give any true history or any useful account either of living animal orders around us, or of the living being *Man*, he must incorporate mind and body—and this, not merely because otherwise his physiology of the body will be unintelligible, but because the history he undertakes to

---

* Sea-Side Studies, p. 389.

† "Some physiologists, indeed, misled by the *a priori* tendency to *construct* the organism, in lieu of *observing* it, speak of the muscles and nerves of the simplest animals; because when they see the phenomena of contractility and sensibility, they are unable to dispossess themselves of the idea that these *must* be due to muscles and nerves. Thus, when the fresh-water polype is seen capturing, struggling with and finally swallowing a worm, yet *refusing* to swallow a bit of thread, we cannot deny that it manifests both sensibility and contractility [both instinct and instinctive motion], unless we deny these properties to all other animals. Nevertheless, the highest powers of the best microscope fail to detect the slightest trace of either muscle or nerve in the polype."—*Ibid. in loco.*

deliver will be incomplete.   For when he professes to give us, as, along with "the physiological anatomy," Messrs. Todd and Bowman do, "the physiology of man," he promises a good deal more than the physiology of man's living body.   "Human physiology," too, includes a good deal more than the physiology of the human body.   The physiology of man is not the physiology of his body only; it is the physiology of his mind and of his body as coëxistent. Nay, it is in very truth the physiology of his mind as existing in his body, and as acted on and acting *by* and *through* the nervous system therein, together with whatever else in the body is either specially subservient to the mind, or is requisite for the sustentation of the entire body as the hand-maid of the mind.   Man's mind and man's body, it is true, are in themselves two distinct *natures*, not one; but they make up together not two but one distinct *being*.   What, therefore, God hath joined together let not the   o o   put asunder.

phys l gist What if consciousnesss, which, from the statement of Mr. Lewes, appears to be a more general fact in animal physiology than the existence of a nervous system—what if, in as far as it is connected therewith, it be coëxtensive with the whole nervous system ? What if the mind—"couched in its den behind its two windows"—sees "*at*" or "*in*" the retina, as well as "*by*" the retina ?

[In this paper, it will be easy to recognize in the perceptive and volitional powers of the spinal cord, and in the universality of sensation throughout the nervous system, that these functions are not solely confined to a sensorial spot in the brain, long denied on experimental grounds and intuitional evidence by the managing editor of the *New Orleans Medical Journal.*]

ART. III.—*Experimental Physiology.*

[*The Glasgow Medical Journal* (July, 1859,) quotes with unqualified approval several passages from Mr. Joseph Lister's late *Contributions to Physiology and Pathology*, reprinted from the Philosophical Transactions.   Mr. Lister's experimental investigations into the parts of the nervous system which are supposed to regulate the contraction of the arteries, and the conclusions which he draws from them, the following paragraphs will serve to show more or less satisfactorily upon this branch of his inquiry.]

Experiment.—On the 8th of April, 1857, I laid open the spinal canal of a frog in its entire length, and divided, as I supposed, all the roots of the nerves coming off from the left side of the cord, from the occiput to the sacrum, and immediately examined the webs of both feet, the frog being under the influence of chloroform. In the right limb the circulation was almost entirely arrested, while in the the left it was going on freely. My attention was then diverted for half an hour, when the arteries of the right foot were found of medium size ; but in all the three webs of the left foot they were extremely dilated, appearing to have two or three times the diameter of those of the right limb. This observation was of itself sufficient to prove that the spinal system, as distinguished from the sympathetic, does influence the contractions of the arteries of the frog's foot. The effects, however, were not permanent. Six hours later, the arteries on the left side appeared smaller than they had been, though still bearing marks of the operation by remaining constant in calibre, whereas those of the right foot exhibited very frequent variations from pretty full dilatation to almost absolute closure. Next day, the same state of things continued; the vessels of the left foot being constant in size for four minutes together, while, in the right foot, an artery exhibited about eight distinct variations of calibre per minute, as observed by micrometer; but, after three days more, they had become both small and variable in the left foot, and seemed to have quite recovered. On the application of galvinism to the cord, however, both legs were thrown into violent spasm, showing that communications still existed between the left limb and the nervous centre ; and it appeared probable that the branches which remained undivided had come, after a while, to supply more or less perfectly the place of those which had been cut.

General Results.—1st, That, of the nervous centres usually recognized, the cerebro-spinal axis is the only part which regulates the contractions of the arteries of the web (of frogs) ; this function being apparently exercised by the whole length of the cord and the posterior part of the brain, operating through fibres which arise from the same region of the cord, as do those through which sensation and motion are effected in the hind legs.

2nd, That there exists within the limb some means, probably ganglionic, by virtue of which the fibre-cells of the circular coat of the arteries may contract in concert with each other, independently of any ganglia contained in the trunk.

And, 3rd, That the local co-ordinating apparatus, though capable of independent action in special conditions of direct irritation, is, under ordinary circumstances, in strict subordination to the spinal system; while a remarkable provision exists for the maintenance of this control, notwithstanding almost complete severance of nervous connection between the cord and limb.

Inflammation.—The effects produced upon the circulation, by the application of an irritant to a vascular part, are twofold, consequent upon two primary changes in the tissues, which, though often concomitant, are entirely independent both in nature and mode of production. One of these is dilatation of the arteries (commonly preceded by a brief period of contraction), giving rise, in proportion to the increase of calibre, to more free flow through the capillaries—the blood remaining unaffected, except in the rate of its progress. This purely functional phenomenon is developed indirectly through the medium of the nervous system being not limited to the part acted on by the irritant, but implicating a surrounding area of greater or less extent. The other change is the result of the direct operation of the irritating agent upon the tissues, which experience some alteration; in consequence of which the blood in their vicinity becomes impaired, losing the properties which characterize it while within a healthy part, and which render it fit for transmission through the vessels, and assuming those which it exhibits when removed from the body, and placed in contact with ordinary solid matter. The first indication of this disorder of the vital fluid is, that its corpuscles, both red and white, acquire some degree of adhesiveness, which makes them prone to stick to one another and to the vascular parietes, and, lagging behind the liquor sanguinis, to accumulate in abnormal numbers in the minute vessels. This adhesiveness may exist in proportion to the severity of the affection, in any degree, from that which merely gives rise to a very slight preponderance of the corpuscular elements of the blood in the part, up to that which induces complete obstruction of the capillaries; and when the irritation has been very severe, the liquor sanguinis also shows signs of participation in the lesion, by a tendency to solidification of the fibrine.

ART. IV.—*Hysterical Anæsthesia.—Catalepsy in Religious Revivals.*

i.—*Anæsthesia of the Skin in Hysteria :* By M. AUG. VOISIN, of Paris. [An abstract of M. Voisin's interesting pamphlet, of 39 pages, on this subject *(De L'Anesthésie Cutanée Hystérique)* was translated for the last September number of this Journal, but was excluded, with the exception of a single paragraph, for want of space. The following analysis, from *The American Journal of Insanity* (for January, 1860), being more complete, will be found below. M. Voisin's ingenious remarks are founded on fifteen anæsthetic cases, together with some cases of hyperæsthesia, paralysis, etc., which he had observed at the Charity and Lariboisière hospitals during his *internat* (*internship*—anglicised by a neologism) in these institutions.]

In a brief historic notice of the principal writers on hysteria, the learned author pays a well-merited tribute to the name of Sydenham. In the very thorough discussion which follows, he makes the following divisions : 1. The relations that may exist between the attacks of hysteria and cutaneous insensibility. 2. The tendency of this insensibility to localize itself in one-half the body. 3. The coëxistence there of excessive sensibility with the entire want of it. 4. The pathology of the sense of touch, and the treatment proper for the class of paralytic symptoms here considered.

Among the many valuable remarks which this paper contains, we notice the following as specially worthy of attention :

"In cases of hysteria, cutaneous insensibility, with scarce an exception, pre-supposes that the attack was attended with loss of consciousness. In other words, loss of consciousness and the anæsthesia are related as cause and effect."

"My grandfather, Dr. Felix Voisin, in his '*Etude sur les Causes des Maladies Nerveuses*,' maintains that the immediate seat of hysteria is in the brain. My own opinion is, that the anæsthesia of hysteria may be traced directly to disturbance in the cerebro-spinal column. So intimate, however, is the connection between this column and the brain, that the two ideas are not far apart."

"The existence in the same subject of insensibility and the liveliest sensibility, appears like a pathologic contradiction. For an explanation of this we are indebted to the careful researches of M. Briquet. According to him, the insensibility belongs to the skin, the excessive sensibility to the muscles."

Amid some curious observations on the different qualities and conditions of the sense of touch, the author mentions a remarkable effect produced by the paralysis of this very part of the human frame. Where this sense is wholly gone, that of sight becomes the sole reliance. Blindfold the patient thus affected, and he cannot even direct his hand to his mouth. An instance came under the eye of M. Briquet at La Charité, in which the patient, having her eyes blinded, was taken out of bed, placed on the floor, and then put back into bed, without the slightest consciousness that anything had been done to her. Another described her sensations when deprived of light, by saying that "she felt as if she had been plunged into utter emptiness."

The treatment of hysterical anæsthesia is involved in difficulty. Few efficacious remedies have as yet been found.

"For hysteria itself, preparations of iron and other tonics, belladonna, and the anti-spasmodics, are the means in common use, though often unsuccessful."

"For the paralytic affections, we use friction, kneading of the flesh, strychnine, brucine, and the water-cure. Quite recently, M. Duchenne, of Boulogne, has applied local electricity in the cure of this disease. We have ourselves seen, under the hand of M. Briquet, several cases suffering from *recent* anæsthesia, restored to feeling in the course of a few minutes, by the electric action. But cases of long standing resisted this treatment, as they had every other."

The author relates fifteen cases of hysterical anæsthesia, giving, with much minuteness of detail, the symptoms, course, and treatment of the disease in each case.

ii.—*Religious Catalepsy, or Nervous Epidemic connected with the Religious Revival in Ireland.* (From *The Am. Jour. of Insanity*)

However imperfectly technical language may describe these manifestations, they are, it is easy to see, governed by well-known physiological laws. Where the epidemic prevails among a people of a low grade of intelligence, the disorder will be manifested chiefly in the functions of the spinal cord, and catalepsy and convulsions will be presented. Epidemics of a similar kind in this country during the past fifteen years, arising among a people of more active intellect, have affected more the cerebral functions, and have developed hallucinations of all kinds, fanatical passions, and the wildest vagaries of belief. Of these, Millerism and Spiritualism are prominent instances. In a more robust and energetic people we have a greater degree of boisterousness and activity in the manifestations. This is illustrated in the history of the so-called "Backwoods Revivals," which occurred in our Western States many years ago. Indeed, the manner in which the nervous contagion is modified in its effects by the condition of its subjects is precisely that which is observed in epidemics of cholera and yellow fever. In both cases, at the first appearance of the disorder, only those in some way predisposed to its attack are affected, and the symptoms are not sudden or severe. But when the height of the epidemic is reached, persons are attacked almost indiscriminately, and with great power.

The relations which this epidemic has attained, through natural causes, or perhaps by a special providence, to evangelical religion, are, however, the most important of all. It is these which have excited, and are still giving rise to much discussion through the pulpit and the press of Great Britain. On the one side, it is claimed that the revival phenomena are almost wholly supernatural, and are to be encouraged in every form and direction in which they may be developed. While on the other hand, they are condemned as physical only, and tending solely to the hurt of morals and religion. A great amount of evidence, statistical, historical, medical and theological, has been brought forward upon the subject, but the best and most learned still differ very widely in their conclusions.

Probably in no country have these epidemics been so frequent and powerful as in our own, and nowhere is there so general an agreement as to their character and their practical treatment. It has been observed that the conditions under which they are developed are similar, whether the manifestations are evangelical, Spiritual, Millennial, or any other. They usually have their rise in a profound stagnation of public concern regarding matters of religious and social interest, or, on the other hand, in occasions of panic or crisis. But while observation proves that they are reäctive in their origin, experience shows that they all have both a retrograde and a corrective tendency. The physical manifestations are only evil in their effects, and we believe much more powerfully so than is generally considered. The moral manifestations have no necessary relations with the physical, and by careful, well-directed effort, especially in the early stages of the epidemic, may almost always be made to tend to beneficial results. Through the great Millennial epidemic many were brought to connect themselves with the evangelical churches, and even that of Spiritualism has, in some communities, been made to advance the interests of true religion. We have little doubt that if the experience of our own religious teachers in these revivals could direct the treatment of the Irish epidemic, it might be made largely productive of good. But to this end a moderate, and above all a united sentiment and action are necessary. Between a gross superstition on the one side, and too great religious nicety on the other, the present opportunity may be sadly misimproved.

These nervous affections, as they have been observed especially in religious revivals, are treated in a most candid and philosophic spirit by a writer in the *Methodist Quarterly Review* for April last, and may, we suppose, be taken as a representative view of the phenomena, among a sect in connection with whose Christianizing efforts they have been most frequently manifested. The writer, treating of "Religious Catalepsy," considers the phenomena "as perhaps in the largest degree physical," and as far as possible to be discouraged. After an analysis of the manifestations, and treating of them from the side of physiology quite at length, he concludes as follows:

"The first inference drawn from the above showing is, that there is danger of placing quite too much importance upon this occasional feature of personal piety and of revivals of religion. We cannot resist the conviction that the cataleptic exercise is the slenderest of all evidences of the genuineness and depth of the work of grace. It is not a criterion of piety. A revival may be genuine which is thus characterised. One may be equally so which is not marked by a solitary example of catalepsy; and precisely so as to individual Christians in every stage of experience. It must not be taken as the test or measure of piety."

Only on one point, perhaps, must the medical observer differ from this experienced and learned minister. He considers that "nothing morbid, or in the slightest degree prejudicial to physical health, is assumed to attend or result from this sort of paralysis." Our own observations too fully confirm the plainest inferences from physiology, that these manifestations tend greatly to impair the nervous functions, and to superinduce various forms of positive disease. The moral exercises, though they may be in some cases dissipating to their subject, we know are oftener salutary in the highest degree. These can only be cautiously and reverently guided, howsoever extraordinary they may appear. But ecstacy, hallucination, hysteria, and catalepsy can have only an accidental relation to a spiritual illumination.—*Am. Jour. of Insanity*, Jan., 1860.

ART. V.—*Notes on Insanity and Cerebral Lesions. General Paralysis.*

i.—*Notes on Insanity, and Cerebral Injuries and Lesions :* By B. DOWLER, M. D.

ESQUIROL, the learned psychiater or alienist (mad-doctor—born, ·

1772; died, 1840), who modeled the lunatic asylums of France, published in 1838, two years before his death, his great authoritative
work, *Des Maladies Mentales, Considerées sous les Rapports Médical,
Hygiènique, et Médico-Légale.* t. ii. It may be of interest to glance at
this representative work, giving a few analytic notes from it and
some other sources, with remarks chiefly in relation to injuries or
lesions of the brain, in their relations to mental maladies, in order
that the prevalent opinions of 1838, and those expressed twenty years
later in France (as will appear in the second part of this article),
may be compared.

As to the nature and the seat of the organic lesions observed in
the bodies of those dying of mental diseases, all is, according to
Esquirol, sterile, or lead to negative or contradictory results. The
lesions found in this class of cadavera, are found equally in other
classes that never suffered from mental derangement, while, in many
long affected with mania and idiocy, no trace of morbid alteration
can be discovered. Again : various parts of the brain may alter,
suppurate, and be destroyed without any chronic affection following.
Hence, he concludes that the immediate cause of mental alienation
has escaped our means of investigation ; but he says, contradictorily
enough, that it depends on an unknown modification of the brain
[how know that which is unknown ?] ; that this modification does
not always take its point of departure from the brain, but often
from the different centres of sensibility in various parts of the body.
M. E. propounds theory in a dubious form. (See vol. i ; 110–114.)
He rejects autopsies, because they do not explain every case of
mental disease. One ought rather to be thankful for what they do
reveal, and hope for more. Having rejected the known methods as
inadequate, he seems to know all about the matter when he asserts
that there is in mental alienation an unknown change produced in the
brain. He quotes Cabanis' assertion, that the brains of the insane
and of suicides possess a greater amount of phosphorus than is found
in the normal condition. (i—640.) Nor does he often hesitate to
define mental maladies by cerebral definitions. He says dementia is
a cerebral affection, in which the lesions of the brain are greater
than in any other mental malady (ii—219–244); that, in melancholy,
there is an alteration which he has often observed in making autopsies;
namely—a displacement of the transverse color, its position being
oblique, and even perpendicular, its left extremity resting against the

pubis, and sometimes hid behind the symphysis—a displacement often observed in the alienated who committed suicide. He considers suicide due to mental alienation, and that autopsic examination affords little information as to its cause. The reading books which glorify suicide, he considers mischievous, quoting Madame de Staël, who assures her readers that Goëthe's Werther has produced more suicides in Germany than all the women of that country. (i—444, 641, 589)

The laws which confiscated the goods of criminals executed under the Roman 'Emperors, multiplied suicides. The same happened during the reign of terror in France. The military government, and the law of conscription, in that country, each served as a great epoch or point of departure for the multiplication of suicides and maniacs. (i—53)

So little is known with certainty in the pathological anatomy characteristic of insanity, that some regard it as strictly a disease of the soul, not of the body. Now, although the medical man has often no peculiar criterion beyond others whereby to diagnosticate insanity, yet, not a few cases occur in which he can clearly trace this affection to material causes and morbid changes in the body; while, on the other hand, those who contend that the disease is due to mental or psychical alterations, cannot confirm their doctrine by a single test or example of this alteration. Hence, a presumption arises in favor of the former doctrine, namely, that insanity is in every instance due to abnormal alterations in the body, though not yet fully ascertained by any existing means of exploration. Sound analogy supports this view, but ignores any purely psychical change, as the cause of mental aberration.

On the other hand it must not be forgotten that the brain has been injured, altered and most extensively disorganized without having impaired, much less destroyed the mind, and without having produced general or local palsy. Dr. Wigan, in his work, mentions a boy whom he attended after the patient had fallen from a tree, fracturing his skull, whereby more than a quarter of a pound of brain was lost. The boy was very intelligent after, as well as before this accident, and so continued until the moment of his death. He had so far recovered as to engage in play, in the hot sun, and having been heated from the exercise, went into the water to cool himself: " The new blood vessels burst, and he died of hæmorrhage ; never having manifested from first to last any loss or perversion of mental power." (39, 40.) He mentions another patient of his in whom "one hemisphere [of the brain] was entirely gone," and yet this man, aged 50, "conversed rationally and even wrote verses within a few hours of his death." (*ib.*) He quotes a case from Dr. Connolly, in which the man possessed his entire faculties quite perfect to the last, yet one hemisphere "was entirely destroyed—gone, annihilated, and in its place a yawning chasm"—a similar case he gives from the late Dr. James Johnson—another from Cruveilhier's *Anat. Path.*, though, in this case, there was paralysis on the opposite. side; another from the same, showing that the right cerebrum had been totally disorganized without any injury to the intelligence; another of a child injured by a blow ten months before death—the left hemisphere had been converted into a soft pulpy mass, *blanc mange*; another from the same author, in which the right cerebrum "was utterly disorganized." This man (Martin, aged 32) was in the full possession of his faculties, and enjoyed the use of all the organs of sense, though suffering the most dreadful tortures—another from Dr. Abercrombie, reported by Mr. O'Halloran, wherein a great part of the brain was discharged; "at each dressing three ounces of brain came away. The cavern was terrible, yet the man preserved his intellect entire till the very moment of his death;" another case by Dr. Abercrombie, in which "the left hemisphere was a mass of indurations and softenings;" another from Dr. Ferriar, in which the whole right hemisphere was entirely destroyed by suppuration." In all these cases the mind was unimpaired.

Perhaps tne most remarkable case on record is that of S. P. Gage, reported by Dr. Harlow, and attested by numerous professional and non-professional witnesses, showing that an iron crowbar, weighing $13\frac{1}{4}$ lbs., was, by the explosive force of gunpowder, intended to blast a rock, 'driven under the zygomatic arch, diagonally through the brain, out at the top of the head, and up into the air, leaving at its emergence a hole in the skull, at the junction of the coronal and sagittal sutures, three inches and a half in diameter. The man fell, but soon got up—mounted a cart and rode home, sitting up unsupported—walked up stairs with but little aid—sat down in the piazza, self-possessed. With the exception of nocturnal fever, delirium and coma, which supervened but yielded readily to treatment some weeks after the injury, this man possessed all his faculties of body and mind, the sight of one eye excepted, from 1848 to 1850, when he was examined by the Medical Society of Boston, whose report is the last that has appeared in the case. An authenticated case which appeared in the *Western Medico-Chirurgical Journal* of a later date is of almost equal interest. A large charge of buck-shot entered a man's head above the ear, and passing through the brain lodged against the skull on the opposite side, where it was found at the post mortem examination. From the wound before death, a tea cup full of brain was discharged; yet the patient's senses and mental powers were unaffected until just before death, which occurred several days after the accident.

A single case of the disorganization or complete softening of the brain or of a great portion of it, without impairing the mental functions, or voluntary forces, is sufficient to throw some doubt upon the whole received system of cerebral physiology and pathology, and, in connection with the experimental decapitation of animals unattended with a complete loss of sensation, volition, and intelligential motion, must overthrow some of the fundamental doctrines of this system, as now taught.

The pivot on which the following pathological discussion turns, is the softening of the brain as the anatomical character of general paralysis in the insane. In commencing this paper, it was intended to inquire into the circumstances which give rise to post mortem softening simulating that of disease, illustrations of which might be taken from books received as authoritative on the pathological anatomy of the brain, in which equivocal examples of this lesion are taken at a lenghtened period after death, in warm weather, under conditions which must, upon physical principles alone, produce the alteration in question, independent of any antecedent malady. But the paper which follows is a long one, and the execution of the purpose mentioned would give undue extension to this article.

I will only add, that about eleven years ago, I made an extensive numerical analysis of the alleged periods which elapsed between death and post mortem examination, in the autopsies reported by some of the most celebrated pathologists in insular and continental Europe, from which it appeared that the mean time is about thirty hours. In many cases the time is not noted at all! In the one case, cohesion, a fundamental test, is thus rendered doubtful; in the other, ignored altogether. Mr. Solly's book on the Brain, which is some times brought into courts of justice as authority in medico-legal investigations, mentions in all seriousness, softenings found as late as eighty-four hours after death " in the summer season." I have found

in a medico-legal investigation before the jury of inquest, that a person who died suddenly at breakfast without previous sickness, who
was buried the same day, and who was disinterred seventy-six hours
after death, had the entire brain softened to the consistence of castor
oil.

ii.—*Distinguished French Alienists on General Paralysis.* (*From the Reports of Discussions by the Medico-Psychological Society of Paris, in the
Annales Médico-Psychologiques,* 1858–9.—*Am. Jour. Insanity.*)

M. PARCHAPPE. * * * In all the cases of paralytic insanity that
have come under my observation, amounting to three hundred and
twenty-two, I have constantly found inflammatory softening, more or
less extensive, of both hemispheres. In many cases, if I had confined
myself to appearances simply, and to the modes of examination commonly employed, I might have overlooked a characteristic lesion. The
membranes were healthy, and easily detached from the surface of the
brain without producing that decortication which commonly reveals,
on the slighetst tractile effort, the softened condition of the cortical
substance. The cerebral surface was not altered in color; its consistence seemed even to be augmented; the brain cut in slices appeared
perfectly sound; but careful examination and recourse to the following procedure have enabled me in these cases to prove positively the
existence of softening of the middle portion of the cortical substance.
The handle of a scalpel, slightly engaged in one-half the thickness of
the cortical substance, enabled me, by gently raising the outer portion
of this substance, to detach it over a greater extent than that in which
the action of the instrument was exercised, and thus to cause that
decortication which is so readily produced in most cases by simple
traction exerted upon the membranes.

The efficiency of this procedure for demonstrating the existence of
softening is also shown in ordinary cases, when decortication is produced by simple traction of the membranes. This result is obtained
principally on the free margin of the convolutions. But it would be
a great mistake to suppose that softening only existed in cases where
decortication is produced by traction on the membranes. Softening
of the cortical substance is quite as marked in many points of the
convolutions corresponding to the anfractuosities, and of the free
margin of the convolutions, from which the membranes may be detached without causing decortication. In all these points, by raising
with the handle of the scalpel the external portion of the cortical substance, the existence of softening may be proved with the utmost certainty. I believe that all the instances of perfect integrity of the cortical substance in paralytic insanity which have been related, can be
explained by an error of diagnosis during life, or the insufficiency of
the examination after death.

In regard to the use of the microscope for determining the portion
of the brain affected in general paralysis, I believe it may be said that
the instrument is not indispensable for the solution of the question.
Doubtless much assistance and many discoveries may be expected

from microscopic researches. I am convinced that the microscope will prove, if it has not already done so, the inflammatory nature of the changes of the cortical substance in general paralysis. But it is not, in my opinion, the province of the microscope to replace ordinary anatomy. The eye aided by the microscope is to me only an auxiliary to the study of anatomy by the naked eye, and by the touch; and microscopic observations, in order that they may have a scientific value, must never contradict but confirm, by explaining, and sometimes by modifying the fundamental doctrines of pathological anatomy.

All the facts afforded by pathological anatomy agree in affirming the inflammatory nature of the characteristic lesion of the cortical substance of the brain in general paralysis. The special character of this lesion is to affect simultaneously both cerebral hemispheres, principally in the anterior and middle lobes, and to be associated nearly always with an inflamed condition of the meninges, frequently with inflammatory softening of the gray substance, of the intra cerebral ganglia, of the cerebellum, and of the medulla spinalis; with a granular condition of the ventricular walls, and with induration of the white substance, and finally very frequently with atrophy of the convolutions.

The development of the disease is peculiar as regards the succession and connection of the symptoms, the structural changes, and the termination of the malady. Mental disorder is constant from the first, at least under the form of impairment of the memory and judgment; and very frequently under that of maniacal or melancholiac excitement. This impairment of the intellectusl faculties goes on increasing until it ends in their complete extinction. The lesion of motion only becomes very apparent after that of the intelligence. It may be entirely wanting at the commencement, so that the most experienced alienists are sometimes kept in doubt during many days or even weeks as to the real nature of the disorder, by reason of the absence of every symptom of paralysis. In most cases the lesion of motion is first manifested in the power of articulation, and afterwards extends to the other voluntary movements, especially to those concerned in walking and standing, though it sometimes happens that the gait is affected, while as yet the power of speech remains almost intact. It is not unusual for the powers of locomotion and speech to be affected simultaneously. Sometimes the paralysis is more marked on one side, simulating hemiplegia. Sometimes the motion of the iris is affected, producing unequal dilatation of the pupils. The muscular lesion always goes on increasing in extent and intensity, as the disease becomes more aggravated. * * *

In general, and except accidentally in the state of congestion, the disease is not accompanied by a true febrile movement, although my investigations of the state of the pulse among the insane have led me to notice a slight increase of its frequency in those affected with general paralysis. But one of the most striking symptoms of the disease, is the important part performed in its development by cerebral congestion. Very frequently an attack of congestion is the first symptom of paralytic insanity, and in that way may be explained the large number of cases of insanity attributed to apoplexy in the

table of causes kept at the Bicêtre, before the disease began to be
recognized. The frequency of cerebral congestion at the outset of
general paralysis is so well established, that I have frequently been
able to foretell the speedy manifestation of paralytic symptoms in
cases where the attack of insanity, as yet unimplicated with paralysis, and sometimes even when very slight, had been preceded or
accompanied by cerebral congestion. These attacks are generally
renewed several times during the course of the disease, and after each
recurrence leave the patient with a considerable aggravation of all
the symptoms   *   *   *   The inflammatory action, which is set
up from the first in the cortical substance of both hemispheres, at
once produces the pathological change known by the name of softening, which softening is constant and unceasing in its progress. In
the majority of cases, and in the first periods of the disease, the softening is found at the surface on the free margin of the convolutions,
and its existence is manifested by flakes and layers of the softened
cerebral substance, which the membranes bring with them when they
are removed. But from the outset of the disease the softening is
invariably found in the mass of the cortical substance, generally in its
middle portion, and the traction upon the membranes, pressure with
the finger, or the introduction of the handle of a scalpel, readily
causes the separation of layers of the cerebral substance, whose
thickness equals about half that of the cortical portion. As the disease progresses the softening may invade the cortical substance in its
entire thickness, in which case pressure with the finger causes complete decortication of the convolutions. The softening of the cortical
substance generally progresses from before backwards, occupying at
first the extremity of the anterior lobes, and extending along their
convex surface, then by way of the middle lobes until it reaches the
posterior surface of the hemispheres. At a more advanced period the
softening sometimes extends to the gray matter of the corpora striata, of the optic thalami and the medulla spinalis, and it not unfrequently affects the cortical substance of the cerebellum.
    The softening of the cortical portion, and the changes of this sub-
stance or of the meninges, offer, in the first or acute stage, all the
characters of an inflammatory condition; a rose, lilac, or even ama-
rauth color of the cortical substance, hyperæmia, pointed injection,
extravasations of blood in the cortical substance or in the membranes,
adhesion of the pia mater to the surface of the convolutions, sometimes separation of the pia mater, and collection of a sanious liquid
between it and the cortical substance. At a more advanced period,
if the patient's life is prolonged, hyperæmia is no longer found. The
softened cortical substance has a pale, dirty-gray or yellowish tint.
At this period of the disease are found atrophy of the convolutions,
serous effusion in the anfractuosities, with thickening and opacity of
the membranes.
    The connection between the symptoms and lesions, which is mani-
fested by the prominent features of the disease, deserves to be attentively studied. The mental disorder, under the form of mania or mel-
ancholia, coincides with the period when the alteration of the cortical
substance is only superficial, and of limited extent. The loss of men-

tal power, as well as the paralysis, is intimately connected with the depth and extent of the softening of the cortical substance. The difficulty of speech is generally dependent upon a lesion of the anterior lobes. I have frequently observed, in cases where the paralysis was more marked on one side so as in some degree to resemble hemiplegia, a greater extent of softening of the cortical substance of the opposite side. Finally, one of the most constant characters of general paralysis of the insane is its fatal termination.

In giving this opinion I do not wish to discourage others more than myself. I believe we ought to treat general paralysis, in its first stage, as we would a curable disease. But though I have conformed to this rule, I have not been so fortunate as to obtain a single positive and certain cure. The fatal termination of general paralysis has this peculiarity, that it takes place more or less suddenly by cerebral congestion, or comes on gradually by a slow decline, towards the end of which gangrenous eschars are frequently formed on all parts of the body subject to pressure, while life is only manifested by vegetative phenomena; a condition which I have designated as *cerebral marasmus*.

This rapid sketch of the principal characters which belong to the essential elements of general paralysis, appears to me to be an unanswerable proof of the necessity of referring it to a distinct nosological species. It is in fact a morbid entity, different from all others, a disease which is produced by causes which bring on over excitement of the brain, generally in men, and during the adult period of life; whose symptoms may be summed up in general and simultaneous lesion of the intelligence, the voluntary motions and sensibility; which has for its seat the cortical substance of the hemispheres, and for its constant anatomical character inflammatory softening of the cortical substance of both hemispheres, which, aggravated by cerebral congestions, causing every day a more marked impairment of motion, intelligence, and sensibility, terminates fatally in an attack of congestion, or by cerebral marasmus.

When, in the course of the year 1838, I became convinced that general paralysis was constantly characterized by inflammatory softening of the cortical substance of both hemispheres, and that the affection constituted a distinct nosological species, I felt strongly tempted to give it a special name, expressive of its seat and nature, and of the pathological alteration which is essential to it. At this period Dr. Bayle had referred general paralysis of the insane to meningitis; Dr. Calmeil had attributed it to encephalitis, of which he could not at first positively determine the seat and character, but which, in 1841, he thought himself warranted in designating as *chronic diffused peri-encephalo-meningitis*. If I had given to general paralysis the name of general cortical cerebritis, I would have indicated the principal result of my pathological researches, and could at once, and without the possibility of confusion, have distinguished the results obtained by my predecessors, and especially those which have led Dr. Belhomme to designate the disease by the name of meningo-cerebritis. I have resisted this temptation, preferring to my own interest that which appeared to be for the benefit of science, and have given to the disease the name of paralytic insanity.

The following considerations have induced me to follow this course: In the first place, I do not think it possible to sever the close connection between the disease and simple insanity, in both of which the predisposing and exciting causes are the same. The disease frequently begins with intellectual disturbance, exempt from all complication with paralysis; and during days and weeks the patient, who may be in the end attacked with general paralysis, can only be considered and treated as if affected with simple insanity. The paralytic symptoms are sometimes developed after a long duration of ordinary mania, and I have met with cases of sudden invasion of general paralysis after the patients had been a long time affected with simple dementia. The disease has the same seat as insanity—namely, the cortical substance of the hemispheres.

Though simple insanity may not be characterized by any constant change in the cerebral structure, nevertheless the alterations which are frequently found in the brains of the insane, and which, as some observers assert, are always found there, have the greatest analogy with the alterations which are met with in paralytic insanity. These are hyperæmia and thickening of the membranes, hyperæmia or decoloration of the cortical substance, induration of the white substance, atrophy of the convolutions, and collections of serum in the anfractuosities of the convolutions. Besides, it is essential that the importance of appreciable organic lesions should not be overrated. Because no constant structural change is found in the cortical substance in simple insanity, which is therefore classed with the *neuroses*, and considered a purely functional disorder, shall we therefore conclude that morbid action can be set up without structural change in the organ? But functional passes into structural disease in the lowest grades of dementia, by atrophy of the convolutions. In my opinion, simple insanity from being a purely functional disorder, becomes organic in those cases in which it becomes complicated with general paralysis.

Moreover, it does not appear to me to be possible to include general paralysis in the class of phlegmasiæ, and in the genus of cerebral inflammation. The disease is apyretic; it is not accompanied at its origin by bilious vomitings, so usual in meningitis, and so frequent in encephalitis. It does present the group of acute febrile symptoms which characterize frank inflammation of the meninges, and that of the white and grey cerebral substance. True encephalitis is generally partial, and occupies only one hemisphere; it affects commonly both the cortical and medullary portions of the brain, or of the cerebellum. The cases of inflammation of the cortical substance of both hemispheres that have been cited in the treatises on encephalitis, are for the most part cases of unrecognized general paralysis. In encephalitis the paralysis is generally confined to one side of the body, and is more marked at the onset than in general paralysis, and is usually accompanied with contractions. The course of true encephalitis is rapid; it continues only a short time, while general paralysis of the insane lasts sometimes for years. These are the considerations which determined me, in 1838, not to refer general paralysis unconditionally to inflammation of the brain, and not to separate it too rigidly from simple insanity, and which still compel me to persist in this determination. *   *   *

M. DELASIAUVE.—I will be brief, and will confine myself to the question as stated—What is general paralysis ? Does the group of symptoms described under this denomination deserve to occupy, with a special title, a distinct place in the catalogue of nervous disorders ? May not the muscular enfeeblement be only a complication of the mental disorder ? Do they alone characterize the affection, or are they not merely the necessary and inevitable, or at least the direct consequence of the nervous lesion ? These questions present only another aspect of the same problem, and their solution will only be another mode of arriving at the same point—that of determining the nature of general paralysis.

Much importance has been attached to the seat and character of the structural changes. That which, according to Bayle, is the result of chronic meningitis, is caused, according to Delayé, by a molecular change of the cerebral tissue, especially of the gray substance, and according to Calmeil, by encephalitis or meningo-encephalitis. M. Parchappe, on the contrary, supported by numerous autopsies, maintains that the pathological lesion consists in softening of the cortical substance. A lesion that corresponded in its phases to all the changes of symptoms, would certainly be a great discovery. A disorder which so speedily becomes general, ought manifestly to depend upon an organic change—a molecular transformation, attacking simultaneously both hemispheres. In what does this change consist ? In an affection which continues for years, and gives rise to such frequent and such formidable congestions, is there not reason to fear that effects may be taken for causes, and that the disease may be attributed to changes of structure, which are themselves only its consequences ? This I am led to believe in regard to the chronic meningitis of Bayle, which does not, however, deprive our lamented brother, who was also my valued friend, of the great merit of having been the first to describe general paralysis, and of having so well traced its history, that, with the exception of disputed points, he has left nothing to be added by his successors. The existence of encephalitis does not seem to be better established. All inflammations are at first local and circumscribed. Extending gradually as in general paralysis, it ought, a long time before extending from one lobe to another, and to those of the opposite side, to be manifested by limited signs. But we see from the beginning the muscular defect, though still obscure, showing itself in different parts of the system. I have always preferred the opinion of Delayé, who, while locating the disease in the cerebral mass, and particularly in its superficial portions, has not ventured to decide upon its nature. In the hospital Bicêtre, where there are so many deaths of general paralysis, I have, in spite of the obstacles often opposed to autopsies, nevertheless had occasion to examine the brains of a great number of subjects. All kinds of lesions have been presented to my observation, but there was nothing constant, and frequently it has been impossible not to remain in doubt touching their existence. My colleague, M. Moreau, must remember two cases which we examined together, in which we did not think ourselves justified in deciding upon the presence of primary lesions. The cortical substance often indeed presents slight softening. But if it does yield to pressure with the handle of the scalpel, in numerous instances probability permits us to attribute this circumstance as well to serous infiltration of the tissues as to morbid degeneration. The wasting of the convolutions, and especially the decoloration of the grey substance, contrasting infinitely less with the white than in the normal condition, were the changes that appeared to me to be the most constantly present. Are these due to latent inflammation? Whatever may be the authority of the recent microscopic researches of M. Calmeil, this question is still, in my opinion, undecided.

It appears to me more probable that this is one of those defects of nutrition, the mystery of which has not yet been unraveled. Every one has observed cerebral congestions, so common among the paralytic insane. It seems probable that this complication has not yet received its true explanation. Most authors consider the paralytic symptoms as dependent upon the congestion, when it occurs in the onset, and attribute to it an aggravating influence over the disease. In my opinion its mode of production is different, and of such a nature, if properly explained, as to throw much light upon some points which are imperfectly understood. For many reasons, I am induced to believe that these congestions differ essentially from those of an apoplectic nature. Caused by a rush of blood, which commonly takes place towards a limited portion of the brain, the latter are of an active kind; and as they attack the patient whilst in full health, when they disappear speedily the intellect does not materially suffer. The congestions of general paralysis, on the contrary, are entirely passive in their nature, and instead of being primary, appear to me to be subordinate to a preëxisting condition of the brain, whose tendency is to produce embarrassment of the circulation, and stasis of the blood in the cerebral vessels. * * *

This leads me to notice some points of the learned discourse of M. Parchappe. Hesitating as to the choice of a name, he inclined to the term cerebritis, but preferred that of paralytic insanity, so as to avoid severing the connection which exists between the mental and physical phenomena. What I have already said will show the incorrectness of the first of these designations. Inflammation is not certainly present, and it may be asked, while recognizing its elements, if they may not be produced by the congestion itself forming by its long continuance a sub-inflammatory reäction? If inflammation were really present, would we have the same consequences? Under whatever aspect we regard them, are there not differences which compel us to make a distinction between the two categories, and to apply a special qualification to the variety we are engaged in discussing?

The term paralytic insanity does not appear to be more appropriate. It has often been remarked that words which have passed into common use are generally the most correct. That of general paralysis is especially of this character. It answers to the prominent symptoms, and sufficiently indicates the mental disorder. Without prejudging the nature of the disease, and being readily comprehended, it has the advantage of realizing the conditions of a good definition, by suiting under its most obvious meaning *soli et toti definito.*

Is it so with the appellation substituted by M. Parchappe ? Without regard to the anatomical lesion, and to the difference of symptoms, does it not confound all cases in which mental disorder coëxists with paralysis ? Our honorable colleague does not seem to have escaped entirely this inconvenience. In a special article on the diagnosis, in the "*Annales Médico-Psychologiques*," 1851, I was the first, perhaps, to attempt to distinguish *pseudo*-general paralysis from the true idiopathic affection. M. Lesègue, in a well-written thesis, has pursued the same course, and M. J. Falret, in his inaugural dissertation going still further, and eliminating under distinct titles all the bastard forms, admits, as the true type of the disease, that only which, supervening at certain periods of life, develops itself in an irregularly progressive manner, and terminates almost invariably after a comparatively brief period in a fatal issue.

M. BAILLARGER—Commenced by remarking that under the name of general paralysis, cases were described, in appearance at least, very dissimilar. It was sufficient, he said, in order to prove this, to compare the two classes of cases in which the symptoms are most opposite: the first of these classes comprises all cases of ambitious mania accompanied by some slight symptoms of paralysis ; the second includes those of simple and primary paralytic dementia. The symptoms in the two cases are as different as possible—exaltation of the faculties opposed to mental enfeeblement, and augmented muscular action contrasted with paralysis. M. Baillarger then compared the anatomical lesions in ambitious mania and in paralytic dementia ; he found in the former case hyperæmia and turgescence of the brain; in the latter, atrophy of the same organ, with grave lesions of its substance. On the other hand, if it is considered that ambitious mania does not terminate inevitably in paralytic dementia, and that it consequently has a separate existence; and that besides paralytic dementia is every day met with, without ambitious mania, the conclusion must be admitted that the two pathological conditions ought to be distinguished, since their symptoms and anatomical characters are different, and they exist separate and independent of each other. In admitting this distinction, the same opinion would be extended to ambitious mania and paralytic dementia which is already received as regards ordinary mania and dementia. The same reasons are applicable in both cases. M. Baillarger therefore concluded by proposing to make of ambitious mania a special malady under the name of *congestive mania.* Congestive mania would then bear to paralytic dementia the same relation that simple mania does to simple dementia.

M. BELHOMME. * * * In 1845, I presented to the Academy of Medicine a memoir of my recent examinations of the brains of the paralytic insane, and I endeavored to show that the structural change, coinciding with the manifestations of the disease, extends successively to all parts of the brain, not only affecting the cortical substance, which is the first to become diseased, but in addition reaching the deep-seated portions of the organ, as the commissures, which are themselves frequently softened.

I reported in detail fifteen cases, which prove that general paralysis depends upon the alterations which I am about to enumerate. Thickening of the membranes, and their adherence to the cortical substance of the brain, which is removed with them; the different layers of the cortical substance are softened, and present various shades of color, red, yellow and brown. The central portions diseased are the medullary substance, which is strongly injected, of a reddish or yellowish tint, softened in different degrees, sometimes only to a limited extent; and very often one of the hemispheres more altered than its fellow. The ventricles, often distended with serum, the arachnoid lining their walls is often thickened, and the medullary matter in contact with it either harder or softer than natural. The central parts constituting the cerebral peduncle, and the commissure are often altered, the septum lucidum destroyed, the fornix softened to a greater or less extent, the corpora striata atrophied or changed in color, the optic thalami, forming the principal wall of the third ventricle, are more or less softened. The cerebral peduncles are less consistent than in the normal condition; the annular protuberance sometimes partakes of the general condition of hardening or softening; in fine, the fourth ventricle and the rachidian bulb present various degrees of unequivocal hardening or softening, and the cerebellum partakes sometimes of the general diseased condition.

I conclude by expressing the belief that general paralysis is an encephalitis of a particular kind, an inflammation which is developed under the congestive form, a disorganizing hyperæmia which is established slowly, producing at first induration, and afterwards softeuing of the cerebral substance. At the same time, there is a gradual impairment of all the functions of the brain, motion, sensibility and intelligence.

It only remains for me to say one word in relation to my cases. After having made out the history of each fatal case of general paralysis, I have reported the autopsy, which was made with the greatest care, and accompanied each case with remarks, observing that the affection which caused the death of the patient was not merely a lesion of the cortical substance of the brain, but that there existed besides material changes of structure in the central portions of the organ. It might be said that the inflammation progresses layer by layer until it reaches the central parts, most essential to life. Thus in the first case, in which the disease ran a rapid course, and in which the post mortem appearances indicated a very active inflammation of the serous membranes, the brain was rather hardened than softened: this is not the first time that I have noticed that softening does not ensue until a later period of the paralytic affection. In this first case the patient died of suffocation, and I found at the autopsy softening of the fourth ventricle at the point of junction of the cerebral fibres with those of the medulla spinalis.

The fifth case perfectly proves the coincidence of the cerebral lesions with the paralytic symptoms. The paralysis came on slowly, progressively, and life was not threatened until the disease reached the cerebral centres. The autopsy showed an altered condition of the cortical substance, and the annular protuberance and the rachidian bulb were softened. On the 9th of May, 1856, I read before the Academy of Medicine the notes of two fatal cases of general paralysis, the autopsy proving that the brain was profoundly diseased. The softening of the central portion was so marked that it was impossible to distinguish the tubercula quadrigemina, the optic thalami, or the walls of the third and the fourth ventricle, the annular protuberance, and the rachidian bulb were softened, and the cerebellum had lost its normal consistence. * * *

Such, gentlemen, are my views of the nature and seat of general paralysis. They go to corroborate the opinions of others who have preceded me, but I claim in addition the demonstration of profound structural changes, and their connection with the functional lesions.

M. BAILLARGER.—M. Parchappe is surprised that I have not mentioned softening of the middle portion of the cortical substance, as one of the morbid changes met with in paralytic dementia. It is well known, indeed, that in the opinion of our learned colleague, this is the only constant change, and that to which the disease ought to be referred, as its anatomical character. According to my belief, the word softening does not convey a correct idea of the alteration which the cortical substance undergoes in paralytic dementia. This portion of the brain, I believe in the majority of cases, and at certain points, is softer than in the normal condition, but it has not, in the greater number of cases, undergone that change which in pathology is designated as softening. Softening, in fact, implies true disorganization ; the molecules glide freely over each other, and the texture of the organ is destroyed. But this is not the case in paralytic dementia, except in a few instances. This opinion was expressed long ago by M. Calmeil. "There is," says he, "a great difference between the condition of the gray substance simply wanting in consistence, and that same substance really in a state of softening."

But, according to the same author, if there is not in general paralysis real softening, even at the points where the gray substance adheres to the membranes, how much less does it exist in cases where there are no adhesions, and which are far from being rare. There is, therefore, properly speaking, no softening. As to the want of consistence presented by the cortical substance, M. Calmeil adds: "A reflection that leads to the conclusion that want of firmness of the cortical substance is of less importance than was at first supposed is, that many paralytics whose brains were found to be of normal consistence, were as deeply affected, as regards their voluntary movements, as those in whom the gray substance was more or less wanting in consistence." (p. 410.)

It may, besides, be concluded from M. Parchappe's own cases, that softening, that is to say true softening, is not the cause of general paralysis. In a passage of his work, he admits, in fact, that when the cortical substance is sliced vertically, nothing is observable, because the cortical substance is firm, and in a vertical section, nothing is seen but the violet or lilac discoloration, which effaces in one tint the distinctive shades of the two planes, so that nothing except the change of color is perceived, different from the normal condition. But, I ask, is this the case where the part is really softened ?

This explains how such skillful pathologists as MM. Calmeil and

Lelut have published cases, in which they declare that they have found no change of consistence ; how M. Calmeil, especially in the passage cited above, could declare that many paralytics had brains of the natural consistence and exempt from every alteration. (p. 140.)

Another objection against the opinion of M. Parchappe may be based on the cases which he has himself published ; in the descriptions which he has given, he does not go so far as to say that the cortical substance is *softened ;* he limits himself to saying that it is soft, or very soft.   In one of the cases he does not even venture to assert that its consistence is diminished; he only says that it *appears* softer than natural.   There are, moreover, six or seven cases in which the condition of the cortical substance is described, without loss of consistence being stated.   In fine, in a number of cases induration was met with, instead of softening.

Genuine softening of the cortical substance is, therefore, far from being always present, and the anatomical theory of paralytic dementia cannot consequently be based upon this alteration, as it has been by M. Parchappe.

Is it necessary that the softness of the gray substance may be explained in most cases by the congestion which terminated the life of the patient, by the time that elapsed after death, by the temperature, etc. ?

It has been perceived that the author assigns the middle portion of the cortical substance, as the seat of the softening.   I cannot on this point either, agree with him.   All physicians who have examined the bodies of the paralytic insane who have died during the first period of the disease, know that in most cases the membranes, on being removed, bring with them only very small portions of the cortical substance.   But if it is admitted that the point of separation is that at which the softening is the greatest, it must be confessed that, in the first stages, at least, this is not the middle portion.   Often, also, when the portions of the cortical substance which remain attached to the membranes are more extensive, they are so thin and so superficial, that it still is not the middle part that is the most softened.   On the other hand, there are cases, far from rare, in which the cortical layer comes off almost entire, leaving the medullary substance bare. M. Parchappe has cited examples of this kind, and I have also seen a considerable number.   It is very true that, in the greater number of cases, it is only the external layer which separates, but it is only necessary to refer to the structure of the cortical substance to perceive that it could not be otherwise. * * *

Esquirol, as M. Parchappe still does, regarded all cases of ambitious mania as simple insanity, as long as they were uncomplicated with symptoms of paralysis. Bayle, on the contrary, and with him M. Jules Falret, considers many of these cases as presenting a special form of insanity, even before the appearance of paralysis.   A case of ambitious mania is reported in the thesis of M. Falret, which was cured after two years' duration, without the patient having presented any evidence of paralysis.   But, according to the author, this patient was not the less attacked with paralytic insanity, very different from simple insanity, in its etiology, in its progress, and in its symptoms. The diagnosis was based, in this case, upon the general aspect, and chiefly on the nature of the mental affection, so that the paralytic symptoms, which doubtless would confirm the diagnosis when they did appear, were nevertheless not necessary to establish it. M. Parchappe, on the contrary, maintains in this respect the opinion of Esquirol, that, in order to constitute paralytic insanity, it is neccessary that paralysis should be actually present, and until it is present, the case is only one of simple insanity. But this difference between M. Parchappe and M. J. Falret is a circumstance of the greatest importance. Having made this explanation, it will be easy for me to state, in a few words, the new opinion which I wish to see adopted. I am firmly persuaded that almost all cases of ambitious mania ought to be separated from simple insanity, but I do not agree with Bayle and M. Jules Falret, that they should be necessarily referred to paralytic dementia, of which they may only constitute the forming stage. They ought, in my opinion, to be referred to a distinct category, under the name of congestive mania. Their relation to paralytic dementia is the same as that of ordinary insanity to simple dementia. * * *

M. Jules Falret.—M. Baillarger has said that there is a wide difference between M. Parchappe and myself. M. Baillarger has stated the question on clinical grounds, and it is thus, doubtless, that it ought to be stated. Among the cases of mania with ideas of grandeur, which M. Baillarger wishes to exclude from general paralysis, it is important to make a distinction. In one class of cases, and these are the most numerous, the embarrassment of speech is present, and M. Parchappe admits them, as I do, into the category of general paralysis; in the other, the difficulty of speech does not exist as yet, and this is the only difference between us; but this even is very slight, for M. Parchappe acknowledges with me that general paralysis, if not actually present, is at least imminent.

M. Baillarger.—I persist, nevertheless, in maintaining that between you and M. Parchappe there is a very important difference. The cases which M. Parchappe considers as simple mania, and which you regard as paralytic insanity, are very numerous, and I can cite them from the work of M. Parchappe himself. I grant that he considers ambitious mania as threatening paralysis, and as a precursor of the disease. In this respect M. Parchappe only adopts the general opinion. To deny that patients affected with ambitious mania are much more liable than others to become paralytic, would at this day be to deny what has been clearly proved. It is from the general agreement as to the formidable character of ambitious mania, that I draw my principle argument in favor of separating it from ordinary mania. How is it possible not to perceive that so great a difference in their prognosis and in their termination is sufficient to prove a difference in their nature? It seems to me that authors who continue to confound ambitious and simple mania, while admitting that the ambitious form announces the imminence of paralysis, are very inconsistent.

ART. VI.—*Do Bad Smells Cause Disease?*

THE tendency of the human mind to rest satisfied with any belief that is authoritatively asserted, is too well known to require any comment. Philosophers of all kinds are no more exempt than other people from this easy style of dealing with difficult problems. Medicine is, we think, especially chargeable with cherishing pet answers to questions that force themselves unkindly on her; and we think that the way in which she has made up her mind as to the causes of various kinds of fevers is an example of this style of cutting the Gordian knot.

Of late years, it must have struck all our readers that pig-styes, dirty pools of water, open privies, ash-heaps, etc., have been declared highly criminal, and on all occasions even adjudged guilty of producing any kind of fever or bowel complaint that may have broken out in their neighborhood. If a child happen to suffer typhus in a farmhouse, it is the mixen at the end of the barton that caused it. If an epidemic of English cholera befall a village, it is traced to the duck-pond by the road-side. If in a wealthy household the inmates are stricken with diphtheria, some open sewer close at hand has, as a matter of course, been the cause. So accustomd are we to hear this sort of reasoning resorted to on all occasions, that one feels a little difficulty in expressing doubts as to the certainty with which the effect is thus unhesitatingly traced to its cause. Nevertheless, we think there is at least sufficient evidence to cause reflecting minds to pause ere they give in their adhesion to the general opinion, and thus shut their eyes to further research and inquiry. Dr. Watson has, we know, stated it as his distinct opinion, "*that neither animal nor vegetable decomposition is sufficient to generate fever of any kind;*" and the researches of Dr. Guy, and other observers have certainly gone some way to support that opinion.

Dr. Guy, in his very interesting contribution to the *Journal of the Statistical Society*, on the health of Nightmen, Scavengers, and Dustmen, gives us a mass of statistical facts which, it must be confessed, run counter to the generally received opinion, that foul animal or vegetable emanations are the fruitful source of disease. This class of men without doubt spend their days in the very midst of filth of all kinds. He says:

"In most of the laystalls or dustmen's yards, every species of refuse matter is collected and deposited—night-soil, the decomposing refuse of markets, the sweepings of narrow streets and courts, the sour smelling grains from breweries, the surface-soil of the leading thoroughfares, and the ashes from the houses."

This heterogeneous mass the scavengers or "hill" people have to sort or to pass through sieves, so that the emanations arising therefrom must be brought into intimate relation with their lungs and skin. If fever and diarrhœa are so clearly traceable to the vicinity of these so-called noxious materials, surely the scavengers ought to be a poor fever-stricken race. A medical examination, however, of this class of workmen as compared with brickmakers and bricklayers' laborers, proves that the scavenger is comparatively exempt from disease. Thus, among a number of men examined in each of the three classes, it appeared that the numbers attacked by fever were, among the scavengers, 8 per cent.; among the bricklayers' laborers, 35.5 per cent.; and among brickmakers, 21.5 per cent.

This result seems extraordinary enough; but it may be argued that these men do not live in the laystalls or dustyards, and therefore that their exemption from fever may be attributable to this; but what can be said, if the master dustmen and their families, who live all their lives in the midst of these heaps of so-called fever-nests, are healthy ? Dr. Guy says:

" I do not think that, whether in town or country, such another body of men (as master dustmen) could be brought together except by selection; and it is not going too far to assert of them that, if the comparison were limited to the inhabitants of London, or our large towns, no score of selected tradesmen could be found to match the same number of scavengers brought casually together."

Unless we suppose that the scavengers get used to this so-called miasmatic atmosphere, or that after a time it no longer affects them, we cannot see how the foul emanation theory can hold water. Nature cannot work in one place differently from another. Nightsoil must be just as deadly in an open yard in London as in the country. But here we have the experiment tried on a larger scale, of a whole class of men subjected to foul emanations, and yet they are far from being an unhealthy race, and are not nearly so prone to fever or bowel-disease as the brickmaker's laborers.

We are far from wishing it to be understood, however, that we do not consider foul emanations as dangerous or baneful under any circumstances. In our opinion, they become noxious when much concentrated. Our houses, for instance, are built on the principle of a bell-glass; and our drains and privies, and all other impurities, if allowed to give off a deleterious miasma, most certainly do become most virulent sources of disease. But, in the open air, we think it very doubtful whether these emanations are ever the cause of injury to man.

Let us watch with Dr. McWilliam a still more gigantic experiment on the health of the Thames waterside people, which has been going on for years, and is still proceeding. The whole sewage of two millions and a half of people has within the last ten years been turned into the metropolitan stream. Year by year its waters have become more contaminated, and its smell more disgusting. It should follow, that the health of the waterside community is proportionately decreasing; that febrile complaints, cholera and diarrhœa, are alarmingly on the advance. But what is the real state of the case ? Dr. McWilliam, in his Report for the year 1858 on the health of the Water Guard and Waterside Officers of Her Majesty's Customs, says:

" As respects bowel affections, in which I include diarrhœa, choleraic diarrhœa, dysentery, etc., the types of those forms of disease, which in this country noxious exhalations are commonly supposed to originate, we find the additions during the four hot months of the past year from this class of complaints 26.3 below the average of the corresponding period of the three previous years, and 73 less than those of 1857."

The quantity of purtescent animal and vegetable matter in the Thames has been going on increasing ; but the illness generally attributed to the emanations arising therefrom has been decreasing ! We know that many will urge that all the combustibles (if we may use the term) being thus accumulated, it only requires the match to be applied, to find epidemics raging like wildfire. But the year before last, cholera did break out on the banks of the Lea, and there died out, apparently from want of sustenance. This year, according to the *Lancet*, cholera, veritable Asiatic cholera, has been on board the *Dreadnought ;* yet it has not spread, and there seems no likelihood of its doing so for this season at least. As Dr. McWilliam truly says, " It is nowhere sustained by evidence that the stench from the river or docks, however noisome, was in any way productive of disease." It is true that one waterman, in June last, was said to have died of Asiatic cholera, and that his death was ascribed to river-poisoning ; but, as the eminent observer whom we have just quoted correctly remarks, "it is opposed to all analogy, and to the usual order of nature, and therefore entirely unphilosophical, to suppose that a cause so extensively diffused should have been so singularly limited in its effect."

Greatly doubting, as we do, the alleged ill effects of foul emanations in the open air upon human life, we nevertheless do not think that the crusade against filth should for one moment be relaxed. A bad smell may be no more unhealthy than a bad taste ; but we should, if possible, avoid the one as much as the other. What we should above all things avoid, however, is the falling into the error of supposing that bad smells are the indubitable sources of many puzzling diseases, and of thus hardening our minds' against investigations of the kind which were instituted a year or two ago by Dr. Barker, and which, when completely carried out, will enable us to decide what the noxious principles are which make all the difference between an unpleasant and a malarious odor.

LETTER FROM ALBERT NAPPER, ESQ.—*Sir :* This is a question more easily asked than answered, but as it is now become a question involving the credit of our profession, it behooves us to return a speedy and decisive reply. The subject has latterly much occupied the attention of the medical profession, as well as of the public, and as is usually the case with all popular subjects of a scientific character, has been taken up with a certain amount of prejudice, resulting in the notion that many diseases do arise from bad smells.

Without going the length of asserting that this never does occur, my observation has confirmed me in the opinion I expressed in a communication inserted in the *Journal* of the 15th of November, 1856, in reply to some remarks of the Registrar-General on the subject, in which I stated my conviction that zymotic diseases are not the result of merely offensive exhalations, so much as of those arising from the products of fermentation and putrefaction, whether with or without smell. I have since had reason to modify this last opinion, and concur with that of Dr. Watson (which I had not seen, before reading it in your leader)—" that neither animal nor vegetable decomposition is sufficent to generate fever of any kind "—I am, however, far from admitting that fevers are not affected, and most materially affected, although not *generated* by them. I have long urged on my poorer neighbors the doctrine that the "bad smells" arising from the cess-pool under their windows, which have been endured so long with impunity, were only waiting for the seeds of fever to be sown in the system of some member of the family, to convert that which otherwise might pass off as a mild form of fever, into the most fatal kind of typhus. It appears to me that fever, of whatever type, must, by some, at present, unknown agency, be in the first place implanted in the system, where it will flourish or decline in proportion to the capabilities of the tissues in which it is engendered to support it; and that these exhalations bear the same relation to the various types of fever as guano and phosphate of lime do to wheat and turnips. I have also remarked, that typhus and remittent fevers appear to be nourished by the emanations of the cess-pool, and by those gases proceeding from the fermentation of stagnant water exposed to atmospheric influences. Intermittent fevers and ague depend on the exhalation of water (let it be ever so pure) contained *in* the soil, but not exposed to the air. Synochus, synocha, and the milder forms of fever being of the same character as typhus, are probably under the same but modified influences.

The thanks of the public are due to Dr. McWilliam for the attention he has bestowed on the subject, but I fear the consolatory feeling of security his statement will engender, may have the effect of turning the tide of public opinion to a do-nothing policy, if not judiciously directed by those best qualified to arrive at correct data, and for the medical profession to maintain this position, it will be necessary to lay aside those extreme theoretical views in which the leaders in some of the branches of medical science have of late years indulged, much to the prejudice of the whole body. Although as yet the disease adapted to be nourished by the filthy effluvia of the Thames has not appeared, the time may not be distant when its destructive powers may be too surely established. I would therefore urge on my fellow practitioners, even though like myself, occupying the humble position of a "village doctor," the necessity of bringing their practical knowledge to bear on this, as yet obscure, but most important subject.

I am, etc.,   ALBERT NAPPER.
—*British Med. Jour.*, *Sept.* 24, *and Oct.* 15, 1859.

Art. VII.—*Treatment of Varicose Veins.—Septic Phlebitis.*

i.—*Varicocele Treated by M. Vidal's Method, under the care of J. E. Erichsen, Esq., University Hospital. (From his Case Book.)*

JAMES J., aged 32, a laborer, was admitted under Mr. Erichsen's care on August 12th, for varicocele. He had suffered for twelve months from pains in the back, and found relief from cupping. He had had

gonorrhœa. Three months ago, he felt an aching pain in the left testicle, and the veins were then found to be much enlarged. He had
since found some relief from keeping the scrotum supported, so as to
be able to go about with little inconvenience; but whenever the support was withdrawn, he felt a severe sense of fulness, with very great
pain extending from the loins downwards.

On examination, a tumor, with the knotty feeling characteristic of
enlarged veins, was found on the left testicle, with its base downwards, and its apex extending towards the inguinal region. It diminished in size when he lay down.

Mr. Erichsen proceeded forthwith to operate, after the method recommended by Vidal. This is thus described by M. Guérin: A silver
wire, in a straight needle, is passed across the skin of the scrotum,
behind the distended veins, and another in front; and their ends are
twisted together, so as to make of the two a single cord. During
this movement of torsion, the veins get finally entangled around the
wires, so as to be pressed upon at several points. A piece of bandage, rolled up, is then laid upon the skin of the scrotum, between the
two ends of the wire; and they are twisted upon it, so as to produce
an amount of strangulation proportioned to the tightness with which
they are twisted. The constriction is augmented gradually every
day, till the skin is at length divided. (Guérin, *Elém. de Chir. Opératoire.* Paris: 1855. P. 514.) In practice, a perforated pin is used
instead of the anterior wire; and the silver thread is tightened by
twisting this. The instrument can be obtained at most of the best
shops.

The tension was increased by twisting up the pin daily till August
21st, when the irritation so produced caused severe pain, extending
up towards the inguinal region, tenderness of the abdomen, full pulse
and severe headache. As the wire seemed now to have done its
work, it was withdrawn.

The patient was kept in the house for ten days longer, and was
then discharged, the tumor having disappeared.

*Varicocele Treated by M. Vidal's Method, under the Care of R. Quain,
Esq. (From Notes by W. L. Winterbotham, Esq.)*

Geo. B., aged 20, was admitted on August 23d, under the care of
Mr. Quain. He had had an attack of gonorrhœa about Christmas,
which was followed by orchitis, aggravated by a blow, and by abscess
in the neighborhood of the testicle. He had also had syphilis, both
primary and secondary. He applied for relief on account of aching
pains in the limbs and head, having no idea that the scrotal veins
were enlarged.

On admission, a large mass of varicose veins was found around the
left scrotal cord, almost entirely surrounding it. There was an excoriated sore on the scrotum, and a large patch of dry mucous tubercle
over the pubes. The patient complained of a good deal of dragging
pain when he stood up, and the pains then became very prominent.

The testicle was supported by means of a **T** bandage, and the secondary symptoms treated in the appropriate manner, when, on September 8th, he was judged sufficiently well to be operated on. The

operation was performed by Mr. Marshall, after the method of Vidal. On the next day, the scrotum was rather swollen; and on the 11th it is noted that the needle was causing some amount of irritation; it was accordingly withdrawn on the 13th, at which time there was a great deal of swelling in the veins and cellular tissue of the scrotum; but the testicle itself was unaffected. The swelling remained almost stationary for some time, but without any prominent symptoms. It decreased gradually, under the use of discutient lotions and hot poultices; and on October 1st it is noticed that it was almost gone.

Remarks.—The advantage of this method, besides its easy application, is, that the veins are obliterated by the previous pressure before being cut through by the wire, and thus the risk of phlebitis is obviated. A similar plan has been used in this hospital by Mr. H. Thompson, in the treatment of varicose veins of the leg; and with good results.—*British Med. Jour.*

ii.—*Septic Phlebitis.*—(*Transactions of the Berlin Obstetr. Soc. Monatschrft. f. Geburtsk*, xiii 6, June.) *By Dr. Senftleben.*

Dr. Senftleben exhibited before the Berlin Obstetrical Society a specimen of phlebitis in a a young girl, which took its origin on the day on which a resection of the left elbow joint had been performed for caries. The wound and surrounding parts were found in excellent condition, progressing favorably towards healing, the veins leading from this point being perfectly healthy. The disease most evidently took its origin from the sexual organs, the veins situated between bladder, vagina and uterus being all filled with purulent deposits, while the left ovary was considerably swollen, dark red, and very much inflamed. Metastatic abscesses were found in the lungs, spleen and left kidney. In the discussion which followed, Dr. Virchow remarked that the foregoing case was very apt to direct the attention to the theory of the so-called pyæmia. It happens too often, he remarks, that metastases occurring after an operation, are accounted for by the operation itself, while a post mortem examination very often reveals a quite different cause. He, himself, has found very often the veins in the neighborhood of resected and carious places quite healthy, while the starting point was in a remote location. (See Gesammelte Abh., p. 570.) Similar modifications have to be taken into account, with regard to phlegmasia alba. As a puerperal disease, it is often, and unjustly so, explained by an affection of the womb, which in many cases is found intact, and the disease very often is unconnected with the puerperal state. In cases of far spread varicose degeneration of the veins, it often occurs that a muscular vein enters the muscle with a lumen of normal size, while the same vessel forms in the body of the muscle saclike enlargements, exceeding the normal size of the lumen four or eight times. Thus hidden entirely in the muscular tissues, these varicosities escape our attention, more especially because the constant muscular exertions are apt to keep up a perfect circulation of the blood, and thus every stagnation is prevented. But if, in consequence of some or other disease, the patient is kept at continued rest, the movement and circulation of the blood in these parts comes to a stand still ; if, moreover, the vital energy is lessened by exhaustion, if in consequence of fever the force of the heart's impulse grows less, it very often happens that thrombi are formed in these sacs of the intra-muscular veins, which may easily decay, and being swept along with the current of the blood into some remote organ, do here give rise to so-called metastatic abscesses. This same process can be often observed in women laid up after delivery, where the uterus is found intact many times, while the entire process is localized in one extremity.—*N. Y. Jour. Med.*

ART. VIII.—*Arctic Hygiene.—Miscellaneous Notes on Climates.*

i.—*Arctic Hygiene:* By DR. HAYES. [In the last number of the Proceedings of the Biological Department of the Academy of Natural Sciences of Philadelphia, Dr. Hayes made the following report, under the head of *Hygiene.*]

Dr. Hayes stated that during the late cruise of the Advance to the Arctic seas, his attention was directed to some facts in relation to the capabilities of men to resist low temperatures, which, at the friendly suggestion of Dr. Hammond, he had grouped together, and, with permission, would submit them to the department.

He thought that there was a great misapprehension existing in the popular mind upon the subject of Arctic life, it being generally thought that Arctic travelers were necessarily subjected to great hardships, in consequence of the lowness of the atmospheric temperatures. This he could but consider a' great mistake. The animal economy everywhere adapts itself with greater or less facility to surrounding circumstances, and this power of adaptation is no where more strikingly exhibited than in the Arctic regions. The appetite and digestive powers are doubtless more intimately concerned than any other of the animal functions, and, in the quantity and quality of the food consumed we are led to look for an explanation of the cause which enables the inhabitants of Polar countries so successfully to resist the cold.

The Esquimaux, with whom he had had communication in the far North, were found living mainly without fire. They have no wood, and no means of creating an artificial temperature, except with a small lamp, using blubber for fuel and moss for wick. The flame of this lamp gives very little heat, and is barely sufficient to melt from the snow the water which they require, and to light their huts during the dark period of the winter. During the coldest season they often live in snow-houses, the temperature of which ranges from zero to the freezing point, being kept thus elevated above the temperature outside, which ranges from —30° to —70°, chiefly by the heat radiated from the persons of the occupants; yet, with this seemingly unendurable temperature, they appear to live in comfort. They do not hesitate to expose themselves to any degree of cold, when engaged in hunting, and often sleep upon the snow, with no other protection than a piece of bear skin, on which they lie. Nevertheless, these people are strong, robust, and healthy. Scurvy is unknown amongst them, and Dr. Hayes had never heard of, or seen, a case of tubercular disease.

Dr. Hayes thought that we must look for an explanation of this wonderful power of resistance to the character of their food. They subsist entirely upon an animal diet, the flesh mainly of the walrus, seal, narwhal, and bear; and the quantity which they consume seems really enormous. He had frequently seen an Esquimaux hunter, when preparing for a long chase, eat from six to twelve pounds, at least one-third of which was fat, and he would place the daily consumption of the men at from twelve to fifteen pounds. In this large consumption of animal food they find their shield against the cold, and he does not believe that they could live upon a vegetable diet under such exposure. The same laws govern the Esquimaux and the white men, and just in proportion as the crew of the Advance accustomed themselves to the diet of the natives, did they gain power to expose themselves with impunity to low temperatures. They found themselves continually craving animal food, and especially fatty substances. The process of acclimation went on in proportion to their ability to eat and digest this kind of diet. During the early part of the cruise, they suffered much from temperatures, which, at a later period, produced no impression whatever upon them.

Dr. Hayes thought it was worthy of more than a mere passing remark, that scurvy and strumous diseases were unknown to the natives of the region, so far, at least, as his observations extended. In relation to the last, he would merely submit the fact; with regard to the former, he would say that wherever scurvy has occurred in the Arctic regions, it has been owing to accidental causes, which experience has taught us to remove or avoid. The long continued use of a salt meat diet had much to do with its development, and, as accessories, the cold, darkness, and excessive exertions. There is now, however, no necessity for the use of such a diet, and with abundant supplies of fish, animal food, and especially of fat, the last mentioned predisposing causes of disease ceased to have existence. Dr. Hayes thought that it was owing to their weakened condition, resulting from the use of salt food—of which they could eat only small quantities—allowing the cold and darkness to prey upon them, that an *epilepto-tetanoidal* disease exhibited itself amongst the men of Dr. Kane's command, and affected similarly their dogs.

While fresh animal food is absolutely essential to the inhabitants of Arctic countries, Dr. Hayes considered alcohol in any shape not only useless but positively injurious; and in this opinion he was fully sustained by the experience of the enterprising and indefatigable traveler, Dr. Rae, whom we had recently the highly gratifying opportunity of welcoming to the Academy. On the other hand, tea and coffee are most useful; and he found himself at a loss to say which is best.   The English and Russians prefer tea, while Dr. Kane's men took most kindly to tea in the evening when retiring, and coffee in the morning when preparing for a day's journey.

In relation to the animal diet used by the Esquimaux, Dr. Hayes observed that they eat it chiefly uncooked and frozen.   This fact had been useful to him, and he would suggest it to his brethren of the profession as having, perhaps, some importance.   He had frequently found that stomachs of scorbutic patients, which rejected cooked meats, would readily take raw meat in this state, or, as they expressed it, "cooked with frost."   By this process the repulsiveness of the uncooked flesh is entirely destroyed.

Dr. Hayes said, in conclusion, that he submitted these facts to the department without comment, leaving for those better qualified to determine as to whether they threw any new light upon the highly interesting and important physiological questions which they involve.

ii.—*Miscellaneous Notes on Climates, gleaned from Travels through Books:* By BENNET DOWLER, M. D.

The influences of climate upon the physical and mental characteristics of man, have been variously interpreted by writers.   According to Aristotle : The inhabitants of Europe, and of most cold countries, abound in strength and courage; but their intellectual powers are feeble or defective.   The inhabitants of Asia, on the contrary, are artful and ingenious, but mean-spirited and dastardly.   (*Ethics and Politics*, ii, 263.   Translated by Dr. J. Gillies.)   Aristotle thinks that Greece affords the most favorable climate, lying, as it does, between the extremes of heat and cold.

In his book on *airs, waters and localities*, Hippocrates gives a most deplorable picture of the physical and mental characteristics of the northern inhabitants of Europe and Asia, as the Scythians, Nomades and others.   He sets out with the general proposition " that Asia greatly exceeds Europe in respect both to its vegetation and its inhabitants."   To the latter, however, he concedes superior courage, as does Aristotle.

Dr. Copland, in his Dictionary of Medicine, written about twenty-two centuries later, gives the preference, not to Grecian skies, but to his own northern latitudes, between the 45th and 63d parallels, which, according to him, " are inhabited by the most robust and enduring of our species, in respect to both physical and intellectual powers."

These boundaries lie far north of the original nurseries of art and science—namely, India, Egypt, Greece, Rome, Palestine.

Sir William Temple (born 1628—died 1699) has a favorable opinion of the hot countries, both as it respects healthfulness and long life. He says: I have sometimes wondered that the regions of so much health and so long lives were all under very hot climates; whereas the more temperate are allowed to produce the strongest and most vigorous. (Works, iii, 280. London, 1814.)

It is within a narrow range of climate that great men have been born. In the earth's southern hemisphere, as yet, not one has appeared; and in the northern they come only within certain parallels of latitude. (Prof. J. W. Draper. *Treat. on the Forces which produce the Organization of Plants.* 8.)

Clapperton, in his Travels in Central Africa, affirms from personal observation, that the negroes suffer from cold whenever the temperature descends to 70° (Fah.)

Professor Graves of Dublin says: "Most animals brought hither from tropical climates die of some form of scrofula. Monkeys die of consumption; so do lions and tigers. Negroes and the natives of warm countries die of phthisis in England.

" Captain Ross, after having spent four years in the Arctic regions, became so habituated to cold, that on his return he found it quite impossible to bear the warmth of a London winter, and was forced to remove to a colder and more congenial situation."

[The following ideas of Humboldt, so far as they regard the influences of the climate of the torrid zone as a retarding cause of intellectual progress, are specious rather than solid. Other things being equal, an abundance of subsistence and the physical comforts, are favorable, because affording leisure for intellectual cultivation, while perpetual manual labor under uncongenial skies must necessarily prove a cause of retardation. Hottentots, Negroes, Indians and their mixtures with Caucasians of the lowest grade, in a word, race, not climate, must be chiefly referred to for an explanation of the mental and moral status of tropical countries. No climate however cold, no soil however sterile, will energize the intellectual organization of inferior races. Neither the Arctic nor Tropical Indian is civilized or intellectual.]

"An immense population finds abundant nourishment on a narrow space covered with plantains, cassava, yams and maize. The fecundity of nature on a small spot of land suffices for the wants of several families. The agriculture of the torrid zone reminds us of the intimate connection that exists between the extent of cleared land and the progress of society. That richness of the soil, that vigor of organic life, which multiply the means of subsistence, retard the progress of nations towards civilization. Under so mild and uniform a climate, the only urgent want of man is that of food. It is the feeling of this want only which excites him to labor ; and we may easily conceive why in the midst of abundance, beneath the shade of the plantain and bread-fruit tree, the intellectual faculties unfold themselves less rapidly than under a rigorous sky, in the region of corn, where our race is in a perpetual struggle with the elements." (HUMBOLDT's *Personal Narrative*, iii, 14.)

In the sittings of the Academy of Sciences (Sept., 1844), M. Gasparin maintained that the climate of France had not changed since the earliest historical records. The most hardy oranges (citrus aurantium) perish, except the trunk of the tree, from a cold below 10° Cent. In the seventeenth century, the cold killed the orange trees seven times; in the eighteenth six times. The orange does not require a hot summer to ripen. The olive trees were killed in 1601, 1658, 1659 and 1680.

In Chambers's "Information," etc., it is stated that "the hogs of Cuba, all of which are descended from an European stock, are twice as large as modern European hogs. The horses which run wild in Paraguay, though from variegated European races, are now of one peculiar color, which we cannot doubt is the effect of some peculiar local circumstances." (i, 59, 63.)

Geographers have estimated, that upon 12,000,000 square miles in the northern portions of Asia and America, the population is only 33,800,000, while, in southern Asia alone, on half as many square miles, the population is 400,000,000, or nearly twenty-four times greater.

Lind, in his work on Hot Climates, says that "women enjoy a much better state of health in the West Indies than men, and are not so liable to yellow fever." 87.

M. Raciborski, in a work written a few years since, on female puberty, maintained that southern climates are the most prolific: "In Portugal there are born 5.1 children per marriage, but in Sweden only 3.62." The Registrar-General of Great Britain, a few years ago, showed that conception in that country was more frequent in the warm than the cold season.

H. Rowe, M. R. C. P., late resident medical officer of the Demerara

Seaman's Hospital, maintains that it is a great desideratum to have medical lectures in all of the college courses, upon the diseases of hot climates, that many otherwise well educated medical men who go to the West Indies, are quite at a loss to know how to treat yellow fever, and that " the knowledge picked up in England is worse than useless, for it is erroneous, being imparted from mere theory." (*Lancet.*)

ART. IX.—*Homœopathy not Recognized in Europe.*

THE following correspondence, which sufficiently explains itself, has been furnished us by Dr. E. F. Smith, the efficient health officer of this city

Messrs. Editors: It will be remembered by the readers of your journal, that in May, 1858, the homœopaths of this city petitioned the City Council of St. Louis to permit a portion of the City Hospital to be set apart for the alleged purpose of testing the so-called merit of homœopathy; the real incentive, as we know, of their petition being, that its allowance might magnify the humbug into some professional consequence. Among the arguments they used in support of their petition, was the assertion that homœopathy was sanctioned by the crowned heads and nobility of Europe, and that European governments recognized it by permitting its teaching and practice in their hospitals. The falsity of this assertion was known to every one conversant with the state of medical affairs in Europe; but that it might receive its emphatic contradiction from an official source, I addressed myself to the American Ministers resident at Vienna and Berlin, and to the Minister of Public Instruction of France, asking from the proper department of these governments a reply to the following questions:

1. Is the teaching of homœopathy authorized or permitted in any of the colleges or institutions of your government? 2. Is the practice of homœopathy permitted in any of the public hospitals of your government? 3. Is the private practice of homœopathy sanctioned in your government?

In reply, I received the following letters, which, as they will prove of interest to the profession, I give you for publication:

LEGATION OF THE UNITED STATES, {
Vienna, July 19, 1858. }

Sir—In the absence of Mr. R. H. Jackson, Minister Resident of the United States at Vienna, I have the honor, in compliance with the request contained in your letter of May 14th, to transmit the following

34

translation of a communication just received from the Austrian Minister of Foreign Affairs:

VIENNA, July 10, 1858.

In his esteemed note of the 21st ultimo, the Minister Resident of the United States, Mr. Jackson, requested the mediation of the Ministry of Foreign Affairs to obtain a declaration from competent authority on these points: 1. Is the teaching of homœopathy authorized or permitted in any of the colleges or institutions of Austria? 2. Is the practice of homœopathy permitted in any of the public hospitals of Austria? 3. Is the private practice of homœopathy sanctioned in Austria?

The Imperial Ministry of the Interior, which was applied to, as it has charge of all medical and sanitary affairs in the Empire, has returned answer—to 1st, that in Austria homœopathy is taught not by publicly appointed professors, but only by private teachers; to 2d, that this mode of cure is practised, not in public hospitals, but only in cloister, criminal and private hospitals; to 3d, that the private practice of homœopathy is permitted to every physician who has a diploma.

In the hope that the above will answer the wishes of the Honorable Minister Resident, the undersigned renews to him the assurance of his perfect consideration.

[Signed]   COUNT BUOL, *Minister of Foreign Affairs.*

As these declarations come from the highest official source, I presume they will satisfy the object of your inquiries.

Very respectfully, your obedient servant,

G. W. LIPPITT, *Secretary of Legation.*

To E. F. SMITH, M. D., St. Louis.

Sir—In reply to your letter of the 5th instant, in which your Excellency asks information upon the instruction and practice of homœopathy, I have the honor to inform your Excellency that homœopathy in Prussia is not admitted into the universities nor hospitals, nor other public institutions. Physicians are allowed, if they please, to exercise homœopathy in private practice.

Returning to your Excellency the letter of Dr. E. F. Smith of St. Louis, I beg you to accept the opinions of my very high consideration.

Berlin, April 15, 1858
[Signed]   RAUMER.

His Excellency, Mr. J. A. WRIGHT, Envoy Extraordinary and Minister Plenipotentiary of the United States.

PARIS, April 22, 1858.

Sir—I take cognizance of the letter which you have written me, demanding of me information upon the subject of the teaching of homœopathy in the faculty of medicine of the Empire.

The exercise of homœopathy is not legally authorized in France. My administration has not authorized me to exercise any measure having reference to the teaching of homœopathy.

Receive, sir, the assurance, etc. The Minister of Public Instruction,

ROULAND.

Dr. E. F. SMITH, St. Louis, Mo.

These letters speak for themselves. Coming, as they do, from· the highest official sources of Austria, Prussia and France, they palpably show that this humbug not only meets with no favor from the scientific departments of those governments, but is completely discountenanced by them.

Respectfully,

E. F. SMITH.

— *St. Louis Med. and Surg. Jour.*

ART. X.—*Mineral Waters.—Hernia.*

IT would appear that the Medical Staff of the French army, during the recent campaign in Italy, while courageously discharging the duties more immediately belonging to them, had not been inattentive to other matters bearing on the sanitary condition of the inhabitants of Lombardy. During their hurried march they had collected some thirty specimens of water, taken from the streams and rivers of the country, particularly in those districts where goitre prevails. These specimens they analyzed with great care on their arrival at Milan, with the view of ascertaining what influence they might have in the production of that curious affection, the causes of which have been for many years the subject of much conjecture, and concerning which so much mystery still prevails. The conclusions arrived at, and which were communicated, in the first instance, by M. Demortain, the Pharmacien-en-chef of the army, to Marechal Vaillant, who afterwards submitted them to the Académie des Sciences, are altogether at variance with the observations made some time ago by Bourchadat. The researches of Bouchardat show that the salts of magnesia are found in abundance in the soil of all districts where goitre is endemic, and to them he is disposed to assign an important part in the production of that disease. The analysis conducted by M. Demortain and his assistants, show, on the contrary, a total absence of the salts of magnesia in the water collected in those districts of Lombardy where goitre, or wen, is most prevalent, as also the simultaneous absence of all muriates. In fact it was only on treating large quantities of these waters at a time with nitrate of silver and nitric acid that even a trace of a muriate could be detected.

M. Gosselin, of the Hòpital Cochin, at the meeting of the Academy of Medicine on the 25th ult., read a very interesting and somewhat remarkable paper on the taxis, and especially its *forcible* and *prolonged* employment in the treatment of strangulated hernia. In this paper, after alluding to some eighty-five cases which had come under his care, thirty-five of which he had treated with considerable success by the forcible and prolonged use of the taxis, he entered into details of his mode of procedure. He commences his manœuvres by exercising on the hernial tumor gentle and moderate pressure, and if at the end of five or six minutes the reduction has not been accomplished, he increases the pressure by using both hands, at the same time leaning over the patient so as to add to the pressure made by his two hands a certain part of the weight of his body, and sometimes even causes the hands of a powerful assistant to be placed over his own.   To this latter manœuvre he gives the name of "*taxis à quatre mains*."   He continues this prodigious force steadily during twenty, thirty, forty or fifty minutes, until the hernia is reduced or until the resistance is such as at the end of this time its reduction appears impossible.   He regards as of little value all the preparatory means usually recommended by authors previously to the employment of the taxis, such as warm baths, lacking the use of tobacco, enemata, etc.; such measures he considers lead only to the loss of valuable time.   He, however, subjects all his patients to the anæsthetic influence of chloroform, not for the purpose of producing muscular relaxation, but to overcome their sufferings, and so permit him to employ an amount of force which the cries and expressions of pain on the part of the patient might otherwise deter him from using.   The conclusions arrived at by M. Gosselin, and which I venture to say will not be generally accepted as orthodox, are, 1st. That the forcible and prolonged use of the taxis is not so dangerous as surgeons generally suppose, and that its utility is far greater than that usually attributed to it; and, further, that it may be had recourse to without any risk during the first seventy hours in crural and umbilical hernias.   2. That the treatment of strangulated hernia is essentially surgical, and should consist in the immediate employment of the taxis when this is possible, or in an operation where prudence does not sanction the use of the taxis.   Temporisation is,. according to M. Gosselin, permissible only when the diagnosis is not complete, and where, for the purpose of clearing up the difficulty, it is necessary to have recourse to a purgative.

Although the opinion of M. Gosselin is, from his position and great experience as a surgeon, entitled to very considerable respect, still I cannot help thinking that in the reduction of strangulated hernia it is an exceedingly difficult, or, I ought rather to say, an extremely thankless task to lay down any fixed rules, either in reference to the amount of force to be employed in the taxis, or as regards the length of time the manipulation should be continued.   On these two points surgeons will, and must, in each individual case, judge for themselves. Besides, by tact and ability, one man will often succeed with one-half the amount of force (and consequently with less risk of doing mischief) than that required by another, who goes about his work clumsily and awkwardly.   I well remember having seen an illustration of the deplorable results of the prolonged and forcible use of the taxis in the service of M. Robert some twelve months ago.   The operation was performed by that distinguished surgeon almost immediately on the admission of the patient, when the mesentery was found so much lacerated, and the gut so much injured in consequence, that a large portion of the former, together with some three or four inches of the latter required to be cut away.   M. Robert at the time expressed his conviction that the entire mischief had been the result of the injudicious and forcible employment of the taxis.—*Medical Times and Gaz.*

ART. XI.—*Pain as a Symptom of Disease of the Stomach:* By S. O. HABERSHON, M. D.

Dr. Habershon commenced his paper by observing briefly on the difference in the value of pain as a sign of disease. As a general rule, mucous membranes were free from ordinary sensation, except at the external orifices, and were capable of undergoing a vast amount of pathological change without an increase of this sensation; the same was the case with the parenchymatous viscera. In serous membranes, on the other hand, almost every change was felt. In acute inflammation of these membranes, pain is often severe, as in pleurisy, peritonitis, synovitis, etc. In these cases, relief was capable of being obtained by rest; and the rest so obtained was not such as to interfere with life. Pericarditis formed an exception; here there was absence of pain, unless pleurisy were also present; and in pericarditis, rest of the organ was unattainable so as to be compatible with life.

With regard to pain as a symptom of disease of the stomach, the author set forth the following propositions, most of which he illustrated by cases. 1. Acute (so-called) inflammatory disease of the stomach may be free from pain, if the mucous membrane alone be affected. It was commonly said that acute gastritis was very rare, and that its most usual cause was irritant poisoning ; but this opinion, Dr. Habershon thought, arose from the comparative absence of pain in the disease, which he regarded as more common than is usually supposed. Even in irritant poisoning, if the mucous membrane alone be affected, there may be no pain beyond that which is produced by the violent muscular efforts of vomiting. In illustration of this, Dr. Habershon related two cases, one of poisoning by oxalic acid, followed by recovery; the other fatal, of poisoning by sulphuric acid, in which pain was absent. In the latter case, the mucous·membrane of the stomach was found to be extensively destroyed; but the deeper structures were uninjured. He also referred to a case of poisoning by chloride of zinc, in which pain in the scrobiculus cordis was first complained of thirteen weeks after the accident. Death took place eight days afterwards; the stomach was found extensively ulcerated, and there was a perforation towards the cardiac end, which was probably connected with the attack of pain. 2. Organic disease of the mucous membrane—*e. g.*, cancer—may be comparatively free from pain. Cancer is often found deposited in the stomach where there has been no symptom of the disease in that organ during life. The author related a case of dropsy, with cirrhosis of the liver, in which the anterior surface of the stomach was coated with a cancerous villous growth ; the orifices were free. He had no pain in the stomach during life, nor vomiting. 3. Disease extending to the muscular and peritoneal coats of the stomach, often produces severe pain, as in perforation. In some cases, Dr. Habershon had found branches of the pneumogastric nerve involved in the edges of ulcers. 4. The stomach is naturally capable of a certain amount of distension without sensation ; but over-distension of the organ produces severe pain. 5. Disease, especially acute, affecting the peritoneal covering of the stomach, is generally accompanied by severe pain. 6. Dr. Osborn has shown that in some cases of gastric ulcer, the position which the patient assumes in order to' obtain relief from pain, shows the seat of the disease. 7. In disease of the lesser curvature, near the pylorus, pain is felt as soon as food enters the stomach, and gives the idea of a disease of the œsophageal orifice. 8. Many conditions of functional disease of the stomach are entirely free from pain. 9. The pain in many so-called functional diseases of the organ is very severe ; but it arises from a mal-condition of the nerve-centres, and the intimate connection of the spinal and sympathetic nerves. 10. The effect of diseased conditions of the pneumogastric nerve, or of its branches, in connection with stomach disease, is a matter of interest. Vomiting has been produced by irritation of a reflex character; for example, in disease of the suprarenal capsules, the irritation here being communicated through the branches of the pneumogastric nerve distributed to these bodies. The dyspepsia of phthisis had been attributed to a similar cause ; but, in Dr. Habershon's opinion, it more probably arose from the general state of mal-nutrition. 11. In functional disease of the stomach, attended with pain after taking food, it is probable that severe disease of the pyloric orifice exists. 12. Pain may be produced by distension of the stomach, by gases arising from the decomposition of food. 13. In lesions of the stomach, where pain may be expected, it is sometimes absent, from destruction of a portion of the pneumogastric nerves. 14. Pain at the scrobiculus cordis, simulating stomach disease, often arises from other causes. It is often present with chronic bronchitis or obstructive valvular disease, being probably connected with an over-filled state of the right heart. 15. Aneurism of the abdominal aorta sometimes produces severe pain, which may be mistaken for that arising from a cancerous disease of the pylorus.

Dr. Gibbon objected to the statement (if he understood the author of the paper rightly) that disease of the muscular or serous coats of the stomach was necessarily attended with pain. He had seen ulceration—even perforating ulcer—attended with little or no pain, even when food was taken into the stomach; but, when the branches of the pneumogastric nerve were exposed, there was pain. He had met with a case of apparent gastritis from drinking iced champagne after dancing. There was at first severe spasmodic pain, almost producing collapse; but this did not continue. The patient invariably rejected his breakfast every morning after taking it. In this case, and in one which he had noticed of poisoning by chloride of antimony, the only food which the patients were able to tolerate was sopped beef.

The Chairman thought he had seen cases of perforating ulcer unattended with pain.

Dr. Mackenzie mentioned the case of a gentleman who for some time had signs of malignant disease of the stomach and digestive organs. In the course of time a supposed cyst formed in the left hypochondriac region ; which, after consultation with Mr. Quain, was opened, and a pint of fluid discharged. The patient was relieved; but no pain was produced. He ultimately died of the cancerous disease, and, on post mortem examination, it was found that the supposed cyst was in reality the stomach, the opening of which had apparently been followed by no injury—the patient dying as he would otherwise have died.

Dr. Habershon said, with respect to the occurrence of pain in perforation, that almost any change, occurring slowly, may be unattended with pain. He had not intended to say that no disease of the muscular or serous coats of the stomach was without pain, but what he had especially wished to say was, that disease of the mucous membrane alone might be unattended with pain. He would ask the opinion of the Fellows of the Society on the question, whether the pain at the scrobiculus cordis in heart disease was to be referred to the distension of the heart or to the stomach.

Dr. Hyde Salter would corroborate the observations of Dr. Habershon as to the discrepancy often existing between the seat of pain and the seat of disease. The place, however, to which pain is referred is not haphazard; but the pain arising from the disease of a viscus in a cavity is referred to the middle line of the body, at a point corresponding with the level of the diseased organ. Thus, in bronchitis, the pain is referred to the breast bone or between the shoulder blades. In disease of the stomach, the pain is referred to the scrobiculus cordis, and to the corresponding point in the spine. Again, in colic, the pain is generally between the stomach and the umbilicus, and also in the spine. This "fore and aft" character of the pain was also observed in other instances. Dr. Salter thought that the transfer of pain to the surface might explain the action of counter-irritants to the external parts in inflammation of the viscera. The pain was probably reflex; and as the external sensation was affected by the vascular condition of the affected organ, through the sympathetic nerve, so, conversely, by the application of an irritant externally, at the seat of pain, a modification might be produced of the circulation of the diseased part.

Mr. Streeter called the attention of the society to the doctrines laid down by Sir Charles Bell regarding pain; and observed, in regard to Dr. Salter's view, that there were two remarkable exceptions—viz., the pain in the right shoulder in liver disease, and the pain and retraction of the testicle in disease of the kidney.—*British Medical Jour.*

ART. XII.—*On the Contagiousness of Secondary Syphilis:* By M. GIBERT, and others. ("Comptes Rendus," May 24th and 31st, 1859.)

MEDICAL men have long been divided in opinion upon the contagiousness and non-contagiousness of secondary syphilis. Clinical facts and experimental researches not a few have convinced the majority of the contagiousness of this affection; but these facts and researches have failed to carry conviction to the minds of a large party, of

which Ricord is the leader. Of this party the dogma was that no
syphilitic affection was contagious unless it was inoculable, and that
secondary syphilis was not contagious because it was not inoculable.
It is but just to M. Ricord, however, to state that he is not entirely
responsible for the most positive rendering of this dogma, and that
he himself always maintained a cautious reserve upon the subject.
What he held was that the primary chancre was alone inoculable in a
person already suffering from syphilis. It is to be remembered, also,
that in experimenting upon the contagiousness of secondary syphilis
he had never ventured to inoculate *healthy* individuals, and that he
never distinctly asserted that inoculation would give negative results
in such cases. Be this as it may, however, M. Ricord has abandoned
his doctrine as to the non-contagiousness of constitutional syphilis,
and the change in his opinion has been thus brought about.

On the 25th of October, 1858, a letter was addressed to the Imperial Academy of Medicine at Paris, by the Minister of Commerce,
Agriculture, and Public Works, requesting an authoritative answer
upon two questions: first, whether constitutional syphilis was contagious; and, secondly, whether, as regards contagion, there was a
difference between constitutional syphilis as seen in infants at the
breast and in adults. This letter led to the appointment of a commission consisting of MM. Velpeau, Ricord, Devergie, Depaul and
Gibert, and these commissioners have reported (and their report has
been adopted by the Academy without opposition of any kind)—first,
that some of the manifestations of secondary syphilis, especially con-
dylomata, are undoubtedly contagious; and, secondly, that there is
no reason to suppose that the case is different in infants at the breast
and in adults.

The commissioners arrive at this conclusion after examining the
clinical facts and experimental researches already on record, and
after four experiments of their own, which were undertaken with
great reluctance on their part. The persons experimented upon were
all suffering from lupus, but free from any syphilitic taint, and these
were chosen from the notion that the treatment for syphilis, if the
inoculation took effect, might possibly be of service in remedying the
lupus. The cases are given in detail, and as the results were very
similar in the four, one will serve as an example.

On a man, whose face had been affected with lupus from childhood,
a raw surface was made on the left arm by strong ammonia, and to
this was applied a piece of lint soaked in purulent matter obtained
from a condyloma near the anus of a person who had had a chancre
fifteen months previously. The condyloma was of fifteen days' standing. Fourteen days afterwards there was slight redness at the seat
of inoculation. Four days later still, a prominent coppery-colored
papule made its appearance in the same part. On the twenty-second
day this papule was much larger, and there was a slight oozing from
its surface. During the week following the oozing, after being purulent, dried up into a thin scab. On the 29th day a gland in the corresponding axilla became enlarged. On the fifty-fifth day, the papule
on the arm had become a real tubercle, with some slight ulceration
in the centre, and several blotches and coppery papules had made

their appearance on the trunk. During the week following, these papules became multiplied on the body, and they spread also to the extremities; many of them also changed into pustules of acne. Two or three days later the patient was put under treatment for syphilis, and in six weeks, at the date of the report, there was still much to be done in the way of a cure.

In addition to asserting the contagiousness of secondary syphilis, the reporters have also arrived at the conclusion that there are characteristic grounds of distinction between the primary and secondary affection, but here M. Ricord is somewhat at issue with his colleagues. The conclusions arrived at, indeed, are similar to those already arrived at—that the period of incubation in the secondary affection is from eighteen to twenty days, or even longer, and that the result is first a papule and then a tubercle, which is finally converted into an ulcer covered with a crust.

Be this as it may, however, the question of the contagiousness of secondary syphilis would seem to be set at rest, for if the evidence in the affirmative had not been thoroughly conclusive, it is certain that M. Ricord would not have read his recantation.—*Ranking Abst.*

Art. XIII.—*On the sickness of Pregnancy.* By Dr. CHARLES E. BAGOT.

In 1846, writes Dr. Bagot, I had had under my care a woman laboring under that extreme form of sickness from pregnancy which placed life in the most imminent jeopardy. I had tried all the usual remedies suggested in such cases, and found them one after another to fail in producing any relief. Although there were no symptoms whatsoever which would make me suppose that inflammation was either the proximate or remote cause of the sickness, I resolved to try the effects of mercury, and having had some experience of the powers of calomel in allaying other forms of vomiting, I fixed on the administration of this preparation, steadily persevering in its use until her gums showed appearances of salivation, which they did in a very short time. This treatment resulted in the best effects. Immediately after slight salivation took place, the vomiting, previously so persistent, at once ceased, food remained on the stomach, the patient rapidly recovered, and was in due time safely delivered of a full grown infant.

After a more than ordinary length of time, and about three years from my publication of her case, this woman again became pregnant, when she was once more seized with the same dangerous vomiting at the fourth month of gestation, and I was again obliged to resort to the calomel treatment before I could succeed in allaying the almost fatal form of sickness under which she was laboring. By the use of the same medicine she, however, was again brought through, but with this difference, comparing this present attack with the former one, that it was found necessary to prolong the salivation for some days before complete relief from her urgent symptoms was obtained, whereas, on the previous occasions, as I have mentioned, the vomiting subsided on the first appearance of mercurialization.

I had a third opportunity of trying the calomel with the same patient, as during her next pregnancy her life was again placed in imminent peril by a recurrence of the same urgent symptoms, the violence of the vomiting and weakness produced by want of nourishment, exceeding, if possible, the state on the two previous occasions, at least such was the account which I received in the country, where I was at that time residing. A medical practitioner by whom she was attended, having heard of my success in producing relief by salivation, administered to her some medicine which had that effect, but I am not aware of the preparation which he used, and only know that his treatment was of no avail, the symptoms continuing with unabated violence. At this juncture I was written to, when I recommended that slight salivation should be kept up by means of small doses of calomel given three times daily, and that with each dose she should have a draught containing fifteen drops of chloroform. This treatment was adopted under the direction of a medical gentleman of my acquaintance, and was attended with almost magical effect; after the administration of a few doses the vomiting ceased, light nutriment lay upon the stomach, she gradually gained flesh, became restored to health and strength, and at the full period of nine months was safely confined.

Since that time (1854) this woman has not become pregnant, for which fact her age will account.

I hope those brief remarks will suffice to call attention to this important subject, and that no man in the profession will again resort to the induction of premature labor without at least giving a fair trial to the treatment I have recommended. The illness of Mrs. F— was of the very worst form; her symptoms were so urgent I despaired of her existence being prolonged; her prostration of strength was excessive; her emaciation extreme; her pulse a small thread; she had no tenderness in the epigastrium; neither had she pain in the region of the womb, nor the least uneasiness on pressure over that organ; she had no febrile nor inflammatory symptoms, and yet the most complete relief followed the exhibition of the mercurial pushed to slight salivation; and this success, I sincerely trust, may induce others to follow the example and fairly test my plan, although my experience is but the result of three trials, practised on the same patient.—*Dublin Med. Press. Ranking. Abstract.*

ART. XIV.—*Acupressure—A New Method of Arresting Surgical Hæmorrhage:* By J. Y. SIMPSON, M. D., F. R. S. E., Professor of Medicine and Midwifery in the University of Edinburg, etc., etc.

At the first winter meeting of the Royal Society of Edinburgh, held on Monday, the 19th December, 1859, Professor Simpson made a lengthened communication on acupressure, as a new mode of arresting surgical hæmorrhage. After describing the various methods of stanching hæmorrhage in surgical wounds and operations, which the Greek, Roman, Arabic and Mediæval surgeons employed, he gave a short history of the introduction of the ligature of arteries, and spoke of it as—with the occasional exception of torsion for the smallest arteries—the hæmostatic means almost universally employed in chirurgical practice at the present day. But he thought that surgery must advance forward a step farther than the ligature of arteries, particularly if surgeons expected—as seemed to be their unanimous desire—to close their operative wounds by the immediate union or primary adhesion of their sides or walls.

To enforce this point, Dr. Simpson recapitulated the arguments which he has already adduced on the same topic in this Journal (see *Edinburgh Medical Journal* for December, 1858, p. 547); urging that since we now know that in obstetric surgery we can, with metallic sutures, produce, with great frequency and certainty, complete union by the first intention of the vivified lips of a vesico-vaginal fistula, (and that, too, in despite of urine, the most irritating fluid in the body, constantly bathing one side of the wound), surgeons ought to heal *their* common surgical wounds by primary adhesion also, provided there were no counteracting circumstances to prevent this desirable result. Yet the complete and entire union by the first intention of surgical wounds left by the removal of a limb, mamma, tumor, etc., was confessedly not very frequently seen in surgical practice. The *ligatures*, by their presence around the cut arteries of the wound, formed the counteracting circumstances or agents, which prevented the primary union of the sides of the wound. They produced this effect in two ways. 1. They acted themselves as foreign bodies in the depths of the wound; and when composed of silk or organic matter, they rapidly swelled with imbibed animal fluids, which soon decomposed, and thus rendered each ligature thread liable to act like an irritating seton. 2. They counteracted immediate union or primary inflammatory adhesion in another way, viz: they always set up in the ligatured points and ends of the tied arteries *higher* stages of inflammation than the adhesive—stages that were indeed destructive of adhesion ; for every ligatured artery, at the point of deligation, has its two inner coats mechanically torn and divided by the ligature, and before it escapes from its hold on the arterial tube the ligature requires to eat through the remaining bruised and strangled coat by the process of ulceration, suppuration and mortification. If two, three, or more arteries are tied in any wound, then there are consequently two, three, or more points in that wound, in each of which there is going on simultaneously an action of ulceration, of suppuration, and of gangrene. Under such circumstances, complete healing of the wound by immediate union by primary adhesion, or by simple adhesive inflammation, is more than can be expected. Surgeons have made various efforts to overcome the two difficulties thus connected with arterial ligatures. (1) In olden times they were in the habit of including portions of the surrounding tissues in the loop of the ligature. But the process of ulceration, etc., by which each ligature cuts through the part it embraces, was thus found to be rendered unnecessarily severe and protracted. Hence arose (2) the rule of including within the ligature nothing but the arterial tube itself. After this important reform was introduced, the arterial tubes were by many surgeons tied (3) by large, and sometimes flattish, ligatures. These, however, cut and ulcerated through the included artery very slowly ; and in practice they were betimes entirely replaced by (4) ligatures as small and slender as was compatible with due strength. To diminish the bulk of the foreign body, or ligature, in the wound, the practice was next adopted of (5) cutting off one end or limb of the ligature after the knot was tied. Others, with the vain hope that the mere loop of a silk ligature might remain buried permanently (though a foreign body) within the depths of the wound, proposed (6) that both ends of the ligature should be cut off ; a practice followed with little or no success. The chances of union of wounds by the first intention have been attempted to be advanced by changing also the constituent materials of the ligature. Instead of vegetable threads of flax or hemp, (7) animal ligatures of cat-gut, silk-gut, buckskin, fibres of the sinew of the deer, etc., have been employed, under the expectation that they would prove less irritating to the wound, as approaching more nearly to the living animal tissues. (8) *Lastly*, Ligatures of metallic thread have also been placed around bleeding arteries with the same hope ; and though not irritating, as far as the material of which they are composed is concerned, yet Dr. S. had found that metallic, like any other form of ligatures which is placed around bleeding arteries, and left there to ulcerate through the constricted tube, usually excited, in the course of their ulcerative progress, too high irritation and inflammation to allow of union of surgical wounds by the first intention.

All the march of modern surgery has thus been in the direction of attempting to increase the chances of the union of surgical wounds by the first intention, by diminishing more and more the irritation derived from the presence and action of the ligatures supposed to be inevitably required for the arrestment of the hæmorrhage. By the new hæmostatic process of acupressure, Dr. Simpson hopes to overcome in a great degree all those difficulties, as by it he expected to arrest the hæmorrhage attendant upon surgical wounds *without leaving permanently any foreign body whatever* in the wound itself. It was an attempt to bring bleeding wounds, in common surgery, to the condition of wounds in plastic surgery, where no arterial ligatures were used, and where union by the first intention was in consequence the rule, and not the exception to it. Sewing up the outer or external lips of a large surgical wound by silver, iron, or other metallic or non-irritating sutures, and yet leaving within the depths of the wound a series of silk ligatures, each producing ulceration, suppuration and gangrene at the tied arterial points, was, he argued, but an illustration of a very paradoxical state of matters—like enforcing cleanliness and the best hygienic measures, as it were, outside a house, whilst within doors there were retained and locked up filth and decomposition, and the elements of destruction and disease.

Dr. Simpson stated that he had tested, with perfect success, the effects of acupressure as a means of effectually closing arteries and stanching hæmorrhage first upon the lower animals, and lately in two or three operations on the human subject. The instruments which he proposed should be used for the purpose, were very sharp-pointed, slender needles or pins of passive or non-oxydizable iron, headed with wax or glass, and in other respects also like the hare-lip needles commonly used by surgeons at the present day, but longer when circumstances required it. They might be coated with silver or zinc on the surface, if such protection were deemed requisite.

At first, Dr. Simpson believed that in using acupressure as a hæmostatic means, it would be necessary to compress the tube of the bleeding artery between two needles, one placed on either side of it. But in his later experiments upon the living as well as the dead body (as in amputations on the latter, and subsequently injecting tepid water through the arteries, in imitation of the flow of blood), he had found that the compression of one needle was usually perfectly sufficient to shut up an artery, and that even sometimes, when two or more bleeding points were near, they could be closed simultaneously by the action of one needle or pin. The whole process consists in passing the needle *twice* through the substance of the wound, so as to compress together and close, by the middle portion of the needle, to the tube of the bleeding artery a line or two, or more, on the cardiac side of the bleeding point. The only part of the needle which is left exposed on the fresh surface of the wound, is the small middle portion of it, which passes over and compresses the arterial tube ; and the whole needle is withdrawn on the second or third day, or as soon as the artery is supposed to be adequately closed, thus leaving *nothing* whatever in the shape of a foreign body within the wound, or in the tissues composing its sides or flaps. To produce adequate closing pressure upon any arterial tube which it is desired to constrict, the needle must be passed over it so as to compress the tube with sufficient power and force against some resisting body. Such a resisting body will be most frequently found, 1st, in the cutaneous walls and component tissues of the wound ; 2d, sometimes in a neighboring bone, or other resistant point, against which the artery may be pinned and compressed by the acupressure needle; and 3d, in a few rare cases, it may possibly be found in practice, that a second needle may require to be introduced to serve as a point against which the desired compression is to be made. Most commonly the first of these three plans seems perfectly sufficient, and that even in amputation of the thigh; a thicker or deeper flap merely requiring a proportionally longer needle. In acting upon this mode, the surgeon may place the tip of the forefinger of his left hand upon the bleeding mouth of the artery which he intends to compress and close; holding the needle in his right hand, he passes it through the *cutaneous* surface of the flap, and pushes it inward till its point projects out to the extent of a few lines on the raw surface of the wound, a little to the right of, and anterior to his finger-tip; he then, by the action of his right hand upon the head of the needle, turns and directs its sharp extremity so that it makes a bridge, as it were, *across* the site of the tube of the bleeding artery, immediately in front of the point of the finger, with which he is shutting up its orifice;' he next, either with this same forefinger of the left hand, or with the side of the extremity of the needle itself, compresses the locality of the bleeding arterial orifice and tube, and then pushes on the needle with his right hand, so as to make it *re enter* the surface of the wound a little to the left side of the artery; and lastly, by pressing the needle further on in this direction, its point reëmerges through the *cutaneous* surface of the flap—the site of the tube of the bleeding artery being in this way left pinned down in a compressed state by the arc or bridge of steel that is passed over it. The needle thus passes first from and through the skin of the flap *inward* to the raw surface of the wound, and after bridging over the site of the artery, it passes secondly from the raw surface of the wound *outward* again to and through the skin. Sometimes the needle will be best passed by the aid of the eye alone, and without guiding its course by the finger-tip applied to the bleeding orifice. It compresses not the arterial tube alone, but the structures also placed over and around the *site* of the tube. When the needle is completely adjusted, all of it that is seen, and that not necessarily so, on the surface of the raw wound, is the small portion of it passing over the site of the artery; while externally, upon the cutaneous surface of the flap, we have remaining exposed more or less of its two extremities, namely, its point and its head. The rest of it is hidden in the structures of the flap or side of the wound. The degree of pressure required to close effectually the tube of an artery is certainly much less than medical practitioners generally imagine; but in the above proceeding the amount of pressure can be regulated and increased, when required, by the acuteness of the angle at which the needle is introduced and again passed out—the cutaneous and other structures of the flap serving as the resisting medium against which the needle compresses the arterial tube. If it were ever, perchance, necessary to produce greater compression than can be thus accomplished by the needle alone, this increased pressure could be readily obtained by throwing around the two extremities of the needle, which are exposed cutaneously, a figure-of-eight ligature, as in hare-lip, with or without a small compress placed between the arc of the ligature and the skin. In practice, however, the pressure of the needle upon the artery will—without any such external aid—be found to err more frequently, at first, in the way of excess than in the way of defect. The process of the adjustment of the needle is difficult to describe shortly by words, but the whole of it is readily seen and imitated when repeated upon a piece of cloth or soft leather. We fasten the stalk of a flower in the lapelle of our coat by a pin passed exactly in this manner. To compress a bleeding artery against a bone is somewhat more complicated, but not much so. In accomplishing it, we have to introduce from the cutaneous surface a long needle through the flap of the wound, obliquely to near the site of the artery, and then compressing against the bone, with the fingers of the other hand, or with the end of the needle itself, the part containing the artery, we make the needle, after passing over this compressed part, and after testing whether it has closed the vessel or not, enter into the tissues beyond, and if necessary even emerge from the cutaneous surface on the other side, at an angle somewhat oblique to that at which it entered; thus taking advantage of the resiliency and resistance of the soft textures to make them push the needle with the necessary degree of force against the artery and bone. Arteries in particular parts require special adjustments and modifications to compress them against the neighboring bone, which only anatomy and experience can point out. There is always sufficient soft tissue on either side of the artery for the needle to get a purchase upon, to compress the arterial tube against the bone or other resistant point ; and a comparatively slight purchase of this kind is generally all that is required. In two cases, Dr. S. had found that branch of the internal mammary artery which so frequently bleeds in the bottom of the wound after excision of the mamma, easily and perfectly closed by a needle passed through the flap to near the artery, then lifted over it and (after compressing it so as to stop the flow of blood) pushed onward into the tissues beyond. Possibly, in some amputations, an acupressure needle or nedles may yet be passed immediately before the operation, half an inch or so above the proposed line of amputation, so as to shut the principal artery or arteries, and render the operation comparatively bloodless. If so, these needles would serve, at one and the same time, the present uses of both tourniquet and arterial ligatures. Perhaps this will be found, in some cases, a simple and effectual means of compressing and closing arterial trunks for hæmorrhage and other practical purposes; as, for example, the artery leading to an aneurism—as the femoral artery in popliteal aneurism—changing the operation for that disease into a simple process of acupuncture instead of a process of delicate dissection and deligation, when in any case the milder methods of compression, manipulation, and continuous flexion of the knee fail. It has been hitherto a difficult problem to obstruct the vessels of the ovarian ligament in ovariotomy, without leaving a foreign body, whether clamp or ligature, upon the stalk of the tumor, to ulcerate and slough through it. If the stalk be transfixed and properly and strongly pinned in its whole breadth to the interior of the relaxed abdominal walls, by one or more acupressure needles passed through these abdominal walls from without, this difficulty may possibly be overcome.

That needles used for the purpose of acupressure, and passed freely through the walls and flaps of wounds, will not be attended by any great degree of disturbance or irritation, is rendered in the highest degree probable by all that we know of the tolerance of living animal tissues to the contact of metallic bodies. Long ago John Hunter pointed out that small shot, needles, pins, etc., when passed into and imbedded in the living body, seldom or never produced any inflammatory action, or none at least beyond the stage of adhesive inflammation, even when lodged for years. Some time ago, when the subject of acupuncture specially attracted the attention of medical men, Cloquet, Pelletan, Pouillet, and others, showed that the passage and retention of long acupuncture needles were attended with little or no irritation in the implicated living tissues. The reviewer of their works and experiments in the *Edinburgh Medical Journal* for 1827 observes: " It is a *remarkable* circumstance that the acupuncture needles never cause inflammation in their neighborhood. If they are rudely handled or ruffled by the clothes of the patient, they may produce a little irritation; but if they are properly secured and protected, they may be left in the body for an *indefinite* length of time without causing any of the effects which usually arise on account of the presence of foreign bodies. In one of M. Cloquet's patients, they were left in the temples for eighteen days; and in cases in which needles have been swallowed, they have remained without causing inflammation for a much longer period. It appears probable, from the facts collected on the subject, that metallic bodies of every kind may remain imbedded in the animal tissues without being productive of injury."—(Page 197.) All the late observations and experiments upon metallic sutures are confirmatory of the same great pathological law of the tolerance of living tissues for the contact of metallic bodies imbedded within their substance. In the operation for harelip, where the whole success or failure of the operation depends on the establishment or not of union by the first intention, surgeons use needles to keep the lips of the wound approximated, often compressing these needles strongly with their figure-of-eight ligatures, and find this measure the most successful means which they can adopt for accomplishing primary adhesion.

The acupressure of arteries, when compared with the ligature of them, appears, as a means of arresting hæmorrhage, to present various important advantages:

1st. Acupressure will be found more easy, simple, and expeditious in its application than the ligature.

2d. The needles in acupressure can scarcely be considered as foreign irritating bodies in the wound, and may always be entirely removed in two or three days, or as soon as the artery is considered closed; whilst the ligatures are true foreign irritating bodies, and cannot be removed till they have ulcerated through the tied vessels.

3d. The ligature inevitably produces ulceration, suppuration, and gangrene at each arterial point at which it is applied; whilst the closure of arterial tubes by acupressure is not attended by any such severe and morbid consequences.

4th. The chances, therefore, of the union of wounds by the first intention should be much greater under the arrestment of surgical hæmorrhage by acupressure than by the ligature.

5th. Phlebitis, pyæmia, etc., or, in other words, trumatic or surgical fever, seem not unfrequently to be excited by the unhealthy local suppurations and limited sloughings which are liable to be set up in wounds by the presence and irritation of the ligatures.

6th. Such dangerous and fatal complications are less likely to be excited by the employment of acupressure, seeing the presence of a metallic needle has no such tendency to create local suppurations and sloughs in the wound, such as occur in the seats of arterial ligatures.

And 7th. Hence, under the use of acupressure, we are entitled to expect both, *first*, that surgical wounds will heal more kindly, and close more speedily; and *secondly*, that surgical operations and injuries will be less frequently attended than at present by the disastrous effects and perils of surgical fever.—*American Medical Gazette, Feb.,* 1860.

ART. XV.—*Hypnotic Anæsthesia.*

[ALTHOUGH the foreign medical journals, especially on the Continent of Europe, teem with notices of animal magnetism or hypnotism as a new and safe anæsthetic, nothing but the respectability of the persons who make the most positive statements of its efficacy and superiority over chloroform and æther, would warrant one in introducing this subject into the pages of this journal. Nevertheless, it may be all true that the placing a bright (or even black) object very near the nose for the patient to look at and fix his attention upon, will produce complete anæsthesia under the severest surgical operations. A few months ago it was pretended that three millions of people in the United States were able and willing to vouch for the reality of spiritualism, table turning, rapping, etc. Perhaps hypnotism in the hands of doctors may not be equally as visionary.

The platform of common sense seems to have broken down under the ponderous weight of illusions, delusions and modern miracle-mongers. The so-called Biologists, and many other progressionists, travel to and fro, from city to city, being more powerful than the ancient gods, genii, astrologers, and enchanters, exercising at will supreme power over their auditors or a portion of them, either annihilating or controlling their sensations, wills, voluntary motions, actions, thoughts, passions or purposes; while the public press for the most part is silent or advocates these wonderful manifestations as true.

It is remarkable that nearly every case of the new marvel of hypnotism reported up to the latest mail as having been put into a cataleptic sleep, has been of the feminine gender. Of the two genders, this is the better one as well as the more fortunate. It was, moreover, this gender that gave birth to the rapping and sundry kindred sciences, including medicine. These sciences having become epidemic, as a matter of course, included the other sex. Hypnotism in like manner seems to have anæstheticised at last one man, as will be seen in the last number of *The Lancet;* from this journal several other passages will be subjoined. B. D.]

Amputation of the Thigh in the Hypnotic State.—M. Guerinau, surgeon to the hospital of Poitiers, in France, has just published in the *Gazette des Hôpitaux*, the case of a farm laborer, of thirty-four years of age, who has had his thigh amputated for white swelling in the knee joint, whilst under the influence of hypnotism. The patient has been ill two years, and experienced such pain in the knee that it could not be touched without exciting cries of distress. So apprehensive was

36

he of pain, that he would not be carried to the operating theatre, but hobbled on crutches until he fainted. This was a case evidently unfit for chloroform, so that hypnotism was tried. A bright spatula was held about four inches from the root of the nose, the patient being recumbent. Strabismus immediately occurred; but when attempts were made to separate his legs he resisted and said it hurt him. Five minutes after the beginning of the experiment, one arm of the patient was raised by the surgeon, but it fell down ; hence it was plain that catalepsy was not being produced, and the man then observed that it would be difficult to put him to sleep in that manner. Great silence was then enjoined in the room ; and after five minutes, the patient being still fixed by looking at the spatula, the flap amputation was performed. It lasted one minute and a half, and to the surprise of all present, not a sign of pain was evinced by the patient, and he made not the slightest movement, though hardly held by the assistants. When asked how he felt, he said he thought he was in Paradise. His eyes remained open the whole time, were somewhat oscillating, and affected with strabismus. About two minutes before the beginning of the operation, a pupil pinched the patient's thigh, asking him whether he felt pain, upon which he answered, "Yes, I feel a little." After the operation, the patient said: "I felt what was done; for, at the time the limb was being amputated, you said to me, ' Do you feel any pain ?' " Now it should be remembered that the limb was removed two full minutes *after* this circumstance occurred, so that the man could not have felt any pain at the time of the actual operation. It is, however, not ·stated how he bore the tying of the arteries and the dressing of the stump.

Failure of Hypnotism.—The excitement produced by the introduction of Dr. Braid's method of hypnotism into Paris, as a proceeding applicable to the operative purposes of surgery, is likely to end in the flattest evaporation, as we predicted. The successes have been less striking, and the failures more numerous, than we expected. Experiments have been made on a very large scale in nearly all the hospital establishments of Paris. It has been clearly proved that only women are affected, except in unusual instances. As regards the male sex the question is judged. With females the results are variable, imperfect and practically useless to surgery. A well arranged series of trials was carried out by Drs. Demarquay and Giraud Teulon in fifteen cases. The temperament of the patients and the results are very impartially related. It is worth while to analyze these cases; the patients were all females, the majority having (cancerous) affection of the uterus. The result was, in No. 1, catalepsy without anæsthesia; 2, no results; 3, no results ; 4, hysteria, with exaggeration of the sensibility; 5, muscular relaxation, sensibility still continuing; 6, no results; 7, no results; 8, anæsthesia; 9 and 10, no results; 11, slight bewilderment—" experienced during the trial voluptuous sensations;" 12 and 13, no results; 14, fell asleep—awoke and cried out when pricked with a pin; 15, anæsthesia. So that, out of fifteen females, there were two in whom anæsthesia was produced. But this is neither profound nor lasting. ·A noise, or the movement of the object before the eye, is sufficient to interrupt the process. Meantime, it is evident that all the forms of abnormality which may be induced by thus forcing the vision are not thoroughly known. Enough is seen to demonstrate that the proceeding can have no surgical value, and that the results attributed to "mesmerism," "animal magnetism," "electro-biology," and the like, are capable of imitation by these means. This was already shown by Dr. Braid's experiments; but, singularly enough, it has been customary to draw very opposite conclusions from his experience. While interest is still felt in the inquiry in Paris, it is very desirable that the physiological relations of the enforced action of the eyes on corresponding parts of the brain should be investigated. The whole series of phenomena incidental to catalepsy, epilepsy, hysteria and induced coma, may be found to be connected with disturbance of the circulation at the base of the encephalon, which is, for the most part, so carefully guarded against by the anatomical arrangements of the beautiful circle of arteries to which Willis has given his name. Meanwhile, the comparative danger of inducing these forms of disease, or of administering chloroform, must be carefully weighed by experiments.

A Revolution in Anæsthetics.—The Paris medical papers are full of the new method of producing anæsthesia introduced by M. Azam of Bordeaux.

It would appear that, about eighteen months ago, M. Azam, had under his care an hysterical young lady, who was subject to cataleptic attacks. Upon this patient very extraordinary phenomena were noticed, which, coming to the ears of M. Bazin, professor at the Faculty of Sciences of Bordeaux, this gentleman advised M. Azam to consult a work published in England in 1842, by Mr. Braid, in which the means of producing catalepsy and artificial anæsthesia were detailed. M. Azam, procured this book, of which Dr. Carpenter has written an analysis in Dr. Todd's Cyclopædia, under the head of "Sleep," and began a series of experiments on his young patient and about thirty other persons. He found that most of Mr. Braid's statements were correct, and that catalepsy and anæsthesia could actually be obtained in the following manner :

The patient, either sitting up or lying down, is put in a convenient position. The operator then, standing either before or behind him, places before his eyes, at the distance of a few inches, but generally nearer than the point which allows of distinct vision, some bright object, upon which the patient should steadily and continually fix his eyes. The bright object should be so placed that the eyes, in looking at it, must be forcibly directed upwards, the contraction of the superior recti being carried to its maximum degree. In this position, the levatores palpebrarum and recti are strongly contracted, and convergent strabismus takes place. After this attitude, which is certainly fatiguing, has been kept up for two or three minutes, the pupils are noticed to contract, and soon afterwards to dilate ; the eyelids quiver rapidly, then fall, and the patient is asleep. Two symptoms, almost always present, are then observed ; they are, however, in different cases, more or less marked and lasting : 1, catalepsy, exactly as described

in books ; 2, anæsthesia, which lasts from three to fifteen minutes,
either complete or incomplete, but which allows of pinching, pricking
and tickling, without any feeling being aroused in the patient, and
without any change in the cataleptic state being produced. This anæsthetic state is generally followed by a very opposite condition—
namely, very remarkable hyperæsthesia, in which the senses, the feeling of heat, and muscular activity reach an unusual degree of excitability. At any moment of the experiment the symptoms may be
suddenly stopped, by rubbing the eyelids, and directing upon them a
stream of cold air. When the patients recover their senses, they
remember nothing of what has taken place.

Several experiments have been instituted in Paris by Messrs. Follin,
Broca, and others ; and M. Velpeau seems so convinced, that he has
presented a short paper on the subject, by M. Broca, to the Academy
of Sciences at the meeting of the 5th inst.

The *Gazette Hebdomadaire*, of the 9th of December, mentions the
following case : A woman, aged twenty-four, rather nervous and
timid, had, in consequence of a burn, a large abscess by the verge of
the anus, and was told that she would be narcotized before it was
opened. A bright brass tube (a telescope made by Bruecke) was
placed five inches in front of the nose. The patient was obliged to
squint considerably in order to look steadily at the object, the pupils
contracting very strongly. The pulse, which before the experiment
was quick, became now weaker, but immediately afterwards weaker
and slower. After a couple of minutes the pupils began to dilate,
and the left arm being artificially lifted up vertically above the head,
remained motionless in that attitude. Towards the fourth minute
the answers became slower and almost painful, but perfectly sensible, and the respiration slightly irregular. At the end of five minutes,
M. Follin pricked the skin of the left arm, which was still held up at
a right angle with the trunk, but the patient did not move. Soon
afterwards a puncture was made, which drew a little blood, but no
feeling was evinced. The right arm was now placed in the same
attitude as the left, and the region where the abscess was situated
brought into view. The patient yielded willingly, saying, very quietly, that she was doubtless going to be hurt.

Finally, about seven minutes after the beginning of the experiment,
M. Follin laid the abscess largely open, and freed a great quantity of
fœtid pus. A faint cry, which lasted less than a second, was the only
sign of reaction which the patient gave. No movement of the muscles of the face or the limbs was observed ; and the arms remained in
the same cataleptic state which they had previously assumed. Two
minutes later, the attitude was still the same ; the eyes wide open
and a little vascular ; the face motionless ; the pulse as it was before
the experiment began ; the breathing quite free ; and the patient insensible. The left heel was now raised, and it remained unsupported
in the air, whilst the cataleptic state of the arms persisted. M. Broca
at this period removed the bright object which had hitherto been constantly kept before the patient's eyes, gently rubbed her eyelids, and
directed upon them a current of cold air. She now made a few
movements, and was asked if she had felt anything ; upon which she

answered she did not know. Both arms and the leg, remained, however, in the artificial position in which they had been put. At this stage the left arm was again pricked, and no sensation thereby excited.

Eighteen minutes after the beginning of the experiment, and twelve after the operation, another friction on the eyelids and another current of cold air were used; whereupon the patient awoke suddenly, the cataleptic limbs all falling together. The patient then rubbed her eyes, came to her senses, remembered nothing that had passed, and was surprised that the operation was over. Her state was somewhat analogous to that of patients who wake from anæsthesia induced by ordinary means ; though the waking was certainly more sudden, and without agitation or talking. The anæsthesia, which had thus been artificially interrupted, had lasted from twelve to fifteen minutes.

Two attempts of the same kind have been made by MM. Azam and Follin, in the same hospital, upon a girl aged eighteen, who was affected with a slight wound of the foot ; but the results have not been so satisfactory as they were in the last case. Two other experiments which were undertaken by M. Azam, on the 8th inst., were more successful. In a young woman, catalepsy began in a minute and a half, and in two or three minutes both catalepsy and anæsthesia were complete. With another woman, suffering from chorea, anæsthesia was well established in less than two minutes. A third experiment was tried in the presence of M. Trousseau, upon a girl who has been for sometime in the hospital for epileptic vertigo. In a minute and a half, by means of a pair of scissors held ten inches from the eyes, she was cataleptic and asleep ; and when awakened, she complained of severe lumbago and much fatigue : altogether she remained in a state of hebetude and stupor much longer than happens after recovery from epileptic attacks.

ART. XVI.—*Epidemics in* 1859.—*Zymosis.* (*Epidemiological Soc., Nov.* 8, 1859. *Med. Times and Gaz., Nov.* 26, 1859.)

i.—*Report on Epidemics which appeared in various parts of the world during the last twelve months :* By Dr. McWILLIAM, Secretary of the Society.

Cholera, we learn, broke out in July last, at Bombay and Poona, and almost simultaneously on the continent of Europe, selecting on this, as on former occasions, the city of Hamburg as the scene of its development. It next appeared at Helsingfors, in the Gulf of Finland, and afterwards in Southern Sweden, and early in September it declared itself in Stockholm, the capital of the kingdom. While cholera was prevailing in these northern latitudes, its appearance was also announced at Murcia, which is situated in the south-eastern part of Spain. The disease, however, soon abated in the town ; but it lingers still on the coast, as Alicante and Valentia are still considered as ports suspected of cholera. More recently the disease had attacked Rotterdam and Bruges, at which latter place its progress was for some time most alarming. There was not, it appeared, any very satisfactory or trustworthy information with reference to the origin of the disease in any of the continental ports ; but it was well known that in the course of the past summer and autumn cholera had been imported into several of the ports of this country by vessels from Hamburg, viz : the river Thames in two different vessels; Hull, Grimsby, Southampton, and North Shields. In the last-named port, the disease was communicated to a lodging-house on shore, when it proved fatal to two of the inmates. From the time that the existence of cholera was known, our Government appear to have been fully alive to the necessity of taking measures against the invasion of this country by that scourge. Quarantine restriction was not resorted to, nor was the freedom of commerce or of intercourse with other countries at all interfered with, but every precaution short of these was taken by the authorities. All arrivals in the ports of this country, more especially in those having intercourse with Hamburg, were carefully watched for cholera cases; and in those vessels where the disease did exist, a certain degree of isolation from other ships, and of limitation of intercourse with the shore, but not such as to cause inconvenience, were recommended, and in all cases followed. Diarrhœa was unusually fatal in London during the past summer, and a death from cholera was occasionally to be found in the Reports of the Registrar-General. Partial outbreaks of cholera, as on the banks of the Itchen, near Southampton, were said to have occurred in some of the country districts; but nowhere in this country, except at Wick, in Caithness, and at Glass Houghton, in the parish of Castleford, near Pontefract, had the disease appeared in an epidemic form.

In the West Indies, yellow fever had been prevalent at several of the islands, more especially at Antigua, Trinidad, and St. Thomas. In the *La Plata*, which arrived last week at Southampton, from St. Thomas, there had been fifteen deaths from yellow fever during the passage home. Much remained to be done in the way of improving military barracks in the West Indies, and, indeed, a thorough and minute inspection of all barracks in these islands seemed absolutely necessary, if we intend to put an end to, or at all events to mitigate, the evils of every-day occurrence in that part of our colonial possessions. Scarlatina and diphtheria had prevailed in most parts of this country, more especially in the rural districts. Diphtheria had also appeared in Australia. The origin and progress of this disease in a country like Australia, which had all along enjoyed a comparative exemption from epidemics, were subjects worthy of careful investigation. * * * The great small-pox epidemic which commenced in 1857, had, within the last twelve months, had possession of this metropolis, within the limits of which scarcely less than one thousand persons have paid in this period by death, and probably ten times that amount by sickness, the penalty of their neglect of, or of the imperfect manner in which they have received the great prophylactic of vaccination. Dr. Babington concluded his address by exhorting the members to zeal, in furnishing papers for the Society, and in regular attendance at the meetings.

ii.— *On Zymosis:* By Dr. RICHARDSON.

He first considered the process of fermentation as it occurs out of the body. He dwelt on the different views which have been held as to the nature of this process, explaining that they divided themselves into three groups : the vital, the physical, and the chemical. In regard to zymosis, or ferment *in* the body, the view generally held was linked with the idea of the vital character of the fermentation process. Having at some length sustained these positions, the author passed on to observe on the objections which might be urged against the vital hypothesis, and then presented a reading of the subject, which, resting on a basis purely chemical, explained much that was obscure and conflicting. He (the author) did not oppose the idea of zymosis; on the contrary, he gave to it a direct affirmative, but he argued in reference to three points : 1st. That the virus exciting the fermentation was simply an albuminous product. 2d. That the virus was not by its presence the cause of the symptoms, but that the symptoms of the epidemics of zymotics were due to the presence of new chemical products, resulting from the new chemical changes. 3d. That the reäppearance in some cases of the virus as an excrete was a necessary result, but that the origin of the virus was purely local. Dr. Richardson next passed on to show that, if the views he had advanced were tenable, they would explain many points which otherwise were all in confusion, would link certain diseases to the zymotici which are not at this moment ranged in that list, and would yet, at the same time, reduce the verbal list of zymotics to a few units. In the first place, he urged the theory of zymosis, as he explained it, disclosed the reason of the analogy which exists between diseases acknowledged to be communicable, and certain other diseases which are not considered communicable, such as dissecting-room cholera. In the next place, it explained the reason why a small, equally with a large quantity of poison introduced into the body, excites the same intensity of effect. Thirdly, the theory suggests an alliance between diseases arising from the absorption of poisons, and diseases produced by changes occurring in the body spontaneously, such as rheumatic fever and tetanus. Fourthly, it explains why the majority of zymotic diseases get well of themselves. If the poisons of these diseases were vital and increased, or multiplied in the body, the reproduction would last so long as the material for the continuance of the reproduction were present. But if the process were simply chemical, as he supposed, there is a direct reason why the diseases ran a limited course, inasmuch as chemical changes having no independent continuance when their causes are removed, cease necessarily after a time, together with the symptoms excited by them during the period of their operation. Lastly, on the theory suggested by the author, an immense field was opened for direct experimental inquiry. Here scientific researches might take two directions—the one towards tracing the action of known poisons on animals, and exciting diseases analogous to the zymotic diseases after the synthetical method; the other, by ascertaining whether diseases so excited could be transferred to subjects previously unaffected. The point which attracted most interest in the paper, was that which had reference to tetanus. This disease Dr. Richardson claimed to be essentially zymotic. His theory of its production in traumatic cases, is that the wound in the process of healing secretes a special albuminous product, which has the property of a ferment. This substance absorbed into the body excites new chemical changes, and as a product of these, there is developed an alkaline or alkaloidal substance, having properties analogous to strychnine. Whether the patient shall or shall not recover, depends, therefore, on the circumstance of this produced poison being or not being eliminated from the system by the excretions, before the tetanic symptoms excited have progressed to a certain degree. If the symptoms are extended, or are moderate, or are moderated by medicinal means, the poison may be eliminated, and the patient may recover, or the reverse. In regard to tetanus, two experimental questions were open for solution; viz : Will the secretion from the wound in a tetanic patient, introduced by another wound into a healthy animal, excite tetanus ? Secondly, are the excretions, say the urine of a tetanic patient, capable, like strychnine in solution, of exciting tetanic spasm in a susceptible animal ?

CORRESPONDENCE.

I.—*Corneous Tumor.*

COLUMBIA, TEXAS, January 28, 1860.

DR. BENNET DOWLER—*Dear Sir :* I inclose to your address this morning a corneous tumor I excised from a negro woman Breline, the property of Mrs. Block of this county. The tumor, as you see, is over three inches long on its external surface, and over an inch wide and half of an inch thick at its base. It is curved like a ram's or goat's horn, and blunt at its point. The woman is about forty years old. The tumor or horn grew from the cicatrix of an old burn. It was situated just below the inferior spinous process of the ilium of the left side, and just over the rise of the sartorius muscle. It turned inwards, and the point had formed an attachment to the skin just over the femoral artery. The woman had torn up this new adhesion before I saw her. She said the point began to pain her before she broke it loose. She says it has been growing six years. I excised it on the morning of the 9th instant, in the presence of Drs. R. R. and S. Porter, Dr. M. S. Stearns, and other gentlemen. I made an incision around its base parallel with the sartorius muscle, cutting through the cicatrix of the burn, and in elevating it to make the inside incision, it broke in two, as you see. The wound is healed up, and I have discharged the case as cured.

Owing to the rarity of such tumors, I send this notice to you for the *Medical Journal*, as a contribution to southern pathology; and request you to place the tumor itself in the museum of the " Medical Department of the University of Louisiana."

Yours, etc.,

GREENVILLE DOWELL, M. D.

II.—*Antidotes against the Bites of Poisonous Serpents.*

LIBERTY, MISSISSIPPI, January 14, 1860.

DR. DOWLER—In the January number of the *New Orleans Med. and Surg. Journal*, there is a communication from Dr. Peake, entitled " Tobacco as an antidote for the poison of the rattlesnake." I myself have, as Dr. P. tells us in his article *he* has, heard of many and very astonishing cures from the bites of the most poisonous of serpents by both tobacco and whisky (or brandy), but all from non-professional gentlemen. Indeed, Dr. P.'s article is the only account of these agents, as antidotes, which I have ever seen in print.

My object in writing this is, to inquire 1st, whether tobacco and alcohol are known by professional experience to be antidotes for the poisons of serpents; and 2d, if they are antidotes, their probable *modus operandi*. It appears to me a little strange that alcohol, one of the most powerful *stimulants*, and tobacco, a very powerful *sedative*, should produce the same results when given to patients bitten by poisonous serpents.

My third inquiry is, why the bites of snakes do not hurt hogs, which, so far as I know, are the only animals not injured by these poisons. Is there any principle in *fat*, so plentifully deposited under the skin of the hog, which neutralizes the effects of the poison ?

Please answer through your journal. By so doing, you will very much oblige,

S. C. YOUNG.

III.—*Case of Monstrosity.*

WEST BOYLSTON, MASSACHUSETTS, Dec. 31, 1859.

Dear Sir—I send you a photograph of a remarkable monstrosity that occurred in my obstetrical practice recently.

It consisted of two female children, *joined together* from the clavicle to the umbilicus, having a sternum on either side, and the ribs of each child meeting in a common sternum.

The thoracic and abdominal cavity was common to both. There was but *one* liver, double in size, with *two* gall bladders, and extending entirely across the cavity from side to side. There was one heart, double in size, and having two aortæ. There were four kidneys, of large size, with two ureters from each.

This monstrosity was still-born, 18 inches in length, each head measuring $12\frac{1}{4}$ inches. The labor was terminated successfully, and the mother is doing well. A copy-right is secured on the photograph, but if you deem it of sufficient importance to the profession, you can insert a wood-cut in your journal, together with a history of the case.

Yours, etc.,

CHAS. A. WHEELER, M. D.

Ed. N. O. Med. and Surg. Jour.

IV.—*Trismus Nascentium.*

FORKLAND, GREENE COUNTY, ALA.

DR. BENNET DOWLER—*Dear Sir :* If you have had any success in the treatment of Trismus Nascentium, do me the favor to furnish a brief statement of your plan of procedure, and much oblige your friend and obedient servant,

H. B. ROBINSON.

[Unable to propose a satisfactory plan of treatment for this most destructive malady of infancy, the editor publishes the above note, hoping thereby to call the attention of readers to the pathological and therapeutic solution of the question which it propounds. During a street conversation with a physician of New Orleans, a few months ago, he averred that he had cured a number of cases by alcoholic stimulants, gradually increasing the dose so as to intoxicate the patient.]

V.—*Delirium Tremens.*

WARRENTON, MISS., Feb. 30, 1860.

DR. DOWLER—*Dear Sir:* Enclosed you will find an account of a case of *mania à potu*, occurring in my practice a few weeks ago, of which the most interesting feature is the remarkable tolerance of chloroform and opium. Should you deem it worthy of publicity, you can give it a place in your journal. Very respectfully,

THOS. T. BEALL.

Case of Mania à Potu.—Having been called to Mr. R. H., I found him with decided symptoms of delirium tremens, which had been slowly increasing in intensity for eight days, without a moment's sleep during that period, despite the pretty free use of opium for several days prior to the one on which I was called to him. His bowels not having acted for several days, I ordered for him an injection, to be frequently repeated until a full fæcal discharge was pro duced. He was then put upon opium, 2 grs. every 3 hours, with a little brandy at alternate intervals of the same duration. Refusing nourishment, it was not pressed.

On returning the next morning I found him a *raving maniac*, much worse than on the preceding day—the remedies having made no favorable impression whatever. I at once gave him 4 grs. sulphate-morphia, and directed 1 gr. to be given whenever there should be a tendency to a return of the restlessness. Two such doses were found sufficient during the succeeding 24 hours. After giving him the 4 gr. dose of morphia, I had him held down by force, and made him inhale chloroform *strongly* for *one hour and a half;* at the expiration of which time his violence was subdued (and permanently); he lay quietly and contentedly in bed, but *no sleep* was induced. Late in the afternoon he dozed half an hour, and during the night slept an hour or so. Towards the next morning (the third of my attendance), symptoms of secondary depression came on, attended with cool, clammy skin, feeble, frequent and intermittent pulse, with unconsciousness, followed by drowsiness, and this again by profound coma, yet without sleep, and with a normal state of the pupils. Morphia was now given him, $\frac{1}{2}$ gr. every hour or two, alternating with brandy in potions of a wineglass full. I was happy to observe the marked effect of morphia in this state of depression—the pulse rising and the skin warming under each dose of it, until by the evening, when his consciousness was restored, the morphia, together with the brandy, was gradually diminished in amount, and finally withdrawn.

From the second morning of my attendance, after the subdual of the maniacal excitement before mentioned, he commenced taking food, and continued to take it in gradually increased quantities (the period of coma excepted) at intervals of a few hours. I would here mention that in my first visit I found him with inflammation (in third stage) of the apices of both lungs, for which he was largely blistered. Now the enquiry naturally suggests itself, what had this to do, if anything, with the resistance manifested to the action of chloroform? for, so far as I could judge, the chloroform was almost entirely without effect.   T. T. B.

VI.—*Geological Letter.*

HOUMA, LA., Sept. 16, 1859.

B. DOWLER, M. D.—*Dear Sir:* At the request of the Houma Scientific Association, I send you three specimens of soil obtained at different depths. The specimens were found about ten miles below Houma, on the Bayou Little Caillou. Seven years ago the spot was about one hundred feet in circumference, and about five feet high. At present it is about four hundred feet in circumference, and about two feet higher than the surrounding land. It is in the centre of a cane field. Until the present year it has produced no vegetation—which at present is very scant. It looks as if pulverized on the top, and is very loose. When walked upon, it trembles like the floating prairies of this country, and it is nearly impossible for a horse to go through it.

Three of us—Messrs. Dunn, Bond and Woods—dug to the depth of two feet, when a sound like a rattlesnake's rattle was distinctly heard—so much so that none of the party were willing to trust their hands in the loose soil. At five feet, the noise was that of water boiling in a steam boiler. At eight feet the sounds were the *fac similes* of a steam whistle ; and at ten and a half feet there were undistinguishable sounds. When we left the place there was a confusion of sounds. And to-day, which is fifteen days after the hole was dug, I am informed that the sounds still continue. There appears by vegetable decomposition, to be vertical veins throughout the whole mound, which you will discover by the specimens sent. At the depth of ten and a half feet we found roots of trees, but unfortunately lost them in returning home. The formation appears to be principally organic. No. 1 was found at a depth of two feet; No. 2 at five feet, and No. 3 ten and a half feet from the surface of the ground.

The surrounding ground is perfectly hard and arable, and produces well.

We have been informed that there are three other mounds of the same species in this parish, but have not yet examined them.

If you will be so kind as to give us your opinion of this formation, you will greatly oblige the members of the H. S. A. We will gladly give any other information in regard to the formation in our power.

Yours, respectfully,   T. A. Woods,
Cor. Sec. H. S. A.

[The answer returned to this letter is, it is feared, inconclusive. The publication of the letter may, perhaps, call forth a better explanation of the phenomena mentioned.]

MISCELLANEA.

MEDICAL CHRONOLOGY.

[In 1824, the editor of the *Æsculapian Register* commenced the publication of a series of chronological tables, giving the chronological history of the world, and that of medicine, in parallel columns, which, however, owing to the discontinuance of the periodical, he never completed. In his preface he says :

" We commence a chronological table, to facilitate a knowledge of the history of medicine. It is translated from the excellent work of Sprengel, who appears to have taken much pains in its construction ; and we can only add, that we wish such encouragement could be given by the medical profession, as would warrant the printing of his whole work. It would amply remunerate every proprietor of a copy, at least, if we may judge from the advantage we have ourselves derived from its perusal. A complete History of Medicine is scarcely to be found in the libraries of any of our physicians ; and the work in question is extremely scarce amongst us. It is in seven volumes, but might be readily included, omitting his notes and references, in about three volumes of five hundred pages each. We have made considerable advance in the translation of the work, but have met as yet with little encouragement to undertake its completion."

It is believed that students (all are students) often have occasion to refer to chronological data, which few libraries contain, or if they do contain them, the data are so scattered that references are difficult and tedious.

The tables above referred to commence with Indian Period, twenty-six centuries before Hippocrates (3100 B. C.), and end A. D., 1603 and, containing as they do the chronology of the world as well as that of medicine, are too much extended to be admitted into the *New Orleans Medical and Surgical Journal* without great retrenchment. It is therefore proposed to begin with the Hippocratic era, omitting the external or non-medical data altogether, giving a condensed medico-chronological synopsis ending about the commencement of the seventeenth century of the Christian era, an ever memorable period, in which letters, science, the mariner's compass, the microscope, printing, copper-plate engraving, the dissection of the human body, pathological anatomy, and many other means were operating energetically, by which general as well as medical knowledge was improved and extended; while governmental, social, and educational reforms were inaugurated in both insular and continental Europe; although, as yet, Harvey's discovery had not immortalized his name.—B. D.]

B. C. 436. Hippocrates becomes celebrated (*Cyrill.* contra Julian, v. 1.)
428. Death of Anexagoras.
425. Plague renewed at Athens.
404. Death of Democritus.
400. Lucina worshipped by the Romans.
396. First Lectisternium, at Rome, on account of an epidemic.
390. Ctesias of Cnidos.

384. Birth of Aristotle.
381. Plague at Rome.
377. Death of Hippocrates 2d, according to some historians.
374. Thessalus, Draco and Polybius, successors of Hippocrates.
371 Birth of Theophrastus.
370. Death of Hippocrates 2d, according to some historians ; Dioxippus of Cos; Philistion of Locra; Petronius.
363. Siennesis of Cyprus; Diogenes.
362. Third Lectisternium at Rome.
360. L. Manlius Imperiosus, named dictator, drives a nail into the right side of the temple of Jupiter, to procure a cessation of the plague. This ceremony, called *clavum figere*, was anciently employed by the Volsiniens, a people of Etruria, to mark the number of years. From them it passed to Rome. The nail was called *clavus annalis.*
354. Diocles of Carista ; Eudoxus of Cnidos.
348. Death of Plato.
345. Fourth Lectisternium at Rome, on account of a pestilence.
341. Praxagoras of Cos.
336. Chrysippus of Cnidus.
335. Aristotle quits the court of Alexander.
331. Callisthenes of Olynthes.
329. A dictator drives a nail into the temple of Jupiter at Rome, to procure the cessation of a strange insanity, which was regarded as the cause of the multiplication of crimes in the city.
327. Plistonicus.
324. Aristoxenes, the musician, mentions the latest philosophers among the ancient pythagoreans. (*Diogen.* viii. 46.)
323. Fifth Lectisternium at Rome, on account of a pestilence.
322. Death of Aristotle.
321. Eudemus of Rhodes.
320. Establishment of the Alexandrian library ; Philotimus ; Mnesistheus; Dieuches.
318. Hippocrates IV, son of Draco.
307. Birth of Zeno of Citium; Herophilus of Chalcedonia; Premigenes of Mitylene.
304. Erasistratus at the court of Seleucus; Cynethus the Homerist.
293. Plague at Rome.
292. Plague at Rome ; ten ambassadors are sent to Epidaurus,
291. Plague at Rome.
who bring to Rome the god Esculapius, under the figure of a serpent.
290. Death of Theophrastus ; Pyrrho of Eleus ; Philinus of Cos.
285. Division of Medicine at Alexandria; Diodorus Cronos; Nicias of Miletus; Strato of Lampsacus; Strato of Beryta.
279. Birth of Chrysippus of Solis; Eudemus the Anatomist; Xenophon, disciple of Erasistratus; Serapion of Alexandria.
276. Mantias, disciple of Herophilus ; Philoxenes ; Demetrius of Apamea; Heron; Gorgias ; Glaucius, the Empiric ; Ammonius the Lithotomist.
274. Plague at Rome; a dictator drives a nail into the temple of Jupiter.
264. Lycon of Troy ; Amyntas of Rhodes ; Apollonius of Memphis; Bacchius of Tanagra.

263. Plague at Rome ; a dictator drives a nail into the temple of Jupiter.

261. Death of Zeno of Citium.

251. Callianax; Perigenes.

246. Callimachus; Cydias of Mylasa.

245. Lysimachus of Cos.

242. Sostrates; Nymphodorus.

234. Birth of Cato the Censor.

230. Chrysermes, disciple of Herophilus.

224. Dreadful epidemic in the Roman army.

223. Artemidorus of Sida; Charidemus.

221. Apollophanes, disciple of Erasistratus.

219. Arrival of Archagatus at Rome.

218. Apollonius Biblas.

212. Great epidemic in the Roman army at the siege of Syracuse.

206. Death of Chrysippus of Solis.

205. Epidemic in the Roman army ; sixth Lectisternium at Rome.

204. Apollonius Ther; Hermogenes of Tricca.

174. Violent plague at Rome.

158. Zopyrus.

149. Death of Cato the Censor.

146. Apollonius Mys of Citium.

143. Death of Antiochus Eutheus. This prince perished under the hands of lithotomists.

138. Nicander; Cleophantes.

123. Gaius.

117. Apollonius of Tyre; Dioscorides Phacas.

100. Arrival of Asclepiades at Rome.

78. Sylla dies of a lousy disease.

68. Themison of Laodicea.

49. Heras of Capadocia; Nicon of Agrigentum, disciple of Asclepiades.

44. Titus Aufidius of Sicily.

42. Marcus Artorius ; Philonides of Dryachium; Clodius; Niceratus.

31. Death of Marcus Artorius.

30. Icecias at Smyrna; Menodotus; Pasicrates; Nileus.

20. Meges of Sidon; Philo the Jew.

B. of J. C. Zeuxis of Laodicea.

A. D. 3–5. Cornelius Celsus.

6. Apulejus Celsus.

14. Eudemus.

23. Birth of Pliny; Menecrates of Zeophleta; Phido of Tarsus; Vettius Valens.

33. Charmis of Marseilles.

37. Servilius Damocrates.

41. Alexander Philalethes; Scribonius Largus.

43. Xenocrates of Aphrodisea.

54. Dioscorides of Anazarba; Andromachus; Thessalus of Tralles; Gaius and Evelpides, oculists; Crinas of Marseilles.

68. Atheneus of Attalus.

69. Demosthenes Philalethes; Apollonides of Cyprus; Menema-chus; Olympicus; Mnaseas; Zoilus.

79. Death of Pliny.

81. Menodotus of Nicomedia; Aretæus of Capadocia; Agathinus; Philomenus ; Marinus ; Crito; Apollonius Archistrator ; Pamphilus; Migmatopoles

96. Death of Apollonius of Tyana.

97. Archigenes; Rufus of Ephesus; Cassius the Iatrosophist; So-ranus, son of Menander; Heliodorus, the Surgeon; Asclepiades Phar-macion; Herodotus.

117. Moschion; Theudas of Laodicea; Artemidorus Capiton; Di-oscurides; Lycus of Naples; Philip of Cæsarea; Acibah and Simeon ben Jochai, founders of the Cabala.

131. Birth of Galen.

138. Marcellus of Sida; Andrew Chrysaris; Julien the Methodist.

152. Galen goes to Smyrna.

155. He returns to his country.

165. Galen arrives at Rome.

166. Magnus of Ephesus.

200. Death of Galen.

211. Ammonius Saccas.

222. Serenus Samonicus.

230. Coelius Aurelianus; Leonides of Alexandria.

237. Serenus Samonicus, the Son.

253. Plotinus.

270. Manes, founder of the Manichean Sect.

282. Porphyry.

296. Edict of Dioclesian against Alchymy.

307. Palatine Archiatri; Jamblichus.

330. Antyllus the Surgeon.

337. Zeno of Cyprus.

357. Ordinance of Constantine against magic.

360. Oribasius; Magnus of Antioch.

363. Cæsarius.

364. Vindicien; Posidonius; Philagrius.

367. Edict against Magic.

379. Theodore Priscian; Sextus Placitus ; Nemesius ; Marcellus of Bordeaux; The *Cyranide*.

400. Death of Martin of Tours.

431. First persecution of the Nestorians at Edessa.

440: James Psychrestus.

541. A general plague.

543. Benoit of Nursia, founder of the convent of Monte-Cassino; Aëtius of Amida; Alexander of Tralles.

565. Small-pox in France.

572. Small-pox in Arabia.

582. Isidore of Seville.

610. Theophilus Protospatharius.

622. Aaron; Hhareth ebn Kaldath.

634. Palladius the Iatrosophist; Paul of Egina.

640. Stephen of Athens; John of Alexandria.

668. Simeon ben Taibutha, the Nestorian.
671. Apsyrtes of Prussia; Theodore, Archbishop of Canterbury.
680. Masardschawaih; Sergius of Rasain; Gosius of Alexandria.
690. Theodorus and Theodunus, Greek physicians in Irak.
702. Birth of Geber.
772. George Bakhtischwah is called to Bagdad; Asa abou Koreisch.
774. Isa abou Koreisch.
775. Bakhtischwah abou Dschibrail.
804. Hhonain ebu Izhak.
805. Dschibrail Bakhtischwah.
814. Iahiah ebu Batrik.
820. Serapion the elder.
835. Birth of Thabeth ebu Korrak.
846. Bakhtischwah 4th.
865. Death of Jahiah ebu Masawaih.
867. Michel Psellus the elder.
872. Death of Sabor ebn Sahel.
873. Death of Hhonain ebn Izhak.
880. Death of James Alkhendi.
886. Senan ebn Thabeth; David ebn Hohain; Hhobaisch.
912. Death of Izhak ebu Hhonain.
923. Death of Rhazes.
936. Theophanes or Nonus; the Hippiatriques are collected.
940. Izhak ben Soliman.
978. Birth of Avicenna.
980. Aladdin al Karschi.
984. Adalheron, Archbishop of Verdun, goes to Salernum to be cured.
994. Death of Ali ebno'l Abbas.
996. Avicenna goes to Dschordschan.
1002. Serapion the younger; Abdorrahman al Hanisi.
1010. Haroun, son of Izhak of Cordova.
1014. Thieddeg, physician to Boleslas, King of Bohemia.
1017. Death of Mesue the younger.
1028. Fulbert of Chartres.
1036. Death of Avicenna.
1040. Berthier, Abbot of Monte-Cassino.
1054. Nicetas; Romuald, Bishop of Salernum; Gariopontus; Hugh, Abbot of St. Denis.
1071. Désiré, Abbot of Monte-Cassino.
1080. Herman, Count of Vehringen; Abou-Dschafar.
1087. Death of Constantine the African.
1095. Death of Jahiah, son of Dschala.
1098. Birth of Hildegarde, Abbess of Bingen.
1100. *Regimen sanitatis Salernitan;* John of Milan.
1110. Nicholas, intendant at Salernum.
1114. Birth of Gerard of Cremona.
1122. Death of Khalaf abou'l Kasem; Synesius.
1131. Mich. Psellus the younger.
1139. Abou Hamed al Ganzali, the philosopher.
1143. Roger gives medical laws to Salernum.

1150. Eros or Trotula; Lucas, Patriarch of Constantinople, interdicts the practice of medicine to the priests; Mathew Platearius;
Abou'l Hassan Hebatollah.
1162. First regulations in England relative to bawdy houses.
1164. Death of Ebn-Zohr.
1169. Egide of Cerbeil.
1180. Obizo, Abbot of St. Victoire; death of Hildegard, Abbess
of Bingen.
1187. Death of Gerard of Cremona.
1193. Birth of Albert of Bollstaedt.
1195. Death of Abou Bekrebn Tofail.
1199. Hugh, the physician, professor of medicine at Paris.
1206. Death of Averrhoës; Roger of Parma.
1209. The philosophy of Aristotle defended at Paris.
1214. Birth of Roger Bacon.
1220. Faculty of medicine at Montpelier.

(To be concluded in next Number.)

THE EXPIRED AIR.

At a session of the Academy of Sciences during the last year, a
prize of 5,000 francs was awarded to M. Doyère for his researches
upon the composition of the air expired by *cholériques*, and upon the
temperature of patients during the last moments of life. M. Doyère
has recorded in this memoir the analyses of 209 products of expired
air, of which 170 were from *cholériques* and 39 from men in health.
Each analysis comprehends the ascertainment of the oxygen consumed
and that of the carbonic acid produced. Previously, in 1832, M. Rayer
had announced that the air expired by *cholériques* contained more oxygen than in the normal state. M. Doyère has confirmed this result, and
has given the following details: He has seen in no case the absorption
of oxygen reduced to zero; he has never seen that the air expired
contains as much oxygen as the air inspired; but he has established,
in the severest form of cholera, that there is most oxygen in the expired air. As for carbonic acid, M. Doyère has constantly met with
a notable decline in the proportion of this gas in the expired air of
cholériques, the mean of which is no more than 1 to 100.

Nevertheless, one may, by analyzing these products of expiration,
measure the severity of the disease. Thus among *cholériques* who are
promptly cured, the oxygen absorbed never falls below the proportion
of 3 per centum, nor the carbonic acid exhaled below that of 2.3. On
the other hand, M. Doyère has never seen a patient recover after the analysis had shown a fall of the former gas to 1.75 and of the latter to

1.45, even in such cases where the amelioration of the symptoms had given rise to great expectations of recovery.

Notwithstanding the diminished activity of the respiratory function, notwithstanding the little combustion of the carbon, the temperature of the body does not a little increase in a notable manner; and then, when nothing escapes from the lungs but a small quantity of carbonic acid, yet in this physiological state one witnesses a temperature in the axilla of 40° C. and over.   At the approach of death, when the circulation is embarrassed and becomes arrested, when the respiratory function becomes every moment less active, the axillary temperature augments among *cholériques* to the elevated point of 43° C., that is to say, it then attains a maximum to which it rarely rises in febrile maladies during their periods of greatest heat.   At the moment when death is taking place, the singular phenomenon of the ascension of temperature ceases abruptly.   [This does not occur in choleraïc cadavera in New Orleans.]   B. D.

PRIZE FOR EXPERIMENTAL PHYSIOLOGY.—M. JACUBOWITSCH.

During the past year the Academy of Sciences of Paris, awarded the great prize for experimental physiology to M. Jacubowitsch, of St. Petersburg, for his work *On the intimate structure of the Brain and Spinal Marrow of Man and the Vertebrated Animals.*

The reporter of the commission says M. Jacubowitsch has undertaken some of the most diffcult problems in anatomy and physiology; namely—the unraveling of the textures of the nervous system, distinguishing their various elementary constituents, with the view of determining their physiological action.   The author recognizes and describes three peculiar forms of nerve-cells, relating to and connecting with three different kinds of nerve-fibres.   He has determined the exact arrangement of these different histological elements in the spinal marrow, medulla oblongata, and the brain ; he has indicated the points among the nervous centres in which these cells or fibres are grouped, accumulated, mixed, separated, appear or disappear. These anatomical researches, made, not only on man, but still more fully upon the four classes of vertebrated animals, are of great importance in physiology; they prepare, in the best manner, the ground on which we may finally establish the most delicate physiological experimentation.   *(Gaz. Heb.)*   B. D.

MORTALITY STATISTICS.

Mortality of the year 1859, *in New Orleans.* (*From the Report of the Board of Health.*)

Total Deaths................6,847	Deaths under 5 years.............2,652
Whites......................5,778	" from 5 to 20................ 710
Negroes.....................1,069	" " 20 to 50 2,781
United States...............4,073	" " 50 to 100............. 694
Foreign.....................2,774	" over 100................. 10

Greatest mortality, in November...........................788
Least   "   in March 438

APOPLEXY.—Last year 114, this year 101; decrease 13. Largest number of deaths in May.

BRONCHITIS.—This year 69, against 74 last year.

CASUALTIES.—This year 59, against 52 last year.

CHOLERA.—Last year 26 deaths.

CHOLERA INFANTUM.—This year 88, 108 last year. Greatest number in July.

CONGESTION OF BRAIN.—This year 172, last year 156.

CONSUMPTION.—This year 869, last year 729. In November 108 deaths.

CONVULSIONS, INFANTILE.—This year 367, last year 521.

CROUP.—This year 87 deaths, last year 126.

DELIRIUM TREMENS.—This year 97, last year 85.

DIARRHŒA.—This year 293, last year 297. In November 40, the greatest.

DROWNED.—This year 87, against 86 last year.

DYSENTERY.—This year 223, against 229 in 1858.

DIIPHTHERIA.—This year 253, chiefly children between two and ten.

ENTERITIS.—This year 140, last year 117.

EPILEPSY.—This year 17, last year 20.

SCARLET FEVER.—This year 121, last year 79.

TYPHOID FEVER.—This year 214, last year 189.

YELLOW FEVER.—This year 91, last year 4,845.

GASTRO ENTERITIS.—This year 67, last year 87.

DISEASE OF HEART.—This year 94, last year 87.

HEPATITIS.—This year 26, last year 231.

GASTRITIS.—This year 52, last year 48.

INTEMPERANCE.—This year 41, last year 44.

MARASMUS, INFANTILE.—This year 169, last year 188.

STILL-BORN.—This year 353, last year 338.

TEETHING.—This year 202, last year 189.

TRIS. NASCENTIUM.—This year 212, last year 222.

It is much to be regretted that mortuary tables in this city are so meagre. The length of time the patient has resided in this city before death is a very important item, and one which few physicians notice in their certificate, although blanks are furnished on application at this office, and every means resorted to to procure full returns. A legislative enactment, not only in this respect, but also to obtain full and complete mortuary returns from the whole State, seems desirable.

H. D. BALDWIN, M. D.,
Secretary of the Board of Health.

REMARKS.—The President of the Board of Health in his annual report observes, "It will not fail to be remarked that yellow fever has occasioned the death of 92 persons," and, "as far as any evidence to the contrary is known, it was incontestibly of domestic origin—the product of soil, season, and susceptible subjects existing concurrently together." These causes are deemed, by a large portion of our physicians, to be ample to account for all our epidemics; and when assigned, by one advocating the importation views adopted by Dr. Axson in his previous reports, as sufficient to explain the existence of yellow fever in 1859, it will be unnecessary to advance any facts to disprove its importation during the last year.

In regard to the assertion that "yellow fever has occasioned the death of 92 persons," we believe it to be incorrect, and that the actual number was much greater. It is well known to many of the physicians in this city that cases diagnosed during life as yellow fever, had their certificates of death written, with the words "yellow fever" unaccountably omitted therefrom. Whether this omission resulted from a fear of injuring the commercial interests of our city, or other plausible excuse, the omission is not to be commended. It may partake of "old fogyism," but we have an abiding conviction that "honesty is the best policy," whether in commerce or medicine.

It will be further observed that although the mortality for the whole city is reported as only 92, yet the Charity Hospital furnishes 84 of these deaths. That is, that but 8 deaths from yellow fever occurred outside of the walls of this Hospital ! The statistics of other years in regard to yellow fever, and of this year in reference to other diseases, lead us to believe that if there were only 84 deaths of yellow fever in the Charital Hospital, it is more than probable that a much larger number than 8 died from the same disease throughout the balance of the city.

However, the report of the Board of Health is based on the certificates of the physicians of the city, and we do not desire to impugn the accuracy of the addition as reported by its President.

S. E. C.

Statistics of Charity Hospital for 1859. (*From the Annual Report, kindly furnished by Mr. H. Vanderlinden, Clerk.*)

ADMISSIONS.		DEATHS.	
Total number	12,775	Total number	1,321
Males	10,785	Males	1,092
Females	1,990	Females	229
Total from United States	2,011	Greatest number deaths, in Oct.	200
Of these, from Louisiana	377	Greatest number admit'd, in Oct.	1,836
Total of foreign birth	10,764	BIRTHS.	
Of these, from Ireland	5,888	Total	110
" " Germany	1,748	Males	61
No. of patients remaining in		Females	48
the Hospital Jan. 1st, 1860	730	Still-born	1

SOME OF THE DISEASES.	ADMISSIONS.	DEATHS.
Yellow Fever	105	84
Typhoid Fever	252	99
Intermittent Fever	3,707	5
Remittent Fever	665	38
Congestive Fever	84	61
Bronchitis	205	8
Pneumonia	148	59
Pleurisy	72	6
Phthisis	429	250
Rheumatism	579	3
Syphilis	498	6
Delirium Tremens	254	56
Intemperance	153	8

Statistics of Insane Asylum at Jackson, Louisiana, for 1859.

Number of patients remaining December 31, 1858.....................................137
    "   "   "   "   " 1859.............................,..................157
    "   "   admitted in   1859................................ 97
    ··   "   who died in   1859................................ 37

Of the thirty-seven deaths, twenty-four were caused by diarrhœa. The average number of patients in the Asylum during 1859, was 164. This Asylum has accommodations for thirty-five paying and one hundred and sixty-five non-paying patients. The former class have contributed $6,710 to the funds of the Asylum during the year.

Mortality Statistics of New Orleans, from December, 1859, to Feb. 12, 1860, compiled from the Weekly Reports politely furnished by Dr. Baldwin, Secretary of the Board of Health.

Time.	Total Deaths.	Children under 2 yrs.	Under 20.	U. States
December (5 weeks)	549	164	259	297
January (4 weeks)	567	151	229	316
February (2 weeks)	242	69	98	124

Principal Diseases.	December (5 weeks.)	January (4 weeks.)	February (2 weeks.)
Apoplexy	9	16	5
Cholera Infantum	2	3	0
Congestion of Brain	13	13	3
Congestion of Lungs	1	57	2
Consumption	56	88	26
Convulsions, Infantile	39	24	19
Croup	5	11	4
Diarrhœa	30	32	7
Dysentery	23	20	20
Diphtheria	12	1	2
Fever, Miasmatic	19	4	7
" Scarlet	8	11	4
" Typhoid	22	17	10
" Yellow	3	0	0
Gastro-Enteritis	6	3	0
Inflammation of Liver	6	5	0
Inflammation of Lungs	42	49	21
Inflammation of Throat	1	2	2
Marasmus, Infant	11	12	3
Measles	0	0	0
Pleurisy	1	1	2
Pneumonia	1	3	0
Small Pox	0	0	1
Still-born	37	20	14
Teething	13	3	4
Tetanus	1	6	0
Trismus Nascentium	19	15	6

S. E. C.

MONTHLY SUMMARY—METEOROLOGICAL REGISTER.—*From the Medical Purveying Office, U. S. Army, N. O.* New Orleans, La., Lat. 29 deg. 57 min. 30 sec. N.; Long. 90 deg. W.　Altitude of Barometer above the level of the sea, 35 feet.

1859.	BAROMETER.			THERM. ATTACHED.			THERMOMETER.		
MONTHS.	Max.	Min'm.	Mean.	Max.	Min'm	Mean.	Max.	Min'm	Mean.
December·	7 A. M. 9th. 30.606	2 P. M. 16th. 29.824	30.196	2. P. M. 6th. 76°	7. A. M. 21st. 44°	60.49	2 P. M. 6th. 77°	7 A. M. 9th. 32°	53.65
1860. January...	7 A. M. 2d. 30.628	9 P. M. 6th 29.962	30.281	2. P. M. 11½&13th 74°	7. A. M. 3d. 46°	63.33	2 P. M. 11 &13th 75°	7 A. M. 2d & 3d. 35°	56.99

1859.	HYGROMETER.			PREV'G WINDS.	WEATHER.		RAIN.	
MONTHS.	Max.	Min'm	Mean		Fair.	Cloudy.	Days.	Quantity.
December.	2 P.M. 6th. 72°	7 P.M. 9th. 30°	51.33	N.W., N., & E.			8	5.09.
1860. January...	2 P.M. 13th. 72°	Several. 33°	54.19	E., N., & N. W.			5	0.64.

T. HARRISON, Clerk.

TO OUR SUBSCRIBERS.

Our subscribers are hereby notified that JAS. DEERING, and his assistants, are the only general agents authorized to collect for the New Orleans Medical and Surgical Journal, for the year ending December 31, 1861.　His authority to collect is limited to the States of Louisiana, Mississippi, Arkansas, Tennessee, Alabama, Georgia, Florida and South Carolina, and to accounts due for three years or more.

To postmasters and others the bills of those subscribers who may reside in their towns or counties are sometimes entrusted, but in all such cases they have our written authority to collect, specifying the names of our debtors, with the amounts due by each.

Any payments due to us which may be paid to parties not indicated above, will be at the subscriber's risk.

Bank bills current at par in the subscriber's State will be received in payment, and if forwarded by mail in letters registered "valuable," will be at the risk of

DRS. CHAILLÉ & NICHOLS,

Proprietors of the N. O. Medical and Surgical Journal.

THE

NEW ORLEANS

MEDICAL AND SURGICAL JOURNAL.

MAY, 1860.

ORIGINAL COMMUNICATIONS. ✓

ART. I.—*Mania à Potu:* By WARREN STONE, M. D., Professor of Surgery in the University of Louisiana.

THIS term is often applied to all the forms of delirium that are caused by the excessive use of stimulants, but it more properly belongs to the acute form, where the violence of the delirium, or mania, is mainly due to alcoholic blood-poison. The term delirium tremens is more appropriate to the more chronic form, where the delirium and tremor are due to the sudden privation of a long-accustomed stimulant. It is the former that I think is generally improperly treated, and is so often the cause of sudden and premature death. Brain fever and apoplexy are terms often kindly substituted as being more respectable; but names do not alter facts. Mania à potu usually occurs with the robust who habitually use alcoholic stimulants, but not to any great excess, except upon occasions, and when they are carried to a certain extent, a necessity for their continuance is created, and their excessive use cannot, or will not, be resisted until the stomach gives way and finally rejects them. During this process the mucous membrane becomes engorged, the digestion, and finally the appetite, entirely fail, and the patient is sustained for some days after by stimulants alone, until furious delirium sets in.

39

This madness is not due to the stoppage of an accustomed stimulant, for it often sets in while the subject is in the full use of it, but it is plainly due to alcoholic poison and .the absence of proper nutritive matter in the blood. I think I may add another cause, which has often something to do in causing the delirium, and certainly much to do in causing death, under some modes of treatment, and that is suppressed excretions. So long as the stomach is intact, and the appetite and digestion are good, an immense quantity of stimulant may be disposed of without serious immediate consequences; but when the organs finally, from constant excitation, become engorged, nutrition ceases, and the alcohol is retained more in the blood, instead of being carried off by excretions, and a wild delirium soon follows.

It is plain, under these circumstances, that the indications are to establish the excretions, disgorge the system of the alcoholic poison, and to introduce proper nutriment. The first two are accomplished by one and the same means. The stomach is generally irritable; at least there is frequent vomiting; but it is owing to the accumulation in the stomach of morbid secretion, rather than from inflammation or even irritation; for calomel in small doses, frequently repeated, arrests it with great certainty. If the subject is governable, and will take medicine willingly, calomel should be given in two or three grain doses every hour, or oftener, if the case is urgent, until fifteen or twenty grains are given; but if medicine has to be given by force, it is best to give a full dose at once; and this is the better, for in the worst cases the stomach is often not nauseated, and the sedative effect of a large dose of calomel calms the nervous excitement, and at the same time produces the appropriate effect upon the excretory organs and mucous coat of the stomach and bowels. It requires some hours for this effect to be produced, and it is improper to give anything to promote its action upon the bowels under ten or twelve hours, and I think even a longer time would be better, if the case is not urgent. Small and frequently repeated doses of saline medicine are the best, after the calomel (sulphate of magnesia is best), which promotes the excretions, disgorges the stomach and bowels, and clears the system of its alcoholic poison, to its great relief. An active cathartic may afford some relief, but the system is not so well disgorged by it; more or less serum from the blood is carried off, causing weakness; while, in the other process, by giving time for the action of the calomel, and then promoting it by gentle but continued means, the organs exercise a selection in excreting, and thereby a large amount of effete matter is discharged, and the patient feels the stronger for it, being freed from an incubus that was weighing it down, and producing apparent exhaustion. After this process, we should lose no time in introducing nutriment, and for this purpose milk is almost universally applicable; and as the mucous membrane of the stomach seems to be denuded of its epithelium, the addition of lime water renders it particularly grateful and soothing. Patients in this condition generally loathe animal substances, but milk is almost always grateful to the taste, and is particularly appropriate, for it furnishes the most innocent solid for the bowels, that have been long deprived of their wholesome stimulus. If it should happen that a patient could not take milk, well boiled corn-meal gruel is the next best diet, most likely to be relished; and for something more substantial, strong, well-seasoned broth, frozen, will be the most likely to agree.

In all acute cases, alcoholic stimulants should be withheld, for they act like a poison, and will often bring back the delirium. Should stimulants be thought necessary (and it is not often really necessary), the carbonate of ammonia, or the aromatic spirits of ammonia, are preferable; or it may be proper, in some cases, to allow malt liquor. Opium, in all forms, should be prohibited, until the system is relieved thoroughly of its alcohol, and even then I find that it can generally be omitted; and when it can be, the patient recovers sooner and better. The patient is not expected to sleep well, but if the blood is renewed by its appropriate nutriment, natural sleep will soon follow.

Occasionally, when, previous to the debauch which immediately caused the mania, a free use of stimulants had been indulged in for some time, we have an exalted state of the nervous system, attended with hallucinations and sleeplessness, which require special attention. Potent stimulants operate badly, and opium alone does not operate well, though in large doses sleep may be forced, though not without some risk, in some cases, to the brain; but equal parts of morphia and tart. antimony, given in small and repeated doses, will soon calm the nervous system and induce sleep, without injury either to the brain or stomach. There is nothing that cools off the heated imagination in these cases like nauseating doses of tart. antimony, and opium in some form may be added, if it is thought necessary.

The too general opinion that sleep is the all-important thing in this disease, has led to fatal errors in treatment. Opium, given freely, as it often and very generally is, while the blood is charged with alcohol, produces an unfavorable effect upon the nervous system, and tends to check the excretions, which are already diminished, and the patient, without being, narcotized, often goes into a stupid state resembling the effects of uremic poison; and if about one-half (about the usual proportion), by the vigor of their constitutions, weather it, in spite of all the poisons imposed upon them, they recover slowly, and their organs are left in a bad condition.

I have kept no record of cases, but within the last ten years a large number have been treated at my Infirmary, by the different house surgeons, under my general directions, and I do not recollect of a single death, unless there was some grave complication more important. In delirium tremens, where it may be proper to keep up the accustomed stimulant to a certain extent, it is generally necessary to attend to the nourishment; for it will be found that the nutritive process is defective, and the stimulant will afford but temporary relief, unless this function is restored; or, if it is persisted in without, it will produce the more acute form of mania. With this view, calomel and other medicine proper to disgorge the stomach and digestive organs, may be proper, and special attention to diet. As in the different forms of other diseases, these two approximate each other in character, and require, in treatment, corresponding modifications. In my early experience in the Charity Hospital, I adopted the opium treatment, and it was not by a sudden change to the opposite extreme that I arrived at my present mode of treatment, but by degrees, as the true nature of the disease became apparent, and the frequent ill-effect of opium warned me of my error.

In the effect of calomel and salines in this disease, in disgorging the abdominal viscera, and particularly in relieving the stomach, when subject to morbid secretions; and in the effect of tart. antimony and morphia in subduing morbid sensibility of the nervous system, we discover a therapeutic law that may be usefully applied to other diseases. In engorgements and effusions resulting from obstructed circulation, particularly from the heart, this method is admirably adapted. From the venous engorgement, the functions of digestion and assimilation are almost suspended, the blood becomes impoverished, the skin becomes of a bronze color, and palpitation and other nervous symptoms result in a great measure from it. The dropsical effusion in these cases is generally looked upon as the chief feature of the disease, or consequence of the heart disease, and active hydragogues and diuretics are usually resorted to, when, in reality, if we disgorge the organs and establish nutrition, the watery effusion will disappear without trouble. In some cases it takes a large amount of calomel to produce the effect, but it is sure, if persisted in. When I say a large amount, I mean fifty or sixty grains, in small doses, such as will not derange the stomach. When the effect has once been produced, it can easily be kept up, and at the same time the stomach be left free to take the much-needed nutriment. The calomel may be given at night, and early in the morning the appropriate saline or hydragogue, and in two or three hours after the patient will digest better than before, by reason of the improved circulation of the digestive organs. In this way the disgorging process can be kept up, and at the same time the impoverished blood renewed.

In many painful nervous affections, the antimony and morphia are very appropriate, and afford the desired relief with much less injury to the system than by opium or any anodyne alone. In nervous or spasmodic colic, where the patient often suffers excruciating pain, this combination, if given early, before organic changes take place, not only gives ease very promptly, but relaxes the organs and prepares them for the action of purgatives, if they should be thought necessary. I have given the antimony, combined with Battley's sedative, in low typhoid or nervous fever, when attended with occasional violent neuralgic pains in the head or elsewhere, with the happiest effect, when the sedative, taken alone in a sufficient dose to relieve the pain, produced bad effects. In exalted states of the nervous system and nervous delirium generally, when interference is thought necessary, it is highly useful.

ART. II.—*The Evils arising from Tight Lacing:* By S. C. YOUNG, M. D.

ALTHOUGH the evils of this pernicious practice are so patent as to be cognizant to every one, yet no one unacquainted with anatomy and diseases of the human system can appreciate them in their full extent. And, indeed, I believe that few even of physicians have considered this subject so fully as its importance demands.

The evils resulting from this practice may be considered as affecting 1st. The osseous system. 2d. The thoracic viscera. 3d. The abdominal viscera. 4th. The pelvic viscera.

1st. The principal parts of the osseous system affected are the spinal column and the ribs. *a.* The spinal column is so firm (though flexible), and so well protected, that it is seldom affected; but it sometimes *is*, and when this happens, the extent of the injury is proportioned to the importance of the part injured. Caries and necrosis of the vertebræ *may* result from this cause. This must cause great deformity, and impair the usefulness of the column, and may be carried so far as to press upon the spinal marrow and paralyze the parts whose motor nerves spring from the seat of pressure.

b. The ribs are more frequently injured than the spinal column. Caries and necrosis may be caused in these just as in the vertebræ, but these are rare.

There is another condition of the ribs, however, which is a very common result of this practice, *i. e.*, what is commonly known as the "chicken-breast." This means a turning inwards of the ribs, from continued pressure from without, which materially diminishes the space occupied by the lungs. By this means the angle of the ribs is made more acute, thus rendering them more liable to fracture. By it, also, their union with the sternum, by means of the cartilages, is rendered less firm.

The sternum and clavicle, also, may suffer injury, but are less liable to it than the ribs and vertebræ.

2d. Injuries to the thoracic viscera. These may be considered as affecting the lungs and heart.

a. The lungs. In these organs are carried on the processes by which the vital fire is maintained, and the venous changed into arterial blood; the objects of which are to keep up the animal heat, and to consume the effete particles of the venous and supply oxygen to the arterial blood. It is plain, therefore, that whatever interferes with respiration diminishes the temperature of the body, loads the blood with effete particles, and prevents the introduction of the requisite amount of oxygen. Instead of arterial blood, which is the food required by the organs and tissues, we have venous blood, which is entirely unfitted to supply their wants. Hence we have, as a first consequence of impeded respiration, general inanition, which in time must result in debility and wasting away of the system, and render it much more liable to the inroads of diseases, especially those of an asthenic character.

The brain, too, is deprived of its supply of arterial blood, and cannot act properly; hence we have debility of mind as well as of body. But the lungs themselves are injured; the parts most compressed may become atrophied and collapsed, which very much favors the deposition of tubercle, while in those less compressed, having the office of the whole lung to perform, the air-cells become enlarged, and incapable of contraction, producing a state similar to what is called "heaves" in horses. Since through the instrumentality of the breath sounds are produced, this cutting off of the supply of air from the lungs must modify the voice.

b. The heart. Compression of the chest may be carried so far that room is not left for the heart to expand properly, hence the current of blood is diminished; and if a full current of blood, vitiated as I have shown it to be by the imperfectly performed functions of the lungs, cannot supply the wants of the system, much less can a diminished current supply them. This assists in the production of general debility.

The call of the system for its accustomed supply of nourishing blood creates an effort on the part of nature to supply the deficiency by accelerated actions of the heart, causing palpitations; each period of this overwork must be followed by a corresponding period of rest; hence we have retarded as well as accelerated action of the heart. This irregularity of the heart's action causes accumulations of blood in some parts, while their usual supply is cut off from others; thus, the former may be attacked by inflammatory diseases, while the latter are wasting away. Looking at it in this light, may it not be that many of the inflammatory diseases to which our fashionable ladies are subject, are primarily caused by this fashion? The heart itself may suffer, first from hypertrophy, caused by an effort on the part of nature to supply the wants of the system by overwork of that organ, but after a while it works itself down and becomes atrophied.

3d. Injuries done to the abdominal viscera are confined principally to the liver, stomach, and intestines.

a. Of the liver. By pressure this organ is prevented from developing in its proper shape, forced in upon itself and back against the spinal column, and caused to grow thicker than, and not so long or broad as, the normal liver. The ducts of the liver may also be obstructed, which prevents the instrumentality exerted by the bile in digestion, and favors the deposition of gall stones. But, perhaps, the worst effect produced on the liver is its displacement. The direction in which the pressure is exerted forces the liver from its natural position down into the abdomen; this causes dragging sensations, as if something were pulling the diaphragm downwards, as, in fact, the displaced liver *is.* The circulation in the liver, both hepatic and portal, is also obstructed, and its glycogenic action interfered with. Thus, in another way, is the production of animal heat interfered with.

The last three effects mentioned, viz: displacement of the liver, obstruction of the passage of the bile, and to the circulation of the organ, tend greatly to the production of irritation and inflammation. These may have been the prime causes of many of the cases of chronic hepatitis, so frequently met with among our fashionable ladies.

The pancreas and spleen may also suffer from tight lacing; but, as the offices they perform in the animal economy are neither so important nor so well understood as those performed by the liver, they need not a further explanation. There is one condition, however, which requires notice. The spleen sometimes becomes enormously enlarged from the effects of frequent attacks of intermittent fever, and when this happens, the organ is materially interfered with, and it, in turn, interferes with the neighboring organs. This may be carried so far as to cause splenitis, though this is a *very* rare disease.

b. The stomach. The stomach suffers in three ways. 1. It suffers with the other organs and tissues in the general debility. 2. It is prevented from developing to its proper size, and if developed before the process is begun, is compressed. 3. Its rotatory and peristaltic actions are interfered with. By these means the gastric juice is vitiated, and the progress of the food through the stomach retarded. This causes sour eructations, spitting up of the food, dyspepsia, and even irritation and inflammation of the stomach. While this is going on, the call of the system, through the sympathetic nerve, on the stomach, for its accustomed nutriment, causes a morbid and vitiated appetite, and this increases the disorder.

c. The intestines. The vitiated mass is carried from the stomach into the intestines, where the processes of digestion and assimilation are doomed to meet with further obstruction from the diminution of the supply of bile and pancreatic juice, already alluded to, and from direct pressure; for the corset is frequently carried so low before as to press upon a large portion of the abdomen.

Pressure over the abdomen produces evil results in five ways. 1. It diminishes the peristaltic action of the intestines. 2. It obstructs the circulation, particularly the portal. 3. It prevents the absorbents from performing their office perfectly. 4. It diminishes the cavity of the abdomen. 5. It forces the abdominal viscera into the pelvis. From the first of these, and especially when it is conjoined with the derangements of the liver and stomach already alluded to, we almost always have constipation, diarrhœa and irregularities of the bowels, and may have irritation and inflammation of the intestines, tubercular enteritis, impaction, and intussusception. The absorbents are not supplied with the proper nourishing material, and, of course, cannot supply it to the circulation; and thus the blood becomes impoverished, as well as vitiated, by the improper actions of the lungs and heart, above alluded to. The evils arising from forcing the viscera into the pelvis will be alluded to when I come to speak of the pelvic viscera.

All surgeons admit that whatever tends to diminish the cavity of the abdomen, so far predisposes to hernia; and the proportion of the human family who suffer from these accidents (estimated by some at one in every eight), and the dangers to which they are subject, are too well known to require more than a passing notice.

4th. Injuries to the pelvic viscera. Those of the pelvic viscera which suffer principally are the bladder and uterus. These suffer not from direct pressure, but secondarily from pressure exerted by the displaced abdominal viscera.

a. In this way the size of the bladder is diminished and it incapacitated for holding the requisite amount, causing a frequent desire for micturition, and dribbling away of the urine; or, it may be that the pressure is exerted on the urethra, where it dips under the symphysis-pubis, which will cause retention of the urine. Retention of urine causes irritation and inflammation of the bladder, and may predispose to the deposition of stone.

b. The uterus. More harm is done by pressure on the uterus than

40

on any other organ. From this cause we have retro- and ante-versions, retro- and ante-flexions, prolapsus, and procedentia uteri, even in the virgin, and very frequently in those who are pregnant. These accidents and their results justly occupy no inconsiderable portion of our works and lectures on obstetrics. If the uterus is displaced before conception, it can hardly be expected to perform its office during gestation properly. During pregnancy the uterus expands (to make room for the development of the fœtus) from three inches long, two wide, and one thick, to eighteen inches long and from twelve to fifteen in its transverse and lateral diameters. This soon fills up the pelvis, and gradually rises into the abdomen, until, at the end of the eighth month of pregnancy, it reaches as high as the umbilicus. If not permitted to take this course, it must inevitably be displaced, or its contents be expelled.

Who can tell how many of the miscarriages and abortions so frequently met with are dependent on pressure on the abdomen? And when we reflect on the terrible consequences of these accidents, both to the mother and her offspring, it becomes indeed appalling.

Having enumerated the principal injuries done to the several parts of the system by this very prevalent but very hurtful fashion, I will close with a suggestion to physicians, for it is mainly through them that the reform must come, if it ever does come. It is the *imperative duty* of every physician to exert his influence against its perpetuation; and this he should embrace *every* opportunity of doing among his patrons. He should impress the importance of this on mothers and on young ladies; should teach them how much easier and better it is to *live* unfashionably than to *die* fashionably. He should impress it on them that this is one of the causes of the degeneration of the human race; that not only themselves must suffer, but in this, as well as in other things, "the iniquities of parents are visited on their children, even to the third and fourth generations."

Men and boys should also be warned, for the practice of going without suspenders subjects them to most of the accidents liable to happen to females; indeed they are more liable to some; herniæ, for instance. There can be no doubt but that, if all men (particularly the laboring classes) were compelled to wear suspenders and loose pantaloons, herniæ and many other diseases would be much less frequently met with.

Liberty, Mississippi, February 4, 1860.

ART. III.—*Strangulated Femoral Hernia. Operation. Cure:* By WM. WOODWARD, M. D.

MESSRS. EDITORS—Will you allow me space in your extensively circulated and valuable Journal to report a case that may be of some importance to the medical profession, and to the public in general?

The patient was Mrs. P., a lady of forty-eight or fifty years of age, and of one of our best families. Mrs. P. has been troubled with an occasional protrusion of the bowel, at the crural ring, for many years ; but she has always (this one time excepted), by her own exertions, been enabled to return the bowel into its proper position; generally either in the sitting or standing position, but sometimes, however, she would be compelled to resume the horizontal position before she could succeed in returning the bowel into the cavity of the abdomen. But she was destined to suffer something more serious than that which is described above. On the 26th of January last (1860), in the afternoon, she being on her feet more than usual, discovered that the bowel had again been forced down, and was protruding through the crural ring. But, for some cause or other, she did not give it any special attention until it began to cause pain and other unpleasant sensations. At this time she took to her bed; but when she attempted to return the bowel, she found the immediate surrounding parts somewhat inflamed, and the tumor larger than it had ever been before, and all her efforts at reduction proved to be useless ; yea, worse than useless, for they would naturally tend to bring on a greater amount of vascular excitement, and to hasten all of the unpleasant and distressing difficulties that we usually have in strangulated hernia. The patient, though suffering very much, was allowed to remain in this condition until the morning of the 27th, at which time the family physician was sent for, who, when he arrived, found all the parts involved in the difficulty very much inflamed, the tumor not large, but hard, the lymphatic bodies of the immediate vicinity considerably enlarged ; though, notwithstanding all this, the doctor was enabled to correctly diagnosticate the case. But after making use of all the various manipulations, and calling to his assistance all the means usually made use of in such cases, he found all his labor to be in vain. The hernia could not be reduced without the assistance of the surgeon's knife. At this time I was sent for; but the patient's residence being some fourteen miles from this place (Clinton), it was late in the evening of the 27th before I was enabled to reach her. After learning the particulars of the case from the doctor, and after making an examination of the patient I thought it would be well enough to make another attempt to reduce the hernia; and to put the patient in proper condition for this, we administered one dose pulv. ipecac, et opii, and a powerful enema of a decoction of tobacco. These produced perfect relaxation of the entire body. I then attempted to reduce, but a very few minutes convinced me that nothing could save the patient's life, except an operation, and even this seemed to promise but very little encouragement, when we took into consideration the patient's age and her general feeble health. But, of course, as there was no other remedy by which the patient's life could be saved, I determined to operate; but it was now night, and I did not like to operate by candle-light, and as the patient was in a perfect state of relaxation, I determined to postpone the operation until morning. The patient rested quite well through the night; slept several hours.

As soon as it was sufficiently light in the morning (which was about forty-three hours after the first positive symptoms of strangulation), the patient was put in position for the operation. Chloroform was administered until perfect anæsthesia was produced. The parts being prepared for the knife, I began the incision, one inch above Poupart's ligament; with one stroke of the knife I divided the skin and superficial fascia for the full length of the tumor, and for nearly an inch below it. The incision was carried parallel with the tumor, and a little to the inner side of its median line. One small artery was severed; a minute's pressure with the finger of an assistant, upon its mouth, completely arrested its bleeding. I next divided the fascia propria, for the full length of the incision. I then tried to return the sack without dividing the ring. This I could not do. I then tried to draw the neck of the sack or tumor sufficiently out of the canal, that I might easily enter a director. This I could not do without using too much violence. The neck of the sack seemed to be firmly adherent to the upper and inner, or pubic side of the ring; so I at once took up the sack proper and laid it open. I found the bowel very much congested and discolored, with frequent dark spots, which gave it very much the appearance as though it was in a state of gangrene. Nevertheless, I felt warranted in returning it. After the sack was laid open, I was enabled to pull the bowel a little out, and by pressing it a very little down, it gave sufficient room for the director to enter, which I entered with the grooved side towards the pubic side of the canal. I then passed in a probe-pointed curved bistury, turning its edge upwards, and a very little inwards. I then, by one cut, divided the neck of the sack into the canal, the canal itself, Gimbernat's ligament, and the conjoined tendon, up, or very near to, Poupart's ligament; after which I found no difficulty in returning the bowel. The sack itself was considerably thickened, and adhered to a portion of the canal; but by a very little trouble I broke up this adhesion, and allowed the membrane to return to its proper place. To make sure that the bowel and the peritonæum had cleared the canal, I passed in and through the canal a female catheter.

There were some lymphatic bodies that were very much enlarged, and which I thought would be in the way when I came to close the wound, and would prevent adhesion by the first intention; and, to save trouble, I extirpated them. Then the wound was brought together, and held in position by two or three sutures and isinglass adhesive plaster. A small compress was laid over the wound, and held in position by strips of adhesive plaster.

The time occupied, from the commencement of the operation until the dressing was finished, was from twenty to twenty-five minutes. The patient was then laid in bed, and perfect quiet enjoined. This was about 9 o'clock, A. M., of the 28th. I then left, with the understanding that pulv. ipecac et opii were to be given in sufficient quantities to allay all arterial excitement, and to give relief from pain; if this should fail to control the heart's action, then recourse should be had to veratrum viride; the bladder to be relieved by the catheter.

I saw the patient next day, 29th. She had rested quite well; had slept several hours in the twenty-four; pulse seventy-four per minute, but very weak. (It should be borne in mind that the patient's general health was *very* feeble indeed.) No swelling or pain of the abdomen; but there was a constant desire to go to stool. An enema of castor oil, turpentine, and salt water was administered, which gave entire relief, but brought way no fæces. We thought it best to let the bowels be quiet just as long as we could with safety; but, if in case there should be feverishness, with much pain in the bowels, and a desire to go to stool, there should be administered castor oil and turpentine, by the mouth, and if need be, assisted by an enema.

Through the course of the night some or all of the above symptoms were present; the oil and turpentine were administered, and in proper time followed by an enema, as directed above. Soon after this there was a copious, natural stool; and by the time I saw her, on the 30th, there had been three healthy stools. Pulse seventy, and everything favorable for a rapid recovery. The bowels were to be controlled by the use of opiates and astringents, if need be. The patient's diet for a few days to be nutritive, but not stimulating.

As this patient was some fourteen miles from my place, and I having several other very important cases under my care, I left her in the care of her family physician, who, I am happy to say, managed the case *well;* and the consequence was an early convalescence.

At this time the patient has entirely recovered from the strangulation and operation.

I have several other patients on hand, upon whom I have operated for burns, tumors, etc., one of which, at least, I consider to be of great importance, a report of which I will write out in the course of a few days. -

Clinton, Louisiana, February 21, 1860.

Art. IV.—*Extirpation of a Medullary Tumor:* By William Woodward, M. D.

About six weeks ago I was called to see a negro woman who had a large, hard tumor upon the side of her neck and jaw. The woman is twenty-seven years of age. The tumor has been upon her neck for about sixteen years. At first, and up to within the last three or four years, it had the feel and appearance of an ordinary soft adipose tumor or wen. But a very few years ago it was examined by a gentleman who bore a good reputation as a surgeon, but for some cause or other he declined removing it. At that time it was not larger than an ordinary hen's egg, and its situation was just back of, and near to, the angle of the inferior maxillary. About two years ago it began to increase in size, and to change from the pulpy feel to that of a fibrous or hard substance. I may here say that since this change began to manifest itself, the tumor has been examined by one or two surgeons of considerable repute, and by quite a number of physicians, all of whom declined operating for its removal; some saying that "an operation ought to be performed;" others saying, *emphatically*, that "the tumor could not be removed without *sacrificing* the patient's *life ;* that she would *die under* the *operation,* or from its *direct* consequences."

As I have said above, for the last two years the tumor has been increasing in size; and as it grew in bulk, it naturally ascended the neck. But in the last twelve months preceding its removal, it had grown fully two-thirds of its whole size; and in the last six months, about one-half of its entire bulk. I will now give its location and condition as it was when I first saw it, some six weeks ago: It was an irregular, oblong tumor ; its anterior superior portion reached to the meatus auditorius externus, and for an inch in front of it, with the parotid gland lying over it. The posterior superior portion extended equally as high, and was firmly attached to the cranium, just back of, and opposite to, the middle ear, by a cartilaginous growth, which extended over and into the tumor for more than an inch. Of course the lower ear was very much pushed up; in fact, there was a partial closure of the meatus extremus. The lower portion of the tumor reached about half way from the jaw to the clavicle, and seemed to be situated beneath the platysma myoides and sterno-mastoid muscles, and appeared to be deeply imbeded back of, and beneath, the angle of the jaw. The whole tumor was slightly movable, except the portion that was attached to the skull. The tumor seemed to be composed, as it were, of two distinct lobes, or bodies, the one slightly movable upon the other; and which divided it into an upper and lower portion. The upper portion was composed of about three-fourths of the whole mass, and the lower portion of one-fourth. The whole mass was about as large as a man's two fists would be if put together. Its weight was just one pound when first removed. The whole mass was hard and inelastic. When I came to consider how long the tumor had been forming, and how rapidly it had grown of late, and its entire change in consistency, and then to see that it was situated beneath the superficial muscles of the neck, which very much impede its outward growth, and would mechanically force it in upon the internal jugular and carotid, as well as the tracha and œsophagus, thereby causing serious difficulty, if not death in a very short time. To prevent all this, I determined to remove the tumor. And in accordance with this determination, on the 25th of January last, with the assistance of four physicians, I proceeded to operate. I seldom operate without the use of chloroform, consequently it was here administered, and until complete anæsthesia was produced. The operation was begun by making an elliptical incision, including all of the integument between the two incisions that I thought I could spare, and have enough left to come together · without stretching, after the tumor should be removed. By this means I was enabled to save a goodly amount of dissecting. I aimed to carry the incision in such a way as to allow the cicatrix, when formed, to be back of the angle of the jaw. I found the tumor, for its lower two-thirds, situated entirely beneath the platysma myoides and sterno cleido mastoid muscles. Its upper portion, which was much heavier and thicker than the lower, protruded out over the two muscles, pushing the one anteriorly and the other posteriorly, and at the same time pushing the external jugular very much anterior to its normal position. I found these two muscles firmly adherent to the tumor; consequently a portion of each muscle was included in the incision. By carefully dissecting up the platysma, I was enabled to leave the external jugular undisturbed, as it was more external to the muscle than it is usually found. I found the lower and posterior portion of the parotid gland adherent to the tumor, which I removed with the tumor, together with some of the descending fibres of the portio dura nerve. On dissecting up the sterno-mastoid, or rather in working our way beneath it, the auricularis magnus nerve was necessarily severed; also the occipital artery. I now found that the tumor was *very* deeply imbeded beneath and under the angle of the lower jaw, pushing the small muscles of the neck out of its way. As I got down beneath the jaw and neck, and to the inner portion of the tumor, I found that it had several rounded bodies, or protuberances, projecting from it; one of which seemed to be of large size, and which was extended further in than the main body of the tumor could get, and which was pressing the internal carotid and jugular well towards the vertebræ, and itself reaching to, or very near, the lateral wall of the œsophagus. The facial artery, and a small branch thrown off by the temporo-maxillary, were severed, and a small artery, which was very deeply situated, and which required a ligature. I think this artery was given off by the internal carotid, as nothing but the ligature could close its mouth. The bleeding from all the rest was easily controlled by the finger of an assistant; and upon the one the ligature was not applied until after the tumor was removed from its long resting place; after which all of the lookers-on *seemed* to *breathe* easier.

After the bleeding was sufficiently checked, the lips of the wound were brought together and dressed. The whole time occupied in removing the tumor was a little over an hour. This may seem long, but when we think of the great amount of dissection necessary, and it being in such a position that it was very difficult to sponge the blood out sufficiently that we might see, and that a very small mis-cut might have given me more trouble than I could have gained in time by hurrying the operation; I thought, as another had said, that any time in which the operation was well done, would be quick enough.

By the time the wound was dressed the patient had sufficiently recovered from the effects of the chloroform as to know all that was going on about her.

I am quite certain that I did not leave any of the diseased mass in the dissection, to reproduce itself; neither do I think that the disease had sufficiently established itself in the general system so as to be likely to reproduce itself in any of the internal organs. But as to this opinion there is, of course, an uncertainty; consequently, I have the patient under treatment for the purpose of completely ridding the body of any possible disease.

[The cut No. 1 shows the facial appearance, and also the outline of the tumor before the operation ; No. 2 represents the appearance of the face at present.]

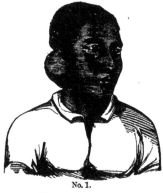 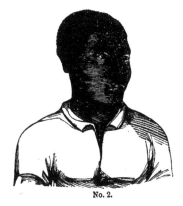

No. 1.   No. 2.

41

This is the thirtieth day after the operation, and while I write the patient is sitting in my office. I have just made a thorough examination of her condition, and especially of the parts that were concerned in the operation. I find that the wound has entirely healed; that there is a firm, healthy cicatrix, perfectly movable; there is no undue tightness of the skin, neither is there any looseness or flabbiness of the part. There is some little induration of the muscles about the cicatrix, but it is daily diminishing. I feel quite well satisfied that we will have no further trouble, so far as regards the old disease. On a close examination of the tumor, I found that it was divided into two parts, a greater and a smaller one, as was its appearance while upon the patient. The two parts were united by a fibrous sheath or band; from the greater and upper portion of which grew several small bodies or processes, one of which was more than an inch in diameter, and which, as I said above, was crowding hard upon the internal jugular and carotid. While the tumor was in position, the smaller bodies were above, and a little posterior to the large one; and had the tumor not have been removed, and had the small bodies continued to enlarge, which they most *assuredly would have done*, they would inevitably (before they were as large as their fellow, that has been described) have come in contact with the internal carotid and jugular. These vessels, and their accompanying nerves, must have been pressed back and against the vertebræ of the neck. I suppose that there can be no doubt in any sane man's mind as to what the result must have been, to say nothing of its pernicious effects upon the system in other respects. As to the vascularity of the tumor, the lower or inferior portion seemed to be destitute of vessels, but the upper portion had both arteries and veins connected with it; and the more recent seemed the growth, the more complete was its vascular system. The rounded projections, spoken of above, showed this plainly. When I cut into the tumor, it was like cutting into a rich cheese, only it was a little more spongy. It was of a yellowish white color. As to its consistency and appearance, it was very much like the human brain, after it had been in alcohol a few days; probably it was a little harder. As I approached the center of the tumor, it gradually grew more soft and spongy. To speak of the tumor as it was situated upon the neck: a little to the inner side of its center, it was more soft and watery than elsewhere, with some bright yellowish streaks running off to its inner edge. I think, after considering the tumor's beginning, its slow growth for many years, then its recent rapid growth and entire change in appearance, and finally, its real condition after its removal, we may safely say it was, as is *implied* at the beginning of this article; or rather, considering it in this wise, at first, and for many years, it was an adipose tumor. But later it changed its texture, or, at least, it became firm and hard; still later it assumed a new growth, and seemed to be of a character differing entirely from its original one, having assumed a *rapid growth*. Its upper portion encroaching upon and coming in contact with the skull, and at once beginning to assume the osseous appearance at the place of union (by the way of exostosis, if you please), while its inner, or still more recent growth, is of the medullary character..

Mr. Editor, have we not here a complication of two or more of the malignant growths? This question I will leave for yourself and others to decide according to your own notions of such things. Mr. Editor, I hope you will pardon me for the lengthiness of this report. The reason why I give so many of the particulars of this case, and of the one that I reported for the Journal a few days ago (in reference to strangulated hernia), is, that I hope to arouse or stimulate the members of the medical profession to action; more especially the country portion of it. Why should we stand idly by, with our arms folded, looking calmly on, while disease of one form or another is absolutely *destroying* our patients.

CLINTON, LOUISIANA, February 24, 1860.

P. S. I should state that I have been requested by several physicians to report this case for the Journal.

I send you two photographs of the patient from whom the tumor was removed—one was taken one day before operation, the other thirty days after operation—which you are at liberty to dispose of as you may see fit.

ART. V.—*Cuba for Invalids:* By R. W. GIBBES, M. D., of Columbia, South Carolina.

THE necessity of a change of climate to northern invalids, to avoid the cold of winter, makes it important that they should know where to go. An indefinite direction, "go to Cuba," is constantly given by their medical advisers, most of whom have no experience of the localities of the Island, and the exposure, inconvenience, and positive dangers of some of them. The want of proper accommodation out of Havana, and the exaggeration of difficulties of transportation, as well as denunciation of the country for want of medical assistance in case of illness, which it is the interest of hotel-keepers to impress upon visitors, induce a large number to remain in that city, which is the worst place on the Island for those enfeebled by disease or with nervous irritability. The hotels are usually crowded, the accommodations forced, the streets filthy, causes of excitement, in the way of amusements and sights, abundant and enticing, the atmosphere loaded with the thick vapors of a large city, and more important than all is the prevalence of cold northers and a varying temperature, so oppressive, uncomfortable, and injurious to the invalid. We say nothing of the expense of living in Havana, which is much beyond that of the country, and as enfeebling to the pocket as its changes of temperature are to the constitution.

After careful examination of many places, and particular inquiry from proper sources, I have become satisfied that the south side of the Island presents the most positive advantages to the invalid during the winter months. A residence at Trinidad, with rapid and steady improvement for several weeks in its delightful climate, enables me to commend it as the most salubrious position I found. It is beautifully situated on the side of a mountain, and the *Hotel de la Grande Antilla* admirably located, about 400 feet above the sea, presenting a view of nearly the whole city, and of the bay and sea beyond. There is a constant breeze of the most delicious air, soft and balmy, and most grateful to fevered systems or weak nervous power—the temperature varying from 73° F. to 82° F. During the past winter, the 18th of December was the coldest of the season, when the thermometer stood at 67° F. Dr. Urquiola, a practitioner of thirty years, informed me that he had never known, during that time, the thermometer as low as 56° but once, and that for a day, in 1842. The temperature is so equable, and the sea breeze so uniform, and, perhaps, strange to say, dry, that the invalid cannot have a more desirable location. The city is the cleanest on the Island, and sloping gradually to the sea, its well-paved streets are washed by every heavy rain. Its freedom from dust and mosquitoes is a great consideration. In addition to the climatic influences, the hotel is a good one, now kept by Mr. Bernard, of Havana, who promises to use every effort to give full satisfaction to his guests.

The importance of proper diet, to make good blood to recruit the failing energies, or to restore them, when reaction commences, from depressing influences, cannot be too highly estimated; and in this point of view there is as much necessity for a good table as for fresh air. Garlic and onions, and Spanish oil, are abundantly used in Spanish cooking, with the constant addition of saffron to color the dishes ; but the French *cuisinière* of Bernard is far preferable, and you get good " biftek " and mutton chops, though the latter are sometimes made of pork. Wild ducks are plenty, and poultry and eggs, with a large variety of vegetables, are well served up. Since the experiments of Beaumont, showing the easy digestibility of crab and lobster, I may venture to say that the latter is far superior and more delicate at Trinidad than the northern specimens. Fish is a constant dish, and the *pargo* equal to any of other regions. Fruits are abundant, though not in as great variety as at Havana.

Cienfuegos is a neat city, situated on the Bay of Iagua, and has a good hotel, but is hot, dusty, and full of mosquitoes. At Cardenas the latter are distressingly numerous and annoying, and you find them at most of the interior towns. The railroad from Cienfuegos to Sagua will enable visitors to cross the Island on their return, though at Sagua there is no inducement to stop, as there is only a *fonda* of the poorest class. At the boka of Sagua, the shipping port, twelve miles below, there is a very fair hotel, built on piles in the river, where one may enjoy a fine sea breeze while waiting for the steamer, which you may take either to Matanzas outside, or among the *Cayos* within. The latter presents a beautiful navigation among the Keys, where flamingoes and other sea birds present a lively addition to the interesting scenery.

At Trinadad the invalid has fine scenery and pleasing walks. From the mountain in the rear of the hotel, the picturesque valley of Trinidad, dotted with *ingenios*, or sugar estates, may be seen for miles, spreading its varied vegetation of sugar cane, cocoanuts, mangoes, and other beautiful trees, under the seeming protection of the royal palm, whose stately crest is so richly ornamented with its plume-like foliage.

The rail car leaves at 6, A. M., and passes through the rich valley of *Manaca*, the ingenio of Senor Isnaga, where the processes of making sugar may be seen, and a fine view had from the tall tower, and the visitor may return by 10, A. M., to breakfast, or in the afternoon. *Volantes* may be had for rides to the beautiful *quintas*, or country seats, in the neighborhood, of which one kept by Mr. Cascelles may be found a quiet retreat for those who prefer a location in the country

Trinidad is a quiet place, but the theatre is occasionally opened, with opera troupes or other performances, and twice a week the fine regimental band, not excelled even in Havana, entertains the citizens in the plazas, and brings out the Cuban ladies to take exercise. The *Plaza de Armas* being opposite the hotel, the exquisite music is enjoyed from its marble halls ; but the *Plaza San Antonio* is only a short walk, and exposure to night air seems to be free from deleterious effects in this delightful climate. The institution of these musical soirées by the Government in the Cuban towns, is productive of much pleasure and advantage to the citizens, and it would be quite a valuable addition to our public amusements to have it introduced into our squares and parks.

To persons with threatened or incipient pulmonary disorder, or broken down by over-work, or recovering from acute disease, a residence in Trinidad may be commended by one who has experienced the benefit of it. In advising it, however, I would impress upon all who go there not to jeopardize their improvement by leaving before April, when northers are divested of their rawness. They may then visit some of the other localities of the Island, which present such scenery as only a tropical region can furnish. The fine city of Matanzas may well attract them ; if not for its own advantages, for the unsurpassed loveliness of the views of the Yumuri valley, from the heights of the Cumbre.

For the benefit of travelers, it may be as well to mention that the morning train leaves Havana at 6, and arrives at Batabino at 10, A. M., where they take a fine steamer (every Wednesday), with staterooms on deck, and arrive next day to dinner at Trinidad. The navigation is in sight of land the whole way, and the scenery quite attractive.

Art. VI.— *Urethro-Vaginal, Vesico-Vaginal, and Recto-Vaginal Fistules ; General Remarks ; Report of cases successfully treated with the Button Suture:* By Nathan Bozeman, M. D., of New Orleans (late of Montgomery, Alabama).

[Continued from page 199.]

Case xxvii.— *Vesico-Vaginal Fistule, complicated with Constriction of the Vagina ; Case operated upon with the Button Suture, at the University College Hospital, London ; Operation successful ; Relapse.—* Soon after my arrival in London, June, 1858, I was told by Prof. Erichsen that there was a case of vesico-vaginal fistule in one of the wards of the above-named hospital, which had been for some time under the treatment of Mr. Marshall, by the electric cautery. He requested that I should accompany him to the hospital and make an examination of the case, which I did, in the presence of himself and Mr. Marshall. My notes of the history of the case I have lost, but this is of no consequence. The woman, according to my recollection, was about thirty-five or forty years old, rather above medium stature, stout and heavily built, and excepting her excessive nervousness, appeared to be in the enjoyment of good health. She had been married a good many years, and had had several children. At the birth of her last she sustained the injury of her bladder for which she was admitted into the hospital.

Examination.—Fistule belonged to my fifth class, first variety; that is to say, it was high up in the vagina, complicating the anterior lip of the cervix uteri, which formed its upper border. It was rather circular, and about large enough to admit easily a No. 10 bougie. Even beyond the limits of the cervix uteri, the edges were hard and unyielding. Across the vagina, just a little below, there were hard and unyielding bands, which had resulted in great constriction of the canal at this point, and contributed largely to the condition of the edges of the fistule above mentioned. This feature of the vaginal canal I regarded as a very serious complication of the case, and so expressed myself to the gentlemen present, not believing, however, but that it could be overcome and a cure effected.

Prof. E. now requested that I should take charge of the case, and at my convenience to operate, as he desired to see me make an application of the button suture. At first I did not feel much inclined to do so, knowing what the difficulty in the case would be, and believing that my instruments would not arrive in time from New York to enable me to carry out the preparatory treatment necessary, before my engagements would require that I should leave London. I consented, however, to operate under the circumstances, and as soon as I could, which was ten days or two weeks after my first examination, I commenced the preparatory treatment. This consisted in making a deep incision upon each side of the constricted portion of the vagina, and then dilating the canal by the use of sponge tents. These were worn as constantly as the patient could bear, their size being gradually increased according to the progress of dilatation. Every day the tent was removed, and the vagina syringed out with cold water.

The above plan of treatment was kept up until the 21st of July, at which time I concluded to operate for the closing of the fistulous opening. The incisions I had previously made in the vagina had not, however, healed up ; a condition of things which I very much regretted, knowing, as I did, that it would militate very much against the permanent success of the operation. But my engagements to leave London in a few days, left me with no other alternative than to operate at once. I remarked to Prof. Erichsen, that these granulating surfaces being in such close proximity to the fistulous opening, were liable to do mischief by their cicatrization and the consequent re-contraction of the vagina. I had before operated under similar circumstances, and had seen a reproduction of the fistulous opening from the above causes ; I was, therefore, prepared to meet with an unsuccessful result.

Operation.—The patient being brought into the amphitheatre, was placed upon a table, on her knees and elbows, and the operation commenced. Present : Professor Erichsen, Mr. Marshall, Mr. I. B. Brown, Mr. Spencer Wells, Dr. Tanner, Dr. Browning, Dr. J. Henry Bennet, Dr. Stone, the distinguished Professor of Surgery of the University of Louisiana, and a number of other medical gentlemen and students. Upon introducing the speculum, I found that the fistulous opening could be but very poorly displayed, owing to the fact of our having a sky-light instead of the light from a side window, which is always preferable. The disadvantage I labored under on this account retarded very much the different stages of the operation, and especially that of paring. I succeeded, however, in completing the operation to my satisfaction in about three-quarters of an hour. Three sutures were required (one of them touching the anterior lip of the cervix uteri), and a button of the usual shape for this variety of fistule. The whole being secured in place, the patient was put to bed, and a self-retaining catheter introduced.

I attended the case for three or four days after the operation, and during this time there was not an untoward symptom—everything went on as well as could be desired.

Upon my departure from London, I left the case in charge of Prof. Erichsen, with directions to remove the suture apparatus on the ninth day, which he accordingly did. Two or three days afterwards he addressed a letter to me at Edinburgh, where I was sojourning, as follows : " I am very glad to say that the case of vesico-vaginal fistula on which you operated last week has gone on most satisfactorily. The wires and plate were removed on Friday, the ninth day after the operation. Union appeared to be firm and complete, and not a drop of urine has since escaped. We may, therefore, I think, look upon the cure as perfect."

As would be indicated by the above report, the result of our operation was entirely satisfactory. I certainly regarded it so, and would not have thought otherwise, had I not received, a couple of weeks afterwards, a letter from Mr. Wilkerson, House Surgeon of the University College Hospital, stating that the cure of our patient had not been permanent ; in other words, that there was leakage of the bladder. This result I, of course, regretted very much to learn, but I cannot say that I was much surprised at it. I recollected the condition of the parts when I performed my operation, and knew very well what had happened. The raw surfaces in the vagina, heretofore mentioned, had cicatrized, and the consequent contraction of the canal had partially pulled asunder the edges of the fistulous opening ; hence the partial or complete failure of the operation, and dribbling of urine. Such a result, as I have before said, was to be expected under the circumstances. Upon my return to London, some six weeks after the operation, I learned from Prof. Erichsen that our patient had gone to the country to recruit her health, and would soon return to the hospital. He remarked that dribbling of urine did not take place for four or five days after the removal of the suture apparatus. This showed very conclusively that there was a reproduction of the fistule there, which can only be explained by the causes above mentioned.

42

This case, therefore, will require to be thoroughly prepared before any operation is likely to be attended with permanent success. I do not regard it as at all difficult, and had I the time to devote to it, I could, at another operation, I am quite sure, guarantee entire success.

Remarks.—This case I have reported at length, giving all the facts connected with it as near as I can. Our operation, although performed under many disadvantages, as is to be inferred from the facts above stated, may very justly be said to have been successful, and yet not absolutely so. The immediate result of it cannot be regarded otherwise than satisfactory, as showing the efficacy of the method adopted. The reproduction of the fistulous opening was, from the very nature of things, to be expected, and should not detract in the least degree from the merits of a successful operation.

Could I have prepared this case properly for an operation, and attended it throughout, it certainly would have been more gratifying to me, and perhaps more decisive of the just claims of our suture, and have saved it from the unjust animadversions which appeared in the London Medical Times and Gazette a couple of months after our operation.

The object of the author of these remarks seemed to be to show the inefficiency of our suture apparatus. This he did by producing the results of our operations in Great Britain, performed, as they all were, under many disadvantages. Thus, in the case of which we are speaking, he puts down the result as a failure, without the statement of a single fact connected with it. Whether our operation was a failure or not, I will leave to others to decide. All the facts of the case are fairly stated.

CASE xxviii.—*Vesico-Vaginal Fistule, complicated with Retroversion of the body of the Uterus and Incarceration of its Cervix in the Bladder ; Case operated upon at the Royal Infirmary, Edinburgh, with the Button Suture ; Death of the patient on the sixth day ; Autopsy.*—The following report is taken from the *Edinburgh Medical Journal* for October, 1858, and is by my much esteemed friend Alexander Keiller, M. D., F. R. C. P., Lecturer on Midwifery and the Diseases of Women and Children in the Medical School, Surgeons' Hall, Edinburgh :

[The pitiable condition of those laboring under vesico-vaginal fistula can scarcely fail to enlist the sympathy even of the least humane ; the state of misery to which the unfortunate subjects of this complaint are constantly subjected being, in most cases, more than

sufficient to excite regret that a structural defect so local and comparatively insignificant should be considered so much beyond the
pale of curative control.

It may be confidently affirmed, that the records of surgical experience sufficiently show that the results of even the most approved
modes of treating vesico-vaginal fistula have been the reverse of
encouraging, if not in the great majority of cases absolutely futile,
and it therefore must be conceded that to the originator of any operative procedure or plan of treatment, calculated to restore the
efficiency of the vesico-urethral canal in urinary fistula occurring in
the female, much credit is due, and a large amount of gratitude will
doubtless be experienced towards those whose persevering ingenuity
and skill may lead to the achievement of such an important practical
result, as the satisfactory cure of that hitherto unmanageable lesion.

It being by no means an easy or gracious task to decide as to
whom such an honor may already belong, it is not my intention here
to canvass the individual merits or special claims of those who may
be entitled to much of our regard in connection with this subject,
my object on the present occasion is simply to relate the particulars
of an unusually interesting case which was recently operated on, at
my request, by Dr. Bozeman, of Montgomery, Alabama, United States,
who is well known to have distinguished himself, not only by the
discovery of what is styled the "button mode of suture," but by the
singular amount of success which, in his hands, has attended this
very ingenious plan of treatment.

As the comparative value and safety of the various modes of
operative treatment, recommended from time to time, can alone be
determined by a correct knowledge of the facts and circumstances
connected with unfortunate as well as successful results, it behooves
the practitioner faithfully to record the particulars of any special
instances of failure, which may in any degree tend to the onward
progress of surgical art.

Besides such cases, the publication of which are often so instructive, there are unfortunate results occasionally occurring, which,
although they cannot fairly be attributed, either to the operation or
the operator, it is not only proper but prudent to make known.

Such a case is the following, which, in accordance with the views
just expressed, and with the concurrence, or rather the solicitation,
of Dr. Bozeman, I will now endeavor to relate.

Catherine M., æt. 28, native of Ireland, first pregnancy, was admitted into the Royal Maternity Hospital at 5, P. M., on the 26th September, 1854. Although symptoms of labor had come on previous to her admission, the first stage was not completed until 9, P. M., on the 28th, and her delivery was not accomplished until the evening of the 29th, when, immediately after being summoned to the case, I applied the long forceps, and with some difficulty extracted a large dead male child. The labor thus having been allowed to occupy upwards of 88 hours, it was not difficult to account for the vesico-vaginal sloughing and fistula which followed. The urine was first observed to come per vaginam, within a fortnight after delivery, corresponding with the period at which the separation of the slough usually occurs ; and subsequent examination, as well as the persistence of the urinary sign, left no reason to doubt that an extensive breach in the vesico-vaginal septum had taken place.

After a very tedious convalescence from her unusually protracted labor, the patient was able to move about ; but, from being originally of a somewhat plump and healthy frame, gradually began to indicate the undermining effects of the constant irritation and discomfort so inseparable from such a condition, more especially among the poorer class of women to which she belonged.

During the years which occurred from her parturition to the date of the operation, I had frequent opportunities of observing the wretched state of health in which she lived. On several occasions she placed herself under my care, with the view to an attempt being made at a radical cure, but because of the large size of the fistulous opening, and the restless, unmanageable character of the patient, no operative measures were adopted.

The nature and extent of the fistula were investigated by several gentlemen accustomed to examine and treat such cases ; amongst others I may mention Mr. Spencer Wells, who, on one occasion, now several years ago, satisfied himself that the opening was situated in close approximation to the cervix uteri, and was capable of admitting the points of three fingers (or about the size of half a crown in circumference), and considered that it could not be cured but by repeated operations (probably three), and, moreover, stated his belief that a preparatory step would be necessary ; viz: that of dividing the whole of the mucous tissue, between the cervix and the fistula, so as to admit of the posterior edge of the latter being sufficiently separated from the anterior lip of the former, in order to allow approximation and union taking place without injurious dragging of the adjoining parts.

I mention this circumstance for the purpose of proving the particular relative position of the parts involved, as seen to exist at the time just referred to, and as compared to their subsequent relation, a change of position having occurred, which led me, along with others, to believe that, in addition to fistula, a state of vaginal occlusion had gradually supervened ; for, on examining the parts on a more recent occasion, we were induced to suppose, from the entire absence of the os and cervix uteri from the vagina (which had now become very much shortened), that occlusion of the latter canal had taken place, and that in the event of an operation being now had recourse to, it would be necessary to get rid of this supposed state of occlusion before the fistulous opening could be properly reached and treated.

Such being our opiuion of the state of matters in this case up to the time of its being seen by Dr. Bozeman, I felt justified in specially referring to it at one of the recent meetings of the British Medical Association, when Mr. I. B. Brown communicated his paper on the subject of vesico-vaginal fistula.

This view, however, of the nature and relative position of the parts, was corrected during a careful examination, subsequently conducted by Dr. Bozeman, who, by the use of a speculum and other instruments, admirably adapted for the purposes of diagnosis, convinced me as to the exact relation of the organs involved.

On placing the patient on her knees, the fistulous opening was readily brought into view by the introduction of the speculum referred to. The os uteri was now found directed forwards, completely through the fistulous opening into the bladder, by which relative position the fundus uteri was pressed downwards and backwards, and by being thus partially retroverted, accounted for the shortening of the posterior wall of the vagina, and the apparent vaginal occlusion before alluded to.

By passing a sound backwards through the ante-verted os, the retroversion of the fundus was distinctly shown, and it was, moreover, ascertained that the whole cervical portion of the uterus had become fixed into the gap formed in the bladder, the *posterior* lip of the os being now the most dependent, and lying in immediate contact with the fistulous opening in the upper and anterior wall of the vagina. By this abnormal position, it became abundantly evident that menstruation had for some time past taken place through the vesico-vaginal opening, from which was seen protruding a portion of the lining membrane of the bladder. This herniated condition of the mucous membrane was in a state of considerable congestion.

Although the parts had thus become unusually situated and fixed, Dr. B. undertook the treatment of the case, according to a plan which he has the merit of suggesting ; and, in several equally complicated cases, successfully carrying into effect ; viz : that of first relieving the vesical incarceration of the cervix uteri, and then restoring it to its normal position in the vagina ; and this he accomplished by a peculiar modification of the more ordinary plan of fixing the button suture. To the nature of this ingenious procedure I shall now refer, and state the facts connected with the operation as they were noted at the time.

August 4th.—To-day Dr. Bozeman operated in presence of Drs. Simpson, Weir, and a number of other members of the profession in Edinburgh. The patient, after being put under the influence of chloroform, was placed on her face, with the pelvis raised, and the head and chest in a depending position, which was maintained by a peculiar arrangement on the operating table, and partly by manual support. Considerable difficulty was, however, experienced in keeping her in a proper attitude, and at the same time continuing the safe and sufficient administration of chloroform. The necessity of having a table specially adapted for the purpose of operating on, in such cases, under chloroform, was very evident. Dr. Bozeman commenced by enlarging the opening on either side by carefully dividing its extremities in a lateral direction by means of an angular bladed knife. By these lateral incisions the cervix uteri became disengaged from the bladder, so as to allow of its being more readily restored to its normal position in the vagina.

Having, by this preparatory procedure, brought the os and fistulous opening, not only into more distinct view, but into a more natural position (the anterior, and not as before the posterior lip of the former, being now in more immediate juxtaposition with the anterior edge of the latter), the operation was proceeded with in the following manner : By means of a small hook, the right angle of the anterior edge of the fistula was raised, and the mucous membrane dissected off transversely towards the left angle. The anterior lip of the cervix uteri was then pared far in upon the vesical side, so as when the sutures were introduced and adjusted, the tendency to the previously existing uterine displacement might be overcome. By means of an ingenious *port-aiguille*, seven silk sutures were passed through the now denuded lips of the fistula; to the end of each silk thread a silver suture was attached, and the former then drawn through, so as to bring the latter into their position. The silver sutures being arranged in pairs, and the parts to which they were attached put on the stretch, Dr. B., after observing the extent and shape of the fistula thus ligatured, cut out a leaden button, shaped and perforated it on the spot, and immediately applied it over the sutures, fixing the former to the latter by means of seven small perforated leaden bars or crotchets, which he squeezed so as to sufficiently compress the sutures—each suture, after being by means of forceps turned over the edge of its corresponding bar, was cut through, and the whole apparatus described left lying so completely against the fistulous opening, as to induce every one present to express their admiration, not only of the ingenuity of the plan, but of the admirable manner in which in this case it was accomplished. In manufacturing the button (which occupied but a few minutes), Dr. B. took care to make a deep notch in its posterior edge, for the purpose of better accommodating and preventing injurious pressure upon the denuded anterior lip of the now replaced cervix uteri. The great advantage of substituting *lead* for silver (or other hard and inflexible material) in the formation of the button, was thus rendered obvious, its soft and comparatively ductile properties readily admitting of its being cut and moulded into the form adopted for the case in hand. The patient was put to bed and placed on her back, a catheter was then introduced through the urethra, but with considerable difficulty, owing apparently to some constriction at the vesical extremity of the urethra.

August 5th.—The catheter introduced into the bladder after the operation was allowed to remain, with directions for its being taken out every twelve hours, and the external parts syringed with warm water and again introduced. One grain of opium to be given every four hours. During the evening the patient became irritable and unruly, constantly trying to withdraw the catheter. In the evening she vomited several times.

At 11, P. M., she was quite drowsy, urine coming freely by the catheter.

August 6th.—Complains of much thirst and paroxysms of pain in the abdomen. Catheter removed, cleaned, and reintroduced ; pulse 100. Slight tenderness on surface of abdomen, tongue dry and dark—skin hot, is very irritable and restless. Opium continued. Menstruation has appeared ; the catamenial fluid escaping from the vaginal canal ; none through the catheter. The urine flows freely through the catheter, none is escaping per vaginam. Ordered lemonade *ad libitum.*

August 7th.—Has not slept through the night ; is very restless, complaining of pain in the abdomen, which is tympanitic and tender to the touch, particularly in the right groin ; pulse 114, full and strong' ; skin hot and dry ; much thirst, tongue brown and parched ; she is still found to be menstruating, all the secretion coming per vaginam. The urine is freely secreted, and flows freely by catheter, which has been regularly removed, and there is no admixture of blood. No urine escaping by the vagina. She has a constant hacking dry cough, and has vomited twice this morning. Hot poultices to be constantly applied to abdomen, and opium continued.

7, P. M.—She is much in the same condition, but the pain somewhat less in the belly, which, however, is more tympanitic.

August 8th.—Menstruation continues, and the urine flows freely, and quite unmixed with any blood. Pulse 122, full, strong, and hard ; no escape of urine per vaginam. Much pain and distension in abdomen. Turpentine stupes applied, and opium continued ; the changing of the catheter has been regularly attended to ; bowels still confined ; tongue dry and dark ; skin hot. This evening she has vomited several times ; ordered mustard poultices to abdomen.

August 9th.—Slept a little during the night ; feels less pain in the belly, which, however, has become still more tympanitic. Pulse 116, but weak ; skin cooler ; much less thirst, but the vomiting continues. Menstruation ceased. Stimulants to be given occasionally. The urine flows freely by catheter, unmixed with blood.

7, P. M.—Appears weak, and still inclines to vomit ; ordered brandy ʒiv. Opium continued.

2 o'clock, A. M.—Has not slept, and is crying out with pain in the belly, which has become much aggravated. Vomiting. Hot turpentine stupes applied freely. Brandy and opium. Pulse very rapid.

6.30, P. M.—The vomiting incessantly continues; pain unabated; pulse irregular, weak, and fluttering. Much tympanites; tongue dry; considerable thirst. All the urine comes by the catheter, but it appears darker, and is less in quantity; she appears sinking. The catheter has been regularly removed and washed out; bowels not moved since operation. During the day the symptoms of peritonitis continued, and death occurred about 7, P. M., on the sixth day after the operation.

Post Mortem Appearances.—The surface of the peritoneum was covered with recent lymph, which glued together the coils of the intestines.

No trace whatever of any wound, or direct injury to the peritoneum in the vicinity of the parts involved in the operation, was discovered, either before or after their removal from the pelvis, which was most carefully done with the view of ascertaining the source of the inflammatory process. The pelvic organs being removed *en masse*, together with the front of the pubis and ischium, with the external genitals, and other soft parts attached, the edges of the fistulous opening were found well approximated, the application and adjustment of the suture apparatus being in every respect perfect.

On opening the bladder, so as to obtain a view of the vesical side of the septum, union was here also found perfect. At the right extremity of the line of union, however, a sloughy condition of a small portion of the mucous coat of the bladder existed, at which point (in all probability consequent on slight urinary infiltration) cellular inflammation had kindled up, extending subsequently into the surrounding tissues, and more especially downwards towards the right ramus of the pubis, where a small quantity of thin purulent matter existed.

From the progress and character of the symptoms during life, and the appearances observed on dissection, it was evident that cellulitis had set in early; that the inflammatory process had commenced in, and was communicated from, the sloughy point referred to, as having been seen at the angle of the fistula on its mucous surface, and that subsequent peritonitis was the cause of the fatal termination. The position of the uterus, as well as the condition of the vesico-vaginal septum, showed that the special mode of operation adopted in this case (a mode which seems sanctioned by the results of Dr. Bozeman's

43

previous experience, *vide* his Pamphlet, pp. 26–7), fulfilled the object intended ; viz : that of excluding the os uteri from the cavity of the bladder, and fixing the cervix into its normal direction towards the vagina, thus overcoming the tendency to ante-version, and at the same time facilitating the approximation and necessary coäptation of the two edges of the fistulous opening.

The two sutures which were specially introduced for this purpose, through the substance of the cervix uteri, were found transfixing the anterior lip to the depth of half an inch from the os ; the paring of the edges of the fistula, their coäptation by the various sutures, and their fixing by the button apparatus, being altogether as perfect as could in any case be desired. ·

I deem it proper to state, that the bodily and mental conditions of the patient were such as to go far to account for the unfortunate termination, she having, for a considerable period previous to the operation, lived in a state of great penury, being ill-fed, wretchedly clothed, and long accustomed to a mode of life which rendered her a most unfavorable subject for an operation.

Although endeavors were made from time to time to restore her bodily health, her weak and singular state of mind usually rendered her very unmanageable, and doubtless had a most injurious influence immediately subsequent to the operation.]

Remarks.—The above case, scarcely need I say, is one of much interest to the surgeon. To me it is especially so, being the first and only one I ever had to terminate fatally from an operation of this kind. When the case was presented to me for an examination, I knew nothing of its previous history. I took it for granted that, as regarded the general health, all was right, and I viewed it only in a surgical light. I saw at once what the difficulty in the case was, and I knew it could be overcome. In deciding upon the course, however, to be pursued, as regarded an operative procedure, it did not enter my mind that I had a broken-down constitution to deal with—a condition of things, according to my experience, seldom met with in the United States. The class of patients we mostly have in this part of the Union—negroes—are well-fed, have good constitutions, and stand operations, perhaps, better than any other population in the world. In Europe, the reverse of this is true. A large proportion of this class of patients, in that country, are reduced to the lowest penury, with broken-down constitutions, from drink and other vices, when they apply for surgical aid. The surgeon's chancés òf success, then, are, as a matter of course, greatly lessened, however skillful he may be. Under such circumstances the simplest case is liable to be attended with the most disastrous consequences from an operation. Such was the character of our patient, and the causes which determined the unfavorable result of our operation. Even a simple incision in the vagina, or in almost any other part of the body, would, in all probability, have been attended by a like result. I had met with the same complication that existed in this case, in my practice in this country, and yet I had never seen an untoward symptom after any of my operations. The pyæmia, therefore, which carried our patient off, I little expected.

This patient, as it seems from Dr. Keiller's account, had been a standing case at the hospital for some years, and from what I could learn, had been given over as incurable. It was, therefore, calculated to excite the deepest commiseration, and to call aloud for the best resources of surgical art. In such a condition, and with no prospect of relief, what was life to this poor creature ! Death was far preferable, and to this end, I have no doubt, she had given herself up ; therefore, almost any attempt to relieve her seemed to be justifiable. Could she have undergone some preparatory treatment before our operation, the result might probably have been different. Should I ever be so unfortunate as to meet with a similar case, I shall take this precautionary step before operating.

As to the post-mortem appearances we found, Dr. Keiller has said all that is required.

The preparation (namely, the parts involved in the operation, with the suture apparatus adjusted just as it was at the time of the operation), is in the possession of my friend Dr. Keiller. So far as the immediate result of the operation is concerned, it must be regarded as entirely successful. Union of the edges of the fistule was found to be complete throughout, and the cervix uteri restored to its proper place in the vagina ; our patient, therefore, lived long enough to prove, we may truthfully say, the success of the operation.

CASE xxix.— *Vesico-Vaginal Fistule operated upon with the Button Suture, at Edinburgh, in the private practice of Prof. Simpson. Operation successful.*—The subject of this case came to Edinburgh to consult Prof. Simpson, just after my operation in the preceding case.

Being in the city at the time, Prof. S. requested that I should make an examination of the case, with a view to an operation, which I accordingly did, in the presence of himself and several other medical gentlemen. The case I found to be plain and simple. My notes of this case enable me to state it as follows : Mrs. W., from Loch Lomond, aged 32, tall, well-formed, and apparently enjoying very good health. She states that she was confined with her third child about fifteen weeks ago, at which time she became the subject of her present affliction. Her former labors were unattended with difficulty. Her last labor lasted twenty-seven hours, and was terminated by opening the child's head and delivering in that way. After this she had considerable difficulty in relieving the bladder ; the catheter was required ; about two weeks after labor, first noticed dribbling of urine, which has continued uninterruptedly to the present moment.

Examination.—Fistule was found in the *bas fond* of the bladder, and accordingly belonged to the third class of Velpeau. It was circular, and scarcely large enough to admit the point of the index-finger into the bladder. Its posterior border was somewhat indurated.

There being no previous preparation of the case required, excepting to clear out the bowels, I proceeded, August 15th, to the

Operation.—There were present Prof. Simpson, Dr. Keiller, Dr. Coghill, Dr. A. Simpson, and Mr. Edwards, of Edinburgh, and Dr. Paul, of Elgin. The patient was placed in the usual position, upon her knees and elbows, before a window, and the operation commenced. The edges of the fistule were easily pared, and the sutures then introduced, four being required. Two of them were of iron-wire, which I introduced at the solicitation of Prof. Simpson, in order that the comparative effects of the two metals might be tested. I was rather averse to doing so, but seeing that there was not likely to be much dragging upon the sutures, I accordingly put them in.

The sutures now being adjusted, a button of the ordinary shape was slid down upon them and secured in the usual way. The patient was then put to bed, and a self-retaining catheter introduced. The after-treatment consisted in keeping the bowels locked up by the free use of opium, cleansing the catheter once or twice a day, and syringing out the vagina with cold water. Diet to be light. Day after the operation patient is doing well. All the urine passes through the catheter.

My engagements to leave Edinburgh now prevented me from seeing further the progress of the case. It was left in charge of Prof. Simpson, with directions to remove the suture apparatus on the ninth day. As to the result, here is what Prof. Simpson says, in a letter addressed to me at Paris, some six weeks afterwards : " The patient you operated on recovered excellently. The two iron stitches were exactly in the same healthy condition as the two silver stitches, when I removed the shield. She has gone home quite well."

Remarks.—The report of Prof. Simpson, as to the result of the above case, was truly gratifying to me, especially so, as my other operation in Edinburgh had turned out so unfavorably. As to his statement of the comparative effects upon the tissues of the two metals used in the case, I do not for a moment question it. It does not, however, accord with my experience, nor that of others who have employed these two kinds of suture. This was a very favorable case for the iron-wire sutures, and being used in conjunction with those of silver, the difference of effect upon the tissues would necessarily be slight. I do not pretend to doubt that, when the fistulous opening is small, the edges coming together easily, as was the case in the present instance, iron-wire sutures may be made to answer, as they will not cut out to a sufficient extent to endanger the tender cicatrix before their removal becomes necessary. But, as I have heretofore said, if the opening is of considerable size, and there is more than ordinary stress upon them, some, especially the middle ones, are almost sure to cut through and cause a partial failure of the operation, as I have seen. Knowing this, therefore, to be a fact, I could not recommend sutures of this metal, and would not have employed them in the present instance, but for the request to do so by my friend Prof. Simpson. There is no metallic suture, in my humble judgment, equal in all respects to that of silver.

CASE XXX.—*Vesico-Vaginal Fistule operated upon with the Button Suture, at the Royal Infirmary, Scotland ; Operation successful ; Case Reported in the Glasgow Medical Journal for October,* 1858, *by* GEORGE BUCHANAN, *A. M., M. D., one of the Surgeons to the Infirmary.*—The above case, I should observe, was republished in this Journal for Jan., 1859, to which I must refer for a full account of our operation, and the after-treatment. As the case, therefore, has been presented once to the readers of this Journal, I shall content myself with introducing here, again, only what relates to its history and the final result, which I prefer doing in Dr. Buchanan's own language, as follows :

Mrs. Mary Cairney, aged thirty-five, was admitted to the Royal Infirmary on the 18th of August, and gave the following history of her case : She has had two children, and on both occasions labor was tedious. At the birth of her first child, which happened ten years ago, she was attended by a midwife, and labor lasted two days. She was delivered without the aid of instruments, the child being born dead. Her recovery was not tedious, and she soon regained her strength.

About nine years ago she had a second child, on which occasion she engaged the services of a medical man. Labor was again lingering, and at the expiration of thirty hours she was delivered with instruments, though of what kind she does not know. During the use of the instruments she suffered great pain, and the child was born dead. Immediately after the birth of this second child, she found herself totally unable to retain her urine and fæces. The dribbling of the urine annoyed her so much that she became a patient in the hospital of Enniskillen, where she was under treatment for five months ; but her health failing, she returned home for awhile. After several months she was readmitted to the hospital, and was again under treatment for a second period of five months, at the end of which time she was dismissed in much the same state as before admission. During her residence in the hospital she was seen by a number of medical men, and various plans of treatment were tried, but of what nature she is unable to explain ; the result, however, was always unsuccessful. Since then, that is, for about eight years, she has remained in the same state, and has not applied for relief to any surgeon, although she has always suffered the greatest inconvenience and annoyance from the urine constantly dribbling away, keeping her clothes moist and foul.

On admission to the Infirmary, examination of the parts disclosed a fistula the size of a sixpence, communicating between the bladder and the vagina, the situation of which was about an inch internal to the orifice of the urethra, and in the mesial line. The perineum was found to be ruptured, and the fissure between the rectum and vagina to extend for about three inches, laying these two canals into one for that extent.

Dr. Bozeman, of America, being in Glasgow on a short visit at this time, he was requested to examine the patient, and he pronounced it a case in which he could nearly insure success by his new plan of operation.

A consultation of the physicians and surgeons of the Infirmary was called, and they unanimously agreed to request Dr. Bozeman to perform the operation. Accordingly, that gentleman, having shown and explained the exceedingly perfect and ingenious instruments which he had brought along with him, proceeded to operate in the following manner, in presence of the hospital staff, and several medical gentlemen who had heard of the case, and were interested in the result.

Here Dr. Buchanan describes the operation—four sutures and a button of the ordinary shape were required.

August 26th.—The catheter has daily been removed, cleansed, and replaced. It remains *in situ* without apparatus, and the patient has remained steadily in one position. The bowels have not been moved, and there is apparently no ulceration around the shield. This being the ninth day from the operation, and the period which Dr. Bozeman recommends, I proceeded to remove the apparatus. The patient was placed on her knees, as at the operation, and the vagina being exposed, with the aid of a bent speculum, I removed the bullets by twisting them a little to one side with a long forceps, and snipping across the wires between them and the leaden shield. When the bullets were cut off the shield fell off, and the wound was seen perfectly cicatrized throughout its whole extent. Three of the wires I easily got hold of with a pair of forceps, and pulled out ; the fourth had got imbedded in the soft tissue, and I could not find it. However, knowing that a metallic wire would produce no irritation, I left it ¯in, rather than disturb the parts by a prolonged search. The patient was again removed to bed, the catheter retained as before, and she was requested to move about as little as possible for a day or two. The opium was discontinued.

27th.—Urine passes entirely by the catheter. Complains of headache and uneasiness in bowels. To have two drachms of sulphur and bitartrate of potash.

September 1.—Bowels moved freely yesterday by a large dose of black draught, after which the use of the catheter was discontinued. She can now retain the urine for some hours, and pass it voluntarily. Dismissed to-day.

On the 7th September I visited the patient at her own house, and found that the cicatrix had become quite firm. She can retain urine for two or three hours in the recumbent position, but not so long in the erect. Still complains of headache and indigestion, with irregularity of the bowels. I ordered some Gregory's mixture, and a small dose of quinine, twice daily.

On the 16th September the patient was stronger, but still had some uneasiness in stomach and bowels. She was ordered to take a little exercise in the open air, having confined herself to the house since she returned home. In examining the cicatrix, which I found perfectly strong, I felt the sharp point of the wire which was left in the tissues when the shield was removed. It had produced no inflammation or ulceration, and I easily seized it with the forceps and withdrew it. The bladder had not yet entirely regained its retaining power when the patient stands or walks, but she has perfect control over the urine for several hours when in bed. The bed is never wet, as it used constantly to be, and both the patient and her husband express themselves as exceedingly happy at the result, and thankful for the success of the operation.

October 4th.—I received a letter, while at Paris, from Dr. Buchanan, to this effect : "The woman is now very comfortable, but still is unable to control the urine when she stands or moves about. The cure of the fistula is perfect, but I presume long loss of vesical muscular action has caused this weakness, which, however, is slowly but gradually improving."

Remarks.—The fistule in this case belonged to my fourth class, first variety ; that is to say, it involved a part of the trigonus vesicalis and the root of the urethra. The loss of substance here accounts for the want of power to control the urine while the patient stands or walks about. The retentive power of the bladder, under these circumstances, may, after a lapse of time, be restored, but it is very questionable in my mind. I have always found that, in this variety of fistule, the want of retentive power of the bladder continues to a greater or lesser extent, however well the fistulous opening may have been closed. So far as the operation itself, in the present instance, is concerned, it could not have been more successful. This fortunate result now places the patient in a condition that she may be operated upon for the ruptured perineum under which she labors, with some prospect of success ; otherwise, an operation for this would be useless.   The irritating effect of the uncontrolled urine being the obstacle to success.

Case xxxi.—*Vesico-Vaginal Fistule of enormous dimensions, in the Hotel Dieu, Paris; Two operations by MM. Verneuil and Robert; Both failures; Case afterwards operated upon with the Button Suture; Fistulous opening closed at the first operation; Case reported in the Gazette des Hôpitaux for January 4th and 6th, 1859, under the head, " Opération de Fistule Vésico-Vaginale Practiquée Suivant la Méthode Américaine," by* M. Robert, *one of the Surgeons to the Hotel Dieu.*— M. Robert's general remarks upon the case, the history, the progress of it after our operation, and the final result, I have translated as follows : For some years the American, and more recently the Eng-lish Journals, have announced to the profession a number of suc-cesses in the operation for vesico-vaginal fistule.   I admit that the recital of these cures left some doubts upon my mind ; doubts rather founded to the effect that, in France, notwithstanding the important works of M. Jobert upon this subject, the success of operations for vesico-vaginal fistule was as yet only exceptional, whilst in America almost as many successes are claimed as operations.

The truth is, I think that I should have the same doubts still as to the results of the operation practised in America and England, but for the fortunate circumstance which brought into our wards at the *Hotel Dieu* Dr. Bozeman, of the United States, one of the principal pro-moters of this method.   By chance, we had then in the ward St. Paul a patient affected with a fistule, very large and very rebellious.   We pre-sented the patient to Dr. Bozeman, who, seeing the considerable dimen-sions of the vesico-vaginal perforation, hesitated a little to operate upon the patient.   I insisted that the American surgeon should operate, agreeing with him that the case was very difficult, and affirming, be-sides, that a failure, under the circumstances, would not, in my eyes, be a sufficient reason to detract from the value of his operative pro-cedure.   Finally, he consented to my request, and performed the operation; in consideration of which he explained to us the advan-tages of the American method, such as is actually used, after the different modifications that it has undergone.

You know the result of the operation performed before us by Dr. Bozeman ; it is very beautiful, very remarkable, and has entirely convinced us of the importance of the method.

44

In fine, one of our *internes*, M. Dubrizey, in a visit which he lately made to London, has had occasion to assist at three operations for vesico-vaginal fistule, performed by Mr. Baker Brown. He followed these patients ; he took notes of them, and then, upon his departure, he was able to state that two of these patients were completely cured ; the third was still under treatment ; but after his return to Paris, he received a letter from Mr. Baker Brown, who informed him of the complete cure of this patient. Thus, in England, out of three operations, three cures were well authenticated by an eye-witness. This is a result truly magnificent, and such, it is proper to say, French surgeons are not accustomed to.

What is the reason of these successes, so numerous in America and England, whilst they are less frequent among us? Evidently this difference in the results can be attributed only to choice of operative procedure. It will be interesting, therefore, to inquire what are the fundamental principles of the French method, compared to those of the American, and to examine in detail the different modifications, the one and the other have undergone since their adoption to the present moment.

We will first say that vesico-vaginal fistules, rather rare in France, are, on the contrary, frequent in England and America, because of the position the patients in these two countries are made to take during parturition, which is to sit upon a chair. The pelvis is, therefore, placed in a declining position, and the head of the child presses strongly upon the anterior wall of the vagina ; thus, fistules are frequent. The surgeons, therefore, have numerous operations to perform ; and it seems, indeed, that Mr. Baker Brown, of London, pays special attention to this branch of surgery.

We will give here the case of the patient upon whom Dr. Bozeman had the kindness to practise before us his method ; then we will examine summarily the principles upon which the French method is founded, compared to those which are embodied in the American. Finally, we will give in detail the operation actually employed in America, and which the English surgeons have of late fully adopted.

At No. 7, ward St. Paul, is lying a woman named Dubocq, aged thirty-five ; burnisher ; entered Sept. 11th, 1858. She is the mother of nine children ; each time delivered easily and without accident. In the month of July, of this year, she was delivered for the tenth time. The presentation was the breech, and the child came dead, after only twelve hours' labor. The lochia was scanty ; the patient had no milk. She remained in bed eleven days, urinating as usual, and having no symptom calculated to lead her to suspect what had taken place during her delivery, and which came to be known afterwards.

The twelfth day she got up, and soon perceived that a quantity of water ran down between her legs. Here is what had happened : The vesico-vaginal wall, strongly compressed by the passage of the child, had become mortified, and the eschar which had resulted from this did not become detached until the twelfth day ; then, the patient being up, the weight of the abdominal viscera pressing upon the bladder, caused a rupture of the last attachments which retained the gangrenous portion of the vagina, and allowed the passage of urine. Since then the catamenia have not returned.

The patient entered the hospital the 11th of September, seven weeks after her confinement. M. Verneuil, who replaced us, then proceeded to the examination, and stated the case as follows : The general health is good ; the patient cannot retain her urine ; she is constantly wet, and never feels any desire to urinate. She is not conscious of the passage of urine through the fistule. Nothing goes through the urethra. We found upon the vesico-vaginal wall, to the right of the anterior column of the vagina, a solution of continuity, about 0.035 millim. in diameter ; the anterior lip of this perforation is situated at 0 m., 04 from the orifice of the vulva, and the posterior, is distant 0 m., 03 from the neck of the uterus*. The vaginal and vesical mucous membranes were entirely united around the whole circumference of the fistule.

September 21st, M. Verneuil operated upon the patient. The scarification was made with care, and the lips of the wound were simply united by suture.

The first days after the operation were marked by a desire to urinate ; but it was soon perceived that reünion had totally failed.

---

* Here I would remark that M. Verneuil was deceived as to the situation and extent of the fistulous opening. At my examination, I found it involving nearly the whole of the trigonus vesicalis and the *bas fond* of the bladder. It extended about as far on one side of the longitudinal axis of the vagina as the other, and measured in its transverse diameter something over two inches. It did not quite touch the root of the urethra below, nor the anterior lip of the cervix uteri above. Its anterior edge was deeply notched opposite the urethra, and could not be carried upwards any, because of its close attachment to the pubic bones. There was less protrusion than usual of the vesical mucous membrane, considering the size of the fistule. The fistule belonged to my fourth class, second variety.   B.

The patient, on the 10th of October, was in the same state as before the operation.

October 18th, I operated myself, according to the autoplastic procedure of Gerdy, which consists in lapping the vaginal mucous membrane over each lip of the fistule, in order to obtain two flaps, which are united by the *suture enchevillée.*

For three days urine passed by the catheter, but on the fourth day some clots of blood escaped from the vagina, and from this moment the desire to urinate disappeared.

November 2d, I examined the patient, and found that the flaps were gangrenous. The fistule presented the same dimensions as before.

The patient was reduced to this state, when, on the 16th of November, at our request, Dr. Bozeman had the kindness to operate upon her. I pass over the details of the operation here. It will suffice to state that ten silver sutures were required to unite the edges of the fistule, and that no lateral incisions were made.

November 18th.—The abdomen is painful and tympanitic. I fear a latent peritonitis. *Onguent napolitain belladoné et cataplasmes sur le ventre ; potion avec camphre et opium,* 10 *centigrammes.* The urine passes by the catheter. This general and local state continues until the 22d, at which time the fever diminishes, the abdomen becomes soft, and the pain ceases. The urine still passes through the catheter. The patient supports opium badly, which causes vomiting. Opium discontinued. The same day she had an action of the bowels, but without any effort.

24th.—General condition very good ; Dr. Bozeman removed the sutures. We could then see that union was complete in 19-20ths of the wound. This small part, not united, was at the right extremity of the wound. Dr. Bozeman recollected, then, that in this place he had seen the orifice of the ureter during the operation, but he did not care to dissect it out.

During the removal, which required nearly half an hour, the urine accumulated in the bladder, and the patient experienced a desire to pass it. Dr. Bozeman, being about to quit France now, recommended us to continue the use of the catheter seven days longer and not to permit the patient to get up under twelve days.

December 5th.—The catheter is removed, and the patient commences to leave her bed. She experiences a desire to urinate.

11*th.*—Examined her with the speculum. The wound seems to be completely united. There is no appearance of the small opening discovered at the time of removing the suture apparatus. Nevertheless, the patient, who urinates seven or eight times a day, and retains perfectly her urine two hours at least, says that she feels wet at times.

Cold injections, as on the preceding days, to be made into the vagina.

Patient continues to get up. She is gaining strength. She can retain her urine for two hours, and passes each time about a wine glass full.

14*th.*—Another examination with the speculum. The vagina is a little moist at the moment when the instrument is introduced. A sponge passed over the walls of the vagina, removes every trace of humidity. Notwithstanding the minutest care and the most serious attention, it is impossible to discover the slightest opening. We looked for some minutes to see if there did not escape a little fluid ; the vagina remained perfectly dry.

How, then, explain this fact, related by the patient, that sometimes, after having retained her urine for two hours, she feels herself wet? There are but two hypotheses possible ; one is, that there exists an opening, a passage very narrow, so small that by the minutest examination it cannot be discovered. In this case we are obliged to inject a colored fluid into the bladder, that we may see it escape in the vagina, when there exists a perforation, but in the case of the patient of whom we are speaking, the vagina, once wiped, remains perfectly dry. We cannot, therefore, admit the existence of an opening. The second hypothesis, the only one probable in the case, is this : Women who have had a vesico-vaginal fistule, preserve, for a variable length of time after the operation, a very small bladder, capable of holding but a small quantity of urine. This fact of retraction of the walls of the bladder upon themselves, in case of perforation, is constant, and, therefore, explains itself very readily ; add to this, then, that the capacity of the reservoir is still more or less diminished, in consequence of the loss of substance which it has undergone. But our patient can retain her urine for two hours ; this is already an immense progress ; but this proves to us, likewise, that the bladder is still very small. It is, therefore, very probable that there is in this woman a little incontinence of urine when the bladder is distended as much as possible ; incontinence which, first, easily explains itself by the weakness of the neck of the bladder in women generally, and, secondly, by the circumstance that, in this particular case, Dr. Bozeman, in his operation, was obliged to implicate the neck of the bladder.

Lastly, 18th of December, I profit by the state of the weather, which gives us a clear light, to examine again the state of the parts. This last examination has not left any doubt upon my mind. There is no incontinence of urine ; nothing passes by the urethra. The vagina, at the moment when the speculum is introduced, and whilst the patient remains quiet, is, and continues, perfectly dry ; but when the patient makes an effort, we see a drop of urine escape in the vagina. There is, therefore, a small opening, but it is so contracted that we cannot discover it, however much care we take. We could make a colored injection into the bladder, in order to determine the seat of this opening, but the patient declares herself perfectly satisfied with her condition. She retains her urine for more than two hours, is very rarely wet, and there is scarcely a drop of urine that escapes.

She asks to leave the hospital. We recommend her to use, night and morning, astringent injections per vaginam, persuaded that this small fistulous opening will disappear completely, as it has already so diminished, after a month, that we cannot discover it to-day.

This is, therefore, a new success to record in favor of the American method—success, the more remarkable in this woman, as there was a loss of substance from 3½ to 4 *centimètres*, and that the operation seemed to offer so little chance of success that Dr. Bozeman hesitated a long time before he would undertake it.

Here M. Robert examines in what consists the American method, prefacing his remarks with a notice of the procedure of M. Jobert, denominated *autoplastie par glissement*. The latter he regards as differing totally from the former, it being essentially an autoplastic operation, whereas the other is not.

The American method he considers the result of a combination of procedures devised by many surgeons, and thus has allowed himself to be led into the error of supposing that the "clamp suture" of Dr. Sims and our button suture differed but very little, not seeming to know that the former had been entirely abandoned by its author.

He next states what position of the patient is preferred in this country, and the kind of speculum in use, after which he proceeds to describe the different stages of the operation, making two only :

1st. Scarification.

2d. Reünion.

These stages, with the various instruments employed in the operation, together with our suture apparatus, he describes very minutely. He then concludes with a supplementary note as to the further progress of our patient, and the conclusions arrived at finally. Here is what he says : At the moment of going out, the patient had an attack of inflammation in the lower part of the abdomen, probably the result of cold. She, therefore, remained some days longer in the hospital, to undergo antiphlogistic treatment, to which the disease rapidly yielded.

Finally, the 30th of December, the patient, on going out, was subjected to a last examination, with this result : With the catheter, the bladder being completely emptied of about 130 grammes of urine, we injected into it 300 grammes of milk. Notice, *en passant*, this considerable increase in the capacity of the bladder. The vagina then being dilated by means of a speculum, we explored this canal. The milk injected in the bladder neither escaped into the vagina nor by the urethra. After prolonging the examination, however, we saw now and then a drop of clear urine escape from the vesico-vaginal wall, at the point precisely where Dr. Bozeman had encountered the right ureter, and which he endeavored to avoid with the suture. This examination, therefore, demonstrates in a positive manner : 1st. That the vesico-vaginal perforation is obliterated, since the milk contained in the bladder does not escape into the vagina. 2d. That the urine which wets the vagina from time to time, is turned directly into the canal by the ureter, which was implicated by the suture, notwithstanding the efforts of the surgeon to prevent it. We would remark that the dribbling of the urine from the right ureter into the vagina, is limited to a few drops, because of the compression that the cicatrix exerts over the former, which is found to be considerably diminished in size. 3d. Lastly, and this is the main fact, that the opening in the vesico-vaginal wall, being 4 *centimètres* in diameter, has been completely obliterated by the simple suture, without having recourse to incisions to permit locomotion of the tissues, and notwithstanding, too, the presence of the ureter between the edges of the fistule.

Remarks.—It may be thought by the reader that M. Robert himself has said enough in connection with this case, but as he has shown himself to be in error in some of his statements, I must be excused for appending these additional remarks, by way of explanation.

First, he says that vesico-vaginal fistule is rather rare in France, but, on the contrary, frequent in England and America. This circumstance he attributes to the position the patient in these two countries is made to take during labor, which is sitting upon a chair. In this, scarcely need I say, he is entirely mistaken. The back and side are the two positions generally recommended in this country, and they are, I think, as a general rule, preferred in England.

The above explanation of M. Robert as to the frequency of vesico-vaginal fistule among us, recalls to my mind another one, equally erroneous, though made with less charity, which I saw a year or two ago in the *Dublin Hospital Gazette*. The writer here says : " One fact must painfully strike us—the frequency of vesico-vaginal fistula in the States ; surely it indicates a great amount of ignorance and rashness in American midwifery." Now, such an explanatien as the latter certainly implies very great wisdom on the part of Irish practitioners, and must strike the reader with peculiar force. If I may be allowed to judge, this sage writer might have given another, and I am inclined to think a truer, explanation of the matter. It is this, namely ; his inability to cure the disease in question, has placed him in a position not to be applied to by this lamentable class of sufferers, of which he can consequently know but little. It is well known that, as yet, comparatively little has been done in Ireland in this branch of surgery ; but because this is so, it is no proof of the disease not being as common there as it is in America. I hold it to be true, that injuries incidental to parturition are equally common everywhere, and that whenever the surgeons of Ireland, France, or any other country arrive at that degree of success in treating these accidents, which has for several years characterized the practice of American and English surgeons, then, and not until then, will they be placed in a position that will enable them to speak knowingly as to the frequency of these diseases in other countries, as compared to their own.

Another point that I would now call attention to, is M. Robert's remarks relative to the small opening that remained after our operation. This, he says, was at the right extremity of the cicatrix. Here he is mistaken again ; it was nearly half an inch from this point, corresponding, though, as he states, with the entrance of the right ureter into the bladder. It was in paring the posterior edge of the fistule that I cut off the end of the ureter. I was not positive, at the time, that it had been done. The cut end was not visible upon the pared surface, as is usually the case ; nor could I discover any urine issuing from it. I had seen the urine escaping from this point before I commenced the operation, and it was owing to this circumstance that I was on the lookout for the ureter in my operation. I remarked to one of my assistants, Dr. Noyes, that I did not understand how it could escape being cut, and expressed my fears as to the consequences, should I not be able to find it. The difficulty, under such circumstances, must at once suggest itself to the mind. The cut ureter opening upon the denuded edge of the fistule, is in a situation to be brought directly against the opposite one, when the sutures are introduced, and approximation comes to be effected ; hence the necessity of the urine coming from the corresponding kidney, forcing an outlet. The resistance being less in the direction of the vagina, the urine very naturally escapes that way, owing to the manner in which the edges of the fistule are pared, and the force with which they are brought together on the vesical side of the septum.

My usual plan of overcoming this obstacle, when I can find the cut end of the ureter, is to slit it up to the extent of a third of an inch on the vesical side of the septum, including, of course, the vesical mucous membrane with it, which can be done without difficulty. In this way an opening to the bladder is made, and the entrance of the urine consequently turned away from the approximated edges of the fistule. Could we have discovered the ureter in this case, and disposed of it as above stated, no difficulty would have been experienced. As our operation was completed, however, the result was inevitable ; namely, a partial failure. Upon visiting our patient a few hours after she had been put to bed, I found only about half of her urine passing by the catheter ; the remainder was going through the vagina. Recollecting, now, my suspicions as to the implication of the right ureter at the time of the operation, I came to the conclusion at once what had happened, and explained it to one of the *externes*, Dr. Whitehead. Had there been any doubts upon my mind as to the correctness of the conclusion arrived at, they would have been removed by seeing the quality of the urine. All the urine that came through the catheter was bloody, as it generally is for several

45

days after the operation, whereas that which escaped from the vagina was clear, showing that it came directly from the kidney.

The morning after the operation, I explained to M. Robert what had taken place, and told him there would be a partial failure of our operation, just at the point where the right ureter entered the bladder. This explanation he seemed to doubt, and expressed his belief that it was impossible for me to tell where and to what extent the operation would fail. Now, M. Robert, in his account of the case and operation does not mention this circumstance, nor does he say anything about half of the urine passing through the vagina immediately after our operation. This I think is a great oversight, as these facts form a very important part of the history of the case, and go to prove, in a very striking manner, with what certainty we can calculate upon a successful result from an operation.

Another fact I should mention is, that the quantity of urine passing through the vagina became less every day, which I could explain in no other way than that the obstacle to its entrance into the bladder gradually gave way, and it changed its course; in other words, that the escape of urine through the vagina after a few days, was the result of a communication direct from the bladder, and not the ureter, as in the first instance.

On the eighth day after the operation, I proceeded to remove our suture apparatus, in the presence of Prof. Nélaton, M. Verneuil, M. Robert, Dr. Hayward, of Boston, Dr. Noyes, of Rhode Island, Dr. Whitehead, of Virginia, Dr. Hoff, of Georgia, and a number of other French, American, and English medical gentlemen. Before doing so, however, I explained what had happened in the outset of our treatment of the case, and stated that I expected to find a partial failure of the operation at the point heretofore designated; namely, at the entrance of the right ureter into the bladder.

The apparatus then being removed, showed that union of the edges of the fistule was complete throughout, excepting at the point above mentioned, where we found a small opening communicating with the bladder, as indicated by the introduction of a probe.

My engagements now to leave Paris prevented me from seeing any further progress of the case. It was left in charge of M. Robert, with directions how to manage it in another operation which I expected, of course, would require to be performed to complete the cure.

The report of the case after this, M. Robert has furnished us with, and we can only judge of the final result from this. It seems that he never attempted an operation for the closure of the small remaining fistule. At his last examination, he satisfied himself, as he states, that there was no communication between the bladder and vagina, which he did by injecting milk into the former until it was distended, none of which escaped into the vagina. By looking closely, and for some time, a drop of clear urine was seen to issue from the vesico-vaginal wall just opposite the end of the right ureter.

Now, M. Robert's test, as to their being an opening in the bladder, was certainly very satisfactory, and proved beyond doubt that none existed. But, admitting this to be true, and that the right ureter, as he says, did open directly into the vagina, we are forced to doubt his statement as to the drop of urine escaping into the vagina from the latter, which could only be seen after looking for some time. With this state of things, according to my observation, there would have been no difficulty in seeing the urine escape from the end of the ureter into the vagina. The quantity coming from one kidney, as was the case here, is considerable, and escapes in drops rather frequent. Again, if it should be said that the ureter entered both the bladder and vagina, and that the quantity of urine from the kidney was divided, why then we would have expected to see the milk injected into the bladder, enter the ureter on this side of the vesico-vaginal septum, and escape into the vagina by regurgitation. I take the position, therefore, that if no opening exists in the bladder, and the right ureter is turned into the vagina, not only the latter would be wet by the escape of urine here, as M. Robert says, but that the patient herself and clothes would be constantly wet ; and furthermore, that no difficulty would be experienced in seeing the point whence the urine issued, as the flow direct from the kidney would be sufficiently constant to enable one to do so.

With these facts before me, therefore, I am forced to doubt the accuracy of M. Robert's statements as to the final result of the operation in this case. My convictions are that no opening in the vesico-vaginal wall exists—that it closed up itself after the removal of our suture apparatus, and that the patient being made slightly wet at times was the result of incontinence ; in other words, the fistule was closed, but that the bladder, at the time of M. Robert's last examination, had not regained its retentive power. The latter condition I have known to continue for months, especially when the bladder had sustained great loss of substance, as was true of this case. In whatever light viewed, however, our operation, as regards closure of the fistulous opening, must be considered entirely successful.

(To be continued.)

ART. VI.—*Contributions to the Temperature of Cold-blooded Animals, together with Speculative and Practical Researches into the Theories of Animal Heat:* By BENNET DOWLER, M. D.

MARCH 31, 1846.—Of five large alligators confined in boxes which contained a stratum of water about three inches deep, exposed to the weather, two of the larger (supposed to be a male and a female) were selected for experiment. These were from ten to eleven feet long, and from four to five feet in their greatest circumference. They were slightly torpid, and constantly inclined to sleep, but when irritated, distended their bodies greatly by inspiring a great quantity of air, which they expelled with loud, angry hissings. Although their lungs, even during sleep, appeared to be constantly distended, yet, when left in quietude, no appreciable breathing could be detected. The shoal water in which their abdomens and the inferior portions of their sides rested, would have produced an agitation of the water, had the slightest respiratory movement taken place. In neither cool nor hot weather do they respire like warm-blooded animals. The experiments which follow, made upon alligators and turtles of various sizes, and, in some instances, weighing about one thousand pounds, involved mechanical manipulations and apparatus for securing the animals, which it would be too tedious to enumerate—such as the opening the mouth with a powerful lever, so as to pass thermometers into the gullet, etc ; also, the duration of the experiments will generally be omitted.

10, A. M.—Air 59°; river 53½°; water in which the alligators lie 56°; flanks (the thighs being mechanically compressed against the sides) each, after many trials, gave 56°. Noon.—Air 62°; water in the boxes 57°; female (forty minutes) 57°; male 57½°. 6, P. M.—Air 61°; water in the boxes 61°; alligators in the flanks, under the tongues, and in the upper part of the gullets, each 61°.

April 1, sunrise.—Flanks ¦59½°; gullets nearly 60°; water 59½°. Noon.—Air 63°; river 54°; water in the ·boxes 61°; flanks 61°. 5, P. M.—Air 67°; water in the boxes (two inches deep) 64°; alligators 65°.

April 2, sunrise.—Air 57½°; the water 58½°; flanks and axillæ 59½°.

April 3, 7, A. M.—Air 64°; flanks and posterior fauces 63°. Noon.— Air 68°; flanks and axillæ 65°. Sunset.—Air 64°; alligators 65°, nearly.

April 4, 1, P. M.—Air 63°; flanks 60½°; gullets (half an hour later, the air growing warmer) 61°. Sunset.—Air 64°; flanks and gullets 64°. These five alligators appeared fat, though they were not known to have eaten anything. Food was offered, but not accepted. They probably had eaten nothing since the preceding autumn.

February 7, 1848.—Air in the alligators' pen 45°; gullet 50°. 8th, sunrise—Open air 52½°; in the pen 52°; gullet 50½°. 9th, sunrise.—Pen 51°; gullet 52°. 10th.—Pen 54°; gullet 55°. 12th, before sunrise.—Pen 58°; gullet 58½°. 13th.—Pen 52°; gullet ·53½. 14th.—Pen 58°; gullet 58°. 15th.—Pen 57½°; gullet 58°. 16th.— Pen 61 deg.; gullet 58 deg. 17th.—Pen 65 deg.; gullet 64½ deg. 18th.—Pen 64½ deg.; gullet 64½ deg. 19th.—Pen 68 deg.; gullet 68 deg. 20th.—In the water at 68 deg.; gullet 68 deg.; air 70 deg. 21st.—Water 68 deg.; gullet 68½ deg. The weather during the day became warm. Air 81½ deg.; the water 75 deg.; the gullet 82 deg. 22d.—Pen 70 deg.; water 68 deg.; gullet 68½ deg. 23d, sunrise.— Air in the pen 69 deg.; water 66 deg.; gullet 56 deg. 24th, sunrise.—Air of the pen 56 deg.; water in which the animal was lying 55 deg.; gullet 55 deg. 25th.—The air and water each 49½ deg.; gullet 49 deg.; sleeps ; nearly torpid. 27th, sunrise.—Air in the pen and the gullet each 56½ deg. 29th.—Air in the pen 53 deg.; the the water and the gullet each 52½ deg.

March 1, sunrise.—Air of the pen 64 deg.; the water and the gullet each 62½ deg. 12th, sunrise.—Open air 61 deg.; air in the pen 57½ deg.; the water and gullet each 56 deg. 14th, sunrise.—Open air, air in the box, and the gullet, each 47 deg.; the water 48 deg. 16th, sunrise.—Open air and the air of the box, each 54 deg.; the water and the gullet each 53 deg. 18th, sunrise.—Open air 63 deg.;

the gullet and air in the pen each 65 deg. 20th, sunrise.—Open air and that of the box 70 deg. each ; water and gullet each 69 deg.

November 1, 1848, 9, A. M.—Gullet 53 deg.; air of the box 54 deg. 2d, sunrise.—Gullet 48 deg.; air of the box 48 deg. 5th, sunrise.— Gullet 43 deg.; box 43 deg.; open air 44½ deg.

July 31, 1850, 8, A. M.—Air 81½ deg.; gullet 81½ deg.; the alligator, in a room, at 83½ deg.; in thirty minutes, gullet and flanks each 82 degrees.

January 27, 1851, 10, A. M.—Air 64½ deg.; pharynx 65 deg.

ii.—*Temperature of the Fish of Lake Pontchartrain.*

In the following experiments on fishes, the thermometer was thrust down the throat the moment the fish was drawn up with a hook from the water :

October 12, 1849, 9, A. M.—River 75 deg.; Lake Pontchartrain, at the end of the wharf, about a quarter of a mile from shore, at 10½, A. M., 71½ deg.; a catfish, taken directly from the water, gave in its gullet and stomach 70 deg.; another nearly 71 deg ; a perch the same.

I believe I have some records (which I cannot now turn to) of similar experiments on the fishes of the Mississippi. It is reasonable to suppose that, if the temperature of these fishes coincides with that of the water from which they are taken, a difference may, nevertheless, exist between individuals of the same species, caught in deep or shoal water, where the animal has been swimming for some time, in hot or cold weather, near to or far from the surface. My experiments, however, are too limited to determine absolutely whether the fishes of the river and lake coincide in temperature with the waters which they inhabit.

iii.—*Temperature of the Turtle.* (*Chelonia Midas.*)

September 23, 1855.—Humid, cloudy ; air 84½ deg. in the shade. Two medium sized turtles, weighing about 300 pounds each, gave in the groin 84 deg. each. (A turtle which I examined weighed 941 pounds.)

September 25, 4½, P. M.—Clear ; air of my office 88½ deg.; air of the room, where four turtles lie, 87 deg. The turtles above mentioned, and two others, much larger, were experimented on. The former two gave each, in the flanks and axillæ, 87 deg.; of the others, one gave 90 deg. in the axilla and 90½ deg. in the flank ; the other 90 deg. The differences here noted are supposed to be owing to position, the sun's rays having fallen on the latter for a few minutes before the experiments were made.

September 26, 9, A. M.—Air at office 83 deg.; the room where the turtles are varies from 83 deg. to 85 deg.; turtle No. 1, axilla 84 deg., flank 84½ deg.; No. 2, axilla 84 deg., flank 84½ deg.

October 3, 1855, 10, A. M.—Air of office 73 deg.; air of the room near the turtles, 72 deg. to 73 deg.; turtle No. 1 (a fresh and large one) flank 73 deg., axilla 71 deg.; No. 2, flank 71½ deg., axilla 71½ degrees.

October 6, 9, A. M.—The weather has become cold within sixteen hours, after heavy rains ; strong wind ; cloudy; office 60 deg.; air of the room where the turtles lie (about three feet above them), 61 deg.; turtle No. 1, axilla 70 deg., groin 73 deg.; No. 2, axilla 70 deg., groin 72 deg.

October 7, 9, A. M.—Air of office 60 deg.; where the animals lie 60 deg.; axillæ 61 deg.; flanks 62 deg.

October 25.—Within two days the weather has changed from warm, cloudy, and wet, to clear, cold, and windy; office 45 deg.; room near the turtle 46 deg.; axillæ 52 deg.; groin 54 deg. The animal, which weighs about 500 pounds, seems in great pain from the sudden cold weather. The ratio of refrigeration in the air and in the animal differs considerably in this case, being slower in the latter, owing (as former experiments indicate) to the rapidity with which the weather changed ; that is, in very sudden changes, turtles and alligators do not fall to the minimum, or rise to the maximum of the air so quickly as the mercury of the thermometer. A sudden cold or hot blast produces a more immediate effect upon the latter, though the minimum, maximum, and mean results are virtually analogous or identical.

November 20, 1855.—The weather for two days has been changing from warm to cool, but is to-day rather changing back to warm, being clear, calm, and delightful, though so cool as to require fires. Office, at 9, A. M., 62½ deg.; where thirty turtles lie on their backs, the air near and above them is 63 deg.; probably the floor and air touching their bodies is 1 deg. less. I took the temperature in the groins of nine, varying in weight from 50 to about 1,000 pounds ; No. 1, 62 deg. (the largest); No. 2, 61 deg.; No. 3, 61 deg.; No. 4, 62 deg.; No. 5, 62 deg.; No. 6, 61½ deg.; No. 7, 61 deg.; No. 8, 62 deg.; No. 9, 62 deg.; being, to all intents and purposes, the same.as the surrounding media, as the floor, air, etc.

5, p. m., same day.—Clear, pleasant ; air of the room 68 deg.; same turtles ; groins 66 deg., 68 deg., 68 deg., 68 deg., 68 deg., 69 deg., etc.; air of office 68 deg.

The proprietor of these animals says that he recently received seventy-five turtles of various sizes ; that a number of them, particularly the smaller ones, which were plump and lively before the late two days of cool weather on the 18th and 19th, have been torpid, and have shrivelled, or "fallen in," as he calls it ; lying on their backs, it was easy to see that the abdominal surfaces had lost their convexity or rotundity, from the collapse or contraction produced apparently by cold.

November 21.—Weather clear, calm ; 9, a. m.; same turtles ; room 64½ deg.; office, 64½ deg.; No. 1, groin, 66½ deg. (largest one about 700 lbs.); No. 2, 64 deg.: No. 3, 64 deg.; No. 4, 64 deg.; No. 5 (large), 65 deg.; No. 6, 64 deg.; No. 7, 64 deg.; No. 8, 65 deg.; No. 9, 65 deg. Afternoon ; same weather, day, and turtles ; air of office and room where the turtles lie, each 79 deg.; experimented on six turtles, in the groin, all being 79 deg., but one, which gave 78 deg.

November 23.—Air of office, 55 deg. Weather has suddenly become cool since yesterday ; room where the turtles lie, 56 deg.; No. 1, 55 deg.; No. 2, 62 deg.; No. 3, 61 deg.; No. 4, 59 deg.; No. 5, 61 deg.; No. 6, 59 deg.; No. 7, 59 deg. The smaller ones (15 to 20 lbs.) were the coolest.

Temperature of turtles, Feb. 27th, 1856 ; 10 a. m.; six turtles, having an average weight of about 250 lbs. Temperature of the weather but little variable for two days ; room where the turtles lie on their backs, 65 deg. No. 1, axilla, 65 deg., groin, 65 deg.; No. 2, axilla, 64 deg., groin, 65 deg.; No. 3, axilla, 65 deg., groin, 65 deg.; No. 4, axilla, 64 deg., groin, 64 deg.; No. 5, axilla, 64½ deg., groin, 64½ deg.; No. 6, axilla, 64 deg., groin, 64 deg.

The thermo-vital zero of the alligator, so far as I have observed, is at least 1 deg. above the freezing point, that is, 33 deg. Fah. Whether it can endure a lower temperature without a fatal result, is doubtful. I lost two in one night from cold, but in these cases they would doubtlessly have escaped congelation and death, had there been sufficient water in their pen for the immersion of their bodies. In the coldest weather I have known since 1836 in New Orleans, I have found that although the air may fall to 14 deg., or 13 deg. below the freezing point, the alligator does not die when immersed in water under ice an inch or more in thickness, in which case, however, the very tip of the muzzle, and, consequently, the nasal orifices are placed above the surface of the water, and when ice forms and even adheres to the muzzle, the tip remains a little above the ice. In this low temperature, in which the animal is torpid, I have not thought it safe to make thermometrical experiments, but have made holes in the superincumbent ice, and have found the water around the body to be 33 deg. Fah., which I am satisfied represents the temperature of the body itself.

In his general account of the Reptilia, Cuvier says : " As the respiration imparts the warmth to the blood, and the susceptibility of the fibre to nervous irritamen, reptiles have cold blood, and their aggregate muscular energy is less than in the mammalia, and much less than in birds." (*An. King.*) This exposition of the origin of animal heat and of muscular force is founded upon received hypotheses rather than upon facts. The muscular powers of some cold-blooded animals rival, nay exceed those of the warm-blooded of equal size. To capture an alligator and secure it during vivisection, will, in the hot, non-hibernating season, convince the operator that its muscular power is very great, though, from its anatomical structure, its locomotive speed is small. The energy and pertinacity of its bite are little less than the lateral force of its tail. If what is generally said by travelers and naturalists of some cold-blooded ophidians or serpents, such as the boæ, be true, the theory which places their muscular energy far below mammalians and birds of equal muscular masses, must be false. The boa constrictor's crushing power and relentless grasp, by which it kills man and large animals as cattle, are prodigious, being an almost peculiar example of mere muscular force, whether in defense or in capturing prey, without inflicting wounds, as do warm-blooded, carnivorous animals. Perhaps few, if any of the warm-blooded animals of equal muscular masses, equal the sword-fish (*Xiphias gladius*) in force—a penetrative force little short of cannon shot*.

---

* While reading the proofs of this article, the following paragraph appeared in the public journals :

The Sword Fish.—A British vessel in the African trade, undergoing repairs at Bristol, shows the extraordinary powers of the sword fish. A fish drove its sword through a double sheeting of copper, a plank two and a half inches thick, and deep into one of the ship's timbers, when the weapon broke short off.

In my earliest experiments upon the alligator, I irritated the animal so as to cause it to inspire and expire air copiously, which it does when offended, but no elevation of temperature could in this way be detected.

I had previously (in 1843) found in human bodies, a few minutes after death, that the lungs so far from being the heating and heated furnace of the whole system, often presented a lower temperature than several other regions both external and internal. At that period, M. Liebig's chemical calculations in formulæ for and reaffirmation of the long accepted theory of pulmonary combustion, were hailed with loud acclaim as demonstrations—fundamental principles of physiology. It is now nearly a score of years since I dissented from this still prevalent theory, and published abundant experimental evidence, conclusive at least to myself, against its validity. Of late, there is an ominous reticence, with an increasing unwillingness to render either an exact bill of the weight of oxygen and charcoal of the heating and heated furnace of the whole animal economy, or the exact number of degrees of heat this fuel will make in the lungs, to be thence radiated or conducted to the remotest parts of the body.

In his Physiological Chemistry (1855), Prof. Lehmann quotes Baron Liebig, as saying, "that as the blood considered as a fluid can mechanically absorb only a very small portion of the oxygen which disappears during respiration must of necessity be chemically absorbed. The very careful and accurate experiments of Liebig appear at first sight to oppose the idea of chemical absorption of the oxygen in the lungs ; for he found that the difference of temperature in the different parts of the circulating system, including both the arterial and venous systems, were solely referable to the physical laws of the radiation of the heat, etc.; and that in the lungs especially, the blood not only undergoes no elevation, *but even a slight depression of temperature*. Here, therefore, we obtain for the first time, a direct confirmation of the early hypothesis, that the blood is cooled in the lungs by respiration." (ii. 475.)

Without following Prof. Lehmann in his dubious explanation of these facts, it may be proper to note that Liebig's experiments are quoted from his publication at Giessen, in 1853. Sixteen years ago I sent to Prof. Liebig, through the German Consul at New Orleans, my two experimental memoirs on animal heat, published in *The Western Journal of Medicine and Surgery*. Prof. Lehemann is not warranted by history in his ascription of priority to Baron Liebig. He was not " the first," as the sequel will show, to offer experimental evidence, " that the blood is *cooled* in the lungs by respiration." No chemico-physiological formula, or even experiment out of the living economy, explanatory of the generation of animal heat, can be comparable to, much less invalidate, the thermometrical test applied before and immediately after death. At the time when the experiments were made in New Orleans, and for years afterwards, Prof. Liebig held doctrines the reverse of those quoted by Prof. Lehemann.

Life, in the language of these chemists, is identical with chemical action. They talk and write in a very business manner about the burning of hydrogen, oxygen, and carbon. They kindle charcoal fires in the lung-furnace, as literally as firemen on steamboats and in founderies, and furnish, withal, numerical tables abounding in figures, and even minute fractions, showing the quantities, qualities, measures, and weights of the fuel consumed, and also the quantity of caloric produced therefrom, leaving, however, out of view the antagonistic contemporaneous processes constantly contending, face to face, with these calorifacient agencies, by which heat is radiated, conducted, dissipated, and lost during the disentegration, liquefaction, volatilization, and evaporization proper to the functional actions of the body itself, not to mention numerous external agencies which contribute unceasingly towards the production, equilibration, and waste of heat. " In every instance," says Prof. Draper, " the production of heat is due to oxidation." Why forget the other side of this assumption, namely : that in every instance of oxidation there is an equal instance of *deoxidation*, etc, going on in the economy to produce refrigeration ?

If it be admitted, contrary to well established facts, that animal heat is developed in an exact ratio with the activity of respiration ; or, in a ratio corresponding to the quantity of food assimilated, it would not necessarily follow that either caused calorification. Either, or both of these, might furnish the condition, without being the cause of animal heat. The soil, warmth, and moisture furnish the conditions, but are not the causes of the vitality of the seeds which have grown up into plants, after an entombment of thousands of years in Egyptian coffins.

With the silent decline of the pulmonary, that of the nutritive theory of animal heat appears to be culminating. The latter, though more probable than the former, is open to formidable objections. An energetic nutrition might, upon theoretical grounds, be regarded as a source of calorification ; but, on the other hand, decomposition or waste would furnish a physiological antithesis or equipoise, upon a principal equally well known as fundamental.

Dr. Carpenter asserts that, "wherever the aëration is extensively and actively carried on, there is a proportionate elevation of temperature, and that, on the other hand, wherever the respiration is naturally feeble, or the aëration of the blood is checked by disease or accidental destruction, the temperature of the body falls." (*Comp. Phys.*, 460,)

Prof. Draper also says : "The production of heat must be connected with the power and precision with which the pulmonary apparatus works.   Heat depends on the power of the pulmonary engine. The absolute temperature will depend on the respiratory condition. Whatever accelerates the introduction and expulsion of the air, increases the warmth.   Animals possessing the highest powers of locomotion, will possess, also, the highest temperature," *et passim.* (*Phys.* 176-7.) And such is the language of all the text books, and such are the logical conclusions which the accepted theory of animal heat warrants, though directly antagonistic to the facts of both physiology and pathology.   Indeed, for anything that the physiological chemists have fairly proven to the contrary, respiration should be regarded as the normal depressor and regulator of that primitive element of the economy by which animal heat is perpetually generated during life, which, otherwise, might accumulate, as is found to be the case when that function is directly or indirectly impaired or obstructed by disease.   Further on, this topic will be examined more fully.

Prof. Draper, one of the best and latest systematic expounders of the prevalent theory, thus sums it up : "Reduced to its ultimate conditions, the evolution of animal heat depends on the reäction taking place between the air introduced by respiration and the food, and as either one or other of these is touched, the result may be predicted." (*Phys.* 182.)

Among the numerous facts which refute the diet theory, not the least striking are those derived from the natural history of the cold-blooded animals, inhabiting both land and water, many of which are most voracious eaters, and digest enormous amounts of food, and yet have no higher temperature than the surrounding media in which they live. "Eight pike," says Mr. Jesse, "of about five pounds weight each, consumed nearly eight hundred gudgeons in three weeks ; and the appetite of one of these pikes was almost insatiable. One morning I threw to him five roach, each about four inches in length ; he swallowed four of them, and kept the fifth in his mouth for about a quarter of an hour, when it also disappeared." (*Mus. Nat. Hist.* ii, 154.) Still more voracious is that cold-blooded, hibernating dipteran, the mosquito, which gorges itself with blood, by which the weight of its body is suddenly augmented perhaps from ten to fifteen hundred *per centum ;* yet such is its enormous muscular power that it can wing its way with its ponderous load, which immediately becomes as cold as the body itself.

That the mosquito is cold-blooded, is easily recognized by the sense of touch, by crushing one that alights upon the skin, especially when the animal is gorged with any kind of fluid ; even the freshly-drawn human blood in its body, will, upon crushing, cause a marked coldness of the part. The penetrative force of its proboscis is, perhaps, a hundred fold greater than that of any mamifer or bird, in proportion to size and weight, passing readily through the thick skin of the alligator, excepting such portions as are protected by osseous plates. The leech, a cold-blooded annelidian, possesses great musculer power, as every leecher must know.

The great quantity of rich animal food required to sustain health and vigor in the arctic regions, even though it should be one of the conditions necessary to the development of animal heat, is not for that reason its direct cause. The withdrawal of this food would, doubtlessly, according to most reliable accounts of starvation, be attended with irritation, thirst, fever, and delirium before death. Starvation is often the forerunner of typhus (one of the hottest of fevers), as has been strikingly exemplified in Ireland, where, during the famine a few years ago, several hundred thousands perished in a single year. Here little food is replaced by much fever or heat.

Prof. Draper, with most other authors of the text books, says : " A starving animal dies of cold" (181); and Prof Dunglison, who advocates the same doctrine, happens upon an illustrative case of starvation from stricture of the œsophagus, reported by Dr. Currie, which is very conclusive the other way; as " parched mouth—scanty, extremely high colored, pungent urine—heat of the body natural from first to last—delirium—*burning heat of the surface and the ex-*

tremities—death, that of a furious maniac." (*Phys.* i, 124.) Nevertheless, this is the only pathological example of which he gives the details.

The excessive and persistent development of heat in many prolonged fevers, especially such as obstruct the action of the respiratory organs, together with the nutritive function, is one of the most frequent occurrences observed at the bed-side. Where the lungs are directly attacked, as in sthenic pneumonia, or even in asthenic typhoid pneumonia, the heat is excessive—far above the normal standard ; and when consumption eats away or obstructs the lungs, excessive heat is generally observed. Dr. Rush designated the three stages of pulmonary consumption as three stages of fever ; namely, the inflammatory, the hectic and the typhus. (*Inq.* ii, 65-6.) Sir James Clark describes what he calls "*febrile* consumption ;" and in his general account of this disease, he maintains, that, "as it advances, the paroxysms of the fever become stronger, especially the hot stage, and that the heat is more generally diffused over the surface." (*Treatise*, pp. 38-78.) M. Louis, in his work on phthisis, says that, "although treatment lessened the rigors, the heat always remained elevated." Without naming other authorities upon this point, I will here add, that my thermometrical observations confirm these statements. Some writers appear to regard consumption as a lung-fever or inflammation, the tubercular deposits and suppurative action in which may be lessened or prevented by the local applications of cold. Which, then, is worthy of credit, the natural history of pathology, or the artificial history of physiology?

Upon this particular subject, the physiologists indulge in eccentricities of ratiocination, which cannot be easily explained. After all their positivism, they relapse into scepticism. Thus, Prof. Lehemann, in the same page (i, 479), sums up his elaborate logic with the following statement : "We will not enter more fully into the theory of animal heat, *since it rests on a very uncertain foundation,* and since a further accumulation of the various facts and arguments bearing upon the subject, would extend our work to an unreasonable size. We ought to observe, however, that the special *heat of every animal organism is merely the result of chemical combinations formed within it.*"

If the reader will turn to the Jan. (1859) No. of the *N. O. Med. and Surg. Jour.,* p. 87, *et seq.*, he will find copious extracts from an interesting article in Blackwood's Magazine upon the subject of animal heat. This article of the Magazine, based chiefly on M. Martins' extensive experimental researches published in M. Brown-Séquard's *Journal de la Physiologie,* and now reproduced in Mr. Lewes's Physiology (the first volume of which appeared in the present year), shows that during the starvation and the full-feeding of animals, their temperatures are about the same, or differ but inconsiderably, especially after the first few days of experimentation, from which Mr. Lewes concludes, " that animal heat is not evolved by the combustion of food."

Thus the nutritive, not less than the respiratory theory of animal heat is negatived by the natural history and physiology of the cold-blooded animals, which, under the maximum of nutrition, possess muscular energy often surpassing the warm-blooded animals, including man and monkey. If some learned casuist would decide the ethical question, whether teachers and text books are warranted in devoting much time and many pages to *ex parte* evidence to prove these theories, a great benefit would redound to the anxious student who is doomed to unlearn these elaborate lessons.

As previously indicated, the calorific differentiation between the thermometer and cold-blooded animals of large size, as turtles and alligators, would, upon theoretical principles, happen occasionally, even though the latter possessed no independent powers of calorification ; for, in sudden changes of the atmospheric temperature, it could not be expected that the increment or conduction of heat from the circumference to the centre of an animal mass of a thousand pounds, more or less ; nor on the other hand, that the decrement or radiation of heat from the centre to the circumference of such a mass, would proceed in a ratio with the velocity of the small mass of mercury in the thermometer. The non-observance of the physical laws of conduction and radiation, and their ratios in different bodies, will probably account for most discrepancies between the cold-blooded animals, the surrounding media, as reported by writers. Cold-blooded animals, though very sensitive to sudden changes, can often maintain vitality under a great but gradual range of temperature. In very rare cases congelation itself does not prove fatal, while, on the other hand, great heat is, though as rarely, borne with impunity. Thus, Mr. Gulliver, in a note on Hewson's works, says : " Sonneret is reported to have seen fishes, apparently not incommoded, in a spring as hot as 187 deg. Fah., in the island of Lugon ; and Cuvier received some fishes from the waters of Cassa and Tozer, which are said to be as high as 170 deg. Fah. (p. 27.)

Both physiology and pathology furnish abundant evidence that animal heat is due neither to pulmonary combustion nor in any way attributable to the energy of respiration. For example : In solar asphyxia (sunstroke of the first degree), which is almost always quickly fatal, respiration is very imperfect, being restricted chiefly to the bronchiæ and trachea and is attended with loud mucous rattlings *(râles)* ; yet this is the hottest of all diseases. As the suffocation, I might say strangulation, increases, so does the heat, which in a few minutes reaches, in some cases, 112 deg. Fah. in the axillæ and other regions. The post mortem heat is equally remarkable, and may be of very long duration. The lesion usually found being either extravasation into the pulmonary tissues or congestion, which illustrates the previous history of pulmonary embarrassment.

In sudden apoplexy *(apoplexie foudroyante)*, as well as in most cases of apoplexy, coma occurs, and as the coma increases the heat increases, and is very persistent after death. Generally, in cases of the comatose form of death from acute diseases, particularly fevers, the close of life is attended with a comparatively high temperature, notwithstanding the embarrassment and infrequency of the respiratory act.

Here it may be allowable to refer to dates, documents, and expositions published nineteen years ago illustrative of the subject under consideration, and the more because they have a practical bearing, and the opinions then advanced were more fully demonstrated by subsequent observation and experiment in many diseases besides sunstroke.

The New York Journal of Medicine for 1846, quotes from my paper published in 1841, on *Solar Asphyxia* (sunstroke in the first degree), the following statement, which I extract, not having a copy of the original publication : "Whether the pulmonary congestion be the primary or secondary condition of insolation, I will not say; but I must remark, that of all morbid appearances of a congestive character, this is the least equivocal, so far as I have examined. * * * Although physiology teaches us that man is endowed with the power of maintaining the same heat of his body in all climates and situations, with few exceptions, still it is possible, under peculiar circumstances, that the body may become actually heated [beyond the normal standard]. A chemico-vital refrigeration, by means of perspiration or evaporation, is constantly going on. 'The fire-kings' themselves, when in a heat of 500 deg. or 600 deg., would roast and turn to cinders, were it not for this refrigerating process, in conjunction with a vital energy which for a time neutralizes the accumulating power of caloric. The solar heat [in sun-stroke] probably accumulates upon the surface [and in the lungs] of the body faster than nature can refrigerate through *the lungs* and the skin by evaporation ; the vital energy being exhausted by the contest as well as by excessive labor [in most' cases], is unable longer to neu-tralize the excess of temperature ; vital chemistry is unequal to the task of preventing the conduction of heat into the body, and death is the consequence. (*N. Y. Med. Gaz.*, vol. i, p. 209.)" Under such circumstances, the air, gases, water, blood, and air-vesicles in the lungs, ought, upon merely physical principles, to expand, thereby favoring extravasation into the delicate pulmonary tissue, and all the symptoms of suffocation or asphyxia which are recognizable in true sun-stroke ; though, perhaps, in mere solar exhaustion, a different explanation may be given.

In the April number, 1843, of *The Western Journal of Medicine and Surgery*, in a paper entitled *Post-mortem Researches*, I applied the doctrine of post-mortem calorification, together with the physical law of refrigeration, to pathological anatomy, as modifying actual pre-mortem lesions. Thus, in noticing the heat of the recently dead body, and the physical influence of the radiation of heat upon pre-existent lesions, I said : "Cold alone may, perhaps, remove morbid appearances, and create mechanical congestions by unequally condensing the solids and fluids of such parts as undergo refrigeration the most rapidly — congestions resembling morbid turgescency. Cold acting on the superficial capillaries and other vessels [and tissues], may force the blood towards the centres and more dilatable parts. Even in the living body, cold, more particularly congelation, causes paleness or bloodlessness upon the surface, and, of course, sanguineous centralization." On the other hand, in reference to the manner of dissecting bodies while the animal heat persists, the following practical remarks are given in the same page (254):

" Another fact which exerts a modifying power over morbid appearances, a fact which has been too generally omitted by authors, is the

47

following : If the body be warm, the blood fluid, a morbid congestion
in one cavity may be removed, or lessened, at least, in some cases,
by severing the blood vessels leading to another, especially after an
acute disease of short duration. Let the jugulars, or the cavas be
cut, or the heart and lungs be removed ; in an hour, or less, the
brain and the abdomen may become more or less bloodless. Though
the blood vessels may have been previously engorged, and their
calibers dilated, now, they may appear in a very different condition,
collapsed, and comparatively exsanguinous. Again, let us suppose,
that in two persons recently dead, we proceed to examine whether
hepatic congestions exist. In the one case we open the abdomen ; we
penetrate the liver with the finger, or open its texture with the knife,
severing its vessels ; the blood wells up rapidly, several pounds may
flow in a few minutes ; engorgement seems to be present ; and yet
this happens when there is no congestion at all. In the other case,
let all the great vessels be divided—let the liver remain in its natural situation, and let it be the last organ examined, and it will probably be found nearly bloodless ; even its parenchyma may not indicate the previous congestion. Without regarding these circumstances, the former liver would be congested ; the latter bloodless or
anemic."

If, as is usual, twenty-four hours elapse after death, before a post-
mortem examination is made, the physical law of cooling bodies obtains, with consequences adverse to the accurate observation of hyperæmic lesions ; for, with the cooling of the extremities and circumference, including muscular rigidity (death stiffness), the centres yet
warm, the last to cool, the most yielding, spongy, and vascular portions of the body must receive, as the external contraction proceeds,
a great quantity of blood, by which the natural history of lesions is
rendered uncertain, in some cases, at least. On the other hand, when
the body gets hot after death—hotter, perhaps, than before death,
and, as sometimes happens, hotter upon the surface than in the
centres—hyperæmic lesions of the interior may be obliterated, or
at least modified. .Hence the pathological anatomist needs a thermometer, as well as the knife and the note book. There is not,
however, a thermometer in use adapted to these purposes, so far as
I know.

In an experimental paper published in *The Western Journal of
Medicine and Surgery* (June, 1844), after having given a summary of

the prevalent but fallacious theories of animal calorification, I have said : "The histories of morbid and post-mortem temperature, which will be given, will show whether these assertions [theories] are stronger proofs than facts themselves, even though unconnected with theoretical fortifications." (491). Again, in alluding to the respiratory and other theories, it is said : "Theorists ascribe animal heat to one or all of these with the confidence of mathematical truth, in defiance of the antagonism of facts." (492.) Once more (June and October Nos., 1844, pp. 472, 296) : "These experiments are quite sufficient, if I may be allowed to judge, to overthrow the doctrine which ascribes the origin of animal heat solely to respiration. Chemistry teaches, it appears to me, a very different doctrine from that which makes the lungs a heating furnace—the calorific focus of the whole body. Ought not the abundance of water and carbon which take the gaseous form in the respiratory act, to cause a perpetual refrigeration to go on in the lungs during life? Transpiration by the skin, or evaporation, performs a similar function—these ceasing at the moment of death ; and for an indefinite, often short period, heat reveals itself, until dissipated by the antagonism of the surrounding temperature," etc.

The reader will excuse the insertion of the following document having the same date, seeing that its pathological import deserves more or less consideration, and not the less so, because its postulates at the time it was written were adverse to the then universally accepted theory of animal heat or "pulmonary combustion," concerning which writers are now beginning to speak doubtingly and even adversely, denying it altogether.

"If we suppose the central, the great vital organs to be as hot during life as they are found to be soon after death, the only wonder is that vitality should maintain its seat for a week or more, under the positive changes that ought, by every law of caloric, to take place in the molecular arrangement of the tissues. Let us suppose the brain in life to become as hot as the thigh is found to be after death, that is 14 deg. or 15 deg. above health ; the cerebral mass to expand faster than its cranial walls ; the fluids would dilate, and perhaps transude ; compression would be the consequence, attended with convulsions, coma, and other effects incompatible with life. Suppose any other organ should become such a focus of morbid caloric only for a moment, would not each vessel from dilatation lose its

healthy elasticity and cohesion, and thus pave the way to sanguineous congestion.　In some diseases, the lesions will afford an average
alteration as great as fatal gun-shot wounds ; as, for example,
dysentery, consumption, cancer.　But in a fever how much is unexplained !　Is not morbid caloric the agent that eludes the knife of
the anatomist ?　To say nothing of its directly poisonous, let us
consider its mechanical effects, as above mentioned, upon the brain.
After dilating its delicate vessels, and establishing a sanguineous
congestion, death follows.　The brain, as we have shown, falls sooner
than other central parts under the law of refrigeration ; the cranium
contracts ; this tremendous force drives the blood down from the
brain towards the warmer and more yielding centres of the trunk ;
perhaps a real apoplexy, without rupture, has disappeared.　The
febrile subject offers many instances of great vascularity of the
vessels of the pia mater, without turgescency ; the veins especially,
are found empty, but flattened as if by pressure.　There can be no
doubt that in the living, as well as in the dead body, foci of caloricity
establish themselves in particular parts, sending off, not always in
right lines, but in deflected currents, morbid heat to certain organs,
passing by others.　Thus the epigastrium and axilla may stand
charged with a positive heat of 109 deg., while the organs of that
part of the chest lying between these points shall be in a negative,
or much lower state of temperature.　I could muster serried columns
of facts illustrative of some other points, but I must omit them
altogether.

"So far as morbid heat can be identified as a cause of disease, we
deal with a positive, not an imaginary agent, where the ground is
not eternally slipping from beneath our feet.　Albumen, which
abounds in the brain and fluids, coagulates at 160 deg. ; hematosine,
the coloring matter of the blood, at 149 deg. ; and moderate increase
of heat vastly augments the solvent powers of the serum over gelatine, so abundant in the body.　The phosphorus in the body, were it
uncombined, would burn in a heat less than 113 deg.*

"Admitting that the whole body be permeated with 10 deg. or 15
deg. of heat, and that it cannot render this heat latent, I ask again,
is it wonderful that death should ensue ?　Which atom has not
undergone a deleterious modification, or a new arrangement in its

---

* William Hewson says : "I think it probable that the precise degree at which the lymph of the
human blood coagulates is between 114 and 120 deg." (Wks. p. 27, Sydenham ed.)

chemical, mechanical and vital laws and relations ?   'Delaroche and Berger prove that animals, in chambers heated to 120 deg. or 130 deg. Fah., have their temperature raised 11 deg. or 16 deg., and die speedily.' If, as some maintain, all lesions may be reduced to those of nutrition, caloric is an agent well adapted to play an important and fundamental part, not only diminishing the elementary cohesion of the tissues, but in debilitating all the organs, thereby favoring intertextural depositions, hypertrophies, softenings, hæmorrhagic, serous effusions, morbid secretions, engorgements, and other alterations, solid, liquid and gaseous.   The whole subject is still in a very unsatisfactory state.   I am very far from advocating the exclusive igneous pathology of fever."   Pp. 297, 298.

One of the most striking landmarks—not excepting structure itself—by which the animal kingdom is characterized, is that of the temperature of the economy, as in the hot and the cold-blooded—a distinction of the widest import.   Even in the diseases which the physician encounters, the temperature is of the utmost importance as indicative of their treatment.   Pyretic and apyretic coïncide for the most part with the sthenic and the asthenic, being indicative of the therapeutics of cold and heat.

The chemical physiologists maintain that animals " during hiber. nation burn up their fat, and come out of their winter's sleep emaciated, lank and lean.   This, so far as I have seen, is altogether visionary; it is certainly false as it applies to the alligator.   The very same theory is applied, as already mentioned, to the human subject during the process of starvation. Dr. Carpenter says, "death by *starvation*, is really death by *cold*" (Phys. 82); That is to say, when the fat is all burned up, cold and death are the results.   An animal already lean, though strong and muscular, would have no fuel, and would speedily die!   Although the physician seldom has an opportunity of witnessing actual starvation, yet, he has many opportunities of seeing in both civil and military practice, that lean muscular men maintain a high temperature, and great vital tenacity during hardship, exposure to cold, and under disease when food is either refused or not digested, or when deprived of food during campaigns, famine, shipwreck, etc.   Death by starvation on shipboard (concerning which not a few authentic narratives are extant, sometimes reported by medical men who had themselves been sufferers), shows that the burning up of the fat is not accompanied with this pretended decline of calorification, at least in the human subject, though of course, the fluids and solids must diminish including the fat, during the starving process.

The fat-theory, as accounting for the origin and perpetuation of animal heat, is visionary. If its presence cause animal heat, its absence causes it to be still more intense, which is not a paradox, but a plain contradiction.

The article *Abstinence*, of the National Cyclopædia (London, 1847), enumerates the calorific manifestations of the economy during starvation, as follows : " During the first two or three days the temperature is natural—subsequently the heat seldom sinks below the natural standard—finally the skin becomes intensely hot—delirium—coma," etc.

M. Londe, in the article *Abstinence* (Dict. de Méd. et de Chir., i., 104), refers to the terrible shipwreck of the *Méduse*, and to the authenticated narrative of the sufferers, given by M. Savigny, who was himself a sufferer on that occasion, who relates his own symptoms, as well as those of others who suffered and died of starvation. The furious delirium, and the monstrous crimes of his compatriots, are staggering to human belief. In his own case, to use a common expression, his blood boiled: " *mon sang* bouillonnait dans mes veines." In his general account of the symptoms which prevailed in others before death, he says : " *La perte du sommeil et l'influence permanente d'une chaleur brûlante me paraissant avoir en plus de part, encore que l'abstinence à la production des symptômes cerebraux.*" Here starvation is accompanied with a burning heat, " *chaleur brûlante !* " and yet this is called death from cold !

But it is time to return from this digression, to a few general remarks, with which this paper, already, perhaps too long for the reader's patience, must close.

Notwithstanding the contrast in temperatures of cold-blooded and hot-blooded animals, and also in the caloric which reigns in the inorganic world, yet all approximate more or less, and conduct themselves in an analogous manner.

Calorification, like consciousness, understanding, will, vitality, matter, and mind, is an original endowment inherent in man's constitution, the immediate cause of which is no more explicable by chemistry than man's color, form, size, altitude, the number of his toes, his appendix vermiformis, bearded women, or the colossal size of

California trees, gravitation, chemical affinity, epidemic diseases, or a thousand things which might be enumerated. But the conditions, phenomena, analogies, laws, and effects of animal heat are important objects of study, classification and practical use. Neither the creation of animals nor their primitive constitutional endowments have been fathomed by the sounding line of chemistry.

The most uncertain, not to say insane kind of philosophy is that which pretends to prove its way throughout the whole circle of the sciences, including intuitions, first principles, self-evident truths. Des Cartes himself was willing to take for granted his own existence, because he thought, " *cogito ergo* sum." Physiologists are obliged to admit primitive elements, self-evident functions, first principles, which chemistry cannot explain, either synthetically or analytically, among which is the temperature of the warm-blooded animals. For aught that has been proven to the contrary, physiology and chemistry are distinct and independent sciences. Notwithstanding their analogies and parallelisms, fundamental antitheses, differentiations, and peculiarities characterize each. As physiology cannot teach chemistry, neither can chemistry teach physiology.

Vitalism (the vis vitæ) or vitality is self-revealed, self-evident, and no more demonstrable by experiment, testimony or reasoning, than consciousness, mind, matter, space, duration. If physiology can claim any vital element or principle, the generation, with the maintenance of animal heat, takes precedence. If this be abandoned to physics or chemistry, chairs and books of physiology are misnomers, and ought to be suppressed without delay, or merged in chemistry.

ART. VIII.—*Antidotes to Serpent Poison.*

DR. DOWLER: In the March number of the Journal is a letter from Dr. S C. Young, on the subject of antidotes against the bites of poisonous serpents.

Dr. Young having read my communication in the January number, on the " Use of Tobacco as an Antidote for the Poison of the Rattlesnake," says he has long been acquainted with the popular notion of its usefulness in such cases, as well as of alcoholic stimulants, and inquires as to their *modus operandi* He seems, and with good reason, to consider this question the more pertinent, inasmuch as one is a powerful sedative, while the other is as great a stimulant. I regret exceedingly my not being able to answer satisfactorily the question proposed. But while this is the case, I am of opinion that we frequently stray from a path that might lead to a useful end in seeking to explain the *modus operandi* of a drug on account of any sedative, stimulant or other effect which it may be capable of producing upon the system. In the matter under consideration, I feel a great amount of confidence (founded somewhat, I confess, upon popular report) that tobacco and alcohol are the best remedies for the bites of poisonous reptiles with which I am acquainted. If the opinion can be proven, by subsequent experience a fact, it will be none the less valuable because one is a sedative and the other a stimulant ; for the truth is, we know very little of the action of but a very few drugs in our materia medica. Yet, of the power of many of them to control morbid conditions of the organism we have no doubt. How, for example, does quinine cure ague ? We do not know ; but if we could cure all other diseases as readily as we can the ague with quinine, we should have a column in our bills of mortality for "death from old age."

That tobacco would prove an antidote against the poison of venomous reptiles might have been inferred, analogically, from the *fact*, known to many persons that the very best remedy for the sting of a hornet, wasp or bee is the immediate application to the wound of a fresh quid of tobacco. This I have experienced time and again in my own person, and witnessed often in others. When applied within] a few moments after the sting has been inflicted the relief is almost *instantaneous*, and tumefaction of the part, in a great degree, is entirely prevented. Applying this *fact* to the solution of the question of the *modus operandi* in snake bite, the probable inference would be, that it neutralized, in some way, the poison. If it were worth the while to speculate as to the manner of its action, we might suppose it barely possible that it acted by means of its sedative property ; lessening the rapidity of absorption and causing the more gradual introduction of the poison into the blood. This supposition might be strengthend a little if we read a report of five cases of snake-bite, successfully treated by grain doses of arsenious acid in the Island of St. Lucie.* These doses were repeated frequently, until abundant vomiting and purging were produced—circumstances which were considered essential for its success. I need hardly say that here must have been a powerful sedative effect. We might also add, as regards alcohol, that the single fact of its being given usually in doses of at least a quart, *might* give slight grounds for the tenure of the opinion that absorption was prevented by that circumstance—the alcohol passing rapidly into the circulation, distending the blood vessels, preventing endosmotic action and absorption. But arrayed against these possibilities is the result of general observation, that neither the alcohol nor tobacco produces its ordinary effect ; that, and the effect of the reptile's poison seeming to be spent upon each other. Again, in so far as the antidotal properties of tobacco are concerned, another obstacle to the view thought possible presents itself in the fact, that the snake-poison produces the most alarming sedative effect, which is relieved or prevented by the tobacco—a powerful sedative. Indeed, we should expect a homœopathist to select it as the proper antidote, in accordance with his principle, " *Similia similibus curantur.*"

Dr. Young asks, also, an explanation of the circumstance that hogs are not harmed by the rattle snake bite, and asks if there is any principle in fat which neutralizes it. The following explanation has always been the one I have given myself : The hog has a very thick skin which is lined with a fleece of fat ; both are traversed by a very small number of blood vessels and absorbents, which would render the absorption at least very slow, if taking place at all.

Very respectfully,

HUMPHREY PEAKE, M. D.

YAZOO CITY, Mississippi, March 17, 1860.

---

* Vide Braithwaite, vol. xxviii, p. 423.

48

PROGRESS OF MEDICINE.

Art. I.—*On Oxygen as a Therapeutic Agent:* By S. B. Birch, M. D.
Read at the Twenty-seventh Annual Meeting of the British Medical Association (held in Liverpool, July 27th, 28th, and 29th, 1859).

The gradually increasing interest which I now find existent in the
profession, with regard to oxygen as a therapeutic agent, induces me
to believe that a communication on this subject may not prove unacceptable at this our annual meeting, particularly if the paper offered
be rendered as practically useful as possible.

Somewhat discouraged by much opposition, passive and active, I
have thus far permitted myself to remain comparatively isolated.
No doubt this has been a grave fault ; yet even now I come forward
with considerable diffidence, and can only hope that due allowance
will be made for imperfections, and any savor of egotism, to a certain extent unavoidable in a position almost unsupported. Long
silence, since I first introduced the subject in the pages of the *Lancet*, may have conveyed the impression that untenable ground was
about to be quietly evacuated. It is desirable, therefore, to enter a
caveat against any such possible assumption, and to give an assurance that (far from entertaining such an intention) the further my
clinical experience of oxygen advances, the greater does its value as
a remedy in intractable disease appear, and the more does the conviction obtain, that ultimately it must be acknowledged as one of our
most approved resources, failing ordinary treatment. Had I, however, been premature, where would have been my collection of facts ?
where my practical knowledge of the subject ? where the basis upon
which I could venture to form an opinion adverse to general
authority ?

A few of my professional brethren in different localities have latterly been induced to promise a fair trial in suitable and carefully
selected cases in private practice ; but to arrive thus at fair results,
will be the work of time in the hands of gentlemen in extensive general practice, who can hardly, amidst their laborious daily duties,
afford the necessary amount of time which a proper trial, entailing
close watching and daily observation, necessitates. Indeed, I almost
feel certain that extended, patient, and impartial trials in several
large hospitals, will be needed, in order to satisfy the professional
mind of the true place which this gas ought to occupy in our materia
medica, and of the necessity of precise rules in exhibiting it.

It may seem presumptuous to imagine that I may succeed where
Drs. Beddoes, Hill, and Thornton (although eminently successful in
their own practice), left no permanent impression ; where hospital
experimenters are reported to have always failed ; where authorities
in general are decidedly adverse. But duty and *esprit de corps* must
urge each of us to promote truth to the utmost of our ability, and
to endeavor to extend beyond our own limited sphere of practice any

assumed improvement in therapeutics. Previously to adducing facts within my own cognizance, it will be right to show that, even ignoring clinical evidence altogether, chemical and physiological experiments are sufficiently conflicting to warrant the medical practitioner in regarding the question of the therapeutic value of oxygen (beyond atmospheric proportions) as *adhuc sub judice*. A very brief outline of the main results hitherto obtained from experimental research may not be *mal à propos*.

In 1807–8, Messrs. Allen and Pepys apparently established the following : 1. That, however much oxygen was inspired in a given time, the carbonic acid evolved, and the oxygen actually entering into chemical combination with the constituents of the blood, underwent so very small an increase, as practically to nullify the idea that even the pure gas could prove useful as a medicinal agent. 2. That the disappearance of an extra amount of oxygen was simply consequent upon its temporarily taking the place of nitrogen as the residuum in the lungs.

Fortified by general opinion, and by such amusing jokes as that of Sir Humphry Davy and his thermometer cure, men of science almost rested on their oars (it would seem), until MM. Regnault and Reiset issued their beautiful series of experiments, with the view to prove that quantity and quality of food, exercise, etc., in a great measure regulate the amount and relative proportions of oxygen absorbed, and carbon given out by the system.

In the *British and Foreign Medico-Chirurgical Review* for 1856, Dr. Harley, reviewing the writings of Magnus, Liebig, and Lebemann on respiration, and adducing his own experiments, concludes that time and temperature are agents which modify the absorption of oxygen, and the chemical changes resulting therefrom.

Dr. Edward Smith has lately carried this matter somewhat further, and in his laborious and admirably conducted investigations, has shown that no experiments can be relied on which do not extend over considerable periods, and which do not include all the variations of diet, exercise, rest, temperature, sunlight, and darkness, to which the animal economy may be subjected during the twenty-four hours.

The late Dr. Snow found that the presence of carbonic acid in atmospheric air acted more deleteriously in proportion as the normal quantity of oxygen had been reduced, and that oxygen being added to atmospheric air surcharged with carbonic acid, renders it respirable for a while, and capable of supporting life. A little practice will enable most of us with little inconvenience to hold the breath for several minutes after taking an inspiration of pure oxygen—a tolerable proof that oxygen may be absorbed, while the exhalation of carbonic acid (except by the skin) is suspended.

Dr. Gairdner's experiments on rabbits go to prove that the inhalation of pure oxygen increases the fibrine and diminishes the corpuscles and albumen of the blood.

Dr. B. W. Richardson, following out this idea, in his admirable work on the *Cause of the Coagulation of the Blood*, details some experiments proving that a condition of hyperinosis, with tough fibrinous concretions in the blood, is induced by prolonged inhalations of pure oxygen.

Mr. Savory, *On Animal Heat*, states that he has found the temperature to be lowered, not increased, by an extra amount of oxygen. My own experience, however, tends to the conclusion that, in healthy, well-fed animals, the animal heat is usually first increased, then lowered; while clinical observation has afforded satisfactory evidence that oxygen, when employed in disease, will raise or lower the temperature *under different circumstances.*

Lastly, I would draw special attention to the highly interesting experiments of Mr. Erichsen, detailed in his monograph on *Asphyxia.* He says: "In a considerable number of experiments that I have performed on this subject, I have never succeeded in reëxciting the contractions of the ventricles by means of the inflation of the lungs with common air, provided they had fairly ceased to act before artificial respiration was set up." He was then led to try oxygen, and in several experiments was successful in restoring the action of the ventricles after the entire cessation of the heart's action.

It would be tedious, and needlessly taking up valuable time, to give more than an epitome of such facts. To comment upon them, *in extenso*, would at present be equally injudicious. I simply wish to intimate that physiology certainly does not negative oxygen in a therapeutic point of view. With a few remarks, as brief as possible, I will pass on to the purely practical portion of this paper.

When we reflect on the acknowledged difficulties and trouble, and probably many fallacies, attendant upon tedious and lengthened experiments; when these are associated with at least uncertainty regarding facts based on chemical researches; when our still imperfect knowledge of animal chemistry in connection with the vital dynamics and the generation of nervous force is taken into due account; when the fact stands forth that we can, if we please, by means of pure oxygen, indúce a state of hyperarterialization and hypernosis; when, further, Mr. Erichsen's experiments are brought into the field of mental vision; it must be acknowledged, that the *dicta* of even the most accomplished chemico-physiologists as to the uselessness of oxygen in medical practice, ought to be received with extreme caution. Then, add to this the recent views put forth by Prof. Schönbein, which a few weeks ago were made the subject of an interesting lecture by Dr. Faraday at the Royal Institution, and the therapeutic question becomes of still deeper import. It may now be fairly inferred that oxygen can exist in no fewer than three allotropic conditions—ozonic, antozonic, and neutral; the two former even possessing the power of assuming opposite polarities with regard to each other. This interesting discovery is highly suggestive, and opens out a new field for observation and investigation, which, it is earnestly hoped, may assist to elucidate this at present obscure inquiry as to the cause of the frequently unquestionable potency of oxygen, when employed in suitable cases *in very small quantity beyond atmospheric proportion.*

Without risking shipwreck upon an obvious yet somewhat vague hypothesis, nearly allied to that so energetically proffered by that acute old physician, Dr. Stephens, but partially illuminated by the discovery of Schönbein, I will here simply trust that sufficient obscurity and doubt exist in the scientific world, on this interesting subject, to afford ample apology for my differing from authority, while on the present occasion I deviate but very slightly from the practical experience of the clinical observer.

Whatever be the true *modus operandi* of small doses of oxygen (irrespective of the purest atmospheric air), when judiciously exhibited, in many intractable forms of disease, abundant evidence can be brought forward to prove beyond moral doubt that, in certain lowered conditions of the vital forces, this gas cannot unfrequently exercise an alterative and tonic influence upon the entire animal economy, which no other medicinal agent at present known can exert. And further, waiving the therapeutic question, instances will from time to time present themselves, during extended employment of oxygen in practice, where certain unexpected, curious, and sometimes unpleasant and serious effects, will so immediately and decidedly manifest themselves as to render it impossible for even the most incredulous observer to impute, *post hoc ergo propter hoc*, expectancy, etc., without ignoring truth altogether.

One mode of casual and limited investigation, for the purpose of testing its action on the system, has often struck me as a fruitful source of error ; viz : impulsive trials made by my professional brethren upon themselves and their friends, *in a state of health*, or at least where there is absence of any actual disease requiring its use, or of that susceptible condition occasionally met with, through disease or natural temperament, in which a *nidus*, as it were, is presented for the exhibition of abnormal sensitiveness to the action of the gas. Now, oxygen seldom evidences its special influence to any marked extent in persons enjoying perfect health, although rare exceptions are met with ; and perhaps it may not be amiss here to add *en passant*, that this fact ought not to be lost sight of, when considering the therapeutic relations of oxygen in derangements of the animal frame. Be it understood, also, that my advocacy of oxygen is exclusively confined to disease otherwise incurable, imminently dangerous, or very intractable.

In employing oxygen in different diseased conditions, it appears necessary to regard its action from two aspects : 1. The alterative and tonic influence which it can exert on the nervous system (apparently irrespective of immediate chemical action *per se*, in the ordinary acceptation of the term), when exhibited in very small doses, and for a very limited period daily. 2. The augmented activity of the normal chemical changes in the animal organism directly induced by bringing a largely increased proportion of the gas in contact with the pulmonary cells ; the duration and frequency of the inhalation being, in this case, an important consideration.

So far as relates to the first suggestion, I have, as before stated, had ample opportunities of observing that oxygen can in many susceptible temperaments, and in certain diseased conditions, exercise a peculiarly powerful influence, rarely met with in persons enjoying perfect health ; and, by taking advantage of this peculiarity, many cases will quickly undergo a change for the better, where the most enlightened and judicious treatment had previously failed to produce any beneficial effect. In such instances, the gas ought to be used with great caution ; for I have known serious and unpleasant (not to say alarming) symptoms arise from what would usually be regarded as a ridiculously small per centage added to atmospheric air. Most of these examples have occurred in sensitive nervous systems— in individuals possessing a very susceptible nervous organization ; or otherwise in those affected with lesions of the brain or spine, from disease or injuries. Fanciful imagination, hysteria, *et hoc genus omne*, may very naturally create misgivings in the minds of those who have not personally witnessed such phenomena. Willingly do we grant a liberal discount to the incredulous, while we add that several of the best exemplifications have presented themselves in men of powerful frames, ignorant of the increase or diminution of the doses that they were being subjected to, and not only devoid of all apprehension of the treatment, but in the highest degree surprised that "a little more pure air" could exert such a perceptible action on the system. The principal symptoms of a disagreeable character, here referred to as occasionally resulting from extremely small doses, are, a sense of constriction of forehead and temples ; a feeling of weight over the center of the parietal bones, and in the occiput ; a rush of blood to the head ; fulness, pain, or oppressive sensation in the nape of the neck and base of the brain ; sudden faintness ; palpitation of the heart ; spasmodic contraction of the affected parts, *e. g.*, violent reflex movements in extremities affected with paralysis of voluntary motion. Moreover, I have seen, on two or three occasions, a state of unnatural excitement of the entire nervous and vascular systems, which has continued for several successive days after one moderate dose. The chief symptoms of a disturbing character observed from pushing very large doses of the gas are, in thin, anæmic persons, sudden or gradual disappearance of pulse, pallor of countenance, coldness and partial collapse ; in the plethoric and sanguineous, the reverse—viz : too excited circulation ; full, bounding pulse ; intense heat of head, face, and skin ; severe, oppressive headache. I have also known the frequent and long continued exhibition of it, when not duly superintended, cause much emaciation.

For individuals, however, to be obnoxious to the extremes of the foregoing symptoms, is only occasional.

On the other hand, certain beneficial effects of oxygen may be mentioned as not unfrequently immediate and well marked, where due judgment has been exercised in selecting cases, and in directing the doses and duration of the inhalation. Such are, complete relief from excessive oppression of the brain ; sight improved in defective vision consequent on venous congestion ; general warmth, even to the ends of the toes and fingers, succeeding to extreme chilliness and collapsed condition ; sudden departure of great nervous depression ; permanent relief afforded to the uterus, ovaries and spine, by sudden induction of long suppressed catamenia, particularly at the change of life ; unexpected diarrhœa, of highly offensive character, with dark inspissated bile, in long continued torpor of the liver and portal system ; cutaneous transpiration suddenly and freely produced. To guard against any possible misapprehension from dwelling upon these special and important points, it must be distinctly understood that, in very many cases, the beneficial alteration effected by oxygen takes place with no characteristic signs of action perceptible to the patient, or even to the practitioner, except general improvement in the constitution, such as may be observed in many debilitated frames undergoing a mild course of chalybeates. Speaking generally, there will be found, in suitable subjects for the treatment, improved appetite and powers of digestion and assimilation, a feeling of being much more " up to the mark," less lassitude, more ability to bear physical exertion, and (that to sex not less so) a clearer, fairer, and softer skin.

The semeiological and pathological indications for the employment of oxygen, with a view to cure or palliation, must next receive some general consideration ; and afterwards will follow certain points contraindicating its use.

The deviations from health in which it will be found most beneficial are those where there has been no very considerable reduction of what may be called intrinsic vital power. Depression or oppression may be extreme ; the nervous and vascular systems may be incapable of receiving more than temporary tone or stimulation by means of ordinary tonics, stimulants, and attention to the best sanitary and dietetic rules ; but, as a rule, there must not be present that permanently lowered condition induced by long continued, insidiously undermining nervous debility (so well known to us all), which, having become almost a second nature, has incapacitated the system for " making life" beyond such amount as is absolutely essential for the maintainance of Psyche in her terrestrial abode.

In some constitutions, with blue noses, congested conjunctivæ and scleroticæ, semi-stertorous breathing on the slightest exertion, hæmorrhoids, etc., all vividly depicting to the mind the internal state of matters—each dose will often cause a slow, labored, full, but very compressible pulse, to become quicker, firmer smaller. In others, with a small, weak, quick, and even irregular pulse (in the absence of much excitement with hyperæsthesia), the quick conversation into a slower, fuller, and firmer pulsation, is sometimes equally well marked. Examples of each (modified, of course, as to rapidity of production and duration of effect) have frequently occurred in my practice.

The diseases *par excellence* in which the gas has afforded me the most gratification are those attended with either local or general venous congestion—a preponderance of the venous over the arterial, and torpidity of the capillary circulation. The good effects have been, as a rule, most decided in persons of a gouty or strumous habit, or otherwise in a state of general *malaise*, with sluggish circulation, either constitutional or superinduced by an atonic and oppressed condition through over-feeding and other luxurious or indolent habits, so prevalent in these artificial days.

The organs which, specially affected, experience the most immediate and sensible advantage from oxygen, are the brain, lungs, liver, and spleen, including the entire portal and mesenteric system, and uterus and ovaries.

In plethoric habits, with chronic local or general congestion interfering with the functions of one or more of these organs, the commencement of the curative process has sometimes been ushered in by sudden and unexpected efforts of nature to throw out peccant matters—efforts for so long a period previously unattainable through the most judicious treatment, and so immediately following two or three large doses of the gas, as to afford almost unquestionable evidence of true sequence. The assistance urgently demanded by the system has been given ; Nature has thus had a starting-point, and a critical discharge has made its appearance. It has been my fortune to see this exemplified in cases of long suppressed catamenia, in torpidity of hepatic functions with pent-up biliary secretion (as evidenced by sudden diarrhœa of most offensive character), and in gouty affections with much cerebral, nephritic, and other distress. In the last, I have known the urine, which had been for many weeks uniformly clear and limpid, become, to the horror of the patient, turbid, dense, and loaded with urates and phosphates.

I would venture particularly to draw attention to the ascendency of oxygen over the cutaneous capillaries, not unfrequently evidenced from the commencement of its use in torpid and unhealthy conditions of the cutaneous function, and cachexia arising therefrom. The benefit afforded will occasionally demonstrate itself in profuse perspiration, when a dry harsh skin had been previously the order of the day ; or a relaxed and moist state of the cutis, with constant chilliness and liability to colds, will give place to a warm, healthy, and comfortable state, to which the invalid had been long a stranger. With reference to extremes which occasionally present themselves, it may be added, although any prompt improvement or disappearance of certain eruptions, previously almost untouched by the treatment, will usually evidence the *suaviter in modo* as well as the *fortiter in re* operation of oxygen ; yet I have met with a few instances where ladies have been disagreeably surprised to find some slight but chronic eruption become very unsightly after a few days exhibition of the gas. To calm the female mind is not very easy under such circumstances ; but a bold assurance of the exacerbation being merely temporary—an effort of Nature to endeavor to rid the system altogether of the disease—has thus far not been falsified by the result.

Even inveterate skin-affections, the history of which points to a congenital origin, and incurable in the permanent sense of the word, may nevertheless receive much benefit from an occasional resort to this remedial agency.

Rapidly spreading ulceration, with sloughing nearly allied to gangrene, has, under my observation, been suspended solely through the influence of oxygen in a few liberal doses. A similar result has followed its employment in malignant anthrax, the most serious symptoms being brought under permanent subordination. And, indeed, I firmly believe, with oxygen as an adjunct, surgeons might regard with much less dread the frequently alarming and even fatal supervention of erysipelas or gangrene in traumatic cases. Conjoined with proper sanitary measures and the usual treatment, abundant stimuli, beef-tea, cinchona, ammonia, etc., the inhalation of the gas might, in some cases of the worst description, prove the salvation of the patient. Perhaps this suggestion might not inaptly be extended to the notoriously fatal effects of badly located hospitals.

The space to which I must necessarily limit myself in this paper, will admit of little more than a glance at those pulmonary and cardiac affections, in which oxygen merits cautious, careful, and judicious trial. I will simply remark, that the palliative effects of oxygen have kept hopelessly phthisical subjects in comparative comfort and freedom from dyspnœa and exhausting cough, up to their dying hour ; while the necessity for opium and other sedatives has been very trifling, and comfortable sleep has been secured, *minus* any disagreeable feelings following the free use of medicines. I know a lady in London who, with fatty degeneration, and probably attenuation of the muscular walls, and enlargement of the cavity of the heart, has been kept alive for the last three years by a dose of oxygen almost daily. On many occasions, in this lady's case, the heart's action, capable of only partial and temporary restoration by brandy and other stimulants, has at once been restored by oxygen in large doses. She lives by exercising great care and avoiding physical exertion, to a certain extent enjoys life, yet cannot do for more than a few days successfully without the renovation afforded by the gas. Again, in asthma, there is a tolerable percentage of cases in which oxygen can either cure or greatly relieve. As a rule, the subjects most benefitted are those in which we can trace no congenital or hereditary predisposition, and where the disease owes much of its origin to chronic bronchitis or partial congestions and indurations of the pulmonary parenchyma.

As to conditions of the organism contraindicating the employment of oxygen, or in which it ought to be exhibited with extreme caution, no stringent rules can be offered. A few hints sufficiently suggestive to the professional enquirer, will alone be needed. *Du reste*, each case must be considered on its own merits.

Both functional and organic affections of the heart, when accompanied with much nervous and vascular excitement, will, as a rule, decidedly negative its use. With a constitutional predisposition to nervous hyperæsthesia, where the slightest causes derange the heart's action, in impulsive and sensitive temperaments, there seldom will be found much satisfaction from oxygen. This obtains especially in subjects who have been the victims of chronic functional derangements calculated to upset cerebro-spinal equilibrium, and to induce morbid sensitiveness. A grave distinction, however, should be drawn between rapid pulse thus almost constantly present, and that arising purely from the presence of disease. It seems almost superfluous to guard the educated practitioner against the use of the gas in acute inflammatory attacks and aneurismal tumors. I have already intimated that cases of long continued spanæmia, in which the *vis vitæ* or *vis medicatrix naturæ* has been slowly and assiduously undermined, would rarely confer any credit upon the practitioner who might be led to make the most earnest trial of oxygen. Indeed, in all chronic cases of extreme debility, with spanæmic condition

49

and imperfect digestion and assimilation, oxygen, if tried as a last resource, must be employed in very small doses. Large ones, even two or three, in such cases, will invariably tend to lower the vital powers, to increase the preëxisting coldness of skin and extremities, pallor, sallowness of countenance, and general lassitude; nor may a patient for many days recover from the effects of one large inhalation.

The following carefully noted clinical facts, which have from time to time came under my personal observation, will, I trust, assist to illustrate my position. They are by no means adduced as testimony of therapeutic success, but simply selected as indicative of the peculiar power to which oxygen may justifiably lay claim.

Case 1. Nearly three years ago, Captain M., long a sufferer from diabetes mellitus, consulted me as to the probability of oxygen proving serviceable in his case. He told me that he had consulted and been for a lengthened period under the care of the most eminent physicians in London and Paris; that he was becoming gradually weaker and thinner; and that forced residence abroad had been the only available means to prevent a rapid progress of the disease, which always became seriously aggravated whenever he remained in England. I advised a trial. In a few days, the harsh, dry, feverish condition of skin, so common in this affection, was removed; and the thirst, as well as dryness of mouth and fauces, were much less distressing. The treatment was continued scarcely three weeks, during which the most marked advantage was derived from it— great improvement in the general health, increase in weight and strength, and great diminution in quantity of urine. Unfortunately, I could not get any samples of the fluid. This gentleman expressed himself as being highly gratified, and then started for France. I have latterly observed his name several times in the public journals, but have had no opportunity of knowing his subsequent history.

Case 2. Miss D., in the last stage of phthisis pulmonalis with respiration from 30 to 40 per minute, pulse 120 to 135, with profuse purulent expectoration, and every two or three days considerable hæmorrhage, with alarmingly increased prostration, found instant relief to the urgent dyspnœa after the first dose of oxygen, which likewise produced a pleasant warmth, and removed the "feeling of sinking" within the chest. During the following night, hæmorrhage again took place; but the blood was more coagulated, and the chest was much relieved by it. No further hæmorrhagic attack occurred for three weeks. For five months I treated her, myself administering every dose for the first six weeks. Vomicæ from time to time opened suddenly, discharged their contents, and then apparently contracted and cicatrised. Improvement was extremely slow, but progressive, as long as she remained in my hands. Her friends then removed her, other practitioners assuring them that she never could recover. She then retrograded, and died six months afterwards.

I ought not to omit naming that the oxygen in one week restored her appetite, and removed her craving for liquids; that her weight (only 5 st. 5 lbs., while her height was 5 feet 5¼ inches) underwent no increase for four months and a half, but then in a single fortnight improved to the extent of two pounds and a half; and that she could at length walk several miles daily, with pleasure and advantage.

CASE 3. A gentleman's coachman came to me, laboring under extreme debility, with constant liability to profuse—alternately hot and cold—perspirations after the slightest exertion; yet compelled, from cutaneous relaxation, distressing chilliness, and icy-cold extremities, to wrap up in a thick great coat in warm weather. He said that he had for twelve months tried several of the principal London hospitals, but without the slightest benefit. He appeared to have no *special* malady, except dyspeptic symptoms and imperfect assimilation. The first dose of oxygen acted almost like a charm, and made him thoroughly and comfortably warm from head to foot, without perspiration. The next day, I found that it had been no transient effect. He took a dose daily for one week, ahd then, feeling himself quite well and up to his work, and not needing his extra clothing, ceased attendance. Unfortunately I forgot to take his name and residence before his somewhat sudden disappearance. Out of gratitude (being a gratuitous patient), he ought to have called again.

CASE 4. Mr. S., a well known Yorkshire gentleman of family and fortune, placed himself under my care three years and a half ago. He was sixty-two years of age; had suffered for several years from paraplegia of the lower extremities, from the loins downwards. In spite of treatment of every possible kind, the gradual diminution of motion and sensation continued. Under my advice, he determined to try a lengthened course of oxygen, in small doses. From the first, there was evidenced some gradual improvement, more decided for the first two months, scarcely perceptible afterwards; yet so firm of purpose and so patient was this gentleman, and so strongly did experience impress him with a feeling of hopelessness regarding his case, if this failed, that he steadily persisted with extreme small doses (depending solely upon it) for two years. He is now perfectly well.

CASE 5. Three years ago, Miss T., a patient of the late Dr. Thornton, who stated that her life was formerly saved by oxygen, inhaled the gas three times under my immediate direction. The result was peculiar and interesting. The first inhalation (six pints of oxygen in eighty of atmospheric air) raised the pulse in frequency, then caused it to become gradually slower and fuller. Towards the end of the administration the pulse again became quicker, and assumed a hard wiry character, the forehead at the same time feeling very slightly constricted. This last sensation passed away in two minutes. Next day this lady came for her second sitting, being much gratified with the agreeable feelings experienced ever since her inhalation of the day previous. She said she felt "two or three inches taller, and as though the nerves were elongated." This day the effects were nearly allied to those manifested before, but with the addition of a "curious fluttering" about the heart. For two days she did not appear. On the third day, she again visited me, and stated she had felt so unnaturally excited during the whole day after the last dose, that she thought it advisable to discontinue for a day or two. The unnatural (though not disagreeable) excitement had left, but she still felt " taller, and nerves elongated." Wishing further to satisfy myself, I now administered three pints in about fifty of atmospheric air. No immediate result of special moment followed, and I arranged for another visit in a few days. A week elapsed before my patient again called; and she then informed me she dare not at present take any more oxygen. Violent palpitation of the heart, with great excitement of the circulation, had supervened a few hours after taking the last dose, and had continued more or less for several days. She had only just recovered from this condition, after resorting to certain sedative measures which I had taken the precaution to recommend in case of absolute necessity.

Now this lady, it should be borne in mind, was entirely prepossessed in favor of the gas, and had no anticipation whatever of such unpleasant consequences. The first two doses had influenced her most beneficially; and the same gas had produced no such effects upon her sister, who had for ten days previously been inhaling daily with great advantage. Moreover, she had no tendency to cardiac affection, no functional derangement of uterus, and had comfortably transited the change of life.

CASE 6. Mr. S., of Waterford, who was for many months under my care, could take twelve pints without any special effect, except gradually increasing warmth and strength of pulse; but invariably the four pints succeeding the twelve would convert this warmth into profuse perspiration. To demonstrate that there could be no fallacy, I repeatedly tried minute doses, and even atmospheric air alone, without his knowledge, ensuring the precise conditions of physical exertion, etc., but no such result followed as with the larger quantity.

CASE 7 occurred in the person of a brother physician in London. He has kindly permitted me to use his name. Dr. C. H. Thompson, of Sussex Gardens, was seriously affected with partial amaurosis, which had resisted the best directed treatment, and had at length rendered him unable to employ the sense of vision for the most ordinary purposes; in fact, professionally, he was becoming almost *hors de combat.* He could only see the largest type in print, and could not read a very few successive lines of that without the greatest difficulty. Fearing total loss of vision from the progressive nature of this serious affection, which had even appeared to advance more rapidly in proportion to his improvement in general health under ordinary treatment, he was induced to request my advice as to the possibility of oxygen being serviceable. The exciting cause was clearly traced to extreme congestion and torpid action in the medulla oblongata, base of brain, and parts adjoining, implicating especially the origin of the optic nerves. To predisposing causes it is needless to refer. I acquiesced in, and indeed, urged, the propriety of immediately resorting to oxygen; but, for special reasons, advised an extremely cautious use of it; the maximum dose to be six pints in eighty pints of atmospheric air. This maximum dose was tolerated very well for the first few days; and a decided improvement in visions, in head-symptoms, and in feeling of strength, at once manifested itself. About ten days or a fortnight, however, after the first dose, this gentleman called upon me, and stated that he had been obliged to reduce the amount of his daily inhalation to the *minimum* which I had suggested, viz: two pints of the gas; yet he had still, a few hours after inhaling, experienced so much uneasiness of head, tremor, lassitude, and exhaustion, as to compel him to omit his inhalation the day before. He added, that to-day he decidedly felt better for the omission, and almost feared any further trial of the treatment, notwithstanding the steady improvement in vision. I explained that I had met with various eccentricities in the action of oxygen on susceptible individuals, earnestly encouraged him to proceed, but recommended a diminution in quantity, and an inhalation only on alternate days. When next I saw him, he informed me that this plan had proved successful, adding, as an example of the benefit he felt, that he had just read without difficulty a long letter—a feat which he had been unable to accomplish for months.

The other day I saw my former patient, after an interval of some months. He stated that, although vision was anything but perfect, he had found no retrogression from the *statu quo* following *first* improvement, which had been of a permanent character. Occasionally he takes, for two or three successive days, a minute quantity of the gas. This is borne very well ; but he cannot persevere longer without producing unpleasant symptoms, which will then arise from even one pint to seventy of atmospheric air.

I may remark, that several cases have occurred in my practice equally demonstrative of idiosyncrasy, yet indicative of a peculiarly alterative, cumulative, perhaps catalytic or electrolytic action on the part of oxygen in extremely small doses. May we not, without rendering ourselves obnoxious to an imputation of undue enthusiasm after a hobby, admit the probability of such an influence being employed wih permanent advantage in obstinate disease ? Is it not our duty to afford an unprejudiced, impartial and extended trial ?

The doses advisable in different cases, as well as the mode of administration, demand a few words of consideration before concluding. General rules only can be laid down ; but, since the axiom, "Nullum remedium quod non tempestivo usu tale fiat," attaches itself especially to oxygen, I will endeavor to be as lucid as possible.

In speaking of small doses, a range is implied of from 2 to 12 per cent. of the gas in a given amount of atmospheric air. Large doses are signified by a *minimum* of 12 per cent., ascending to the *maximum* of pure gas. It is rarely, however, that I use it undiluted. Nine to twelve pints of the pure gas, diluted with about seventy-five pints of atmospheric air, may be stated as a fair medium dose. The inhalation of this quantity should, *mutatis mutandis*, extend over a period of fully half an hour ; and, in the majority of cases to which it is applicable, no inconvenience will be occasioned. The time to be occupied in inhaling a given quantity demands quite as much vigilance and judgment on the part of the medical attendant, as the prescription of a dose. As a rule debilitated and anæmic subjects will not tolerate a lengthened sitting, and then will only bear very small doses ; while the plethoric and congested will receive but an infinitesimal amount of benefit, unless they are compelled to expend a full hour on each occasion. Of the latter class, some will need thirty or forty pints of oxygen (diluted according to circumstances) during the hour ; others will experience unpleasant effects from sixteen pints. Everything, in fact, depends upon the greatest attention to minute details in management, presuming, of course, that proper judgment has been exercised in selecting the case. If the practitioner desire success from the use of the gas in very bad cases, he must not lose sight of either point. Above all, he must carefully superintend, and in many instances himself administer and anxiously watch throughout the inhalation.

And now, gentlemen, it is incumbent on me to draw your attention to a fact which doubtless is known to some, but perhaps to few, viz: that the mechanical difficulties which formerly militated against any extensive trial of this remedial agency no longer exist. The mechanical means to which I would refer, and by the assistance of which oxygen may be used with perfect facility, are an apparatus, and condensed gas supplied by Mr. Barth, 217 Piccadilly, London. Any gentleman in the profession by simply writing to him, could by the next train receive supplies, with every requisite information as to their manipulation. In private practice, this plan is undoubtedly the least troublesome, and almost as economical as for the practitioner to employ a druggist, or prepare the gas himself (of course, uncondensed). It likewise insures purity, which is an important consideration; for the patentee has informed me that there are only two or three manufacturers of pure chlorate of potash in the kingdom; and that he has frequently had to return large quantities, too impure for the purpose, though sent by eminent firms. The authorities of large hospitals, who would naturally prepare their own gas, should note this point.

In conclusion, permit me to observe, that it has been my wish carefully to avoid hypothesis, and any undue parade of success, while I have endeavored to preserve the simple position of the impartial and careful clinical observer, appealing to an experience of some years duration, almost exclusively gained by experiments, and trials in diseases either intractable or incurable. The animal organism, though no doubt subject to certain laws of chemistry, is amenable to higher laws than those practically known in the laboratory. A physician if he see the sudden change of a pathological condition—a long continued unpleasant entity—must accept the fact, notwithstanding that the *rationale* be unascertained by the chemist. Certain observed effects become the basis of a law. Opium causes sleep; aloes purges; antimony is diaphoretic. May not oxygen claim admission into the list of our therapeutic agents? Splendid as are the achievements of chemistry, there is a boundary beyond which it cannot pass; yet every medical practitioner knows that he must cross this Rubicon every day in practice.

Not deeming myself competent to undertake an extensive series of chemical analysis, it would be presumptuous to present any such crude experiments of my own, in opposition to accomplished chemical analysts. I venture to hope that, by bringing the subject (however imperfectly) forward, I may enlist the coöperation of gentlemen well versed in chemico-physiological investigation, and derive mental profits from their further researches. A second and not less weighty consideration urges me to trust that so much interest may be created in the minds of practitioners generally as to induce extended and fair trials.—*British Med. Jour.*

ART. II.—*Yellow Fever of Lisbon in* 1857.

[DR. R. D. LYONS, who went voluntarily to Lisbon to investigate the nature of this epidemic, presented to both houses of Parliament, by command of Her Majesty, a report of one hundred and twenty-seven pages upon the same. The British and Foreign Medico-Chirurgical Review (Jan., 1860), in a commendatory notice of this work, gives sundry statements from this report, among which are the following :]

That the epidemic was true yellow fever, is shown by the author in the clearest manner ; indeed, so well marked were its symptoms that there was no room for question respecting its nature. The first cases of it occurred on the 19th of September, the last early in January. During this period, according to the most reliable returns, between 16,000 and 17,000 of the population of the city were attacked—about 1 in 12·125 of the whole—of whom about 5,500 died— one in three—which is near the average mortality from the disease as it has occurred at different times in the West Indies, the Continent of America, and the south of Europe. Though the disease was generally considered to have been imported and contagious, and this not only by the people at large, but by many of the educated class, and by many respectable members of the medical faculty ; yet the author sought in vain for satisfactory proof ; all his inquiries had negative results. His words deserve to be quoted.

Dr. Lyons enumerates as causes of insalubrity of the city, a lack of water, deficient sewerage, badly constructed houses, etc. Upon this subject the reviewer says :

These local circumstances, so unfavorable to health, so favorable to the production of disease, and of such a disease as the dire one in question, on cursory consideration, may appear adequate to account for its origin ; but, if we keep in mind that all of them are of a persistent kind, liable to little variation from year to year, and yet the malady, as an epidemic, has been of rare occurrence, the last being only the third recorded, formally and by name, from the year 1191 to the present time, as having broken out in the Portuguese capital, we cannot be satisfied with this ætiology. The author, with great industry, has brought together a large amount of information respecting the climate of Lisbon in connection with the appearance of the epidemic. The results as expressed in tables, including most meteorological phenomena which can be measured by instruments and tests, are not without their value,.but they do not appear to throw any satisfactory light on the invasion of the disease. Little else is shown than that at the time it occurred, and whilst it lasted, the atmospheric temperature was a little above the average, and the degree of atmospheric moisture a little higher than usual, that following a fall of rain a little in, excess of the ordinary quantity. We express doubt in this matter, reflecting on the appearance of the disease at other seasons and in other countries, and under climatological conditions the opposite of those just referred to, especially in our West India colonies. One of the most severe epidemics there was that of 1847–48, in Barbadoes, where it broke out without any grounds for supposing that it was imported, and was entirely confined to the garrison, which was in constant communication with the town, and this at the coolest season of the year, and when the weather was very agreeable, and it might be supposed favorable to health. In seeking for causes, especially of diseases, how much caution is required! If the inductive method is needed in one inquiry more than another, it is surely in this, in which the imagination is so apt to overpower the reason, and amidst the panic of dread any plausible circumstance is likely to be seized on as the *causa mali*. At present we are of opinion that, on the inductive plan, the only conclusion we can arrive at is, that we are ignorant of the immediate cause of the disease, and that our sound knowledge is limited to the conditions, such as those described by the author, conducing to its production ; conditions of the first importance, insomuch that, if corrected or removed, the great probability is the public health will be secured. In justice to Dr. Lyons, we must say that the caution we hold to be necessary, has been observed by him, he having pointedly forborne fixing on any one cause, or combination of causes, excepting as auxiliary, for the origin of the epidemic. As in most other epidemics, the disease exhibited many varieties. The most characteristic of these, according to Dr. Lyons, were the following : 1. The algid form. 2. The sthenic. 3. The hæmorrhagic. 4. The purpuric. 5. The typhus form.

Under the head of general phenomena common to all the forms, the following are described as worthy of note : 1. A constipated state of bowels, which the author considers peculiar to the inhabitants of Lisbon. 2. In some cases an almost complete suppression of urine, whilst in others it was normal and abundant—normal in specific gravity and reaction ; in others loaded with lithates; in others coagulated by heat and nitric acid ; and was occasionally brownish-red, smoke-colored, or variously tinged, from more or less admixture of blood elements and of bile. The suppression of urine was confined to the algid cases ; the abundance of lithates and other secretions to the sthenic cases ; the albuminous condition was not special to any one class—it was found more or less in all of them ; and the same remark applies to the presence of bile. 3. A swelling of one or other of the parotid glands, of an inflammatory kind, ending in suppuration, often exhausting and fatal.

On the treatment of yellow fever the author is very concise, having but little confidence in any of the very many modes hitherto tried. Quinine and bark, which were largely used, he thinks unfavorably of. From the reported efficacy of the former in the epidemics of British Guiana, the atmosphere of which is more or less malarious or productive of ague and remittent fever, we are disposed to have faith in it under similar climatic influences. As a palliative, the author reports favorably of the perchloride of iron in checking the hæmorrhagic tendency.

The deaths of males, it would appear, were nearly as two to one to those of the females. The mean age of those who died, calculated on two hundred and ten successive entries into the hospital, was 33·5571 years. Very few children under ten were attacked, and few old persons over seventy. The mean duration in hospital was six days ; of those cured, eight days ; of fatal cases, four days. The negro race were in a great measure exempt, seeming to enjoy their usual immunity from attack. In the worst quarters of the town the mortality was forty-two and forty-three per cent.; the mean mortality being about thirty-three per cent. of those attacked.

The immunity enjoyed by the shipping in the Tagus, notwithstanding the great and most constant intercourse with the town, is very remarkable. The author adds : I know of but one instance of a British seaman (master of a brig) having become a victim to the disease. The individual in question had been drinking on shore ; he died in the British Hospital.

THE YELLOW FEVER AT LISBON.—The municipality of Lisbon have had above two hundred silver medals struck, for the purpose of honoring the acts of devotion and charity manifested during the prevalence of yellow fever in that capital in 1857. They are to be distributed among those persons whose services were most eminent during the epidemic. On one face of the medal is an allegorical upright figure, symbolising the town of Lisbon; and on the other side is the legend, " To humane devotion," surrounded by a crown of oak. A diploma or certificate will accompany each medal. Pensions, not exceeding 200,000 *reis* (about £58), are also to be granted to medical men; priests, and other persons, who, after having distinguished themselves in the epidemics of 1853 and 1857, have become incapacitated from continuing their profession.—*Brit. Med. Jour.*

ART. III.—*The Ætiology and Treatment of Peritonitis:* By S. O. HABERSHON, M. D., London, F. R. C. P., Royal Medical and Chirurgical Society.

DR. HABERSHON first alluded to the value of a knowledge of the causes of disease as a guide to right treatment, and to the importance of considering local disease as connected with a constitutional or general origin. In reference to peritonitis, he remarked that, although written and spoken of as an idiopathic disease, we did not find any proof that the malady really existed in that character. An analysis of the records of 3,752 inspections after death at Guy's Hospital, and extending over a period of twenty-five years, was brought forward as confirming this statement, and as an indication of the general plans of treatment. Five hundred and one were instances of peritonitis, and they were divided—first, into those in which the disease is set up by mischief extending to the peritoneum from without, as from adjoining viscera, injury, or perforation ; secondly, those which might be called blood diseases, connected with albuminuria, with pyæmia, or puerperal fever or erysipelas ; and thirdly, those in which general nutritive change in the system is followed by acute or chronic peritonitis, as in struma or cancer, or after continued hyperæmia of the capillaries of the serous membrane, as in disease of the liver or heart, where very slight exciting cause suffices to produce acute mischief.

Of the *first* division, there were two hundred and sixty-six instances, and one hundred and two of these arose from internal or external hernia, or mechanical obstructions, nineteen being of the internal kind. Reference was made to the mode in which the extreme tension of the intestine leads to intense congestion of the mucous membrane, diphtheritic inflammation, and ulceration in the direction of greatest tension, leading to perforation in many cases. In thirty-five cases, peritonitis arose from injuries or operations directly affecting the serous membrane, and in fourteen had followed tapping ; this number was lower than might be expected. In fifty-six cases there was perforation of the intestine ; in ten from hernia, in nine of the appendix cæci, in two of the cæcum, four from cancerous disease of the colon, nine from disease of the stomach, fifteen from typhoid disease of the ileum, four from struma, two from ovarian adhesions, and one from cancerous disease of the vagina. In five other cases of fever, peritonitis had resulted, in two of which the perforation was not complete ; one was of doubtful character. In nineteen cases, fæcal abscess had taken place. In forty-two cases the peritonitis was caused by extension of disease from the bladder, uterus, or pelvic viscera ; ten from lithotomy, six from ovarian disease, and fourteen from calculus in the bladder, cystitis, or stricture. In eleven cases, disease of the liver or gall-bladder had led to direct extension of disease to the serous membrane, and in three other cases it followed acute inflammatory disease of the colon, and from disease of the cæcum, not previously mentioned, in three instances. Thus two hundred and sixty-one cases of the five hundred and one were produced by disease not commencing in the serous membrane, but propagated to it from adjoining parts ; and the author stated that in each of these instances as far as medicinal treatment could be of service, he believed that the plan suggested by Drs. Stokes and Graves, in instances of perforation of the stomach, was of the greatest value in promoting rest to the intestines, the localization of the mischief, and the acceleration of reparative changes ; in many instances, that local depletion and the external application of anodyne remedies might be combined with advantage ; but that mercury, in the form of gray powder or calomel, with opium, was injurious rather than otherwise, as tending to prevent adhesions, exciting action from the bowels, or rendering their contents more fluid, and increasing the depressing effects of the disease on the nervous system.

The *second* class of cases consisted of those in which peritonitis was set up by a changed condition of the blood, as in albuminuria, pyæmia, etc. In sixty-three instances, the peritonitis was connected with Bright's disease, in nearly all of an acute kind. The peritoneum was rarely the only serous membrane affected. The treatment of the general disease was regarded as best calculated to remove the local affection, assisted sometimes by counterirritants ; but that the ready salivation produced by mercurials did not afford corresponding benefits. Ten were puerperal in their origin ; in thirteen, pyæmia followed operations, local suppuration ; and five others were with erysipelas. Instances were alluded to in which serous membranes became simultaneously affected, perhaps from pyæmia or rheumatism, or renal disease ; and three of those were mentioned, one where peritonitis was connected with pericarditis and pleurisy, a second with pneumonia and dysentery, and a third with pericarditis, pleuropneumonia, and obscure renal mischief. In the treatment of these cases, the local affection must be almost lost sight of in the general treatment, and local depletion and mercurial preparations would not promote the cure.

The *third* class of peritonitis consisted of cases connected with general nutritive changes, as cancer, struma, etc., or where, with continued hyperæmia of the peritoneal capillaries in cirrhosis, or heart disease, a very slight exciting cause suffices to produce acute disease. Seventy cases rose with struma ; twenty-two acute and forty-eight chronic and acute. The varieties of the strumous form of disease were mentioned, leading sometimes to serous effusions, to general adhesions, to perforation, or fæcal abscess. The ages were stated not to be limited to early life, many occurring between thirty and forty years of age. It was urged that in all these cases the same general rules of treatment should be observed as in ordinary strumous disease, sometimes assisted by counterirritants, very cautious local depletion, anodyne applications, and opium ; but the avoidance of purgatives and of mercurial preparations was recommended. Forty instances of peritonitis with cancer, besides those already mentioned, were next referred to ; nine in males and thirty-one in females. In men, glandular organs were generally affected ; and in women, the ovaries or uterus ; but, in twenty instances, the disease consisted of tubercles upon the peritoneum, generally with dropsical effusion ; nineteen of these were women, and one a man ; the average age of the former fifty-two, and evidently coming on after the cessation of ovarian functional activity. The inutility of diuretics, and the inadvisability of depressing measures, as mercurials were spoken of ; and it was stated that paracentesis was often followed by increased effusion of lymph, and the best treatment consisted in sustaining the ebbing powers of life by every means in our power.

The *last* cases were those of peritonitis associated with hepatic or heart disease. In thirty-two of the hepatic complication, fourteen were chronic, twelve acute, and six acute and chronic ; five had been previously referred to as rendered acute by tapping. In some instances pneumonia was present, and slight exposures to cold and wet evidently sufficed to induce acute changes. The degenerative arterial changes often found with cirrhosis were mentioned ; this chronic state should be borne in mind in the treatment of the acute disease. In early cirrhosis, the usual treatment of peritonitis by calomel and opium was more serviceable than in any other form of peritoneal disease, on account of the stimulating effect of mercurials on the glandular organs of the abdomen ; but that even here it was not necessary to produce salivation to ensure the beneficial effects. Nine cases were connected with heart disease.

The general causes of peritonitis were :

Hernia (nineteen being internal)..	102
Injuries—operations, as tapping, etc...................................	35
Perforations of the stomach, ileum, cæcum, appendix, colon, etc. (Other 13 included under hernia, etc.) And leading to fæcal abscess (2 otherwise mentioned)............................	17
Ulceration, with fever, without perforation.............................	5
Disease of the bladder or pelvic viscera; operations, as lithotomy, etc..	42
Abscess of the liver, gall-stone, etc.......................................	11
Acute disease of the colon..	3
Other diseases of the cæcum..	3
	261

Bright's disease..	63
Pyæmia, puerperal fever, etc...	31
Strumous disease..	70
Cancer (12 before mentioned)..	40
Hepatic disease (and 5 acute, from tapping)........................	27
Heart disease..	9
	240

The author concluded with the following propositions :

1. Peritonitis is never idiopathic in its origin, and we do not find any such instance as acute disease of the peritoneum coming on from mere exposure to cold ; in such case, the cold tends to render acute an already existing morbid state.

2. The consideration of the origin of the disease, either in a local or general source, is the best guide to treatment ; whether—first, from extension of disease from adjoining viscera, as the ovaries,

bladder, intestines, perforations, or injuries ; secondly, from blood-changes, such as occur in albuminuria, pyæmia, or erysipelas ; and thirdly, from almost imperceptible changes, or deficiencies, in general health, as in struma, or cancer, or climacteric changes, or as a consequence of the hyperæmia of cirrhosis, or heart disease.

3. In the first form, perfect rest, the avoidance of food as far as possible, and the mode of treatment recommended by Dr. Stokes, in producing rest to the ˙intestinal canal and peristaltic action, and diminishing the collapse and prostration consequent on disease—constitute the best mode of treatment ; using, as far as need be, other means, as anodyne applications, local depletion ; and, in many instances, also˙ seeking to remove the exciting cause, as in˙ cystic disease, etc.

4. Where peritonitis is a symptom of blood-change, as Bright's disease, pyæmia, etc., it may be best relieved by the treatment of the primary disease ; but here opium is sometimes of great value, and more effective without mercurial combination.

5. In the treatment of the third class, the consideration of the cause is also our best guide ; strumous and cancerous disease should be regarded in their general relations ; and in those connected with hepatic disease, the remembrance of .the condition prior to the supervention of peritonitis should prevent us from using means calculated to increase the primary mischief ; and any benefit due to mercurial action may be attained without mercurial salivation.

6. In general, the benefit ascribed to mercury in the treatment of peritonitis, is not established, and may, perhaps, be correctly attributed to the opium with which it is combined.—*Brit. Med. Jour.*

ART. IV.—*Puerperal Fever—Dead-born Children.*

i. Puerperal Fever.—*A Contribution to the Microscopic Investigation of the Blood in Puerperal Fevers:* By D. SCHULTEN. (Virchow's Archiv., xiv, 5, 6. *The Pathological Anatomy of Puerperal Fever:* By BUHL. (Monatsschr. f. Geburtsk., July, 1859.)

1. DR. SCHULTEN has undertaken the difficult, but useful, task of tracing the influence of the poison of puerperal fever on the blood. The following is the case that gave rise to his researches. A strong woman, twenty-four years old, was taken thirty-six hours after her second labor with a violent shivering, followed by heat and profuse sweating. On the fourth day, renewed shivering, heat and sweat, after which restlessness and delirium ; face red, eyes glistening, speech quick. Pulse 140–145 ; abdomen painless on pressure, but somewhat distended. Lungs and heart free ; no enlargement of

liver or spleen ; great thirst, swimming in the head, anxiety. She had several doses of calomel, nitrate of soda, and was cupped. The symptoms became aggravated. She had quinine ; the pulse fell to 95–100 ; the shiverings ceased. Under the use of quinine recovery progressed.

The first examination of the blood was made three hours after being drawn. The cupping was performed four hours after the second shivering fit, before the use of any remedy. Before the serum had completely separated, a drop of blood was put under the microscope. The serum was a little turbid. The blood-globules were scanty. On the other hand, the whole field was covered with those little ball-like, yellow-colored corpuscles which are but seldom seen in healthy blood. Without forming *rouleaux*, they lay thickly together ; between these imbedded were white corpuscles, in great number and of various sizes ; but the smallest were scarcely half the size of the blood-corpuscles, whilst the largest were twice or three times the size.

Two days later, when the impetus of the fever had already remitted, a second blood-test was made. The serum was quite clear ; the blood-globules were of normal size, and formed sharp-outlined rouleaux.

White corpuscles were still frequent in bundles of 5–8 ; but their size was no longer various. Of blood-cells no more were to be seen. On the other hand, there appeared in the inside of most of the corpuscles small fatty vesicles, reflecting the reddish color of the surrounding fluid. Single white corpuscles appeared to have passed into fatty substance.

Three days later another sample was examined. A drop of serum showed a crowd of fat-globules of every size. White globules were not in greater abundance than in healthy blood. The blood-globules were normal, but had a tendency to shrivelling. After fourteen days, another examination of the blood and milk was made, to determine whether the child might be suckled without danger. Still there appeared single fat-globules, but nothing else abnormal could be found. Even the tendency in the blood-globules to shrivelling had ceased.

Analysing these observations, we discover two interesting appearances. First, the great increase of white corpuscles in the blood of a person before in health, in whom there was no indication of leukæmia. These could not be regarded as pus-globules. We are driven to conclude that, in this case, there was a special *disease of the normal white corpuscles of the blood*. Secondly, the appearance of fat-globules in the later tests, which, as they were wanting in the first examination, exhibited only traces in the interior of the white corpuscles in the second examination, and presented in abundance in the third examination, contemporaneously with disappearance of the white corpuscles, was probably the result of a change of the white corpuscles in the course of the disease. Schulten has recognized similar appearances in three out of four other cases in which he has repeated his examinations.

2. The practice of hospital lying-in, so prevalent abroad, supplies

an experience of childbed-fever on a scale which is fortunately impossible in this country. Dr. Buhl has the unhappy privilege of relating the autopsies of fifty patients who died in the Munich Hospital in the three years 1854 to beginning of 1858. He says there is one constant and characteristic appearance—a pulpy, dirty red or black-brown mass, which here and there has a mildewy, and here and there a putrid smell. This condition leaves no doubt that in it is to be found the starting-point of the development of puerperal fever. It is an infection disease, and the infecting poison lies in the inner wall of the uterus. On the cause of this putridity or decomposition we are not clear. Whether it be the immediate conveyance of a poison into the womb, or whether it be the preceding empoisonment of the blood by miasmata, which produces a secondary decomposition in the womb. In preventive or curative therapeia the distinction is important. There are two principal forms of the disease—1, puerperal pyæmia ; 2, puerperal peritonitis. These forms are clinically distinct in prognosis and in treatment. The usual terms, oophoritis, uterine croup, uterine dysentery, uterine putrescence, metrophlebitis, lymphangioitis, phlegmasia alba, and so on, may all be classed under the two heads named.

In the cases observed, *puerperal pyœmia* killed usually not before the ninth day, and sometimes even not under three weeks. It appeared most frequently when there was no epidemic—or, at least, but a slight epidemic ; and in eighteen of the fifty cases, the path of infection was the veins. The pyæmic form is characterized by not sequestrated, purulent plugs in the veins of the placental seat of the uterine walls, in one of the pampiniform plexuses, or in one of the spermatic veins. We never found both spermatic veins plugged ; and only once was the inferior vena cava filled with adherent coagula. In two cases (lasting three and six weeks), the pus in the vein-plexus was cheesy. The so-called metastatic deposits were found fresh in the lungs in one case, cheesy in one case. The pleuræ mostly exhibited ecchymoses. Three times purulent exudation was in the pleural cavity without pyæmic infarction of the lungs. The kidneys in one case showed purulent deposits ; and twice fructiform ecchymoses. In two cases there was hypopyon ; three times pus in joints ; and twice phlegmasia alba.

Puerperal peritonitis was more frequent, more violent, and killed more rapidly than pyæmia ; out of thirty-two cases, only two ended fatally, after six and eight weeks. There was always purulent exudation. In eighteen cases, pus was found in the Fallopian tubes of one or both sides ; fourteen times there was sub-serous pus in the uterus, especially in the vicinity of the neck ; also in the lumbar-glands. Disease of the veins has no relation to peritonitis. Peritonitis may be etiologically and anatomically discriminated—1. In cases in which through the direct passage of the poisonous material out of the womb through the tubes, peritonitis is set up ; and 2. In those cases in which, through the reception of the poison from the inner surface of the womb into the lymphatics, the peritonitis has been excited. Peritonitis through tubal-pus is much the more ready, purely and primitively inflammatory form ; the other, on the contrary, is the more severe, and occurs chiefly during epidemic diffusion. The principal changes observed were—œdema of the ovaries ; the spleen (ten times) enlarged ; liver always pale ; the kidneys pale ; the peritoneal exudation mostly in small quantity ; the intestinal walls mostly œdematous, their canal filled with gases and watery contents ; œdema of the lungs and hypostatic blood-filling ; twice fibrine on the pleura ; one, hydrothorax ; often pleural ecchymoses ; three times capillary bronchitis.

Pyæmia and peritonitis had the following properties in common : 1. An almost constant slight swelling and watery infiltration of the recto-peritoneal, inguinal, and mesenteric glands.   2. Osteophites in the inner table of the skull.   3. In most cases, especially in those of pyæmia and lymphatic resorption, a swelling of the capsules of the kidneys, and an acute stage of Bright's disease.

ii. *Some Observations on Dead-born Children:* By DR. AUGUST BREISKY, Assistant in the Lying-in Clinic at Prague. (Vierteljahrssch., 1859.)

Dr. Breisky's paper on dead-born children is a valuable contribution to a subject which, on many grounds, demands extended and careful investigations.   We will give first a condensation of his observations, and then a summary of his conclusions.

CASE 1.—*Prolapsus of the Funis : Aspiration of Liquor Amnii.*— A woman with a well-formed pelvis was in labor with her second child.   Head in first position ; a small knot of funis prolapsed within the thin membranes.   In endeavoring between pains to replace cord, pulsation was felt.   The indication was taken to be that the membranes should be ruptured to afford a better opportunity of replacing the funis and rescue the child from the threatened danger of interruption of the placental circulation.   The rupture of the membranes let out a great quantity of turbid fluid, much discolored with meconium.   The funis was carried down in a long loop ; it was pulseless.   The pains were strong, and a dead boy was born.   [We regret that we are unable from the author's history to fix the lapse of time from the cessation of the pulse in the cord to birth.—REP.] The *dissection* showed—paleness of the skin, with cyanosis of the face and extremities ; bloodvessels and heart cavities full of dark fluid blood ; atelectasis of the lungs ; the lower part of the trachea, the bronchi and their branches, as far as they could be followed, were filled with fine mucous, yellowish brown contents, which under microscope was determined to be a mixture of mucus, meconium, and liquor amnii.

CASE 2.—*Menconium in the air-passages.*—A woman with a roomy pelvis in labor at term.   Head presenting ; *funis not pralapsed.*   At 3·30, A. M., liquor amnii, discolored with meconium, ·escaped, and quickly thereafter a fully-developed girl was born.   *Dissection* showed—paleness and light cyanosis of the skin ; paleness and relaxation of the muscles; formation of skull normal; the kidneys without trace of uric acid infarction ; much dark blood in the large veins; both lungs atelectasic; the mucous membrane of nose, mouth, and laryngo-tracheal canal covered with a thin yellow layer ; the bronchi, down to the smallest ramifications, filled with a yellow mucous fluid, determined under the microscope to be meconium mingled with liquor amnii.

Case 3.—*Menconium in air-passages; slight dropsical effusion in serous cavities; intermeningeal extravasation; laceration of the left tentorium cerebelli..*—The dead child of a primipara, born after twenty hours' labor. Head lay in first position; the fœtal heart had been heard during labor; green-colored and somewhat offensive liquor amnii discharged; funis came down. *Dissection*—An unusually large child; skin pale, and slight cyanosis of face and extremities; the end of the funis discolored yellow; between the skull and pericranium were small extravasations; the sinuses were uninjured in their walls, and gave vent to dark fluid blood; the tentorium cerebelli on the left side was slightly torn; there were small, fresh ecchymoses near; brain and meninges full of blood, and infiltrated with watery fluid; the large veins of the neck, thorax, and abdomen filled with fluid, dark-red blood; the heart cavities also contained dark blood; in the pericardium, pleuræ, and in peritoneum, was some clear, bright yellow serum; the lungs contained a few small lobuli filled with air, but the great mass was in a state of complete atelectasis; a small lump of meconium was found in the trachea, and in the minute bronchi was a slimy mixture of liquor amnii and meconium; no trace of uric acid infarction.

Case 4.—*Narrow pelvis; large child; natural delivery after thirteen hours; rent of the left tentorium cerebelli and of the sinus transversalis; intermeningeal hæmorrhage; meconium in the air-passages.*—A primipara, aged twenty-nine, with a contraction of the pelvis, was in labor in the hospital; the fœtal heart was heard; the liquor amnii tinged with meconium; but still the heart was heard; the head-swelling was very large; the child was born apparently dead, after strong labor. The heart and funis continued to pulsate, but all attempts at resuscitation were fruitless. *Dissection*—Slight cyanosis of face and finger-ends; the head was lengthened in the direction of the diagonal diameter; under the external periosteum, in the course of the sagittal suture, were flat, dark-red extravasations. In the arachnoid cavity, especially in the region of the left hemisphere and at the basis, was a very dark fluid extravasation; several ecchymoses on the tentorium of the right side; on the left side, near the falx, was a rent; the transverse sinus was opened. The brain was much infiltrated, and full of blood. The bronchi contained a thin, yellow, somewhat frothy mucous mixture. The lungs were small, deep-sunk against the spine; the edge of one lobe contained a little air, and gave out a little frothy fluid on cutting. The pulmonary vessels, the vanæ cavæ, and heart cavities were filled with dark fluid blood. In the pericardium was a little serum; no ecchymosis. Kidneys without trace of uric acid infarction. Under the microscope the bronchial contents showed the yellow-colored elements of the meconium, some cholesterine crystals, and the epidermic cells of the vernix caseosa.

In his commentary on these cases, Dr. Breisky observes that the presence of liquor amnii in the air-passages, in the first case, was the effect of prematu\r^e intra-uterine inspiratory effort, excited by the interruption of the placental circulation. We may also learn from this observation, that the cause of the first respiration of new-born children consists in the breaking off of the placental circulation, which gives rise to the *besoin de respirer*. Connected with this is the indication always to tie the cord immediately after the birth of the child ; this is the more urgently required in the case of apparently dead and weakly children, in order by suddenly cutting off the intra-uterine respiration to compel an inspiratory effort.

The etiology of the respiration in the remaining three cases in which there was no compression of the cord is not so clear ; but here also the author, relying on Schwartz's experiments, maintains that it was produced by an interruption to the interchange of elements between the maternal and fœtal blood. He believes that the in-draught of liquor amnii is facilitated in head presentations, where some liquor amnii is always ponded up behind the head, allowing freedom for the chest to expand ; and he says he has found this not to be the case in breech-presentations, which allow the liquor amnii to run off.—*British and Foreign Medico-Chirurgical Review, Jan.*, 1860.

Art. V. — *Obstetrical Practice.* (Reports of the Obstetrical Society of London.)

A case of Craniotomy, in which Delivery was readily effected by Turning, after Perforation, when Instrumental Extraction was found impossible, etc.: By F. W. Mackenzie, M. D.

The conjugate diameter at the brim was only two inches and three-eighths. As the woman had arrived at the full term of gestation, it was thought necessary to perforate the cranium ; but all subsequent attempts at extraction by the crotchet and craniotomy forceps failed. Turning was, however, easily performed, and the child brought away. The mother died, apparently from exhaustion, a few hours afterwards. The paper concluded with the suggestion that turning should be had recourse to in all cases of craniotomy similar to the one detailed.

On the Statistics of Midwifery, from the Records of Private Practice
By Robert Dunn, Esq.

In this paper was comprised a summary view of the author's midwifery records for twenty years. He began by expressing his conviction that the records of private practice might be usefully and advantageously contrasted with the statistics of lying-in hospitals and public institutions ; and that, while his own experience could only be brought to bear upon the working and middle classes of society, he hoped—seeing how important was the influence which the different modes and habits of life had upon the parturient process—that other Fellows of the Society would not be wanting to supply the desiderata in relation to the other grades and ranks of social life; not only to the highest, to those living in the lap of luxury, surrounded by the elegancies, and enjoying all the indulgences of life, but also to the lowest, to those sunk in the depths of indigence, ignorance, and penury, and often without even the ordinary comforts of life. The author considered that what had been said of statistics in relation to medicine in general, applied with peculiar force to obstetrics in particular ; for what we wanted in midwifery "were facts, comparable facts, numerous facts, well observed, carefully arranged, minutely classified, and acutely analyzed."

From 1831 to 1850, a period of twenty years, he had registered 4,049 cases of midwifery as occurring in his practice. Of these, after deducting 228 for premature births, there were 2,133 male and 1,688 female children. In regard to plurality of infants, there were two cases of triplets and forty-five of twins. He had met with three cases of monstrosity, one of which was worthy of notice, and had been put upon record in *The Lancet* for April 27th, 1844. It was that form of monstrosity which Dr. A. G. Otto has designated *monstrum humanum sereniforme*. He had met with one instance of the hydatidiform, or vesicular mole, and several cases of cranial blood-swellings, three of hare-lip, four of cleft palate, three of spina bifida, and five of imperforate anus. In one of the last, Amussat's operation for artificial anus in the left lumbar region was attempted, but was not successful. The descending colon was found to be impervious, and not larger than a crow-quill.

There were one hundred and seventy still-born children in all, from various causes, and in thirty cases death was attributable to the pressure of the cranial bones upon the brain in tedious and difficult labors. There were sixty instances of preternatural presentations. Of eleven cases in which there was a prolapsus of the funis, eight were born dead ; and of these, in three instances, the cord came down with the head, in two with the head and arm, in one with the foot, and in two with the shoulder. Of twenty-five breech presentations, nine were still-born ; and of these, five were putrid. There were three face presentations, one child dead ; eleven cases face to pubis ; two head and arm, both dead ; three hand, and three footling cases.

In the use of the forceps the author confessed to have had but slender experience. Impressed with the importance of the maxim, that "a meddlesome midwifery is a bad midwifery," he had always, in the absence of danger to the life of the mother, and when convinced in his own mind that the natural efforts would effect delivery, been content to wait, and had avoided instrumental interference. He had had ten cases of craniotomy ; two proved fatal to the mothers—one from sloughing of the bladder, the other from a tumor at the neck of the womb. Once satisfied that the child was dead, he had never hesitated to have recourse, without delay, to craniotomy. The use of the stethoscope, in such cases, he considered of paramount importance. Of placenta prævia, six cases had occurred in his practice; three since the promulgation of Dr. Simpson's views and mode of treatment. He gave a brief narrative of two of these; one as having presented evidence to his own mind that the detached portion of the placenta, from its appearance and condition, had afforded the channel through which the blood had gushed; and another as being an instance of the instantaneous arrest of the hæmorrhage as soon as the placenta had been entirely and completely separated from the uterus. He had met with thirty cases of adherent placenta requiring the introduction of the hand into the uterus; and four instances of the hour-glass contraction. He had witnessed two fatal cases from sheer exhaustion after delivery, where the hæmorrhage before the birth of the child had been great; and one fatal case of internal flooding. Other fatal cases of exhaustion he referred to, which were unconnected with the loss of blood. One interesting and instructive case had come under his notice, in which, while the mother lay in a state of coma from an apoplectic seizure, and the phenomena of life were reduced to a mere series of automatic movements, a fœtus of five or six months was expelled from the womb. Of twelve cases of puerperal fever which had occurred, three were acute, and terminated fatally. In one of these, the placenta had been found adherent, with hour-glass contraction of the uterus, and great hæmorrhage. In all, excepting where a hereditary tendency existed to mental disease, the loss of blood had been great. Of puerperal convulsions, he had met with four cases—none fatal; of phlegmasia dolens, six, and two proved fatal; of scarlatina, three, and one died.

Dr. Barnes made some brief observations on Mr. Dunn's treatment of his cases of placenta prævia, to which Dr. Waller replied, as he had partly been responsible for their management.

Dr. Tanner remarked that the ruling law in Mr. Dunn's practice seemed to have been the old proverb, that "meddlesome midwifery is bad." Dr. Tanner considered that this rule was the cause of a great deal of mischief. In practice, it was not only necessary to consider the life of the mother, but also to how great an extent we might beneficially mitigate her sufferings. A lingering labor could hardly be otherwise than injurious to both mother and child. Although his practice had been much smaller than Mr. Dunn's, yet during the last twelve years he had employed the forceps much more frequently than this gentleman, and had obtained only the happiest results from such a proceeding. He had never found the slightest mischief result from it, either to offspring or parent.

Mr. Baker Brown was glad to hear the opinion just expressed by Dr. Tanner. In almost all the cases of vesico-vaginal fistula which had come under his care, this accident had happened from the long retention of the fœtal head in the pelvis, giving rise to inflammation and sloughing. In reply to an observation from Dr. Graily Hewitt, that he had traced cases of vesico-vaginal fistula to the improper use of instruments, Mr. Brown stated that he had only known of one such instance.—*Brit. Med. Jour.*

ART. VI.—*On Bloodletting.* *(British Medical Journal.)*

IN the following letter Dr. Markham disputes, to a certain extent, the correctness of some remarks in a paper recently published in this Journal, by Dr. Handfield Jones, on the efficacy of local bloodletting in relieving inflammations of internal organs. The question whether local depletion is really *per se* efficacious in relieving congested states of viscera separated from the outer wall by a serous space (as the pleura or peritoneum), is one which may well lead to much consideration ; but it is one which we, and probably many of our readers, remember to have seen examined several years ago, by Dr. John Struthers, of Edinburgh. A paper on the subject was published by that gentleman in the *Monthly Journal of Medical Science* for April, 1853 ; and an abstract, illustrated by wood cuts, kindly lent by the author, appeared iu the *Association Medical Journal* for the. 20th of the same month. The propositions laid down by Dr. Struthers were briefly these : The relief in local bloodletting is through the blood-vessels or vascular system ; and there can be no special relief from local bloodletting, unless the bloodvessels of the affected part communicate with those of the part from which the blood is drawn. But, according to this statement, such communication, in the case of the thoracic and abdominal viscera, is wanting, except in the case of the anastomosis between the vessels of the rectum and the parinæum, which gives a rational explanation of the French practice referred to by Dr. Markham. Dr. Struthers believes that local bloodlettings in inflammations of the internal viscera do good only in the same way as general bloodlettings—by relieving the general circulation. His object, however, is not to depreciate local bleedings, which he rather supports, on the ground that the blood may as well be taken from one place as from another, and that, perhaps, the inflammation being of a serous lining of the parietes, the benefit may be direct. We would again commend Dr. Struthers' essay to the attention of our worthy contributors, Drs. Jones and Markham.

Local Bloodletting in Inflammation. Letter from W. O. MARKHAM, M. D.

SIR—Will you allow me a few lines of remarks on a point referred to by Dr. Handfield Jones, in his very valuable papers on inflammation, etc.?

Dr. H. Jones maintains that abstraction of blood from the skin which lies over certain inflamed internal organs, where there is no direct vascular connection between the skin and the internal organs, is a practice whose utility remains unquestioned. He instances the cases of leeching at the epigastrium in gastritis, of cupping the back of the chest to relieve pulmonary hyperæmia, and of the loins to relieve congestion of the kidneys. Now, without denying the fact, I would gladly hear from my friend the evidence upon which he founds his assertion of it. Is it clear and indubitable that such abstraction of blood really does relieve these congestions? To *prove* the fact, it must be shown that all those *other* remedies which are invariably used in the treatment of these diseases were dispensed with in such cases. In congestions of the kidney, in which cupping over the loins is practised, are not other still more powerful remedies always resorted to at the same time—viz: warmth, rest in bed, purgation, and ·opiates? And so, in pulmonary congestions, we invariably use other remedies besides the cupping ; and how are we to distinguish between the effects of these on the congestion, and the effects of the cupping?

Besides this, do not these local abstractions of blood, in the cases referred to, very often fail to give the relief expected from them? This much, at all events, seems to me as undeniable ; viz: that, in all such cases, the relief which follows upon the bleeding is never so certain, so constant, so manifest and undoubted, as the relief which follows in those cases in which there is a direct vascular communication between the skin and the inflamed part beneath—as, for instance, between the skin and an inflamed parietal pleura. I do not pretend to give any explanation of the fact, but I take it as one which every one will admit ; viz: that the withdrawal of a small quantity of blood from an inflamed part—say, by leeches from a sprained ankle— will diminish the chief phenomena of the inflammation—the pain, the heat, the redness, and the swelling. We all see this effect too constantly follow to doubt the relation of cause and effect. Now, taking this fact, I apply it to the case of internal organs ; and I cannot but think that, in all those cases in which there is a distinct vascular connection between the skin and the inflamed internal organ, we have much more certain proof of the efficacy and benefit of the remedy than we have in those cases in which there is no vascular connection—in cases, for instance, referred to by Dr. II. Jones. And I would observe that, in some of those cases in which there is no vascular connection, relief to pain may undoubtedly be given by local bleeding, and in a way which has not been referred to. For example, in some cases of pericarditis, when there is much local pain, local abstraction of blood gives relief, as I believe, by its action on the pleurisy which almost always accompanies severe pericarditis. So, again, in liver diseases, when leeching over the hepatic region gives relief (which we know·it very often fails to do), may we not very fairly ascribe the beneficial action to the influence which it has had over the inflammation which has been excited in the parietal peritoneum over the liver? The proofs of the existence of such inflammation are frequently shown to us in the deadhouse, in the adhesions between the surface of the diseased liver and the parietal peritoneum over it.

In inflammation of the lungs, local bleeding is of service, because it acts upon the pleurisy which usually accompanies pneumonia. Is, I might add, the French system of leeching the parts around the anus, to relieve abdominal congestions, a mere farce ? I should be too much trespassing upon your space, if I were to prolong this note; but I would just venture to say, also, that I believe the vascularity of the new formed adhesions, which unite internal organs to the parts around them, may in some cases create a new and direct vascular connection between the skin and these organs.

Altogether, I think my friend will himself admit this much—that the benefit of local bleeding in internal inflammations is much more sure and manifest in those cases in which there exists a direct vascular connection, than when no such vascular connection exists.

I am, etc.,   W. O. Markham.

Art. VII.—*On the Medulla Oblongata, the Pons Varolii, and some parts of the Spinal Cord, in their relations with Respiratory Movements, with Vertiginous or Rotatory Convulsions, with the Transmission of Sensitive Impressions and of the Orders of the Will to Muscles, and with the Vaso-Motor Nerves and Animal Heat :* By E. Brown-Sequard, M. D.*

Since the time of Galen, most of the physiologists, and particularly Lorry, Cruikshank, Lorenz, Bartels, and Legallois, have ascertained that a sudden and deep injury to the lower part of the medulla oblongata, in animals, causes immediate death, and many cases observed in man have shown the same thing. It has been almost universally admitted that death is then due to the fact that respiration ceases. because the lower part of the medulla oblongata is the center for respiratory movements. But if we study carefully what takes place in most of the cases of immediate death caused by a sudden and deep injury to the lower part of the medulla oblongata, we find that it is impossible to explain this curious mode of death by admitting that it is only due to a sudden arrest of respiration. If we take two living animals of the same species, and decapitate them by a section passing, in one of them, on the nib of the *calamus scriptorius*, and in the other, on the fourth or fifth cervical vertebra, and cutting, also, in both, the principal nerves of the neck, and avoiding the section of the carotids, we find that the first one has no convulsions, or, in other words, no agony ; while the second almost always

* *Course of Lectures on the Physiology and Pathology of the Central Nervous System.* Delivered at the Royal College of Surgeons, of England. Lecture XII.

has very violent convulsions in the four limbs and in the trunk.   In both cases the medulla oblongata is taken away and respiration is stopped ; we cannot, therefore, attribute to the cessation of respiration the absence of convulsions in only one of the cases.   We will see in a moment what is the cause of this absence of convulsions. Before we come to this explanation, we must say that a physiologist who has attained a very high situation in France, M. Flourens, one of the perpetual secretaries of the Academy of Sciences, to explain the sudden death after the destruction of a small part of the medulla oblongata, has proposed a theory of which we ought to take notice, on account of the standing of its author.   M. Flourens imagines that life depends on a force springing from a very small part of the medulla oblongata, which small part he calls the *vital point* or the *vital knot*.   If this hypothesis were true, certainly it would be very easy to understand why there are no convulsions, and hardly any signs of life in the heart and in other organs after the extirpation or destruction of the pretended vital knot.   Unfortunately for this theory, the part which is supposed to be the *focus* or the *source of life*, may be taken away, and life, persist, without any marked trouble.   My experiments not only show that life may last long after the extirpation of a much larger part of the medulla oblongata than this small amount of gray matter erroneously considered as the source of life, but that neither any part, nor the whole of the oblong medulla, can be considered as the source of a pretended vital force.   In the first place, a sudden irritation of the spinal cord, as well as that of the medulla oblongata, may cause a sudden death, without agony or convulsions, although in both cases, and especially in the first one, the pretended *focus of life* remains almost or entirely uninjured.   In the second place, the extirpation of this pretended only source of life, when made carefully by slow and partial sections, at a certain distance from it on the spinal cord and the pons varolii, is followed by the most violent convulsions and by energetic movements of the heart, the bowels, the bladder, etc.   In the third place, if the par vagum has been divided in a living animal, any kind of operation may be performed upon the medulla oblongata without destroying quickly or suddenly the movements of the heart ; and, in this case, the convulsions of agony take place with energy.

From the above-mentioned facts, and from several others, I have drawn the conclusions that the irritation of the oblong medulla, and of some parts of the spinal cord (a great portion of the cervical region), is able to produce a sudden stoppage or diminution of the movements of the heart, and that it is, in a great measure, to this influence on the heart that is due the absence of agony in most of the cases of sudden destruction of the oblong medulla.

More than ten years ago, I found that certain animals may live for many weeks, and, in more recent researches, for eight months, after the extirpation of the whole medulla oblongata.   In these animals all the functions of organic life, except pulmonary respiration, continue without any apparent alteration, showing that these functions do not depend upon the medulla oblongata, as some physiologists have thought.   The persistence of life in these animals was possible on account of the cutaneous respiration ; but in animals in which the skin absorbs but a small amount of oxygen, such as birds and mammals, death is said to be always rapid after the extirpation of the medulla oblongata, even when care is taken to avoid the influence of the operation upon the heart. It seems, therefore, that the medulla oblongata is an organ absolutely necessary to respiratory movements.   Against this view I will remark : 1st, that Dr. Bennet Dowler, of New Orleans, has seen thoracic respiratory movements continuing in decapitated alligators ; 2d, that Dr. B. W. Richardson has observed the same fact in young mammals ; 3d, that I have seen it also in birds, and in kittens and puppies.

It seems, therefore, quite certain that the respiratory movements do not depend only upon the medulla oblongata.   I have already tried to show, in 1851, that many parts of the encephalon are employed in respiration, and, since then, I have collected a great many pathological facts proving, I think, the correctness of this view.   It is known that the only two appearances of proof that the medulla oblongata is the only center of respiratory movements, or, in other words, the only source (direct or reflex) of these movements in the cerebro-spinal axis, are—1st, that a transversal section of the lower part of the medulla oblongata causes a sudden cessation of respiration ; 2d, that when transversal sections are made on the encephalon, from its front to its back, taking away layer after layer, it is said that it is only after the greatest part of the medulla oblongata has been taken away that respiration is destroyed.   As regards the first of these two assertions, we have already shown the objections against it—objections which are also very good against the second assertion.   When, after a series of transversal sections of the encephalon, we have reached the medulla oblongata, just above the upper roots of the par vagum, we find that respiration continues almost normal.   If now we cut away the part of the medulla giving origin to this pair of nerves, we find, in most cases, that respiration is suddenly stopped.   This certainly *seems* to prove that the small part to which the par vagum is attached is the nervous center for respiration.   But is it truly so ?   I will try to prove that it is not.

1st. In weak animals, after many parts of the encephalon have been taken away, the whole of the medulla oblongata and of the pons varolii remaining, respiration sometimes continues normal, but it certainly stops after a small part of the pons is removed.   It would be wrong to draw from this experiment the conclusion, that this small part is the central organ of respiration.   To draw such a conclusion, however, would be to employ the same reasoning which has been adopted concerning the part of the medulla oblongata giving origin to the par vagum.   The stronger an animal is, the more of its encephalon can be taken away before we destroy respiration.   It is in animals in which the spinal cord is rich in gray matter, and possesses a powerful reflex faculty, that we find respiration persisting after the whole of the encephalon, including the oblong medulla, has been extirpated ; such is the case in alligators, in birds, in young dogs and cats.

2d. In the strongest animals, death occurs in a few hours, and from

52

insufficiency of respiration, after the ablation of the encephalon except the whole of the medulla oblongata ; and so it often is with the encephalic monster. These facts show clearly that, although respiration may be carried on almost as well as in the normal con-dition of the central nervous system, when only the medulla ob-longata and the spinal cord exist, these organs are insufficient for a long persistence of this function. A series of experiments on pigeons has given me the following results : With the spinal cord alone, respiration continues a few minutes ; with the spinal cord and the part of the oblong medulla giving origin to the principal excitors of respiration—the vagi—this function continues many hours (the longest duration we have seen is thirteen hours) ; if there is also a great part of the base of the encephalon left, respiration continues longer, but I have never seen it last more than a day and a half ; if the cerebrum alone is taken away, respiration remains undisturbed ; and if death occurs, it is not on account of an insufficiency of the parts left of the cerebro-spinal axis to carry on respiration.

3d. In man, hæmorrhage in the various parts of the base of the encephalon, near the median line, or upon it, produces a trouble in respiration, which is more and more marked the greater the amount of effused blood, and the nearer it is to the medulla oblongata. Cer-tainly, in many cases, the trouble of respiration may be partly attributed to pressure on the medulla oblongata, but it is not always so ; and, at any rate, in several cases of softening of the pons va-rolii, in which it cannot be said that there was a pressure on the oblong medulla, there has been a trouble in respiration. From the ex-amination of a great many cases, I have been led to the conclusion that the whole base of the encephalon is employed in respiration.

4th. Many cases have been observed in which the medulla oblongata has been so much altered, that almost all its actions as a nervous center ought to have been destroyed, and, nevertheless, respiration has continued to take place ; in those cases there was still, however, a more or less free communication between the pons varolii and the spinal cord, and probably several of the filaments of the par vagum continued to act as excitors of respiratory movements.

All the facts just mentioned, and many others of which I have no time to speak, have led me, first, to abandon the view so generally admitted, that the medulla oblongata is the essential source of the respiratory movements in the nervous centers; and, secondly, to propose the view that these movements depend upon all the *incito-motory* parts of the cerebro spinal axis, and on the gray matter which connects those parts with the motor nerves going to the respiratory muscles. I must add that, according to the theory I have arrived at, the principal cause of respiration is in the lungs, as Dr. Marshall Hall has tried to prove ; but that excitations coming from all parts of the body, as shown by Volkmanns and Vierord, and also direct irritations of the base of the encephalon and of the spinal cord, almost constantly taking place, contribute to the production of res-piratory movements.

It seems, indeed, wonderful to see animals, sometimes after a slight puncture of some part of the encephalon with the point of a needle, *turn round,* just like a horse in a circus, or *roll over and over* for hours, and sometimes for days, with but short interruptions. The same phenomena having been often observed in man, I think it may prove interesting, if not useful, to point out the parts of the encephalon which may produce virtiginous or rotatory convulsions. The convulsions differ a great deal, according to the place injured and the depth and size of the injury. If we suppose that the right side of the encephalon, in the places I will name, has been injured, we find that the animal *turns* or *rolls,* and that in the first case the side on which it turns is either the left or the right ; while, if it rolls, the rolling begins either by the left or right side.

Parts producing turning or rolling after an injury on the right side :

Turning or rolling by the right side.	Turning or rolling by the left side.
1. Anterior part of the optic thalamus. (Schiff)	1. Posterior part of the optic thalamus. (Schiff.)
2. The hind parts of the crus cerebri. (Schiff.)	2. Some parts of the crus cerebri, near the optic thalamus. (Brown-Séquard.)
3. The tubercula quadrigemina. (Flourens.)	3. Anterior and superior parts of the pons Varolii.
4. Posterior part of the processus cerebelli ad pontem. (Magendie.)	4. Anterior part of processus cerebelli ad pontem. (Lafargue.)
5. Place of insertion of the auditory and of the facial nerves. (Brown-Séquard and Martin-Magron.)	5. Place of insertion of the glossopharyngeal nerve. (Brown-Séquard.)
6. Neighborhood of the insertion of the lower roots of the par vagum.) (Brown-Séquard.)	6. Spinal Cord, near oblong medulla. (Brown-Séquard.)

While rotation takes place, it is easy to ascertain, 1st, that it is not its production by contractions resembling those of voluntary movements which causes the rolling or the turning ; 2d, that some muscles are in a state of tonic contraction ; 3d, that the trunk and neck of the animal are bent by a spasmodic action on the side of turning if it has a circus movement, and that it is bent like a corkscrew, as much as the bones allow, in cases of *rolling* ; 4th, that sensibility and volition may remain, and there are frequent efforts to resist the tendency to turn or roll. It seems clear from these observations and several others, that these rotary movements depend chiefly upon the fact that certain muscles are in a state of spasm.

The persistent spasmodic contractions, due to a mechanical injury to certain parts of the nervous centers, are always curious, but never so much so as when they result from some irritation of a part like the auditory nerve, which we were accustomed to consider simply as a nerve of sense. M. Flourens has found that the section of the semicircular canals, in certain animals, is followed by a strange disorder of movements, and sometimes by a rotation (circus movement). I have ascertained that the phenomena, observed in these experiments do not depend on the section of these canals, as this operation may not cause these phenomena, but that they are the results of an irritation of the auditory nerve, from the drawing upon it by the membranous semicircular canals at the time we divide them. In frogs and in mammals, the direct irritation of the auditory nerve is followed by the most interesting phenomena. It is well known that in frogs the peripheric extremity of this nerve is enclosed in a bag containing carbonate of lime ; as soon as this bag is laid bare and slightly touched, and still more if it be punctured with a needle or a bistoury, the anterior limb, *on the opposite side*, is thrown into a state of slight convulsion, and kept almost constantly in a spasmodic pronation ; and almost at every attempt to move forwards the animal turns round on the side injured. As long as it lives (many days, or even many months), these phenomena may be observed, although not quite so marked as immediately after the injury, or after the first twenty-four hours. In mammals, the least puncture of the auditory nerve causes *rolling*, just as after the irritation of the processus cerebelli ad pontem ; violent convulsions then occur in the eyes, the face, and many muscles of the neck and chest. The doctrine that the nerves of the higher senses are not endowed with general sensibility (i. e., are not able to cause pain) seems not to be true with regard to the acoustic nerve ; at least, the signs of pain given after an irritation of this pretended nerve are often as great as those observed after an irritation of the trunk of the trigiminal nerve.

In man, also, the auditory nerve seems to be able to act as it does after an injury in animals. 1st. Any one who has received an injection of cold water in the ear may know that it produces a kind of *vertigo*, and that is difficult to walk strait for some time after this irritation. 2d. A sudden noise makes the whole body jump, particularly in old people, or in persons attacked with anœmia, chlorosis, epilepsy, chorea, hysteria, hydrophobia, in certain cases of poisoning ; in a word, in all circumstances in which the control of the will over reflex actions is lost or diminished. 3d. Vertigo and various convulsive movements, in cases of irritation of the acoustic nerve, have been observed in adults and children. Rotatory movements have taken place in cases of suppurative inflammation of the ear, and twice immediately after an injection of a solution of nitrate of silver.

The parts of the base of the encephalon, which are capable of producing persistent spasms, seem to be different from those employed in the transmission of sensitive impressions or of the orders of the will to muscles, at least in the medulla oblongata and the pons varolii. They constitute a very large portion of these two organs, and perhaps the three-fourths of the first one ; they are placed chiefly in the lateral and posterior columns of these organs ; many of their fibres do not decussate, and produce spasms on the corresponding side of the body ; they seem to contain most of the vaso-motor nerves, by which, directly or through a reflex action, they may act on other parts of the nervous system, as I will show hereafter ; they have much to do with the phenomena of several, if not most, of the convulsive diseases ; and, lastly, I will say that the history of their properties and actions throws a great deal of light on the effects of extirpation or diseases of the cerebellum.

The small number of fibres in the anterior pyramids, on the one hand, has appeared to be insufficient for the conveyance of the orders of the will to all the muscles of the trunk and limbs ; and the existence of paralysis on the side injured in the encephalon, on the other hand, has contributed to lead to the actually-admitted opinion that the voluntary motor fibres make a part of their decussation in the medulla oblongata, and the other part in the pons varolii, and also higher up between the two sets of tubercula quadrigemina and the two cerebral peduncles.

Suppose an alteration in one of the crura cerebri. According to the theory, as a part of the decussation of the voluntary motor nerve-fibres takes place there, we should find that voluntary movements are diminished on both sides of the body—more, I acknowledge, on the side *opposite* to the alteration, but partly, also, on the *same* side of the body. This is not what exists. One side only of the body is paralysed ; and it is the *opposite* side. A number of cases prove that this is the rule. The hemiplegia may be complete or incomplete, according to many circumstances, and particularly the extent and the nature of the alteration, and the rapidity of its formation ; but there is something constant, together with these numerous varieties; it is that the seat of paralysis is on the side of the body opposite to that of the disease. It is evident, in consequence, that the decussation of the voluntary motor nerve-fibres has entirely taken place before they reach the crura cerebri.

The same thing may safely be said of the corpora quadrigemina. Although the cases relative to these organs are much less numerous than the cases relative to the crura cerebri, there are enough of them on record to prove that the crossing of the voluntary motor nerve-fibres must have taken place entirely before they reach the base of the corpora quadrigemina. Besides some other cases, there are two very interesting ones which have been published, one by Mohr and the other by Burnet—both of which I have already quoted.

As to the pons varolii, the question is much more interesting, because this is the place where the decussation of voluntary motor fibres, according to Foville, Valentine, and Longet, more particularly takes place. Here, according to the theory of these distinguished anatomists, we ought to find different symptoms in these three different cases : 1st. Alteration limited to the superior part of the organ. 2d. Alteration limited to the inferior part (the nearest to the medulla oblongata). 3d. Alteration occupying the whole of a lateral half of the organ. In the first case we should see an incomplete paralysis on both sides, but greater on the side of the body opposite to the side of the disease ; and, in the second case, we should see, also, an incomplete paralysis on both sides, and almost to the same degree in both. Many cases are on record proving that it is not so, and that whatever is the part of the pons altered (the superior, the inferior, or the middle), the same effect is produced on voluntary movements. When paralysis is produced by the disease, it exists exclusively on the *opposite* side of the body ; and when the alteration is not limited to one side of the pons, and extends on the other, then the side most paralysed in the body is the one *opposite* to the most altered side of the pons.

I might prove that I am right by relating here many pathological facts ; but as I have already mentioned some (see Lecture VI, p

296), and as I shall have in a moment to mention several others, I will merely now affirm again that there are many.

It seems absolutely certain, from the above facts and reasonings, that there is no decussation of the voluntary motor fibres of the trunk and limbs above the crossing of the pyramids.

From the preceding remarks, and from the facts and reasonings contained in our lectures (the third and seventh) on the decussation of the conductors of sensitive impressions, it results that, as regards anæsthesia and paralysis, three different groups of symptoms may be observed, according to the place of the alteration in a lateral half of the cerebro-spinal axis : 1st, above the decussation of the pyramids, a lesion on either the medulla oblongata, the pons varolii, the crura cerebri, the optic thalami, the corpora striata, or the brain proper if it produce anæsthesia and paralysis, produces them both in the opposite side of the body ; 2d, below the decussation in the pyramids, a lesion in the spinal cord produces paralysis in the same side, and anæsthesia in the opposite side ; 3d, at the level of the decussation of the pyramids, and upon the decussating fibres, and also behind them, a lesion produces paralysis in both sides of the body, and anæsthesia only in the opposite side. So that *wherever the lesion in a lateral half of the cerebro-spinal axis may be—below, above or at the level of the crossing of the pyramids—if it produces anæsthesia, it is in the opposite side ; while paralysis, in these three cases, is either in the same or the opposite side, or in both sides.*

To complete, as much as time will allow, the exposition of my views on the physiology and pathology of the central nervous system, I have now to speak of the condition of animal heat in cases of alteration of the spinal cord and the encephalon. The following conclusions may be drawn from a great many facts bearing on the subject : 1st, that usually anæsthesia is accompanied by a diminution of temperature ; 2d, that hyperæsthesia almost always co-exists with an increased temperature ; 3d, that in paralysis, without either a notable hyperæsthesia or anæsthesia, the temperature is nearly normal. I must remark that the state of heat of a part is due to the amount of blood, the degree of heat of this fluid, the exposure of the part to the influence of the temperature of the surrounding medium, and the temperature of this medium. Now, in anæsthetic parts the bloodvessels are usually contracted, and, therefore, there is less blood in them, and also a lower temperature. In hyperæsthetic parts the reverse exists.

Table of symptoms in the trunk and limbs, according to the seat of a lesion in one lateral half of the cerebro-spinal axis.

1. Lesion in the brain proper, the optic thalamus, or the corpus striatum.

	On the opposite side.	On the same side.
Sensibility	Diminished or lost	Normal
Voluntary movements	ditto, ditto	ditto
Temperature (even without fever)	Increased	ditto

2. Lesions of the pons varolii or the medulla oblongata above the decussation of the anterior pyramids.

	On the opposite side.	On the same side.
Sensibility	Diminished or lost	Increased
Voluntary movements	ditto, ditto	Normal
Temperature	Diminished	Increased

3. Lesion of the medulla oblongata at the level of the decussation of the anterior pyramids.

	On the opposite side.	On the same side.
Sensibility	Diminished or lost	Increased
Voluntary movements	ditto, ditto	Diminished or lost
Temperature	Diminished	Increased

4. Lesion of the spinal cord.

	On the opposite side.	On the same side.
Sensibility	Diminished or lost	Notably Increased
Voluntary movements	ditto, ditto	Nearly normal
Temperature	Diminished	Increased

It is unnecessary to say that nothing is more variable than the degree of temperature of paralysed or anæsthetic parts, and that, therefore, what is stated in the above table ought to be considered as the most frequent condition, and not as a constant one. Paralysed bloodvessels may contract under the influence of cold, and the temperature and the hyperæsthesia of a part may, in this way, diminish for a time. On the other hand, contracted bloodvessels will necessarily relax after a long period of contraction, because they lose their power of contraction by a persistent and somewhat spasmodic action, and, in this way, anæsthetic and cold parts may temporarily become warm.—*Savannah Journal of Medicine. March,* 1860.

ART. VIII.—*Metallic Ligatures.*

On the 21st of March, 1829, Mr. HENRY S. LEVERT, of Alabama, now Dr. Levert, of Mobile, in the same State, graduated in medicine in the University of Pennsylvania, having presented a thesis entitled "*Experiments on the use of Metallic Ligatures as applied to arteries.*" This paper was published as the leading article of *The American Journal of the Medical Sciences* for May, 1829, the experimental portion of which will be found below. This paper, simple, unpretending, and conclusive in its experimental character, and significant in its physiological and surgical import, was altogether demonstrative, so far as the analogical evidence derived from surgical operations upon dogs is applicable to man. These experiments excited much attention, but made no converts. Surgeons, biased in favor of silk and similar ligatures, did not choose those of metal, but sought for arguments which cast doubts upon the superiority of the latter. If they failed to verify the new experiments, they did not fail in defending themselves against even an appearance of favoring an innovation, which virtually proved that an important branch of operative surgery was not practised in the best manner. Each defended himself, as far as was prudent, until, at length, the subject was almost wholly forgotten.

Let us look at a few text-books—the first which come to hand—in order to ascertain what was said, for nothing was done, in relation to Dr. Levert's experimental investigation :

In his Principles of Surgery, Prof. Miller says, nature regards metallic, as well as other forms of ligature, as "foreign substances to be extruded by suppuration."

Prof. Fergusson, in his Practical Surgery, says : "The ligature which I generally make use of is small, smooth, and well-spun twine. * * * Some practical surgeons have been far too nice regarding the size and material of ligatures," etc.

M. Velpeau sums up the various kinds of ligatures, including those of Dr. Levert, in the following words : " From these inquiries it results, as I conceive, that the nature and the form of ligatures in the treatment of aneurisms, are not so important as they have been generally thought," etc. (Operative Surgery.)

In the 11th vol. of the Dict. de Méd. et de Chir., M. Bégin (art. ligature) notices Dr. Levert's experiments upon animals with metallic ligatures. But M. Bégin throws into his appreciation doubt and dissent, thinking that man and animals differ, and that metallic ligatures are not so good as some other kinds, especially those of animal substances.

In his Surgical Dictionary, S. Cooper, art. ligature, no mention is made of Dr. Levert's experiments, or of metallic ligatures. Prof. Henry H. Smith, of Philadelphia, in his treatise on Practical Surgery (1856), says: "Experience has shown that any ligature that is strong enough, and that is properly applied, answers equally well."

Lisfranc, a great, though somewhat eccentric surgeon, in the second volume of his surgery (*Médecine Opératoire*, Paris : 1846), after giving a summary of Dr. Levert's experiments with ligatures of lead, gold, platina, and silver, virtually rejects them, because he had neither seen metallic ligatures employed, nor did he know that they had ever been applied directly upon the human subject. ("*Je n'ai pas vu employer ces ligatures ; je ne sache même pas qu'on les ait appliquées sur l'homme.*" (805.)

Tacitus has somewhere said, that if the reward of investigation be taken away, study will be neglected : "*Sublatis studiorum pretiis, etiam studia peritura.*" Now, without having either a personal acquaintance with Dr. Levert, or any information as to his own attitude in regard to his claims, it is reasonable to assume that he exexpected his experiments should be tested, and if found to be a great step towards the advancement of surgery, that he should have the satisfaction of a just recognition in the Republic of science, and the more so, because, at the present moment, the silver suture which he had so fully tested as being upon an experimental basis "free from danger, and productive of peculiar advantages," is proclaimed and otherwise appropriated, as the greatest discovery of the nineteenth century. This is what has been called playing Hamlet with the part of Hamlet left out altogether. If even the half of the merits now claimed for the silver suture be conceded, Dr. Levert did not write in the sands ; nor will the waves of the third of a century wash out his record. Documents and dates, thanks to the art of printing, are more powerful than the Roman Lictors, who, bearing *fasces* and axes, marched before Kings and Consuls, enforcing respect and punishing the refractory. It is the pen of history "which is mightier than the sword" or the Lictor's axe.

Without affirming that the suture of silver, or other metal, is what its advocates have recently claimed for it, the greatest discovery of this century, there seems to be already extant considerable evidence, which daily increases, in favor of its superiority over those ligatures which have been, and are still usually employed. Hence, whatever merit the former may possess attaches itself chiefly to the experimental investigations of Dr. Levert, as the following document will show.   B. DOWLER.

Experiment I.—On the 16th of May, 1828, I laid bare the right carotid artery of a dog, and after separating it carefully from its accompanying nerve and vein, I passed under it a lead wire, and tied

53

it firmly. Both ends of the wire were then cut off with a pair of scissors, and the sharp points bent down with a common dissecting forceps. The wound was now drawn together with a few stitches of the interrupted suture, and over these were laid some adhesive strips. This animal was not confined, but suffered to run at large : when I examined him several days after, I found the stitches ulcerated out, and the wound open ; it had filled up from the bottom with granulations, but the edges of the skin were separated to a considerable distance : with light dressings it healed entirely by the 5th of June.

June 28th.—I killed this animal and dissected with care the neck. A small cicatrix existed in the skin ; the lead was found in the situation in which I had placed it, by the side of the vein and nerve, perfectly encysted ; the artery at this place had been removed entirely, for the space of half an inch.

Both ends of the vessel, caused by this removal of its central portion, adhered by loose cellular substance to the surrounding parts, which appeared to be in a perfectly natural state. The end towards the heart was not at all increased or diminished in size ; it was sealed up for three-eights of an inch in extent, by an organized substance, resembling a coagulum of blood in color, but not in consistence, it being much firmer. The end towards the head resembled the one just described, in all particulars : the substance, however, which filled its extremity was of greater extent, and occupied the whole space up to the next branch, which was rather more than half an inch.

Not the slightest trace of inflammation existed in the neighboring parts ; on the contrary, they appeared perfectly natural. The lead itself was enclosed in a dense cellular substance, which formed for it a complete cyst.

Experiment II.—The right carotid artery of another dog was separated from its contiguous parts on the 17th of May, and a lead wire placed around it, as in Experiment 1. The lips of the wound were kept in contact with sutures and adhesive strips. I examined it three days after, and found that it had united by the first intention, in the whole of its course, except in those points included by the stitches ; these I cut loose and dressed it simply with adhesive strips. When I looked at this dog again, I found that from the itching of the wound the animal had scratched off the dressings, and broken up the new adhesions ; I washed it carefully to remove the dirt, and dressed it with simple dressings. It healed kindly, and was entirely well on the 6th of June, at which time I killed the dog, and made a careful dissection of the parts. The cellular substance here was much thickened and indurated, forming a strong bond of union between the nerve, vein, and artery. The two former were in their natural condition ; the artery was pervious its whole extent, to within three-eighths of an inch of the wire ; at this place the calibre was entirely obliterated ; a firm substance, resembling bruised muscle, filled its cavity ; between the ligature and the head the artery was impervious, and much diminished in size, having the appearance of a mere cord, not exceeding one-fourth the original dimensions of the vessel. The lead preserved its situation around the artery; it had become entirely encysted, and not the slightest remains of inflammation existed.

Experiment III.—I cut down on the left carotid of a third dog, on the 29th of May, and proceeded as in Experiments I and II, differing in no respect, except in dressing the wound ; I used no stitches, but merely adhesive plasters.

June 1st.—I examined the wound, and found that it had united through its whole extent ; but as I supposed the union not to be very firm, the strips were reäpplied, and suffered to remain on until the 5th, when they were removed altogether.

June 27th.—The animal was killed, and a minute examination made. The lead wire was found around the vessel, which was impervious for an inch or more, as in the former experiments. The surrounding parts healthy.

Experiment IV. June 9th.—The dog which was the subject of the last experiment, having entirely recovered from the first operation, now became the subject of a second, which was performed on the carotid of the opposite side. This was conducted exactly as the preceding ; the wound united by the first intention without the least difficulty; no constitutional symptoms manifested themselves. On the 27th, at which time this dog was killed, an examination was likewise made of this side of the neck ; the appearances corresponded exactly with those of the preceding experiments.

Experiment V. August 5th.—I performed a similar experiment on the carotid of another dog. I killed him on the 3d of September, and found that the appearances differed in no respect from the foregoing.

The lead having answered my expectations so well in these cases, I felt a great inclination to ascertain whether that substance alone possessed the property of remaining in contact with the living tissues, without exciting irritation or any unpleasant consequences, or whether similar results might not be obtained by using other metals. I accordingly continued the subject, using gold, silver, and platinum, instead of lead.

Experiment VI. August 12th.—The right carotid of a dog was separated neatly from its surrounding parts, and tied firmly with a small gold wire ; the wound was kept closed with adhesive strips, and by the third day had united firmly. *September 2d.*—The dog was killed, and I examined his neck ; I could perceive no difference in the appearances exhibited here from those produced by the lead.

Experiment VII. October 13th.—I exposed the left femoral artery of a dog, and placed around it a gold wire. *15th.*—I examined this dog, and found that from his restlessness he had removed the dressings, and had torn open the wound; I replaced them, and he recovered in a short time. *Oct. 30th.*—I examined the subject of this experiment, and found that the results corresponded in every particular with those above related.

Experiment VIII. October 16th.—The above experiment was repeated on this dog ; the wound healed very kindly by the first intention, etc. *Oct. 30th.*—I found the result to coïncide with the last in all particulars ; there was a slight appearance of ecchymosis around this ligature, which, no doubt, would have been removed in a few days more, only fourteen days having elapsed between the operation and the examination of the result.

Expeiment IX. October 5th.—I passed around the carotid of a dog a piece of silver wire, and united the wound by the first intention, which had taken place on the 9th, at which time I examined it. *Oct. 30th.*—I found that the silver had become encysted, and had left no remains of irritation.

Experiment X. October 5th.—The same experiment on another dog. *30th.*—The results the same.

Experiment XI. October 13th.—I passed a silver wire around the right femoral artery of a dog. *15th.*—Wound healed. *30th.*—Wire encysted. No traces of inflammation remaining.

Experiment XII. August 29th.—I cut down on the left carotid of a dog, and passed around it a platinum wire. This animal made his escape, and I did not see him again until the 16th of October, when I examined his neck ; the wound had united so nicely that its former situation could scarcely be recognised; the cellular substance beneath was slightly thickened and indurated ; the artery was obliterated for an inch and a half or two inches ; the middle portion resembled a small cord, around the center of which I found the platinum wire enclosed in a mass of condensed cellular substance, which formed for it a cyst; the inside of this cyst was smooth, and adhered closely to the platinum ; no traces of inflammation remained.

Experiment XIII. October 15th.—Another dog was subjected to an experiment resembling the above in all particulars. *Oct. 30th.*—I killed him, and found no other difference in the appearances than that the cyst which enclosed the platinum was not so perfectly formed ; it however existed.

Experiment XIV. October 16th.—This experiment was conducted precisely as the two last ; the appearances upon examination were the same. This dog was the subject of Experiment VII, and was examined on the 30th of October.

Experiment XV. June 15th.—I enclosed the humeral artery of a dog in a ligature made of a single stran of silk, previously waxed. In applying the ligature I drew it barely tight enough to place the opposite sides of the vessel in contact, without dividing the internal and middle coats. Both ends were then cut off, and the lips of the wound placed in apposition ; it did not unite, however, by the first intention, the dressings having been removed by the animal ; it was now dressed in the usual way, and soon healed perfectly by granulations. On the fourteenth day after the operation I made a dissection of the parts ; the artery was filled with a firm coagulum, both above and below the place of the ligature, which prevented the possibility of hæmorrhage, so firmly did these coagula adhere to the parietes of the vessel.

The ligature was found in the center of a small *abscess,* loose and detached from the surrounding parts ; the artery was ulcerated through, the ends being separated a short distance.

Experiment XVI. August 15th.—I repeated this experiment on the femoral artery of another dog ; the wound was united by the first intention. *Sept. 2d.*—Upon dissection, an *abscess* as large as a pea was discovered immediately under the skin and above the artery ; the loop of silk was found in its center, and offered no resistance when I attempted to remove it.

Experiment XVII.—I passed under the femoral artery of a dog a piece of gum-elastic, previously stretched and rolled to render it of a proper size, and tied it with a single knot. This operation was performed on the 15th of August ; the wound united by the first intention. *Sept. 3d.*—An examination was made of the result of this experiment. The ligature was found encysted ; the inner side of the cyst was uneven, and not in close contact with the gum-elastic ; from its appearance I thought that pus had existed, but was now absorbed ; the artery was obliterated to the next branch, both above and below.

Experiment XVIII. August 20th.—The same experiment repeated on the right carotid of another dog. *23d.*—Perfectly united by the first intention. *Sept. 2d.*—The gum-elastic was found contained in an abscess as large as half a nutmeg ; the artery was impervious both above and below the ligature, and ulcerated through at the place of its application.

Experiment XIX. September 1st.—The experiment with gum-elastic was repeated on the femoral artery of another dog, and the wound united in the usual manner. This dog was the subject of Experiment XII ; consequently I had not an opportunity of examining him until the 16th of October, when he was again caught. The cicatrix in the skin was to be seen plainly. On making an incision at this place, I perceived a small lump about the size of a pea, immediately under the skin, and at the lower angle of the wound. I opened this, and found it to contain the gum-elastic ligature, surrounded by a small quantity of yellowish-looking pus ; the vessel was removed for the space of an inch and a half, both ends obliterated. Just above the place of the ligature, several small arteries, not distinguishable in the healthy condition of these parts, were observable, and appeared to be spent upon the contiguous muscles.

Experiment XX. August 25th.—I cut down on the left femoral artery of a dog, and tied it firmly with a grass ligature, such as is used for fishing-lines. *27th.*—It had healed by the first intention. *Sept. 2d.*—The grass was found encysted, but the inner side of the cyst was moist and uneven, and did not appear to embrace the ligature closely ; no appearance of inflammation.

Experiment XXI. August 25th.—The same operation performed on another dog. *Sept. 3d.*—It was examined, and found to correspond with the twentieth in every particular.

From the experiments now detailed, we may, I think, conclude that the plan of tying arteries with lead and the other metals is free from danger, and may be productive of some peculiar advantages.; more experience and a greater number of experiments are necessary to establish this point thoroughly, and it is to be hoped that some one fully competent to the task will prosecute the subject.

Art. IX.—*Lectures on Experimental Pathology and Operative Phy-siology.* Delivered at the College of France, during the Winter Session, 1859–60. By M. Claude Bernard, Member of the French Institute ; Professor of General Physiology at the Academy of Sciences.

[The following extracts made from eight lectures, which appeared as original in the *Medical Times and Gazette* (January to March, 1860), possess so many intrinsical merits that the large space assigned to them in the present issue of this journal cannot, it is believed, be better occupied. Although only a comparatively small portion of these lectures will be copied, yet the most striking, suggestive, and valuable, will be reproduced, and will sufficiently show that their author possesses a skillful hand as an operator, and what is more important, a logical mind.   B. D.]

What is Medicine ? This is, doubtless, no new question ; it is one which has been asked for centuries past, but it has not yet re-ceived a satisfactory answer. Is Medicine an art or a science? Does it form a part of natural history? or does it enjoy an inde-pendent existence of its own ? Each of these different points of view has had its partisan, as is abundantly proved by the various definitions handed down to us by classical authors. According to Hippocrates, Medicine consists in the taking away all that which is in excess, and in supplying of all that is defective in the economy : in a word, it is the art of restoring equilibrium to the human body. According to Herophilus, Medicine is the science of health, and the knowledge of all the agents that can either injure or improve it. According to Hoffmann, it is the means by which the sciences of Physics and Chemistry are rendered subservient to the preservation of health. Pitcairin, regarding the question in an exclusively prac-tical point of view, has given it a totally different definition. The science of Medicine, in his estimation, has no other end than the solution of the following problem : "*For a given dieasse find its remedy.*" Viewing it from a diametrically opposite point, Pinel com-pletely changed the conditions of the problem—the question with him is: "*For a given disease find its place in a nosological classifica-tion*" ("*une maladie etant donnée, trouver sa place dans un cadre nosologique.*")

Not one of these definitions completely satisfies the tendencies of the present age ; in fact, medicine consists in the application of a great number of sciences—anatomy, physiology, therapeutics ; even physics and chemistry, each in its turn pays its tribute to the healing art.

Considered in this point of view medicine no longer exists as an isolated science ; properly speaking, there exist only medical sciences (*sciences médicales*). Such is, at the present day, the view most generally adopted. Whether medicine be a science or an art is a question of but minor importance, seeing that in every branch of human knowledge, art and science are found closely interwoven. The doctrinal and purely theoretical part of all human knowledge is altogether an abstraction *(absolument impersonelle)*; it is truth viewed under a peculiar aspect; but in its practical application we find the personal qualities of the individual necessarily blended with it. "Art is action," said Aristotle.

Let us, therefore, content ourselves by directing our attention to the only point which really merits our consideration; let us consider art and science in their mutual relations, and as exercising an influence one on the other. It seems at first sight, impossible to call in question the impulse which theory had given to practice: in the physical sciences a discovery cannot be made without its furnishing to industry generally a multitude of useful applications; but in medicine such is not as yet the case; thus the progress or the modification of theories exerts but a very limited influence on the practice of the healing art, and we see a goodly number of practitioners isolating themselves entirely from science, as if it were of no importance to follow it in its various fluctuations, and content themselves with endeavoring to cure their patients on purely empirical principles.

Ampère has divided the history of a science arrived at its fullest degree of development into four periods. To each of those periods or states he has given a particular name. Science is in the first period *Autoptic* or purely descriptive: when, without penetrating beyond the mere surface of things, we confine ourselves to a description of what we observe in the external world. Later, we inquire into the hidden springs which give rise to these phenomena; we desire to penetrate beneath the surface of things; this is the *Cryptoristic* period. But we must also become acquainted with the changes which take place in beings—the modifications, so to speak, which they present; this is the *Troponomic* period. At last, we arrive at the highest degree of knowledge to which it is possible to attain; this is called the *Cryptologic* period. It consists in a knowledge of the laws of succession which regulate all natural phenomena in a given order of things. It is then that knowing the general law, the starting point, as it were, we are enabled to predict the phenomena which are to take place, and even to indicate the disturbances which may modify their development. Such is the highest point, such the extreme limit to which the human mind can attain—we can go no further.

Now in biological sciences, animals and natural objects were first described; later they were classified; then diseases were described, and efforts were even made to cure them without any exact notion existing as to anatomy or physiology. Later we reach the second period of science which in zoölogy is represented by anatomy, and in medicine by pathological anatomy. But in biology, the anatomy of the dead body, pure and simple, is equally insufficient as it is in medicine. It is the anatomy of the *living* body which we require: recourse has consequently been had to vivisections; but it is evident that, taken by themselves, vivisections do not constitute an experimental method ; it is necessary that the physiologist should possess a knowledge of the sciences requisite to enable him not only to observe, but also to explain the phenomena which he has induced. It is here that medicine ceases to satisfy the parallel which we establish with regard to physiology ; medicine remains in the second period ; it has not yet reached the third.

It becomes necessary, therefore, to have recourse to pathological experiments on the living subject *(vivisections pathologiques)*, in order to arrive at a knowledge of what takes place in the diseased body in which the tropological conditions of physiology are manifested. But as in the study of physiology healthy subjects are required, so in the study of pathology subjects in a state of disease are necessary—we must even render them diseased by artificial means ; we must, in short, introduce into experimental pathology a knowledge of exterior agents, together with their effects on the constitution. This is assuredly rendering an immense service to therapeutics.

What are the animals best suited for this class of experiments ? Physiology has no other definite object in view than that of contributing to the progress of medical science. All our experiments have man for their object, and we should select, as far as it is possible, in prosecuting our studies, those animals which approach most closely to man ; but it is often difficult in practice to follow this precept, hence we shall often make use of animals of a very inferior type.

It is indispensable, in all experiments, to have recourse to counterproofs. The grand method adopted in physiology consists in suppressing an organ, and in comparing what then takes place with the natural and ordinary phenomena of life ; but we must put aside, in such a case, all the immediate results consequent on vivisection—surgical accidents, so to speak. If, for example, we divide a nerve in an animal, we must, at the same time, make a counter-proof on another ; the nerve must be exposed without being divided, and we shall then distinguish the disturbance which results from the section of the nervous cord, from the simple accidents which are the consequence of the preliminary operation. It is impossible to imagine how many unexpected services this method has rendered to science. It is by this proceedure that I myself succeeded in discovering the glycogenic function.

Is man justified in torturing innocent animals for the mere purpose of extending the domain of scientific knowledge ? Many philosophers think not ; and you have all heard of the Quaker who crossed the Atlantic for the purpose of expostulating with Magendie on the cruelty of his experiments. In this respect phosiologists have been ably defended by Legallois. If man is the lord of the creation, and has the right to make animals serve for food, has he not *à fortiori* —the right to use them for the purpose of acquiring knowledge ? The progress of an art, which alleviates the sufferings of humanity is, after all, the final object of all our endeavors : we are, therefore, no more guilty of cruelty in having recourse to vivesections than is the surgeon who amputates a limb in order to save the life of his patient.

In order not to inflict unnecessary suffering on dumb animals, we may, however, have recourse to anæsthetics, exactly as in the case of man ; these agents having, at the same time, the property of suspending for a moment, all the animal movements, render the operator's part a matter of less difficulty ; we shall, therefore, frequently have recourse to them ; but in certain experiments it becomes altogether impossible to do so, on account of the great perturbations which the inhalation of chloroform creates in several important functions of the economy.

Domestic animals are those which principally serve for our experiments ; they are more easily obtained. The dog, the cat, the rabbit, the guinea pig, the horse and ass, are almost exclusively employed in vivisections. Among the lower animals the frog is generally found the most convenient for the purpose.

In order to maintain the animal invariably in the same posture while undergoing an experiment, artificial means, with a view to restraining its movements, cannot be dispensed with. Veterinary surgeons have long been familiar with their use, and various contrivances for this purpose have been invented by MM. Blondlot, Pirogoff, Schwann, and others. The easiest and most expeditious way is to operate on a table perforated with numerous holes, through which cords are passed ; the animal is then tied down, so as to render all motion impossible*. Such was the *modus faciendi* adopted by De Graaf, in his experiments on the canine tribe ; he used also to open the windpipe, in order not to be annoyed with their cries. We generally succeed in obtaining the same result by dividing the recurrent nerve.

M. Bernard's sixth lecture, which relates to the salivary glands, and which is chiefly operative, so to speak, will be subjoined almost *in extensò.*

The parotid gland in the horse is situated partly beneath, and partly before, the external ear. The numerous ducts which arise from its granulations gradually coalesce into a considerable trunk, which, after descending for a certain space, and then rising again towards the mouth, penetrates into the oral cavity in front of the second molar tooth. A curve is thereby described, the concavity of which embraces the ascending ramus of the lower jaw. The facial vessels and nerve, which pass over the duct, must be carefully avoided in dividing it. In order not to injure these important parts, the anterior edge of the masseter must serve us as a guide in performing the operation. Let the incision be carried along its lower third, and the duct will be at once discovered, on the very point where it changes its direction, and rises towards the mouth. It may there safely be divided so as to allow a slender tube to be introduced. The one we are about to make use of is a small silver pipe containing a probe, which serves to clear it when obstructed, and makes it easier to be introduced. The excretory duct is then tied over the canula, just above the point where it has been introduced.

* I have found that a firm, narrow plank, to which the alligator should be bound with bandages, is a convenient mode of securing this animal during vivisection. B. DOWLER.

(After demonstrating the operation on the head of a horse, M. Bernard performs the experiment on a living animal ; not a single drop of saliva escapes at the moment when the tube is introduced into the ductus stenonis.)

The same proceeding is applicable to most of the herbiverous animals. The rabbit, however, offers a totally different arrangement; the ductus stenonis in this species presents the same relations as in the dog ; it therefore becomes indispensable to operate as in the case of this latter animal.

The parotidian duct in the dog passes through the muscular fibres of the masseter, and following a direct course, opens into the mouth in front of the second molar. In order to practise the same operation as before, the lower edge of the zygomatic arch must be felt for and followed from its posterior to its anterior extremity ; a slight depression will thus be discovered ; at this very point the duct passes into the mouth. Let a horizontal incision be made over this point, the duct will be easily discovered ; but the facial vessels and nerve, which lie before it, must be previously dissected with care, and then drawn aside with a curved probe ; the duct immediately appears beneath them ; nothing remains but to open it and plunge a tube within its cavity.

(M. Bernard performs the experiment on a middle-sized dog. At the moment when the duct is laid open, the animal utters a few plaintive cries. This proves, according to M. Bernard's remark, that the parotidian duct is sometimes endowed with sensibility, although the reverse is usually the case.)

You see, gentlemen, that not a single drop of saliva escapes at this moment from the tube ; in general the fluid is only secreted during the process of mastication and deglutition, or under the impression of acute pain, or of a powerful sapid sensation. You are well aware that various moral influences are capable of exciting its secretion ; the fact is a well-known one in man, and can be equally verified in the lower animals. The horse which has just undergone the operation we have performed in your presence, has been fasting for several hours ; the mere sight of his food will immediately bring on an abundant secretion.

(A bundle of hay being brought in, the animal exhibits great excitement, and a jet of saliva flows from the tube.)

Acids, however, are, of all the agents that can be brought to bear upon the salivary glands, the most powerful. Berzelius had remarked, several years ago, that alkaline secretions were excited by acid substances, and *vice versa ;* now saliva, being an alkaline secretion is likely to be elicited by the action of acids upon the gustative nerves, while alkalies remain comparatively inefficient.

(The experiment is tried on the dog, into the parotid duct of which a tube had been previously introduced. A few drops of vinegar being poured into the mouth, saliva flows from the tube drop by drop ; an alkaline solution being then substituted, no sensible result is obtained.)

Let us now examine the saliva we have obtained from both animals. In the dog, as you see, it is a limpid and colorless fluid, the reáction of which is strongly alkaline. But this is not always the case. We find in Tiedemann and Gmelin's great work on the digestive fluids, that, after dividing the parotidian duct in a dog, they plunged its extremity into a small glass case, so as to obtain ten grammes (180 grains) of a viscous fluid, strongly resembling albumen in its general appearance. Such are, therefore, the properties which these celebrated observers acknowledge as characterizing the parotidian secretion—a conclusion widely different from that which we have just arrived at ; and, in repeating the experiment on ten or twelve different animals, you would probably meet once or twice with the same result. How is this apparent contradiction to be explained ? A peculiar anatomical distribution is its real cause. It sometimes occurs that, before opening into the mouth, the ductus stenonis receives the excretory canals of two or three little mucous glands, which impart the properties of their own secretion to the parotidian fluid. Nothing is easier than to prove this. In the animals which offer this peculiarity let the duct be laid open above the point where it is joined by these tributary canals, and the normal and unmixed secretion of the gland will be ascertained to be exactly similar to that which we have just exhibited to you. In man the anatomical peculiarity we have noticed as an anomalous exception, in the dog is normal. The parotidian saliva, as poured into the mouth, always, therefore, enjoys a certain degree of viscosity in our own species. In this respect we find the dog approaching closer to our own organization than other animals.

· As to the saliva obtained from the horse, you see it offers, on the contrary, a viscid appearance ; as in the dog, its reáction is strongly alkaline ; but the action of heat, or the addition of nitric acid, precipitates an albuminous substance, which appears to be peculiar to the equine genus, although its chemical composition has not yet been precisely ascertained.

Let us now consider a few of the more important characteristics of the secretion itself, viewed apart from the nature of the fluid produced.

A tube being introduced into the parotidian duct, in a living animal, it may be easily ascertained that the saliva only flows at intervals ; in the horse, which during mastication emits prodigious quantities of it, the secretion now and then ceases in an abrupt manner, although the triturating process is still going on. The reason of this singular phenomenon long remained uncertain ; we are now aware that the gland which lies on that side of the mouth where mastication is going on, almost entirely suffices for the insalivation of aliments ; when the animal (as in the present case) has had both ducts laid open, and a tube passed into them, it becomes evident that during mastication the two parotids are alternately called into action ; while the one secretes, the other is at rest. The horse we have operated upon is at present satisfying its hunger, and you perceive that the saliva, however abundant, only flows on one side at a time.

In the normal state, the chemical composition of saliva, as secreted by each gland in particular, remains invariably the same ; it may, however, accidentally contain foreign substances. We gladly seize this opportunity of exhibiting, in a strong light, the elective action of glands ; the secretion we are investigating at the present moment offers a remarkable instance of this singular property. Among the various bodies introduced into the blood, we find some which almost instantaneously pass into the saliva ; iodine and its various compounds enjoy this property. Other substances cannot penetrate without the greatest difficulty into this secretion ; the salts of iron belong, for the most part, to this latter class. A direct experiment will enable you to judge for yourselves. The crural vein of a dog being opened, the extremity of a small syringe is introduced into the vessel ; a determinate quantity* of a solution containing 1-100th part of the yellow prussiate of potash is then injected into the torrent of circulation, together with an equal amount of a similar solution of iodide of potassium ; this latter substance will almost instantaneously be met with in the animal's saliva, while none of the usual tests exhibit the slightest vestige of the yellow ferro-cyanuret of potash. In the animal's urine we shall, on the contrary, discover it in considerable quantities ; a fact which amply demonstrates the penetration of this substance into the system, although the salivary glands refuse to eliminate it.

(These various experiments are all tried on the dog, and meet with perfect success. It is necessary, before employing the usual tests, to neutralize, by adding a few drops of acetic acid, the alkaline reaction which saliva naturally presents ; the chemical actions might otherwise be impeded.)

You therefore see, gentlemen, that iodine and its compounds will readily pass into the saliva, while the principal salts of iron are not to be found in that fluid, under ordinary circumstances. We possess, however, various means of overcoming the resistance (so to speak) of the salivary glands. If, in the first place, we combine one of the refractory substances with another body that enjoys the property of passing into the saliva, the difficulty is overcome ; iodide of iron, for instance, passes readily into the saliva, on account of the iodine it contains.

In the second place, if a direct injection be had recourse to, the salivary glands may be compelled, as it were, to eliminate the obnoxious substances. The largest doses of prussiate of potash may, for instance, be poured into the animal's veins, without giving the slightest indication of its presence in the saliva, even when recourse is had to the most sensible tests ; but if, by means of an injection into the common carotid artery, we create, in a manner, a local plethora in the atmosphere of the salivary glands, we succeed in obtaining the desired result, which, under any other circumstances, we should invariably have failed in producing.

It therefore remains an established fact, that the so-called affinity of glands for certain bodies, only expresses the greater facility with which they gain admittance into the fluid secreted ; all substances are capable of passing into the secretions, provided that a sufficiently

---

* Five cubic centimetres.

large quantity of them be conveyed into the blood that furnishes the elements of these various fluids.

The affinity of the salivary glands in particular produces, however, a great many singular phenomena. If, for instance, iodide of potassium be administered to a dog, vestiges of that substance will be discovered in the saliva for several weeks together. A sort of *circulus* is, in fact, established ; iodide passes into the saliva through the elective affinity of the glands ; but the animal, which keeps on swallowing its own saliva, impregnated as it is with iodine, absorbs new quantities of the substance, and the process might last indefinitely ; but if the animal be strongly purged, the iodine is at once evacuated by the intestinal discharge, and appears no longer in the saliva.

It now remains for us to perform the inverse experiment. The internal surface of glands is endowed with a considerable power of absorption, provided the substances injected into their cavity belong to that class of bodies for which the gland exhibits a certain elective affinity. But when the secreting process is in full activity, absorption is almost entirely suspended : thus (as we have already informed you), if a strong solution of strychnia is injected into a dog's parotid duct, the animal is almost instantaneously poisoned, if the gland is in a state of rest ; but if the secreting powers have been previously called into play, the animal resists for a pretty long space of time.

In order to convince you of the rapidity with which absorption takes place in the glands, we shall now inject into the parotid duct of the horse, which has already served for our previous experiment, a solution containing 1-100th part of iodide of potassium ; the duct being then tied over the canula, we shall almost immediately discover iodine in the secretion of the parotid on the opposite side—a fact which proves that after passing through the vast extent of the entire circulatory system, the substance injected has been eliminated again by the glands, in an incredibly short space of time.

(The experiment is tried on the horse, and succeeds perfectly. The reactions of iodine are not, however, distinctly perceived before a few seconds have elapsed after the injection.)

You see, gentlemen, that, although rapid, the elimination has not been altogether instantaneous ; but in the horse the circulation is known to be particularly slow ; by injecting prussiate of potash into the jugular vein, and testing the blood drawn from another point, Hering has proved that in this animal the blood does not accomplish its entire circuit in less than twenty-five seconds—a fact which sufficiently accounts for the comparative slowness of the process of elimination. In the dog the same result would be more rapidly attained to.

In his seventh lecture *on catalysis, or the chemical agents of disease in the living body*, M. Bernard says : septic bodies, or specific poisons are almost invariably organic substances, and are produced within a living organization ; here, we have, no doubt, a peculiar and characteristic biological action ; we need not, therefore, be surprised to see pathologists endeavoring to withdraw this class of phenomena from the domain of physiology, in order to make them the exclusive property of medicine.

We must not, however, in my opinion, give up all hope of connecting, one day, these morbid phenomena with the laws of physiology. If at present unable to do so, we shall, no doubt, succeed at some future period. Is it not, in fact, quite possible that in animals certain physiological conditions may arise which would give birth to virulent poisons? We are aware that in a perfect state of health, several creatures are venemous; that is to say, they possess a peculiar virus which Nature has given them for the purpose of killing their prey, and defending themselves from their enemies. Here, then, we have a physiological virus; how is it produced within the system? The difficulty is quite as great as with regard to morbid poisons.

It would appear that in several cases the noxious substance prevails throughout the economy; in other cases we only discover it in certain fluids. The virus which occasions hydrophobia belongs to the latter class; it resides exclusively in the animal's saliva. We are not yet aware whether any one of the salivary glands is its peculiar seat, or whether it is indifferently secreted by all of them. No experiments have been tried on this point; but it has been experimentally proved that the peculiar venomous principle does not exist in the blood; transfusion does not convey the disease from a mad dog to a healthy one.

It is a singular fact, and one which preëminently deserves our attention, that in so general a disease the virus, which alone is capable of transmitting the affection, should be exclusively localized within one single apparatus, without existing in the blood at large. Yet, if we reflect upon the question, we discover, in the physiological state, a great many similar dispositions; the principles which concur in a vast number of physiological functions; pepsine, ptyaline, and the active principle of the pancreatic juice, are they not created by special glands? and is not the venom of serpents, which does not exist within the blood, produced by a special apparatus? Viewed in this light a mad dog resembles a viper or a rattlesnake.

But, on the other hand, there exist several virulent diseases, in which the blood really appears to contain the morbid principle. This is the case with the glanders; and it is a well known fact that healthy animals may be infected with the blood of a diseased horse, as well as with the slimy matter that escapes from the nose and mouth.

But another particular which will, perhaps, excite your astonishment, is that the normal secretions, bile, saliva, gastric juice, and so forth, do not appear to contain the slightest vestige of this poison; while, on the other hand, the pathological fluids appear to be impregnated with it, and possess the property of transmitting the disease to sound animals—a fact experimentally proved with regard to pus, the fluid contained in a hydrocele, and various other 'morbid secretions. For this reason alone are the autopsies performed on animals that die of the glanders attended with so much danger; the virus pervades the whole system, and the slightest wound is sufficient to inoculate the complaint.

You need not, however, be astonished at this singular property;

you have already witnessed the repulsion which the salivary glands evince for certain substances introduced into the blood ; and why should not certain morbid principles be in this manner rejected from all the secretions in which the normal conditions remain unimpaired? The same thing appears to take place with respect to the contagious pneumonia of horned cattle. We are aware that volatile emanations transmit the morbid principle ; but experiments have been tried (in Belgium) for the purpose of inoculating it directly to animals, as a preservative against the disease. Something similar to the process of inoculation in the small pox was expected to result from this ; it was then discovered that neither the animal's blood nor any of the fluids of the economy was endowed with the property of propagating the complaint. It appears to have chosen the lung for its exclusive seat, and the liquids therein contained, pus, lymph, etc., are alone endowed with the property of transmitting the complaint. The intense local inflammation which follows the operation sufficiently testifies to the noxious properties of this virus ; and when, in order not to spoil the animal's flesh the tail is selected as the point where inoculation is to be performed, the subsequent inflammation frequently causes it to mortify.

Here, then, we have another virus which exclusively resides in the tissue of the lungs, and is not found in the blood at large ; but even in the normal state a great many substances are found in various tissues, which do not exist in this fluid. Thus, muscular flesh contains a large amount of salts of potash, while scarcely any trace of them is found in the blood : in a word, the various bodies found in different parts of the economy are not invariably represented in the torrent of the circulation.

The history of specific diseases offers therefore, nothing which cannot rationally be explained ; it now remains for us to discover the physiological process by which a virus may be originated. Nothing is easier than to produce putrid affections in sound animals. Thus, when transfusion is performed under the ordinary conditions —when the blood is conveyed directly from one animal into the veins of another—no accidents whatever are produced ; but if the blood is allowed to remain for a short space of time in contact with the atmosphere, and if the serum is then injected into the vessels, all the symptoms of putrid resorption are observed, and the animals die after exhibiting all the characteristic symptoms of putrid infection.

The blood is therefore capable of acquiring toxic properties without the intervention of any foreign principle, merely through the modifications which takes place in its composition when life is extinct. The same results may be attained to without even drawing blood from the veins. If the blood of a fasting animal is directly injected into the veins of a healthy one, the latter is poisoned exactly in the same manner as before ; and yet the blood in this case, has not undergone any previous decomposition.

The introduction of foreign principles, of course, acts upon the blood with still more intensity ; nearly all the substances known under the name of *ferments*, are endowed with the property of communicating a deleterious influence to this fluid. When yeast is introduced into an animal's veins, passive hæmorrhage, and other adynamic symptoms, are immediately produced, and death takes place within a few days. Now, if the animal's blood is transfused into another's veins, all the phenomena previously described take place in rapid succession, exactly as if yeast, and not blood, had been directly poured into the vessels.

It seems likely that in this case a series of decompositions take place within the blood, which give rise to other *ferments*. The well known experiment related in Pringle's work on Army Diseases, appears to tally with the result of our own experiments.

(In order to prove the influence of putrid emanations, even at a distance, on the chemical phenomena of life, he plunged a thread into the yolk of a rotten egg, and then suspended it in a jar containing the yolk of another egg, and under these circumstances, decomposition took place with far greater rapidity than usual.)

We, therefore, perceive that all this series of phenomena holds intimate connection with that mysterious chemical process known under the name of *catalysis*. The theory of fermentation is at present so imperfectly known—and organic chemistry has in this respect made, as yet, so little progress—that it would hardly be fair to reproach medicine with its deficiencies on this point. There exists a whole series of diseases which evidently result from the chemical actions which take place within the body. It is, therefore, chemistry alone which, in its future progress, can teach us the physiological laws which embrace this particular branch of medicine.

In his eighth lecture *on diseases arising from the vitiated development of cells*, M. Bernard says :

Consider the morbid manifestations of this [developmental or vital] power, which never suspends its action within the living body ; we allude, of course, to those peculiar tissues which have been styled heteromorphous—an expression utterly condemned by German micographers ; for morbid tissue is generated within the economy in strict conformity with the laws that preside over fœtal development. But, as we have previously seen, both nervous influence and catalytical agency give rise to a variety of diseases when deviated from their proper course ; thus, also, in certain given cases, the power of histological evolution may create positive disorder in the system. An immense and uninterupted movement takes place within the organs of which the body is composed, for the purpose of supplying new tissues, in the place of those which are no longer fit to accomplish the functions devolving upon them ; let this unceasing activity be diverted from its proper channel, and the production of tubercle, cancer, and all kinds of morbid deposits, will be the immediate consequence. We find here, as usual, an evident connection between the phenomena of health and disease, between physiological activity and pathological influence. The question which lies before us must evidently be viewed in this light ; and such is the principal object of Virchow's labors on cellular pathology, the leading features of which it is our purpose to make known to you. But, before entering into the study of this particular point, a few general notions on the subject cannot safely be dispensed with.

Some diseases, in the first place, result from total absence or considerable deficiency of normal evolution on a given point. The mucous coat of the intestinal tube affords us a fine example of incessant development. New layers of epithelium are continually being secreted, to line its inner surface ; but a living medium, or blastem, is necessary to their production ; and whenever this blastem itself happens to be altered in its essential properties—a modification which always occurs in inflammation—the epithelium disappears, and is no longer regenerated. Cholera also exhibits another instance of this; for it has been indisputably proved that, in this disease, the vessels which ramify on the internal surface of the intestines are completely laid bare. In his admirable researches on the intestinal mucous membrane, Professor Goodsir has established that, after each meal, when absorption has taken place, the epithelium which covers the villosities falls off, and is renewed during the interval which elapses before food is again introduced into the digestive apparatus—a remarkable instance of the rapidity with which the reproduction of tissue frequently takes place. But when, through some pathological agency, epithelium is no longer secreted, what results from its absence ? No obstacle is henceforth opposed to serous exudation from the vessels ; no protecting surface resists the introduction of various poisons into the economy ; and, lastly, no regulating power of absorption any longer exists. In this manner innumerable diseases may be traced back to the suspended activity of normal evolution as their primary cause. The chronic inflammation of the trachea and bronchial tubes likewise destroys the vibratile epithelium, the utility of which is too well known to be expatiated on.

But we meet, at the same time, with other diseases, which arise, not from interrupted, but from perverted, evolution. You are, of course, well aware that cells which pursue a regular course in their development comprise three distinct elements—firstly, an envelope, or cellular paries, the physical properties of which take a prominent share in its action ; secondly, liquid contents, the importance of which is principally derived from their chemical composition ; and, lastly, a nucleus, in which the powers of development appear to reside. As soon as a morbid state of nutrition supervenes, the contents of the cell are liable to alteration. Whether pigment, or fatty substances, or calcareous salts are therein deposited, morbid tissues are gradually formed, and disease is introduced into the system; and, even in similar cases, no pathological entity, no abstract principle of disease, is required to explain the fact. The deviation of physiological activity is its only cause. It is, therefore, evident that, in their successive phases of development, heteromorphous tissues entirely resemble the normal ones, and are subject to the same natural laws. To Müller belongs the honor of having been the first to proclaim this great principle ; and he may therefore be deservedly styled the creator of cellular pathology. He was the first to open that path in which Virchow now treads with so much success.

The intercellular tissue, or blastem, is the medium from which the cells derive the elements of their formation ; it is, according to Virchow's picturesque expression, their territory. Now there exist va-

rious conditions in which the blastem no longer contains the principles required for the normal development of cells ; it is, for instance, indispensable that it should always contain glycose, albumen,
and fat ; the absence of a single one of these three substances is an
insuperable barrier to cellular evolution ; and we, therefore, constantly find them existing as well in the tissues of the embryo as in
those of the adult. But a variety of other conditions, essentially
injurious to histological growth, may casually arise ; and the existence of morbid blastems, which give birth to all tissues endowed
with abnormal properties, may easily be conceived as of possible
occurrence. Such are, no doubt, those very general dispositions of
the economy, known under the name of diatheses, and which, when
once they have firmly established their hold on a previously sound
individual, are capable of being transmitted to his posterity ; we
must evidently consider them in the light of conditions of existence
entirely new, which, in the first instance, are accidentally produced
(for disease must evidently begin somewhere), but which, when once
called into existence, exhibit a strong tendency to maintain themselves in being. Thus, when food, insufficient in quantity, or of an
unwholesome kind, has ultimately reduced to a consumptive state an
animal previously enjoying perfectly sound health, its offspring often
inherits the morbid disposition which, in the parent, was entirely
accidental ; and syphilis, that well-known and fruitful source of heteromorphous productions, is similarly transmitted from parent to child.

Such pathological dispositions, or diatheses, result from causes
various in their nature, but which concur in one point, viz : the disposition which opposes all modifications favorable to the patient's
health. Sometimes they are the result of a profound change in the
fluids of the economy ; sometimes they originate in the introduction
of peculiar poisons, which, after having once penetrated into the system, can in no way be expelled ; if there existed, for instance, a
poison which none of our organs could eliminate, it is clear that
after penetrating into the torrent of the circulation, it would nowhere
find an issue, and would in consequence become the origin of permanent modifications in the economy. The possibility of a similar case
may be rationally conceived, by referring to the singular fact already
mentioned, that iodine, when once introduced into the blood, is not
eliminated before a long space of time, on account of the affinity
which the salivary glands exhibit for this substance ; we have, therefore, in this case, an instance of a body which cannot (for a time, at
least) be expelled from the system ; the animal is, therefore, during
that period, laid under an iodic diathesis.

Viewing the subject in an entirely physiological light, it may be
contended that individuals affected with local cancers are not properly, so to speak, in a state of disease, as long as the organs affected
are not altogether essential to life ; but when cancer attacks the
limbs, the possibility of a surgical cure may at least be presumed, if
not expected actually to take place ; and the patient is not really diseased—that is to say, life is not directly brought into danger. Thus,
when cancer attacks the liver, if a disease is not too extensive, the
morbid productions are separated by large tracts of sound tissue,

which fulfill, as in the healthy state, their physiological duties ; bile is secreted as usual, and grape-sugar exists within the glandular tissue.   But when, at a later period, the disintegration of the elements which constitute the morbid production have poisoned in some measure the whole economy, by pouring into the torrent of the circulation fluids impregnated with the noxious principle, then, indeed, the affection becomes a general complaint, and its nature entirely changes.   Cancer is not a diathesis in itself ; but the subsequent cachectic state is evidently diathetical.

To conclude the history of these morbid evolutions, there yet remains one to be described ; and this is imperfect nutrition.   It is evident at the present day that the anatomical conditions, brought so prominently forward in Bichat's celebrated work* are quite insufficient to explain all the various modes of dying.   Experince has taught us that patients often die without offering, in the post-mortem examination, the slightest modification in the anatomical condition of their organs.   In the course of our physiological experiments we often see dogs arrived at the very last stage of emaciation, although the appetite continues unimpaired till the last moment.   They sink from sheer exhaustion, while the lacteals are gorged with chyle ; and, when opened, their bodies offer no trace whatever of pathological alterations.

The latent cause of this singular process is, that nutrition, when considered within the depths of our organs is, in fact, nothing more than a peculiar mode of evolution.   The economy produces within itself substances indispensable to life ; glycogenous matter affords us an example of this : formed within the body by a special process, it plays an immense part in histological phenomena.   As soon as it fails to be supplied, epithelium is no longer produced ; various diseases are the immediate result ; and, under similar circumstances, life is inevitably brought to a close.   The physiological act called nutrition, comprehended, therefore, two distinct parts : formation of cells is the first ; creation of blastems is the second ; and the latter is no less indispensable to our existence than is the former ; as soon as pathological influences arrest either the one or the other, death is the consequence.   There exist, therefore, two distinct modes of dying : sometimes life is cut short at once by an important injury to some essential organ ; sometimes, on the contrary it gradually fails through imperfect nutrition ; and this latter termination is the ordinary result of acute diseases, when they prove fatal.   In certain cases, for instance, glycogenous matter is no longer produced ; and after a given space of time the patient dies, although the appetite remains unimpaired till the last moment.   In making the autopsy the lacteals will be found in a state of repletion ; but when analyzed the fluids of the economy no longer present the slightest vestige of sugar.   Death then supervenes, and is the mere result of suspended activity in organs for which proper nourishment is no longer provided.

You therefore see, gentlemen, that to create laws especially for the

---

* " Recherches Physiologiques sur la Vie et la Mort."

the use of pathology cannot in case be justified ; and that physiology furnishes, in every possible condition of health or disease, a key to the interpretation of vital phenomena.   These general notions I look upon as indispensable to the study of particular points : it now re-mains for us, in order to complete this general survey, to examine the all-important question, "Whether medicines act on a sick patient in the same manner as on a sound individual ? " and how far the results obtained in one case are fit to be compared with those observed in the other.   It is our intention to examine this subject in the next Lecture : its study is an indispensable introduction to the various investigations we are about to undertake ; for, after pro-ducing artificially—no matter how—a morbid state in an animal, we shall have recourse to the counter-proof, by seeking for therapeutical agents to effect its cure.

Art. X.—*Military Surgery.*

[Since the eventful days of Napoleon I and Larrey I, the army sur-geons have contributed comparatively little towards the advancement of surgical science.   The military memoirs of Baron Larrey (father of the present surgeon-in-chief of the French army), is a work of great value, notwithstanding its composite character, into which the most desultory historical and non-professional topics enter largely.

Of the late war with Mexico no complete surgical account has yet appeared.   Of the more recent wars in the Crimea, India, and Italy, little that is professional is known in the United States, or perhaps elsewhere.

The following extracts from two recent works by Drs. Williamson and Fraser, on military surgery, are cited from *The Br. and For. Med. and Chir. Rev.* for Jan. 1860.   B. D.]

Large number of cases of gun-shot compound fracture of the femur, in the Indian mutiny, where the patients recovered with good useful limbs, as compared with the number of thigh stump cases, and the total, by all wounds, Dr. Williamson says: this very satisfactory feature in the classified return of invalided, wounded by the mutiny, appears to me, perhaps, not uncommon for Indian wars, but certainly very much so for European wars, as far as records enable us to make the comparison.   This difference in favor of results by Indian wars I believe to be mainly due to the facilities afforded by the dooley for the successful treatment of this severest of all forms of compound fracture.

The following passages contain the principal information which Dr. Williamson's work conveys on the subject of resection of each of the larger joints.

Hip.—Excision of the hip-joint for gun-shot injury has been performed eleven times. Of these, but one recovered, that of a soldier wounded by a shell at Sebastopol, and operated upon by Dr. O'Leary. The patient was twenty-five years of age ; the head, neck, and trochanter of the femur were removed.

Of the eleven cases recorded, six occurred in the Crimean war, one occurred in the Schleswig-Holstein war, one by Dr. Ross, one by Oppenheim, one by M. Seutin, and one by Schwartz. In the Crimean war, excision of the head of the femur was performed six times, and all but one were primary operations. One of the patients survived the operation and recovered—viz : private Thomas M'Kenna, 68th Regiment. On his arrival at Chatham, the limb is reported to have been about two and a-half inches shorter than the other, and capable of bearing some considerable portion of the weight of the body. He could swing it and advance it, but the knee could not be bent. Rotation was admitted to a very limited extent, but performed with considerable pain. The wound was soundly healed.

So far as the Crimean war goes, it clearly proves the superiority of the excision of the head of the femur over amputation at the hip-joint. * * * No doubt in any future campaigns, excision of the hip-joint will be much more frequently employed, and great attention paid to the selection of cases.

Knee.—As yet our experience of excision of the knee-joint in cases of gun-shot fracture is not extensive, and the means necessary for after treatment in military practice are not encouraging ; but the success which has followed it in cases of disease of the joint, makes military surgeons also wish to extend it to the field. The absolute rest and quiet after the operation, which are so difficult to obtain with an army in the field, is the chief and only objection to its adoption.

There are two cases recorded of excision of this joint for gun-shot injuries—one in the Schleswig-Holstein war, and the other in the Crimean war. Both died.

On the subject of resection of the shoulder, Dr. Williamson says—Only one case of resection of this joint was admitted from India ; but there is another case where a secondary operation was performed at Fort Pitt, in a patient who is returned as a wound of the joint.

In the Crimean war the head of the humerus was removed twice as a primary operation during the first period of the war, or that ending March, 1855, and eight times during the second. One of the two first mentioned ended in death, and of the eight subsequent operations only one proved fatal. The head of the bone was five times removed as a secondary operation, without a single casualty. In addition to these there was a case in which the head of the bone, and a large portion of the scapula, broken into fragments, were removed.

Out of the total number, then, of sixteen cases, three deaths took place or 18.9 per cent. Had this operation not been resorted to, amputation at the shoulder-joint, it is believed, would have become necessary in all.

Of resection of the elbow, the return stands thus : In the Crimean war twenty-two operations in all were done on the elbow joint, of which three ended fatally, and two more deaths took place after secondary amputation—in all a total of 5 deaths, or 22 per cent. of the cases treated. This per centage slightly exceeds that of resection of the shoulder joint, but in both instances resection afforded a much more favorable result as to the mortality than amputation.

Dr. Fraser makes the following extraordinary statement : That in the human subject, as well as in animals, an actual wound in the substance of the lung is always, sooner or later, mortal ; not from the effects of inflammatory action, but, in recent cases, from a sudden cessation of proper aëration in either the whole or portions of one or two lungs, or sudden hæmorrhage.

In opposition to this, Dr. Fraser himself says : There are cases in which recovery has taken place when the substance of the lung was wounded ; and refers to a case related by Larrey, in which recovery took place, and there was no doubt that the lung was wounded. A very interesting case, and one which would have been very valuable to Dr. Fraser had he met with it before the publication of his treatise, is found at p. 31 of Dr. Williamson's work, with a beautiful representation of the parts, in which the lung had been wounded, but the patient survived eleven months, and then died of gangrene of the opposite lung, from some unexplained cause, but influenced as Dr. Williamson supposes, in some manner, by the old wound, which had never soundly healed. The track of the ball was found still open and lined by a membrane, on which the bronchial tubes opened ; the exit of the ball had been kept open by necrosed bone. We may notice that here, if anywhere, according to Dr. Fraser's reasoning, tromatopnœa should have been absent, since the wound communicated directly with the air tubes, and consequently there was no resistance to the passage of air by the natural way ; yet it is stated distinctly that air escaped on expiration and coughing.

Upon the treatment of wounds of the chest, Dr. Fraser reasons strongly against the necessity of the copious and indiscriminate bloodletting which is, or was lately, prescribed for such injuries ; and we must say that the cases he has adduced, together with the notes of those reported by Dr. Williamson (so far as the latter are fully reported), are enough to create some little doubt, at any rate, whether bleeding can be so necessary to the cure of these wounds as some would still have us believe. Many cases may be found here in which wounds of the chest, which would by most people be diagnosed as involving the lung, recovered without bleeding ; and others in which the fatal progress and the distressing symptoms seemed little affected by copious bloodletting. Dr. Fraser seems opposed to bleeding altogether ; but we have no doubt that his theoretical reason for it—viz : because pneumonia is, as he believes, a rare complication of wound of the lung—is erroneous. There is every reason however, to believe that the pneumonia which follows a wound of the lung is often, perhaps usually, only as much as is sufficient and necessary for its closure, and that if bleeding would affect it at all, it would be injuriously. On this subject, as on so many others, the truth seems to lie between the extreme partisans on either side, and the symptoms of each case will doubtless furnish the best guide to practice. With the limited experience that we have in London of gun-shot wounds, we cannot affect to give any opinion on this subject ; but we can entertain no doubt of the relief which we have seen from *small* and *cautious* venesection in cases of fractured ribs with wound of the lung, and should certainly expect similar results in gun-shot injuries.

ART. XI.—*On the Mechanism of Sinuous Ulcers.* By Professor ROSER. (*Archiv für Physiol. Heilk.*,1859.—*Br. and For. Med. Ch. Rev.*1860.)

PROFESSOR ROSER observes that the practice of cutting away undermined portions of skin, although an old one, is far from being resorted to so frequently as it deserves to be, and is scarcely alluded to in the most recent text books. Those who do resort to it do so for the most part as a mere empircal procedure ; and can give no account of why these undermined portions of skin will not heal, or why an ulcer, which may have remained for months unhealed will take on reparative action only a few days after excision of such portions has been performed. So, too, there is wanting the means of determining the cases in which the undermined portions should not be cut away, and the healing brought about by means of suitable compression. In this state of things it is Dr. Roser's object in the present paper, to explain the mechanism of sinuous ulcers, in order to furnish something like a scientific explanation of the mode of treatment which has been found practically so useful.

Sinuous ulcers are most frequently met with in the scrofulous suppuration of the cervical glands. By the prompt opening of such abscesses we may anticipate the undermining process, and do much to hasten healing and prevent disfiguring cicatrices. And when even the skin has become undermined, if we cut it away, we may, with few exceptions (as when the infiltrated glandular substance is laid bare), still secure a quickly formed and proportionally well looking cicatrix. But if we leave these abscesses quietly to themselves, waiting for spontaneous perforation, the undermining suppurative process leads to a gradual thinning and atrophy of the skin, one hole opens after another, and after tedious discharge, a wrinkling of the skin takes place, and hideous irregular scars result. The undermined skin, in a condition of atrophy from disturbed circulation and innervation, and from venous stasis, is not in a condition to undergo the healing process. On cutting such portion of skin away,

it is found remarkably void of blood (as indeed its blue color already
indicated), a small portion of dark venous blood alone flowing away.
Its sensibility, too, is almost entirely lost. It is true that, after a
very long period these ulcers will heal of themselves, the undermined
skin first retracting at its base, converting the irregular into a
simple ulcer, which then cicatrises from its circumference. The
tedious part of the healing is the retraction of the undermined skin,
and the process is immensely hastened by the removal of this part,
which after all is lost whether removed or left.

If however, the removal of this skin is advantageous in simple
subcutaneous abscess, which by perforation or dividing in the middle
has become a sinuous ulcer, it is of far greater utility in undermining
abscesses having numerous perforations. Such multiple perforations
are common in the undertermined and atrophied condition of the
skin, and they are sometimes even advantageous, as the fusion of
the several holes into one will promote the gaping of the opening
and the retraction of the undermined tissue. But in a great number
of cases these multiple perforations give rise to the production of half
isolated, bridge formed, or tongue-like slips of skin, which are quite
incapable of undergoing the process of healing. When they do not
entirely disappear from the influence of progressive ulceration or
atrophy, they gives rise to a peculiarly ugly form of cicatrix,
termed by the author the "bridge-cicatrix," and the "lappet-cicatrix."
The skin, cicatrising behind these bridge-like slips of integument,
they remain stretched over it as projecting cords, and are especially
observed in the cervical and inguinal regions. Their disagreeable
appearance renders it necessary to cut them smooth off with the
scissors, an operation which, on account of their bloodlessness and
little sensibility, give rise to but little inconvenience. In like manner when the small tongue shaped lobules of skin following multiple
perforation are not removed by the knife, they give rise to the production of small projecting lappet-cicatrices, attached by a pedicle,
and resembling warts, or having a broad basis. These also must be
cut off with the scissors.

What has already been said will indicate the circumstances under
which the undermined skin may still be considered as capable of adhering again. When it has become thinned and blue, its nutrition
may be considered as arrested ; but as long as any of the *panniculus
adiposus* remains, it is capable of healing. Frequent division is the
best treatment for threatened integument, the edges of the wound
retracting and becoming thicker, and the nutrition and circulation
being facilitated. When the undermined skin continues well
nourished, the healing may, under favorable circumstances, be
brought about by compression ; but these cases are rare, as various
complications, such as exposure of bone or fasciæ, infiltration of the
cellular tissue, the retention of decomposed pus, or dyscrasis, may
furnish contra-indications. Compression, too, is in some regions
difficult of application.

What has here been said of the skin will also apply to the *mucous
membrane*. Undermining of this certainly is a much rarer occurrence ; but it is met with, as in the case of the rectum, and more

rarely the entrance to the vagina ; and if the undermined portions are not removed, endless suppurations and the formation of the bridge cicatrices will be the result. Many cases of fistula in ano are nothing else than this undermining process, affecting the skin and mucous membrane in common ; and to secure rapid healing, excision of the atrophied membrane—not a mere incision—is required. When there is a mere fistulous tract without undermining, simple incision is alone required.

ART. XII.—*On the Duties imposed on Practitioners by Lithotrity:* By M. CIVIALE. (*Moniteur des Hôspitaux. Brit. and For. Med. Chir. Rev.*)

M. CIVIALE took the occasion of two favorable lithotrity cases to make the following observations to his class at the Necker Hospital : As long as cystotomy constituted the sole surgical resource in a case of stone, the conduct to be followed by the surgeon was distinctly marked out. The rule was, at least as regards the adult and the aged, to delay the operation as long as life continued supportable. It was founded upon the fact that any cutting operation on the bladder, independently of the circumstances under which it may be resorted to, gives rise to real perils, and that under the most favorable conditions, both as regards the size of the stone and the state of the patient, the hopes of the practitioner may be belied. Under these circumstances, a prudent and experienced practitioner, suspecting the existence of stone, pursued a judicious course in not communicating his suspicions to the patient as long as the pains were slight and of short duration, and capable of being rendered very bearable by the use of internal remedies ; and a very great number of facts prove : 1st, That the stone may remain stationary, and many patients who would have succumbed to an operation performed at an early stage, have lived for a long period without suffering excessively ; and, 2d, that the operations performed at a later period, when functional disturbances have rendered them necessary (and always before the condition of the patient has become seriously deteriorated), are not followed by notably more unfavorable results. This rule constituted the basis of all rational practice, and has received the sanction of experience and the consent of the greatest practitioners. No serious arguments can be opposed to it ; and some exceptional cases or isolated opinions, founded on an insufficient experience, do not possess this character.

Since lithotrity has become the general method of treating stone, this rule of conduct has undergone a change ; for all is different, both as regards the manner of proceeding and the result obtained. The operation succeeds with greater certainty in proportion to the small size of the stone, a few days' treatment then securing the patient an easy and durable cure, unattended by unfortunate consequences. All calculous patients are in these conditions at one part of their malady, and may then rely upon the benefit of treatment. Lithotrity, too, presents the invaluable advantage of saving the patient from suffering from stone; and especially of preventing the development of the organic lesions of the bladder, which constitute a long series of complications, involving the operator in uncertainties and mistakes.

Looking at these general results, it might naturally be expected that every enlightened and conscientious practitioner would make it a rigorous duty to carefully study the early rational signs of the presence of stone, and have recourse to the new means of explorations which art has furnished for establishing an exact diagnosis. It is much to be regretted that this is not the case, the same line of conduct being now pursued with regard to lithotrity which formerly was properly applicable to lithotomy. Practitioners of high repute may be daily found not making a stand at the early symptoms, and without assuring themselves as to the presence of stone, merely palliating these by the use of sedatives. Such means succeed all the better, inasmuch as the symptoms of stone are often interrupted, especially at an early period; and when these return, the same means are again prescribed, the patient is sent to Vichy, or appropriate regimen is directed—the idea of stone never being raised for fear of alarming the patient or his friends. Every practitioner is aware, that in order to establish the diagnosis of a calculous affection, a direct exploration is essential; but on the patient exhibiting any signs of fear, this is indefinitely adjourned; and thus both patient and practitioner live in ignorance of what really exists, both seeming to fear recognising the true condition of things, and remaining in a state of deceptive calmness and security. In M. Civiale's "Traité de l'Affection Calculeuse," he has related a great number of curious facts, each more melancholy than the other, which only too plainly exhibit the deplorable censequences of this mode of procedure, which leads the patient fatally to his end, and involves the practitioner in the most painful errors. In the present paper he adduces additional instances of the mischief accruing from this temporizing practice—the stone in some of these having acquired such a magnitude as to be no longer amenable to lithotrity, while in other cases death ensued upon operative procedures too long delayed. M. Civiale finally observes that it is impossible to relieve a practitioner of the responsibility of events, the occurrence of which he might easily have prevented, had he made or caused to have been made a careful exploration at the period of the first appearance of the symptoms. In some instances the patients have been nearly on the point of bringing this point of medical responsibility before the legal tribunals.

Art. XIII.—*Fragmentary Notes on the Epidemic Yellow Fever of Texas in* 1859, *with brief Remarks :* By Bennet Dowler, M. D.

In the hope, perhaps an illusory hope, that the following imperfect memoranda may be the means of calling the attention of the Texas physicians to the necessity of giving a history of the recent epidemic yellow fever of their State, I venture to give such fragmentary data as were accidentally met with in the public journals, which have fallen under my observation, and, which, though devoid of satisfactory historical details and statistical continuity, are, nevertheless, frought with great interest and suggestiveness.

During the past year the valley of the Mississippi was, perhaps, almost wholly exempt from epidemic yellow fever, with the exception of a slight one in New Orleans. The deaths from this disease in the city, will be found duly noted in the mortality tables of this journal. The whole number according to the official report is ninety-two.

It may be proper, before proceeding further, to remark, that up to the 9th of October, 1859, according to the official report of the Board of Health, ten deaths from yellow had occurred in this city. The first case is thus noted by the same authority :

" If this case be a case of yellow fever, it originated on a steamboat at Vicksburg, coming down the river. . The patient had been sick two days before admission into the Hospital."

This, the first case, thus provisionally admitted as possibly yellow fever, was attended by James A. Jones, M. D. The patient, Wm. King, born in Pennsylvania, aged 21, had black vomit, and died comatose. His case was pronounced genuine yellow fever by his medical attendant, already named.

It is remarkable, that all of the deaths from yellow fever in 1859, with the exception of nine, occurred in the Charity Hospital. The office of this journal is indebted to the kidness of Wm. H. Sprague, M. D., for a very complete copy of the statistical and other data which the official record of the Hospital furnishes, of all the yellow fever cases of the year. For the present the following data only will be given :

Admissions...................................102
Deaths..................................... 83
Discharges 19
The periods of sickness of these patients, respectively, when admit-

ted were—5, one day ; 16, two days ; 13, three days ; 22, four days ; 8, five days ; 4, six days ; 15, seven days ; 3, eight days ; 1, nine days ; 8, after two weeks ; 4, with chronic disease ; 3, unknown. Of those admitted, the first two had been resident, respectively, seven and eight years, and were last from Liverpool, England ; the third and fourth, last from St. Louis, resident three days and three weeks ; fifth and sixth, from the same city ; resident two and a-half years and one week, respectively ; seventh, eighth, nineth, tenth and eleventh— from New York, nine months ; from Cincinnati, two months ; from St. Louis, ten years ; from Chicago, eleven months ; from St. Louis, three months, respectively. The oracles of contagion in New Orleans, give no responses for 1859.

From these and other facts which the sequel will develop, it will appear that this malady did not show itself either in New Orleans or in Galveston, the great seaport of Texas, until late in the season— later, indeed, by two months, than in some interior parts of the latter State—facts that must puzzle quarantinists, contagionists, and other expounders of the essential cause of yellow fever.

In some districts of Texas, even in the interior towns, remote villages, and isolated hamlets, the disease occasionally attacked all, and sometimes killed more than half of the inhabitants, as, for example, in Cypress City. Were an epidemic, thus unsparing, to invade the great city of New York, where the present generation is destitute of the protection which a previous attack of this fever affords, no language could enumerate the disaster, dismay, and bereavement that would ensue. North of Charleston, all of the cities of the Republic, except Norfolk, in Virginia, are equally susceptible, should epidemic yellow fever revisit the old localities which it had desolated before it appeared (in 1796) in New Orleans.

The epidemic at Norfolk, in 1855, swept to the realm of death about one-third of all that remained in the city, including a similar proportion of the resident physicians, and an extraordinary number of medical men who hastened to aid the sick from almost all of the Atlantic cities. Such calamities, like the shock of contending armies, and the whelming of cities by earthquakes, furnish the historian with events which fill the imagination and move the passions of mankind ; but the scientific ætiologist finds a greater interest in contemplating the causes and conditions which are concerned in producing " the pestilence which walketh in the darkness," and suddenly strikes down a remote village or isolated plantation, because such events, which unfortunately have occurred in numerous instances since 1853, as well as towards the close of last century, in the North, show the insufficiency of crowding, filth, contagion, disturbance of the soil, and other alleged causes of the disease.

In view of all this, the mere history of yellow fever, independently of its pathology and therapeutics, is a desideratum. If the subject were not too serious to allow of any mirth, the many grave, positive, but contradictory and fanciful explanations of the cause of yellow fever, would be altogether facetious. If the solution of this problem shall ever be achieved, a careful study of the history, geography, and conditions of this disease, affords the most promising route ; and if it should fail to reach this hoped-for result, its facts, divested of theory, must serve as the best landmarks and guides for the prevention, avoidance, or mitigation of evils, the cause of which may elude human research.

July 15–20, 1859. Yellow fever prevails on the Rio Grande in both Mexico and Texas. At Reynosa, in the Mexican State of Tamaulipas, the number of deaths variously reported at from 130 to 230. All remaining in the town suffer an attack from this disease.

Many die (some in the spring season) along the river, above Brownsville.—*Goliad Messenger.*

At Edinburgh, a village in Hidalgo county, on the Rio Grande, Texas, thirteen die.

August 4. At Brownsville, Cameron county, Texas, on the Rio Grande, below Reynosa and Edinburgh.

August 28. Aurora Borealis. Reäppears September 2d.

September 17. Houston, Harris county, forty-five miles inland, eighty-two miles from Galveston, one death.

September 19. Galveston. Mr. Hudgkin, from Houston, dies.

September 21. Richmond, an interior town, Fort Bend county, establishes quarantine : The Board of Aldermen, at Richmond, passed an ordinance establishing a quarantine, to prevent citizens of Houston from entering Richmond until ten days from the time of their leaving, and also prohibiting woolen goods being brought there packed in Houston. The fine for violating the ordinance will be not less than ten dollars, nor more than one hundred dollars.

September 23. Galveston. Mr. Gaskin dies. The journals affirm the great salubrity of the city, and the absence of yellow fever.

September 23. Houston. There are to-day, as far as we can hear ight cases of yellow fever under treatment in town, of which four, or five have been taken since our report on Wednesday, and the balance are convalescing. There have been in all five deaths reported by the city sexton of this disease. It does not, as yet, appear to be spreading, and we certainly hope it may not spread. The names of the persons who have died are A. W. Holman, Catrina Stoffle, Geo. Baker, John Day, and one other, whose name we have not ascertained.—*Houston Telegraph* (newspaper).

September 25. Galveston. Mr. Grimes dies.

September 25. Houston. Five deaths. Total, 9.

September 26. Houston. Dr. Pullium dies.

September 29. Galveston. On the 29th, Drs. Heard, Hill, and Welch publish a statement affirming that cases of yellow fever exist in Galveston.

September 30. Galveston. Several deaths reported.

October. Early in October, Montgomery, an interior town of East Central Texas, together with Hempstead, begin to suffer from the yellow fever. The Galveston News says, of this latter village :

Hempstead has suffered greatly from yellow fever ; and Mr. Marschalk, of the Courier, has come in for his full share of affliction, having lost all the hands employed on the paper, including two of his own sons. The editor of the Telegraph learns from Mr. Marschalk and others, that there have been in all seventy-two cases of yellow fever in Hempstead this fall, of which thirty-two have died. Mr. Marschalk had five sick in his own family, every one of whom died.

Oct. 16. At Cypress City, " a station on the Central Road, twenty-five miles from Houston, out of fifty-four persons then in the place, thirty-three, including the doctor were sick with yellow fever. Assistance sent to the sick from Houston."

All persons who remained in the village subsequently, took the disease. About ten days after its invasion the *Houston Telegraph* (newspaper), gave a list of the names of the victims at this village, amounting to 20. Up to the 23d of October the following persons had died of yellow fever at Cypress, namely : Mrs. Loper, Mrs. White, Thomas Gregory, Mrs. M. C. Rowan, Paul Mitchell, J. T. O'Bryan, Charles Meenck, Ann Gregory, Elizabeth Gibson, Calvin Gibson, H. Harris, Tim Kelly, George Meenck, A. Smith, Dr. A. B.

Hart, Martha Gregory, Mrs. Meenck, L. D. White, C. Meenck, Thos. White (infant out of the city), John Fogg, Mike Griffin, Mrs. Mickelborough.

Oct. 6. Houston. The whole number of deaths yesterday, was 5, and the number las night was 4, making now 34 in all.—*Houston Telegraph*

Oct. 7. Up to 10 o'clock this morning there were six deaths since yesterday morning reported to the sextons. The whole number is now forty. We would caution people about repeating street rumors of the number of deaths. We get our reports from the sextons, of which there are two, and are bound to believe they are correct.—*Ibid.*

Oct. 8. Galveston. The health of our city continues the same. There is undoubtedly something more than an average amount of sickness, and yet there have been but five or six well ascertained cases of yellow fever during the season, and all but one or two of these have been brought from abroad, and most of them taken directly from the steamer to the Hospital.—*Galveston News.*

Oct. 13–14. Deaths, 11.

Oct. 12–14. Houston, 11, including Dr. Dewey.

Oct. 19. Galveston, 5, including Dr. Hartman.

Oct. 20. Galveston, 4.

Oct. 21. Galveston, 5.

Oct. 22. Galveston, 6.

Oct. 21–24. Houston, 17, including Dr. Kelly.

Oct, 25–26. ———— 20 ?

Oct. 25. Galveston, 8.

Oct. 27–28. Galveston, 7.

Oct. 29. Galveston, 8.

Oct. 30. Galveston, 8.

Oct. 28. Sugarland, Fort Bend County. Mr. Dunlavy loses every member of his family—6 in all.

Oct. 29. Yellow fever at Brazoria and Indianola.

Cypress City. The Galveston News of Oct. 25th, says, that "Judge John Dean returned last Friday from a journey to the interior, and passed through Cypress City, on Wednesday; and when there he informs us, he took particular pains to ascertain the number of inhabitants in that place, immediately after the first alarm of yellow fever, and when many had left. The number at that time was 45; and of this number 27 have since died; two of the remaining number were dying when he was there, and 15 others were sick! It will be seen that this leaves but one well person in the place, except those who are there as nurses from Houston! Such mortality, we think, is entirely unprecedented. We are glad to learn that there is now no want of medical and other aid.

Nov. 2–5. Galveston, 8.

Nov. 6. Galveston, 4, including Dr. Williams.

Nov. 12–14. Galveston, 10.

Nov. 17–18. Galveston, 5.

Nov. 5. Houston, 4. The disease seems to have persisted more than a month later—having lasted, perhaps, nearly three months.

MISCELLANEA.

Art. I.—*Pharmacology in France.*—*Impurity of Drugs.*—*Hypophosphites in Consumption.*

i. *Chair of Pharmacology in the French School of Medicine.*—Mr. Dumas in his report to the Minister of Public Instruction, proposes that the pharmacological course shall comprehend : 1. A general exposition of the processes for the preparation of medicaments. 2. The special study of medicinal substances, including their natural history, physical and chemical characters, pharmaceutical forms, and their adulterations. 3. The art of prescribing. 4. The history of mineral waters, both natural and artificial. 5. The history of pharmacy among the ancients, and also among the principal nations of the present time.

ii. *The Appointment of a Chair of Pharmacology in the Faculty of Medicine of Paris.*—Napoleon, by the grace of God and the national will, Emperor of the French, to all whom these presents shall come, saluting : We have decreed and do decree as follows : The chair of Pharmacy in the Faculty of Medicine at Paris shall henceforth take the title of the Chair of Pharmacology. M. Regnault, doctor of medicine, doctor in the sciences, pharmaceutist of the first class, *agrégé* to the Faculty of Medicine of Paris, is nominated professor of pharmacology in the Faculty of Medicine of Paris. Our minister, etc. Done at the palace of Compiègne, Nov. 13, 1859.— NAPOLEON.—*Gaz. Heb.*

iii. *Imprisonment and Fines for Neglecting to Test Drugs.*—A country practitioner in France recently prescribed santonine for some children who had worms. The eldest, aged 7, who was the first to take the medicine, died in convulsions at the end of a few hours. On being analyzed five-sixths of the supposed santonine were found to be strychnine. The shop where the drug was bought was in a deplorable state ; poisons were mixed with other substances, and the sale of the drugs was entrusted to a most illiterate shopman. The case was brought before the correctional tribunal at Tongres. The charge alleged against the practitioner was, that he had not analyzed and verified the purity of his drugs. The tribunal condemned the druggist to a month's imprisonment, a fine of 200 *francs* (£8), and half the costs ; the shopman to fifteen days' imprisoment, a fine of 100 *francs* (£4) and one-fourth of the costs ; the practitioner to a fine of 50 *francs* (£2), and one fourth of the costs. The former two had appealed against the sentence.—*Brit. Med. Jour.*

iv. *Dr. Churchill and the Hypophosphites in Pulmonary Consumption.*—Dr. Churchill, curer of consumption, writes a reclamatory letter to the editor of the *Gazette Hebdomadaire*, demanding justice to be done to himself and his hypophosphites. The following is the editor's reply :

" M. Churchill having ingeniously discovered, as he has been kind enough to tell us before several persons, that our appreciation of the facts which he laid before us was wanting in good faith, and had no other object than that of pleasing the Faculty, we are surprised, rather more than honored, by finding him again asking our opinion. It would be easy enough for us to show that four deaths out of twelve patients in less than two years, show a result not particularly satisfactory, when we recollect that of the twelve who did not appear to us to be phthisical at all, and that five were apparently affected with tubercle, but only in the first stage, presenting merely correlative symptoms, bronchitis, and pulmonary congestions, and belonging to that class of patients whose life may be prolonged ten, twenty, or thirty years. We may add that the carelsss way *(peu de riguer des notes)* in which M. Churchill takes his notes of the stethoscopic signs, does not inspire us with perfect confidence in the cures which he announces. But he cannot wish us to make him, a second time, victim of our partiality and base flattery. All we can do for him, in declining his offer, is to recall to him the offer we made in the conversation above alluded to : 1. To submit fresh patients to the examination of competent physicians ; and 2d. To submit to the test those patients only who are incontestably the subjects of pulmonary consumption."—*Med. Times and Gazette*, Feb. 25, 1860.

Art. II.—*Academical Degrees.   Science and Practice.*

i. "The use of academical degrees, as old as the thirteenth century, is visibly borrowed from the mechanic corporations, in which an apprentice, after serving his time, obtains a testimonial of his skill, and a license to practise his trade and mystery." *(Memoirs of Gibbon, 61.)*

Other authorities say that the degree of doctor was first conferred on the continent of Europe, at Bologna, in 1130, and in England in 1209.

ii. *French Degrees in Medicine, anno* 1860.—A few months ago the Government reïnaugurated the degree of A. B., as a necessary preliminary before graduation in medicine, and now the new chair of Medical History is established in the Medical Faculty of Paris, as a part of the regular course of instruction.   Chairs devoted to *specialities* have been prohibited by authority.

While it must be admitted that, upon the whole, these academical regulations cannot but promote the learning, dignity, and usefulness of the medical profession, it is melancholy to think that, if they had been rigidly enforced a few decennia ago, some of the greatest lights now in the Parisian heavens would have been "hid under a bushel."

B. D.

iii *Scientific versus Practical Instruction.*—The following testimony of Liebig as to his famous school at Giessen, is worth considering in these days of schools of practical science : "The technical part of an industrial pursuit can be *learned* ; principles alone can be *taught*. To learn the trade of husbandry, the agriculturist must serve an apprenticeship to it ; to inform his mind in the principles of the science, he must frequent a school specially devoted to this object. It is impossible to combine the two ; the only practicable way is to take them up successively.   I formerly conducted at Giessen a school for practical chemistry, analysis, and other branches connected therewith, and thirty years' experience has taught me that nothing is to be gained by the combination of theoretical with practical instruction.   It is only after having gone through a complete course of theoretical instruction in the lecture-hall that a student can with advantage enter upon the practical part of chemistry.   He must bring with him into the laboratory a thorough knowledge of the principles of the science, or he cannot possibly understand the practical operations.   If he is ignorant of these principles, he has no business in the laboratory.   In all industrial pursuits connected with the natural sciences, in fact, in all pursuits not simply dependent on manual dexterity, the development of the intellectual faculties by what may be termed school-learning, constitutes the basis and chief condition of progress and of every improvement.   A young man with a mind well stored with solid scientific acquirements, will, without difficulty or effort, master the technical part of an industrial pursuit ; whereas, in general, an individual who is thoroughly master of the technical part may be altogether incapable of seizing upon any new fact that has not previously presented itself to him, or of comprehending a scientific principle and its application." — *American Journal of Sciences and Arts.*

ART. III.—*Medical Scepticism and its Evils.*

[Professor Skoda, of Vienna, has made himself conspicuous by his ultra scepticism in therapeutics. It is worthy of remark that the greatest sceptics may be the greatest bigots, believing in unbelief, searching for the doubtful, dissenting from the certain. Nevertheless, the physician, during the first years of actual practice, when his positivism is usually greatest, might, on the other hand, gain knowledge with more facility and certainty, by a moderate indulgence in scepticism. A provisional scepticism, anterior to abundant observation and experience, useful as a means, pernicious as an end, may be advantageous, instead of dogmatism, which closes the door to further investigation. A continuous experience with inductive reasoning, must generally lead either to probability or certainty. B. D.]

"Dr. Gallavardin, who recently visited Skoda's clinique observes: That which essentially distinguishes the originality of Skoda from that of all the other clinical observers of Germany is his scepticism. A doubter so absolute, so fervent, has rarely, if ever, been seen in medicine ; so that with the German Skodism is synonymous with Pyrrhonism in physic. Every year at his clinical lessons he tries, successively, upon his twenty-eight patients, all the medicines, the most vaunted, of the pharmacopœia. And with what intention, think you ? Simply to convince his pupils that all these medicines are invariably inefficacious. If, by chance, a prompt and marked amelioration follows the employment of any treatment, he bestows all the honor upon the natural progress of the disease. For instance, a young and very robust man, 19 years of age, entered the hospital on May 11, for pneumonia of severe type. On the 13th and 14th, Skoda prescribed infusion of digitalis, which produced six evacuations daily. On the 15th he bled. On the 16th, the pulse which was 106 the preceding evening, had fallen to 66. To explain this prompt and obvious modification of the pulse, Skoda thus expressed himself : "It may be the effect of the bleeding ; such a result has occurred. It may be the effect of the digitalis ; that has been also observed. But it may be equally considered as due to the natural progress of the disease ; for that result has also been seen." This is Skoda's habitual mode of argument—invariably indirect. In this manner he gradually insinuates doubt into the minds of his pupils, and eventually leads them to lose all practical faith ! "

In a recent treatise on Domestic Hygiene, by M. Devay, of Paris, the author says, in reference to scepticism and its accompanying evils:

"We have already stated elsewhere what we now repeat, there is a fault which causes as much serious injury in our profession as ignorance itself—namely, scepticism and systematic doubt of the value and bearing of the art of medicine. We allude here especially to the weakening of belief in medicine in the opinion of the public, that public which reverences no deities, gives way to no illusions, and watches with malicious interest the conflicts of our vain theories, oscillating with equal indifference in either direction. This evil is among us, and is at its height; it makes us regret a time now far distant, when the physician was encompassed with dignity; a time when the family welcomed him with pleasure, tempered with deference, and when his presence alone offered the first fruits of recovery. The medical man was then accepted, not indeed as an oracle, but as a man marked out by a special character, which there was no gainsaying. And does not the defect arise, in great measure, from the little influence which medical men exercise on the family? Does not their mission almost terminate in our times with the superintendence of accidents, and of illness actually in progress? The power of physic is brought to bear after the evil has burst forth, never as a means of prevention. The medical man, summoned, like the handicraftsman or the public official, at the moment of a catastrophe, treats more patients than he in reality cures; because to cure the evil he must fathom it, and he requires to fathom it—a confidence which is usually refused him. Generally he is ignorant of the pathological history of the family to which he is sent for, and lacks that guiding clue without which it is impossible to bring the treatment of chronic disease to a good result. On one side and the other medicine is thus too lightly treated. In return, the man of science, considered in some sort as a stipendiary, soon contracts a corresponding tone of feeling—namely, indifference and coolness. When his business is done he departs, without giving the family the advantage of useful advice, arising out of the emergency, and on matters which he has observed perfectly, but on which he has not been questioned. Thus, in presence of mutual suspicion, the internal hygiene of the family is neglected, the most serious diseases silently spring up, and the medical man, who should be a daily adviser, has only a limited and occasional function."

ART. IV.—*Medical Chronology.* (Continued from page 299.)

1225. Foundation of the University of Naples; Richard of Wendmere.

1227. Nicholas Myrepsicus.

1235. Birth of Raymond Lully.

1238. Frederick 2d gives laws to the schools of Salernum and of Naples.

1243. School of medicine at Damascus.

1248. Death of Ebn Beither; Gilbert of England

1250. The scurvy ravages the army of Louis 9th; Birth of Peter of Abano.

1252. The Emperor Conrad endeavors to improve the school of Salernum; Brunus of Calabria; John de St. Amand.

1263. Demetrius Pepagomenes.

1264. Death of Vincent, Abbot of Beauvais.

1271. College of Surgery at Paris.

1277. Death of Peter of Spain.

1281. William of Salita.

1282. Death of Albert of Ballstaedt.

1283. John, son of Zacchary, surnamed Actuarius.

1285. Bernard Gordon; Arnoldde Villanova.

1287. First appearance in Europe of the Plica polonica.

1295. Lanfranc goes to Paris; death of Roger Bacon and of Thaddeus of Florence; Simon of Cordo

1298. Theodoric, Bishop of Cervia.

1302. William of Varignana.

1304. William Baufet, Bishop of Paris, and physician to the King of France.

1305. Bernard Gordon writes his Manual.

1306. Peter of Aichspalt, Elector of Mayence.

1308. Torrigians.

1311. Great privileges ceded by Philip le Bel to the college of St. Come, at Paris.

1312. Vitalis of Four, Cardinal; death of Arnold of Villa Nova.

1314. John of Gaddesden; Mohammed ebn Achmad Almarakschi.

1315. Mondini; first public amphitheatre for dissections; death of Raymond Lully.

1316. John Sanguinaceus regarded as a sorcerer.

1317. Matthew Sylvaticus writes his Medical Pandects.

1320. Death of Peter of Abano.

1325. Death of Mondini; death of Dinus of Garbo, and St. Roch.

1328. Francis of Piedmont.

1340. Gentilis de Foligno.

1342. Cecco of Asculo; death of Nicholas Bertrucco.

1343. John de Dondis.

1347. Regulation of Queen Jane respecting the houses of ill-fame at Avignon.

1349. Death of Gentilis de Foligno; James de Dondis.

1363. Guy of Chauliac.

1365. Confirmation of the regulations of the School of Salernum, by Queen Jane.

1369. Death of Thomas de Garbo.

1373. The necessary conditions are fixed, by which a cure should be deemed miraculous, and the physician canonized.

1374. Epidemic dance of St. Guy, on the borders of the Rhine; St. Catharine of Sienna.

1376. Permission granted to the School of Montpelier to open dead bodies.

(To be continued.)

CORRESPONDENCE.

I.—*Sewerage and Drainage of Cities.*

At the meeting of the American Medical Association, held in Louisville, May, 1859, the undersigned was appointed chairman of a committee to report on the influence of *"Sewerage and Drainage of large cities on public health."*

Any facts, suggestions, documents, reports, or other matter in reference to this important subject, will be thankfully received and duly acknowledged.

As the permanent residence of the undersigned will be fixed in the city of New Orleans, La., all communications must be addressed to him at the above city.   A. J. SEMMES, M. D.,

Chairman of the Committee.

II.—*Removal of the Coccygeal Bone.*

EDITOR N. O. MEDICAL AND SURGICAL JOURNAL—In the last (January, 1860) number of Ranking's Half-Yearly Abstract, page 227, Prof. Simpson, of Edinburgh, reports an operation for the removal of the coccygeal bones for the cure of coccyodynia—pain in the coccyx.

We do not know that amputation of the coccyx had been resorted to for the cure of the disease in question, before Prof. S. performed it; but the operation had been performed on this side of the Atlantic for relief in cases of fracture of the coccyx, as Prof. J. C. Nott, of Mobile, distinctly stated to his class in the University of Louisiana, during the winter of 1857-58. Dr. Nott had operated in two cases. In both these cases fracture occurred during labor, and the females were ladies who had married late in life, and the coccygeal bones were anchylosed. Dr. N. was the attendant accoucheur in one of the cases, and heard the "snap" when the fracture occurred. Permanent relief followed both operations. We state this for the information of those who are ignorant of the fact that the operation has been successfully performed in the United States.

Respectfully,   GEORGE S. D. ANDERSON.

SIMMSPORT, LA., Feb. 24, 1860.·

III.—*Decennial Convention for the Revision of the Pharmacopœia of the United States.*

THE following appointments of delegates to the Convention for revising the Pharmacopœia, to meet at Washington on the first Wednesday of May next, having been duly made known to me, are hereby announced, in compliance with a provision of the Convention of 1850:

From the Massachusetts College of Pharmacy, Messrs. Theodore Metcalf and Charles T. Carney. From the New York Academy of

Medicine, B. W. McCready, M. D.; E. H. Davis, M. D., and E. R. Squibb, M. D. From the College of Physicians, of Philadelphia, Geo. B. Wood, M. D.; R. P. Thomas, M. D., and Robert Bridges, M. D. From the University of Pennsylvania, Joseph Carson, M. D.; R. E. Rogers, M. D., and Jos. Leidy, M. D. From the Jefferson Medical College, of Philadelphia, Franklin Bache, M. D., and T. D. Mitchell, M. D. From the Philadelphia College of Pharmacy, Messrs. Wm. Proctor, Jr, Edward Parrish, and Alfred B. Taylor. From the Medical Society of the State of North Carolina, Wm. G. Thomas, M. D.; Peter E. Hines, M. D., and Edward Warren, M. D.

By order of the Convention of 1850,

GEO. B. WOOD, *President.*

PHILADELPHIA, Feb. 14, 1860.

IV.— *American Medical Association.*

THE *American Medical Association* will hold its thirteenth annual meeting at New Haven, on the *first Tuesday of June,* 1860.

The Secretaries of local societies, colleges, and hospitals are requested to forward to the undersigned the names of delegates, as soon as they are appointed.

STEPHEN G. HUBBARD, M. D., *Secretary,*

New Haven, Connecticut.

TO OUR SUBSCRIBERS.

Our subscribers are hereby notified that JAS. DEERING, and his assistants, are the only general agents authorized to collect for the New Orleans Medical and Surgical Journal, for the year ending December 31, 1861. His authority to collect is limited to the States of Louisiana, Mississippi, Arkansas, Tennessee, Alabama, Georgia, Florida and South Carolina, and to accounts due for three years or more.

To postmasters and others the bills of those subscribers who may reside in their towns or counties are sometimes entrusted, but in all such cases they have our written authority to collect, specifying the names of our debtors, with the amounts due by each.

Any payments due to us which may be paid to parties not indicated above, will be at the subscriber's risk.

Bank bills current at par in the subscriber's State will be received in payment, and if forwarded by mail in letters registered "valuable," will be at the risk of

DRS. CHAILLÉ & NICHOLS,

Proprietors of the N. O. Medical and Surgical Journal

Mortality Statistics of New Orleans, from February, 1860, to April 8, 1860, compiled from the Weekly Reports politely furnished by Dr. Baldwin, Secretary of the Board of Health.

Time.	Total Deaths.	Children under 2 yrs.	Under 20.	U. States.
February (4 weeks)	522	166	265	297
March (4 weeks)	540	125	296	343
April (1 week)	165	52	95	107

Principal Diseases.	February (4 weeks)	March (4 weeks.)	April (1 week.)
Apoplexy	7	3	3
Cholera Infantum	2	2	0
Congestion of Brain	8	9	1
Congestion of Lungs	4	1	0
Consumption	68	65	25
Convulsions, Infantile	27	32	8
Croup	9	10	1
Diarrhœa	16	18	8
Dysentery	23	11	3
Diphtheria	16	23	9
Fever, Miasmatic	12	10	7
" Scarlet	14	20	6
" Typhoid	18	6	2
" Yellow	0	0	0
Gastro-Enteritus	4	5	2
Inflammation of Liver	1	5	1
Inflammation of Lungs	47	48	15
Inflammation of Throat	1	1	0
Marasmus, Infantile	9	14	4
Measles	0	7	4
Pleurisy	5	2	1
Dropsy	11	15	0
Small Pox	2	11	2
Still-born	34	28	4
Teething	6	4	4
Tetanus	6	2	1
Trismus Nascentium	15	12	3

Monthly Summary—Meteorological Register.—*From the Medical Purveying Office, U. S. Army, N. O.* New Orleans, La., Lat. 29 deg. 57 min. 30 sec. N.; Long. 90 deg. W. Altitude of Barometer above the level of the sea, 35 feet.

1860.	Barometer.			Therm. Attached.			Thermometer.		
Months.	Max.	Min'm.	Mean.	Max.	Min'm	Mean.	Max.	Min'm	Mean.
February..	7 A. M. 25th. 30 544	2 P.M. 18th. 29.700	30.202	2. P. M. 17 & 22d 73°	7. A. M. 2d & 3d. 52°	63.93	2 P.M. 15th. 75°	7 A. M. 2d 38°	59.51
March......	7 A. M. 11th. 30.426	7 A. M. 17th 29.932	30.212	2. P.M. 7th & 8th 78°	7. A.M. 14&29th. 58°	66.72	2 P. M. 7th. 80°	7 A. M. 13th 52°	64.97

1860.	Hygrometer.			Prev'g Winds.	Weather.		Rain.	
Months.	Max.	Min'm	Mean		Fair.	Cloudy.	Days.	Quantity.
February..	2 P. M. 17th. 70°	7 A. M. 2d. 36°	56.30	E., N., & S. W.			10	8.61
March......	2 P. M. 7th. 74°	7 A. M. 13th. 46°	60.40	N. E., E.. & S.			2	0.76

T. Harrison, Clerk.

THE

NEW ORLEANS

MEDICAL AND SURGICAL JOURNAL.

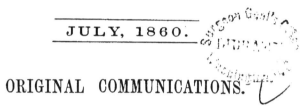

JULY, 1860.

ORIGINAL COMMUNICATIONS.

ART. I.—*A Case of Stricture of the Œsophagus, with Cancerous De-position, terminating fatally :* By Drs. Scales and Gilmore, Craw-fordville, Mississippi.

A Mr. J. F., of spare make and medium size, about thirty years of age, called on us the 22d of July last, complaining of his throat, and stating that he had been under medical treatment for some time, and had received no relief, after a free and prolonged application of caustic to his throat and tonsils. On examination we found the fauces injected, the tonsils a little enlarged, and the uvula slightly elongated. We excised a portion of the uvula hoping an emeliora-tion of the symptoms would follow, but on the 31st of the same month our patient called on us again, still complaining. We then scarified the throat freely, and put him on the use of the iodide of potassium, and saw him again on the 4th of August, when he com-plained of some difficulty in swallowing. The left tonsil was much enlarged, a portion of which we excised, and turned out a considera-ble quantity of creamy looking matter. After this simple operation the swallowing became easy, and we supposed we had succeeded in relieving the local difficulty. We advised, however, the use of the

58

compound syrup of sarsa to be added to the iodide of potassium, and taken three times daily, with instructions to inform us, if there was any future trouble in swallowing. On the 12th of August he called, still complaining, when we made an examination for stricture of the œsophagus. We attempted to pass a probang which we could not make enter the tube.

We met with the same fate in the use of a stomach tube, but passed a No. 12 male catheter through the stricture. On the 19th and 27th August, respectively, we passed stomach tubes, and gave him different sizes, with directions to pass them at intervals of six to ten days. On the 9th of September he called again, and was much worse than on any previous occasion. The throat was very tender, and discharging, occasionally, an ashy looking mucus, streaked with blood. There was great difficulty in swallowing solids or fluids —both being thrown back in the effort. We advised him to lay aside the instruments until the excessive tenderness subsided, when we would take the future dilatation of the case into our own hands. The next thing we heard of our patient, he had gone to New Orleans to seek the aid of a distinguished Professor, in one of the medical Schools of that city ; but after a stay of a few days or weeks he returned unimproved. While in the city or on his way home, an abcess formed in his throat, and discharged a large quantity of matter by the mouth.

October 30th. We were again sent for and resorted to dilatation, as before, which we kept up regularly once a week, till the last of November ; when another abscess formed on the opposite side of the throat, and discharged by the mouth as did the first. After this the emaciation and debility increased rapidly, and on the 18th December, for the last time, we passed a No. 5 rectum bougie through the stricture. As we became satisfied that the disease was malignant and the treatment unavailing, we simply made an occasional visit in January, about the last of which month he died.

Dr. Gilmore obtained permission, and removed the larynx and the trachea, with the diseased portion of the œsophagus attached. On laying open the tube we found a narrow hard ring surrounding it, and producing, as we supposed, the first symptoms of stricture. Above and below this ring, was, for some two and a-half inches, a cancerous deposition extending from just below the glottis downwards and encircling the entire tube. It had rather a dark or dirty white appearance, a papillary or watery surface, and about the consistence of soft cheese, easily broken down or torn up by the finger nail. The mucous surface or membrane was entirely destroyed or concealed by the deposition. In alcohol it has rather a flocculent or shaggy aspect. At the upper end of the tube the cancerous deposition detached itself from the wall of the œsophagus, and mounted upwards about three-eighths of an inch all around, except at the glottis (where it reached its opening), and was, in this projection or rim, about one-fourth of an inch in thickness. There was frequently a difficulty in introducing bougies, which this explains, the end of the instrument passing between this fold or projection and the wall of the tube. The lower edge of the diseased mass projected downwards, detaching itself, as above, from the tube's entire circumference, but was not so thick. On the right and left sides, about the middle of the deposition, the œsophagus was ulcerated through, and the deposition of cancerous matter extended through the ulcer, but did not involve the larynx. One of these openings was as large as a pea, and we supposed them to be the seats of the abscesses before mentioned. We think the specimen a very fine one, and fills perfectly the description of epithelial cancer as described by Mr. Paget and others.

April 18th, 1860.

ART. II.—*Extra-Uterine Pregnancy. Hæmorrhage. Death :* By N. F. SCALES, M. D., Crawfordville, Mississippi.

ON the 8th of August, 1856, I was called to see a negro woman, a house servant of one of my patrons, a few miles from town. She was upwards of twenty years of age, had no husband and no children. After investigating her symptoms, and learning she had not menstruated for two months or more, I came to the conclusion that she was pregnant. There was considerable mental disturbance ; hysterical symptoms were most prominent. At the same time, however, there was slight tumidity and tenderness of the lower part of the abdomen, for which I applied cupping glasses and a mustard plaster, and gave instructions to follow the mustard plaster

with poultices, till the tenderness subsided, or I saw the patient
again. I also directed that the bowels should be moderately moved
by laxatives. I gave it as my opinion that the woman was pregnant,
in which she concurred, but her mistress thought it was not possible,
and was of the opinion that her symptoms grew out of a suppression
of the menses from some imprudence or exposure to cold. On the
next day I visited my patient again, and found the abdominal tenderness much lessened, and learned from her that she had discharged
blood, moderately, *per vaginam*. Her mind was more quiet than the
day before, and her symptoms generally improved, except the
hæmorrhage, which I viewed as threatening abortion, but which her
mistress viewed as returning menstruation. The ordinary symptoms
of pregnancy were so manifest, that I still adhered to the opinion
expressed the day before, and made a vaginal examination, but could
gain nothing satisfactory, as the mouth of the womb, I thought, was
natural, and in its proper position. I prescribed such remedies as I
supposed best calculated to compose the system, and prevent flooding.
I left, with a promise to repeat my visit next day, which I did, and
found my patient so much improved that I considered further attention on my part unnecessary.

On the 13th of the same month I was sent for in great haste, and
on my entering the room, I found the woman tossing herself about
on the bed, and seemingly in great agony. The abdomen was very
much distended, and tender, the breathing difficult, the lips purple
(she was a bright mulatress), and the tongue very pale, indicating
a great loss of blood. She did not remain in this condition
long before death terminated the scene. I informed the owner I
thought a blood-vessel had given way, and that the abdominal cavity
was filled with blood. He expressed a wish that a post-mortem
examination should be made, and on the evening of the same day,
with the assistance of three medical friends, I proceeded with the
examination. As soon as the wall of the abdomen was laid open, a
large quantity of fluid blood was discharged, and after finding no
ruptured vessel in its cavity, I ran my hand down into the pelvis—
raised the uterus, and found a mass superimposed on its upper
extremity, with a rent in its apex, whence the blood had been discharged. One of our assistants pushed his finger into the rent and
pulled out a fœtus about two month's old. This superimposed mass
was made up of a membranous covering, the placenta, and its

contents ; the fœtus being removed, a portion of the umbilical cord was left attached to the placenta. The end of the left fallopian tube was merged in the placenta, and its covering spread out in a broad surface that covered over the left side, and a part of the front of the placental wall. The remaining portion of its front, and its posterior aspect were overlaid by the outer membrane of the womb passing up on it. As this membrane ascended the top of the placenta or ovum, it became so thin that it scarcely afforded any support, and just across the apex, where it was thinnest, the rent occurred. The substance or wall of the placenta was not attached to the apex of the uterus, but was maintained loosely in its position by the membrane that ascended and covered it from the uterus. Had that been severed, the ovum would have fallen off suspended to the end of the left fallopian tube. The left ovary had degenerated into a mere sac, and was resting against the body of the ovum, above, and that of the uterus, below. The body of the uterus was something thicker and larger in its various dimensions than in the unimpregnated state. The mouth was not closed by a plug, nor did the cavity contain any deciduous membrane. The previous loss of blood possibly may account for these facts. It is rather singlar that a larger proportion of unmarried than married females should be subject to this unfortunate conception, and of the number conceiving, that the left ovary should be so much more frequently involved than the right. I have no doubt that the tumid and tender state of the abdomen, in the first instance, was produced by partial hæmorrhage, and the arrest, till its fatal termination, was accidental.

In Ramsbotham's System of Obstetrics, page 570, and plate 63, will be seen an excellent drawing of a case of extra-uterine fœtation, in which the fœtus lies off from the body of the womb, involving the left ovary and fallopian tube.

[To the above interesting case, it may be allowable to add the following, as reported in the Obstetrical Society of London (March, 1860), published in the *British Med. Jour.* :]

" *Case of Fallopian Pregnancy.*—By HENRY GRACE, Esq. (Communicated by GRAILY HEWITT, M. D.) The patient was six or seven weeks advanced in pregnancy, and died from rupture of the tube. At the post mortem examination, about three pints of blood, partly coagulated, were found within the peritoneal sac. The source of this was a rupture of the left fallopian tube, which was enlarged about its middle to the size of a walnut. On cutting into this enlargement, a layer, resembling the decidua, presented itself within the tube connected with the chorion ; and on a deeper incision being made through the amnion, about a drachm of liquor amnii escaped, and an ovum of about six weeks was seen. The uterus was neither enlarged nor congested, and had no decidua. A corpus luteum was present in the left ovary."

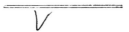

Art. III.—*A Case of Strangulated Omental Hernia:* By Gilbert T. Deason, M. D., Elyton, Alabama.

I sometimes think that the proneness of some practitioners to evade public censure and ridicule, is as great a crime as the strong inclinations of others to bring themselves into notice. The former, through timidity, withhold from public inspection many practical observations, although simple, yet involving, both practically and theoretically, many useful lessons. While the latter, induced through selfish motives and self-aggrandisement, imbue medical proficiency with many discreditable stains. And when public sentence is passed upon this humble effort, to introduce a simple case of omental hernia, I know not in which class my lot will fall. But, however that may be, if I can but induce one of my profession, although he may be as young and as inexperienced as myself, to boldly step forward, when duty calls, and save the life of a fellow being, I shall have, at least, accomplished some good.

With this view I offer. the following case: F. M. S., had been troubled several times with inguinal hernia, but at each succeeding protrusion, he was able to make the reduction by his own manipulations. But eventually, while in the act of carrying some poultry, swinging them from each hand, he again felt the sudden protrusion of the abdominal viscera through the inguinal canal, but which, at the time excited no pain. Not wishing to release his poultry, he delayed for some time making the attempt at reduction. But as soon as convenient, he commenced his usual manipulations, but to his great dismay found it of no avail. After many succeeding and fruitless attempts, a messenger was dispatched for assistance. I arrived in about thirty-six hours from the time of the protrusion, and found him laboring under the most excruciating pain imaginable. The tumor apparently was about the size of a hen's egg, with considerable congestion of the vascular tissue around. On inquiry, I found he had had several operations from his bowels during that day, which was a satisfactory diagnostic of omental hernia. After the usual mode of anæstheticising, nauseating, taxis, etc., I was convinced that nothing would afford relief short of an operation.

Never having seen a case of hernia before (much less having operated on one), and being, I might say, alone, twenty miles in the country, I must acknowledge I was somewhat at a loss to know how to proceed. I proposed to send for another physician who was six miles off, that I might at least have an assistant. But my patient avowed that he would die before that assistance could be obtained, and persisted in wishing that I should operate immediately. So seeing no chance for help, or rescue for the man, but by an operation, I made the necessary preparations, and put him under the influence of chloroform, which I considered hazardous in the extreme, having to guide both the pulse and my knife at the same time. However, I soon cut down upon the tumor, and found, as I suspected, that a portion of the omentum had pushed the peritoneum through the canal, and had formed an oval-shaped tumor enveloped in the peritoneum. Opening this sac by means of a sharp pointed bistoury and a grooved probe, there was a small amount of bloody water collected in the sac, together with the omentum. On further examination, I found the omentum to be greatly congested, with dark, and apparently coagulated blood, from the fact that the strangulation was so great that there was a complete obstruction in the circulation of the blood. I further found that perfect adhesions had taken place in the folds of the omentum, cementing the parts into a globular shape, thereby causing an utter impossibility of reduction. I here brought to mind the valuable lectures of Dr. Stone, while I was in New Orleans, in the winters of 1856-7, and 1857-8. His instructions were to cut the mass entirely away, and tie the bleeding vessels. This plan I adopted, and after cutting the mass off even with the external ring, I found that the bleeding vessels even in the mouth of the orifice were blocked up with coagulated blood, which obviated the necessity of ligatures. I then passed the mass back through the orifice into its natural cavity, and made a deep suture `down immediately over the mouth of the orifice, and brought the lips of the wound together and secured them ; one more suture on each side of this, completed the operation. I heard from him ten days after, and he was hauling corn.

One question in relation to this case, and I will have finished. Could this reduction have been made in its gangrenous state, would it not have acted as a foreign body, irritating the part around, and thereby produce a fatal peritonitis ? Or would the vital powers have been sufficient to have absorbed it, reïnstating vitality and thereby rescue the man ? Again, as this man has had no symptoms of hernia since (having been operated on twelve months ago), I consider it a permanent cure ; and notwithstanding all the writings of Wützer, Gerdy, Cooper, Wood, etc., and their different plans of operation, it stands to reason that a simple incision down to the orifice, and a deep suture over its mouth, is as little painful as any operation, and will certainly excite inflammation and adhesion sufficient to constitute a radical cure in every .case of hernia, either before or after strangulation.

ART. IV.—*Observations on Military Surgery, translated and condensed from the German :* By FREDERICK STRUBE, M. D.

The Military Hospitals in Brescia after the Battle of Solferino.

IN the Austrian Journal for Practical Medicine, we find an article by Professor Patruban on the report of Dr. Gualla, Surgeon-in-chief of the Austrian Military Hospitals in Brescia, which contains some interesting items on the surgical and medical treatment after the bloody battle of Solferino.

Brescia, a city of Lombardy, of 30,000 inhabitants, received in the first days after the horrid carnage on the heights of San Martino and Solferino, the enormous number of 33,000 sick and wounded, who were distributed in forty different provisional hospitals. Churches, barracks, the vast palaces of the rich, monasteries, school houses and country residences were charitably thrown open for the relief of the sick and wounded. The physicians were nobly assisted by the inhabitants in their arduous task, and both did their best to afford every possible help and comfort to the soldiers wounded on the battle field. To give an idea of the immense labor the surgeons had to undergo, we add that their number amounted to only 140, and that they were occupied continually during fifteen hours of the day.

Of the above mentioned number of 33,000, there were 13,250 wounded on the battle field by all possible kinds of arms ; 19,750 being medical cases. According to nationality this number divides itself into 17,400 Frenchmen, 14,000 Italians, and 1,600 Austrians. The amount of deaths was 1,270, which gives the favorable result of not quite four per cent. of the total amount treated.

A. Of the 13,250 *surgical cases*, only 453 required amputations, of which 180 ended in death, six ligatures of the larger arteries with two deaths, four cases of trephining, of which three were successful, twenty-five disarticulations, of which only five proved unfavorable to life. The course of the incised and penetrating wounds, as compared with gun-shot wounds, was remarkably advantageous and of short duration.

1. *Amputations,* performed shortly after the injury was done, showed a much more favorable result than those undertaken later in the stage of advanced suppuration—a delay mostly owing to the refusal of the wounded to submit to surgical operations. The proportional result in favor of life was nearly two to one. The importance of a firm, immovable provisional bandage showed itself in every case, and as such, prevented the access of air, and kept the displaced parts in a firm position during the transportation from the battle field, over a rough ground, on the " sanitary wagons," saving to the wounded a great deal of pain and loss of blood. The purulent infection frequently combined with eruption of miliaria crystallina, was very much feared by the surgeons wherever it showed itself, and few cases of pyæmia were saved.

2. *Tetanus* appeared in. seventy-six cases of gunshot wounds, and the great danger of this grave complication is proved by the deaths of seventy-one of this number. The director of the hospitals in Brescia accounts for this great mortality by the sudden changes of temperature during the day as compared with the night. Let it be remembered that the battle of Solferino was fought in the latter part of summer. The heat in the plains of Lombardy, where the rays of the sun are reflected from and increased by the neighboring Alps,

59

rising many thousand feet, almost perpendicularly from the plains, is, during the summer days, as high, if not higher than with us in New Orleans, and the cool nights produce there, as well as here, in the later summer months, tetanus after wounds, particularly in the crowded hospitals, where ventilation had to be kept up in the night as well as in the day.

The recorded observations in the Crimea show only thirty cases of tetanus among many thousand wounded, whilst in the barricade battles of June, in Paris, not a single case of tetanus is remembered. The application of chloroform was, indeed, the best and most useful mitigant—lessening the attacks in frequency and duration ; but in no case did it prove any real cure. The same has been observed in *eclampsia parturientium.*

3. *Conservative surgery* had great success in the treatment of the wounded. Many limbs were saved by careful examination of the wounds, by removing from them bullets, bone-splinters, and other substances, by attentive bandaging, by the use of the inclined plane, by permanent extension, which otherwise would have been lost by the amputation knife. Many resections (the number is not given) were made successfully.

4. Amongst the four *trepannings,* one is interesting, as the total paralysis of the right part of the body was immediately relieved after this operation.

5. The *penetrating shot-wounds* caused, as may be imagined, the most fatal cases, and particularly the thoracic wounds proved more fatal than those penetrating the abdominal cavity. One case is recorded where the injury of the bowels was cured by the spontaneous formation of artificial anus.

6. The *extensive destruction and crushing of the facial bones* mostly succeeded well, although in the beginning the prognosis seemed very unfavorable. One case of a Turco is mentioned, where the ball had entered the ophthalmic cavity, and had made its exit behind the processus mastoïdeus, and where, after a dangerous meningitis, life was saved. In another case the ball entered by the left "ala nasis," crushed the bones of the superior maxilla, went down to the angle of the right under jaw, and had imbedded a quantity of bony fragments in the muscles of the tongue ; the ball itself remained here also, for in the course of the suppuration which followed, the Turco one day spit the ball away. Cases of shot-wounds, where the

ball had traversed the facial bones, fracturing and crushing them all, were healed, in single instances, in the short space of six weeks.

The general treatment of the wounded by Dr. Gualla was anti-phlogistic. The Italian physicians were strictly opposed to the opinions of some French surgeons, to keep up the strength of the patient from the beginning by a stimulating and nourishing diet.

Chloroform was extensively exhibited, not only as anæsthetic during operations, but also in after-treatment, to give relief of severe pains, and to relax the muscles when they were spasmodically contracted by reflex action.

B. *Internal Diseases.*—In Brescia, as well as in many other cities where great numbers of sick and wounded soldiers were accumulated, the observation was made that most diseases which appeared assumed a typhoid character. The malaria to which the troops were exposed in their cantonments, the unusual heat of the season, the excitement in the numerous skirmishes and fights, which frequently continued for several days, and the consequent fatigues, the reception of the weak and exhausted into crowded rooms and localities filled with patients having suppurating wounds, are sufficient evidence of the correctness of this observation. The physicians did their best, by very energetic measures, to cut off as quickly as possible the first symptoms of any apparent typhoid fever, by removing the patients to better localities, etc., and in this way succeeded in postponing an epidemic of this kind, which often in campaigns kills more soldiers than the arms of war. We also here remark, as in all former great campaigns, that the psychical influences on the different bodies of troops have a marked effect on the intensity of their diseases. It had been already observed in the campaigns of Napoleon I, that wounds, when an army is victorious, always took a healthier and more favorable appearance than when the contrary was the case ; the same with other diseases. The typhoid fever generally set in with the eruption of a papulous exanthema, the appearance of which frequently gave some relief, whilst its sudden disappearance was mostly an unfailing symptom of approaching dissolution. Sometimes bronchial catarrhs appeared a few days before death, and the sputa, thrown up during the spasmodic attacks of cough, were intermixed with very dark blood, whilst those parts of the skin where a mustard poultice had been applied, soon appeared erysipelatous, becoming gangrenous, as also the bed-sores, and all these were sure symptoms of rapidly approaching death. The French were, however, more subject to these forms than the Italians.

In these cases the best practice was found to consist in small venesections, leeching of the epigastrium, the fossa iliaca, and the umbilical region, soothing poultices, cool drinks, and if inflammatory symptoms appeared, tartar emetic in refractissima dosi. In other cases, where bilious symptoms prevailed, cathartics, emetics, and acids were given with the best result. Putrid fevers required tonics, in the shape of wine, peruvian bark, quinine, etc. Where cerebral affections prevailed, an antiphlogistic treatment was instituted, tartar emetic in larger doses, and different narcotic sedatives, as opium, etc. When the fever began to subside a little, the use of quinine did wonders towards a rapid cure. Frequently these typhoid fevers left behind them an infiltration of the mesenteric glands, exudations in the different cavities, ulcerations and suppurations, and particularly very extensive bed-sores, which were treated with decoctions of peruvian bark and camphor, and the local application of caustic ; furthermore, bad colliquative diarrhœas, œdemas, etc. At the post-mortem examinations were found infiltration of Peyer's glands and of the follicles, ulceration of the same, inflammation of the mucous membrane of the stomach, softening of the spleen, hypostatic pneumonia, bronchitis, exudations in all parts, as also in the ventricles of the cerebrum. An immense number of intermittent fevers were treated, as usual, with quinine, the dose being, however, not mentioned. Dysentery and diarrhœa were very prevalent, as usual in campaigns, sometimes degenerating into real cholera. These cases were treated with antiphlogistics, ipecac, mild purgatives, particularly tamarinds, whilst other medicines, as colombo, tannin, bismuth, and particularly opiates, proved very injurious.

We here may add some remarks on the different nationalities which came under the observation of Dr. Gualla during the campaign. The Italian soldiers had a great advantage in some respects over the French, as they fought on their native soil, in their native climate, in their full vigor and health, not exhausted by fatiguing and long marches, whilst the French, weakened by the dangerous route over the cold Mount Cenis in the Alps (for only few brigades were transported by sea to Genoa), subjected to a rich and unusual Italian diet, and drinking at "*discretion*" the heavy, thick Italian wines and liquors of all kinds, lost great numbers by inflammation of the bowels in this hot season of the year. A rich diet was even allowed to surgical patients by the French physicians, so Dr. Gualla says, and they lost many in consequence, by extensive suppurations, and by pyæmia, whilst the Italian treatment in these cases was the contrary, keeping all surgical cases on low diet, with a much more favorable result, according to this authority. The Austrian prisoners in the hands of the French showed a very great mortality, as they frequently repudiated all medical assistance, however kindly offered, partly from hatred, partly from mistrust, and preferred dying to being assisted by French physicians and surgeons. Such was the hatred in this mortal combat, undoubtedly kindled and supported by all kinds of false rumors and lies.

In regard to statistics, we have to add to the above given numbers, that the proportion of deaths in seven hospitals was, for medical cases, 190 to 9,148, *i. e.*, 1 to 48 discharged, and for surgical cases, 352 to 4,189, or 1 to 12.

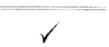

ART. V.—*Death from Chloroform:* By HUMPHREY PEAKE, M. D., of Yazoo City, Mississippi.

ON Friday, May 4th, I was sent for to visit one Peter Phillips, for the purpose of amputating his thigh. I found him the mere skeleton of a man—a miserable looking object and picture of protracted and intense suffering. This·was the result of an old ulcer upon the left leg. He had led an irregular life and was intemperate. Of late, his health had been steadily declining, and for weeks his only rest had been procured by taking immense doses of morphine. Meantime, the ulcer had extended rapidly, so much so as to have involved nearly the whole of the muscles of the leg from near the petella to the malleoli. On the outer aspect of the leg, a ribbon-like strip of integument extended from that above the upper border of the ulcerated surface, and connected it with that of an almost gangrenous foot. The exposed muscles seemed literally rotten, and exhaled an odor, if possible, worse than that from a gangrenous lung.

It seemed almost useless to attempt an operation, but he was clamorous for it, and his friends insisted also, notwithstanding I informed them of the possibility, nay, probability, of his dying under the knife. Moreover, death was certain without it, albeit his chances for recovery with it were not two in a thousand. Let it be remembered here, that there is a difference in the practice of rural surgery, if I may so speak, and that of a city or metropolitan hospital. In the former case it may take a ride of twenty miles over a miserable road to bring you to the cabin of your patient, as was so with me ; while in the latter, the days during which a patient may be braced up and prepared for an operation are not permitted to pass by, if, indeed, it is deferred so long. But thus it was with the patient whose case I am reporting, and the operation was to be done at once. So I concluded to operate, having the advice and assistance of a brother physician, Dr. Ingersoll. The patient was placed upon a table, and chloroform administered by Dr. I. Col. Wm. Bataille, an intelligent gentleman, was also present and assisted me. A couple of minutes' inhalation had placed him sufficiently under the influence of the anæsthetic, when I proceeded to make my first cut for the circular operation at the junction of the lower with the middle third of the thigh. I was turning up the in tegumentswhen his breathing and pulse suddenly stopped. I at once resorted to artificial respiration, and kept it up for some time, but to no purpose. He was dead.

MAY 11, 1860.

ART. VI.—*Observations on General and Cardiac Hypertrophy:* By
BENNET DOWLER, M. D.

THE word hypertrophy (from two Greek words signifying excessive nutrition) as commonly defined, seems to be generally understood in its literal sense as not necessarily including the idea of morbidity. In its most active form, nutrition, that is, the digestion, assimilation and appropriation of nutritive matter without the introduction of any new solid, fluid, or modified element foreign to the special,

normal tissue or organ hypertrophied, would seem to be the antithesis of disease, the realization of health. Drs. Jones and Sieve-
king, in their Pathological Anatomy speak of " uncomplicated hypertrophy, where we have to deal with *no morbid product*," etc., and
most authors adopt a similar phraseology. From this point of view,
might it not be assumed that health may be excessive as well as
nutrition ? Is it not worthy of further inquiry whether the present
vague application of the term hypertrophy should not be abandoned,
and its use be restricted to a morbid condition alone, and the more
so because the postulate that in hypertrophy no new, foreign, or
altered element is ever introduced into the organic tissue of the
part, is but an assumption? The contrary conclusion is not without
probability, especially when an organ is undergoing an active alteration in volume, consistence, or configuration. Even in cases where
no visible augmentation or other change can in the early stage be
detected, the elements of morbidity may be, nevertheless, active,
and for a time elude the most careful research.

In treating of diseases of the heart, some writers place organic
alterations in the foreground, and functional disorders in the distance as merely secondary, and *vice versa*. This has been the case
in regard to hypertrophy. But this collocation is not altogether
satisfactory in a pathological point of view, because it is generally
impossible to draw *ab initio* a distinct line of demarcation between
organic lesion and functional disorder. They often really or apparently constitute a unity rather than a duality, being coëxistent and
so blended as to be virtually inseparable ; nevertheless, the general
tendencies of physical, physiological, and anatomical phenomena,
seem to favor the priority of the former.

Active exercise as the cause of the increased size of an organ,
has been generally appealed to as the type, *experimentum crucis* and
argument illustrative of normal hypertrophy. But exercise, whether
moderate or excessive, does account for even the physiologically en-
hanced development of some of the animal tissues. Inertia or indolence affords, on the other hand, an equally valid explanation of
alterations of a kindred character, as in the case of obesity, in which
the fatty or adipose tissue is often enormously developed as the
effect of inactivity and luxury. Galen, in his book on tumors, explains these preternatural enlargements principally " as the products
of actual disease," but alludes to the increased adipose tissue in

obesity as a natural increase, which is, perhaps the best example that has ever been given of the normal enlargement—one which, indeed, is sometimes either directly or eventually morbid from its excess or infiltration of certain organs, as the liver, heart, etc.

In the second volume of his Physiological Chemistry, Professor Lehmann says in reference to the fattening of agricultural stock, that "the process which consists essentially in the augmentation of the fat in the organism, very often assumes a course very different from that of normal nutrition ; for we cannot regard the development of a fatty liver in geese, or the frequently observed partial disappearance of the nitrogenous constituents of organs, as, for instance, the muscles, in certain modes of fattening, as normal processes. Unfortunately, however, we are not entirely in possession of the conditions necessary to give one special direction to the process of nutrition, by which we might be enabled to determine the relations already indicated. The difficulties which the unequal development of heterogeneous organs oppose to the determination of the metamorphosis of matter during the period of growth, depend upon the circumstance that we are not able to make nutrition assume any special form, either by means of food or any other external relations. The ingenious combinations of Liebig, have sufficiently shown us the conditions under which, independently of proper food, a more abundant deposition of fat may be formed in the animal organism."

This author candidly admits, with many other histologists, that there is very little certainty in the calculations and conclusions already extant upon the nature of hypertrophy. Such being the case, small must be the basis for the usual classification of hypertrophies into normal, true, false, and other varieties.

Although speculative and analogical reasonings appear favorable to the doctrine that functional disorders are but sequents of antecedent lesions, either in the solids or in the fluids, or in both together, yet, in a practical point of view, this fundamental distinction cannot always be ascertained ; that is, the present means of research do not furnish reliable criteria by which these probable lesions may be invariably recognized. The hypothesis which assumes that lesional and functional disorders are inseparably conjoined and mutually react on each other, though in various degrees, is not without probability, though much may be said on the other side. How is it possible to form a conception of agency without an agent, of office without an officer, of diseased function without diseased structure ? Is it by any means absurd to suppose that functional disease is *ipso facto* proof of primordial or coëxisting organic alteration ?

Hypertrophy, a materialistic alteration never necessary to health, always suspicious or morbid, whether it be such *ab initio*, or such as secondary result of a known or an unknown antecedent, is, or ought to be, a point of departure—an indelible landmark in pathology and pathological anatomy ; and if its functional symptoms and their order of succession cannot always be connected with simultaneous organic changes, it must be remembered, that in most medical deductions the same difficulty occurs in tracing the essential relations of final causes.

The definition of hypertrophy by even those who do not regard it as a pathological condition, is really adverse to the assumption that it is altogether a normal one.   Excessive or preternatural nutrition, if not the antithesis to, must be different from the natural or normal, and *à fortiori* the healthful state of the organism.   Even a preter-natural excess of the elementary constituents of an organ, wherein no new or foreign element is introduced (a postulate which histolo-gists have not proved), still excludes the fundamental idea of perfect normality, as in hypertrophies of the thyroid, parotid, lymphatic, hepatic, mammary, testicular and other glands—of the uvula, tongue, muscles, bloodvessels, spleen, bones, cartilages—of the skin in ele-phantiasis and some other affections—also of the cuticle, as in cal-losities, corns, and even horns ! not to name numerous other analo-gous examples, in all of which, as well as in some hypertrophies of a malignant character, the primordial aberration probably exists in the nutritive fluid ; that is, the blood and its cells.   If histological research, both normal and pathological, has not established this view, it has at least rendered it probable.

The increased volume and weight of the uterus during pregnancy, place this organ in a kind of middle ground, or limbo, between health and disease, physiology and pathology, growth and hypertrophy.   A natural growth is not disease, but its excess, that is hypertrophy, even though temporary, might, and usually does, produce symptoms more or less severe during gestation at least, the original curse clinging to woman from conception to child-birth : " I will greatly multiply thy sorrow and thy conception ; in sorrow thou shalt bring forth children."

M. Larcher has recently announced that, as far back as thirty years, he had discovered hypertrophy of the heart as its normal condition during pregnancy. Without affirming or denying this proposition, it is evident from M. Larcher's own statement that this so-called normal condition is rather dangerous :

"The point the author here wishes to bring under the notice of the profession, he has had ample means of investigating at the Paris Maternité, for his investigations have been extended to one hundred and thirty pregnant women, the great bulk of whom succumbed to puerperal fever—no lesion having preceded or given rise to the condition of the heart observed in them. The conclusion he comes to is, that the *heart is normally in a state of hypertrophy during gestation.* The walls of the left ventricle become increased by at least from a fourth to a third in thickness, its texture being also more firm and its color more bright—the right ventricle and the auricles retaining their normal thickness. These observations, made by M. Larcher, date back some thirty years, and have been confirmed by subsequent ones, made with great exactitude, by M. Ducrest, upon one hundred other women ; but why this paper has been so long in being published, no explanation is given. Within certain limits this condition of things may coëxist with the maintenance of health ; but it none the less may be taken to express a predisposition to congestions and hæmorrhages. If, as the general rule, the hypertrophy gradually disappears after parturition, it may be otherwise in exceptional instances, especially where the recurrence of pregnancy has been frequent, and with short intervals. Is this not a cause of the varied lesions of the circulatory apparatus so commonly met with in women who have borne many children, either at too premature an epoch, at too brief intervals, or during an unfavorable condition of health ? There is every reason, too, to believe that the bronchitis, which is so common during pregnancy, derives much of its character of persistency from this condition of the heart. Again, may we not attribute to this the greater danger of pneumonia when developed in pregnant women, and the frequency with which abortion then occurs ? The various forms of hæmorrhage met with in pregnancy, as epistaxis, hæmoptysis, metrorrhagia, and apoplexy, are likewise predisposed to by this hypertrophy, normal though it be.

Although pregnancy may, in the majority of cases, suspend or render slower the progress of pulmonary consumption, the progress of this affection becomes accelerated after delivery, and the still hypertrophied heart increases the perturbation of the respiratory apparatus."—*Archives Générales, tome* xiii, pp. 291-306.   *Med. Times and Gazette.*

Here will be seen something gratuitous, and much that is too dangerous to be admitted within the pale of normal physiology— gratuitous, in assuming that those who died of puerperal fever or peritonitis, had, neither from that nor any preceding malady, any lesion which could have given rise to the alleged hypertrophy of the heart—dangerous, because this condition predisposes or gives rise to "congestions, hæmorrhages, epistaxis, hæmoptysis, metrorrhagia, bronchitis, pneumonia, consumption, apoplexy ; the still hypertrophied heart increases the perturbation of the respiratory apparatus." This (cardiac hypertrophy) topic may be resumed in the sequel.

Vicarious developments and functions, as in cases where one kidney or lung is destroyed, obstructed, or impeded, may be referred to growth rather than to hypertrophous alteration ; such development being neither excessive nor injurious, but physiological and beneficial. Now, this favorable character cannot be applied to some hypertrophies, which, in a certain sense, may be termed almost normal, or at least common, as in the case of the prostate gland, which, in advanced life, often is hypertrophied, and, though not malignant, causes suffering by obstructing the emission of the urine, etc.

That hypertrophy, how simple soever it may be, is but a mere augmentation of the normal or healthy tissue, without any morbid alteration in such tissue, without hyperæmia, interstitial infiltration, increased or diminished cohesion, induration, softening, or other transformation, is scarcely a warrantable assumption, although it may be true that the histological characters of such changes are as yet unknown. In speaking of hypertrophy, Prof. Bennett, in his recent elaborate work, *Clinical Lectures on Medicine*, says : "A cultivation of histology excited the hope that, by studying the ultimate structure and mode of development of morbid growths, distinctive elements, and thereby a new foundation for their classification would be discovered. But extensive researches long ago convinced me that this hope was vain, and in a special work, published in 1849, I pointed out what were the ultimate elements of all morbid growths, and that no one of these was characteristic of any special kind of organic formation. The structural elements of morbid growths may be reduced to six, viz : 1st, molecules and granules ; 2d, nuclei; 3d, cells ; 4th, fibres ; 5th, tubes (especially vascular ones); and 6th, crystals, or irregular masses of mineral matter. Now, no combination of these elements will serve to characterize morbid growths, such as fibro-molecular, fibro-nucleated, fibro-cellular, fibro-vascular, etc., for the simple reason that tumors very unlike in their external characters and natures, may be composed of the same elements. For instance, cystic, glandular, cartilaginous, and cancerous growths are all fibro-cellular. It is not, then, from its showing the existence of one or more elementary structures, but from its pointing to their *mode of arrangement*, that the microscope is destined to be of infinite importance in pathology and diagnosis."

A statement so positive, yet so despairing, from Prof. Bennett, whose microscopic researches during the current decennium have illustrated what he has denominated *Leucocthemia*, and which have contributed so much to his reputation as a histologist, could not have been anticipated. The most skeptical in regard to the utility of the microscope need not go so far in unbelief as this author, who has elaborately worked out a *non sequitur* in the above exposition. It by no means follows because the " distinctive elements of morbid growths" are not yet known by means of the microscope, none can exist ; that "no one of these is characteristic of any special kind of organic formation," and, therefore, that all " hope is vain " in this behalf. A change is not the less real because its intimate nature or elements cannot be made amenable to any combinations of glasses. In neither the organic nor inorganic world can either the purely dynamic or materialistic changes which occur be always explained by recognizable elements of a peculiar kind, as being adapted to produce one specific effect exclusively.

Assuming that in hypertrophy no morbid element has any place (which, however, the prefix *hyper*, or *excess*, does not warrant), too much of a good thing, whether drink or diet, flesh or fat, it has been said, is injurious. If, as some writers aver, hypertrophy, particularly of the left ventricle of the heart, is a good thing, both in purpose and action, some very grave charges have been laid at its door, as apoplexy, pulmonary and intestinal hæmorrhages (which I have witnessed), dropsies, and other accidents.

Much has been said of the benefits of cardiac hypertrophy in valvular disease, or insufficiency, and the principal argument in support of this view has been deduced from the fact that the muscular tissue is augmented in size and energy by increased exercise, as witnessed in the blacksmith's arm, in the dancer's inferior extremities, and in others, as the result of repeated muscular exercise ; but these are not really hypertrophies, nor permanent, but cease with the exercise, and ultimately return, for the most part, to the original state, being limited, symmetrical, physiological, and no more abnormal than the growth of the body. Such growth or development is, therefore, natural in origin, progress, result, and permanency.

The natural growth of the body and heart ; the temporary growth of the pregnant uterus and of the cuticle of the laborer's palms belong to the domains of physiology far more than to those of pathology. It is remarakable that Mr. Paget, whose pathological discrimination is usually admirable, should, in his late work on Surgical Pathology, continue to classify such growths as hypertrophous—a misnomer which would perpetually require the clinical physician and pathological anatomist to clog his nomenclature with the epithet *morbid or abnormal hypertrophy*, while the pure anatomist and physiologist would, in like manner be compelled to say *healthful, normal or natural hypertrophy*—an ambiguity calculated to augment existing obscurity and disorder in both science and its language.

While weights and measures give but limited approximative standards of the normal condition of the heart in several important respects, they do not include other fundamental properties, as color, vascularity, consistence, etc. *A priori* conceptions and the best physical descriptions cannot be relied on as sufficient to give the indisputably distinctive characters of either the natural or altered conditions of this organ independently of experimental investigation. Even volume and density, unless excessive, must be determined by the ideal resulting from ocular inspection, as differentiations may exist without greatly transcending the more rough outlines of normal organization.

Enlargement of the heart or alterations of its valves cannot be isolated and separated from morbidity, as sthenic or asthenic hyperæmia, inflammation, etc. Hypertrophy of this organ, which, doubtlessly arises from antecedent hyperæmia or other changes of

the valves and orifices, cannot be otherwise than a morbid alteration, unless, perhaps, in cases of congenital abnormities or monstrosities. Although hypertrophy of the ventricles may sometimes be
beneficial in obstruction and deficiency of the orifices and valves, by
preventing, to some extent, sanguineous accumulations and regurgitations, and sustaining the general circulation, still these benefits
are accidental only, being the result of the hyperæmic irritation,
excessive stimulation, and reäction. The violent cardiac and arterial
pulsations consequant upon hypertrophy of the left ventricle are
abnormal, and may give rise to pulmonary, cerebral and intestinal
hæmorrhages and sundry other lesions including dropsical effusions,
as already mentioned.

Hypertrophy of the heart *per se*, independently of positive disease,
is an ideal conception, rather than a clinical fact. Dr. Flint, himself, in his recent and able work on the Heart, allows this : He says,
" cases of simple, uncomplicated hypertrophy are so rare that its
clinical history can hardly be said to have been established by observation. The symptomatic phenomena which are described as
distinctive of it have been determined inferentially rather than by
facts observed in well authenticated cases. Rationally considered,
it is clear that the symptoms would be those indicative of abnormal
energy or power of the heart. Undue determination of blood to the
head might be expected to occasion certain phenomena, such as
cephalalgia, flushing of the face, throbbing, vertigo, etc. These
symptoms have relation to hypertrophy affecting the left ventricle.
Assuming the absence of aörtic obstruction and of mitral regurgitation, the pulse would represent the power of the ventricular contractions by its force, fullness, and incompressibility. Dyspnœa, when,
from any cause, the action of the heart is increased, as, for example,
after exercise, would denote that the hypertrophy affected the right
ventricle. Of the powerful action of the heart the patient would be
conscious when his attention was directed to it, and it would be
apparent from the movement of parts of the body and the dress." 33.

Prof. Flint's views of the pathological anatomy and pathological
antecedents or causes of hypertrophy are thus expressed : " With
few, if any exceptions, this process is a result of undue exercise of
the muscular power of the organ. Pathologically considered, it is
difficult to account for the production of muscular hypertrophy of
the heart, except as a consequence of some anterior abnormal con-

dition which has induced, for a considerable period, augmented muscular power. The principle is the same as in the familiar examples of voluntary muscles becoming disproportionately developed when inordinately exercised." 24-5.

"The pathological effects of hypertrophy," he continues, "are to be disconnected from those of concomitant affections and accompanying dilatation. Thus *isolated*, it is not easy to impute to it any special or very important pathological effects." 34. Is not this isolation of hypertrophy from the pale of pathology a refinement? Hypertrophy is, or ought to be, considered intrinsically morbid, or the effect of morbid action. If its epigenises or antecedents have escaped diagnosis, its development is not the less abnormal than a hypertrophied liver, spleen, etc., and it moreover affords, at the least, the strongest presumptive evidence of anterior, present, and future disease, if it be not *ipso facto* pathological.

In reference to the difficulties incidental to the nature of hypertrophy of the muscular system, Prof. Rokitansky says: "The examination of hypertrophied hearts, for which the opportunity is frequent, offers but little assistance towards the solution of the problem, more especially where the increase of mass is considerable. A new accession of muscular fibres is not manifest. On the contrary, in proportion to the diminished energy of the organ, their fibrils are found in the progress of reduction to a partially dark-colored molecule, and of gradual extinction. One thing alone is evidently adventitious, namely, irregular aggregations of an amorphous fibro-laminated blastema, copiously interspersed with nuclei in different grades of development into areölar tissue, and of areölar tissue itself, together with a large proportion of free fat and adipose tissue." In summing up the causes of hypertrophies, this author gives the whole group a pathological character, the ground work being "*a constitutional vice of nutrition and an anomalous blood-crasis*"—an explanation which is sufficiently vague and obscure.

In his Pathological Histology (Sydenham edition, 1855), Wedl says: "Hypertrophy of the *striped muscular fibre* is usually studied in hypertrophied hearts, with respect to which we would make the preliminary remark, that, except in a few cases, hearts so *diseased* are presented for observation at a stage when the hypertrophied parts have already, here and there entered into a state of retrograde metamorphosis. The color of the muscular substance is usually tawny, often of a rusty brown ; its consistence sometimes so much diminished as to admit of its being separated with as much ease as if it had been soddened ; sometimes more tough, as if the fibres were glued together with a more tenacious substance. Occasionally, even, a remarkable succulence is observable in many places. The reality of a substantive or primary hypertrophy cannot be called in question." 194, *et seq.*

Professor Andral in his *Clinique Médicale,* says : " A certain number of hypertrophies of the parietes of the heart, with or without modification in the calibre of its cavities, appear to me ,to recognize for their commencement an acute or chronic inflammation, either of the pericardium, or of the internal membrane of the heart, or of the aörta." " We are right then in inferring what might be admitted, *à priori,* that under the influence of internal carditis, the fleshy subsubstance consecutively or simultaneously irritated, may be hypertrophied." " When the parietes of the left ventricle, being very much hypertrophied, contract with unusual energy, there may thence result some morbid phenomena more or less serious, which depend on the unusual force with which the blood is driven into the arterial capillaries—more particularly felt towards the head," etc.

Mr. Paget sums up his elaborate account of hypertrophy (which coïncides with that of Prof. Flint and many others) in the following words : " The conditions which give rise to hypertrophy are chiefly only three, namely : 1. The increased exercise of a part in its natural functions. 2. An increased accumulation in the blood of the particular materials which a part appropriates to its nutrition or in secretion. 3. An increased afflux of healthy blood." Now, on the contrary, " the exercise of the natural functions" may increase an organ in size, yet naturally, not morbidly, as in hypertrophy. The other two propositions only apply as secondary effects following the primary cause of hypertrophy, be that a poison, an irritant,. mechanical injury, or whatsoever it may. ' In cardiac hypertrophy that condition should not be ascribed to an " increase of its natural function," but to an excessive or morbid increase of blood in its cavities and tissues, thereby causing irritation partly as a foreign body : " *Ubi stimulus ibi affluxus.*"

Prof. Miller, in his excellent work on *The Principles of Surgery,* says : " When the capillaries of a part deposit an amount of plasma simply sufficient to supply what is dissipated by the current expenditure, the result is normal ; the condition is that of health. *When more is exuded than is required to atone for waste, there is necessarily accumulation of the excess; the condition is a morbid one, and termed hypertrophy.* When, on the contrary, deposit from the capillaries is insufficient, by deficiency of arterial supply ; or when absorption exercises its function to excess, the condition of the deposit remaining unaltered from the state of health—the result is of an opposite kind—still morbid—and called atrophy." (257.)

The celebrated Prof. Bouillaud, of Paris, who has written the most elaborate treatise on Diseases of the Heart, and who is always able and self-reliant, whether in the right or wrong, gives a very theoretical definition of hypertrophy, that it is an enlargement without any physical or chemical alteration in the intimate or special composition of the tissues hypertrophied (*sans altération dans les qualités physiques et chimiques ou la composition intime des tissues hypertrophiés*), a postulate, the reality of which the best and latest microscopists and chemists would not swear to in open court, and one which does not accord with M. Bouillaud's therapy. For, how can he be justified in the treatment which in hypertrophy he adopts, that is, enormous bloodlettings and other antiphlogistics, if this hypertrophy be nothing more than healthy, unaltered nutrition ? His formidable treatment to effect " *la résolution de la maladie* " (hypertrophy), indicates a most dangerous alteration in the tissues of the heart, which, notwithstanding the alleged absence of all physical, chemical, or structural changes, is not the less positively mortal for all these negations so confidently and unwarrantably assumed.

Bertin maintains, in the very simplest form of hypertrophy, that " the parietes of one or more cavities of the heart is, for the most part, rather a morbid than an organic lesion. It is not mortal of itself, but becomes so in consequence of the affections it produces, and which it determines or complicates"—of which he reports, at length, three cases, with autopsies ; in the first, there were— "pulsations of the heart, strong, concentrated, and dull ; apoplexy ; simple hypertrophy of the left ventricle ; effusion of blood into the ventricles of the brain ; second, hypertrophy of the left ventricle, without dilatation of its cavity ; cerebral hæmorrhage ; third, simple hypertrophy of the left ventricle ; apoplexy from congestion." Again, he says : " Hypertrophy recognizes for its immediate and proximate cause an irritation applied to the heart." This irritation,

61

according to him, has its source in "too great a quantity of blood, violent exercise, and the passions."

In the decline of life, the muscular forces, including that of the heart, diminish. Some authors quoted above adopt the following statement, which conflicts with the prevalent theory, that the "increased exercise of a natural function" causes hypertrophy of the heart! "M. Bizot and Dr. Clendinning have proved, of the heart and arteries, that their average size regularly increases, though with a decreasing ratio of increase, from childhood to old age, provided only the old age be a lusty one. And this is a real growth; for the heart not only enlarges with advancing years, but its weight augments, and the thickness of its walls increases; so that we may believe it acquires power in the same proportion as it acquires bulk," etc. The enlargement of the heart during old age has not been noticed, as usual by myself, in numerous dissections in New Orleans. It is believed that experience shows a diminished force in the heart and arterial pulsations, as generally attendant upon the decline of life, and, consequently, the assumed hypertrophy of old age cannot be due to "increased exercise of its natural functions," or an excessively vigorous circulation.

Pathologists who deny the possibility of functional disorders without antecedent organic alteration, will readily accept the following statement from Prof. Flint: "It was formerly supposed that prolonged functional disorder of the heart eventuated in the development of hypertrophy. This opinion, sanctioned by Corvisart, is not sustained by clinical experience." 29. If this functional disorder be increased action of the heart, then, according to the explanation already given of uncomplicated hypertrophy (that of "the undue exercise of the power of the muscular organ"), it may, nay, must, "eventuate in hypertrophy;" while, on the other hand, by a parity of reasoning, anæmia, general and prolonged debility, and a feeble action, would eventuate in atrophy, attenuation or emaciation of this organ. The double assumption that functional disorder never eventuates in hypertrophy, and that functional disorder can exist without antecedent alteration, may be distrusted upon clinical grounds. The whole course of general analogy, experiment, and observation, tend to a contrary conclusion. It may be assumed as a clinical axiom, that "prolonged functional disorder" of any organ, affords a strong probability of an antecedent or an already existing lesion, an accomplished fact whence originates the so-called functional disorder, the eventualities of which react upon, augment, and complicate the original malady or alteration. Lesions, before and after death, in a majority of disorders, may be ascertained and serve to account for the latter by materialistic criteria, and these anatomical, chemical, and micrological tests are progressively enlarging the boundaries of demonstrative knowledge, thereby affording good reason to suppose, from past experience, that morbid changes in the fluids and solids exist even in that class of disorders or cases whose special lesions still elude observation, as mentioned above. As there are intermitting changes in the so-called functional disorders, so there may be a series of periodical or alternating changes in structural disorders, which, like the persons of the drama, appear reappear, and finally disappear before the curtain falls, "leaving not a track behind." Intermitting lesions in paroxysmal fever are palpable before death or recovery, as all know, because all can see them upon the exterior, and although the same may happen in the internal organs, they cannot be so absolutely taken for granted without ocular proof, or post-mortem examination, which is the great verifier, or, it may be, falsifier of the previous diagnosis. What Swift said of his physicians applies here, perhaps, in some cases :

> " They rather choose that I should die
> Than their predictions prove a lie."

The physical diagnosis of hypertrophy, though comparatively easy in the advanced or fully developed stage, is usually of small value in regard to the chances of cure, being secondary, both in a diagnostic and ætiological point of view. Were its antecedents even curable, the opportunity for medication would seldom be presented, because the patient seldom applies for aid until the mischief has been done.

The negro population is by no means exempt from hypertrophy and other forms of cardiac disease. These are virtually, if not expressly, recognized in the courts as redhibitory maladies, and often give rise to litigation. The enormous value of slaves, not less than twenty-four hundred millions of dollars in the Southern States (valuing each at only six hundred dollars), gives a pecuniary importance to all the redhibitory causes of action mentioned in the civil code, and to many not so mentioned. Cardiac diseases, often obscure or difficult to ascertain in their inception, afford, more than any of the maladies expressly enumerated in the code of Louisiana, just grounds for redhibition, and present an impossible barrier to an honest guarantee, as such slaves are not only useless, but often a burthen.

In the incipient stage of hypertrophy, which even then is usually coïncident with or secondary to valvular affection, an affirmative diagnosis is, or ought to be, redhibitory in the case of a slave. A mere external inspection, the feeling of the pulse, and the like, might convey but little positive information. Those physicians or others who are either incompetent or unwilling to make a careful physical diagnosis, might readily obtain presumptive evidence of value, by causing the individual to run up a stairway, or take other active exercise. It should be borne in mind, that, in the absence of physical diagnosis, serious and even incurable cardiac lesions may exist, unrecognized for indefinite periods, without any emaciation, pain, or very marked symptom of disease, especially if the patient does not undergo any hard labor. He may even appear to be fleshy and strong, and may be purchased as such, under full and an apparently honest guarantee, which his appearance may seem to justify, while, at the same time, active exercise cannot be borne without dyspnœa, palpitations, exhaustion, and imminent danger to life. The prominence which field labor gives to these symptoms, soon or late arrests the purchaser's attention. A physician is consulted, who, by a physical examination, ascertains the existence of hypertrophy or other disease of the organ, which a course of treatment will probably fail to cure ; whereupon the slave is returned to, but refused by, his former master. A lawsuit is the result. Although law, that is, equity, seems infinitely easier of comprehension than the multiform science of medicine, yet the uncertainty of the former is as great as that of the latter. The question of redhibitory action, in cardiac disease, gives rise to great difficulty, both to jurists and medico-legal witnesses. Is the disease curable ? Has a cure been attempted ? Did the malady exist at the time of sale ? or did it arise subsequently ? What is the period required for the development of the disease, etc.? A scientific diagnosis carefully made. in all sales of slaves, would doubtlessly prevent or diminish litigation. If the medical witness shall testify, as I have known to be the case, that a certain lesion, say of the tricuspid, mitral, or semi-lunar valves, requires a specified time to arrive at a specified condition or alteration, what could the most learned jury, bar, or bench determine understandingly in the premises? So little was known of the diagnosis of heart-diseases when the civil code of Louisiana was formed, that they are not named at all as proscribed maladies, vitiating the sale of slaves, and, therefore, redhibitory, void, and fraudulent.

The duration, as well as the termination, of hypertrophy is very uncertain. Early in my professional life, I examined a middle-aged lawyer, whose case presented the physical signs of hypertrophy of the left ventricle, who lived about thirty years afterwards, as I have learned, without any serious symptoms, until the last few years of life, when several apoplectic fits at long intervals, together with paralysis, proved fatal at a good old age. I have observed hypertrophy, which, coëxisting with tuberculosis, and pulmonary and serous inflammations, nevertheless, subsided for months or years, but which returned and proved fatal, the tubercular affection having remained apparently latent, hæmorrhage, cyanosis, and asphyxia having predominated at the close of life. I think it probable, from even my own limited experience, that clinical proof may be adduced to show that the left ventricle may be sometimes hypertrophied without recognizable lesions of the valves or orifices, the heart's impetus being powerful and extensive, the pulse strong, and, perhaps, regularly slower by half than in the normal condition, etc.; while, at the same time, if the patient avoids excessive exercise or hard labor, his health may be either good or only slightly affected with dyspnœa, etc., at prolonged intervals. Without affirming or denying that agricultural and other laborious occupations give a higher ratio of heart-diseases than are met with among the affluent, sedentary, and idle, there is reason to fear that when these cardiac affections already exist, violent exercise will prove dangerous. In such cases, however, the current of medical opinion is now in favor of moderate exercise and a liberal diet. Thirty years ago the diet was restricted, the horizontal position directed, and bloodlettings and calomel often prescribed. The abandonment of large and repeated doses of calomel in general practice, is most commendable. But it is worthy of serious inquiry, whether the great modern increase of cardiac diseases, especially such as have an intercurrent, or recent origin during the progress of thoracic affections, might not be prevented, or cured, by the moderate and timely use of that drug, the power of which, in arresting inflammatory exudations and hypertrophous thickenings of serous membranes, as the pericardial, endocardial, and valvular, as well as the peritoneal, is probably equaled by no other.

At the period above mentioned, the then unrivaled work of Bertin, on *Diseases of the Heart*, edited by Bouillaud, appeared. The cardiac ætiology, pathology, and therapy of this work (which is supposed to coincide with those of the French school), will be sufficiently indicated by the few lines which follow, concerning valvular vegetations, hypertrophy, indurations, etc.: "A multitude of considerations have influenced us to believe that very frequently the morbid changes in the valves take place, in fact, under the influence of the phlegmasia. * * * The only success we can expect from the best regulated means, is to relieve the patients a little, and to prolong for a certain time their painful existence." His remedies are : "Sanguine evacuants, diuretic, aperient, anodyne medicines, pedeluvia, revulsions, etc., seconded by absolute repose of mind and body, and by a vigorous diet. But this cure, although it appears somewhat wonderful, is only momentary. The symptoms are again renewed, whenever the patients give themselves up to any kind of excess whatever. · We cannot too often repeat, that perfect repose is indispensable in the case of contraction of the orifices of the heart. It is still more requisite, when the patients are oppressed by the least exercise ; as we can safely assert, that the principal cause of diseases of the heart may be traced to violent and forced exertions, such as the chase, dancing, and all the professions which require energetic and prolonged endeavors. * * * An invincible difficulty in the treatment of diseases of the heart, in general, is the continued action to which the organ is subjected. The first indication, when an organ is diseased, is to place it in the most complete repose ; but this indication it is evidently impossible to put into practice in diseases of the heart. The absolute repose of this organ would be at once an inevitable cause of death. * * * The agents which we ought to employ against the hypertrophy itself, must, for the most part, be sought for amongst the debilitants and antiphlogistics."

ART. VII.—*Treatment of Snake-Bite.*

DR. DOWLER—In the January number of the Journal, Dr. Humphrey Peake, of Yazoo City, Mississippi, calls the attention of the profession to the remedial properties of tobacco in the bites of poisonous reptiles and insects. I have used it in two or three cases of snake-bite, with marked benefit. I use it internally and locally. My observation leads me to a different conclusion from Dr. Peake ; in every instance it has produced nausea and vomiting. It is due to truth to state, however, that its use was accompanied by the free administration of alcoholic stimulants. I regard either as efficacious, when administered in time, and both together more prompt than either separately. Their effect on the animal organism is very much alike ; both are narcotic ; both produce nausea and vomiting in most persons, when taken in sufficient doses. Tobacco may be primarily a sedative—the secondary effect of large quantities of whisky or brandy is also sedative. This being true, the effect on the poison is not so difficult to explain.

I always regard my patient as safe, whenever I can get him nauseated or intoxicated. There are some persons whom neither of these substances will nauseate, under any circumstances. This may have been the case with the individual mentioned in Dr. Peake's communication, in the May number of the Journal ; or it may have been on account of mental emotion or excessive pain. I have so much confidence in these remedies that I feel no fears of a fatal result in a case of snake-bite, if I have enough whisky and tobacco at hand.

I shall rely, in future, on the internal administration of alcoholic stimulants, and the local application of tobacco, either as a cataplasm, decoction, or infusion. The local application of the tobacco greatly relieves the pain consequent on the swelling, and tends to arrest the swelling itself.

As regards the *modus operandi* of these remedies, I will not venture a suggestion. We should not discard any remedy because we cannot give a rational account of the precise mode of its action on the human system. While this would be desirable in all instances, we are bound to admit the fact that we are utterly unable to account for the effect produced by some of our most important remedial agents. This being the fact, we must take these two remedies for a painful and dangerous disease, as we find them, and not discard them because of any difficulty in harmonizing their effects, either on the disease or the animal economy.

Yours, truly,   W. D. JOHNSON, M. D.

HERNANDO, Mississippi, May 10, 1860.

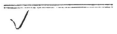

ART. VIII.—*The Position During Parturition.*

B. DOWLER, *M. D., Editor N. O. Medical and Surgical Journal.*— What position is best for woman in labor? This is a mooted ques. tion, and will not, perhaps, be settled at a very early day. In the United States and Great Britain, accoucheurs advise their patients to lie on the left side, with the knees drawn up and separated by a pillow ; whilst the French prefer that their patients should lie on their backs. This, they say, is the only natural position, being that in which labor is easiest, with least danger to the patient. Both positions are defended by the highest authorities.

We should not ourself obtrude, nor enter the list of disputants, but for a remark of M. Robert, of Paris, as it appears in the *N. O. Medical and Surgical Journal,* May, 1860, p. 346. Speaking of Dr. Bozeman's operative procedure for the cure of fistule, he says : "We will first say that vesico-vaginal fistules, rather rare in France, are, on the contrary, frequent in England and America, because of the position the patients in these two countries are made to take during parturition, *which is to sit upon a chair.*" The italics are our own.

It seems to us difficult to understand how so erroneous a statement as this could have been made by one occupying the position of M. Robert, who, it is presumed, has access to libraries in which are to be found the treatises of the most eminent English and American writers on obstetrics. We are sure, if he had taken the trouble to have turned to the works of Dewees and Meigs, of the United States, and Churchill and Ramsbotham, of Great Britain, he would not have made a statement that is without foundation in fact, and calculated to reflect discredit upon American and British obstetricians. The works above mentioned are standard authorities in both countries, and are text books in the medical schools of note in this country.

There is nothing, therefore, taught in our medical colleges contrary to the principles laid down in these treatises.

We are well aware of the fact, however, that there are American practitioners who prefer the position of the French—that is, on the back. We prefer this position ourself, though our experience is probably not sufficient to enable us to speak authoritatively on this subject. We look upon it as the *natural* position. We have invariably found the negroes and the lower class of white women to occupy this position when left to themselves; and we have not seen many accidents happen during their labor. In no case have we seen fistule following a labor in this position. We think it an unnecessary refinement to compel a woman to assume a certain position, because somebody thinks himself a correct interpreter of nature, and becomes her spokesman. There is what we call instinct in animals, and we find this in all animals, from man, "the lord of creation," to the most insignificant of animated beings. Nature directs about everything that pertains to ourselves as animal beings, pointing with unerring aim to those things necessary for the preservation of the individual and of the species. Copulation takes place in a certain position; parturition takes place in a certain position, also.

Under the weight of authority, most American practitioners, so far as we are aware, recommend to their patients the side position. But we have yet to hear of a well-educated physician making his patient sit in a chair. It is very true, we have heard of this practice among ignorant midwives; but this has been many years ago, before we had attained to manhood, or had become a student of medicine. We considered the practice then, as we certainly do now, as barbarous, and unworthy the countenance of an enlightened community. It is possible that, in some portions of the United States, where the practice of midwifery is still in the hands of this class of individuals, that patients are made to sit in a chair, but we are quite sure such is not the practice among medical gentlemen.

As to the cause of vesico-vaginal fistule being more common in England and the United States than in France, we are not prepared to speak. "Meddlesome midwifery" may have something to do with it. Unnecessary operative interference, by contusing the soft tissues, may be one cause of it. Or making the patient sit in a chair during labor, where such is the practice, may cause it.

As to which is the best position, the American or the French,

62

experience alone can determine. We prefer the latter, and always allow our patients to take it, which they seem instinctively to do.

Hoping this communication may not be uninteresting,

I am, respectfully,   GEORGE S. D. ANDERSON.

ALEXANDRIA, Louisiana, May 10, 1860.

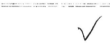

ART. IX.—*Positions in Parturition:* By B. DOWLER, M. D.

THE postures of parturient patients, and the attitudes of their assistants, as practised a quarter of a century ago, and perhaps still in North-western Virginia, have not, so far as I know, been made public. These, consist, as the sequel will show, chiefly of two groups, as witnessed during the last stage of labor—a stage easily recognized, not only by a digital examination, but by the cries or language of the patient, by her deep inspirations, with the holding of the breath, or a long breath, to give greater force to the extrusive actions of the expiratory and abdominal muscles ; congestive flushings of the face, distention of the frontal, facial, and jugular veins ; general muscular tension ; the holding to and pulling by anything within grasping distance during the expulsive pains, etc. These and other kindred phenomena, precursors of the impending crisis, show that the mental and bodily strain of child-birth has arrived ; the sympathies of friends and attendants are excited. All, not accepting the accoucheur, wish that this stage of the labor (agony it might be called) should be completed with the utmost speed consistent with the well-being of mother and child. The fœtal head no longer recedes, but produces more or less pressure, even in the intervals of the paroxysmal throes, the unusual prolongation of which give the medical attendant a degree of uneasiness which the preceding stage, however protracted, seldom, if ever, excites. Hence, every facility, in any wise calculated to aid the natural forces of the patient, is put in requisition. Even the appearance of physical help, though it may be intrinsically powerless, will, if harmless in itself, be highly beneficial, from its psychical influence in inspiring courage, confidence, and hope. With this view, the following plan was often adopted, particularly in rural practice, in the country above mentioned, and it probably still prevails.

The husband is now called in, sits on a chair, his wife on his lap ; his knees separated, sometimes bound with a cloth, so that this separation may be the less fatiguing ; two chairs are placed before the patient, some distance apart ; she places her feet, having shoes on, so as to rest upon the rounds or frames of the chairs ; two female assistants sit on these chairs, causing them to be immovable during the expulsive pains, while the helpers press with one hand or with chest against the patient's knees, with the other hand each takes one of the patient's hands, who pulls during the pains, and also presses her feet against the chairs, and her back against her husband, her knees being supported by her assistants, the accoucheur sitting before the patient and between the assistants—a most convenient attitude, should his services be required.

During the expulsive throes, and, indeed, all the time of the labor, the patient takes neither the horizontal nor vertical sitting posture, but is reclined or semi-recumbent, except when, during the intervals of the pains, she rises or changes her attitude to prevent fatigue.

This plan (which owes its origin, so far as I know, to the people) appears to give the woman a complete control over all the voluntary forces auxiliary to that of the uterus itself. But it fatigues all her attendants, except the doctor, and if the labor be not rapid, the husband is the greatest sufferer, next to herself, sometimes turning pale and faint, unless relieved by some of the attendants, who are always ready to aid in such emergencies.

When the child is born, the patient is carried to bed, even though the placenta may not be delivered.

Another procedure is often adopted, by which the labor is conducted in bed. A bed is doubled up against inverted chairs, the bed being placed behind and next to the patient, a mattress being under her, upon which she rests in the half-recumbent sitting posture, her feet resting against the foot-board ; two sheets or towels are fastened to the two bed-posts at the foot of the bed, for her to pull by during the pains. Here, however, the foot-board is a barrier in the way of the accoucheur, and to obviate this, the bed or other supports are placed against the wall, the patient lies semi-inclined across the mattress, her limbs flexed, her feet resting on two chairs at the bedside ; upon the latter two assistants sit, to aid, as in the former position, the chair of the accoucheur being placed between the latter, but a little in advance.

With proper arrangements, which need not be detailed further, in either of these positions the inferior limbs are flexed, the perineum and outlet unimpeded just as much as in the horizontal attitude, whether resting on the back or side, while, in the former, to use common sense phrase of experienced matrons, the woman "helps herself" by the abdominal and expiratory muscular power to a greater extent than by simply lying down on her back. There is no more danger in the one case than in the other. In all positions, good, bad, or indifferent, labor will "pursue the even tenor of its way" to a successful termination, with rare exceptions.

In the middle period of labor, the patient squeezes—in the last stage, pulls whatsoever she can take hold of—a mechanical advantage which she instinctively seeks, and which a physiologist of a different gender has no right to ignore or condemn as altogether superfluous. The obvious, materialistic muscular actions, both voluntary and involuntary, of parturition, afford the physiological obstetrician data illustrative of that vital and mechanical process infinitely more intelligible than the fanciful expositions of the so-called reflex actions of the "true spinal cord," or even the false.*

From a common sense point of view in the lying-in chamber, the "parturient acts," whether voluntary or involuntary, seem *direct muscular acts*, which take place about nine months after conception, by primary or inherent laws of the living economy, which neither the parturient subject nor her accoucheur can fathom, being ultimate, fundamental, self-evident, and not explicable by obscure language.

Neither danger to the child nor to the mother are likely to occur, whenever labor can be expedited by the natural forces of the mother ; while, on the other hand, ergot, manipulations, and instrumental applications are more or less perilous to both, and, perhaps, in rare cases, the same may be said of even natural labor, when the head remains for many hours fixed or impacted in the pelvic bones, although, probably, the danger, if any, cannot be so great as is generally apprehended.

May I not here add a few words on this subject not originally

---

* "The act of parturition never had been, and never could be, studied properly until the discovery of the physiology of the spinal marrow, by Dr. Marshall Hall. All the uterine motor actions are *reflex*," etc.— *W. Tyler Smith, M. D.*

intended in commencing this article ? Although isolated individual experience may generally be of little import in opposition to that of the many, yet, judging from my own observations, I must say that, in cases wherein the presentation of the fœtal head is normal, or rather in that which is usually considered the most favorable position of the vertex, no danger to mother or child has resulted from severe and prolonged labor, in which the child's head has rested apparently fixed low down, just within the perineum, and ready to make its exit—I say apparently fixed, because in the intervals of the pains the pressure of the head must necessarily intermit, though the head may not sensibly recede. The anatomical conformation of the mother, the position of the child, and the force of the pains being faultless, can anything be more trying to human patience and the moral sympathies, than a continuous series of pangs and disappointments, which, in rare cases, last perhaps an entire day ! The accoucheur, relying upon nature, abstaining from all active or instrumental interferences, regulating the hygienic conditions of the chamber, attending to the conditions of the bladder, etc., inspiring hope, and sacrificing his valuable time, may suffer reproach, his skill being distrusted ; but when a living child is born, and the patient has a quick recovery, he will have an approving conscience, and may have an undamaged reputation among the judicious and right-thinking witnesses of his professional conduct. But, as the world goes, glittering forceps, bloody craniotomies, and violent, quick deliveries will usually pass for skill and superior qualifications. For the most part, the greatest use that an obstetrician can be put to, is to do nothing himself, and to prevent others from doing anything, mere placebos and " pious frauds" excepted.

Early in my professional life I had opportunities of witnessing or learning the natural history of prolonged labor, in which no active interference had taken place, in remote settlements in Harrison, Tyler, and Lewis counties, Virginia, at distances sometimes more than forty miles from my residence, in Clarksburg. In some cases active labor had existed several days before my visits. In one of my first cases, I witnessed with dismay the active hard labor of a woman apparently in the last stage, the head of the child being fixed or locked during twenty-four hours after my arrival ; fortunately, I had no instruments with me. The child was born alive, and the woman was wholly uninjured. I might detail other still more remarkable examples, in none of which accidents occurred. On the other hand, the unwarrantable interferences of some bold and ignorant midwives, and others, under apparently such circumstances, have resulted most deplorably, as I can testify.

ART. X.—*Medical Notes and Observations*, in a letter from STANFORD E. CHAILLÉ, A. M., M. D. (one of the editors of this Journal), now in Europe.

[MANY readers of this Journal will be surprised to see that the following letter comes from beyond the Atlantic, while all, doubtlessly, will be delighted with its perusal, and the more so, because this is, it is believed, but the precursor of numerous letters of a kindred character, should the writer remain abroad two years, as he intended when he left his native land in the South. A young physician in full practice, a proprietor in an established private hospital, already distinguished for his professional and classical learning, officially connected with the anatomical department of the University of Louisiana—Stanford E. Chaillé goes off, nevertheless, *con amore* for professional observation, to take the parallax, that is, the difference between the apparent and the true places of the great luminaries in the medical heavens, as viewed, not from distant America alone, but under their native skies. From his qualifications and independence, readers may expect an impartial account of medical men and measures.

These allusions, however unacceptable they may be to Dr. Chaillé, are made to show the friends of the Journal, that the latter will not lose, but gain by his absence, which, indeed, releases him for a time from the onerous duties of practice, and affords him an opportunity to contribute more fully to the Journal. Besides, I have the most indisputable evidence of his ardent wish, I might almost say passion, to make this periodical useful to its patrons—a wish which neither absence nor distance is likely to abate. J. J. Rousseau mentions the case of a lover who often left his fair one in order to enjoy *the pleasure of corresponding* with her. "*Absence*," says Hume, "destroys *weak* passion, but increases the *strong*; as the wind extinguishes a candle, but blows up a fire." So in the case of the Journal.   B. D.]

PARIS, May 1, 1860.

To BENNET DOWLER, M. D.—*Dear Doctor*—It has been written, that when one has nothing worth saying, he had best remain silent. Mankind might gain by the practical application of such a rule, but medical journals would be often at a loss for the manuscript necessary to fill up the promised pages demanded by their subscribers. Having pledged myself to contribute my quota to our periodical, I shall fulfill the pledge, though the judicious may have reason to conclude that so many blank pages would be as instructive as those filled by my publications.

On my way here, I passed two days in Philadelphia, and as many weeks in New York. My visit to the former was rendered most agreeable, by the courteous hospitality of Dr. Gross. With him I visited their great hospital, Blockley's, and saw in the five or six large wards under his control, many interesting cases, a few cancers, a few cases of scrofula, and, as usual in all surgical wards, a vast number of sore legs. There was also a case of double vagina in the hospital, which I unfortunately did not have an opportunity to see. To the kindness of Dr. Gross I was also indebted for an invitation to one of the famous Wistar parties, given, on this occasion, by Dr. Dunglison, where I had the pleasure of meeting the authors of many of those books which have been so often thumbed by every medical man in America. These Wistar parties were, as you doubtless know, instituted by Dr. Wistar, who was in the habit of assembling at his house, once a week, those of his professional brethren who were distinguished for their attainments. Since his death, these social meetings have been continued. They are now given by a society of some twenty-six members, each of whom, in regular succession, gives a supper at his own house, to which are invited, not only the members of the society, and other medical men, but also those who have attained some eminence in any branch of science. This custom is worthy of imitation, and it is to be regretted that the physicians of New Orleans have not adopted some plan for the cultivation of more intimate social relations. Destitute of social meetings, destitute of any medical society (worthy to be so called) is it surprising that we should be also destitute of a healthy professional opinion ; and that some who claim high position should be unblushing advertisers of their own merit?

Dr. Goddard took me to see the microscopic stand which he has

invented. It certainly surpasses all others in the neatness and simplicity of its mechanism, when compared with the complexity of its
motions, and its adjustability. In fact, almost every part of it can be
made to move easily, in any direction the most exacting microscopist
could desire. He has the most complete collection I have ever seen,
of not only all the essential, but also of all the accessory instruments made use of in microscopy.

In New York I called on three medical men, Dalton, Sims, and
Green. The first has, in his recent work on Physiology, written the
most readable and intelligible chapter on embryology which I have
ever read ; and after he had shown me the collection of specimens
prepared by himself, illustrative of this subject, I could readily
understand, that, knowing well what he was writing about, he could
not easily fail to make himself comprehended. I examined with
particular interest one of his specimens, a normal womb, at about
the eighth month of pregnancy, which demonstrated the identity of
the decidua vera with the mucous membrane of the womb ; a new
mucous membrane was apparent, growing under the old one, and
ready to replace it when discharged.

I have never met a man with whom I was more pleased, after a
brief acquaintonce, than with Dr. J. Marion Sims. However, as personal traits of character are not, perhaps, a proper subject for a
medical journal, I will not offend good taste by descanting at length
upon either his frankness and cordiality, or the simplicity of his
manners and hospitality of his home. I had an opportunity to see
the precision, neatness, and facility of his manipulation in operations
within the vaginal canal. The case was one of anteversion of the
womb, of long standing, and the third case of this character which he
had attempted to remedy by a surgical operation. Encouraged by
the success of the first two cases, he undertook this without fear as
to the result. The principle of the operation is to shorten the
anterior wall of the vagina, thus draw down the cervix, and thereby
elevate the fundus of the womb. The process of the operation was
as follows : The patient was placed on her left side, the thighs flexed
at about a right angle with the pelvis, the chest thrown forward, and
the left arm behind. An assistant introduced Sims's speculum, by
which, and the atmospheric pressure, every part of the vagina was
brought fully into view. The operator now thoroughly scarified
about an inch in length, transversely, of the anterior wall of the

vagina, at its uterine extremity, and a portion, also, of the adjacent cervix ; then a scarification was made an inch and a half lower down the anterior wall of the vagina, which corresponded in extent to that made above. The two scarified surfaces were then accurately applied to each other by six or eight interrupted silver sutures, and the operation thus completed. The pain experienced by the patient was so trifling that no movement was made which interfered in the least degree with the operation, and Dr. Sims informed me that he was not in the habit of resorting to anæsthetics, as the pain inflicted was not sufficient to require their use. He insists upon the necessity of never leaving scarified surfaces free, but of always having them accurately adjusted to each other throughout their entire extent, as even a small portion left free and unapplied suppurates and interferes with union by the first intention in the remaining denuded surfaces, which are properly applied to each other. I was surprised to find that a great diversity of cases were apparently remediable by operation, and that Dr. Sims by no means limited his surgical cures to vesico-vaginal and recto-vaginal fistulæ. He has an operative procedure to relieve anteflexions, as well as anteversions ; but though the principle is sufficiently simple and rational, I doubt my power of describing the operation so as to be comprehended, unless assisted by drawings or plates. He relieves some cases of prolapsus, also, by operation. This is effected by so diminishing the size of the vaginal canal that the womb cannot protrude through it. Two parallel lines of the vaginal mucous membrane are scarified in the course of the length of the vagina, the two scarified surfaces united by the silver ligature, and the vaginal canal thus diminished in size in proportion to the distance of the two parallel lines from each other.

Dr. Emmet, who, as resident physician of the Woman's Hospital, has been for some years associated with Dr. Sims, has a record, in which has been kept, not only the history of every interesting case, but also drawings illustrating the pathological condition of the parts, and the operation performed to remedy it. He showed me several cases, where the posterior *cul de sac* of the vagina was unusually deep, and the os uteri, therefore, further removed than is normally the case from the uterine extremity of the posterior wall of the vagina. These cases had all been sterile for years, but pregnancy had succeeded an operation by which the os uteri had been incised posteriorly, so as to throw the mouth of the womb backwards, and near the extremity of the posterior wall of the vagina, from which it had been so far removed. This description may not be intelligible ; it will be better understood when I give you the reasoning upon which the operation is founded. Dr. Emmet supposes, and I presume his opinion reflects that of Dr. Sims, that copulation seldom results in conception, unless the os uteri be in such a position as to fairly receive the discharge of semen from the meatus urethræ of the penis. If the impulse of the semen in the act of coition be not directed fairly into the womb's mouth (in consequence of its faulty position), then sterility may result. Dr. E. asserts that, notwithstanding those exceptional cases where pregnancy has apparently occurred without even penetration of the virile member, it is none the less true that the wives of those men who have had an abnormal termination of the urethra (the meatus being situated, not on the glans penis, but somewhere in the course of the urethra), have been sterile, which would tend to establish the assertion that impregnation usually requires something more than the simple introduction of semen within the vagina.

The profession will, no doubt, be gratified to hear that Dr. Sims is now preparing for publication a monograph upon the application of the silver suture to all the accidents and lesions resulting from protracted parturition ; and that a most competent artist is now engaged in the preparation of plates to illustrate handsomely and accurately the subject. I may assert, in anticipation of this work, that Dr. Sims's hospital-record abounds in material which, properly arranged, will add to his reputation, and furnish his professional brethren with much valuable and curious information.

Having long desired to see the larynx and trachea probanged and catheterized, I concluded I could not do better than visit Dr. Horace Green, who, as everybody knows, was the first to introduce this practice, which has now for its advocates such men as Trousseau, Bennett, etc., etc. My visit was at his hour of consultation, so that I found several patients present, who were undergoing treatment for laryngeal and bronchial affections. So far as the probang was concerned, I saw what I came to see ; the instrument was introduced, in two cases, into the larynx, and *not* the œsophagus. It was made, not simply to touch the upper portion of the larynx, but was passed downwards five inches at least, and evidently into the trachea, and this without the least difficulty, so far as the operator was concerned, and without annoyance or pain to the patients. Dr. Green pointed out to me the edge of the epiglottis, curling upwards, and demonstrated its comparative insensibility. He asserts, and, I believe, correctly, that the epiglottis presents no impediment to the introduction of an instrument, that both it and the vocal cords are nearly insensible ; but that there is a narrow zone of exquisitely sensitive mucous membrane which covers the lips of the glottis, and that the least irritation of this is quickly communicated to the constrictor muscles of the glottis (the arytenoid muscles), and the aperture of the glottis is as quickly shut up. Before introducing an instrument, it is necessary, therefore, that the sensitiveness of the glottic aperture should be diminished, which is generally effected to such a degree, by daily cauterizations with nitrate of silver for a week, that the instrument may be readily passed. I regret much that I did not have an opportunity to see the bronchi catheterized, and the lungs injected with a solution of nitrate of silver, an operation which is performed almost daily by Dr. Green, and which he promised to show me the next morning, if I would call, which I could not do. He asserts that, "in cases of bronchitis, in asthma, and in early phthisis pulmonalis even, the use of injections into the bronchi, once or twice a week, operate to diminish the cough, expectoration, and dyspnœa with great certainty, and very many cases of these diseases have recovered under local treatment, after other measures had failed," and that, "if he were required to relinquish all other known therapeutic measures, or topical medication in the treatment of thoracic diseases, he should choose the latter, with hygienic means alone, in preference to the entire class of remedies ordinarily employed in the treatment of these diseases." Bennett, of Edinburgh, does not use language as strong, but recommends injections into the bronchi in phthisis, laryngitis, and in chronic bronchitis, with severe paroxysms of asthma. Trousseau has "often injected into the trachea and bronchial tubes, after tracheotomy, in cases of croup, large quantities of caustic solutions, repeating this operation four, five, and six times a day, and many days consecutively." Loiseau and Depaul, of France ; Greisenger, of Germany, and other men of reputation, pronounce the operation easy of execution, and free from danger. A practice recommended by such authorities should at least be generally understood by the physician ; and when we consider the obstinate character of the diseases in which this local treatment is recommended, we must conclude it deserves a careful and impartial trial. That the *modus operandi* may be understood, I send you for. publication directions which have appeared in Bennett's Clinical Medicine and elsewhere, but not in our Journal. Dr. Green writes:

"The instruments I employ may be obtained at any surgical instrument maker's shop. They consist of an ordinary flexible or gum catheter, and a small silver or glass syringe. The catheter is Hutching's gum-elastic catheter (No. 11 or 12), which is twelve and a half inches in length; and, as the distance from the incisor teeth to the tracheal bifurcation is, ordinarily, in the adult, about eight inches, if this instrument is introduced so as to leave only two inches of the catheter projecting from the mouth, its lower extremity must, of course (if it enter the trachea), reach into one or the other of its divisions. I first prepare my patients by making applications, with the sponge-probang and nitrate of silver solution, for a period of one or two weeks, to the opening of the glottis and the larynx, until the sensibility of the parts is greatly diminished. Then, having the tube slightly bent, I dip the instrument in cold water (which serves to stiffen it for a moment, and obviates the necessity of using a wire), and, with the patient's head thrown well back, and the tongue depressed, I place the bent extremity of the instrument on the laryngeal face of the epiglottis, and gliding it quickly through the rima glottidis, carry it down to, or below, the bifurcation, as the case may require. It is necessary that the patient continue to respire, and the instrument is most readily passed during the act of inspiration. The tube being introduced, the point of the syringe is inserted into its opening, and the solution injected. This latter part of the operation must be done as quickly as possible, or a spasm of the glottis is likely to occur. Indeed, if the natural sensibility of the aperture of the glottis is not well subdued by previous applications of the nitrate of silver solution, or if the tube, in its introduction, touches roughly the border or lips of the glottis, a spasm of the glottis is certain to follow, which will arrest the further progress of the operation. The *epiglottis, which is nearly insensible* (and this you may prove on any person, by thrusting two fingers over the base of the tongue, and touching, or even scratching, with the nail, this cartilage), should be our guide in performing the operation. The strength of the solution, for injecting, is from ten to twenty-five grains to the ounce of water. Commencing with ten or fifteen grains to the ounce, its strength is subsequently increased, and the amount I employ is from one-half to one and a half drachms of this solution.

"Latterly, in commencing the injections, I have used a solution still weaker than above denoted. When my patients are prepared for catheterism, by repeated cauterizations of the opening of the glottis and larynx, to reduce the normal sensitiveness of the parts, the tube is then introduced, and a drachm of a solution of nitrate argent, of the strength of from five to ten grains to the ounce of water, is injected through the trachea. Afterwards, the solution may be gradually increased in power ; but, at the present day, I seldom employ the remedy, in bronchial injections, of a strength above twenty grains of the salt to an ounce of water.

"Should a spasm of the glottis occur on the insertion of the tube into the larynx, the instrument should be promptly withdrawn, and no further attempt be made to proceed with the operation, until the irritation has fully subsided. It is necessary that the applications of the sponge-probang be continued in the intervals of the employment of the tube."

Where the operation has been completed, notwithstanding spasm of the glottis, alarming symptoms have in several instances ensued, similar to those thus described in one of Dr. Green's cases : "The whole chest seemed thrown into a violent spasmodic action ; a convulsive cough, with dyspnœa, followed, which continued during several hours, but was finally somewhat relieved by the use of chloroform, and the administration of anodynes. The cough and dyspnœa, however, with increased expectoration, and pleuritic pains, continued for several days ; and although the patient became, in the course of a week, quite comfortable again, under general treatment, yet she never entirely recovered the favorable state she was in before the occurrence of the spasm." In experimenting upon animals, Dr. Green found that a solution of one ounce of water to thirty grains of nitrate of silver, injected at once into a dog's lungs, resulted in pneumonia and death, although a weaker solution, in smaller quantity, was borne with impunity.

Dr. Green describes the immediate effects produced by these injections in terms similar to those of Bennett, who says : "I have been surprised at the circumstance of the injections not being followed by the slightest irritation whatever, but rather by a pleasant feeling of warmth in the chest (some have experienced a sensation of coolness), followed by ease to the cough, and a check, for a time, to all expectoration."

Among other matters which excited my surprise, was the very positive assertion of Dr. Green, that prior to the development of pulmonary tuberculosis, there is invariably a deposit in the tonsils, which, to the close observer, foretells infallibly the impending deposit in the lungs. If not true, no harm will be done in drawing attention to the subject.

Altogether, I was much gratified by my visit to Dr. Green, whose unostentatious manner was so perfectly free from everything like charlatanism that my preconceived opinion in regard to him was more than modified. I had entertained a prejudice against him— where it came from I do not know—founded on the supposition that he had overstepped, at times, the bounds of professional propriety, and claimed more for himself than was consistent with modest merit. I know nothing in reference to the truth of such assertions ; but must we not concede, that, even if his local treatment of the aërian passages possess less merit than he claims,' he has still done something in proving the facility with which the larynx may be subjected to local applications, and the comparative inocuousness of the intro- duction of a catheter through the trachea into either branch of its bifurcation, and the injection of solutions into the bronchial tubes ?

You, Doctor, and those who read this, may be pleased to find that I have nothing more to say in regard to Dr. Green ; but I am sure you will not be dissatisfied that I have not yet concluded with his anatomical speciality, the larynx. My dear sir, I have *seen* it—not the outside of it, but the inside, including the vocal ligaments, su- perior and inferior—and this larynx was not that of a dead body, not preserved in a bottle of spirits, not carefully dried and labelled in a museum, but was the personal property of a *living, healthy*, and *unmutilated* man, which he made use of just as you and I use our larynges ; and this sight I saw, not "in a glass, darkly," but, though in a glass, yet just as distinctly as I ever viewed it in a dis- section made for the purpose—and better, too, for it was a living, healthy larynx, with its mucous membrane colored with the red blood coursing through it, its epiglottis capable of motion, and its vocal cords, when performing their function, opening and shutting like the blades of a pair of scissors. And just as plainly as I have seen the interior of the living larynx, so have I seen the pharyngeal extremity of the eustachian tube, and the posterior nares. This statement will not astonish you, for, before this reaches you, you will have read in your exchanges, that Prof. Czermak has invented a laryngoscope, the use of which he is exhibiting to the M. D. P's., to their great astonishment, and equally great delight. Before seeing the application of the instrument, I inquired of Dr. Czermak its power. He replied that, under favorable circumstances, the bifurcation of the trachea had been seen. Politeness forbade a *visible* smile of incredulity, but I rewarded my own forbearance by wondering, mentally, at the astonishing development of the imagination in some, and the blindfold enthusiasm of men in regard to their own inventions. I then took a look, and although I did *not* see the bifurcation, I still did see the trachea so far below the larynx, that, if others had not been waiting to take my place, I should have commenced, in stupid astonishment, peering out for even the air-cells of the lungs. The instrument is most simple, both in its construction and application, still it requires practice to use it ; and still worse, it requires that the soft palate of the subject should be inured by custom to the presence of a foreign body, and that the subject should be at least docile, if not intelligent. The instrument, therefore, is no more likely to come into general use than the ophthalmoscope, nor can it generally be employed when the subject is young and refractory. It will, however, serve a most useful practical purpose in the diagnosis and treatment of diseases of the larynx and the surrounding parts in the adult. Out of some fifteen of these to whose throats the instrument was adapted for the first time by Dr. Czermak, in one of the hospitals of Paris, he informed me that in only three cases did he fail to render the interior of the larynx perfectly visible. But, apart from the service which will be rendered by this instrument to practical medicine, surgery, and physiology, it is such a gratifying optical curiosity that I have ordered one, with the intention of learning its use, and then sending it as a present to my very dear friend, and our coëditor, Dr. Jones, knowing how highly it will be appreciated by him, and that, in his hands, the hundreds of medical men and students who throng the halls of the medical department of the University of Louisiana, will have an opportunity to see its application and learn its use. The manner of using this instrument, the instrument itself, and the services already rendered and to be rendered by it, are of sufficient importance to be well understood, so I gladly resort to the pen of another, instructed by a better opportunity to see the use of the laryngoscope than I have had, to make these points comprehensible. I translate from the *Gazette Médicale de Paris*, of April 14th : "Every-one is now acquainted, if not with the mechanism and use of the ophthalmoscope, at least with the instrument, and the nature of the services which it renders every day ; with the progress it has been the cause of in ophthalmology, and its great merit in a diagnostic point of view. The only difficulty which its general application in practice encounters, is the delicacy of its employment, and the study of its mechanism, which, unfortunately, remains an object of indif-ference, or laziness, to too large a number of practitioners. This is a sad thing for the general knowledge of deep-seated diseases of the eye.

"This difficulty, this obstacle, need not be feared in the employ-ment of a new instrument of the same kind, which an ingenious and laborious German has just sent us, and the object of which is to inves-tigate by the eye the interior of the larynx. With a large number of physicians assembled on this occasion, during the present week, we have assisted, at the *Municipal Maison de Santé*, together with all the scientific men connected with this establishment, in demonstra-tive experiments made by the inventor, Dr. Czermak, Professor of Physiology at the University of Pesth.

"Imagine a concave mirror, similar to the one used in the ophthal-moscope, only with a larger surface, and a much longer radius of curvature *(rayon de courbure)*, and pierced like the latter, with a small ocular hole in its center. A lamp placed behind, or by the side of the subject to be examined, at about the height of his mouth, sends its rays upon the mirror, which, in its turn, sends them back, concentrated, upon the plain of the back-throat of the subject ; into whose mouth, widely opened, the tongue being depressed by a spatula, the observer introduces, exactly beneath the uvula, and in contact with its inferior surface, a little mirror, placed as are those of which dentists make use to examine the posterior face of the incisive teeth. This little mirror is mounted on a long, slender stem, so inclined as not to be in the axis of the mouth, and upon which the plain of the mirror is adjusted at an angle of 45°.

"Supposing the subject docile, and familiarized beforehand with the very inoffensive position of the mirror between the posterior pil-lars of the veil of the palate, a flood of light enters horizontally into the mouth of the subject, encounters, at the passage of the isthmus of the throat, the plain (at 45°) of the mirror, and is by it reflected from above, downwards, vertically. All the parts situated in the course of this reflected beam of light are thus magnificently illuminated.

And then—this is all." [The author has omitted to mention the necessity of warming the little mirror to blood-heat before introducing it into the back-throat. By this precaution the moisture exhaled in respiration does not deposit a film on the glass, and thus impair or destroy its reflecting power. S. E. C.] "The mechanism is assuredly simple : the larynx widely opened for respiration, the epiglottis raised up, present themselves in the mirror to the eye of the observer, upon even the passage of the incident rays. The larynx is seen (theory of reflection on plain surfaces) upon the prolongation of the horizontal axis of the mouth, opposite to the observer, in virtue of the simple equality between the angles of incidence and reflection. The parts which compose the larynx are naturally seen outward (à l'envers), that is to say, the part of the larynx which is nearest the observer, appears the most distant, and vice versa. It is not an image absolutely reversed, like that of the ophthalmoscope ; for that which is on the right remains on the right, on the left is that which is to the left ; but an inversion takes place from before backwards only, and in relation to the plain of the laryngeal mirror, as a symmetrical plain.

"It may be seen how simple the thing is in theory ; for there is not a word to add to this description in order to render it perfectly intelligible to the most elementary knowledge of physics. But this thing, so simple in theory, is truly marvelous in practice. One who has not seen cannot imagine the size of expansion which the open larynx assumes—the sort of eagerness with which it offers itself to the view. It exposes itself so completely and readily, that at first one doubts, so astonishing does it seem that *there* is truly seen *the larynx*, that organ which to this time has been so concealed, and which revealed itself by its sounds only ! But the doubt soon ceases ; the subject makes sounds, and the vocal cords are seen opening or shutting, exposing at once one of the chief elements of the mechanism of the voice. In the mirror may be perceived the rima glottidis formed by the inferior vocal cords, which, in accordance with the difference and intensity of the sounds, opens exactly like a pair

64

of scissors, the summit of whose V would be turned towards the observer. If the opening gapes widely, the tracheal tube may be perceived, and in very docile subjects, habituated to the use of the instrument, it would appear that the sight can even penetrate as far as the bifurcation of the trachea.

"There is no need of insistance to make comprehensible the extreme importance of such an acquisition ; to furnish the eye with the means of exploring the larynx, the interior of the glottis, all the points of the laryngeal opening, the epiglottis, with all of its neighboring parts—is not this rendering to art a most signal service ? There is no alteration whatever of tissue, though it be as small as a lentil, from simple redness to ulceration, which can escape examination. But, independently of diagnosis, therapeutics has, also, its share. Thus enlightened on the condition of the parts, any instrument whatever, directed by means of the mirror, can be made to convey a topical application upon the exact point desired. A false membrane, an ulceration, an œdema of the glottis, become directly accessible, and without fear of injuring a healthy part, instead of attacking the part diseased. We will not speak of physiology, which has everything to hope from the new researches that the employment of this precious instrument is about to permit.

"Already several points in regard to the mechanism of the voice and of respiration, have been directly and immediately established. It has been so far admitted in physiology, that the glottis enlarges itself during inspiration, and diminishes during expiration. Numerous observations which Prof. Czermak has made on himself, has enabled him to conclude that this belief has been badly founded. In calm respiration, without effort, the superior and inferior vocal cords are more or less widely distant, but perfectly immovable during inspiration and expiration. It is only in case of *blowing* that are seen, at *expiration*, the superior vocal cords approaching each other a little, and separating at the expiration as by a spasmodic motion ; just as the nostrils may be seen, in the same case, to dilate and then to contract with an oscillatory movement. Excepting this case, the larynx remains open and motionless during the entire act of respiration. There is a second state of the glottis which has never been able to be well studied, and of which the laryngoscope permits us to follow all its phases, which are more complex than would be believed *à priori*. It is the mechanism of *the effort*. The effort consists in

maintaining the pectoral cavity and its walls fully expanded, by im-
prisoning all the air which this cavity can contain. An essential
condition of this is the hermetrical closure of the glottis. Now, it
cannot be imagined, without seeing it, with what care this closure
is effected. In the first place, the inferior vocal cords may be seen
approaching each other, and placing themselves in immediate contact—first closure. Immediately above these the superior vocal
cords also join, and contract, the one against the other—second barrier. Thirdly, above this double closure, and perpendicularly to the
joints of this double gate, with its two folds, is applied an inferior
protuberance *(renflement)*, in which the epiglottis terminates below,
and of which the destination and employment had never so far been
suspected, if even any use whatever had been assigned to it. Now,
this protuberance performs the function of pressing upon the two
barriers which we have just seen close, one after the other, and rest
there, as the stone which seals up the lid of a well. The complex
exactitude of this triple precaution was assuredly far from being
divined."

I translate only the following extract on the investigations made
in reference to the singing tones made in running through the gammut: "In accordance with the observations of M. Czermak, the
only supposable changes made in forming the gammut, would be
modifications of the tension and density of the ligaments called the
inferior vocal cords, since the eye perceives no other motion than one
of vibration; their length and thickness appearing invariable, as
also their separation."

"But the application of this instrument to investigation is more
extensive still. If a smaller mirror be taken, and turned so as to
incline the contrary way (so as to reflect the parts above the velum
instead of the larynx below it); if at the same time the veil of the
palate be slightly elevated with a small blunt crotchet, or hook, then,
instead of the larynx, the posterior nares present themselves to view,
and on each side of them may be seen the entrance of the eustachian
tubes. By means of this simple instrument, then, may be explored,
like the open heaven, all the parts which surround the isthmus of the
throat. The study of any tumors whatsoever of this region, and in
particular naso-pharyngian polypi, ought evidently to be greatly
benefited by this method. We have witnessed the examination of a
pathological case, in which the anatomical condition could certainly

never have been affirmed without the aid of this instrument. The
case was one of aphonia, of some ten days' standing. M. Czermak
demonstrated to the eye, and caused several of those who stood by
to see, that the impossibility of rendering sounds audible arose, in
this case, from a considerable swelling of the superior vocal ligaments, which prevented vibrations in the inferior vocal cords. By
this they were reässured as to the posssibility of the existence of an
ulceration, and this diagnosis will certainly influence the treatment
which was proposed to be instituted by the chief of the service,
the Hon. M. Vigla, to whom the patient belonged.

"There are evidently cases where it will be difficult or impossible
to apply this new instrument. With infants and unruly persons
it will be evidently impossible. It is very difficult, or demands preparatory attempts sufficiently long, with many endowed with a very
sensitive uvula and velum. In regard to these latter, it was suggested, in the *reünion* assembled around the ingenious inventor, to
employ the bromide of potassium, which, as a special anæsthetic of
the pharyngeal region, has rendered service to Prof. Gosselin in
staphylorraphy. This assuredly is a very wise indication for new
experiments upon the properties of this substance. In fine, the way
is open ; but whatever destiny may be reserved for this ingenious
process of investigation, the first idea of which originated with Mr.
Liston ; whatever advantages science and art may obtain from it,
homage is due from this day to the simplicity of the means put in
use by M. Czermak, in the invention of an instrument easy in application and marvelous in its results. . . . To M. Czermak is
still due the happy idea of a small supplementary mirror, which,
placed in the course of the incident and emergent rays of light, inter-
cepts one-half only of these rays, and permits the observer to be the
subject of his own observations. This addition has enabled the
learned Professor of Pesth to make on himself a large number of
curious investigations, from which will certainly flow innumerable
advantages."

Dr. Czermak has presented his work, which is well illustrated by
plates, and contains ample details of the manner of using the
laryngoscope, to the Academy of Medicine, and he informed me that
its translation into French was in progress, so that its publication
would appear in a month. As soon as it can be obtained, I shall send
both it and the instrument to Dr. Jones, who will, no doubt, place
them both at your service and that of the Journal.

Besides the laryngoscope, I have seen, since in Paris, Velpeau, Bouchut, and Claude Bernard. Velpeau talks like a practical man ; Bouchut as fluently as your periods flow ; Bernard with an occasioual hesitation, which leaves the close of many of his sentences indistinctly heard. The latter has commenced his summer course, and takes up the nervous system. He has very kindly invited me to his laboratory, where I am at work assisting in the experiments illustrative of his lectures, and sincerely trust I may serve both him and myself.

I have often heard our students at the University complain of their hard seats, etc. I trust to see the day when spring-cushions and brocatelle will yield a welcome to the gluteal region of all those who may there labor for their degrees. But, in the meantime, if the amphitheaters of the Parisian hospitals could be seen by the disaffected, they would conclude they had much cause for rejoicing. They are not dirty, but filthy, wretchedly small, a board six inches wide for a seat, with your vertebral column to support your back, and if that proves tiresome, one may, by way of relief, stand up and lean against the wall. Such is a flattering description of Professor Velpeau's amphitheater, where were assembled some seventy-five students, the day I heard him, and which, under no circumstances, could contain over double that number.

This renowned surgeon was guilty of a joke, which led me to inquiry, and that to the information that he was one of the best punsters in France. As this talent has been so far overshadowed by his surgical skill as to remain unknown in America, I shall retail to you the joke, which, if you deem unprintable, you will please run your pen through. He operated for hydrocele, and while the fluid was flowing into the basin, turned to his audience, and observed, without a smile, " this is what they do every day on the *rue Vivienne*, empty a man's *bourse*." (Bourse means a bag, whether for a man's money or his testicles ; and on the *rue Vivienne* is situated the City Exchange.) It sounded to me very much like an *annual* joke, such as professional lecturers will habitually perpetrate ; but it would be too exacting to require men, whose minds are striving to fathom the depths of science, to concoct new jokes for every new class.

Brown-Séquard has, as you are doubtless aware, removed to London, so I have had no opportunity to present your letter. This pleasure I, however, promise myself in August, when I shall visit England.

Now, my dear Doctor, I must conclude this epistle, which I must send with its many faults, or not at all ; for I have not the leisure to rewrite it, as it should be, nor to condense it. I place it in your hands, and give you full power of attorney to correct the orthography, improve the style, embellish the good, and repress all or any part of it which, in the exercise of a wise and friendly discretion, you may judge calculated to promote the interest of our Journal, or of

Yours, very truly,   STANFORD E. CHAILLÉ.

ART. XI.—*Application of the Button Suture to the Treatment of Vari-cose Dilatation of Veins:* By NATHAN BOZEMAN, M. D., of New Orleans (late of Montgomery, Alabama).

VARIX, scarcely need I say, has engaged the attention of surgeons since the time of Hippocrates to the present day. There are, indeed, many living surgeons, whose names I could mention, commencing with those of Sir Benjamin Brodie and Velpeau, who have paid special attention to the subject, and who, as is well known, have presented it in all its bearings. Had I the time and inclination, it would be interesting to set forth the views of these eminent teachers, as to the causes and pathology of this disease, before entering upon the treatment ; but as this part of the subject is treated so fully in every systematic work upon surgery, I shall pass on to the latter, with the object of offering a few practical remarks in reference to the employment of silver ligatures.

In calling attention to this principle of treatment, which, so far as I know, has not been done heretofore, I appeal only to a few results, based upon my own experience.

Let us, then, first inquire, what are the objects of an operation in the *radical treatment* of varix ; and what the dangers attending such an operation ?

The treatment, according to the best authors upon the subject, is divided into *palliative* and *radical.* Every one knows in what consists the former. The latter, which has for its object the obliteration of the affected vein or veins, is generally, and very justly, too, viewed with great circumspection, because the operation, though simple in its execution, is liable to be followed by consequences sometimes highly disastrous to life. Phlegmons, erysipelas, purulent abscess, phlebitis, etc., are not uncommon results, and we are always taught to consider well the chances of their occurring, before deciding on any operative procedure.

Various have been the plans suggested of attacking the vein, as best suited to the end in question, and least liable to the dangers above stated ; namely, acupuncture, incision, transfixion, compression, section, resection, actual and potential cautery, simple ligature, twisted suture, etc. All these methods have had their advocates, and their advantages pointed out. While some have long since fallen into merited neglect, others have been maintained in practice, and are the established procedures of the day. Of the latter, I may mention the subcutaneous section of the vein, the simple ligature, the twisted suture, and the potential cautery.

Without stopping now to inquire into the claims of these several methods, which are familiar to all, I come at once to the object of our remarks ; namely, the adoption of the silver ligature or button suture method.

The idea of the above plan of treatment occurred to me several years ago, knowing, as I did, from experience, how little irritation followed the use of silver sutures. The ill-consequences of the operation usually had recourse to, I thought, might be obviated by this means to a very great extent, and the life of the patient thereby be less endangered. It was not, however, until the early part of last year that I adopted this principle of practice.

The three following cases I adduce in support of my views :

CASE 1.—I state this case from recollection, my notes having been mislaid. The subject was a negress, the mother of six or eight children, aged about fifty, and of rather delicate constitution. She stated that the enlarged condition of the veins of one of her legs had existed for several years, and now and then, especially after standing any considerable time, she suffered much pain from their distension, which would frequently force her to take her bed.

Upon examination, I found the saphena interna, and a few of its branches above the ankle, the seat of the difficulty. The dilatation of the vein extended as far up as the middle of the thigh. At a point just below the knee, the vein was very large and tortuous. There had never been any ulcer of the leg. The skin was very smooth, and showed no indications whatever of disease.

All the palliative means had been tried effectually, but with no permanent good. The radical treatment, therefore, was the only alternative left me. In deciding, now, upon a plan, I determined to employ the silver ligature at a few points, and see what the result would be. Accordingly, after due preparation of the system, the operation was performed.

For the operation, the patient was placed upon her back, and the ligatures of a suitable length then introduced with a curved needle. (I prefer a needle with a short curve, held in a porte aiguille.) I entered the point of the needle through the skin as far in front of the vein as I could, to allow of its being carried beneath the latter, and out at a corresponding point in the skin. It was my intention, at first, to completely encircle the vein, and in that way to have the two ends of the wire to pass through one opening in the skin; but this I found to be entirely unnecessary. The narrow bridge of skin intervening between the two perforations, as above introduced, is not at all in the way of effecting constriction of the vein.

The ligatures, five or six in number, having been introduced, I next tied the ends of each over a couple of pieces of bougie, in the same manner recommended by Mr. Erichsen in his use of the silk ligature. I was not pleased, however, with this arrangement. I found that I could not tie the wire sufficiently tight to insure occlusion of the vein, without the risk of breaking it. I arranged all of them in this way, however, and put the patient to bed. The after treatment consisted in quietude, elevation of the limb, light diet, etc.

The patient went on remarkably well—had little or no fever. The swelling and pain around the several points of the ligatures were very slight. On the ninth day, I removed the ligatures; found the most of them quite loose, and the bits of bougie, over which their ends had been tied, almost ready to fall out of place, thus showing that the vein was cut through. The skin on which the bits of bougie rested was ulcerated at several points, which I had occasion to regret. The patient was kept in bed several days longer, and then allowed to get up. The hardness, now, along the course of the vein, as far up as the ligatures had been used, proved pretty conclusively that consolidation had taken place. After being up for some time, the patient expressed herself greatly relieved, and desired to have the cure completed, which I promised to do, should she be troubled again.

Case 2.—Jane, a colored girl, aged about thirty-four, the mother of four children, large and stout, was sent to me the 21st of September last, for the purpose of treating her for an ulcer on her right leg. She stated that she first became pregnant in her sixteenth year, and that just before confinement the veins of her right leg became enormously enlarged. After labor, says she had "milk leg," from which she did not recover for several months. The veins in this leg remained large. Two years afterwards she became pregnant the second time, when the veins in this leg again increased very much in size, and caused great inconvenience. After the birth of her child they diminished somewhat in size, but still caused some annoyance, especially after standing a long time. Soon after this she received a slight scratch on the front part of her leg, three or four inches above the ankle. This resulted in the formation of an ulcer, which, after attaining a considerable size, gave rise to profuse bleeding. This ulcer went on increasing in size for five or six years. A physician, then, after a long time, succeeded in healing it up, but it remained so but a little while. She says that, as soon as she began to walk about again, the newly-formed skin gave way, resulting directly in an ulcer as large as ever. In this condition she remained until sent to me.

Upon examination, I found the ulcer situated as above stated, and half the size of my hand. The whole leg was very much swollen, and apparently all the superficial veins were dilated. The main trunks of the saphena interna and externa, were quite large and tortuous. The former, just below the knee, was so large and tortuous that its course could not be traced. Above this it was not so tortuous, but largely dilated nearly up to the saphenous opening. With this condition of things I thought of nothing short of the radical treatment. As a preparatory step to this, however, I determined to reduce the swelling of the leg, and to cure the ulcer, if possible. The patient was accordingly placed upon her back, and the limb bandaged up to her groin, twice a day. The ulcer was dressed with the following salve at the same time

R. Pulv. Rhei. Ɔi.   Pulv. Opii, gr. x.   Ung. Cetacei, ℥i.   M.

65

Under this treatment the swelling rapidly diminished, and in the course of three weeks the ulcer was completely cicatrized.

The patient I now considered in a good condition for an operation on the veins. I determined to limit my procedure only to the largest ones below the knee, reserving the saphena interna, above this point, for a subsequent operation. Five silver ligatures were accordingly introduced, as in the preceding case, they being principally applied to the saphena interna. This being done, I next proceeded to adjust them. Being dissatisfied with the bougie arrangement in the preceding case, owing to the ulceration of the skin occasioned by it, I determined to effect adjustment this time on our button suture principle, in order to ascertain the result. With this view, the two ends of each wire, commencing with the lowest, were now put together and passed through the hole of our *suture-adjuster*.* These being firmly held between the thumb and forefinger of the left hand, the instrument was slid down upon them until complete constriction of the vein was effected. All the others were arranged in like manner. This being done, a disk of lead, with a hole through its center, was put on the wires and slid down to its place. Upon this a shot was next slid down. This now being grasped by a pair of forceps, and held firmly against the plate of lead, the requisite amount of force for the constriction of the vein was then applied to the ligature, and thus secured by compressing the shot upon it. The ends of the wire were next cut off close to the shot, which completed the operation. The patient was then put to bed, the limb elevated, and quietude enjoined. The case progressed well; no fever occurred, and there was but little swelling or pain. Some of the sutures I removed on the eighth, and the remainder on the ninth day after the operation. The patient was kept quiet a few days longer, and then allowed to get up. There appeared now to be pretty general consolidation of the veins upon the front and inner side of the leg. The large bunch just below the knee was quite hard. The patient, after going about for several weeks, experienced so little inconvenience from the enlarged veins remaining, that I concluded not to perform another operation for the present. It has now been about seven months since the operation, and the greater part of the time this woman has been employed as cook, washer, and ironer, using no laced stocking or bandage.

---

* Gross' System of Surgery, vol. ii, fig. 568, p. 1047.

A few days ago I made an examination of the affected limb, and found it the same size of the other. The cicatrix appeared firm, not showing the least indication of breaking at any point. There are a few branches of the saphena externa, and the trunk of the saphena interna, above the knee, still dilated. It is my purpose to operate again upon the case, and complete the cure.

CASE 3.—Elias Smith, plasterer, aged nineteen, of medium stature, and rather sparely built, was sent to me in February last, by my friend Dr. J. C. Batchelor, of this city, to have his leg examined, with a view to an operation. He stated that, ever since he could recollect, there had been an enlarged condition of the vein on the inside of his right leg, and of late it seemed to be increasing in size. He said that it gave him no pain now, or inconvenience, but he feared it would, and ultimately might force him to give up his trade.

Upon examination, I found that it was the saphena interna which was involved, the dilatation extending from the ankle nearly to its passage through the fascia lata. At a point just below the knee the dilatation was greatest, and here the vein was also very tortuous. Having considered the case in all its bearings, I took the view that the man was a laborer, his occupation requiring him to be almost constantly upon his feet, thereby increasing the difficulty, and that, if the disease could be radically cured, now was the time to attempt it. Everything favored a satisfactory result. Accordingly, after such preparation of the system as was necessary, I proceeded to perform the operation, in the presence of Dr. Batchelor, Dr. Frazier, of Arkansas ; Dr. Gilmore, of Mississippi, and several medical students.

The two preceding cases, it will be recollected, were operated upon in the recumbent position. This patient I placed in the erect—and I now greatly prefer this position, for the reason the vein is distended, and the needle can be entered and carried around it with more facility. I introduced five ligatures, two below, one opposite, and two above the knee. This was easily and quickly done. The patient was now made to lie down, in order that the vein might be emptied of as much blood as possible before adjusting the ligatures. The lowest one was arranged first, and the others, then, in regular succession. The disk of lead and shot were next slid down and secured, as in the preceding case.

After-treatment the same as heretofore pointed out. The patient had no fever. On the seventh day I removed two of the sutures, and on the ninth the remainder. On the fourteenth day after the operation the patient went to work, experiencing no inconvenience from it whatever.

I examined this case a few days ago, it being nearly three months after the operation, and I was astonished to find that the obliterated vein had so nearly disappeared. It could be seen only at one point, just below the knee, and here it felt perfectly hard, and was quite movable beneath the skin. The consolidation had extended entirely up to the saphenous opening. The result could not have been more satisfactory.

Varicocele.—Being so well pleased with my first application of the silver ligature to enlarged veins of the leg, I felt very anxious to make a trial of it in varicocele, believing that it would have advantages over the ordinary methods pursued.

It was not long before an opportunity offered. A gentleman of Donaldsonville, in this State, aged about thirty, consulted me in reference to the disease in question, which he said he had had since he was fourteen years old. An examination proved his statement, as to the existence of the disease, to be correct. It was, as is almost always the case, on the left side. Associated with it was an enormous elongation of the scrotum. It hung down, especially on the left side, nearly to the middle of the thigh. An operation, therefore, not only for the varicocele, but for retrenchment of the scrotum, was called for, which I performed in the order mentioned. That for the varicocele was performed upon the button suture principle, the ligature being introduced in the same manner recommended by Prof. Gross, in the use of the silk *cord*.* In this way the veins were completely encircled, and both ends of the wire left hanging out at the same opening in the skin. The ligature was next adjusted, and the button and shot secured as in the second and third cases of varices. The patient was now put to bed, and the scrotum raised up and supported with a suspensory bandage. Cold water dressings ordered. There was the usual amount of swelling below the seat of constriction, and on the fifth or sixth day considerable pain. On the seventh day the suture apparatus was removed, when consolidation of the veins appeared to be complete. After a few days the patient was allowed to get up. The next thing was to retrench the scrotum,

---

* Op. cit., vol. II, p. 956.

which, after the patient began to walk about, was as long' as ever. This operation was performed in the usual way, only a couple of small arteries requiring to be tied. The edges of the wound were brought together by a number of interrupted silver sutures. The patient was then put to bed, and the parts supported by means of a suspensory bandage. Cold water dressings directed.

A day or two afterwards, hæmorrhage took place from a small artery, and before it could be controlled the patient lost a considerable amount of blood. Excepting this, he got along remarkably well. On the seventh day I removed the sutures, when union of the parts appeared complete, excepting at one point, where the edges of the wound had not been closely approximated. This filled up in a few days, however, by the granulating process, and the patient was then discharged cured.

I examined this case a few weeks ago, it being about eight months after the operation, and the condition of the parts could not have been more favorable. The veins all appeared to be completely occluded, and reduced to mere threads. Our patient expressed himself entirely relieved of his former troubles.

Remarks.—Although the cure was not completed in the first two cases of varix, still the result of our operation proved itself, I think, sufficiently successful to establish the superior advantages of silver ligatures over the ordinary methods recommended.

The result of our third case could not have been more satisfactory. It is needless to comment on the result of the operation in the case of varicocele. Suffice it to say, it could not have been more satisfactory The advantages of the button suture principle, in the treatment of the diseases of which we are speaking, may be thus briefly stated :

1st. The inocuousness of the silver wire.

2d. The protection afforded by the button against undue pressure upon the skin in front of the vein.

3d. The facility of adjusting the apparatus, and the great power given the surgeon over the vein, without risk of the wire breaking, as by tying.

4th. The certainty with which the vein or veins can be cut in two, and their occlusion effected, with evidently less risk of the dangers in the usual modes of operation.

ART. XII.—*Medical Correspondence.* Two Letters from S. L. BIGE-
LOW, D. M. P., of Paris.

PARIS, February 14, 1860.

To WARREN STONE, M. D.—*My Dear Doctor*—M. AMÉDÉE LATOUR,
Rédacteur en chef de l'Union Médicale, sent me to-day the January
number of the *New Orleans Medical and Surgical Journal,* containing
the letter I wrote to you in October, giving very briefly my own
views with regard to membranous sore throat. It must be that my
chirography is detestable, and it proves to me a double evil; first,
it gives wrong impressions of my medical sentiments, and of
knowledge of my native language. Your "setter-up" not only
makes me say "intemperatively" instead of "intempestively," and
several other things of the same caliber, but he makes me give ten
grains of chlorate of potash alternately with ten grains of the bichlorate, instead of permitting me to alternate with the bi-carbonate
of soda. Humanity may not suffer by it, but my personal feelings
ought to be regarded, and I am tempted to inflict a due reward of
merit upon him, by giving him another in reclamation, for the last.
As for the homicide of the English language he places at my door
(you know the law-distinction between homicide and murder in the
first degree), I forgive him, for you will not believe that I have forgotten my own tongue to an extent which would permit me to tell
you that certain remarks in my letter would "*pale*" instead of
"*pall*" upon your ear. As for the literary style those *little* vagaries
and other invest me with, I mind it but little, for I am the first to
admit that nature, in the first place, did not endow me with the gift,
nor art, in the second place, inspire or instruct me to compete with
Bennet Dowler, yourself, or Amédée Latour in pen and ink sketches.
Doctors can't, one in ten, tell half they know—nor one in a thousand,
and tell it well; if they could, how much science would gain!—perhaps at somebody's expense, but probably for the public weal—so
the public lent a willing ear. One word more to fill an omission,
and a very important one in my eyes, which I observe in my views
upon the treatment of diphtheritic sore throat, as given in my letter to you, and which has since been expressed by a man well skilled
in medicine, Dr. Bouchardat, and I have done with the subject. It
relates to amputation of the tonsils in the disease, when enlarged and
covered, or touched, even, by the diphtheritic deposit. He advises
their immediate removal—so do I, and I go even further, and advise

their immediate amputation, under *whatever* form of inflammation one finds them enlarged—for it is an immediate, simple, and *radical* cure in simple hypertrophy, and of the greatest benefit in the disease in question. I go further still—remove them if they are enlarged, whether they are inflamed or not. I observe that the physicians in America are, for some reason or other, which I cannot make out, opposed, in the majority, to removing enlarged tonsils, and especially when inflamed. If I could, by my weak pen, do away with this repugnance, which costs so dear to so many, especially children, in our community, I would write you a monograph for publication upon the subject, which would fill an entire number of your Journal; but this is not the time or the occasion. But I will say, do let a child, when he is at an age to require fully all the elements, oxygen not excepted, requisite to his growth, strength, and general development, get his full amount of air demanded by the involuntary respiratory muscles, without forcing him to distort his thorax in getting *too little* air for his purposes, by calling into extraordinary action the accessory *voluntary* respiratory muscles, when it can be done so innocently, easily, and radically. To go fully into the subject would, as I said before, occupy too much of your time, and these few words will suffice to give you my profession of faith. The idea of "outgrowing" them, or curing them by general treatment or nitrate of silver, is just exactly absurd. While "outgrowing" them, the child or adult is even more busy in deteriorating permanently his general health, strength, and consequent manliness, usefulness, and comfort in life; and he, only at that, "outgrows" them by repeated ulcerated sore throats, which finally result in their demolition, and each one of which is a thousand times the guillotine. As for nitrate of silver, or any other but *potential* or *actual* caustics, which no one would think of applying, you might as well apply it to the sole of your boot. Alteratives and antiscorbutics the same—just as well pour them into your boot, as far as the tonsils go; though, as general treatment, conjoined with the guillotine, they are of great value. No—remove the tonsils at the tenderest age, just as quickly as you would take a peach-stone out of the throat; they constitute quite as much a foreign body, and would do infinitely more mischief, if allowed to remain, for they are there as fixtures.

The spiritual article in your Journal of January, upon the speculum and diseases of the womb, has given an itch to my fingers which will only be cured by inflicting another dose of my chirography upon your " setter-up." It is excellent, but sectarian, and I desire to give you, at a later day, a few remarks upon the subject. This word sectarian recalls to mind another portion of my letter to you, in which I am made to say that " I don't believe a religious sectarian can be a religious man." I did not mean that at all, and if the idea passes, I shall pass in the community for one of the medical atheists, or something worse, which we hear and read so much of, but which, upon my word, I have never seen. I believe that no class in the world, ministers of the gospel, perhaps, in some cases, excepted, is so truly religious, after its fashion, as the medical profession. The sea-serpent may exist, for aught I know, and I have no objection to pass for a believer in it, but I do protest against a belief that atheism and medicine have anything in common between them—quite the reverse. What I meant to say was, then, that I believe the soundest doctors, as well as the soundest christians, are those whose opinions are the most thoroughly winnowed from sectarian dogmas. Religion is born in the human heart, and only asks to live and grow; just as well give lessons in love as in religion—they both know how to take care of themselves, and prosper, better than we know how to guide and train them. Conscience is the tell-tale of the one, and sentiment of the other, and we have only to listen to them. If we can do better than God, we shall do well to interfere—if we think. we can't, better follow, instead of lead.

The truth is, dear Doctor, that I sat down to-night to tell .you about a case of hypertrophy of the liver, and so far have spent my time on literature, love, and religion.

One word will tell you the case, and it is among the dozen remarkable ones a physician encounters in his life. Mr. ——, of New York, fifty years old, an active business man and good liver, without excess, had been suffering ten or fifteen years with constipation, indigestion, and occasional jaundice. Five years ago he began to lose flesh, was always yellow, with pains in the region of his liver, etc. Fell from 180 pounds weight to 130 ; and last September, by advice of his homœopathic physician, who had never felt of his abdomen but once, he came to Liverpool, for the sea-voyage, intending to return immediately ; grew more feeble on the voyage, and was only able (by a journey of *three days*) to get to Manchester, where he had intimate friends. He did not leave the house for a month, and finally, being unable to get home, and expecting soon to die, he sent for his family—not thinking to live, as he says, until they arrived. They concluded to come to Paris, and made the twelve hours' journey in seven days, bringing him on a bed. When I saw him for the first time, which was the day after his arrival, he looked like a moribund. I had already received a letter from his Manchester physician, informing me of his entirely hopeless condition from organic disease of the liver. I examined his abdomen at once, and found the left lobe of the liver extending three inches to the left of the median line, the right lobe in the right hypochondrium, and the middle lobe proportionately enlarged—an enormous mass filling the right portion of the abdomen, which contained, also, as near as I could judge, three or four quarts of liquid. His face was cadaveric and jaundiced ; pulse 120 ; unable to walk ten rods, and then not without leaning on his servant's arm ; night sweats, etc. In fact, his condition was such as to give me no idea of affording him even temporary relief. I declined to advise for him before consulting with another doctor, and in the afternoon of the same day met Prof. Trousseau in consultation. When we retired alone, after examining the patient, his first movement was a shrug of the shoulders, and his first words, " *voyez vous, mon cher, c'est un homme perdu.*" We advised as follows : a tepid alcaline bath, of an hour's duration, every night before going to bed ; a large flax-seed poultice covered quarter of an inch thick with a paste of powdered conium leaves, to cover the entire abdomen, every night ; a glass of Vichy water daily, an hour before his repasts ; a laxative pill, p. r. n., to keep his bowels freely opened, daily ; a full, substantial, plain, varied diet, with fruit, vegetables, and Bordeaux wine, and many hours' daily carriage exercise, with as much foot exercise as he could take—to go out, rain or shine.

His treatment commenced the 13th of December, 1859. His first walking exploit was to go from the Hotel Bristol, where he resided, to the Bureau of Galignani's Messenger, not more than ten rods, aided by a servant, and feeling, when he got there, that he could not get back. His treatment has not been changed from that day to this, in any particular. He has never ceased to progress in appetite, good digestion, good sleep, strength, color, and weight, and ten days ago he had gained thirty pounds in flesh. His liver had lost five inches in depth and two in breadth ; his night sweats

66

had long since left him, and his daily walk was from his hotel to the
Barrière de l'Étoile, thence to the Place de la Bastille, and back to
the hotel, by the Boulevards, a distance of nine or ten miles, at least,
in addition to several hours' drive daily, with his family. His liver
now extends only two fingers' breadth below the false ribs, and his
abdomen does not contain an ounce of fluid. He is, in fact, cured,
although I advise him to remain in Paris till June, then to go to
Carlsbad, Vichy, or Hambourg, for a month, to consolidate his cure.
If the success of the treatment in this case proves of service to you
or my professional brothers at home, in similar cases, my object in
giving you a brief outline of this case will be attained. I would
add, that, since three or four weeks, his bowels have become perfectly regular, without the use of the laxative pills, and that he is
ashamed, as well as his family, of the amount he eats daily. But they
dine at the Three Frères, and pay for each dish in restaurant fashion,
so it is no one's business but his own. Urine and fæcal matter perfectly natural.

Since treating the above case, one has fallen under my observation, though not in my own practice, of a similar nature. It is the
case of a French lady, forty-nine years old, Mme. Alexandre, wife of
the inventor and manufacturer of the " piano-organs," which are
now so much in vogue. I was first called in consultation with the
family physician, a French doctor, seven weeks ago, and found the
history of the case to be as follows (I speak of this case at this
time as having a direct bearing upon the preceding, so far as the
treatment is concerned, and the probable results): Mme. A.'s digestion had been for many years impaired. She had borne for many
years the whole weight of the immense establishment upon her
shoulders, had eaten irregularly, hurriedly, and what she could get,
sometimes taking a soup or cup of coffee in the morning, and nothing
again until late at night. For many years, then, as in Mr. ——'s
case, she had suffered from the symptoms of dyspepsia ; cramps in
the stomach, relieved by food ; burning sensation at the epigastrium
and in the course of the œsophagus ; regurgitation of food, and
liquid regurgitations, etc. Eight months ago, in June last, she had
an exacerbation of her pains and symptoms, accompanied by intense
pain in the region of the liver, hepatic colics, as near as I could determine, lasting six or eight hours at a time, and then ceasing *suddenly.* The urine and fæcal matter were not at this time examined.

These symptoms were accompanied by a jaundiced condition of the skin and sclerotic. Andral was called, at this time, in consultation, who, finding a yellowish tint of skin, pains in the epigastrium, vomiting, etc., gave the benefit of a doubt regarding cancer of the stomach. Ricord was then called, who gave his opinion that there was no grave lesion, and advised her to go to her country seat for the summer, or to Vichy. Andral was again called, who was, this time, of the opinion of Ricord, that there was no organic lesion, but advised against Vichy. Ricord was again called, who retracted his former opinion, and considered it probable that there was organic disease of the liver, which was hypertrophied. She went to her country seat, passed the summer, and improved considerably. Her complexion became less jaundiced, digestion better, less pain, increase of flesh, etc. Returned to Paris in October, when she had another attack similar to the one in June. Gendrin was called in consultation, who diagnosticated "dyspepsia, gall stones, engorgement of the liver." She continued better and worse in symptoms, until January, when, upon the occasion of another attack, I was called in consultation to the case, and found it certainly difficult and delicate of diagnostic. She was one of those nervous and exaggerating patients, who inform you they pass a gallon of urine a day, when it is but a pint—that it is the color of blood, instead of high colored—that their pain is everywhere else, and where it is, too—that she eats *nothing*, when the sum-total through the day, upon strict investigation, proves a very respectable allowance—that "nothing passes the stomach," where, in fact, it all goes, etc., etc. After a careful examination, I formed an opinion, which coincided exactly, as I found afterwards, with that of Gendrin ; but not satisfied with my opinion as a last word, desired, of my own accord, to return in consultation in a week—in the meantime, the urine to be observed, and all the fæcal matter to be passed through a sieve. My second visit confirmed me in my first opinion, and I advised the same course of treatment as in the former case (the liver was four fingers' breadth below the ribs), with the addition of one grain daily, in three doses, of the extract of belladonna, to modify, if possible, the pains in the region of the liver, which she compared to labor pains ; also, because I have been pleased with its effects upon the action of the liver and bowels. The following week Professor Trousseau was called, at my request, as the case was really delicate, and we both met the family physician, and went over the ground fully again. The gall stones had been passed, in the meantime; the urine was still high colored ; fæces *good* color, and skin yellow. He arrived at the same opinion as Gendrin and myself, but was like my-self at my first visit, so dissatisfied with the solidity of his opinion that he, in turn, asked to come again in consultation in a week—which fact is enough to convince you that the difficulties of absolute diagnosis were great, as consulting physicians of Prof. Trousseau's standing and merit do not invite themselves to consultations. He advised to continue the treatment. We all met again the following week, his opinion was confirmed, and the treatment continued. Daily alcaline bath of an hour ; Vichy water ; extract of belladonna; daily drives to the Bois ; generous, plain, and varied diet, etc. From the first she has continued to improve, and has passed three weeks without hepatic pains, or tenderness on pressure; though the cramps in the epigastrium, *always relieved* by food, have returned at intervals. No gall stones found yet, and perhaps there are none (that is left an open question, as we can find no positive evidence by palpation); the liver diminishes constantly in size ; the skin has rapidly lost its yellow color ; urine and fæces good. This case, although more com-plicated in symptoms to confound, is still, at the bottom, the same as the former, and appears to be going on to the same results. We saw the patient together on Friday last (five days ago), the last time ; and everything was going on for the best.

These cases may not offer much interest to you. They are cer-tainly of no interest, except in a purely practical point of view; but you may find benefit in like cases, even in the extreme simplicity of the treatment adopted, with such marked results. It is not new—there is nothing new, except hypnotism, under the sun, and by dint of striving to take the merit of a poor discovery, each from the other, they have found that even hypnotism dates back some hun-dreds of years. I have given this very brief outline of these cases, their *apparently* simple treatment, and the marked results, more with a view to divorce the ideas of liver and mercury, united under no divine protection, than to parade them as cases. Mercury is a very good thing in its place, no doubt, and so is the liver, but I think the one is abused and the other "picked upon." Mercury and Venus are certainly better matched, as a couple, than blue pill and bile. Five, ten, or twenty grains of calomel are very sensible in their proceedings with a man in delirium tremens, or bordering upon it, when nothing else can be kept on the stomach, but one-tenth of a grain is much the best dose, often repeated, in ordinary cases, where its use is indicated. No one in this nineteenth century, *who has passed through a faculty of medicine*, and received his " *Vir ingenio ac scientia*," etc., etc., will be disposed to call into doubt, from these remarks, my high opinion of mercurial preparations, in time and place, but I believe that they may be used with much more good effect and discrimination than they have been in times past. Not a day of my life passes that I do not make use of calomel or some other preparation of mercury, but I do not consider it to be my duty to give a dose of calomel or blue pill because a patient tells me he needs it. As a cathartic, in delirium tremens, or as a vermifuge, than which none is better, I do not care to weigh my dose, but divided doses are infinitely best in cases where its exhibition is the most frequently desired. I don't know whether the doctors have given the idea to the world, or if the world has beaten it into the doctors, that blue pill and calomel are the natural enemies of the bile, but of one thing I am convinced, that they have been pitted like game cocks too long. If nobody else understands me, I am sure that you will, so I take my full of comfort in closing this wearisome epistle, which certainly merits the name of " Causerie " or " Feuilleton," rather than of "original article" or "communicated." You will please make what use of it you see fit, always remembering that its intention is strictly personal to yourself.

I am, truly, yours, S. L. BIGELOW.

PARIS, April 2, 1860.

My Dear Doctor—Since I wrote the above letter I have been too much occupied to think of it, and it has laid in my portfolio unnoticed. I am not sorry, as I can to-day make an addition to it of an important character. Mr. —— now weighs *one hundred and seventy-six pounds*, and is in *perfect health*—as he said to me day before yesterday, when I met him accidentally in the street, "I have no complaint to make ; there is nothing the matter with me." Trousseau says of the case what is perfectly and literally true : "Tell it to any one, doctor or plebeian, and they will tell you it is a medical exaggeration, but I say that a man may honorably win gray hairs, as I have done, and not see in his life two cases as remarkable as this." Now, dear Doctor, this is high language from a high source. Instead of going to Carlsbad or Vichy, as was proposed at the date of my letter, Mr. —— leaves for home the 28th of this month. We consider it unnecessary that he continues his treatment longer.

As for Mme. Alexandre, whose case I alluded to briefly, there have been *ups* and *downs*. Rayer has been called since I wrote, who agrees fully in the opinion expressed by Trousseau and myself. She has since passed gall stones. Her case is more grave than that of Mr. ——. I will keep you posted, as I see her in consultation every week.

I gave five grains of calomel to a little child of our minister of the gospel, a few days since, who had passed a lumbricoides. He had been in the habit of taking calomel in divided doses ever since he was born. He had an attack of muguet afterwards (three or four days), which the family and myself attributed to the calomel. A few days after, a little daughter, with a spina bifida, after taking two grains of calomel, was attacked with the same trouble, and she had been taking calomel all her life. What influence shall I attribute to the calomel in these two cases ?

Yours, truly,   BIGELOW, D. M. P.

⌣

ART. XIII.—*A Case of Snake-Bite.*

DR. DOWLER—In the last two or three numbers of your Journal I observe some communications on the antidotes to the poison of serpents.

Being desirous of casting in my mite, and adding my humble testimony to that of those who have preceded me, I transmit for publication the following case which occurred in my practice :

A man, aged about forty-five years, was bitten by a snake, while plowing in the field. About an hour and a half after the accident I saw him. He was lying in bed, holding his foot up in the air, complaining of most intense pain, and occasionally vomiting. The bite had been inflicted between the inner malleolus and the heel. The foot and leg had swollen considerably. I endeavored to apply a cup to the wound, but owing to the swelling and the unfavorable position, I succeeded very indifferently.

A short time after I arrived he was seized with one of the most severe chills with which I have ever seen a man suffer. His pulse sunk to a mere flutter, and the surface became cold and livid. In a word, he presented all the appearances of a man dying from congestive chill. I gave him a dose of aqua ammonia, and commenced the liberal administration of whisky, which, fortunately, was at hand. In the course of two or three hours he had taken about a pint or a pint and a half of whisky, and two or three doses of the ammonia. By this time he was thoroughly intoxicated. With the drunkenness, every symptom of the bite ceased. I saw him again the next morning, and but for the effects of the whisky, he could have resumed his work. Being fond of the liquor, he kept intoxicated for several days ; but the bite presented not another bad symptom.

One thing in this case is worthy of remark. Writers on materia medica say that aqua ammonia counteracts the effects of alcoholic liquors. Dr. Peake, in his communications to your Journal, says that a man cannot be intoxicated while his system is laboring under the influence of the poison of a serpent. Contrary to all this, I saw as fine a specimen of intoxication in this man as ever was presented to the world.

In reference to the *modus operandi* of this agent, I do not pretend to know a great deal. I offer it, however, as my *opinion*, that its efficacy lies entirely in its stimulating property. But, according to Dr. P., tobacco is as good an antidote as alcohol. How, then, can these things be reconciled ? I would ask, may it not be a fact, that, in many instances of snake-bite, a good constitution is capable of ridding itself of the poison without any foreign aid ? If so, this will explain why there are so many antidotes among the common people, from whom Dr. P. received the most of his information in reference to tobacco. Again, we are all aware of the fact that some habitual *chewers* of tobacco can *swallow* the plant without any deleterious effects resulting. May not these considerations throw some light on the case of Dr. P.'s chain-bearer ? The tobacco was administered, the patient recovered ; therefore, the tobacco cured him. *Post hoc ; ergo propter hoc.*   J. J. LYONS, M. D.

PLAQUEMINE BRULÉE, St. Landry, La., May 22, 1860.

ART. XIV.—*Observations on the Hygienic Influences of Buildings and Hospitals:* By BENNET DOWLER, M. D.

THE style of building in New Orleans has, for the most part, little reference, either to salubrity, or to the peculiar topographical requirements of the alluvial formation on which the city stands.

Many houses are constructed in a manner that must be condemned in any climate, but in none more so than in this city, depressed, as it is, below the high water mark of the river almost everywhere, being in the rear nearly on the sea level. The lower floors rot about three or four times in ten years. A great majority of the floors, especially in the stores, rest on the humid soil, sometimes at a lower level than the streets, no air being admitted underneath.

Fluviatile, alternating with lacustrine deposits (containing organic remains, as shells, wood, etc., approximating the newer pliocene), extend to unknown depths, as seen in the lately abandoned artesian well which had penetrated nearly 700 feet. The superficial deposit is chiefly fluviatile, which, when moistened or flooded by rains, and saturated on all sides by the filtration water of the river, gutters, and swamps, generates perennial crops of *algæ, fungi, infusoria,* blight, mildew, mould, etc., which abound in, under, and around the lower story of low, unventilated houses, where, indeed, crops of mushrooms would flourish, were they not repressed by the tread of the tenant. Hence, some goods rust, others become spotted, their delicate colors being discharged. Health, too, is deteriorated from moist and insalubrious exhalations during the day, and at night, as many persons sleep upon these decaying, humid floors.

Physicians, in visiting the poor, especially in depressed portions of the city, must have found the flooring of houses sometimes, after rains, wet, or covered with water too filthy and offensive for description—laboratories for generating carbonic and other deadly gases, predisposing to disease, and rendering recovery from any kind of sickness tedious—too often impossible. What drug can supply the place of pure air, pure water, dry sleeping and business rooms ?

The lower floors (on which the principal business of the city is done, and on which is stored much valuable merchandise) resist decay but a few months, whereas the most perishable kinds of wood, and even cotton and linen fabrics, with their original colors, will, if kept dry, last for thousands of years, as witnessed in the tombs of Egypt, where the cerements of the dead are comparatively sound,

while their coffins (made of sycamore, a wood that speedily ro
where moisture is present) are as sound as they were thousands
years ago, although they had been placed in excavations, often litt
elevated above the inundations of the Nile.

It would appear from a cursory glance at many new busines:
houses now going up in New Orleans, that instead of having one oɪ
two feet of free air circulating under the lower floors, the latter have
been sunk to the lowest level of the oldest houses.

In some cities, even deep cellars are dry. The depressed, inclined
plane on which New Orleans stands, below the high water line
the river before, the swamps behind, subject to sudden inundatio
from enormous rains, all combine to prove that floors ought not t
be placed directly on the mud, though in other cities this mode o
building may be less injurious. In New Orleans it ought to be interdicted by law. It is to be regretted that the two conditions most
desiderated are the most neglected—the two conditions most necessary to the preservation of health and merchandise, namely: elevation and dryness—drainage and the free circulation of air in and
under houses.

Enough is already known of the science of hygiene to warran
the conclusion that overcrowding filth, a want of ventilation, incomplete drainage, and humidity, must be injurious to the health and
detrimental to the physical comforts of the citizens. Healthy individuals, and still more the sick, need pure air and a thorough ventilation in their dwellings, the sites of which should always admit of
drainage.

Two thousand years ago, Dr. Hippocrates, in his book on "*Airs,
Waters, and Localities,*" described certain places and conditions as
highly insalubrious : "The waters of marshes are not clear, but
stagnant, muddy, thick, smelling badly in summer ; as they have no
current, and are maintained by rain alone, they must be of a bad
color [green ?], heavy and bilious," etc. "Rain water readily cor-
rupts and acquires a bad smell, owing to its being constituted of
emanations from all sorts of bodies, whence a great disposition
to putrefaction results." Of the residents in such places, he
says : "Their complexion is bad, and they have little vigor ;
they are liable to every disease I have mentioned, without exception ; their voice is hoarse, owing to the air infected with the
miasmata." Of bad waters, he says : "They enlarge and indurate

67

ιe spleen ; they heat and constipate ; they cause a shrinking of ιe shoulders, the neck, and face ; the flesh seems to disappear, in rder to augment the spleen ; hence they become thin, though great :aters, etc.; they are subject to dropsies, dysenteries, diarrhœas, and ɔbstinate quartans are common in summer, etc.

Modern, especially living writers, have not only ιeäffirmed these general views, but have enlarged and illustrated them so much that hygiene occupies the front rank in the medical sciences. To preserve ' ∩alth, to prevent or ameliorate disease, by means of what the an- ꞓnt physicians called, one might say miscalled, the *non-naturals* (as r, diet, exercise, sleep, passion, mental management, etc.), now :omprehended under the terms hygienic and sanitary means and ɔrinciples ; in other words, all the physical, physiological, psychical, and moral agents and influences conducive to health and longevity, without direct recourse to medicinal drug, pill, potion, or apothe- cary. Benevolence never assumed a more disinterested attitude than it now does in the medical profession, seeing that the medical mind is bent on every measure calculated to render the writing of prescrip- tions and the practice of physic unnecessary, or, at least, of but lim- ited application, by which professional emoluments must be restricted in a corresponding ratio. And when preventives fail, and sickness overtakes one, "nature in disease," the *vis medicatrix*, repels and displaces the doctor, and cures the patient, according to the new faith.

As the prevention of disease, together with the abnegation of self interest incidental to the same, constitutes the highest claim to the gratitude of mankind, it is of great importance that the practice of hygiene should be in accordance with the theory. Hence, without wishing to indulge in censure, it is the duty of the sanitarian to notice both the sins of omission and commission in matters relating to health : "*Salus populi suprema est lex.*" In view of these premises, it may be proper to inquire whether these fundamental principles of hygienic science have not been greatly neglected in New Orleans. The law, as well as the logic, requires that the best evidence which the case admits of shall be produced. Expediency, if nothing else, indicates that animadversion upon a public measure is almost always impersonal, because what is everybody's business is nobody's business, just as the law says, that a bastard is no man's son, but every man's son. ("*Bastardus nullius est filius, aut filius populi.*")

In seeking, therefore, for an example, whether it be of a synthetical or analytical kind, the most recent, public, and appropriate one will be alluded to as reflecting the existing state of sanitary science in New Orleans, namely : the United States Marine Hospital, now nearly completed, at an expense, as I learn, of nearly one million of dollars—a great palace, altogether of iron—one of the most remarkable edifices in this city—unrivaled, perhaps, upon the continent of America. With the lights of science to guide the General Government, it might reasonably be supposed that this hospital would serve as a model, comprehending all of the elements and improvements of the advanced science of hygiene.

The old United States Marine Hospital, the building of which was expensive, commenced more than a quarter of a century ago. It was, however, thought or discovered, when too late, that this edifice was on the wrong side of the river ! It was, therefore, abandoned, but upon what principle of sanitary science this took place is not known. It is more than a mile nigher the heart of the city than its successor. But its splendid turrets still rise above the city and the river to reflect the first and last beams of the sun. Picturesque sentinel of the "Father of Waters," nothing more !

The new Marine Hospital, now nearly, or, perhaps, quite complete, will very well reflect, as already mentioned, the practical appreciation of the sanitary principles too often adopted in this city. This grand *sanitarium* for sick seamen and river boatmen, is situated more than two miles from the river, and nearly that distance in the rear of the inhabited portion of the city of New Orleans, being nearly on the sea-level, the declivity to the latter being, probably, not over three inches, and, in view of the colossal grasses, weeds, and other obstructions, virtually nothing at all. The hospital rises in solitude in the center of a vast desolate swamp region, which is subject to submergence by every heavy rain, and is exposed to the continuous saturation by the filtration water from the river. This hospital, thus situated in the midst of a basin which is a reservoir for the filth of the city, the haunt of aligators, frogs, and mosquitoes, presents a picture not altogether unworthy of Milton's description : "Lakes, fens, bogs, dens" [alligators'], "and shades of death ; a universe of death ; where all life dies, death lives, and nature breeds perverse, all monstrous, all prodigious things, abominable, unutterable, worse than gorgons, and hydras, and chimeras dire."

If filth washed from a great city be injurious; if malarial exhalations from a loathsome, fermenting morass, everywhere treeless, and exposed to the intensity of the solar rays, be deleterious to health, then it must be admitted by the impartial observer, that all these alleged elements of disease are concentrated, to an unparalleled degree upon this hospital site, excepting density of surrounding population. No honest patient, not under sentence for manslaughter or other felony, ought to be condemned to enter it, to breathe malaria, to fight mosquitoes as well as disease. Ought not the Grand Jury to visit this sanitarium at once, seeing that, owing to the unparalleled low water of the river at this season, and drouth also, the institution is now very accessible, by means of a kind of planked-road bridge. A century may, perhaps, roll away before New Orleans and its environs shall again be so waterless as at the present. If it be conceded that filth, marshy soil, and mosquitoes are not insalubrious, still the ineligibility (one might almost say inaccessibility) of its location is a fundamental objection to its occupation by the sick or well, especially as the old Marine Hospital is still standing, which, compared with the location of the new, is paradisical, being only a few paces from the river bank, always the most salubrious portion of the valley of the lower Mississippi, and consequently the best, though most expensive site for hospitals.

The construction of palatial hospitals and asylums of brick, stone, marble, or iron, three or four stories high, at an enormous expense, is, without doubt, a line of policy not only inexpedient, but positively injurious to the well-being of the sick, and adverse to the utilitarian maxim of science and charity, namely : to do the greatest good to the greatest number of the destitute and afflicted. The same sum that is required for a palace of this kind, would build cheap, comfortable, isolated, well ventilated houses, which would, for the same money, accommodate more than double the number of persons without crowding and without the risk of spreading contagious diseases, and with a greatly diminished proportion of mortality, and with a shorter detention in the convalescent period. If the crowding of healthy persons in ships and houses be deleterious, how much more so must this be to delicate children, the infirm, and the sick. Two hundred thousand dollars spent in the erection of a splendid architectural pile, would build two hundred salubrious cottages—a complete village—adapted to the comforts and hygienic wants of their inmates.

Very recently, statistical researches into the site, construction, and influences of hospitals, have led to conclusions adverse to the general economy of these institutions, as hitherto conducted. From the reliable data already accumulated, it is reasonable to suppose that a revolution will take place in the arrangement and administration of these receptacles of the afflicted, so as to diminish the ratio of mortality, facilitate convalescence, and prevent, to a great degree, hospitals from actually causing diseases, which they now do.

Without the remotest wish to detract from the unrivalled excellence and general usefulness of the hospitals of New Orleans, I may be permitted to say, that if the accepted principles of hygienists be well founded, the sites of some hospitals in this city are ill-chosen. Most recent writers are now convinced that the sites and construction of hospitals hitherto in use, are bad, with few exceptions. As it may at first view appear scarcely credible to those who have not reflected upon this subject, that these noble institutions (thanks to Christianity!) intended for, should be ill-adapted to the wants of the sick; some important data and reasonings will be subjoined for the reader's consideration, and the more so, because these data in ragard to ventilation, etc., apply more or less to all dwellings, asylums, factories, colleges, schools, etc.

The British and Foreign Medico-Chirurgical Review (April, 1860), has given a summary from numerous statistical works of late dates, showing, "that the *ratio* of mortality in any given hospital increases whenever there is any great increase in the number of patients; that the more patients that pass through the same hospital, the greater the ratio of deaths per cent. It is now known that brick and mortar, disposed in the form of a building, seven hundred feet square and three stories high, can accommodate with safety 800 to 1,000 patients (*e. g.*, Barrack Hospital, Scutari). But it is now known that the same materials could have built a hospital, differently placed and constructed, to have accommodated easily 3,000 patients, *with good recovering conditions.* It is indeed ruinous to build hospitals after the former plan. The "Report of the Sanitary Commission on the Army,' and the 'Builder' newspaper, have been the first to enunciate the principle in our day, or rather to propound the essential question for consideration in the construction of all hospitals. It is a question economical as well as sanitary. It is *to find that construction which will accommodate the greatest number of patients upon* *a given area, with the greatest facilities for economy, administration, and recovery in the shortest possible time.* Pernicious nosocomial influences indicate the defective sanitary state of a hospital much better than its mortality returns. Medical men are beginning to recognize this fact; but we do not think that such pernicious nosocomial influences have been sufficiently brought into notice. Indeed, it is often difficult to point out any single in-instance, in any single hospital, of special pernicious influences at work; but cumulative evidence of the same general character soon makes the seat of the mischief apparent to the intelligent observer. * * * The statistics of hospitals show that, other things being equal, a hospital in a town yields not only a higher mortality, but fewer permanent recoveries, a longer duration of sick cases, and, therefore, a greater current expense to the administration, than a hospital in the country would do for the same number of cases. Within the last century and a half most of the hospitals in this country have been built; and the demand for them has been supplied. Once done, therefore, there they remain, and if bad, they are generally irremediable. As a profession, therefore, we have not many opportunities of projecting a new hospital, nor of interfering by our good advice in matters relating to hospital hygiene. Moreover, when we do interfere, our influence for good is generally overpowered by the majority in committees and boards of directors, or by the superior influence of Quartermasters-General, or some such similar heads of departments. The Commissioners, in their Report, also most justly exonerate those of us whose fate connected them with army hospitals and their management. The evils of them so much complained of 'have been the subject of constant, though fruitless, representations on the part of the medical officers.'

"*Hospital Construction.*—The first point to be attended to is undoubtedly the selection of the site. Climate here is the first consideration. We must seek to obtain a pure, dry air for the sick, to the exclusion, therefore, of damp climates. In the more damp localities of the south of England, for example, it is now well known that certain classes of sick and invalids linger on without recovering their health. The climate is intimately related to the nature of the ground. Clay is highly retentive of moisture, and where it forms the subsoil, it will keep the air over large districts of the country always more or less damp. Soils of this character are, therefore obviously unfit for hospitals. Soils which extend to a considerable depth in gravel and sand, with a good foundation below of consistent marl, and which are so far self-draining, are the best possible for hospital sites. Valleys, marshy and muddy ground, ought, therefore, to be avoided. It may seem superfluous to state that a hospital should not be built over an old graveyard, or on ground charged with organic matter. Such, however, has been done again and again ; and camps, also, have been pitched on similar spots. If the subject of ventilation is a difficult one as regards buildings in general, it is greatly more so in regard to hospitals. The emanations from sick people are given off in increased abundance, and with increased rapidity, compared with those from the healthy, so that the air of a ward is vitiated with much greater rapidity when filled with sick, than if it were filled with the same number of healthy people. It is still more excessively vitiated if all the sick are fever cases—if the hospital is a fever hospital. Many gases, we know, are also diffused with great rapidity, as when liberated from decaying animal substances and fermenting organic matter, by chemical decompositions of various kinds. The diffusion of these gases takes place with a rapidity proportioned to the square roots of their densities ; and no artificial cements will prevent such diffusion. Many gases also pass through fluids and so-called solids. Hydrogen gas and its compounds easily pass through the pores of stucco ; so that plastered walls and ceilings are no barrier to the diffusion of cesspool emanations. Hence the intolerable and incurable nuisance of them. Latrines, therefore, as generators of this gas, ought not to be placed in contact with hospital wards. In spite of many popular fallacies, we believe that every sick ward should be capable of being flooded with sunlight. Obviously, wards for the treatment of eye diseases are excepted. The windows, therefore, should bear a large proportion to the wall-space in all hospitals—not less than one to two. * * * 'If the recovery of sick is to be the object of hospitals, they will not be built in towns. If medical schools are the object, surely it is more instructive for students to watch the recovery from, rather than the lingering in, sickness. Twice the number of cases would be brought under their notice in a hospital in which the sick recovered in half the time necessary in another. According to all analogy, the duration of cases, the chances against complete recovery, the rate of mortality, must be greater in town than in country hospitals. Land in town is too expensive for hospitals to be so built as to secure the conditions for light and ventilation, and of spreading the inmates over a large surface-area, conditions now known to be essential to recovery, instead of filling them up three or four stories high, a condition now known to be opposed to re-covery.' The sick must be distributed over a large area, in a num-ber of separate buildings, rather than one large one."

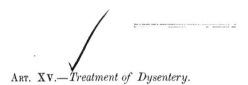

Art. XV.—*Treatment of Dysentery.*

ABERDEEN, Mississippi, May 28, 1860.

DR. B. DOWLER—*Dear Sir.*—As dysentery is at this time prevailing throughout this prairie country (where I am engaged in practice), I have thought it not amiss to call the attention of the profession to the potassæ chloras as a remedy in that intractable and distressing disease. I am using it now daily, with very satisfactory results, and I consider it decidedly preferable to the sulphates of soda and magnesia, creosote, the terebinthinates, etc., etc. I shall not go into the details of treatment, as the pathology of the disease is well understood, as well as the general therapeutic application of the drug. I use it in every and all cases of the disease in some of its stages, as there are various complications and modifications of the disease, that, of course, have to be treated according to general principles. I shall speak only of the chlorate of potassa, premising that, where from torpid liver or other conditions requiring the use of mercury, the potassæ chloras must be withheld during its adminis-tration, as they are antagonistic. My habit is (the preparatory steps having been taken) to order potassæ chloras, gr. xv, in ℥ij iced or coldest water, to be taken at a draught, which I repeat every four or six hours, according to circumstances. When the tormina and tenes-mus are distressing, I alternate the dose by giving pot. chlor. ℈iss, iced or cold water ℥iv, by the rectum, which invariably relieve those troublesome symptoms instantaneously. I have seldom had occasion to continue this treatment longer than one or two days before con-valescence was established. Without stopping to inquire how much

of its action is due to its specific influence on the blood, to its properties of generating chlorine, or to its acknowledged and universally
known effects upon the mucous surfaces, I venture to recommend its
trial to the profession, regarding it, as I do, much superior to any of
the routine remedies handed down to us through the books, or as
taught in the medical schools. I am aware that any suggestions
from a country stand-point pass as other bubbles upon our swelling
tides of gratuitous medical suggestions, yet, as the remedy is cheap,
measurably harmless, so little restriction is required upon the size of
the dose, together with the fact that the disease has heretofore been
so unsatisfactorily managed, all offer a reason for its trial. I will
not burthen your columns further, hoping ere long to see its recommendation from a source that will carry conviction with it.

Truly, yours,   JOHN W. MOORE, M. D.

PROGRESS OF MEDICINE.

ART. I.—*Observations on Digestion, made on a Case of Fistulous
Opening into the small Intestine.*

PROFESSOR BUSCH, of Bonn, has availed himself of the opportunity
afforded by a case in which a fistulous opening into the intestine
existed, of studying several points in regard to the physiology of
the digestive process.

A woman, aged thirty-one, in the sixth month of her fourth pregnancy, was tossed by a bull, one of whose horns lacerated the abdominal wall. At first there seemed to be no injury of the intestine,
but at the end of three days a perforation appeared, resulting in the
establishment of an opening through which food escaped. In six
weeks the woman, although she eat much, had become extremely
emaciated and weak. She was then taken to Bonn. Between the
umbilicus and the pubes, there was an aperture in the abdominal
walls more than an inch and one-fifth in length, the bottom of which
was formed by the posterior wall of the intestine ; the upper and
lower ends of the intestine were represented by two orifices at the
angles of the wound. The position of the wound, the size of the
intestine, the existence of valvulæ conniventes in large number, the
fluidity of the chymous material which exuded from the upper end,
and its grass-green aspect, led to the inference that the injury had

68

affected the upper third of the small intestine. Nothing whatever passed from the upper to the lower opening ; and several attempts to establish a communication proved fruitless. The patient was allowed to eat as much as she wished ; but, as this was not sufficient, food—principally protein, as soups, eggs, etc.—was thrown into the lower opening ; frequently, also, pieces of cooked eggs and meat were thrust into it by the finger. Her general health improved under this treatment ; and, after a time, the supply which she received by the stomach was sufficient.

Hunger.—The patient at first had a most voracious appetite ; she never felt satisfied. She continued to eat, even when the first portions of food which she had taken were escaping through the opening. She then would say that she felt better, but was still hungry. Professor Busch infers that hunger is composed of two separate sensations ; one general, the other local ; the former resulting from the want of material to repair the waste of tissue.

Movements of the Intestine.—The bottom of the opening was formed of a long portion of the posterior wall of the intestine, the anterior wall having been destroyed by gangrene ; there was also a large ventral hernia, the coverings of which were so thin that the least modification in the size of the intestine was as clearly perceived as if it had been laid bare. During the ordinary peristaltic movements, it was not possible to observe any difference between those which took place in the portion of intestine covered by skin and in that which was exposed to the air. When, on the other hand, the upper part of the intestine became invaginated in the opening, this portion contracted much more actively, and was sometimes the seat of a tonic contraction, which stiffened and raised it like a solid body.

The intestinal movements were not continuous ; there were often intervals of complete rest during more than a quarter of an hour. During these intervals, neither exposure of the part to the temperature of the room, nor the careful introduction of the finger, would excite peristaltic action ; even the taking of food would not excite it at once. There was no regularity in these intervals of action and rest, except during part of the night. Up to 10 or 11, P. M., there was a flow of chymous material or of liquids from the upper end of the intestine, so that, at first, the patient was always wet in spite of all care. No discharge then took place until 4 or 5 o'clock in the morning. When she made a hearty supper, a part escaped at once ; but the rest remained in the digestive canal until the next morning. This pause in the intestinal action did not arise from sleep, for it was observed when the patient lay awake at night ; and the matters escaped in the day time while she slept, as well as when she was awake.

The escape of the matters contained in the intestine was not continuous, but jerking ; and a propulsive movement of the intestine was even observed in the neighborhood of the opening. It is possible, however, that this was only the result of the adhesion of the intestines to the abdominal wall, which furnished a *point d'appui.*

Reversed peristaltic movements existed, and frequently impeded the experiments. Thus the aliments introduced into the lower opening of the intestine were often rejected after some hours, and fatty matters even after some days.

Observations on the Lower End of the Intestine.—*The Intestinal Juice.*—As the lower end of the intestine received nothing whatever from the upper end, it was possible to study in it the intestinal secretion in its pure state. The quantity of this, in the physiological condition, was not great. On introducing a bivalve speculum, the intestinal mucous could be plainly seen between the valves; it was white, or of a very slight rose tint. Sugar, tied up in a net bag, and introduced into the intestine, was not completely dissolved in a quarter of an hour. Under pathological irritation, the quantity of juice was increased; this was ascertained on two occasions. It was then thick and consistent. The reaction was always alkaline. The quantity of solid matter contained in it varied, according to numerous observations, from 7.4 to 3.87 per cent.; the mean being 5.47 per cent.

Digestive action of the Intestinal Juice.—The digestive property of the intestinal juice has been denied by some, while others have, correctly, admitted it. At the commencement of the treatment, the state of the patient began to be improved only when she was fed through the lower opening of the intestine. Into this were introduced soup, beer, gruel, hard eggs, and meat cut into small pieces. During the six weeks previous to her entrance into the hospital, the woman had only two small, hard stools. After being fed in the way above described, she had at first an abundant evacuation every twenty-four hours; but later it became necessary to use enemata. The evacuations resembled ordinary fæcal matter in form and consistence; but the color was grayish white, and they emitted a repulsive, putrid odor. No portions of egg nor of meat were found in them.

In order to study the digestive action of the intestinal juice on different foods, a weighed portion of food was enclosed in a net bag, and introduced into the intestine through a speculum. To ascertain the quantity dissolved, the loss of solid matter was sought. For this purpose, a known quantity of the same food was dried, and the amount of solid matter estimated; from which, on drying at the same temperature the portion removed in the bag, it was easy to calculate the loss which the latter had sustained.

Protein Matters.—Coagulated albumen and cooked meat always lost substance; and the morsels, when drawn out, presented traces of decomposition. The angles of the cubes of albumen were rounded, and the surface had a cheesy aspect, and peeled off in grumous masses when washed with water; the meat was flabby, soft, and pale. The masses had a penetrating, putrefactive odor; and the presence of hydro-chloric acid evolved ammoniacal vapor. This was not the result of ordinary putrefaction from moist heat; for none of the experiments lasted above seven hours, and decomposition commenced at an early period. The cause can only be sought for in a peculiar ferment furnished by the intestinal juice. Of albumen, the percentage quantity digested varied from 35.35 in six hours and a half to 6.5 in five hours and a quarter ; that of meat varied from 29.9 in seven hours to 5.5 in five hours.

Starch and Sugar.—Starch, dried at 212°, was introduced. The percentage loss varied between 63.53 in five hours and a half, and 38.5 in six hours. After injecting a solution of starch into the lower end of the intestine, the stools were found to contain neither starch nor sugar, but only traces of dextrine. The starch underwent conversion into grape-sugar, which was always found in the bag. Cane-sugar was not changed into grape-sugar ; a large portion was found in the fæces in the state of cane-sugar, and the urine contained no trace of it.

Fats.—These were submitted to experiment on two occasions. On the first, more than three ounces (avoirdupois) of melted butter were introduced, in small portions, into the intestine. After ten days, the patient spontaneously had a white very fetid stool, of the consistence of *bouillie*. On being examined, after cooling, it was found to be covered by a layer of solid fat ; the subjacent portion, under the microscope, appeared chiefly composed of large fat-drops and fat-crystals, mixed with epithelial cells. The evacuation had an acid reäction ; and the vessel in which it had been treated by ether evolved an odor of butyric acid. A little more than one-sixth of the quantity of fatty matter administered was found. A large portion, however, of the butter had been expelled from the intestine by reversed peristaltic movements ; so that probably little or none of it was absorbed. The second experiment, which was made at the end of a fortnight, with cod-liver oil, gave precisely the same result.

Observations on the Upper End of the Intestine.—Alimentary matters, contrary to the general supposition, did not remain long in the stomach. In the morning, when the intestine was empty, the peristaltic movements expelled frothy mucous. On giving food which could be readily recognised, the first portions appeared at the opening in about a quarter or half an hour ; and, after a copious meal, three or four hours were sufficient for the expulsion of the whole.

The reäction of the mixture of digestive fluids, expelled in the fasting state, was almost always neutral, rarely faintly acid or alkaline. The intestinal juice, when carefully washed from the fistulous opening, was constantly found to be alkaline. After a meal, the chymous mass gave very variable reäctions ; at first, protein compounds seemed to produce an alkaline or neutral liquid, while fat, starch, and sugar gave an acid one ; but repeated observations showed so great variations in these respects, that no fixed result could be arrived at.

The solid aliments contained in the chyme did not appear much changed on simple inspection ; but, on touching the surface of coagulated albumen and pieces of meat, they were found to be more friable than in the fresh state. The muscular fibres of meat were divided both longitudinally and transversely, as is already known to be the case ; and this was observed more when the meat had been very finely cut up. These solid alimentary matters floated in a large quantity of biliary fluid ; but, after the eating of large quantities of cabbage, turnips, and potatoes, a small layer of liquid separated only after the mixture had been allowed to rest a considerable time. Whenever the diet during the day was confined to a single article of food, the chymous mass was more consistent towards the evening than in the morning ; while, after a variety of food, the quantity of liquid was the same at different hours.

After the injection of feculent food, the chyme contained a large amount of starch and sugar ; while, after cooked protein compounds, a slight turbidity was very rarely produced on boiling the liquid.

The digestive fluids were rejected in such a mixed state that no definite result could be derived from their examination. The absence of indications of the presence of sulphocyanide of potassium showed that saliva was not present. Besides bile and pancreatic juice, there must have been a large amount of fluid supplied by the stomach, for the total sum of solid matters was very small ; the average was 2.48 per cent., the extremes 2.56 and 2.34. This is remarkable, since in man the gastric juice itself gives three per cent. of solid residue.

Cane-Sugar.—After having ascertained that the fluids passed from the opening in the morning, when the patient had been confined to an exclusively animal diet on the preceding day, gave no reaction with the potash and copper test, she was made to take, fasting, solutions of cane-sugar. In the fluid which escaped, only a small part of the sugar was found—as grape-sugar, never as cane-sugar. This observation confirms the opinion of M. Bouchardat.

Raw Albumen.—In the morning, the albumen of four eggs, beaten up with a little water, was given to the patient. After four hours, there was collected a moderately large quantity of an alkaline liquid, thready, mixed with bile, and containing no coagulated albumen. If the gastric juice had solidified this substance, portions of it would have been found. The quantity of albumen excreted was found to be 36 per cent. of the amount taken in.

Gum Arabic underwent no change, and escaped almost entire from the opening.

Gelatine.—Of this substance, nearly two-thirds were absorbed ; the remaining third, which escaped, had the ordinary chemical characters, except that it did not gelatinize, and that its warmed solution was rendered turbid by acetic acid.

Milk.—After milk had been taken, an acid liquid escaped, in which the casein had been coagulated by the acids of the stomach, not in large masses, but in fine particles. The filtered liquid contained a portion of uncoagulated casein.

Fats.—A large dose of cod-liver oil was given to the patient in the morning ; and, on each occasion, the quantity of liquid that escaped was relatively very large. Its reaction varied ; most frequently it was acid, rarely alkaline. In the latter case, the fat was so finely divided that it could not be recognized by the naked eye ; but, under the microscope, oil-globules were found in the molecular state. When the reaction was acid, the greatest part of the fat formed a similar emulsion ; but on the top there floated a smaller quantity of oil, in large drops. When the alkaline emulsion had been kept during twenty-four hours, it became acid, and a part of the oil floated on it in large drops.

Digestibility of certain Articles of Food.—Professor Busch endeavored to obtain information on this subject, by examining the quantity of ingested aliment which arrived at the opening in the upper part of the intestine. In one experiment, in which two ounces of sugar were taken, only one-thirtieth part reäppeared ; in another, in which three ounces were taken, one-fifteenth was found. Of albumen, the proportion of the quantity absorbed to that found in the discharged chyme was as seven to four ; of gelatine, almost as two to one.

Professor Busch has drawn up a table which shows the proportion between the weight of the material ingested and that of the chyme thrown out.

	Food taken.		Chyme.
Fat	1		6
Gelatine	1		3.675
Boiled eggs	1		2.73
Meat	1		1.73
Milk	1		1.25
Turnips	1		1.2
Cabbage	1		0.91
Potato soup	1		0.7

With regard to the latter two articles, the quantity of juices secreted is too small to make up for the loss caused by absorption into the stomach and the commencement of the small intestine ; while fat and gelatine give rise to a considerable secretion of fluid.

In examining the relation between the quantity of solid matter taken in and that found in the chymous mass, the loss representing the quantity absorbed, the following results were arrived at :

	Solid matter taken in.		Solid matter rejected.
Gelatine	1		0.94
Boiled eggs	1		0.76
Milk	1		0.62
Cabbage	1		0.58
Potato soup	1		0.53
Turnips	1		0.49
Meat	1		0.35

Although these numbers cannot be supposed to possess an exact mathematical value, they, nevertheless, afford important instruction.

Two experiments were made during periods of twenty-four hours; once with a varied animal diet, and at the other time with a mixed animal and vegetable diet. As far as the results of these experiments showed, the amount of matter absorbed from the mixed diet was about ten times as great as that absorbed from the purely animal diet. While the patient was taking the animal diet, the matters which escaped from the opening consisted, at first (as always), of a liquid in which floated fragments of meat and of egg ; gradually, however, the quantity of fluid diminished, the mass became more consistent, and at last, especially on the following morning, there escaped a mass having the appearance and smell of pure fresh meat, not colored by bile. Under a mixed diet, the chyme preserved its liquid consistence throughout, except in the middle of the day, when it became more consistent after the patient had taken some legumes at dinner.

Digestive Properties of the Fluids discharged from the Small Intestine.—In the course of his researches, Professor Busch observed that the liquid which escaped from the opening, especially after the ingestion of protein aliments, passed very slowly through the filter, and that the fragments of meat and egg continued to diminish in size while lying on the filter, so that at the end of the operation small portions only of solid matter were left. This proved that the digestive influence of the mixture of gastric, pancreatic, and intestinal juices, and bile, was exerted on the protein compounds from the commencement of the small intestine ; and this occurred, whatever was the reaction of the fluid. But the aliments had been in contact with pure gastric juice in the stomach ; it was, therefore, interesting to ascertain whether the mixture of digestive juices possessed equal power on food plunged directly into it. Experiment on this point showed that coagulated albumen and roast veal, placed for a period varying from six to eight hours, at a low temperature, in contact with the alkaline fluid which escaped from the fistula after the ingestion of fluid albumen or of meat, lost a small quantity of solid matter, and were slightly disintegrated. But this action was incomparably less than that which was exerted by the mixed juices on matters which had been submitted to the action of pure gastric juice. It follows from this, that alimentary matters leave the stomach while imperfectly digested, and that their digestion is performed in great part in the intestines. (*Archiv. für Pathologische Anatomie und Physiologie*, Band xiv ; and *L'Union Médicale*, 15 et 20 Mars, 1860.)—*Brit. Med. Jour.*

Art. II.—*Sub-Arachnoid Fluid. Water of the Brain.*

i. *Sub-Arachnoidean Fluid.*

M. Jobert de Lamballe publishes the following singular case, tending to prove that Magendie erroneously considered the loss of the sub-arachnoidean fluid as a cause of functional disturbance to the cerebro-spinal system.

A person of strong constitution, who was admitted into the Hôtel Dieu on the 11th of December, 1858, and died eleven days later, on the 22d, had been stabbed with a dagger by a man who was in the habit of paying her frequent visits. The blow was struck with great violence, and the blade had broken off, close to the handle of the poniard, the base corresponding to the skin, while its point penetrated into the vertebral cavity. The large blood vessels had escaped injury, and the haemorrhage was therefore unimportant; but a continuous discharge of a serous fluid, analogous to the serum of blood, was observed oozing from the oblique wound of the integument. The sheets and bedding were wet through, so great was the amount which exuded daily, and the fluid, on examination, was found to consist in serum, containing a few blood corpuscles. It was impossible to remove the foreign body before the third day of the patient's sojourn in the hospital, and when it was withdrawn, a considerable rush of the same liquid took place. No muscular collapse, or diminution of muscular contractility, was observed at any time, notwithstanding the escape of the cerebro-spinal fluid, nor any change in the mental powers. The patient having died from spinal meningitis, a post-mortem examination showed that the body of the sixth and seventh cervical vertebræ had been grazed by the instrument, the inter-vertebral substance injured, and the parietal dura mater and arachnoid perforated by the point of the blade.

The case is favorable to M. Longet's view, who, repeating Magendie's experiments, demonstrated that the withdrawal of the cerebro-spinal fluid does not materially affect the gait of animals.—*Journal of Practical Medicine and Surgery. Dublin Hospital Gazette.*

ii.—*On the Water in the Brain-Substance.*

M. Marcé has made some observations on the proportion of water in the white and gray substances of the brain, and on the power which the organ possesses of absorbing fluid.

In order to determine the normal quantity of water contained in the cerebral substance, the white and the gray matters were separated, then dried and weighed. The following were the general results of experiments made on the brain of man, the sheep, calf, ox, rabbit, pheasant, and owl: 1. In the healthy state, the gray substance in man contains 80 per cent. of water, while the white substance contains 70 per cent. 2. In animals the figures vary; but in all there is a greater proportion of water in the gray substance than in the white.

In order to ascertain whether the brain can absorb water and become œdematous, M. Marcé injected brains with pure water, and then dried them; and also steeped portions of cerebral substance in water for twenty-four or forty-eight hours, or even longer. He found that brain-substance (not dried) was capable of absorbing half its own weight of water. He also dried brains in cases where the membranes were infiltrated with serum, and found, especially in the gray matter, that the percentage of water was 85 or 90, instead of 80.

The fact that the brain is capable of absorbing water is regarded by M. Marcé as of pathological importance. In comparing the weight of the two hemispheres, it must not be forgotten that a simple serous infiltration may so increase the weight of one hemisphere as to cause the other to appear atrophied. The symptoms of cerebral compression attributed to serous effusion, are produced not only by the effused liquid, but by the increase of the brain arising from the absorption of fluid by the gray matter. Finally, the drying of the brain substance, as the means of recognizing œdema, ought to be applied in pathological inquiries ; and, in this way, we may perhaps arrive at an explanation of some of those cerebral phenomena which have been classed as neuroses.—*Journal de la Physiologie*, Janvier, 1860. *Brit. Med. Jour.*

ART. III.—*Effects of Irritating or Removing the Medulla Oblongata or Spinal Cord.*

IN the *Journal de la Physiologie* for January, 1860, Dr. Brown-Séquard seeks to show that all the results observed to follow entire or partial removal of the medulla oblongata, may be produced when no portion of this part of the nervous system has been removed ; and that the entire medulla oblongata may be taken away without producing any of the effects which are attributed to its removal.

With regard to the heart, Dr. Brown-Séquard finds the following results : 1. Irritation of the spinal cord in the cervical region sometimes produces a remarkable diminution, and even an arrest, of the movements of the organ. 2. The nearer to the medulla oblongata the irritation is made, the more frequent is this effect upon the heart. 3. Irritation of the medulla oblongata itself, not at the so-called vital point *(nœud vital)*, but near the emergence of the roots of the pneumogastric nerves, produces, more frequently than irritation of the spinal cord, arrest of the heart's movements. 4. Diminution of these movements is never produced on irritating any part of the cord in the neck or of the medulla oblongata, after the pneumogastric nerves have been divided. 5. Removal of the medulla oblongata, or of the cervical portion of the cord, very frequently does not produce immediate diminution of the action of the heart.

As to the respiratory movements, the author finds that, in certain cases and in certain animals, they go on after the removal of the medulla oblongata. This has been observed in crocodiles, by Dr. Bennet Dowler, of New Orleans ; by Dr. Brown-Séquard, in birds ; and by Drs. Richardson and Brown-Séquard, in new-born mammalia. On the other hand, irritation of the medulla oblongata, or of the neighboring parts, often does not produce suspension of the respiratory movements. Besides, he has often found that irritation of the spinal cord near the medulla oblongata does not produce the respiratory movements of the nostril and face, which are observed in the ordinary death-agony.

In the death-agony, the epileptiform convulsions may be very feeble, or entirely absent, in animals in which the medulla oblongata has been removed. The convulsive movements are seldom if ever present under the following circumstances : 1. When the blood in

69

the veins is red (indicating diminution of carbonic acid). 2. In death by syncope, in cases where the motion of the heart is more or less completely arrested by galvanism of the pneumogastric nerves, or by crushing the semi-lunar ganglia, etc. 3. Where a prolonged disease, a hæmorrhage, or exhaustion from violent galvanism, have caused a remarkable diminution in the excitability of the cerebro-spinal axis. According to Dr. Brown-Séquard, the convulsions or rigidity which generally take place at the moment of dividing the cord, have the effect of exhausting it in such a way as to prevent the occurrence of convulsions in the death-agony. In some animals, however, especially in rabbits, removal of the medulla oblongata produces neither convulsions nor rigidity. Dr. Brown-Séquard explains this by saying that death does not take place here by asphyxia, but by syncope ; and that convulsions do not occur, because they are dependent on the circulation of black blood, for which asphyxia is necessary.—*British Medical Journal*, April, 1860.

ART. IV.—*Experimental Pathology—Rational Principles of Therapeutics.* Lecture xii. Delivered at the College of France, during the Winter Session, 1859–60, by M. CLAUDE BERNARD, Member of the French Institute ; Professor of General Physiology at the Faculty of Sciences.

GENTLEMEN—We have considered the two opposite points of view from which medical men regard the healing art ; one class, as we have seen, recognize the existence of a *vis medicatrix naturæ*, or healing power in nature, to the influence of which they invariably attribute the return of the sick to health ; the other class, indignantly rejecting this hypothesis, ascribe the honor almost exclusively to the medical man of all the cures which happen to be effected ; and these two different opinions, it is not difficult to foresee, must of necessity become apparent in practice. The partisans of the *vis medicatrix naturæ* maintain the principle of expectation, while their adversaries have recourse to a practice more or less energetic and varied.

Both parties have, to a certain extent, truth on their side ; though it would be dangerous for medical men to attach themselves exclusively either to the one or to the other opinion. It is true that nature frequently exerts herself in the cure of diseases, but her efforts, often impotent and ill-directed, stand in need of the assistance of art.

It is by means of medicinal agents that man interferes, for the purpose of modifying the course of disease ; it is by means of medicinal agents that he accelerates or retards its progress ; it is, therefore, indispensable for every medical practitioner who desires to be unfettered by the trammels of a slavish empiricism, to ascertain their precise action, in order that he may be in a suitable position to use them when an occasion shall present itself.

But scarcely have we embarked on the consideration of this subject, when a new question presents itself, and which it becomes our duty to solve before proceeding farther. What are medicines ; and what is the difference which separates them from aliments and from poisons ? On this subject the following definition is usually accepted : Medicines serve to reëstablish health; aliments serve to support life ; poisons destroy it.

But we are evidently, in this respect, under the necessity of confining ourselves to generalities somewhat vague. Every definition which is of too precise a nature is apt, on that very account, to become inexact. Not to spend too much time on this point, we will merely say that medicines are foreign substances, introduced into the economy there to determine such and such phenomena ; it is, therefore, the nature of their action which it is our duty to specify. We see from this that all medicines are in their nature poisons, the only difference between the two consisting in the extent of their action ; for they act only in virtue of their toxic properties, being naturally substances foreign to the economy. Those substances which already exist in the physiological state in the system, are null in their effects, being neither useful or otherwise in the reëstablishment of health when it is deranged.

We know, however, that chlorine, iron, phosphorus, and many other substances, for example, usually employed as medicines, already exist in the body ; but they are never found there in a state similar to that in which they are exhibited as medicines. Phosphorus, in its pure state, is an energetic poison ; whereas, phosphates are found in abundance in the normal condition of the body. Thus, therefore, all substances, whether medicinal or toxic, are foreign to the system, either by their nature, or in consequence of the particular form in which they are prescribed.

As the greater part of poisons belong either to the mineral or to the vegetable kingdom, it is not surprising that medicine borrows the greater number of the agents it employs from the one or the other of these two. Sometimes these agents are vegetable alkaloids, sometimes they are purgative salts, sometimes they are metallic salts ; now these different substances, once introduced into the economy, exercise on it a perfectly well-defined action ; the salts of quinine combat the periodicity of diseases ; mercurial compounds exercise a specific influence over certain virulent affections ; how, then, are we to understand the *modus operandi* of each medicinal agent ? For a long time it was believed that the medicinal substance, penetrating to the interior of our organs, addressed itself directly to the morbific principle, with a view to neutralizing it ; mercury addressing itself to the syphilitic virus, acids to the principle which generates scurvy, alkalis to that on which rheumatism depends ; an attempt has even been made to treat lead-colic by the administration of sulphuric acid to those suffering under that affection, with a view to rendering the morbific agent insoluble, and consequently inert in the body of the tissues. These examples will suffice to enable you to understand what has been attempted to be realized by the aid of medicines.

It is easy to prove, by the simplest possible physiological notions, that this theory is altogether false. It is manifestly impossible to produce the sulphate of lead in the torrent of the circulation, and it is equally impossible to render the blood acid, for the animal dies a long time before the circulating fluid has ceased to be alkaline ; in fact, in all animals, whether red or white blooded, this fluid is invariably alkaline, although it becomes acid spontaneously after death, when the sugar in it becomes changed into lactic acid.

The chemical combinations which are usually observed to take place in our laboratories, cannot be produced in the blood, but actions of a different kind are readily produced in this fluid ; I allude to fermentations. Introduce yeast into the veins, and you will see alcoholic fermentation follow in spite of all the conditions inherent in the vital principle. But fermentations are not, as we know, chemical combinations ; they are simply actions. Yeast does not combine with the sugar, it only decomposes it, and herein lies the secret of its poisonous action.

It will be easy to give you a still more striking example of these particular reactions. We know that amygdaline, a substance of organic origin which is found in the bitter almond, has the property, in presence of certain ferments, of undergoing double decomposition, giving origin to glycose and hydrocyanic acid. Emulsine, the particular ferment which decomposes the amygdaline, exists in the sweet as well as in the bitter almond ; but this latter alone contains the principle of amygdaline ; hence the characteristic difference, which we know so well, between the odor and the flavor of these two fruits, which in every other respect resemble each other.

Let us now suppose that we inject into the veins of an animal either amygdaline or emulsine separately, no accident follows ; but if we inject these two substances simultaneously into the blood, at two different points more or less distant the one from the other, the animal almost immediately dies, as if struck with lightning ; the reaction which brings about the decomposition of the amygdaline is effected in the blood contained in the veins ; prussic acid has been engendered, and its poisonous effects have not been slow in manifesting themselves. Here, then, is a reaction to which the presence of albumen, of fibrine, and other substances held in solution in the blood, have offered no obstacle—conclusive evidence that, in opsing themselves to the ordinary chemical reactions, the albuminous substances of the blood act simply in virtue of their chemical properties, and do not in this respect exercise any vital influence. If it were possible, by introducing into the blood certain ferments for the purpose of determining reactions of an analogous kind, but of a nature not unfavorable to health, the medical art would doubtless have availed itself of this method of action ; but it is unfortunately impossible to do so in practice—in fact, ferments are not generally capable of absorption ; at least, up to the present time we do not know of any one that can be taken up by the stomach ; it would be necessary to introduce them directly into the blood. The action of emulsine on amygdaline again furnishes a proof of this. Inject some amygdaline into the veins of an animal, while at the same time you introduce emulsine into the stomach, no reaction whatever takes place, for an impassable barrier opposes the passage of the emulsine into the blood. But when the two substances are simultaneously introduced into the stomach, so that they there combine, reaction follows, prussic acid is set at liberty, and the animal dies of poison. This is what takes place ninety-nine times in a hundred to those who are guilty of the imprudence of eating a large quantity of bitter almonds. If, however, half an hour should elapse between the ingestion of emulsine and that of amygdaline into the stomach of a dog, no accident is observed to take place ; the ferment digested in the stomach has descended into the intestines, and has lost all its characteristic properties. We do not, up to the present moment, know any ferment susceptible of being absorbed by the digestive tube.

It is, therefore, impossible to explain the action of medicines on purely chemical grounds ; an explanation has, consequently, been sought for by appealing to notions borrowed from the physical sciences. It is thus, for example, that an attempt has been made to explain the action of diuretics. M. Poiseuille has proved that if distilled water flows with a given rapidity in capillary tubes, we can, without modifying the conditions of temperature or pressure, increase or diminish the rapidity of the flow by the addition of certain substances. If, for example, we add to distilled water a small proportion of hydrochlorate of ammonia, of nitrate of potash, or of some salt of iodine, the flow becomes accelerated ; alcohol, the sulphate of soda, and several chlorides, produce the opposite effect of this. M. Poiseuille thought that the diuretic action of the nitrate of potash could be explained by the increased rapidity in the circulation in the capillaries of the kidneys to which it gives rise ; while alcoholic intoxication could, he thought, be explained by the diminished rapidity of the cerebral circulation, and might be dissipated by the salts of ammonia, in virtue of the acceleration they produce in the movement of the blood in the capillaries. In repeating his experiments, whether on individual organs of the body or on living animals, M. Poiseuille was able to satisfy himself of the fact that the capillary circulation was influenced by sundry agents which accelerate or retard the flow of water in glass tubes.

These are not the only examples of this nature that might be cited; for instance, an attempt was made to explain the special action of purgatives, which give rise to a very abundant serous discharge from the surface of the intestines by the simple principle of endosmose ; it is true the sulphate of soda, and several other saline purgatives, possess endosmotic properties in a very high degree ; therefore, it cannot be denied that, in many of these cases, the reasoning is somewhat specious ; but there are other cases, much more numerous, where this augmentation does not hold good. Purgatives, for instance, in many cases, present but a very feeble endosmotic property, the greater part of the drastic kind being derived from the vegetable kingdom.

There is a third way in which the action of medicines may be understood, and which is more in accordance with physiology. It is admitted that there exists in each organ an elective action, which renders it more apt than the others to be influenced by certain medicinal agents. The different ways by which a substance, introduced into the economy, can escape from it, are, as we have seen, extremely variable. Well, then, medicine acts precisely on that organ by which it is eliminated. Reasoning thus supposes that the medical action is essentially different from the toxic one ; such a manner of viewing the question is, however, quite erroneous, as we shall see by and by ; but in order to better discuss the theory to which we have just alluded, let us proceed to consider it on scientific grounds. According to this hypothesis, the substances introduced into the economy exercise on the organs which serve for their elimination an action altogether specific, and experimental physiology furnishes us with numerous examples of this.

Ether, we know, when it penetrates, by no matter what passage, into the torrent of the circulation, escapes by the lungs ; the characteristic odor of the breath proves this. Well, then, if the quantity of ether introduced into the economy be sufficient to bring about toxic effects, we find at the autopsy traces of an action altogether local, which has been exercised on the lungs.

But, in the case of phosphorus, the fact is still more evident. It is generally by dissolving the substance in oil that we obtain it in a convenient form for injection into the veins ; and when the dose is not of sufficient quantity to produce toxic effects immediately, recourse may be had to the following experiment in order to demonstrate that it is eliminated by the lungs : Place the animal in a dark room, and you will see flames escaping from the mouth and nostrils; this is the well-known result of the phosphoresence of the gases given forth by the lungs. When, after having subjected the animal to this experiment, we kill it, we discover in the lungs lesions of the most serious description ; everywhere their tissues are congested, and a peculiar yellow hepatization is remarked at different points.

There are, besides, several other examples of a particular action exercised by different medicinal agents on the organs which they traverse on making their escape from the economy. Almost all the secreting organs are capable of being modified, in a particular way, by the action of certain substances found in their secretions. We shall content ourselves by pointing out the influence which is almost immediately exercised by cantharides on the urinary organs. We know, in fact, that such is the sensibility of the organs in this respect, that the simple application of a blister suffices, in certain subjects, to bring about a very well-marked irritation in the entire urinary apparatus. The effects of cantharides are still more marked when the substance is taken into the stomach ; it then gives rise to inflammation of the bladder, and to acute nephritis, which are not unfrequently followed by the abundant production of false membranes, and in some cases by accidents of the most serious kind.

But in this entire series of phenomena we cannot recognize any other than a purely local action exercised on the particular organs affected. At the time phosphorus and sulphuretted hydrogen traverse the lungs in making their exit from the body, it is found that they have lost nothing of their irritating properties; it is not, therefore, surprising that they develope in the center of the organ itself, which serves for their elimination, an inflammation more or less intense. The same holds good as regards cantharides; this substance, in traversing the urinary apparatus, acts as a blister on the mucous membrane which lines its internal surface, and there determines acute inflammation.—*Medical Times and Gazette.*

ART. V.—*Synthesis of Cataract.*

AT a meeting of the Medical Society of London, March 26, 1860, Dr. Richardson brought before the society animals presenting cataract in various stages. In the *American Journal of the Medical Sciences* for January, 1860, there was a paper by Dr. S. Weir Mitchell, who, in performing experiments on osmosis, had made the remarkable observation that, when syrup was injected into the subcuticular sacs of frogs, a curious form of cataract was produced. The conclusions at which Dr. Mitchell arrived were: that sugar, in large quantities, destroys the life of a frog; that an abundant supply of water frequently enables the frog to eliminate the sugar and escape death; that the formation of cataract is one of the most striking symptoms of the sugar-poisoning; that the cataract is due to mechanical disturbances of the form and relative position and contents of the compound tubes of the lens. Dr. Richardson, since reading this paper, had performed a series of experiments, amounting now to forty-six in number, which were not only entirely confirmatory of Dr. Mitchell's observations, but were an extension of them. The leading facts adduced by the author may be thus summed up: 1. When from one and a half to two drachms of syrup are injected under the skin of a frog, the body of the animal first becomes enlarged from exosmosis; and afterwards, in from twelve to thirty-six hours (the enlargement having meanwhile disappeared), cataract—usually in both eyes—is the result. This was confirmed by twenty experiments, and is identical with the result previously obtained by Dr. Mitchell. 2. If the frog, after injection, is freely surrounded with water, it recovers without cataract—a fact observed also by Dr. Mitchell. 3. If, immediately after the lens becomes opaque, the animal is surrounded by water, the cataract may be made to disappear. This was confirmed by three experiments. 4. The cataract, being fully developed, remains permanent; the

animal apparently recovering its general health, but being entirely
blind. 5. When the cataractous lens is removed from the animal,
the opacity may be seen to have commenced, either at the posterior
part of the lens, spreading circumferentially, or at the anterior part,
spreading backwards. The opacity is diffused, but it does not reach
the center of the lens. Similar observations had been made by Dr.
Mitchell, except that he traced the opacity from the posterior surface
in all cases. The capsule of the lens seems clear (Mitchell). A
similar opacity of the lens may be produced in the eye of a sheep,
immediately after death, by the injection of syrup into the anterior
chamber. In these conclusions, the results of both authors were, in
the main, the same ; and, having described them, Dr. Richardson
referred to observations of his own. 6. All varieties of sugar—
cane, grape, and milk—produce the same result ; and frogs were
presented with cataract induced by the injection of syrups of each
of these sugars. 7. The form of cataract did not vary in any case.
8 After several experiments, it was found that a syrup of cane or
grape-sugar, of specific gravity 1150, was the most practical ; and
of milk-sugar, that of specific gravity 1120. 9. Injection of gumwater does not produce cataract. In one case, after the injection of
albumen, it was believed that some opacity was produced ; but a
second experiment did not confirm this result. 10. Sugar-cataract is
producible in other animals. In a fresh-water fish, placed in water
brought to the specific gravity of 1070 by cane-sugar, perfect cataract was produced on one side, the other side seeming to escape
altogether. A second fish, placed in the same solution, lived in it
for several hours, but showed no cataract. In guinea-pigs, rabbits,
and dogs, attempts had been made to produce the sugar-cataract by
injecting syrup into the peritoneum. Great difficulties, however,
were experienced in these experiments ; for it was found that, if an
overdose of syrup were injected, the animal died rapidly, as from
hæmorrhage, through rapid transudation of water from the blood
into the peritoneal sac. If, again, small quantities were introduced,
the sugar was rapidly eliminated by the urine ; in which it was
found present in one case within an hour after the injection of grape-
sugar syrup. But, by throwing an ounce of grape sugar into the
peritoneum of a rabbit, and repeating it after ten hours, distinct
opacity of both lenses was produced. The animal, however, died
after a third injection, the opacity increasing till death. The rabbit
was presented to the Society. As to the cause of the cataractous
condition, Dr. Richardson considered it purely osmotic ; that is to
say, it was due to an excessive transudation of water from the lens
to the surrounding fluids, upon which the component parts of the
lens were disarranged, and opacity was the result. This form of
cataract, while it presented the appearance of common cataract, connected itself intimately with the facts which had been made out in
the etiology of the disease, as to the coëxistence of diabetes and
cataract. Dr. Mitchell, at the conclusion of his paper, had noticed
the same circumstance ; and Dr. Richardson thought its importance
could not be overestimated. The coëxistence of diabetes and cataract had been pointed out by Mr. France, by Cohen, Lohmeyer,

Gunzler, Mackenzie, and Duncan ; but especially by Von Gräfe, who had stated that, after examining a large number of diabetic patients in various hospitals, he had found about one-fourth of them affected with cataract. In Dr. Richardson's opinion, however, it was not necessary that the general manifestations of diabetes should always be presented for diagnosis when sugar existed in the secretions; and it might be that there was such a condition as a temporary diabetic state, during which cataract might be developed. Any way, the synthesis of cataract by one process was demonstrated ; and the first rational step towards the pathology of the disease had been made. As a point bearing on the treatment of cataract, Dr. Richardson said that, inasmuch as temporary opacity, produced by exposure of the lens to syrup, was removable by an after exposure to water (*i. e.*, by changing the position of the medium surrounding the lens), it was worthy of consideration whether an operation for letting out the aqueous humor by a small opening, and refilling the anterior and posterior chambers with distilled water, might not lead to removal of the cataractous condition in the *earliest* stages. The author concluded with some complimentary remarks on the important labors of his transatlantic brother, Dr. Mitchell.

Dr. Chowne said that, many years ago, he had read of experiments in which dogs had been fed with sugar, and had ulceration of the eye, and became blind.

Dr. Richardson was conversant with the experiments of Magendie on feeding dogs with sugar. There was no mention of cataract, and the ulceration appeared rather the result of starvation.

The President asked whether in any cases the cornea was affected.

Dr. Richardson said that, in the first case, the cornea was opaque, but he had not seen this since.

Mr. Rogers-Harrison suggested that other diseases besides cataract might be produced by the absorption of sugar.

Dr. Richardson was inclined to think that the effect of the sugar was specific.

The President suggested that the difficulty of inducing cataract in warm-blooded animals was connected with the higher development of the kidney.

Dr. Leared and Dr. Chowne had not observed the connection of cataract with diabetes.

Mr. Hulke said it was quite an exception in the Ophthalmic Hospital to see the connection of diabetes and cataract. When they did occur together, the cases were not favorable for operation.

British Medical Journal.

ART. VI.—*On the Method of Measurement as a Diagnostic Means of Distinguishing Human Races, adopted by Drs. Scherzer and Schwarz, in the Austrian Circumnavigatory Expedition of the "Novara:"* By JOSEPH BARNARD DAVIS.

WEIGHT and measure have been very frequently applied as means to

70

determine the physical proportions of different human races, and to ascertain their essential diversities. But it may well be doubted whether they have ever been employed in that systematic and comprehensive manner, which will afford the results they are capable of yielding. Travelers have generally contented themselves by speaking in indefinite comparative terms of the people with whom they have come into contact. But few have submitted any considerable number of these people to the test of measurement, and thus ascertained their dimensions. Anthropology stands in need of many more accurate and extended observations, to derive the full results from these sources of knowledge.

The subject itself is a large one, and some have confined themselves to one branch of it, some to others. Where actual measurements have been carried out, many have contented themselves with taking the *stature* of a few or a number of the people ; others have, besides, ascertained the length of the *limbs*, and a few have subjected the *head* to a series of superficial measurements. As we are fully assured that this latter division of the body is the seat of those faculties which lie at the base of all the peculiarities of human races, bearing essentially and intimately upon their manners and customs, all their institutions, their religious impulses, their capacity for civilization, and the development to which it has attained, it is not surprising that it should have attracted the chiefest attention. Besides the superficial measurements of the head, a more extensive series of observations has been made upon the bony skull itself, with a view of determining its relative proportions, for comparison in the same race, or among different races. Many observers, advancing a step nearer, have endeavored to ascertain, by measure and by weight, the *internal capacity* of this marble palace. And, lastly, some have laboriously devoted their inquiries to the great central mass of the nervous system, and availed themselves of the opportunities that have occurred to them, to determine the size and the weight of the brain, and its different parts. As this last investigation comes nearest of all to the specialties of human beings—who are so finely discriminated by Professor Owen as *archencephala*—it is to be regretted that the occasions for research among distinct races are so few, and have been so tittle availed of, and the investigation itself is so elaborate and nice, that hitherto this most interesting part of anthropological anatomy is, as it were, a *tabula rasa*, to use the language of one of the most laborious inquirers in this branch of science— Prof. Huschke, of the University of Jena. It is, however, fortunate that gauging the internal capacity of the skull should afford the means of so accurate an approximation to the volume and the weight of the brain ; and thus, for the comparison of these important points among the different families and tribes of men. Hence the labors of Tiedemann, the distinguished physiologist, who, with a very amiable design, undertook to show that the brain of a negro was not smaller than that of the European—an attempt similar to that of the late Sir William Hamilton. Tiedemann might have succeeded in impressing us with his own conclusion, had he not published the tables on which this conclusion was based, and which themselves refute such an erroneous opinion. To Tiedemann succeeded Professor Morton, of Philadelphia, Professor Van der Hoeven, of Leyden, and others. Among the most recent is Professor Huschke, of Jena, one of whose results of whose own estimation of the capacity of the skull and of the size of the brain, is, that the Germanic races, among whom, through our Anglo-Saxon forefathers, we rank as one great branch, have the largest brains of any people. They distinctly exceed the French in this respect.

That great diversities, capable of metrical appreciation, prevail among human races, is very well known. Some of the tribes of North American Indians are remarkable for their great stature. Catlin assures us that the men among the Crows, whose hair will frequently reach the calves of their legs, are most of them six feet or more. Other tribes are of a decidedly lower stature. Of the gigantic Patagonians of South America, the most extravagant accounts have been given by travelers. But Capt. King affirms them, upon measurement, to be from five feet ten inches to six feet high, which is supported by the statement of M. D'Orbigny, that some are six feet three and a half inches, and the medium stature is above five feet eight inches English. On the contrary, the average height of the Bushmen is only four feet four inches. This gives a range of very nearly two feet between the tallest and the shortest races of men we are acquainted with. The other races of mankind are comprised within these limits of difference. Some tribes of the Negritos average about four feet eight inches ; the so-called Malay races ascending to a mean of five feet three inches. But among the Negrito tribes of the Pacific there is, as that eminent ethnologist, Mr. Crawford, has clearly shown, a great diversity of stature. They dwell in islands scattered over a large extent of ocean, and although some tribes do not reach five feet in height, others, as those of New Caladonia, attain to six feet, and individuals among them even more. In the recent expeditions to the Andaman Islands, for the purpose of selecting a spot for a penal settlement, the inhabitants are spoken of as "dwarf Negrillos," and as "men of middle size." An individual who was measured gave a stature of four feet nine and a half English inches. (Selections from the Records of the Government of India, No. xxv : the Andaman Islands.) Thus, in stature alone, a very great diversity prevails. And it is remarkable that tribes in close proximity to each other frequently exhibit startling contrasts. Dr. Livingstone, whose opportunities, had he been an ethnologist, were so extraordinary, observed in the plains of the interior of South Africa, scattered among the Kafirs, who are a tall, fine, and robust race, the hordes of the diminutive Bushmen. He was deeply impressed with what he saw, so contrary to all his preconceptions ; and expresses his great surprise that such dissimilar races should be everywhere scattered about the country without being mingled, where they have dwelt for unlimited ages, exposed to all the same influences of air, climate, food, etc. The tall Patagonians, and some tribes of the Fuegians distinguished for their dwarf stature, afford a similar example of contrast.

The brothers Schlagintweit, following in the train of Mr. Hodgson, carried on an extensive series of metrical observations on the tribes of the Himalaya and of India. Many curious results, chiefly pointing to the different proportion of the parts of the bodies and limbs of these people from those of Europeans, have been attained, which will be published in the ethnological portion of their projected work. After ascertaining the weight of the individual and his strength, by means of the dynamometer, they made from twenty-five to twenty-eight different measurements, chiefly of the head, and of other parts of the body and limbs. But Drs. Scherzer and Schwarz have striven, by a more complex and complete system of observation and measurement, to gain an image of the size and form of the individual, and of all his parts ; thus, not merely to subserve the purposes of the anatomist, the physiologist, and the ethnologist, but those of the artist also. Their more ambitious object of obtaining, in this way, to a natural classification of human races, is an evidence of laudable zeal ; but we can hardly hope that their labors can do more than contribute towards the solution of this difficult problem. Although, it ought to be mentioned that the late Baron Humboldt, a short time before his death, expressed his great satisfaction with the system of measurements of Drs. Scherzer and Schwarz ; by which, he thought, we may at length arrive at a safer result in distinguishing and determining human races than by any other means.

After recording the age, weight, height, strength, color of the hair and eyes, and number of the pulsations of the radial artery, they divide their measurements into three sections, those of the *head*, the *trunk*, and the *extremities;* and of these they take no less than seventy different dimensions in all, by means of different instruments.

Their external measurements of the head are the most complete that have ever been employed. They embrace the face, as well as the other parts of the head, and by means of a perpendicular line with plummet, and a small metre scale, they are able to ascertain pretty correctly the profile of the countenance. The number of their different measurements of and about the *head*, consisting of superficial distances, diameters, circumferences, etc., amount to thirty-one, those of the *trunk* to eighteen, and those of the *extremities* to twenty-one.

When the frigate Novara reached Sydney, these gentlemen printed an account of their system of measurements, "for private circulation" among men of science, which is preceded by a number of ingenious observations. In these they dwell upon the case with which travelers intuitively discriminate the different nations and tribes of mankind ; and yet the difficulty in some selected individuals and cases to carry out this diagnosis, especially when the eye is deceived by a substitution of dress ; and express great confidence in a more minute examination by a systematic method of measurements. They insist with equal confidence, that nature must recognize a definite plan by which man's different types are formed and distinguished, and conclude that we should dedicate the same amount of study and inquiry to the systematic arrangement of our own species, as has long been applied to thousands of species of the vegetable and animal kingdoms.

In the course of these introductory remarks, they mention their examination of the Chinese inmates of the prison at Hong Kong. Among these they found persons belonging to the *Hakka Tribe*, with stout and vigorous constitutions, fine, well-shaped aqueline or long and straight noses, and a form of the eyes not resembling the specific obliquity of other Chinese. As criminals, they had been deprived of their tails, and Drs. Scherzer and Schwarz affirm that they had such a resemblance to the figures of some Europeans of the lower class, that, by a change of dress, they might pass amongst us without being recognized. They also mention how successfully Gützlaff, Medhurst, Huc, and others have traveled the Empire in a Chinese dress without detection. And, no doubt, there are individuals so capable of assuming, and, as it were, substituting the manners and expressions of others, that the ordinary and slight attention which is paid to persons on a journey and among numbers, does not suffice to discriminate them.

Still, *the rule* must run counter to such a confusion, or the statement of the Austrian voyagers could not be true—that an anthropologist on the Island of Java is able, at first view, to classify most of the Malay tribes inhabiting the larger and smaller islands on the Indian Archipelago, without ever mistaking. And the very remarkable account of the Abbé Huc proves that, if there are differences among the races of men too subtle to be detected by the eye, yet they are not the less certainly appreciable. He informs us that he and his companion successfully eluded the detection of the unsuspecting or inattentive Chinese, but that to the Chinese *dogs* they always stood at once revealed as Europeans, by their peculiar smell. "The dogs barked continually at us, and appeared to know that we were foreigners. This is not the proper time to refer to the distinguishable odors of the different races of mankind, which travelers allude to. Huc said he could easily distinguish those of the Negro, the Malay, the Tartar, the Thibetan, the Hindoo, the Arab, and the Chinese. Indeed, it is the same, with those having a delicate sense of smell, as to the French and other European races. And with respect to the fact of the penetrating and offensive scent attached to man, more especially to civilized man, Mr. Galton and others, who have traversed desert countries teeming with wild animals, give distinct and prominent testimony—which testimony is, in truth, not very complimentary to us.

We have been informed, on the authority of one who has seen much of the North American Indians, that they describe an odor to them peculiarly disgusting, as being attached to the Jews. A fact, which, if correct, is little accordant with the extraordinary hypotheses which would derive the Indians themselves from the lost tribes.

Finally, it may be mentioned that, by a recent communication from Dr. Scherzer, we are informed that, during the cruise of the Novara, about two hundred individuals of different races, but of about the same age, males and females, were subjected to measurement. The whole number of measures taken amount to nearly twelve thousand. Dr. Scherzer adds, that he does not consider these observations sufficient, but merely as a commencement of a system of thorough metrical examination ; that the paper on measurements has been translated into different languages, and copies of it left in the hands of physicians and other men of science, in the different places and islands visited by the expedition, who promised to complete the observations on the aborigines, and to forward the results to Europe ; that the measurements already effected embrace those made on Negroes, Malays, Mongols, Papuans, and Indians ; and that the greatest number were taken on individuals in the Nicobar Islands, Batavia, where natives of almost all the islands of the Indian Archipelago were met with ; Manilla, Hong Kong, Sydney (Austral negroes), New Zealand, Tahiti (where were the aborigines of New Caledonia and Norfolk Island), Chili, and Peru.

The results obtained by the extensive series of measurements thus procured, will shortly be published to the world, in the volumes now in preparation at Vienna. The History of the important Voyage of the Novara, a popular illustrated work, from the journals of the commanders, Commodore Wüllustorf and Dr. Scherzer, may be expected to be issued from the Imperial printing office, in Vienna, to be followed by an English translation, in the early part of the present year. It is proposed that this shall be succeeded by a number of other volumes on distinct subjects. 1. Those on nautical, astronomical, meteorological, magnetical, and other observations relating to Physical Geography, by Commodore Wüllustorf. 2. Geology, by Dr. Hochstetter. 3. Zoölogy, by Messrs. Fraunfeld and Zelebor. 4. Ethnography, by Dr. Scherzer. 5. Statistics and Natural Economy, by the same. 6. Medicine (Pathological and Pharmacognostical Researches), by Dr. Schwarz. And lastly, 7. An Album selected from nearly two thousand five hundred sketches made by Mr. Sellery, the artist of the expedition. Whenever this grand programme, which will have the best wishes of men of science in all countries. shall have been completed, the rich results of the first Austrian Circumnavigatory Expedition, placed, as it has been, in able and well-instructed hands, will, we have no doubt, vindicate the national character in a new and much nobler field of enterprise, and give to that country a far more lasting and more dignified fame than any she has hitherto acquired.

Note.—Such is the inconvenience resulting from the use of a variety of metre scales, and such a number of methods of measurement, frequently taking quite different points for measures bearing the same name, as in the case of the skull especially, that the distinguished Prof. Von Bær, of St. Petersburg, has just proposed a Congress of Anthropologists, to determine upon one uniform scale, and to establish one system. By this means all the results of measurement of the human body would be rendered of universal applicability.—*Nachrichten über die ethnog. craniol. Sammlung zu St. Petersburg. S.* 81. *American Journal of Science and Arts,* May, 1860.

ART. VII.—*On the Action of the Auriculo-Ventricular Valves of the Heart:* By. W. T. GAIRDNER, M. D., Edinburgh ; Physician to the Royal Infirmary, Edinburgh ; Lecturer on the Practice of Medicine, etc.   Read before the British Association.

MY object in this communication is to call attention to certain points in the mechanical arrangement of the auriculo-ventricular valves ; I shall leave the members present to draw, to a great extent, their own conclusions as to the bearing of these points on the physiology and pathology of the valves.   The manner in which my own attention has been attracted to the subject was as follows :   I have been for many years in the habit of observing that cases occurred, not unfrequently, in which indications appeared during the life of the patient of regurgitation through the mitral orifice, but in which, afterwards, the valves appeared by no means insufficient.   In many of these cases there was, no doubt, some slight degree of thickening of the valves or widening of the orifice ; but, in some of them the amount of disease and of deformity appeared so trifling, as to necessitate the conclusion that the source of regurgitation was to be sought in the muscular structures, rather than in the orifice itself. Pursuing this line of inquiry I was led to the conviction that certain morbid conditions of the ventricle, and particularly dilatation of its apex, exercised a much more considerable influence on the condition of the valve than was commonly supposed ; and, in particular, that the relative position of the carneæ columnæ had not been sufficiently studied in relation to the action of the valve.   In proof of this, I may mention that in some of the most recent and authoritative works on physiology these structures are represented in diagrams as being, during the ventricular systole, in a position which I believe to be totally inconsistent with the closure of the valve.

I will now proceed to demonstrate the true position, which was rightly apprehended by Bouillaud, when he described the insertion of the chordæ tendineæ into the fleshy columns, as the apex of a cone of which the valve formed the base.   If the heart of a sheep or bullock be chosen, of which the left ventricle is in a state of firm tonic contraction, the ventricle being empty of blood ; and if such a heart be cut into transverse slices, or opened in such a way as to show the relations of the large fleshy columns which connect the chordæ tendineæ with the opposite sides of the ventricle, it will be seen that the columns of opposite sides lie most accurately in apposition, and that the surfaces are fitted to each other with almost as much nicety as the opposite molar teeth of the upper and lower jaw. The effect of this arrangement is, that the contraction of the apex of the ventricle completely obliterates the interspace between these columns, and gathers all the ends of the chordæ tendineæ into one single point in the middle of the ventricle.   Nothing can be more beautiful and regular than this arrangement in the left ventricle ; in the right it is, perhaps, not so perfect—at all events it is less easily demonstrated.   Now, let it be remembered that the first act of the ventricular contraction is precisely this contraction of the apex, and the effect of the mechanism in question will become obvious.   In fact, if the contraction of the heart be carefully observed in a cold-blooded animal, or even in an animal under artificial respiration, and when it is becoming slow, it will be seen that the contraction of the auricles is propagated not to the ventricles in all parts simultaneously, but to the back part and apex first, and then to the conus arteriosus, or front and upper part of the ventricle. Accordingly, the systole of the conus arteriosus, or cavity, properly speaking, of the ventricle, is preceded by a movement among the fibres of the apex, which brings the columnæ carneæ, and therefore the tendinous cords of the opposite sides, into the closest possible apposition. Is this mechanism, or is it not, essential to the closure of the valve? That it is so, in all probability may be shown by an experiment on the left side of the heart. It is well known that John Hunter, followed by Dr. Adams, of Dublin, and Dr. Wilkinson King, of London, held the view that the tricuspid valve was naturally an imperfect one. They admitted however, that the mitral was a perfect valve, and might be made to act in the dead body. On repeating this experiment, however, I found that the competency of even the mitral valve was essentially dependent upon the condition of the ventricle. The moment that the ventricle became distended so as to separate considerably the opposite sides of its apex portion, leakage of the valve began. I am by no means satisfied that the right auriculo-ventricular valve is, any more than the left, an imperfect one, in the normal state of the ventricle ; but undoubtedly its competency is more easily overcome, and is not to be demonstrated after death in most instances.—*Dublin Hospital Gazette.*

ART. VIII. — *Chloroform in Neuralgia and Rheumatism:* By MR. LITTLE, F. R. S. C. E., of Singapore. (Medico-Chirurgical Society of Edinburgh, March 7, 1860.)

A NEW APPLICATION OF CHLOROFORM IN NEURALGIA AND IN CERTAIN RHEUMATIC COMPLAINTS. — During my residence in Singapore, East Indies, I was at one time in the habit of using liquor ammoniæ to produce an immediate blister, when instantaneous counter-irritation was thought necessary in certain cerebral affections, etc.; a piece of lint, soaked in ammonia, being applied to the part, and covered with oil-silk, when in a few minutes so much irritation was produced as to raise a blister. In administering chloroform to my patients, I noticed that their lips were often partially blistered by it ; and recollecting the mode of using the ammonia, I thought of trying the chloroform in the same way, but found that neither oil-silk nor gutta percha tissue would answer. I then used a watch-glass to cover the lint soaked in it, and with the best effect.

The manner of application is to take a piece of lint, a little less in size than the watch-glass to be used (which need not be more than two inches in diameter), put it on the hollow side of the glass, to pour on it a few drops of chloroform sufficient to saturate it, and then to apply it at once to the part affected, keeping the edges of the glass closely applied to the skin by covering it with the hand, for the purpose of keeping it in position, as well as of assisting the evaporation of the chloroform. This may be done from five to ten minutes, according to the amount of irritation wished for.

The patient, during this time, will complain of the gradual increase of a burning sensation (not so severe as that produced by a mustard sinapism), which reaches its height in five minutes, and then abates, but does not entirely disappear for more than ten minutes.

To insure the full operation of the remedy, it is necessary that the watch-glass be rather concave, that it be closely applied to the skin, and that the hand applied over it be sensibly warm. The immediate effect of the application is to remove all local pain in neuralgia, and relieve that of rheumatism.

Its effects on the skin are at first a reddening of the cutis, which, in some cases, is followed by desquamation of the cuticle; but this depends on the part to which it is applied, and also upon the susceptibility of the individual. In some cases, if the application has been prolonged, a dark brown stain remains even for a week or ten days, the same effect as sometimes follows the use of a mustard sinapism.

In Singapore I have used chloroform after this fashion in various neuralgias of the face, in inflammations of the eye and ear, in one case of angina pectoris, in several cases of neuralgia affecting the abdominal parietes, in lumbago, dysmenorrhœa, and in pain attending congestion of the ovary, etc.

Personally, I can testify to its great efficacy in two severe attacks of rheumatic inflammation of the eyes, in which the pain came on periodically about 3, A. M., with such severity that I thought the loss of sight itself would be preferable to its continuance. All other remedies, such as blisters, leeches, opium externally and internally, belladonna, etc., were of no avail in soothing the pain; water almost boiling, applied by a sponge, giving only a little relief. I then thought of this use of chloroform, remembering how much it had benefited my patients in other similar affections. The first night, the application of it to the temple relieved the pain in ten minutes; on its return the next night, the application again relieved it; and four times only was it required to remove completely the local pain; allowing, in the meantime, constitutional remedies to produce their effect. Since my return to this country, I have recommended this remedy on several occasions to persons suffering from neuralgia of the face and head, and always with the same good effects as in India; and the other evening one of my domestics was quickly and effectually relieved by it of a painful spasmodic contraction of the platysma myoides muscle, which prevented her raising her head from her chest. The chloroform was applied as directed, with immediate benefit, and next morning she was quite well, though in previous attacks several days elapsed before relief was obtained. I have mentioned this method to several medical men of this city, who have found it of great benefit ; and that it may be more extensively known, is my reason for now bringing it before the profession.

Dr. Keiller mentioned that this plan had been tried with success in his wards.

Dr. Wright had used chloroform for similar purposes, by pouring it into a bottle containing blotting paper, and applying it over the affected painful part. He has found it sometimes produce vesication, and leave a mark on the skin ; but it had been effectual in removing pain.

[Mr. Little has received the following letter from Dr. Sclanders, House Physician to Dr. Keiller, in the Royal Infirmary :

ROYAL INFIRMARY, March 14, 1860.

My Dear Sir—I have much pleasure in giving you the result of my experience in regard to the external application of chloroform in the way proposed by you. Soon after you made me aware of it, I saw a friend of mine who suffered frequently from neuralgia of the left forehead. I proposed the remedy to him, and with the effect of immediately removing the pain. Owing to my having kept it too long applied, vesication ensued. Since then he has had no return.

I have since used it in several cases of neuralgia of the ovary and pleurodynia, as also in two cases of rheumatic pains in the joints, with marked benefit.

I am yours, truly, ALEX. SCLANDERS.

DR. LITTLE.]—*Edinburgh Medical Journal*, April, 1860.

ART. IX.—*On a New Method for Effecting the Radical Cure of Hernia :* By JOHN WOOD, F. R. C. S., Eng. (Royal Medical and Chirurgical Society.)

THE author commenced by a brief sketch of the *anatomy of the inguinal region.* The peculiarities of structure of the parts concerned in inguinal hernia, of which especial advantage is taken in the operation proposed and practised by the author, are : 1st. The mobility and sliding power of the skin in the groin, owing to the synovial character and loose areolar meshes of the deep layer of superficial fascia. 2d. The total absence of fat from the areolar tissue of the scrotum, its density, elasticity, toughness, and great vascularity, enabling the surgeon to invaginate it into the inguinal canal, to retain it there by stitches, and cause it permanently to adhere to its sides and to the cord. 3d. The protection afforded to the peritoneum and vessels (epigastric and circumflex iliac) by the intervention of the fascia transversalis, and its connection with the deep surface of Poupart's ligament. 4th. The formation by the conjoined tendon of the internal oblique and transversalis muscles, and triangular ligament of the greater portion of the posterior wall of the canal, and the feasibility of raising the former by the finger passed into the canal behind the lower edge of the internal oblique muscle, so as to pass a needle through it and the internal pillar of the external abdominal ring together. The author then stated that the methods respectively practised by Ragg, Bonnet, Gerdy, and more lately by Wützer, of Bonn, and Rothmund, of Munich, most frequently fail in producing a permanent cure, chiefly by their not obtaining a hold upon the posterior wall of the canal, and their securing only the anterior portion of the fold produced by invagination, leaving the posterior half of the fold ready for the reception of a fresh portion of intestine. The objections to the introduction of a hard dilating plug into the invaginated fold of skin, and its retention, by Wützer's method, are, that the skin and fasciæ, intervening into two layers between the compressing hard surfaces and the serous laminæ of the invaginated sac, ward off from them, in great measure, the effect intended—that of adhesive inflammation ; while the absence of counterpressure behind the posterior fold renders the dilating force of the plug almost nugatory, unless sufficient expanding power to cause sloughing be employed—to the great distress, not to say danger, of the patient. The dilating action of the plug upon the canal and external ring, leaves the latter in a worse condition than before, in case of the failure of the operation. The principle of plugging up a dilatable aperture, like the inguinal opening, is false. The invaginated skin invariably descends when the consolidation is absorbed, the latter being temporary only in its duration. The principle of the author's operation is directly opposite to that of dilatation—namely : that of drawing together and compressing the anterior and posterior walls of the canal in its whole length, and their union by the adhesive process with the invaginated fascia of the scrotum, which is detached from the skin and transplanted into the canal, the skin being left to adhere below to the approximated margins of the external abdominal ring. By this means the posterior wall of the inguinal canal is made to act as a valve to prevent any future descent of the bowel, shutting up the superior opening by becoming united to the anterior wall through the medium of the scrotal fascia, which thus affords a very highly organized and vascular connective tissue between the tendinous surfaces, which it would be very difficult to cause to adhere together otherwise. The fascial invagination becomes likewise firmly adherent to the spermatic cord. This continues to be effective, even when the temporary effusion of lymph is reäbsorbed.

The Operation.—This consists, first, in detaching the scrotal fascia from the skin over the lowest part of the hernial protrusion, with a tenotomy knife, and then invaginating the fascia into the canal with the forefinger ; secondly, in passing a strong, well-curved needle, fixed in a handle, armed with a stout, thick thread, and guided by the finger, through three points in the canal, viz : the conjoined tendon and the triangular fascia (forming the posterior wall), and the external pillar of the ring close to Poupart's ligament (forming the anterior wall of the canal). The ends of the ligature are left in the two former punctures, and a central loop in the latter, passing though the pillars of the external ring, and through the same aperture in the skin of the groin. This may readily be done by sliding upon the subjacent aponeurosis. Thirdly, a cylindrical or flattened compress of glass or box-wood, two inches and a half long by one inch wide, is tied firmly upon the axis of the canal, by passing the ends of the ligature through the loop, and tying over the compress. Before tightening the ligature, the surgeon should satisfy himself, by passing the forefinger through the external ring, that the ligatures draw upon the posterior wall. The opening in the scrotum should be tucked well up to, but not within, the external ring.

In recent cases of hernia, in which the sac is small and possesses an intimate vascular connection with the peritoneum, and a very slight one with the cord, it may be pushed back into the superior opening, and the ligature applied altogether external to, and without puncturing, the sac, thus diminishing very much the chances of peritoneal inflammation. But in old and large herniæ, the sac has a more intimate vascular connection with the scrotum and cord, and constitutes, as it were, a separate structure, distinct from the peritoneum. In these cases the sac is necessarily invaginated with the fascia, and the ligatures pass through it. In these the inflammation set up in the sac is much less liable to spread into the abdominal cavity, especially when the upper orifice is closed by the ligature. In a large sac the adhesive process is necessary to complete obliteration of the canal, and to prevent future complications.

The compress is removed from the fourth to the seventh day, according to the degree of action set up. The ligatures may be left in a week or two longer, to act as conductors for the discharges, and to keep up consolidating action as long as may be desirable. When the sac is punctured, serous fluid flows from the wound in greater or less quantity during the first three or four days.

The author called attention to the action of the rectus muscle upon the inguinal canal, through the conjoined tendon, in drawing backward the posterior wall of the hernial canal, thus aiding the dilating action of the protruding bowel in the production and growth of the hernia. The effect of the ligatures, and consequent adhesions, in his operation, directly counteracts this action of the rectus. He considers that the first tendency to oblique inguinal hernia, so often hereditary, is owing to deficient development of the lower fibres of the internal oblique producing an imperfect covering to the internal ring. In some of the cases operated on, he has succeeded in supplementing this deficiency by passing the scrotal fascia well up in front of the internal abdominal ring, and securing it to Poupart's ligament in that position.

He considered that the chief source of failure in the performance of his operation, especially in large and old cases, is in not securing a hold upon the posterior wall. By simply attaching the fascia to the pillars of the external ring, and drawing the latter together, the hernia, though prevented for a time from descending into the scrotum, still occupies the canal, and will, sooner or later, again dilate the external ring, unless constantly bolstered up by a truss. The closing of the external ring by the lower ligatures, in this operation, contributes much, however, to secure in its new position in the canal the transplanted fascia.

In small cases of direct hernia, the closure or obliteration of the external ring only may be effective in producing a cure, if care be taken to obtain a hold with the inner end of the ligature upon the triangular fascia covering the border of the rectus, immediately behind the opening of the external ring. In noticing the objections to the plan, the author showed that, by properly protecting the point of the needle with the finger, and keeping in front of the fascia transversalis, all danger of wounding the epigastric and circumflex iliac vessels or the bowel was guarded against.

The fear of peritonitis is avoided in recent cases (in which it is most to be dreaded), by not puncturing the sac at all, but closing up the tendinous opening external to it. In old cases, adhesive action may be set up in the sac without fear of its spreading to the peritoneum, as the results of numerous cases have shown. The objections made to the limited incision into the skin of the scrotum (which is little more than a puncture), he considers to be puerile: Its advantages in permitting the escape of discharges are evident.

Reports of fifteen cases of hernia (all inguinal) were appended. One of the cases was a boy of eight years of age; the ages of the others ranged from fifteen to fifty-four and fifty-eight years. One was a female with bubonocele; the rest were males. Three were cases of direct, the rest oblique hernia. Thirteen were scrotal; four of large size, and three with very large and lax internal openings. Two were congenital and two complicated with vericocele (cured also by the operation). In only one case were the symptoms at all severe, or gave suspicion of peritonitis. In this case the patient was in King's College Hospital eight weeks; the symptoms were produced by burrowing of matter between the oblique muscles, following a diarrhœa then prevalent in the hospital (in July last). This patient made an excellent cure, was treated entirely without truss, and was one of the cases shown to the Society. The hernia had a very large internal opening, and the subject was cachectic and ill-nourished before the operation. In one other case the patient was in bed a month; in another there was partial sloughing of the sac, which was a large and long one, with a very pendulous scrotum, and a large vericocele. This case was treated also entirely without truss, and both hernia and vericocele were cured in eighteen days. The duration of treatment in the rest of the cases varied from nine to twenty-one days. Eight were treated entirely without truss. Thirteen are good and persistent cures, and have remained firm ever since, extending over the following periods of time: one (the first), very nearly two years (this case was published in the *Lancet* of the 29th of May, 1858); another one year; two ten months; four nine months; three eight months; one two months. Three of the cases had been before operated upon by Wützer's and Ragg's methods :

one case was operated on twice; one is doubtful ; one was reruptured by indiscreet and early hard lifting without truss.

Six cases of cure were exhibited. Of these, four had been treated entirely without truss, and all had been well, and some severely, tested by lifting and heavy labor. The first case (operated on nearly two years ago) was amongst those exhibited. No difference whatever was apparent between the groins of the two sides. One had been cured in a year, three in nine months, and one in eight months. One of those treated without truss was congenital, in a young man aged twenty years ; another was of five years' standing, in a man aged fifty-eight. The rest were of eighteen, sixteen, and three months' standing respectively. All were scrotal herniæ, and two direct. Two had chronic bronchitis (at times severe) after the operation, and one during the progress of the cure.

The paper was illustrated by diagrams.—*Brit. Med. Jour.*

ART. X.—*Disinfection of Wounds and Ulcers.*

WHILE M. Velpeau has been testing, at the Hospital of La Charité, the efficacy of MM. Carne and Demaux's disinfecting powder, other surgeons have been experimenting elsewhere with similar agents, proposed by various individuals, and submitted to the different medical boards for approval or investigation.

M. Boys de Loury, surgeon-in-chief to the Hospital of St. Lazare, has recently published some experiments on the comparative efficacy of the powder of plaster and coal tar of the Central Pharmacy (Pharmacie Centrale), and the compresses, papers, charpie, and other carboniferous preparations of MM. Pichot and Malapert. The following is a resumé of his observations :

Eight patients, affected with ulceration of the whole circumference of the cervix uteri, were every day treated by applying to, and keeping in contact with, the uterus a carboniferous pessary ; and, when the ulcer began to assume a better appearance, touching it with nitrate of silver. Eight other patients, affected with only partial ulceration of the cervix, were treated by applying pessaries impregnated with the powder of plaster and coal tar. The advantage of the former mode of treatment over this, was in the proportion of the first series of eight being cured respectively in 18, 19, 20, 22, 25, 32, 41, and 45 days, to the second series in 30, 33, 35, 40, 44, 49, 60, and 67 days.

The following examples refer exclusively to the effects of MM. Pichot and Malapert's carboniferous preparations : A woman of fifty-five years old, after having been three times admitted to the hospital on account of a fungous ulcer on the left leg, and who each time had been at least three or four months under treatment, was admitted a fourth time, and treated on this last occasion by the carboniferous plan—the "charpie carbonifere" being applied to the ulcer. She was discharged cured in five weeks.

A girl from the country, suffering for a long period from syphilitic tubercles, extending over the labia and part of the anus, and much exhausted by pain and the disease itself, was put upon the prot-iodide of mercury and the local application of charpie carbonifere. The insufferable odor of the ulcers was rapidly lessened, the ulcers themselves improved, and the constitutional symptoms removed, under this treatment.

In a young girl, convalescent from typhus fever, the same application was made to ulcerations over both trochanters, with the effect of inducing a rapid cure.

In the case of two patients affected with cancer—one in the breast, the other in the uterus—the employment of the "sachets carboniferes" removed the odor, and diminished the quantity of the purulent secretion, but did not seem to influence the fatal progress of the disease.

Lastly, in a case of encephaloid cancer of the uterus, where the discharges were so offensive as almost to prevent any approach towards the patient, a paste, formed of the powder of plaster and coal tar, previously mentioned, was introduced into the vagina, with the perfect removal of all disagreeable odor, and with the patient enabled, in this way, to see her friends during her last moments, all other disinfectants having failed.—*Gaz des Hôp. Edinburgh Medical Journal*, May, 1860.

Art. XI.—*Account of the Results of Amputations Observed at Constantinople during the Crimean War:* By M. de Salleron. (Recueil Mémoires de Médecine et de Chirurgie Militaires, deuxième série, tome xxii, pp. 262–420.)

This is another testimony to the enormous sufferings of the French army during the Crimean war, and a silent protest against the disparaging comparisons heretofore instituted between it and the British army. M. Salleron was in charge of the Dolma-Bagtche Hospital, at Constantinople, which he represents as of faulty construction and defective in hygienic appliances. Any mischief which would have resulted from these circumstances alone, was augmented by the unavoidable over-crowding of its wards with the wounded soldiers.

The immediate object of the author's paper is to give an account of the amputations performed and treated under these painful circumstances, and especially to point out the greater amount of mortality that attended secondary amputations. He selects the period from the 1st of May to the 1st of November, 1855, as being that during which the comparison he desires to institute may be best made. During it, 2753 gun-shot wounds were admitted, of which more than one half were of a very severe character. Of the 2753 patients, 2009 were either discharged, or more often transferred to France for ulterior treatment, and 744 died. After great engagements, the subjects of amputation were usually evacuated upon Constantinople as soon as possible, arriving there three or four days after the performance of the operations, with the stumps, as regards dressing, bandages, and cleanliness, in a most unsatisfactory condition. These operations and those performed in the trenches, are entered in the hospital registers as immediate amputations, the secondary ones being those performed afterwards at the hospital itself. The bulk of these latter were also performed from five to ten days after the accident. The total number of amputations was 639; *i. e.*, 490 amputations in continuity and 149 disarticulations. Of the 639, 419 were primary operations, furnishing 221 recoveries and 198 deaths ; and 220 were secondary operations, furnishing 73 recoveries and 147 deaths. Thus, among the 639 cases there were 294 recoveries and 345 deaths, the primary operations yielding more than a half of cures, and the secondary operations yielding but a third.

M. Salleron next examines into the immediate causes of this great mortality after amputation—a result so opposite to that which he and the other French surgeons had been accustomed to in Algeria, where amputations succeed very well. Omitting causes which only operated on a few cases, we find that of the 345 deaths, 65 resulted from gangrene with emphysema, 45 from hospital gangrene, and 228 from purulent infection.

Gangrene with Emphysema.—The author met with gangrene under two forms—*œdematous,* or mild form, and what he terms the *emphysematous or instantaneous* form. No case of the former proved fatal, but rapid death occurred in 65 instances of the latter ; 46 of these had been amputations in continuity, and 19 disarticulations. Among 220 amputations performed in the hospital, 36 cases of this form of gangrene occurred, while among 419 performed in the Crimea, only 29 cases occurred. Those about to be attacked seldom properly rallied after the operation, and were the subjects of great nervous irritation. The attack itself was quite sudden, the limb became rapidly and immensely distended, and soon after blackened, the general symptoms undergoing frightful aggravation. It was not, indeed, peculiar to persons who had been operated upon, as it proved in some of those suffering from wounds rapidly fatal. The progress of the disease was always rapid and continuous, no kind of temporary suspension of its course ever being observed, and its mean duration in the sixty-five cases was from twenty-five to thirty hours. The chief feature was an enormous emphysematous distension, which induced compression of the deep-seated veins. The superficial veins were distended with gaseous fluid, which also separated the fibres of the muscles from each other. These last were pale, but not disorganized. The patient always died, a state of indifference or stupor coming on, and all remedies proving useless. Perhaps the affection should rather be called *emphysema of the stump* than gangrene, for there was not the disorganization of tissues met with in ordinary gangrene—on the contrary, they remained distinct and recognizable, and preserved their consistency, relations, and organization.

Hospital Gangrene.—Besides the well-known ulcerative and pulta- ceous forms of the disease, the author met with a small number of examples of another form, hitherto unknown to him, and which he designates as *caseous,* which attacked stumps nearly healed. The lower angle of the stump became violaceous and engorged, and a small excavation formed, which soon filled with matter of a sabace- ous consistency and of a grayish color. This constantly increased in quantity as the excavation, which was lined by a soft membrane, rapidly augmented in size. The progress of the affection was at once arrested, while it yet seemed local in its operation, by the actual cautery or nitric acid. Hospital gangrene, in the two other forms, affected many patients besides those who had undergone am- putation ; and the author regards it as a manifestation of a general pathological rather than a local condition, the air-passages being the ordinary vehicle of its transmission. He found local treatment of little or no avail, unless the overcrowding could be diminished and ventilation secured, which, under the circumstances, was rarely possi- ble. Of the great number of local applications tried, the *perchloride of iron* succeeded best. In 30 cases, where all other treatment seemed unavailing, amputation was performed, 14 of the patients dying, and 16 recovering. In none of the 30 cases was there relapse of the gan- grene, nor did one of them die of the immediate effects of the operation.

Purulent infection.—This prevailed in the Constantinople hospitals from the period of the battle of the Alma to the end of the campaign, and proved the principal cause of death after wounds and operations. It especially manifested itself in the case of osseous lesions, however slight these might be. Fractures of the shafts of the long bones were always rapidly followed by pyæmia, rendering any subsequent operation useless and mischievous, inasmuch as this but accelerated the progress of the general affection, as of 490 amputations performed in continuity, 192 terminated fatally, while but 32 of 49 disarticula- tions exhibited a like issue. The author has found no description of treatment useful, and recommends only that symptoms should be combated as they manifest themselves.—*British and Foreign Medico- Chirurgical Review*, April, 1860.

ART. XII.—*Acupressure in Surgical Operations.* (Medico-Chirurgical Society of Edinburgh, Wednesday, 4th April, 1860.)

DR. ALEXANDER SIMPSON showed a cast of the first stump, in which acupressure had been applied in England after amputation. In reference to it, Dr. Simpson read the following extracts from letters from Mr. Dickenson Crompton, Senior Surgeon to the Birmingham General Hospital, addressed to Professor Simpson :

17 Temple Row, Birmingham, March 8, 1860.

Dear Sir: According to my promise, I write to tell you that last Wednesday week (February 29) I removed a young man's knee, for strumous disease in the femur, and consequent degeneration of the cartilages of the knee-joint, using two only of your acupressure needles—one to press upon the femoral artery, and piercing the skin in two places, through the short flap, about half an inch from the cut extremity of the artery ; and the other needle was passed through the long anterior flap, to press upon *two* small muscular branches. The operation was the one recommended by Mr. Teale, of Leeds ; no dressings being applied, but metal sutures at intervals. The bleeding was entirely controlled ; and, after fifty-two hours, I oiled, and then rotated the needles before and during their withdrawal. I had perceived strong pulsation against the needle which pressed upon the femoral for some hours after the operation ; but by the third day, in the evening, when I went to withdraw them, the motion communicated to the needle was hardly perceptible, and *I believe* the *profunda* was pulsating more strongly where it is given off than any part of the femoral below it. The man has progressed thus far excellently well, though there appeared every prospect of matter forming on the inside of the thigh, two or three inches *above* where the needle was inserted.

Last Wednesday (that is, March 7) I removed the arm, above the elbow, of a man æt. 65, at his own wish and request, on account of a large cancerous ulceration affecting the cicatrix of an old and very extensive burn. I used two of your needles, and found, what experince will teach others, that the loose structures in elderly people will require more care in applying the needles so as to make sufficient pressure. Two small muscular arteries were secured by passing a common harelip needle through the skin on one side, and deeply into the muscular structure of the flap, on and over the arteries, not again penetrating the skin, which did not seem necessary. The old man has a bad cough, but at present there has been no bleeding. I shall remove the needles to-morrow night, and will keep this note open to give you the result.

At present I see no reason to return to the use of the ligature, though I should be sorry to find that too much will be expected from the more extensive use of the needles ; for I cannot believe that we shall be so fortunate by their use alone to escape altogether from that bane of surgery, "pus poisoning," after amputations, because I am certain that, at least in two-thirds of these cases, the mischief begins in the bone, and not in the cutaneous or more deeply seated veins, and is thence communicated to them, more particularly to some branches of the profunda veins after amputation of the thigh. Too many *post-mortem* examinations have taught me *that.*

Excuse this long story, and accept my thanks for the promptness with which you responded to my request.

The second letter, dated March 29th, was as follows :

17 TEMPLE ROW, BIRMINGHAM, March 29.

My Dear Sir—I hope you will excuse the liberty I am about to take in sending you a basket (not of game), but containing a cast of my first *stump*, at exactly the four weeks' end. It is the thigh case, and Teale's method, with your needles. The young man is well, and the stump has never had a bit of plaister or a roller on it. The old man's arm is nearly well also. And last Monday I was obliged to remove the knee and leg of a young man who had suffered compound fracture into the knee-joint, from a railroad truck passing over his leg. There was great shock, which continued to agitate his pulse till the present time. Nevertheless, I amputated by the circular method ; and using one only of your needles, I controlled the bleeding from both the femoral and a smaller branch in the lower third of the thigh. I intended to have removed the needle at the end of forty-eight hours ; but I felt an artery beating to the very needle, if not just over it ; and the pulse being 130, I was afraid I might not find a clot sufficient to prevent bleeding ; so I waited till this morning (Thursday, 12 o'clock), the amputation having taken place at 12 o'clock on Monday last. The stump looks very well, metal sutures being used, and no plaister, though I put a roller round the thigh to within two inches of the end, but which I intend to remove to-morrow. The stump is laid flat on the bed, with a waterproof cloth under it ; and I intend to treat it as Teale recommends. I may mention that one other small artery was pricked and *torsioned*, and so only one needle was necessary. I have no doubt you will hear of the needle being generally adopted ; and I can only say, I am so pleased with the facility of its use, that, with the *usual* professional feeling, I wished I could have speared *your* thigh, in spite, that you, a "no surgeon," should have hit us purblind surgeons so hard on our own ground. I was sure, as soon as I read your paper, that the *physiology* was right, and that experience only is needed as to how long or how short a time the needles need be allowed to remain *in situ*.

Dr. Simpson also showed a portion of the posterior tibial artery, and read the following letter from M. Foucher, Professor Agrégé of the Faculty of Medicine, and Surgeon to the Necker Hospital, addressed to Dr. M'Gavin, of Paris :

"The 18th March I was called, in the course of the day, to the Necker Hospital, the surgical service of which I am at present charged with, to see a patient whose left foot had just been completely crushed by a wagon passing over it. I deemed it necessary to amputate immediately; and, after having examined the state of the parts, I decided on performing amputation at the lower third of the leg (amputation *sus-malleolaire*) by the double-flap method. The patient having been subjected to the influence of chloroform, I cut from without inwards an anterior flap ; the anterior tibial artery being divided, I immediately raised the flap, and passed a needle from the skin towards the bleeding surface, then from the latter towards the skin, thus bridging over the vessel according to the method of Professor Simpson ; the bleeding stopped immediately

I then cut the posterior flap by transfixion ; and the posterior tibial and peroneal arteries having been divided, I placed a needle over each of them, as I had already done in the case of the anterior tibial artery. The needle which compressed the posterior tibial artery having traversed the posterior tibial nerve, I judged it proper to withdraw it, in order to replace it by another, which should compress the vessel only. The section of the soft parts having been completed, I sawed the bones ; and the interosseous artery giving forth some blood, I transfixed the member obliquely with a long needle, which compressed the vessel against the fibula. It was evident to me, as well as to the internes of the hospital present at the operation, that acupressure constitutes a hæmostatic method speedy and easy of application (un moyen hæmostatique prompt et facile à appliquer).

"An hour after the operation I dressed the stump, bringing together the flaps by means of the twisted suture. The following day two of the needles were removed, and not a drop of blood was observed to follow. I must, however, add, that the general state of the patient is bad ; from the moment of the operation he has been agitated and slightly delirious ; the flaps are swelled and blackish ; the limb is infiltrated with gas ; and my belief is that he will die.

" I do not for a moment entertain the idea that the unfortunate state of the patient is in any degree due to acupressure. Such an idea would be simply absurd. I am too well acquainted with the results of amputations in cases of traumatic lesions ; I know too well what the general disturbance of the œconomy is in such cases, and how often contusion of the soft parts brings about gangrene of the stump ; so that, far from being shaken (by this circumstance) in my conviction that acupressure is a useful measure, I am now in a position to demonstrate that it, as a hæmostatic, has a positive action, and offers as much security as the *ligature;* and I trust that, when I shall meet with a case of amputation of a more favorable kind than the above, that I shall be able to bring about the most incredulous to my manner of thinking.

"These, my dear sir, are the important details which I conceived it my duty to transmit to you, and which you will perhaps have the goodness to communicate to Professor Simpson, to whom is due the honor of this discovery. You may further assure him that I, in adopting this method, am resolved to keep a good watch over it (faire bonne garde autour d'elle), that no one, French or foreigner, shall dispute with him its priority."

In an accompanying letter Dr. M'Gavin adds :

" While I was in the wards of the Necker on Thursday morning, a man was brought in with a formidable scalp-wound, bleeding most profusely. On examining it, it was found that the temporal artery had been divided. Acupressure was employed by Foucher with perfect success."

The further history of the case of amputation is contained in the following letter from Dr. M'Gavin, dated 28th March, 1860 :

" Foucher sends me this morning the following details regarding the patient operated on at the Necker Hospital; and as I consider them, in more respects than one, as of the very greatest interest, I hasten to make you acquainted with them. The enclosed is the lower portion of the posterior tibial artery, which will enable you to judge of the ossified condition of the vessels. Let me hope it may not be crushed in its transit through the postoffice. By gently macerating it, you will be the better able to judge of its real condition.   J. D. M'GAVIN."

" *Cher Monsieur*—As I had foreseen, my patient at the Necker died, and the autopsy took place yesterday. The mortification which threatened the soft parts of the leg increased during the latter days of the patient's life; and foreseeing a fatal issue, I allowed the acupressure needles (those of the under and posterior tibials) to remain, the two others having been removed the morning of the third day after the operation. At the autopsy we were enabled to satisfy ourselves that the two needles compressed firmly the anterior and the posterior tibial arteries; that, on a level with the needles, the walls of the arteries had not undergone the slightest alteration nor destruction. In the interior of the vessels was found an obliterating clot, which, in the case of the posterior tibial, was firmly adhering to the extremity of the cut arterial tube. I may add, and this appears to me a new point in the history of acupressure, that the two arteries were ossified for a considerable distance above the wound, and that their walls *were rigid and friable*.

" This disposition or condition of the vessels, which is altogether unfavorable to the employment of the *ligature*, did not interfere in the slightest degree with the success of acupressure, which, up to the last moment, gave us all we asked of it—to-wit: complete arrestation of hæmorrhage.   Yours always,   FOUCHER.
" à M. le Doct. M'GAVIN, etc."

Dr. M'Gavin adds:
"P. S.—As the needles used here are abominable, from the tendency they have to *oxidize*, I should esteem it a favor to myself, and a duty to Foucher in the cause of acupressure, if you would forward by post a few at your earliest convenience. In a few days we shall have another amputation."

Dr. P. H. Watson asked whether, in any of these cases, union had taken place by the first intention.

Dr. A. Simpson replied, that he knew no more regarding the cases than was contained in the letters which he had read to the Society.
                    Edinburgh Medical Journal, May, 1860.

ART. XIII.—*On Special Position and the Obstetric Binder as Aids in the Treatment of Impeded Parturition:* By ROBERT HARDEY, Esq. [Obstetrical Society of London, March 7th, 1860.]

THE position advocated in this paper was the sedentary on chairs, to which the author's attention had been first directed in 1827, under the direction of the late Mr. R. M. Craven, Sen., of Hull. From that period to the present he had adopted this mode of management (and had recommended the same to his obstetric class at the Hull and East Riding School of Medicine) in all cases where the difficulties to be overcome demanded more than ordinary efforts for the accomplishment of the delivery. The author observed that in our treatment of labor generally we were apt to ignore the important fact, that the activities of parturition were dependent altogether on muscular power—*ergo*, all agents which sustained and increased motor force were real benefits to the parturient female, and *vice versa*. Of these excitors of motor power, two of the most valuable were the sedentary posture and the obstetric binder.

Mr. Hardey next pointed out the advantages and disadvantages resulting from a variety of parturient positions, viz : standing, reclining on the back, prone, and horizontal postures, and concluded this part of his subject by a strong recommendation of the sedentary posture on or between two chairs. The plan adopted was to secure the fronts of two chairs to each other, and then separate their back parts from one and a half to two feet ; to place the patient well over or between these, with her knees firmly pressed against the side of the bed, her chest fixed by holding on to the foot-post of the bed, and her feet placed firmly on the floor. The accoucheur sat or knelt behind his patient, who remained on the chairs till the difficulties in the case had been overcome, which was evidenced by the emerging of the parietal bones from behind the perinæum. The woman was to be then removed to bed, and finally delivered in the ordinary position. Before seating the patient, her abdomen was to be carefully sustained by a broad binder, to which Mr. Hardey attached far greater importance than is conceded to it generally. The views advanced were illustrated by diagrams and drawings. In every case, before adopting the sedentary posture, the part presenting should be somewhat within the pelvis, and the os uteri half dilated. The practice was contraindicated by—1st, impending systemic exhaustion ; 2d, inflammation in any vital organ or part more immediately associated with parturition, serious uterine hæmorrhage, previous puerperal convulsions, version presentations, a pulsating funis, and extreme pelvic obliquity. The agents named, the author maintained, secured to the parturient female in impeded labors—q, the very important aid derived from gravitation in the uterine ovum; b, the putting forth under the most favorable circumstances the highest amount of motor energy of which nature is capable ; c, the bringing the abdominal and pelvic axes into the same obstetric plane ; and d, the imparting great support to the fundus uteri in its contractions by the obstetric binder. He strongly recommended the use of the binder before delivery in a variety of cases, independent of its connection with the chairs, as an agent which usually accelerated the birth of the infant in a remarkable manner. The parturient conditions demanding the use of the chairs and binder were those arising from both mother and infant, in which unusual delay or difficulty presented themselves. The treatment of these was illustrated by cases, illustrative of the efficacy of the plans advocated. The period required for the delivery varied with the obstacles to be overcome, from one to two hours being ordinarily sufficient, with an interval of repose on the bed.

In conclusion, Mr. Hardey commended the practice to his professional brethren from the following considerations : 1st, its great simplicity ; 2d, its entire freedom from danger *per se ;* 3d, its very great potency; 4th, its testing the ability of nature to accomplish the delivery at a period sufficiently early to enable the accoucheur to decide on the use of instruments before material damage had been sustained by the maternal tissues ; 5th, the conscious satisfaction experienced by the woman at feeling her labor is progressing towards completion ; and lastly, its being a great economist of professional time, which, to medical men, is property of the most valuable description.

Dr. Granville was not a sufficient adept in mathematics to understand clearly the diagrams which had been handed round. But the author, by his description of cases, had shown that a practice which it was the fashion to laugh at throughout a part of Europe, might be very usefully adopted. He believed that it was a most common custom for women to be delivered in a sedentary posture in Russia, Greece, Algeria, and some portion of Switzerland ; and also in Germany, when midwives were in attendance. Had, therefore, this practice, which was that adopted by the ancient Greeks and Romans, been found otherwise than useful, it would long since have been abandoned.

Dr. Druitt thought the paper was a valuable one ; for, although it advocated nothing new, yet it was advisable to remind the fellows of the advantages to be derived from adopting the practice recommended by Mr. Hardey. The publication of the paper might also be useful in removing much of the pedantry by which the practice of midwifery was at present surrounded, as well as by showing that the British school was not altogether faultless. He believed that the instincts of most women would lead them voluntarily to adopt the sedentary position, if they were allowed to do so ; and certainly this would very often be the case in difficult labors.

Mr. Pollock said that he could speak from an experience of thirty years ; and he believed that the occasional adoption of the sedentary posture often rendered the use of instruments unnecessary.

Dr. Graily Hewitt wished to know the number of cases in which the author had adopted the method now recommended.

Mr. Hardey was not prepared to give an exact answer.

Dr. Rigby remarked that the adoption of the sitting posture in labor was of the greatest antiquity. He need only remind the fellows of the words of the King of Egypt, as recorded in Exodus : " When ye do the office of a midwife to the Hebrew women, and see them upon the stools." In the present day he believed it was not an uncommon custom amongst the Irish poor for the husband to be called in to the lying-in room, so that the woman might sit upon his knees.

After some further observations by Dr. Tanner and Dr. Tyler

Smith, the author replied to the various remarks which had been made ; and at the same time impressed upon the meeting that he only recommended the sedentary posture in certain cases attended with difficulty, inasmuch as the ordinary position on the left side was admirably suited for the greater number of natural labors.—*British Medical Journal.*

ART. XIV.—*Puerperal Convulsions Successfully Treated by Subcutaneous Injections of Morphia:* By Prof. SCANZONI, of Wurtzburg.

SINCE the attention of the medical profession was first directed by Dr. Wood, of Edinburgh, and more lately by Hunter and Béhier, to the advantageous effects of subcutaneous injection, especially of narcotics, Professor Scanzoni has employed this method with success in numerous cases of neuralgia, hyperæsthesia, etc.; but he attaches especial importance to the following case of puerperal convulsions, because it seems to prove, in accordance with the views laid down by Hunter, that the subcutaneous application of narcotic agents furnishes a means of acting on abnormal irritations of the brain with greater rapidity and certainty than the administration of the same remedies by the mouth. It will, doubtless, be admitted that opium, and its different preparations, deserve the first place in the treatment of puerperal eclampsia. In his own experience, the observation of a large number of cases has convinced Professor Scanzoni that a kind of intoxication produced by opium leads with more certainty to a favorable termination than any other means recommended in this terrible disease. But, unfortunately, it is not always possible to administer a sufficient quantity of opium or morphia ; sometimes the comatose condition of the patient, at other times the rapid succession of paroxysms, prevents administration by the mouth ; and opiate enemata are occasionally rejected as soon as they are received. The subcutaneous injection, however, supplies the means by which these difficulties may be overcome, and a sufficient quantity of opium introduced into the system to render its effects certain. Numerous experiments have convinced the author that, although the effect of this method is not always persistent (the neuralgiæ, for example, are not always cured by it), yet there are constantly produced—within a very short time, often a few minutes, after the injection—certain phenomena, which can leave no doubt as to the action of the opium upon the brain. Such symptoms are drowsiness, giddiness, headache, sickness, feeling of constriction in the throat, even vomiting, and depression ; or, if the dose is large, somnolence. These facts, taken along with the known effects of the subcutaneous application in delirium tremens, mania, chorea, tetanus, etc., induced him to try the same treatment in puerperal convulsions, and with the most satisfactory results. After three injections of the meconate of morphia there occurred only two attacks in nine hours, while previously there had been three attacks in an hour and three quarters. This diminution of the convulsions after the injections is so much the more remarkable, since experience has shown that, as a general rule, the paroxysms become not only more violent, but follow at shorter intervals as the labor advances. And although the author does not imagine that he has discovered in the subcutaneous injection an infallible panacea for this dreadful malady, he is of opinion that the following case should induce physicians to give this means a trial :

Case.—D., aged 21, primipara, strong and robust, was brought into the lying-in ward at a quarter to eight o'clock on the morning of June 8th, 1859. Labor had commenced in the night, and she had been seized with nervous paroxysms and loss of consciousness; no account was given of the nature of the attacks ; the patient remembered nothing of what had occurred during the night. The whole body, and especially the lower extremities, were œdematous ; on the right side of the tongue showed marks of being bitten by the teeth ; the uterus corresponded to the pit of the stomach, and seemed sufficiently consistent ; sounds of the fœtal heart distinct. On examination, the os uteri was dilated to the size of a sixpence, the bag of waters was partly formed, and the head presented ; the urine was very albuminous, and exhibited under the microscope numerous fibrinous cylinders. At eight o'clock she was seized with a second convulsive attack, which was of a very marked character, and lasted for some minutes. On recovering consciousness, she could answer questions, although slowly. A third attack succeeded at a quarter to nine, a fourth at a quarter to ten, a fifth at a quarter to twelve, and a sixth at five o'clock—the last the most violent. After the fourth paroxysm consciousness did not return, and the breathing became stertorous. At ten o'clock she was bled to about eight ounces, an enema with twenty-five drops of laudanum was given, the body was put into a warm bath, while cold irrigation was applied to the head. As opium could not be administered internally, a solution of the meconate of morphia was now, at three different times, injected under the skin, the quantity amounting in all to about ten grains (seventy-five centigrammes) of opium. The labor advanced very slowly. At three o'clock next morning the membranes burst; the os dilated to the size of a half crown; the head still high up above the brim ; sounds of the heart very distinct. After this period the dilatation went on more quickly; at seven o'clock the os was larger than a crown piece, very extensive and dilatable, the head high up and immovable ; complete loss of consciousness, profound coma. In these circumstances, which left little hope of saving the patient, and in spite of the high position of the head and the incomplete dilatation of the os uteri, it was decided to employ the forceps. Their application was by no means easy, but the extraction presented no difficulty. After a few tractions, a fœtus was born, which breathed feebly at first, but soon began to moan vigor-

ously ; the placenta followed. During the operation there was no
paroxysm. Some wine and ten drops of tincture of amber and musc
were now given to the patient, which revived her a little, but did not
restore consciousness. At eleven o'clock, a seventh attack came on,
but was slight and short ; after which she became excited and tried
to escape, but towards morning she grew calm. At nine in the
morning she could answer questions put with a loud voice. During
the whole day she remained like a drunk person ; pulse 128. The
musc was stopped ; nothing but lemonade given. Towards evening
the abdomen was somewhat painful. During the night there were
several slight attacks of mania ; she constantly attempted to escape. In the morning she answered rationally : pulse 108. The
œdema had diminished, the abdomen was still tender ; there was
difficulty of breathing ; and numerous râles, fine and coarse, in the
lungs. Warm bath, lemonade, expectorants, were prescribed. In
the evening the patient was completely herself again ; pulse 132.
June 11th and 12th—She slept well during the night, the expectoration becoming easy, and the pain of the abdomen relieved by fomentations and poultices ; pulse 120; the urine contained little albumen,
and no fibrinous cylinders. June 13th—Good condition ; œdema
gone ; abdomen soft ; some incontinence of urine during the night
was relieved by leaving in a catheter. All medicines were now suspended ; the patient was put on good diet, and ordered to take
every morning a glass of chalybeate mineral water. On the 17th
there was no albumen found in the urine, and on the 21st the patient
left the hospital with her child, being advised to continue the use of
steel for a considerable time.—*Bull. Gén. de Thérap.*, March, 1860.
Edinburgh Medical Journal, May, 1860.

Art. XV.—*Parisian Medical Intelligence.   Iodism.*   (Correspondence
of the *Lancet.* Paris, May, 1860.)

At the last three meetings the Académie de Médecine continued the
discussion on iodism. A letter was read from M. Boinet, who says
that he himself had taken iodine for eighteen months for the relief of
rheumatic pains. The cure being completed, he was, eighteen
months ago, about to discontinue the drug, when he received a communication from M. Rilliet, respecting some cases of iodism in
Geneva, caused by small doses ; he, therefore, continued it until
now. For the last three years he had been taking it, sometimes in
the form of iodide of potassium, forty-five grains in ten ounces of
water, a teaspoonful morning and evening ; sometimes in that of
iodine biscuits, or the tincture rendered soluble by four grains of
tannic acid ; and he finds his health improved by that *régime.*

Prof. Piorry has for the last fifteen years administered iodine in its various forms for syphilis, scrofula, and mall de pott ; internally, the iodide of potassium, from fifteen to twenty grains per diem ; sometimes the substance, by inhalation, or the tincture burned like punch, according to Mallez's system ; but he never observed those symptoms referred to by M. Rilliet, and consequently cannot help thinking that all the apprehensions are founded upon incorrect observations. Many a phenomenon has been attributed to the action of the medicine, which properly belongs to the symptoms of the disease for the relief of which it had been administered. Its immoderate use may give rise to some disturbance of the system, but the symptoms are too transient to merit the designation of poisoning. It would be falling into the absurdity of homœopathy to maintain that it is only small doses that produce poisonous symptoms, whilst large ones are innocuous. The action of arsenic cannot be brought forward as an analogy, because arsenic in small doses is absorbed and accumulated in the system, whilst large doses are expelled by vomiting. An attempt has been made to account for the different phenomena observed in Paris and Geneva by the difference in the constituent elements of the water, soil, and atmosphere ! When shall we renounce such theories, which put science into an unfavorable position of incertitude ? When will medical men confine themselves to strict and correct observation ? If we observe attentively, and study the nature of our patients and the modifications which medicines produce in the different states of organo-pathique, we shall see therapeutics rising above chaos, hazard, and fantasy, and assume a scientific and rational basis.

M. Chatin said that to study goitre it is not necessary to go to Switzerland, for there are some goitres in the neighborhood of Paris, in the valley of Montmorency. Now, in analyzing the water of that district, we find it to be silicious, containing very little or no iodine. From numerous researches which he has made for a number of years, in various countries, at different seasons, he is convinced that iodine is a constituent of the soil, water, and atmosphere, which is constantly introduced into the system by respiration and aliments. It is not necessary to the health of animals and vegetables ; the human economy is peculiar in this respect. All discussion on this subject will prove sterile, unless we first establish the fact, which ought to be the basis of the discussion, namely : whether iodine is a constituent of the atmosphere. He accordingly proposed that the Académie appoint a commission of the chemical section to examine the subject.

M. Gibert thought that there must certainly be an illusion, either in M. Boinet's or in M. Rilliet's observations. His experience enabled him to submit the following formula : Pure iodine, as the liqueur iodinée de Lugol, produces very easily gastro-intestinal irritation, so that its effects must be watched. Iodide of potassium is always harmless, if not exceeding forty-five grains per diem, and is an excellent antisyphilitic. It is better, however, in its combination with mercury, as the biniodide ; the protoiodide acts as an irritant upon the gums and intestines. He agreed, however, with Van Swieten, that the bichloride deserves the first rank as an antisyphilitic. The virtue of the internal exhibition of iodine as antiscrofulous, has been greatly exaggerated, but its topical action is useful in lesions produced by scrofulous diathesis. Iodism, as described by M. Rilliet, is almost unknown in Paris.

Professor Velpeau stated that during his long practice he cannot have administered iodine and its preparations, *intus et extra*, to less than fifteen thousand patients, and he never saw a single case of iodism as described by M. Rilliet. He could adduce some instances where it caused intestinal irritation, and sometimes coryza and ptyalism ; two instances, also, of loss of flesh, without its being, however, accompanied by *bulimia* ; but he never observed any case of atrophy of the mammæ or testicles. Several hypotheses have been proposed to account for its different action at Geneva and in Paris ; but there is a preliminary point which must be settled first, namely : in what proportion do those cases of iodism occur in Geneva ? M. Rilliet reported only twenty-three observations of constitutional iodism. Now this number is insignificant, when we remember the fact that the number of patients submitted to the daily treatment of iodine is very great. Suppose, then, that those twenty-three cases occurred in forty thousand patients, it would not be at all surprising. The small doses given at Geneva may have something to do with its peculiar action. Large doses are eliminated from the system, whilst small doses produce those effects referred to. He recollected a case in which several drops of acid nitrate of mercury applied to a wound caused profuse salivation and mercurial stomatitis.

M. Baillarger. The question of iodism is as old as the employment of iodine for goitre. At first it caused some accidents, which had been exaggerated, and that exaggeration produced the reaction in its favor. Iodism had not been observed everywhere, so that Vienna and Berlin physicians called its existence into question. Dr. Carrs, of Vienna, treated one hundred and fifty goitres without observing a single accident. The different constituents of the atmosphere in different localities is an inadmissible cause as a modification of its action, for M. Chatin did not find more iodine in the water of Vienna than at Geneva. He agreed with Professor Velpeau as to the importance of ascertaining the proportion of the accidents.

M. Bouchardat suggested that M. Rilliet's memoir was based altogether upon exceptional cases, and had consequently more interest in a physiological than in a pathological point of view. Iodism is very rare, even in Geneva. In spite of the occurrence of these symptoms, the goitre disappears in a few days ; hence it ought not to deter any one from employing it in goitre, syphilis, and scrofula.

M. Ricord. Some confusion has been occasioned in the discussion, in not keeping the consideration of iodine distinct from iodide of potassium. His remarks, on a former occasion, referred exclusively to iodide of potassium. As to the former, he was convinced that its internal exhibition produced only local irritation. He must, however, defend the protoiodide of mercury as an antisyphilitic against the opinion of M. Gibert. He was sure that it causes less salivation than mercurial friction. The protoiodide produces only a little diarrhœa, whilst the bichloride, recommended by Van Swieten and M. Gibert, determines sometimes true gastro-enteritis.

Dr. Quain's excellent paper in the *Lancet*, "On the Use of the Hypophosphites in Phthisis," has given general satisfaction here. I am told by M. Becquerel, of La Pitié, that he offered Dr. Churchill his patients to try his treatment, which he refused. Now, M. Becquerel obtained the drugs from Dr. Churchill's chemist, and made two series of experiments—the first upon twenty-five, and the second upon forty patients of La Pitié, and, besides, upon five private patients, and the result was the same as Dr. Quain's. I am also informed that Dr. Churchill tried the efficacy of his phosphites at the Lariboisière, and that the result was—*nothing*.

VITAL STATISTICS.

ART. I.—*Vital Statistics of Massachusetts.*

[From the Seventeenth Registration Report (a document of 147 large octavo pages) for the year 1858, being the official report of the Hon. Oliver Warner, Secretary of the Commonwealth, compiled under the general advice of Dr. E. Strong, with observations by Dr. Josiah Curtis.]

The records for the year cover 34,491 children born alive, 21,054 persons (10,527 couples) married, and 20,776 deaths, besides 747 still-born ; or facts which in the aggregate relate to upwards of *seventy-seven thousand individuals.*

There has been, on the average, each day in the year, no less than 94 births, 58 persons married, and 57 deaths. Besides these, there was a daily average of two still-births. June, as usual, was the least fatal month, in which there was an average of 48 deaths a day ; and in September, which is generally the most fatal month, there was an average of 77 deaths a day, being nearly thirty a day more than in June.

The most fatal cause of death, according to the records, was consumption of the lungs, ascribed to which there was an'average of 25 deaths every two days during the year. It seems worthy of serious consideration that in a given population in Massachusetts the records show three deaths from consumption, while in an equal population in England only two deaths take place from this disease.

In a population somewhat less than 1,250,000 the deaths amounted to 20,776.

After the financial disturbance and distress which broke out towards the close of 1857, it was to be expected, as predicated in our last Report, that there would follow a diminution in the number of marriages in 1858. The result is quite marked, the number registered in the latter year being somewhat less than *nine-tenths* of the number registered in 1857.

Typhus fever is not so excessive among those of particular ages, unless, perhaps, of early adults. 901 deaths were reported from this disease (including infantile fever) in 1858, being slightly below the annual average of the last five years, during which period about one in 20 of all the deaths from specified causes have been attributed to it. Dysentery has been the ascribed cause of 4,687 deaths within the past five years, 752 of which occurred in 1858. This zymotic is particularly severe in the late summer and early autumnal months. Its fatality is about coëqual with typhus.

Constitutional Diseases.—This class comprises two groups, which combined proved fatal in 5,402 cases in 1858, which is 30.76 per cent. of the deaths from all specified causes in the year. Of those under the head of tubercular diseases, pulmonary consumption is particularly severe. It caused 4,574 deaths in 1858, and 23,280 during the five previous years. This was 22.35 per cent. of the deaths in that period, against 21.78 per cent. of all the deaths in 1858, being the most fatal, year after year, of all the maladies that afflict the citizens of Massachusetts.

The registered deaths from consumption to the total population in Massachusetts, in 1858, was 376 in 100,000, and in the five years previous (1853-57) it was an annual average of 411 in 100,000 living. This is a much higher rate than is shown by the English records, to take place in England and Wales. There, the number of recorded deaths from consumption to every 100,000 persons living was, in each of the five years, 1853 to 1857 inclusive, as follows : 303, 279, 282, 260 and 263 respectively ; the annual average being only about two-thirds as high as in Massachusetts. What causes out of equal populations, three deaths from consumption to occur in this State where there are only two in England is a question worthy of further and serious investigation. Climate, perhaps, has something to do in effecting such results, and habits doubtless have also much influence. Of the latter class of causes, fashion unquestionably produces its full share upon her vain votaries. It has been justly said that the difference between the effects of a cord around the waist and around the neck consists principally in a question of time. Consumption proves more fatal to the female sex than to the male. In every 100,000 males living in 1858, there were 342 deaths of males attributed to consumption, while in every 100,000 females living, there were 407 deaths of females from this disease.

Deaths from cholera infantum for the year, 341. In the English reports, no deaths are stated to be from our indefinite term of " cholera infantum," but quite a large number are ascribed to atrophy and debility, which may in many cases include such as we charge to the vague term before mentioned. Of the 15,608 deaths attributed to atrophy by the English, in 1857, no less than 11,411 were under the age of five. Again, the English do not use the term "infantile," but in 1857 they ascribed 19,144 deaths to premature birth and debility, of which 17,802 were under the age of *one year*.

The highest rate of mortality in the tabulated classes, falls upon physicians (2.03 per cent. or one death in 49 living), and the next upon lawyers (2.01 per cent. or one death in 50 living), yet the average age at which physicians (55) and lawyers (56) die is much higher than that of several other classes.

It has been stated that three wet days in London bring 30,000 street people to the brink of starvation; and it is also a well established fact, that a fall of the thermometer of but a few degrees, is attended with an increase of mortality.

The zymotic class of diseases as a whole, has a much larger proportion of deaths attributed to it in Massachusetts than in England; that the same is also markedly the case with consumption and dysentery, while bronchitis and some other diseases are given as causes of much larger proportional numbers of deaths in England than in this State.

Of zymotic diseases, whooping-cough as well as croup, have been the cause of many deaths among children during the year. The latter, which is somewhat more fatal to boys than girls, seems, as before stated, to have been gradually abating during the past five years, but whooping-cough, which produces more deaths of girls than boys, has increased from 277 (125 boys and 151 girls) in 1855 to 347 (146 boys to 190 girls) in 1858 (there being one in each of these years whose sex was not stated).

Scarlatina produced the greatest number of registered deaths, among zymotic diseases, in 1858, and also in the aggregate of the last five years. In 1855, there were only 347 deaths recorded from this cause, but in 1857 the number was augmented to 2,013; in 1858, however, it fell to 1,051.

ART. II.—*Vital Statistics of South Carolina.*

[SOUTH CAROLINA (one of the immortal thirteen which achieved national independence) has taken the lead among the Southern States, being surpassed only by Massachusetts among the Northern States, in carrying into effect a systematic plan for ascertaining the vital, sanitary, and mortuary history of its population. Louisiana seems to have adopted, in vital statistics, Talleyrand's maxim in politics, namely : " Never to do to-day what you can put off until to-morrow." · As the climate of South Carolina assimilates to that of Louisiana, and as the latter is statistically poor, it is proposed to borrow from the former, that is the richer of the two, which is natural in such a case.   B. D.]

According to the Fifth Registration Report of South Carolina, being for the year 1858, Robert W. Gibbes, Jr., M. D., Registrar, the total deaths for the year were 8691, of these 28 were aged 100 or more.

Extreme Old Age.—According to the United States Census of 1850, there were living in South Carolina 206 persons, aged 100 years and upwards, and our Registry Returns for 1858 exhibit twenty-eight deaths at that advanced period of existence. Of these the eldest were, a white female, aged 110 years, who died of old age, in St. John's, Berkeley parish, in the month of January; the next, a white female, aged 107 years, in Fairfield, in June, and the third a female slave, aged 105 years, dying in Abbeville, in the same month—all three of the same *cause.* Out of the whole number, only four were whites, and the rest slaves.

The following table gives the locality, race, sex, age, date, and cause of death, with reference to all of them:

DEATHS AT ADVANCED AGES.

DISTRICTS.	COLOR.	SEX.	MONTH.	AGE.	CAUSE OF DEATH.
Abbeville..................	White.	M.	May........	102 y'rs.	Inflammation of bowels.
Abbeville..................	Slave.	M.	May........	100 "	Old age.
Abbeville..............	"	M.	Sept........	100 "	"
Abbeville..................	"	F.	June.......	105 "	"
Barnwell..................	"	M.	August....	100 "	"
Barnwell..................	"	M.	Unknown.	100 "	Debility.
Chester....................	"	M.	June.......	100 "	Old age
Edgefield..................	"	M.	February.	100 "	"
Edgefield..................	"	M.	October...	100 "	Convulsions.
Edgefield..................	"	M.	July........	100 "	Dropsy.
Fairfield..................	White.	F.	June.......	107 "	Old age.
Lexington.................	Slave.	M.	November	100 "	"
Newberry.............	"	F.	May........	100 "	"
Orange Parish..........	White.	M.	January...	101 "	Gastritis.
Prince George Winyaw	Slave.	M.	August....	100 "	Old age.
St. George, Dorchester	"	F.	April.......	100 "	"
St. Helena................	"	F.	March.....	100 "	"
St. James's, Santee....	"	F.	March.....	100 "	"
St. James's, Santee....	"	F.	Sept........	100 "	"
St. John's, Berkeley...	White.	F.	January...	110 "	"
St. John's, Berkeley...	Slave.	F.	Dec.........	100 "	"
St. Mathew's............	"	M.	Sept........	100 "	"
St. Mathew's............	"	M.	October...	100 "	"
St. Mathew's............	"	F.	July........	100 "	"
St. Paul's................	"	F.	Dec.........	100 "	"
Sumter....................	"	M.	Dec.........	100 "	"
Sumter....................	"	F.	Sept........	100 "	"
York......................	"	F.	Unknown.	100 "	"

                                                            [pp. 82–3.]

CAUSES OF DEATH IN 1858.

Pneumonia	804	Convulsions	197
Typhoid Fever	757	Catarrh	109
Dropsy	475	Burns and Scalds	150
Dysentery	279	Croup	157
Diarrhœa	162	Suffocated	147
Old age	343	Congestive Fever	111
Measles	290	Remittent Fever	104
Teething	282	Accident	119
Consumption	289	Cholera Infantum	84
Fever	196	Apoplexy	120
Bowels, disease of	160	Childbirth	90
Worms	287	Quinsy	22
Brain, disease of	166	Paralysis	64
Scarlatina	310	Yellow Fever	209
Whooping Cough	221		

Of *pneumonia*, 804 persons died, being 9.84 per cent. of the deaths in the whole population, 11.12 of those among slaves, and only 6.16 per cent. in whites. There was a large excess of males in both races, viz : 67 males to 58 females in whites, and 361 males 312 females in blacks. December, March and February, gave the largest mortality from this disease, nearly one-third dying under 5 years, and one-sixth between 20 and 40 years of age, etc.

Zymotic Diseases : for 5 years ending with 1858.—We find that in 1858 the mortality from this class was 34.65 per cent. of all the deaths in the State from known causes, which was less than for either of the four preceding years. If all the deaths from *yellow fever*, however, (716 instead of 209) had been reported as in Dr. Dawson's mortality report for Charleston city, the per centage from Zymotics in the State would have risen to 40.37. On referring to my reports for 1853 and 1854—which did not embrace the Lower Division of the State, where alone yellow fever ever prevails, I find that the higher mortality from this class was due to a greater prevalence of epidemic bowel affections and malarious fevers than we have had since ; and this is also in accordance with my own professional experience. Except, then, for the violent yellow fever epidemic in Charleston last year, it would rightly have appeared to be the healthiest of five years. *Croup*, which heretofore occupied a place in this class, has now been removed to the 4th, where it more properly belongs. *Typhoid fever* we find standing highest in this class, having destroyed 9.27 per cent. of the whole number of deaths from known causes, giving the enormous mortality of 10.76 per cent. in whites, but only 0.87 per cent. in slaves. This excess of fatality in the white race was not near so marked in 1857. *Scarlatina* killed 7.21 per cent. whites, and 2.60 per cent. slaves, and the preceding year 2.77 of the former and 1.84 of the latter. Of course, *intermittent, remittent* and *yellow fevers*, were most fatal to the white race in both years, as also were *thrush, dysentery, diarrhœa* and *cholera infantum*, but in a less degree. *Whooping cough*, on the contrary, as well as *small pox* and *syphilis*, always goes harder with negroes. *Measles* killed about the same proportion in both races last year, but in 1857 was more than doubly fatal to slaves.

74'

CLASS IV—*Diseases of the Respiratory Organs.*—This class comes second in order of fatality, giving 19.49 per cent. of the deaths in 1858, and 18.51 of all of those from known causes in five years.

On the whole, it affected the two races in about similar proportions for the two years. *Consumption, croup, quinsy, bronchitis* and " *diseases of lungs,*" were more fatal to whites, while *pneumonia* was quite the reverse, giving a proportion of but 6.16 among them and 11.12 per cent. in slaves. The latter also die more of " *cold,*" which is about as definite a term as " bowel complaint."

The next class in order is Class VI, or *diseases of the digestive system,* which gives a per centage of 10.87 in our present returns, and an average of 9.70 for the five years. It was always far more fatal to blacks, having destroyed 13.27 in 1857, and 12.32 per cent. in 1858, but in whites only 8.65 and 6.68 per cent.

The chief causes of death in this class are *teething, worms* and " *diseases of the bowels,*" all of which seem to be especially bad for slaves.

Class II, *of general or uncertain seat,* gives 10.94 per cent. for 1858, and 8.89 per cent. for five years.

The only causes of much consequence we find here, are included chiefly in the three vague terms " *dropsy,*" " *scrofula*" and " *debility,*" which have a good deal to answer for. Of course *they* affect slaves the most, as the whole class did in both 1857 and 1858.   .

Class III, or *diseases of the nervous system,* comes next, giving 9.15 per cent. for the year (a high proportion), and 7.42 per cent. for five years. It was most fatal to whites in both years, *diseases of the brain, apoplexy* and *paralysis,* predominating amongst them, and *trismus nascentium, convulsions, tetanus* and *epilepsy,* among slaves.

Class XII, *External Causes* or *Violence.*—This gives 6.50 per cent. for the year, and 6.64 for five years—proportions far above what they *ought* to be. As might well be expected, negroes die in double the numbers of whites, from this class of causes, the principal mortality being due to *burns, suffocation* and *accidents not specified.*

Class XI—*Old Age* furnished 4.22 per cent. in 1858, and 4.64 in five years, the variations from these figures, within that period, being very slight. The greatest mortality appears here among slaves, being 4.58 per cent., and in whites only 3.08. I am inclined to doubt the correctness of these figures. It being often extremely difficult, nay, impossible, to ascertain the cause of death in "old niggers," many of them are hastily and carelessly enterred as " died of old age," when, in fact, some disease was really the guilty cause. The proportion returned as dying from this class in 323,023 deaths, according to the mortality statistics of the last U. S. Census, was only 2.79 per cent. Probably greater pains were then taken to inquire into the causes of death.

In *diseases of the generative system,* or Class VIII, which gives 2.32 per cent. in 1858—a little above the five years average—and only 1.18 per cent. according to the United States returns, we find the whites dying in larger proportion than the blacks, from *child-*

birth, puerperal fever and *affections of the womb,* while *premature birth* indicates, as it did last year, the highest mortality in slaves.

The next class, or *diseases of the circulatory system,* gives 0.64, which is a little below the average—0.99 per cent. being the proportion in whites, and 0.64 in slaves. For the preceding year it was 0.97 in the former, and 0.79 in the latter. The U. S. Census Report gave 0.78 in the whole population.

The remaining three classes are the lowest in order of fatality everywhere ; they are *diseases of the locomotive, urinary and integumentary systems,* and give 0.42, 0.40 and 0.19 per cent. respectively, the few causes included in them indicating a somewhat greater proportional mortality in the white race, although but seldom directly fatal in their effects.

Population.—According to the United States Census of 1850, the population of South Carolina consisted of 668,507 individuals, of whom 274,563 were whites, 8960 free colored, and 384,984 slaves—the proportions of each race being, whites 41.07, free colored 1.34, and slaves 57.59 per cent. * * * The rate of increase in each race during each decade of the last sixty years, shows, that, whilst our population has increased slowly, the rate of increase almost steadily diminishing,* at the same time the proportion of slaves to the whole population has advanced regularly ; that of the whites has fallen off correspondingly, and the free colored have remained nearly stationary. In 1790 the population of this State formed 6.34 per cent. of the total population of the Union, but in 1850 it had diminished to 2.88 per cent.

With respect to the proportion of sexes,.137,747 were white males, and 136,816 females, or 99.32 females to 100 males. Of the free colored, 4131 males, and 4829 females, or 116.89 females to 100 males. Of slaves, 187,756 males, and 197,228 females, or 105.04 females to 100 males. In the total population there was a preponderance of 2.80 per cent. for females—a very unusual condition of things, except in the New England States, where the females have always been in excess, as shown by every census. In all other parts of the United States, the males are in excess from four to ten per cent. In 1850 the total white population of the United States including New England, gave a male excess of 5 per cent., and the total slave population of the Southern States only .05 per cent. The free colored population, however, gives a female excess of 8.16 per cent. The proportion of the sexes is a subject of curious interest, and has received considerable attention from statisticians.

---

* Vermont and New Hampshire are the only two States in the Union whose rate of increase during the last ten years has been lower than that of South Carolina. The rate for the whole United States for sixty years has been pretty constant, viz : from 32.67 to 36.44, which is a little less than occurred in South Carolina from 1790 to 1800, but much greater than at any time since.

DOCTORS AND PHYSIC.

Hear me, my friends ! who this good banquet grace ;
'Tis sweet to play the fool in time and place .

                                        POPE. HOMER. *Odys.*

" A little nonsense now an l then,
Is relished by the wisest men."

GERONTE—*It is impossible to reason better, Doctor. But, dear sir, there is one thing which staggers me in your lucid explanation. I always thought, till now, that the heart was on the left side and the liver on the right.*
MOCK DOCTOR—*Ay, sir, so they were formerly ; but we have changed all that. The College at present, sir, proceeds upon an entire new method.*
GERONTE—*I ask your pardon, sir.*
MOCK DOCTOR—*Oh, sir ! there is no harm—you are not obliged to know so much as we do.*
GERONTE—*Very true, Doctor, very true.*   MOLIÈRE.

1. PROVERBS AND SAYINGS ON DOCTORS' DOINGS.—" If the Doctor cures, the sun sees it ; if he kills, the earth hides it." " The earth covers the mistakes of the physician." "Bleed him, and purge him; if he dies, bury him." "The doctor is often more to be feared than the disease."—*Italian, French, Spanish.* Sir W. Hamilton said : " Medicine in the hands in which it is vulgarly dispensed is a curse to humanity rather than a blessing." Sir Astley Cooper avowed : "The science of medicine was founded on conjecture, and improved by murder." "The Doctor seldom takes physic," says the Italian. The German wit writes : "Physic does good always, if not to the patient, at least to the apothecary." The Spaniard tells : "It is God that cures, and the doctor gets the money;" and " if you have a friend who is a doctor, take off your hat to him, and send him to the house of your enemy."—*Proverbs of all Nations.*

2. THE PUZZLED DOCTOR.—"The Seranes," Borden writes, "father and son, were physicians at the hospital at Montpelier. The son was a lively theorist, who knew by heart and was continually re-peating, all the written documents about inflammation, just as children repeat in their silly way : 'The grasshopper has chirupped all the summer, etc.;' or, 'Mr. Crow sits perched on a tree, etc.' Serane, the father, was a good soul, who had studied under great masters. He had learned to treat fluxions of the chest with emetics, giving them at least every second day, with or without the addition of two ounces of manna ; they were his great *chevaux de bataille.* I have seen him fire them off a thousand times, everywhere and to everyone. The son resolved to convert his father to the fashion of the day ; that is to say, to inspire him with a salutary dread of *phlogosis, erethismus,* and the rupture of the small vessels. The good father consequently fell into a most singular kind of indecision : he knew not how to act. However, he held out firmly against bleeding ; and when he came to a patient, he would murmur awhile, and then pass on without ordering anything. I have frequently known him apostrophise his son with earnestness, and to cry out, when he was desirous but yet afraid of administering an emetic : 'My son, you have ruined me (*Mon fil, m'abès gastat*) !' Never shall

I forget this curious scene. I am greatly indebted to it, and so also were the patients of the Hospital. They got well without being bled, because old Serane did not like the bleeding, and without taking emetics, because young Serane had proved to his father that these remedies increased inflammation. The patients got well, and I learnt a profitable lesson. I concluded that the numerous bleedings with Seranes, the son, practised, when alone, were at least as useless as the repeated emetics to which Seranes, the father, was so much attached."—*Medical Times and Gazette.*

3. Dissecting a Quack.—"To puzzle a Philadelphia lawyer," is a common saying with Transatlantic brethren ; but the following is related of the manner in which one of these gentlemen puzzled a quack, who was bringing a suit for medical services. *Counsel*—Did you treat the patient according to the most approved rules of surgery? *Witness*—Certainly, by all means, I did. *Counsel*—Did you decapitate him ? *Witness*—Undoubtedly, I did that as a matter of course. *Counsel*—Did you perform the Cæsarean operation upon him ? *Witness* Why, of course ; his condition required it ; and it was attended with great success. *Counsel*—Did you, now, doctor, subject his person to autopsy ? *Witness*—Certainly ; that was the best remedy I adopted. *Counsel*—Well, then, doctor, as you first cut off the defendant's head, then ripped up his body, and afterwards dissected him, and he still survives it, I have no more to ask.—*Edin. Med. Jour.*

4. Pinel.—When Pinel undertook the management of Bicêtre, the Revolution was at its height. The notorious Couthon presided over the dreaded *Commune* of Paris, and when Pinel came to him to obtain permission to remove the chains from the madmen, went himself the next day to the asylum, fearing lest in such an act there should be some hidden attempt against the Democratic Government. When he saw the madmen, he turned to Pinel and said : "Are you not mad yourself, to wish to deliver these *bêtes féroces* from their chains ! " " No," answered Pinel, " for I am certain that their chains make these wretched people thus violent." " Do as you like," said Couthon. From this time the good work commenced. The following day he removed the chains from fifty, and from thirty more a few days afterwards. The Academy of Medicine has adorned one of its rooms with a picture of this scene of humanity. Shortly after this we are told that Pinel was seized by some of the ruffians of the day, under the pretext of being an aristocrat, and hurried off " *à la lanterne ;* " and that his life was saved by an old soldier, one Chevigné, whom he had delivered from his chains in the Bicêtre, and who had become his servant.

Pinel states, in letters of his lately published, that he was enabled to live decently on what he obtained by the translation of English works. "At this moment," he says, " I am engaged in the translation of Cullen's ' Institutes of Medicine," for which I receive one thousand francs. I would give up physic altogether, if it were necessary for me to be running about all day in the streets. I wish for only a very small practice—to see little and observe much."

Lunatics in the Good Old Times.—It is impossible for us to imagine the condition of lunatic asylums before the days of Pinel. Dungeons, wet and infected, without light and air, called *loges*, containing a wretched mattress, or some rotten straw strewed on the ground. Human beings, naked or covered with rags, almost always furious, chained to each other, and shut up in these abodes of desolation and misery—actual tombs, out of which they came to be carried to their last dwelling-place. Their brutal keepers, selected from those who had been condemned to punishment, treated them like brutes, and used them most barbarously, abusing and ridiculing them, striking them cruelly, and continually fighting with them, throwing them their deficient and coarse food, keeping their water from them when thirsty, and their clothes when cold ; exposing them to the jokes of visitors. Such were the inhabitants of Bicêtre at that time— wretched beings thought incurable, abandoned by their friends, deprived of all medical treatment, pale, wasted, wallowing in their own filth, groaning under the weight of the chains which tore their wasted limbs, raving under the horrible sufferings to which they were subjected by their inhuman keepers.—*Gaz. Hebd. Med. Times and Gazette.*

5. "THEY MANAGE THINGS BETTER IN FRANCE."—The dryness and want of animation which usually illustrate debates in our own English Medical Societies, have been often cast in their teeth ; it is well, therefore, to hear what a French critic thinks of some of those brilliant outbursts of eloquence which we are often inclined to envy in listening to the prosaic humdrum way of doing business which John Bull usually indulges. "They manage these things better in France !" Let us see. Here are the general remarks, made *à propos* of the particular occasion on which M. Trousseau indulged the French Academy with an hour's burst of eloquence :

"And this leads us to a remark of more general application. Oratorical struggles in an Academy of Medicine have rather a *beautiful* than a *good* effect. They give animation, piquancy and *popularity* to the meeting. But people come to them to hear an orator, not for instruction. Those long brilliant discourses, which refer more *ad hominem* than *ad rem*, or which have no direct reference either to the matter or the person, are like so many beautiful solos executed on different airs. They frighten away from the discussion many a modest but stedfast man, who would speak his mind freely in private society or in his seat, but who has not the courage to mount up to a tribune still vibrating with the echoes of an eloquent peroration. We merely signalize the fact without deducing any consequence from it. There is no other way of curing the evil than by limiting the length of the discourses, but whenever this has been tried it has been given up. Generally speaking, the orators whose voices the Society thus wished to stifle, have complained so loudly that in the end it was necessary to let them have their full swing." *Medical Times and Gazette.*

6. CHANGE OF TYPE.—The change of type theory of disease does

not appear to have advanced much in Italy, if we may judge from what we hear concerning the sanguinary therapeutical code still in vigor there.   The following, we believe, is a daily example of the practice carried on in the way of venesection by our Italian brethren:

"The President opened the sitting by the announcement of the death of General Quaglia, in consequence of the fit of apoplexy with which he was struck in the House the other day, or perhaps of the doctors, who drained the poor aged gentleman to the last drop of his blood—four bleedings in twenty-four hours, three of them after his recovery from the fit."

A propos of this incident, we would like to hear how those gentlemen who argue of the truth of this change in type of disease, from the fact that skillful physicians did bleed in other days but don't bleed now, reconcile with their argument this unceasing love of the lancet—to-day just as in other days—by the skillful Italian physician.

"Let me say to those who think that inflammation has changed its type during these last years," says Professor Forget, "that I believe nothing of the kind.   How can this be when nothing around us has changed ; when all the local and general phenomena of inflammation remain the same ; whilst irritants still preserve the privilege of engendering inflammation, and other remedies of soothing it ; when we see at the same time, in the same town, in the same Hospital, at La Charité for example, enlightened practitioners combatting inflammation by opposite means, we are told that inflammation once sthenic has now become asthenic !   The fact is that it is now what it always has been, and if anything has changed it is not the Medical constitution, it is the Medical heads that have turned."—*Ib.*

7. Gratuitous Services.—The profession has often heard of the abuses of our system of gratuitous hospital advice, and of the manner in which well-to-do persons impose on our public charities.   It seems, however, that on the other side of the world impudence is carried even to a greater extent than in this country.   A writer on charitable institutions, in the *Australian Medical Journal* for January, 1860, concludes his article with the following paragraph :

"It is no uncommon thing for persons with a rental of two or three hundred a year to send their wives and children to the hospital for relief ; that in like manner, store-keepers, who take their £50 or £60 a week, are patients ; that we have heard one of the medical officers stating that he has known a man with a rental of £1000 a year attending as an out-patient ; that it is a common practice with these very persons to say to their friends, 'why do you pay for medical advice, when you can get it from the hospital for nothing ?'   There are to be daily seen, in the out-patients' waiting-rooms, persons seeking advice who are better dressed and adorned with more jewelry than the wives and daughters of many of the subscribers, and it has but lately happened that a man who, upon paying a small account as a private patient, handed a £50 instead of a £5 note, protesting that it was the last money he had in the world, and in a few days after was recognized in one of the wards of the hospital, having obtained admission on the false pretence of poverty."—*British Medical Journal.*

8. Iodine, according to M. Boinet, preserves, cures, strengthens, and modifies the constitution, removes diatheses, and impresses a new energy in the organism. Iodine, according to M. Rilliet, weakens, deteriorates, wastes, destroys, atrophies, and kills !

Last year M. Beau discovered that lead was an excellent remedy for phthisis. M. Broeckx, of Antwerp, has tried the mineral extensively, and has found it worse than useless !

M. Chatin lately informed the French Academy, *à propos* of iodine, that Coindet had by its use reduced so many women to the condition of Amazons, and had brought such a number of men into the state described by M. Ricord under the term "haricocele," that he dare not show himself in the streets of Geneva, through dread of suffering the martyrdom of St. Stephen.—*Ib.*

9. Medical men are found in every part of the earth ; and they do not always confine themselves to ministering to physical maladies. As an example, we may call attention to the fact that at a recent "Missionary Conference" at Liverpool, Dr. Lockhart, of Liverpool, late a medical missionary in China, in an interesting speech, recounted his experience in China. He spoke highly of the system of employing medical gentlemen as missionaries ; its success in China had been marked and satisfactory. He had been in the north of China, where the face of a European was almost an object of fear and surprise, but alone he had succeeded by degrees in winning the confidence and affection of the natives. Surgery was in a low state in China, so that a properly-qualified medical man soon obtained great influence. At Shanghae he opened a hospital, which was attended by three hundred or four hundred natives—at one time by the wounded pirates, Imperialist soldiers, and citizens together. His introduction of vaccination opened the houses of the influential to him to an unexpected degree.—*Med. Times and Gaz.*

10. Severe Wounds—Slow Death.—The following facts appear to be authenticated by Mr. Surgeon Hill, as well as by non-medical witnesses in the ease of the murder of Jno. Groundwater, by Butterworth and Jenison, in 1794 ; they struck him with their shovels three blows upon the skull causing a double handful of his brains to fall out ; they then struck with the same upon the neck intending to severe his head from the body. He lived eighteen hours afterwards ; the pulse was strong and the respiration continuous the whole eighteen hours. (*Celebrated Trials.* Lond. 1825, vol. v, 282.)

11. The Niger Expedition.—Dr. M'Cormac, of Belfast (in *Edin. Med. and Surg. Jour.*, Oct., 1845), says, in article on the Niger Expedition : " Of 158 negroes employed in the Niger expedition, only eleven were attacked with fever—all recovered. Of 145 whites, 130 contracted the fever, 40 perished, 15 escaped from it.

12. Scrofula.—Dr. Gregory, of Edinburgh, asserted as his belief that there was not a single family in Great Britain in which scrofula did not exist.

13. Criminals Condemned to Death.—In the *Celebrated Trials* (6 vols. Lond. 1825), a number of cases are recorded of persons condemned to death who died on the way to execution from remorse, sorrow and fear ; while others hailed death with pleasure. It is a remarkable fact often mentioned in this work, that criminals frequently sleep profoundly the night before their execution.

14. The Torture in the Criminal Jurisprudence of the 19th Century. In the work last mentioned, it is shown that, in 1806, the British Governor of Trinidad, repeatedly inflicted the Torture on Louisa Calderdon, a girl aged 11 years, suspected of robbery. (Vol. vi, p. 1).

15. Consolation for Sciolists.—A physician once said to Barthez, "Your book is much too difficult to be understood." "Patience," replied Barthez, "I am preparing an edition which will be so clear that every ass will be able to drink from it."

16. Systems.—The celebrated Bordeau said : "I was dogmatic at 20, an observer at 30, an empiric at 40, and now at 50, I no longer have any system."

MISCELLANEA.

Medical Chronology. (Continued and Concluded from page 453.)

1380. Peter Argelata.
1406. The Emperor Venceslas grants privileges to the establishers of public baths.
1410. Peter of Tussignana.
1413. Death of James of Forli.
1414. Whooping Cough in France; Ali ben Abi'l Hazaw Alkerschi ben Nasis.
1418. Valescus of Tarentum; James Ganivet.
1420. Birth of Peter Pinctor.
1425. Leonard Bertapaglia.
1428. Birth of Nicholas Leonicenus.
1438. John Concorregio.
1439. Death of Hugh Bencio.
1440. Death of Anthony Guainer.
1441. Death of Cermisoni; Mengo Bianchelli.
1447. Saladin of Arezzo.
1458. Birth of Sebastian Brandt.
1460. Death of Bart. Montagnana the elder; birth of Francis Giorgio
1461. Thomas Linacer; birth of John Widmann, or Salicetus.
1462. Death of Mich. Savonarola; birth of John Manard.

1463. Birth of Alexander Achillini.

1464. Hans of Dockenbourg.

1465. Death of James Despars.

1468. Hans of Dockenbourg cures Matthew, King of Hungary, of a wound; birth of Peter Baiero; Gregory Volpi.

1470. John Platearius.

1472. Death of Matthew Ferrari de Gradi; Birth of Symphorian Champier.

1473. Death of Segismond Poleastro ; Birth of Augustine of Niphus.

1474. Birth of Martin Curtius.

1475. Germain Colot, a lithotomist, operates on a criminal for the stone.

1477. Birth of Bartholomew Maggi.

1478. Vincent Vianio practises the art of fixing artificial noses; birth of Peter Brissot.

1481. Birth of Benoit Victorius.

1483. Birth of Jerome Fracastorius.

1484. Death of John Arcularius.

1485. Birth of John Lange and of Jason of Pratis.

1486. Sweating sickness in England; birth of John Fernelius.

1487. Birth of John Gonthier of Andernach.

1488. Pacificus Maximus publishes his poems.

1489. Birth of John Baptiste Montanus.

1490. Birth of Gabriel Fallopius.

1491. Birth of Victor Trincavella ; John of Cube and Arndes, Burgomasters of Lubeck, give the first figures of planets ; and Kethan publishes the first tables of Vegetable Anatomy.

1492. Birth of James Sylvius; the French disease shows itself in Italy, according to Fulgosi.

1493. Birth of Paracelsus and of Francis Arcæus.

1494. Birth of Randolph Agricola ; William Copus.

1495. Magnus Hundt, Marcellus Cumanus, Conrad Schellig, Wimpheling, and Widmanu, the first writers on syphilis.

1496. Sebastian Brandt and Grunbeck write on syphilis.

1497. Conrad Gilinus, Gaspard Torella, Montagnana the younger, Montetesauro, and Sebastian Aquilanus write on syphilis.

1498. Literary dispute at Leipsic, between Simon Pistor and Martin Pollich; birth of Andrew Lacuna and John Cario.

1500. Publication of the work of Peter Pinctor; birth of John Cornaro.

1301. Birth of Leonard Fuchs.

1502. Death of Anthony Benivieni.

1503. Death of Peter Pinctor; birth of Charles Stephen.

1504. James Cataneos; Birth of Jeremiah Thriverius and James Milich.

1505. The physicians of Paris write against the surgeons; a petechial fever in Italy; the Faculty of Paris take the barbers under its protection; death of Gabriel Zerbi; birth of John Gorreus, of Levinus Lemnius, and of Achilles Pirminus Gassarus.

1506. Birth of Julius Alexandrinus of Neustain, and of Fernelius; Alexander Bonedetti.

1507. Birth of William Bondoletus.

1509. Guiacum introduced into England ; birth of Ambrose Pare and of Michel Servitus.

1510. Whooping Cough in France ; birth of John Cajus, of Volcher Coyter, of Bernard Dessenius, and of John Struthius.

1513. Death of Martin Pollich ; birth of John Argentier, and of William Arragos.

1514. The surgeons of Paris reinstated in their privileges, and received into the Faculty ; Whooping Cough in France ; Brissot proposes his new method of bleeding in Pleurisy ; birth of Andrew Vesalius.

1515. Birth of John Wyer ; Arret declaring the Surgeons to be members of the Faculty of Paris.

1516. Birth of Conrad Gesner.

1517. Birth of Rembert Dodoens ; Sweating Sickness in England.

1519. Guaiacum begins to be known ; birth of Andrew Cesalpinus, and John Crato, of Craftheim.

1520. Death of Sebastian Brandt ; Blenorrhagia begins to connect itself with Syphilis.

1522. Birth of Peter Foreest ; death of Peter Brissot.

1523. Birth of Gabriel Fallopius, and of Thomas Erastus.

1524. Death of Thomas Linacer, and Nicholas Leonicenus.

1525. John of Romaine discovers the mode of operating for the Stone by the great apparatus ; Birth of Ulysses Aldrovandus ; death of Alexander Achillini, and of Andrew Torino.

1527. Petechial fever in Italy ; birth of Louis Duretus, of Horace Augenius, and of John Moibanus.

1528. The sweating sickness in Holland and in Germany ; birth of Anuce Foes.

1529. Birth of Laurence Joubert.

1530. Birth of Julius Cæsar Aranzi, of Jerome Mercurialis, of John Schenk of Graffenburg, and of Leonard Thurneisser ; introduction of Sarsaparilla into Europe.

1531. Birth of Henry Brucæus.

1532. Charles Stephens discovers the valves of the veins of the liver ; Nicholas Massa discovers the lymphatic vessels of the kidneys ; death of William Copus ; birth of Martin Ruland.

1533. Birth of Theodore Zwinger, of Balthazar Brunner, of Claudins Dariotte, and of Andrew Laguna.

1534. James Dubois and Andrew Vesalius discover the valves of the veins ; birth of Volcher Coyter and of Cornelius Gemma.

1535. Description of the Scurvy by Cartier ; Pleurisy of bad character at Venice ; introduction of the root of Smilax Aspera into Europe ; birth of Symphorien Champier.

1536. Death of John Manard, and of John Ingolstetter.

1537. Birth of Jerome Fabricius of Aquapendens, of Henry Smetius, of Felix Plater, of John Posthius and of James Horst ; inoculation already known at Corfu.

1538. Death of Augustin Nifo ; birth of James Grevin, and of William Baillou.

1539. Laurence Colot practises with success the operation of the stone by the great apparatus.

1540. Birth of Thomas Jordan and of Peter Severin Francis Giogio ; death of Mariano Santo of Barletta.

1541. Birth of Paracelsus, and of John Bauhin ; Amatus Lusitanus makes known the utility of bougies against the Caruncules of the Urethra.

1542. Birth of John Nicolas Stupani.

1543. Susius maintains that the Venæ Cavæ derive their origin from the heart ; birth of Constantine Varoli and of John Heurnius.

1544. Death of Matthew Curtius.

1545. William Valvayseur, Surgeon of Francis the 1st, separates entirely the bathers of the body from the Surgeons ; birth of Julius Casterius ; the College of Surgery, at Paris, obtains the participation in all the privileges of the Universities ; establishment of the Botanical Garden at Padua ; epidemic Phrenitis in France.

1546. John Philip Ingrassias discovers the Stapes ; birth of Tagliacotius.

1547. John Baptiste Caunani discovers the valves of the Vena Azygos.

1548. Birth of Scipio Mercurius ; Aranzi discovers the elevator muscle of the superior eyelid.

1549. Mathew Cornax operated for the stone on the Emperor at Vienna.

1550. Birth of Gaspard Bauhin, and of Emilius Campolongo.

1551. Sweating disease, Epidemic Pleurisy in Switzerland ; annulling of the Decree of 1515, which declared the surgeons members of the Faculty of Paris ; death of John Baptiste Montanus ; birth of Hercules of Sassonia.

1552. Anatomical Tables of Eustachius ; Dissecting Amphitheatre at Pisa ; death of Bartholomew Maggi, and of Benoit Victorius ; birth of Louis Settala.

1553. Michal Servetus points out the small circulation of the blood. He is burnt alive at Geneva.

1553. Death of Jerome Fracastor ; birth of James Guillemeau, and of Prosper Alpinus.

1554. Gabriel Fallopius discovers the valve of the colon in monkies; death of Jeremy Thriverius and of John Echt; birth of John Baptiste Cortesi.

1555. Death of James Dubois; Diaz of Isla publishes his work upon syphilis; birth of Henry of Bra.

1556. Epidemic scurvy in the Brabant; anatomical amphitheatre at Montpellier; birth of Archibald Piccolhumoini.

1557. Whooping cough in Germany and France; Petechial fever in Poitou.

1568. Death of John Fernelius, of John Cornarius, of Lucas Ganrico, of Jason of Pratis, and of Peter Bairo; Birth of John of Colle.

1560. Death of Oddus of Oddis; birth of Stephen Roiz of Castro.

1560. Peter Franco practises lithotomy by the high operation;

Whooping cough at Zurich; death of Andrew Laguna, of John Dryander, and of Amatus Lusitanus; Posthius perceives at Montpellier the valves of the crural vein; birth of William Fabricius of Hilden.

1561. Birth of Sanctorius.

1562. Eustachius discovers the thoracic canal upon a horse; death of John Moibanus and of Thomas Houlier.

1563. Birth of Charles Pison; death of Gabriel Fallopius.

1564. Epidemic pleurisy in Switzerland; death of Charles Stephen and of Andrew Vesalius.

1565. Death of John Lange and of Conrad Gesner.

1566. Hungarian disease; death of Leonard Fuchs and of William Rondelet.

1567. Birth of Thomas Fyens.

1568. Birth of Thomas Campanella and of John Hartmann; death of Victor Trincavella, of Levinius Lemnius, and of Joseph Struthius.

1569. Death of Nicolas Massa and of Guido Guidi; birth of James Zwinger.

1570. Death of James Grevin; birth of Antony Ponce of Santa Cruz.

1571. Cesalpin partially discovers the great circulation.

1572. Death of John Argentier; birth of Daniel Sennert, of Gaspard Hoffman, and of Rodolph Goclenius.

1573. Death of Joseph Cajns and of Christopher of Vega; birth of Theodore Turquet of Mayerne.

1574. Birth of Robert Fludd; death of John Gonthier of Andermach, of Bartholomew Eustache, and of Bernard Dessenius; Fabricius of Aquapendente observes the valves of the veins.

1575. Death of Constantine Varoli; birth of Zacutus Lusitanus.

1576. Birth of James Gohory.

1577. Birth of John Baptiste Vanhelmont, of John Riolan, and of Fortuna Licet; singular syphilitic disease at Brunn, in Moravia; death of Achilles, Pirminus Gassarius, of John of Gortis, of Reald Columbus, and Adam of Bodenstein.

1578. Birth of Adrien Spigel ; death of Antony Mizaud, and of Nicholas Manard.

1579. Birth of William Harvey, and of Cæsar Magnati ; death of Cornelius Gemma, and of Francis of Arce ; Bauhin observes the valve of the cœcum ; privilege of the Pope granted to the surgeons of Paris.

1580. Whooping-cough at Rome ; birth of Marcus Aurelius Severinus, and of Claudius Nicolas Fabre of Peirese ; introduction of sassafras into medicine ; death of Francis Valeriola, and of John Philip Ingrassias.

1582. *Cereal* convulsion in the country of Lunebourg ; death of Andrew Ellinger, of Laurence Joubert, and of Thomas Erastus.

1583. Birth of Thomas Raynard.

1584. Death of Simon Peter.

1585. Death of Rembert Dodoens, of John Fyens, and of John Crato, of Craftheim.

1586. Death of Louis Duret, and of James Aubert.

1587. Birth of Ren Moreau ; petechial fever in Lombardy.

1588. Birth of Olaus Wormius ; Death of James Dalechamp, of John Wyer, and of Valentine Weigel ; *cereal* convulsion in Silesia.

1589. Birth of Lazarus Riverius, and of Peter of Marchettis ; death of Jerome Capivacci, and of Julius Cæsar Aranzi.

1590. Death of Julius Alexander, of Neustain, of Ambrose Pare, and of John George Trumph.

1593. Discoveries of Julius Casserius, in the organ of hearing ; death of Henry Brucæus ; birth of Nicolas Tulpius.

1594. Amphitheatre of Anatomy at Padua ; death of Claudius Dariotte.

1595. Birth of Frederic Spee, and of James Scultetus ; death of Annee Foes, and of Leonard Thurneysser ; history of the golden tooth.

1596. *Cereal* convulsiou in Hesse ; death of Al. Bodin ; prohibition of the exercise of surgery to the barbers of Paris.

1597. Creation of the health service of the armies of France ; death of Peter Foreest, and John of Posthius.

1598. Birth of Athanasius Kircher, of Peter Gassendi, of John Vesling, and of Henry Regius ; Harvey goes to Padua.

1599. Death of Tagliacotius ; birth of Werner Rolsink.

1601. Death of John Heurnius ; birth of Guy Patin, and of Vopiscus Fortunius Plemp.

1602. Birth of Peter Severinus ; death of Martin Ruland ; privileges of còllege of surgery, of Paris, confirmed by Henry IV.

1603. Death of Andrew Cæsalpinus, of John Costœus, and of Horace Augenius ; birth of Simon Pauli, and of Kenelm Digby.

―――――――――

MUSINGS ON RAILROAD TRAVEL,

From a Hygienic Point of View, during a Recent Journey of about Four Thousand Miles: By BENNET DOWLER, M. D.

Wieland says : " One could easily amuse people, if they were only amusable."
Goethe says : " He who is not led abroad by a great object, is far happier at home."
Travel in the younger is a sort of education ; in the elder a part of experience.—LORD BACON.

MUCH has been written, many schools and professorships have been established with a view to teach and practise gymnastics, and show their hygienic advantages. Such exercises are noted in the earliest records of the Greeks. In the 23d book of the Iliad, some of these exercises are enumerated at great length as practised in the army. Achilles, in his address to the aged Nestor, says :

> "Though 'tis not thine to hurl the distant dart,
> The quoit to toss, the ponderous mace to wield,
> Or urge the race, or wrestle on the field," etc.

Galen inquires whether the preservation of health is owing to medicine or to exercise, and refers to ancient authorities, including Hippocrates, upon gymnastics.

These exercises which tend to the development of the muscular system chiefly in the limbs, are very often adapted neither to the sick nor the debilitated invalid, to whom, indeed, they would be positively injurious from their active character.

Of the hygienic influences of railroad travel and of the special maladies to which it is adapted as more or less beneficial or curative, I intend to refer, should the remaining space of the Journal permit; if not, I may resume the subject hereafter. Of the supposed injurious effects of this mode of locomotion, I will merely mention that not long ago several French writers, upon theoretical grounds, asserted that the peculiar motion of a railroad train *(trépidation de la machine)* causes a softening or disintegration of the brain, spinal marrow, and nerves, with debility of legs, among the firemen, operatives, and employees of the roads. On the other hand, the physicians actually employed on these roads, who had every means of knowing whether these and other alleged affections do or do not result from this mode of life or occupation, maintain that no special malady whatever is thus produced.

Entertaining a favorable opinion of the hygienic influences of railroad locomotion, I must say, nevertheless, that two cases of locomotive-sickness exactly the same as sea-sickness have fallen under my observation. Of these I will not here write anything further at present. I will give a few desultory thoughts and remarks upon generalities of this topic.

The physiognomy of railroad travelers, particularly after one or two continuous days' and nights' travel, is temporarily damaged. Vivacity and loquacity are reduced to a low ebb. The countenance assumes an aspect of rigid repose, but not that of intellectuality or supreme happiness. This fixity or quietude bears marks of apparent wear, tear, and care, which cannot be referred to any previous or present disturbance of mind or body, being accompanied with a craving appetite and sometimes with positive suffering from hunger, when meals are "few and far between." Everywhere beyond the region of the stomach there is an unwonted passivity, except in seeing, but the visual and intellectual organs, in spite of the most enchanting scenery, are apt, in most cases, to relapse into passionless passivity, not to name noddings, snorings, and dreamings. Among those who may feel neither torpor nor sleepiness, connected trains of thought cannot be maintained without unusual efforts. The supremacy of the stomach (for vision is less potent), is an important hygienic feature of railroad traveling. The peculiar motion of railroad cars seems superior to any other for promoting digestion without the excessive fatigue of manual labor, hunting, etc. There is to some extent an antagonism between the simultaneous and vigorous actions of certain organs. If the mental organs be actively engaged immediately after the taking of a full meal, the digestive powers will, in most cases, be embarrassed ; or if the latter be actively engaged, the former will, for a time, be impeded in many cases.

Railroad traveling is not adapted to conversation, on account of the noise; nor to reading, on account of the motion; nor to connected trains of thought or ratiocinations, because the eye, a semi-passive organ, perceives an innumerable series of objects and pictures. The peculiar effects of railroad motion itself seems unfavorable to trains of connected thought. All of these circumstances are, however, favorable to the supremacy of the digestive powers, and are, therefore, favorable to the physical and physiological ends of the economy, a little mental torpor to the contrary notwithstanding.

Of all modes of traveling, that upon railroads is the best for ventilation, so desirable in the hot season. A sailing vessel, becalmed at sea, in hot, sultry weather, is very oppressive and uncomfortable, and when under full sail, with high wind, the close berths and cabins are generally very imperfectly ventilated, and the same may be affirmed to a considerable extent of steamboat voyaging in hot weather, and carrying large fires. But, however stagnant the air may be, the velocity of railroad cars virtually makes the current of air nearly half as active as that of a tornado. The change of air or scenery is never wanting in this mode of traveling. A degree of latitude or longitude is passed over in two hours, more or less, and such velocity is, therefore, equal at least to a strong breeze.

I will not venture upon a description of the picturesque scenery which for thousands of miles opens, draws near, recedes, and disappears, to he followed by another, another, and another equally beautiful and sublime—forests, farms, villages, cities, spires, rivers, lakes, blue mountain chains, whose rocky walls and towering pinnacles seem outliers of the realm of eternity. Neither pen nor pen cil can portray the varied landscapes which a single hour often brings successively into view, without fatigue to vision, unless it be directed to objects very near to the observer. I will here mention a fact new to me, and not the less valuable because it happens to be personal. During a travel of less duration than three weeks, my habit of looking at objects comparatively distant, removed a short-sightedness which, though slight, had been of long duration—I have said distant as compared to books, manuscripts, etc. I have never used the glasses for near-sighted persons, except for distant vision—for these, however, after a few days' travel, I had no use, having been able to see perfectly as others at the usual distances. This long-sightedness I still retain, though slightly diminished by pen-work and proof-reading, which often extend far into the night.

Extensive journeys, rapidly performed, seem ever and anon to reproduce the cherished idea which often prevails among business and professional men, statesmen and even politicians, namely, retirement if not absolute solitude, where the waves of passion, selfishness and violence are hushed or heard only in the distance. One sees in the repose of the quiet farm-house, girt with green fields, orchards, and woodlands with its flocks and silver-flowing streams, repose, a charming quiet, "solitude sweetened." The same idea is suggested by the rich, wild and uninhabited vales, slopes, and streams, where a sublime stillness reigns, broken only by the clanking cars, singing birds, or solemn waterfalls; the colossal trees and blue heavens above, and the flowery earth in repose below. I repeat the idea, that whether "solitude, with that inward eye which is the bliss of solitude," be sweet or bitter, all imaginative people who arc doomed to busy city life, feel, at least occasionally, an almost irrepressible desire "for a lodge in some vast wilderness, some boundless contiguity of shade," every variety of which is presented to the eye of the railroad traveler from the deep uninhabited forest

76

to the solitary cottage in the gap of some wild disrupted rocky ridge, or in the isolated valley gemmed with waving corn, flowery meadows and orchards, winding streams and gushing fountains, where odors blow from pines, magnolias and many such as salubrious as those "from the spicy shores of Araby the blest."

> Here cooling fountains roll through flow'ry meads,
> Here woods, Lycoris, lift their verdant heads:
> Here could I wear my careless life away,
> And in thy arms insensibly decay.   VIRGIL. ECL. X. WARTON.

But without even the fair Lycoris, it may reasonably be assumed that in such retreats up hill and down dale, on the mountain top, or sloping hill, the elements of health are more easily obtained than in the fashionable crowded hotels and ball-rooms usually resorted to in the hot season by southern people. Railroads throughout the country afford easy access to these natural *sanitaria*, amid every variety of rural scenery, waters, air and isolation from the crowd.

Goethe makes Dr. Faust say, that "man's proper element is restless activity, and that to spend one's days in solitude one must be either above or below humanity." Nevertheless, the temperate use of solitude strengthens both soul and body. Those who cannot discriminate between *ennui* and solitude, between crowded saloons and the ineffable beauties of nature everywhere present, ever varied and charming, should, perhaps, dwell with and look upon the fashionable mob, instead of wild lands, valleys, hills, streams, lakes, rocks, plants, birds, domestic flocks and plodding farmers. However, Samuel Johnson affirmed that "there is no solitude so awful to the stranger as London."

Those who cannot endure their own company will be miserable without that of others. But the poet Cowley has truly said :

> Who loves not his own company,
> Will feel the weight of't many a day.

The present utilitarian generation has consigned to the irrevocable past the hygienic benefits which their predecessors reluctantly enjoyed from long journeyings on foot, on horse-back, and in carriages, at the rate of thirty days for one thousand miles, ere steamboats, railroads and electrical telegraphs had triumphed over space and time, and in regard to the telegraph, utterly distanced beyond all comparison the velocity of the earth and her swiftest associates of the solar system. With a railroad conveyance Moses might have slept on the Nile and taken an early breakfast the same day on the Jordan, thereby saving forty years' travel. But in view of all these victories, the cuttings, and scarrings, and perforations of the rocky summits and slopes of the Alleghanies, and the making of viaducts over deep chasms to facilitate travel, it may be asked, has there not been physical and physiological deterioration, particularly among the misses, and matrons, and even the men of this broad Republic as consequences of the abandonment of the more active modes of travel ? But the remaining space will not permit of the detail of facts and reasons which would go to show the law of compensation enveloped in the steam engine which gives hourly ten thousand shocks, con-eussions, percussions, succussions, and oscillations (whether on the seats or in the sleeping cars), to the whole colony of organs crowded together in the cranial, thoracic, and abdominal prison-houses, causing the whole to wake up, to dance, hop, balance, swing, swim, wrestle, box, fence, and march to and fro, vertically, laterally, and horizon-tally—a gymnastic excitement not attainable in the more elegant mode of travel on luxurious steamboats—an exercise, it may be as-sumed, often curative in certain chronic non-inflammatory affections— as anæmia, hypochondria, hysteria, dyspepsia, general debility, with debility of the intestinal and uterine organs. It is neither a para-dox nor a contradiction to affirm that this is the most powerfully passive exercise for the invalid yet invented, and is precisely the one most desiderated, seeing that all the world seemed bent on de-veloping the voluntary muscles of the limbs and circumference to the neglect of the involuntary or central system.

COMMENCEMENT OF THE MEDICAL DEPARTMENT OF THE UNIVERSITY OF LOUISIANA.

The Annual Commencement of this institution was held at Odd Fellows' Hall, March 20th, 1860. Diplomas for the Degree of Doctor of Medicine, were awarded to one hundred and twelve of the candidates for graduation. There was one graduate in the Department of Pharmacy.

Dr. James Jones, Professor of the Practice of Medicine, addressed the class in an able speech. Dr. S. G. Guchett, of Canton, Miss., delivered the valedictory oration.

Greater success was never promised the Medical Schools of New Orleans, than during the past session. The rapid increase in the annual list of matriculates is the best evidence of prosperity. The number of students in the Medical Department of the University during the session of 1859 and 1860 was four hundred and two, being an increase of sixty-seven above that of last session.

The following is a list of the graduates at the University :

William C. Murphy...James W. Frazer.....Wm. H. Cunningham..
Robert F. Moody.....Samuel L. Bonner ....John Cameron ....
John R. Montgomery..George Badger.......James V. Cook.......
John A. McCreary....George Wyche ......John P. Davis ....
William E. Maddox...John N. Elliott......Moses R. Denman ....
Vandy M. Neal......Samuel N. Caston ....Augustus L. East ....
Samuel Parker.......Wm. F. Robertson, Jr.Augustus W. Egan...
Daniel Parker........Thomas B. Harwood..Peter R. Ford........
William A. Portwood..Walter Lewis........Fountaine D. Garrett..
William A. Robertson.Elam J. Hope........John B. Ginn ....
Birland Shields ......John T. Smith........William G. Gamble...
Frederick L. Sherrer..Jefferson S. Little....Miles W. Goldsby....
William H. Sprague ..Orlando A. Hobson...John W. Guerrant....
Jonathan H. Stroud...Ephraim A. Brevard ..Erasmus F. Griffin....
William H. Statham ..Franklin G. Johnson..James Harper........
Richard G. Turner....William T. Sawyer ...Charles W. Hill......
William C. Trabue....John H. Brack.......Leander G. Hunt......
Peyton W. Vining....George W. Tosey ...'.James M. Holcombe ..
John L. Waglay.....William M. Guice ....James T. Johnson....
James W. Wright....Richard T. Packwood.Derrick P. January...
Patrick H. Wright....Benjamin F. Brown...John Jordan.........
Lemuel Rhodes ......Eugene M. Kidd .....Nathan B. Kennedy ..
Rufus K. Stevens ....Martin L. Smith......Sherrod G. Luckett...
Benjamin F. Passmore.John B. Howell ......Robert L. Luckett....
Frank Rainey........Titus T. Holliday......Samuel P. Lewis.....
John M. Nuckolls ....John W. Jones ......Robert A. Lee ....
Jack Phillips........Alexander S. Delec....Thomas M. Marks ....
John Frost ....Edwin A. Bonneau....William McCord .....
Uriah C. Tate........Alfred A. Alston......Joseph W. Thompson.
William B. King.....James Purviance.....Samuel S. Noel ......
William Weathersby..Richmond P. Austin..Thomas B. Cook......
Frank Nailer ....Jones C. Abernethey..John J. Gardner......
John A. Stewart......Edward W. Britton ..Stephen E. Cuny .....
Jackson M. Gilbert...Preston E. Buckner...Sanford S. Riddell....
Franklin M. Gilbert...Sidney R. Chambers..Benjamin A. J. Avent.
Cicero C. Bates ......John W. Collins......William J. Lee.......
Lemuel Richardson...Charles M. Curell.....Charles W. Gibson....
James W. Jackson...

Graduate in Pharmacy ....Joseph A. La Neuville.

TO OUR SUBSCRIBERS.

We have enclosed in the present issue of the Journal the accounts of our subscribers, specifying all arrears due by each, and requesting an advance to the year 1861. We hope these bills will elicit an immediate response, and thus prevent pecuniary trouble.

We accept in payment of accounts, any bank bills current in the subscriber's State, and take such notes at our risk when enclosed in letters registered as "valuable." There is, however, less loss when sums due are sent by Order on Commercial Firms in this city or Mobile ; and we solicit subscribers to adopt this mode of remitting whenever it is practicable.

JAMES DEERING, and his associate, E. W. WILEY, are authorized to collect the accounts of this Journal. Bills for collection are occasionally entrusted to Postmasters and others, who have the written permission of one of the proprietors ; and such authority should always be demanded by the subscriber before payment.

All business communications should be addressed to

DRS. CHAILLÉ & NICHOLS,

Proprietors of the N. O. Medical and Surgical Journal,

New Orleans, La.

Mortality Statistics of New Orleans, from April, 1860, to June 10, 1860, compiled from the Weekly Reports politely furnished by Dr. Dirmeyer, Secretary of the Board of Health.

Time.	Total Deaths.	Children under 2 yrs.	Under 20.	U. States.
April (4 weeks)	633	230	344	368
May (4 weeks)	646	206	343	230
June (2 weeks)	382	157	210	193

Principal Diseases.	April (4 weeks).	May (4 weeks).	June (2 weeks).
Apoplexy	11	10	8
Cholera Infantum	17	17	17
Congestion of Brain	8	7	5
Congestion of Lungs	1	5	0
Consumption	76	74	28
Convulsions, Infantile	33	28	22
Croup	7	3	4
Diarrhœa	40	36	28
Dysentery	17	26	10
Diphtheria	20	16	5
Fever, Miasmatic	8	25	13
" Scarlet	15	21	14
" Typhoid	19	14	7
" Yellow	0	0	0
Gastro-Enteritis	7	9	5
Whooping-Cough	7	8	7
Inflammation of Liver	6	5	1
Inflammation of Lungs	48	26	10
Inflammation of Brain	0	2	6
Marasmus, Infantile	14	15	8
Measles	17	12	16
Pleurisy	3	0	1
Dropsy	0	0	0
Small Pox	7	2	0
Still-born	19	32	15
Teething	13	20	20
Tetanus	13	8	0
Trismus Nascentium	7	2	1

The Board of Health has reported no cases of Yellow Fever up to the present date, June 15th.

MONTHLY SUMMARY—METEOROLOGICAL REGISTER.—*From the Medical Purveying Office, U. S. Army, N. O.* New Orleans, La., Lat. 29 deg. 57 min. 30 sec. N.; Long. 90 deg. W. Altitude of Barometer above the level of the sea, 35 feet.

1860.	BAROMETER.			THERM. ATTACHED.			THERMOMETER.		
MONTHS.	Max.	Min'm.	Mean.	Max.	Min'm	Mean.	Max.	Min'm	Mean.
April.......	7 A. M. 13th. 30.360	9 P. M. 3d. 29.872	30.132	2. P. M. 9 & 10 83°	7. A. M. 28th. 66°	75.50	2 P.M. 10th. 86°	7 A. M. 27th. 59°	76.04
May..........	7 A. M. 2d. 30.300	7 A. M. 28th 29.990	30.155	2. P. M. 27 & 28 88°	7. A. M. 2d. 67°	79.40	Several. 64°	7 A. M. 1st 65°	80.03

1860.	HYGROMETER.			PREV'G WINDS.	WEATHER.		RAIN.	
MONTHS.	Max.	Min'm	Mean		Fair.	Cloudy.	Days.	Quantity.
April	2 P. M. 9th. 79°	7 P. M. 27th. 57°	70.53	E., S., & S. E.	days. 21	days. 9	4	2.42
May.........	2 P. M. 24th. 81°	7 A. M. 1st. 58°	73.57	S. W., & S. E.,	27.33	3.66.	3	1.26

NOTE.—Comparing the above with the corresponding months for the last four years, shows that this year is warmer 4.46 degrees, while the difference in Hygrometer shows that the atmosphere is about 2 degrees dryer. The force of winds much greater, and only about half the quantity of rain.

T. HARRISON, Clerk.

EDITOR'S OFFICE—NOTICES.

[Managing Editor's Office and Residence, 89 Constance, between Melpomene and Thalia streets; box 106 D, Post Office; box of the Journal at Mr. Morgan's book store, same place, where communications, etc., may be received.]

JULY, 1860.

NEW MEDICAL JOURNALS.

Georgia Medical and Surgical Encyclopædia—Edited by Horatio N. Hollifield, M. D., and Tom. W. Newsome, M. D. No. I, May, 1860. Pp. 48. Sandersville. Georgia.

The Cincinnati Medical and Surgical News—Edited by A. H. Baker, M. D., Professor of Surgery, etc.

BOOKS AND PAMPHLETS RECEIVED.

Clinical Lectures on Certain Acute Diseases—By Robert Bentley Todd, M. D., F.R.S., author of Lectures on Diseases of the Urinary Organs, etc. Pp. 308. 8vo. Philadelphia: Blanchard & Lea. 1860. From Mr. T. L. White, bookseller, 105 Canal street, N. O.

The Diseases of the Ear: their Nature, Diagnosis, and Treatment—By Joseph Toynbee, F. R. S., etc.; with 100 engravings on wood. Pp. 440. 8vo. Philadelphia: Blanchard & Lea. 1860. From Mr. T. L. White, bookseller, 105 Canal st., N. O.

Lectures on Diseases of Infancy and Childhood—By Charles West, M. D., author of Lectures on Diseases of Women, etc. Third American edition, from the fourth revised and enlarged London edition. 8vo. Pp. 630. Philadelphia: Blanchard & Lea. 1860. From Mr. T. L. White, bookseller, 105 Canal street, N. O.

The New American Cyclopædia : a Popular Dictionary of General Knowledge— Edited by George Ripley and Charles A. Dana. Vol. IX. Hayne : Jersey City. Pp. 784. Royal 8vo. New York: D. Appleton & Co. MDCCCLX. From Mr. Samuel Colman, publisher, general agent South, 60 Camp st., N. O. [Medical contributions to this volume, by Drs. Brown-Séquard, J. W. Francis, R. S. Fisher, L. Reuben, S. Kneeland, C. Kritser, J. G. Holland, O. W. Holmes, S. G. Howe, J. Jackson, and others. B. D.]

De L'Hématocèle Rétro-Utérine et des Epanchements Sanguins non Enkystés de la Cavité Péritonéale du Petit Bassin, Consideres comme Accidents de la Menstruation— Par le Docteur Auguste Voisin, Ancien Interne des hôpitaux de Paris, Lauréat de la Faculté de médecine et de la Société de chirurgie, Membre de la Société de la anatomique, de la Société médicale d'observation, de la Société de médecine du département de la Seine. Avec une Planche. Pp. 368. 8vo. Paris: J. B. Ballière et Fils. 1860. From the author, through Dr. Strubé, N. O.

Des signes propres à faire distinguer les Hémorrhagies Cerebelleuses des Hemorrhagies Cerebrales : Considérations de physiologie pathologique éclairant l'étude de la paralyse générale des aliénés. (Leçons de M. le professeur Bouillaud.) Paris. 1859. in-8. Recueillies par M. le Docteur Auguste Voisin, ex-interne des hôpitaux.

Galvanisation par Influence Appliquee au Traitement des Deviations de la Colonne Vertébrale, des Maladies de la Poitrine, des Abaissements de l' Utérus, etc—Par le Docteur J. Seiler. Pp. 157. 8vo. Paris: J. B. Baillière et Fils. 1860. From the author.

Urethro-Vaginal, Vesico-Vaginal, and Recto-Vaginal Fistules. General Remarks. Report of cases treated with the Button Suture in this country, and in London, Edinburgh, Glasgow, and Parisian Hospitals—By Nathan Bozeman, M. D., of New Orleans (late of Montgomery, Alabama). (From the New Orleans Medical and Surgical Journal for January, March, and May, 1860. Pp. 56. 8vo. New Orleans: Printed at the Bulletin Book and Job Office. 1860. From the author, 90 Baronne street, New Orleans. [Probably at no epoch and in no language has a memoir appeared upon this department of operative surgery equal to this. Simple in style, concise in narrative, successful in results, it bears all the internal marks of authenticity, and is, even in its unfinished state, a splendid contribution to practical surgery. From a note in the pamphlet edition, the author gives assurance that he will report the residue of his cases in this Journal. B. D.]

Dental Anomalies and their Influence upon the Production of Diseases of the Maxillary Bones—By Am. Forget, M. D., C. L. D., etc. Memoir crowned by the Academy of Sciences, at its meeting of the 14th March, 1858. Translated from the French. Pp. 32. Plates VI. Paris: Victor Masson. Philadelphia: Jones & White. 1860. From the publishers.

Pathology of Paralysis of Motion, with its treatment by Specific Exercises—By Charles F. Taylor, M. D. Pp. 32. New York: 1860.

Seventeenth Report of the Legislature of Massachusetts, relating to the Registry and Return of Births, Marriages, and Deaths in the Commonwealth, for the year ending December 31, 1858—By Oliver Warner, Secretary of the Commonwealth. Pp. CXLVII. Boston: 1859.

Pathological Phenomena Generalized—By H. Backus. Pp. 42. Selma, Ala.: 1860.

Announcement of Brigham Hall, a Hospital for the Insane—Canandaigua, N. Y.: January, 1860. Pp. 16.

Dr. Horace Wells, the Discoverer of Anæsthesia, with a Portrait—Pp. 15. From Mrs. Elizabeth Wells, widow of the discoverer. New York: 1860.

An Epitome of Braithwaite's Retrospect of Practical Medicine and Surgery—In six parts. Parts II and III: By Walter S. Wells, M. D. Published for the author. Through Mr. Samuel Colman, 60 Camp street, N. O., general agent for the States of Louisiana, Texas, Mississippi, and Arkansas.

To our Subscribers, Correspondents and Contributors.

All payments should be made, and business letters addressed to Drs. CHAILLÉ and NICHOLS, proprietors; and *not* to the publishers; all literary contributions to Dr. BENNET DOWLER.

Office of the Journal at the University Buildings, on Common street, near Baronne street.

Office hour, from 11 to 12 o'clock.

Copies of the Journal may be purchased, and the Journal subscribed for, at J. C. MORGAN & Co.'s, Exchange Place, at BLOOMFIELD, STEEL & Co's Book Store, No. 60 Camp street, and at T. L. WHITE's, 105 Canal street.

This Journal will be published bi-monthly, each number to contain 152 pages.

The Journal will be sent a second time to those who have not received it one month after the time for its appearance, if the subscriber write that he has not received it.

Those once ordering the Journal to be sent to them, will be considered subscribers until they order its discontinuance, which should be at least two months before they wish it discontinued.

No subscription discontinued unless at the option of the proprietors, until all arrears are paid up.

Numbers of the Journal sent as specimens to gentlemen who are not subscribers will not be continued, unless a written order to continue it is forwarded, with $5 enclosed for the first year.

Payments should be made to those only who bear the written authorization of one of the proprietors. When sent by mail it will be at the proprietor's risk, if registered as a valuable letter.

No personal matters, unless of general interest to the profession, will be published, except as advertisements, and as such must be paid for.

All communications for publication must bear the signature of the writer.

Original articles should be sent two months in advance, should be written on only *one side of the paper*, and those which are short and practical will be preferred.

Postmasters and Booksellers are requested to act as agents both in collecting debts, and procuring new subscribers. To collect debts a written authority will be forwarded upon their application, and they will be allowed to deduct a liberal percentage on any payments passing through their hands.

The contributors to this Journal can have forwarded, to their address, at small expense, 100 copies or more of their articles, in pamphlet form, provided the order to this effect accompany their articles.

TERMS OF THE JOURNAL—Five Dollars per annum, in advance.

TERMS OF ADVERTISEMENTS—always in advance—

> One page, per annum, $50; one insertion, $10.
> Half page   "   30; "   "   5.
> Quarter page, "   15; "   "   3·

Special arrangements will be made for inserting a few lines, cards, etc.

THE

NEW ORLEANS

MEDICAL AND SURGICAL JOURNAL.

SEPTEMBER, 1860.

ORIGINAL COMMUNICATIONS.

ART. I.—*Contributions to Comparative Anatomy and Physiology:* By BENNET DOWLER, M. D.

NUMBER ONE.   Eye of the Alligator *(Crocodilus Mississippiensis).*

General Remarks.—From the days of the great Cuvier, to the present, few animals have been written about so copiously, so learnedly, and yet so erroneously as the crocodile or alligator. Cuvier's authority throughout the world of science though unrivalled in the science of organization in general, is often erroneous as to the anatomy, physiology, and habits of this animal, but has been implicitly followed, and consequently no progress therein has been made. His errors have been faithfully copied by his successors. For example, osteologists follow him in affirming, as he has frequently done in his *Anatomie Comparée* and other works, that this and other saurians have no clavicle ;* whereas, in truth, no animal has a better one than the crocodilians.

In the present paper, it is proposed to bring together a few general observations casually made and widely scattered through

---

* Even in the recent work of Mr. Broderip (*Leaves from the Note Book of a Naturalist*), it is said of the *crocodilidæ,* " true clavicles there are none, but as in the rest of the saurian tribe, the corocord apophyses are attached to the breast bone ! "

7'

several MS. volumes, concerning the Eye of the Alligator. These observations, though less complete upon this organ (which was not an object of special study) than upon most others of this animal, may be, nevertheless, not altogether unworthy of the attention of the student of comparative anatomy and physiology, notwithstanding their imperfections. Owing to insufficient leisure to examine and collate all of my notes, it is probable that some facts recorded illustrative of this topic (the eye), may be unintentionally omitted. A mere outline of the special and reïterated records examined, is all that this paper is intended to give.

But before proceeding with this task, a few general remarks may not be misplaced.

Natural science, especially comparative anatomy and physiology, have for their fundamental aim the investigation of the organic structures and functional laws of animated Nature, not only interesting in themselves, but useful in tracing the relations of man to Nature, as well as in developing the laws which are essential to life, health, longevity and well-being. Comparative anatomy, physiology, pathology, and morbid anatomy have contributed, and are contributing beyond all calculation to the progress of medical science, being emiently experimental in their character. In this vast field many investigators already see, and now more clearly than ever, that with due cultivation, a rich harvest may be reaped. There is reason to think, that finally the schools of medicine will adopt this sort of experimentalism as a fundamental part of their courses of instruction upon the structural, functional and pathological history of man in health and in disease. Such materializing researches are not only more likely to elicit practical hints and principles than mere abstract reasonings concerning dynamism or immaterial forces, the nature of which eludes the grasp of the senses, but they also afford a counterpoise to the vain attempts so often made to build systems upon words, dogmas, and assumptions,

> " ——— As imagination bodies forth
> The forms of things unknown,
> Turns them to shapes, and gives to airy nothing,
> A local habitation and a name."

Without anticipating special descriptions, I will remark in general, that the typical position, or anatomical, physiological, and classificatory significance of the alligator possess far more value than has hitherto been recognized. In fact, it combines a greater number of the classificatory criteria of three out of the four departments into which the animal kingdom has been divided, namely, the vertebrata, articulata and mollusca, than perhaps any other single animal. As a vertebrate, its spine (neuro-skeleton) is the beau ideal or archetype of this great primary class—a kind of nucleus, central figure, or axis of mammals, birds, reptiles and fishes. The osseous plates of the skin (dermo-skeleton), the physiological anatomy of which has been wholly misconceived, and which form a exo-skeleton, not an armor of defence, as naturalists pretend. They serve for the insertion of numerous muscles (as will, perhaps, more fully appear hereafter). The alligator represents, to a considerable extent, the molluscans. Thus, the skin, with its infixed, carinated osseous plates, approximates the shell of the testacean, while, at the same time, the symmetrical arrangement, both longtitudinally and transversely, of the epidermic and dermoid tissues and plates resemble the articulata, as insects and crustaceans, bugs, crayfish, crabs, etc., forming a regular series of external articulations, a kind of peripheral skeleton. This animal is quadrupedal or four-footed—therein differing from the footless serpents or ophidians. It has claws like a bird. On land it moves like a quadruped ; in the water like a fish, by means of the tail and webbed feet which act as fins. Along with a most extraordinary peculiarity of structure of the heart, this organ has two ventricles and two auricles as among mammalians. It has numerous and perfect canine teeth, and is carnivorous. It would be tedious to enumerate all of its points of resemblance and typical agreement among the numerous groups alluded to above. At least it will be difficult to name any member of these groups which combines more extensively the common characteristics, varied functions, and close connections of the whole.

Rich as it is in structural and functional capital and typical comprehensiveness, it presents but a limited analogy to, or homological affinity with, the very group to which it has been assigned by zoölogists, namely the reptilia or amphibia (of the branch vertebrata) seeing that it differs much from batrachians, chelonians, ophidians, and even from most members of the order of saurians themselves. As a type, its many-sidedness, however, fills up some chasms in comparative physiological anatomy, and the classification founded on structure and function.

Taking the Linnæan criterion of classification, that is, the circulatory organism, for a guide, the alligator should be a warm-blooded mammalian ; for, as already stated, it has two auricles and two venticles—a double heart as in man, quadrupeds, and birds ; whereas this great naturalist and physiologist agreeably to this cardiac basis, classified the cold redblooded animals, as reptiles with fishes, etc., constituting an altogether distinct class, because they all had, as he mistakingly affirmed, but one auricle and one ventricle as their most striking anatomical characteristic.

The collateral medical sciences (the practical uses of which are not always immediately perceptible) have been too often, and with little reason, viewed with distrust, if not aversion by practical men as they term themselves,. Utilitarianism, however, does not create science, but science utilitarianism. Know all you can and apply what you can. The first is deemed by some scientific societies and investigators the fundamental aim and sole limit of their action— " to discover, not to apply," being their motto.

Professor Agassiz justly says on this subject : "When, in the past century, natural philosophers were studying the physical properties of amber and other resinous bodies, they discovered that on rubbing them singular effects were produced, and while they amused themselves in raising bits of paper, or causing paper dolls to dance upon a plate filled with wax, almost every one looked with ironical smiles upon the doings of these philosophers. Nobody could have guessed in that stage of scientific progress that out of these experiments would grow the most important improvements in the art of gilding, that new branches of industry would spring forth from the same source, in the shape of electrotyping, that lightning would be controlled in the hands of man, that telegraphs would bind nations in a network of instantaneous communication, that the methods of surveying and even those of observing the stars would be placed on a new foundation, and yet such were the results of the seemingly puerile experiments which led to a better acquaintance with electricity. But before such a mighty agent could be made subservient to useful purposes, it must be studied, and for a long time. While it was so studied, nobody foresaw its practical application. So it is with chemistry, so it is with geology, so it is with zoölogy. The most important applications of science to the useful arts may be traced back to some seemingly insignificant experiment, and it is a point which the community at large does not yet fully appreciate in its whole bearing. But while it is the function of science to point out such objects—to investigate the nature of those that have already come into use, to furnish well authenticated specimens of all for the inspection of everybody, it is a current misapprehension to expect from scientific men the practical application of their knowledge. They have fulfilled their task when they have furnished to others the knowledge required for such practical purpose, since their investigations call for peculiar mental qualities with special training, and the number of those who are well qualified to carry the knowledge already acquired into the sphere of its application is always greater than that of those who are best qualified to pursue original researches. For my own part, 1 have always made it a rule to stop my interest in any subject of inquiry which had reached the point where in any way it could be made practically useful, knowing that there would be many ready to take it up at the point where I leave it."

EYE OF THE ALLIGATOR.

Without purposing to give a description of the individual bones which enter into the composition of the orbit, I may remark, that the supra-orbital ridge which is composed of several bones besides the frontal, can afford little, if any protection to the globe, as it is not situated over but to the inner side of the eye. This ridge which is very salient and curves rapidly upon its cranial and inner aspect towards its fellow on the opposite side, but more gradually as it approaches the lachrymal bone in front.

A cranium whose outer posterior articulating processes connect with the articulating surfaces of the inferior maxilla, measuring five and a half inches in horizontal diameter, has an orbital longitudinal (antero-posterior) diameter of about two and a half inches, a transverse orbital diameter one and three quarter inches, with a depth to the palatine bones of about two inches, while the distance between the supra-orbital ridges of the orbits is but one inch.

The globe is large, deep and but feebly attached to the walls of the socket, being fixed in its place chiefly by the large optic nerve, by a little loose areölar or cellular tissue, and by several delicate muscles (about four or six). In the living animal the globe is nearly motionless.

The great capacity and depth of the orbits which are not apparent in the living animal, become evident, enormous, upon removing the supra-orbital integument with its osseous plates, the globes and soft tissues. The two orbits have a thin partial septum of bone for a very short distance which is replaced by a large membraneous partition ; a portion of the floor of the orbits consists of a dense oval membrane, forming a part of the palatine roof.

Owing to the absence of cranial protection to the eye, and the great but virtually concealed size of the orbits exteriorly as well as to the slight muscular or other connections of the globe to surrounding tissues, there can be little difficulty in allowing that the numerous accounts yearly appearing in the public journals concerning the gouging of alligators, to make them relax their hold of persons whom these animals have seized as enemies or prey, are not altogether fabulous. The eye of this animal is like the heel of Achilles, the most vulnerable point. Gouging probably compresses painfully the optic ganglion or bulb which expands greatly on passing the posterior orbital fissure or strait—a subordinated brain (so to speak) thrown out in advance of the brain proper, to which it is united by an isthmus at the base of the cerebrum.

I will here allude to two examples of gouging, the first which come to view among a number of which I have made records as being more or less authenticated. A young man, named Norton, was bitten by an alligator in the hand and arm. He was much injured and had a bone broken. He gouged the animal, which then let go its hold. The alligator, which was captured, measured nearly ten feet. (*Jackson Courier*, Florida, 1835.)

Park, the celebrated traveler, in his second expedition to discover the termination of the Niger, relates that his guide, while crossing a river, was seized by the thigh, by an alligator, and dragged under the water. The man gouged the animal, which released his hold, but soon after it seized him by the other thigh, whereupon the guide took the same method to save himself, and succeeded, having, however, suffered two bad wounds.

Herodotus (father of history and some fiction, too) maintains that when in the water, the crocodile is blind. This would be a great impediment, seeing that it lives chiefly upon animals which inhabit the water, as fish, etc. It can use the naked cornea under water. The nictitating membrane, though not wholly opaque, must diminish rapid and accurate vision. It can hardly be supposed that fish would accidentally, or by design, 'enter into the mouth of such a formidable enemy, however blind.

In the *Histoire Naturelle* de Lacépède, edited by Desmarest (Paris, 1844), it is affirmed that the crocodile has two strong eyelids, both of which are movable. The author quotes, but discredits Pliny, who says (in his *Historia Naturalis*), that the inferior eyelid alone is movable (i, 161). Here the Roman naturalist is right, and M. De Lacépède wrong. There is, as will be stated, but one eyelid proper, the lower one, which alone is movable, and which rising vertically against the fixed, rudimentary one, closes the eye in a horizontal direction.

Cuvier *(L'Anatomie Comparée*, iii, 453) says that crocodiles have three eyelids, " trois paupières," two of which are horizontal, closing exactly, the third being vertical, each having an enlargement along its borders. There is no upper eyelid, but a dense, passive, dermoid tissue, not deserving to be called a rudimentary eyelid, enclosing osseous plates above, especially on the anterior upper aspect of the globe, which forms a semilunar protective structure, serving as the vault of the orbit, and incapable of downward motion in the closure of the eye, although there is sometimes a slight upward curve or recession from any violent contractile action of the under or true lid, as when an irritant is applied to the latter so as to threaten injury to this organ. The inferior is therefore the true lid which closes and covers all the free or exposed portions of the eye, while the strong nictitating membrane acting perpendicularly, also covers the same more immediately. It is a misnomer to designate the latter the third eyelid.

The muscles which elevate the inferior eyelid are inserted partly into the orbitar bones of the head and partly into the immovable upper lid at the palpebral commissure. The bony plates of the so-called upper lids must prevent them from acting as such. Nevertheless, among the several fanciful criteria by which writers seek to differentiate the crocodile and the alligator, MM. Duméril and Bribon enumerate " a bony plate in the substance of the upper eyelid," as characterizing the former. *(Mus. Nat. Hist.*, ii, 82.)

The cornea is large, compared to the globe, and reflects the light brilliantly, appearing less convex than the human cornea. The sclerotica is not white, but apparently of a deep black color; but after washing away the black pigment from the choroid coat on the interior surface of the sclerotica it becomes nearly as transparent as the cornea itself. The iris, the hyaloid, the retina, choroid, the lens, the capsule, etc., are beautiful microscopic objects, which I will not attempt to describe. Several tissues and organs, as the capillary, pulmonary, and muscular, are less opaque in this than in the warm-blooded animals.

In his *Traité élémentaire d'Anatomie Comparée* (1838), Carus says that the choroid and iris of the crocodile are greenish *(verdâtre)!* The iris is sometimes grayish or silvery. I do not find it mentioned in my notes as being green.

The mobility of the iris, and, consequently, the sensitiveness or excitability of the retina, are very great. The form and size of the pupil are very variable, agreeably to the greater or lesser intensity of the light, with the exception of its vertical diameter, in which there is scarcely any appreciable change, while the horizontal diameter undergoes remarkable alterations, varying from the linear to the ellipse. The utmost degree of contraction of the pupil presents an almost perpendicular straight-lined appearance, very little wider in its horizontal center than in its most acute angles above and below. With a diminished light, the horizontal central diameter may attain enormous proportions, which give this irian aperture, in rare cases, a form almost circular.

From the great mobility of the iris and expansion of the pupils, it is highly probable that the alligator can see in comparative darkness, and can easily take its prey in the night, on land, or in the water, giving it an advantage over animals which either see little or none except in daylight, and the more so, because it acts stealthily and by strategem, and lies in wait, rather than pursues, owing to its incapacity for either swift locomotion or sudden turning to the right or left.

The alligator does not appear to require the simultaneous use of both eyes for complete vision. Thus, it appears to see objects on the right and on the left with the corresponding eye. On irritating an alligator, he left the water, walking deliberately to the remotest part of his pen, where he crouched, lying with his head diagonally towards me, so that with one eye he could watch my movements, leaving the other for emergencies in another direction. I have frequently observed one eye next to a closed wall, as if sleeping, while the other appeared to be keeping watch on the exposed side. They appear sometimes to affect sleep, as opossums affect death, when in danger of capture or death, though they do not, like the latter, fall into despair, non-resistance, and passive obedience.   Thus, alligators watch sometimes with only one eye, when that is sufficient or best adapted to their purpose, while the other eye may be shut and apparently sleeping.   They seldom, perhaps never wink, unless with a view of guarding against injury.   While the visual axes of both eyes are probably susceptible of acting in concert upon a single object, yet, in certain positions, under different circumstances, each eye may be capable of independent action, especially laterally—a dual or binoculor vision, with or without the blending of two images into one.

OBSERVATIONS AND EXPERIMENTS ILLUSTRATIVE OF THE PHYSIOLOGY OF THE EYE OF THE ALLIGATOR*.

In thirty minutes after the exhibition of five grains of strychnine to an alligator, the symptoms of poisoning being fully developed, the pupils dilated considerably, but unequally, their centers rolled upward, towards the orbital vault—a rare occurrence even in the agony.

The globes move but little in vision, and deviate but slightly from their parallelism, either in health or during vivisection.   This animal, an hour later, nictitated during dissection.   While progressively slicing away the brain in another vivisection, the ires were little changed until after the division of the olfactory and optic nerves, when the pupils dilated, but the eyes still winked when touched.

May.—An alligator which was somewhat feeble, was vivisected. A portion of the convexity of the brain having been sliced off, the eyes were closed.

May 22.—An alligator, four feet nine and a half inches long, having been decapitated and lost much blood, appeared to possess distinct vision for an hour afterwards.   It closed the eye when a foreign body approached—opened its eyes to watch—the pupil contracted and dilated alternately, according to the intensity of light or darkness, much as in the normal condition.

---

* I ought here to mention that these observations on the eye, though not casual, were incidental or secondary, having been made chiefly in connection with vivisections.

June 5.—The separated head of an alligator was observed for some hours ; the eyes were open, but closed on being touched.

November 1.—Air of the pen 53°; alligator's gullet 54°. This animal, when a loud noise was made, moved its head, but did not open its eyes until it had been manipulated.

In hot weather, for fifteen to twenty-five minutes after tying the trachea, the pupils remained normal, but in from forty to forty-five minutes, and at the time of apparent death from strangulation, the ires dilated enormously.

The head of an alligator, which had been cut off for some time, appearing to be dead, the eyes having been closed, I attempted to open the latter, when the animal closed them more firmly, as if by a voluntary power. This occurred in a hot day of July.

November 23.—During five days the temperature at sunrise has ranged from 39° to 57°. The alligators are in a deep hibernating sleep, and quite torpid, but may be aroused from sleep for a time on being touched, though unable to move ; the nictitating membrane being drawn over their eyes, the pupil of which appear strongly contracted.

November 26.—Air, 7, A. M., 70°; cloudy; the weather has changed suddenly from cold to warm. Upon an alligator, still torpid, a bucket of water was poured. This caused it to open its eyes, the pupils of which were enormously dilated.

December 3.—Weather warm (minimum 70°); the alligators sleep profoundly, with closed eyes.

February 5.—Minimum of the day 50°; alligators sleep, being motionless. On disturbing them, some opened the eyelid, and then slowly retracted the nictitating membrane, but soon sunk again into stupor. In sleep, both the lower eyelid and nictitating membrane appear to close.

At 40°, the alligator in the water, the tip of the muzzle being out, sleeps profoundly, but on being disturbed opens his eyes with difficulty, the pupils of which are contracted to the extreme, presenting straight, vertical lines, which, as the eyes slowly shut, seem to continue thus contracted. In the hot season, the ires often contract also, forming the pupil from twenty to thirty times longer in its vertical than in its horizontal diameter.

When the external air is 26°, the immersed body at 33°, cannot open the eyes when irritated.

MEMBRANA NICTITANS.

The nictitating membrane, which is semi-transparent, occasionally winks, though this is rarely the case. This fibro-muscular web is dotted over with oval but flattened and rather opaque spots, which are probably glandular. This, however, is merely a conjecture. What has been so often said of crocodilian tears is fabulous. I have irritated the eye and witnessed severe traumatic ophthalmia without seeing tears or the watery exudations usual in inflammation of the human eye.

Prof. Carus, who always calls this nictitating membrane of the crocodilians, the third eyelid, says, that "it is found in the *anterior angle* of the eye and acts horizontally" *(Anat. Com.)*; while Dr. Carpenter says, that "this third eyelid is formed by an additional fold of the membrane at the *inner angle.*" *(Comp. Phys.,* § 723).

In examining my notes, I have, as yet, found only one description of the course of action of the nictitating membrane, from which it appears that it acts from the anterior towards the posterior angles of the eye.

As the above distinguished writers of our text books give contradictory statements on this topic, I subjoin the note referred to, and, although my recollection coïncides with it, still I do not wish to be considered as making a positive statement : Alligators wink or shut the eye by rapidly passing the nictitating membrane from *before,* backward, over the cornea ; its advancing margin is straight, though somewhat inclined to the horizon ; but when they sleep, or wish to avoid the contact of a body against the cornea, they close the eye completely, by raising the lower, in fact the only true, lid of the eye. There is a slight rudimental palpebral line above the globe, forming the outer margin of the orbit, being straight, without any motion. The margins of the closed lids form nearly a straight line, which passes in the longitudinal direction of the animal ; that is, forwards or backwards, nearly on a level with the skull, presenting itself above or over the eye, and not laterally, so that in opening the eye the lid descends from this line, which overlies the globe.

June 13.—One of three alligators has lain apparently asleep, under water, without any change of position, for several days, as it has done repeatedly before, having only the nictitating membrane drawn over the cornea, the inferior eyelid not closing over the eye.

In his *Personal Narrative of Travels to the Equinoctial Regions of the New Continent* (6 vols., 8vo.), the late Baron Humboldt, in describing the llanos and pampas of South America, where often thirty square leagues present an ocean of grass, without a single elevation of the ground a foot in height, mentions that, in these regions, the alligators and great serpents bury themselves in the mud, and fall into a lethargy or hibernating sleep on the approach of the summer, or dry, hot season. (iv, 297.) This statement, which he reïterates, and which nullifies much of the reasonings of physiologists upon cold as the direct cause of the hibernating sleep, does not, however, receive any confirmation in Louisianian alligators, whose activity generally corresponds with the climatorial increment of heat. Here cold and torpidity coïncide, and assume the appearance of cause and effect. " It is," says Humboldt, " a curious physiological phenomenon, to observe the alligators of North America plunged into a winter sleep by an excess of cold, at the same period when the crocodiles of the llanos begin their *siesta* or summer sleep—habits that appear essentially linked with their organization. (*Ib.* 501–2.)

Systematic writers on physiology, who live in high latitudes, have an apparently easy way of explaining, after a fashion, the hibernating sleep of animals as being the natural effect of cold, and the diminished respiration is spoken of as diminished combustion, which explains the inability of generating heat, which is reasoning in a circle. Now, if cold is the essential cause of this sleep, it is very fortunate that hibernating animals breathe but little or none for long periods, as breathing would tend to lower their temperature (which, indeed, it does in warm-blooded animals). A hibernating, cold-blooded animal breathing air below the freezing point, would probably be itself congealed, not heated, in extreme cold.

This blowing hot and cold in the same breath is not a good method in physiology, neither is *ex parte* evidence in physiological chemistry the surest mode of establishing a valid theory. If the logic of cold accounts for winter hibernation, how can summer hibernation be explained by its antithesis, heat? Mr. Woodward, in his work on shells, says : " The fresh-water mollusks of cold climates bury themselves during winter, in the mud of their ponds and rivers. In warm climates they become torpid during the hottest and dryest part of the year. Those genera and species which are most subject to this ' summer sleep,' are remarkable for their tenacity of life." 18. In such a case, it were better to assume, provisionally, that hibernation is a primary law infixed or blended with the constitution of certain animals in certain climates, and no more explicable by respiration, cold, or heat, than their instincts, forms, sizes, gravity, color, etc.

The alligator of Louisiana sleeps from necessity during cold weather, cold being at least the condition, if not the cause, of this sleep ; but in hot weather, when supplied with food, it often appears to sleep from choice or laziness—a sleep, however, which is never profound, being more apparent than real.

When recently captured, it is wakeful and anxious. It examines its pen repeatedly (and with great skill, examples of which I might detail); if no avenue of escape above ground can be found, it usually attempts to undermine the enclosure by digging ; but on finding escape impossible, it makes no further attempts with that view, but becomes a great day-sleeper, taking little or no exercise. If the weather be uncomfortably hot, it either sleeps in the shade, or more generally in the water ; if, during the warm season of the year, a sudden chilliness takes place, it sleeps in the sun, or in the water, should the water be warmer than the air. When a number inhabit the same enclosure, they usually sleep together in a closely-packed group, doubling or lying on each other most lovingly.

The latitudinarian, not to say contradictory, explanations which physiological chemists usually give of the cause and effects of hibernation, are neither self-evident in themselves nor clearly deducible from facts. The chemical burning out of the fat, and the consequent emaciation ascribed to the hibernating sleep, are absolutely visionary in regard to the alligator, which is as fat in the spring, after several months' sleep, as it was at the close of the previous hot season. How could a lean animal, one already thin in autumn, keep up the fire of fat for half a year? No fat, no combustion ! Does not Professor Lehmann, in his Physiological Chemistry (which is regarded the ablest extant), forget the orthodox doctrine, when he concludes that "the weight of the body is increased during hibernation ?" He says : "As a large part of the oxygen remains in the body of the sleeping animals (since only a small quantity is expended in the formation of carbonic acid, and the water which is formed does not evaporate, owing to the low temperature of the animal), and nitrogen is absorbed, *we have an explanation* of the fact first observed by Sacc, that the *weight* of the body is generally, though not constantly, *increased during the hibernation of marmots.* These inquirers (Regnault and Reiset) arrived at similar results in reference to the influence of hibernation, or the sleep induced by exposure to cold, in their experiments on *lizards.*" (ii, 457.)

Now, if lizards (that is, the order sauria, which includes a vast assemblage besides crocodilians) increase in weight owing to the influence of cold and the hibernating sleep, and in the meantime eat nothing, and apparently breathe none, surely physiologists ought to reconsider their postulates, and students ought to write on the margins of their text books, on many pages, "*not proven.*" Todd and Bowman, in their excellent Physiological Anatomy, give, as do others, the following general account of the hibernating sleep : "Previous to becoming torpid, the animal accumulates a quantity of fat, which is, as it were, laid up as in a storehouse, to be consumed slowly, while the period of annual sleep lasts." (739.) These learned writers give, in the same paragraph, one illustrative example of their doctrine, namely : that of the marmot ! affirming of this mouse, that when hibernating, "the pulse falls to about 15 beats in a minute, and the respirations to about 14 in an hour, while in the waking state these are respectively 150 and 500 ; " and yet the learned Professor Draper says, that "the sleeping *marmot* exhibits the remarkable phenomenon of *increasing in weight by respiration alone.*" (Phys., 172.)

Does any mouse in the group of the *muridæ* bring forth such a mountain of physiology as this, especially when fast asleep ? It is well, however, for the student to consider, in view of such logic, Lady Capulet's words to the nurse, in Romeo and Juliet—

> " Aye, you have been a *mouse-hunt* in your time ;
> But I will watch you."

Physiology, the guiding star of Medicine, requires additional experimentation in order to verify, or expurgate much (that has found admission in existing text books), which, in the meantime, should be provisionally rejected or received as hypotheses to be tested by further researches.

Art. II.—*Treatment of two Cases of Convulsions, one of which was attended with Cutaneous Anæsthesia.*

Eagle Creek, Bradley Co., Ark., June 5, 1860.

Dr. B. Dowler—*Dear Sir:* If you consider the following reports of two cases, taken from my journal, of sufficient importance, you are at liberty to publish them.

Yours, very respectfully,

Wm. D. Barnett, M. D.

February 22, 1860.—Called to see Simon, negro boy, belonging to the estate of D. F——. He was complaining yesterday morning; took a dose of castor oil and turpentine. He had complained several days ago of pain in his bowels. He had a slight attack of scarlet fever about three weeks ago. Last night, between twelve and one o'clock, he was taken with a violent spasm. McLean's vermifuge was given him. I saw him at 3 o'clock, A. M. Pulse full and strong; some heat of the skin; tongue coated yellowish, and red at the tip; bowels flaccid; oil and turpentine had operated twice; coughs occasionally. I bled him freely, and gave a dose of calomel and ipecac; 3 grs. calomel and 2 grs. of ipecac, to be repeated every two hours. At 5 o'clock, A. M., immediately after the second powder was given, he had a convulsion, and immediately after, another. I ordered injections of spirits turpentine, and a blister applied to the nape of the neck; gave another dose of calomel and ipecac, and put his feet in hot mustard-water. At 9 o'clock I gave him a full dose of calomel, and morphine half a grain, with directions to give the calomel and ipecac, and spirits turpentine injections, every two hours, also to rub the spine with turpentine.

This boy is about fourteen or fifteen years of age, stout and robust constitution.

Are the convulsions in this case dependent upon effusion in, or congestion of, the brain?

Three o'clock, P. M.—He is not any better; has had frequent convulsions since 2 o'clock; breathes heavy, attended with a gurgling noise. Coma; skin warm; pulse full and intermittent; bowels appear somewhat distended. I bled him again; gave another dose of calomel and ipecac. As there had been no action of the bowels, I ordered, at half-past six, to use castor oil and lac assafœtidæ as an injection, for two or three times, at intervals of two hours. If the bowels are not thoroughly moved by these means, to use one drop of tiglii oleum every three hours, until they are. Applied warm poultices over the bowels, and as the heat of the skin had greatly diminished, and the pulse become much weaker, blisters to the extremities. I also ordered the calomel and ipecac to be given after the bowels are opened.

February 23.—I saw Simon again this morning ; he had frequent convulsions during the early part of the night—in fact, up to three o'clock this morning. At five o'clock he had two copious operations from the bowels; he has had no convulsions since; intellect returned ; pulse regular and soft, about 80 ; skin pleasant. During the night he lost a considerable quantity of blood, owing to the accidental removal of the bandage from his arm during the convulsions. The croton oil was administered before the bowels would act. I ordered the oil and assafœtida injections to be given every three hours, in order to keep the bowels open, and if two injections failed, to use the croton oil again.

Saw Simon again this evening. Has not been purged in six or eight hours. I ordered the injections to be commenced with immediately. At five o'clock, R. M., bowels were open, and he appears to be doing well. I. ordered calomel and ipecac to be continued at intervals of four hours, for four doses ; quinine to be given this evening, but if it produces much elevation of the pulse, or heat of the skin, to discontinue it, and keep the bowels open with the means already directed. From this time he improved rapidly, and in a few days was at his daily vocation.

CASE 2.—*May* 16, 1860.—Saw negro boy Ellis, aged sixteen years, belonging to W. D. M. He was discovered, two days ago, in a peculiar condition, in which there was loss of sensibility and muscular power ; and while in this state, to all appearance he was unconscious, yet he remembered everything that was said or transpired during the paroxysm. Pulse full, and slower than natural ; respiration slightly accelerated ; skin cool, with the exception of the head, which feels hot. He has had several paroxysms ; two yesterday and one to-day, while at my office. The first two days they came on about noon ; to-day at about nine o'clock, A. M. The one I saw presented the same appearance as the former ones. He said he was conscious of everything that went on around him ; heard me say bring water, and knew when the tobacco was taken from his mouth.

He was totally insensible to pain, as he manifested none when I pricked him with a pin.

When he came to himself it was suddenly, commencing with yawning and stretching, as though awakening out of sleep, and suddenly jumping up, as though nothing had been the matter. During the paroxysms, his muscles were relaxed, and the pupils of the eyes contracted on exposure to the light. He stated that he tried to speak when spoken to; and I noticed, a few seconds before arousing, a slight tremulous motion of the lips, as though he was endeavoring to speak. There were two teeth in front much decayed, which I extracted.

Ordered a cathartic of blue mass and ext. col. comp., every other day, and the use of oxide of zinc and quinine. I could learn nothing as to the cause of the paroxysms; he says he is as healthy as he ever was, and his appetite good; also has good digestion and regular action from his bowels. The paroxysms mentioned are the first of the kind he has ever had.

May 28.—I hear that the boy Ellis has had no return of the paroxysms. Two or three days after I saw him, I learned that recently he had become a very hearty eater, and had fattened very fast since his present owner had him, which is about six months. His intellect is not very strong. His peculiar nervous state may have been produced by portal congestion, and the operation of the mercurial cathartic removing this, recovery ensued; or it may be that the oxide of zinc and quinine, or the removal of the necrosed teeth, or all combined, produced the effect.

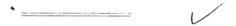

Art. III.—*A Case of Triplets:* By E. Mason, M. D., Wetumpka, Ala.

The occurrence of a triple birth, is worthy of record on account of its rarity, if no other circumstance of interest attend it ; for, according to the most favorable estimate, triplets occur only once in every three or four thousand cases of labor. Collins states, that in 129,172 cases of pregnancy, there were only 29 triple births, or 1 in 4,450 ; Ramsbotham's table of 29,489 cases, gives only one of triplets ; and Churchhill's record of 448,998 cases, furnishes but 77 triple births, or 1 in 5,831.

CASE.—Harriet, colored woman, ,aged 23 years, third pregnancy, property of Mr. H. Zeigler, of Autauga County, was taken in labor on the afternoon of the 18th of February, 1860, and at 8 o'clock, P. M., was delivered of a male child, being attended by a colored midwife. The placenta not coming away in due time, the midwife reported that she could not " clear " the woman, and desired me to be sent for. I arrived about 3 o'clock, A. M., and, upon examination, found the head of a child presenting, instead of a retained placenta. Finding that the midwife had used only one ligature in securing the cord of the child she had delivered, I immediately tied the placental end. The woman being very much exhausted, and the uterine pains having almost ceased, I gave her some ergot, and about 5 o'clock, A. M., delivered her of a living female child. The hypogastric region remained large, and, on further examination, I discovered the head of a third child presenting, which was delivered in half an hour ; but was still-born. This was a female also, and was apparently as well developed as the other two, and there was no abnormal appearance, except that it seemed to be entirely bloodless.

The second child was attached to a separate placenta, which was quite small ; while the first and third children had a common placenta. This accounted for the death of the third child, for it evidently perished from hæmorrhage through the untied end of the cord of the first. The following table shows the sex, weight, and presentations :

1st. Male — weight, 5½ pounds—breech presentation—living.
2d. Female   "   5½   "   vertex   "   "
3d.   "   "   5¼   "   "   "   dead.

ART. IV.—*Contributions to the Pathological Anatomy and Natural History of Typhus Fever:* By BENNET DOWLER, M. D.

NUMBER ONE.

I.

1848 ; Feb. 9, 11, A. M.   J. H., aged 31, born in Ireland, resident thirteen weeks, apparently of good constitution and stout frame, now emaciated from six* weeks' sickness, hair long, black, and coarse ; face dusky copperish color, being sometimes cyanosed ; insensible ; mouth constantly open ; eyes injected, prominent, and suffused with tears, half open, and turning askance without maintaining their parallelism ; breath fœtid ; pasty sordes on the teeth and gums ; tongue tumid, retracted, tremulous, dry, of a dark cherry red, and covered on its dorsum, except near the tip, with a black crust like a large cracked scab ; pulse variable, rapid, irregular ; respiration rapid, laborious, noisy, accompanied with moanings or mutterings, alternating with screamings ; sudaminia on the trunk, though slight ; dusky discolorations in small spots on the arms ; abdominal tension (muscular ?); bedsore as large as the hand, black and gangrenous, on the sacro-lumbar region ; skin dry and dusky ; lies on the back ; unable to change his position ; universal muscular tremblings particularly in the muscles of the eyes, mouth, neck, arms, and fingers; the latter undergo repeated semi-flexions and clenchings ; pupils somewhat contracted ; bend of the arm $104\frac{1}{2}°$, axilla 105°.

Such is a general picture of the last stage of a case diagnosticated typhus, which the medical attendant for six days before death treated with foot baths, cold applications to the head, and also with quinine and opiates.

Feb. 10 ; 10, A. M. Autopsy thirteen hours after death. The sudaminia and dusky discoloration of the arms above mentioned, have disappeared. The dark mixture of bluish copper color gone from the face and neck ; neck limber; jaws rigid (and so continued during the dissection, near 2, P. M.); the skin of one side of the face and neck, as well as of the other dependent parts, nearly black from cadaveric hyperæmia ; moderate but declining rigidity of the limbs; abdomen rigid, not convex ; adipose tissue scanty ; muscles firm, but slightly darkened ; the animal heat not yet dissipated, being natural, excepting the extremities which are growing cold ; not a trace of coagulated blood in the body ; the blood fluid like water, and nearly black—a portion taken in a cup in a few minutes almost resembled ink ; the arteries everywhere empty ; lice on the body, but dead.

Head.—The scalp discharged a few drops of liquid, black blood ; frontal sinus natural but extremely large ; dura mater or its arach-

---

* This is supposed to be an error of the pen, as I find a note at the end of the case, stating that the disease run its course rapidly. Six days, not six weeks, may be assumed as correct.

noid firmly adherent for two inches square upon the superior surface
of the hemisphere of the brain. A slightly opaque, subarachnoid
gelatinous exudation upon all parts of the brain ; universal vascularity, with complete injection and distension of the pia mater
chiefly peripheral and venous ; the ventricles and the substance of
the brain approximate the same state ; the large arteries collapsed ;
the firmness of the brain, especially of the medulla oblongata, increased ; the serosity of the ventricles natural, that of the arachnoidal sac augmented, perhaps an ounce and a half ; the sinuses
rather collapsed ; the latter contain a little blackish fluid blood.

Chest.—Lungs distended, greatly congested, less anteriorly, but
still everywhere loaded with blood ; about eight ounces of black
liquid blood had transuded into each pleural sac, though the lungs
are crepitant in all parts, having a little brittleness and great engorgement ; no other alteration, excepting in the tracheo-bronchial
membrane, which is dark and vascular. The pleura and diaphragm
natural ; the pericardium contains less serosity than usual ; the
heart collapsed, thin, flabby, and non-resilient, its tissue scarcely
brittle ; it is empty—the right side contains a few drops of liquid
black blood ; cardiac and aörtic valves and aörta, etc., natural.

Abdomen.—The peritoneum, including the outer coat of the intestines, unctuous and adhesive to the touch. Omenta greatly attenuated, portions having a dark red hue. The epithelium of the
œsophagus thickened and transformed into a mealy, crustaceous,
or cheesy brittle matter. The stomach small, contained a few
spoonsful of dirty sanguinous liquid, the pyloric half excessively
vascular and injected, pink colored ; mucous tissue had either disappeared, leaving the arborized stems, twigs and leaflets of the
vessels (for such was their general appearance) exposed, or softened
into a muco-sanguineous jelly, leaving the stomach very thin ; serous
coat natural ; the omental connection of the great curvature with
the colon, red and vascular. The duodenum not softened ; its sub-
mucous tissue vascular, injected, loaded and darkened with blood.
The jejunum contains some chylous and yellow pasty matter, being
in some portions injected and softened in the mucous tissue ; the
upper third of the ileum has a firm intussusception about three
inches long ; 12 inches of the bowel from above had descended,
forming an oblong firm mass of a dark color ; above and below this,
the bowel is small and attenuated for two or three inches ; the in-

vaginated mass impacted very firmly as if portions had entered each other like a nest of pill-boxes, the whole appearing to be impervious. The contained portion has an elliptical (Peyerian) plate, many of which were found at intervals to the valve of the colon, sometimes an inch or more in length, but often less, being semi-transparent, non-vascular—an eruption like dusky pits and cells rather than like elevated pustules ; vascularity surrounds, but does not tra-verse these plates ; they are brittle, rather than soft ; and when scraped come away like scraped melon in consistence, rather than like mucous matter ; the soft, velvety mucous tissue natural to the bowels is completely altered, often condensed so as to appear sunk and lost in the muscular coat. The whole of the mucous tissue of the appendix veriformis had this non-vascular, cell-like arrangement ; the centre of these depressed pustules has a dusky point or nucleus as large as a pin's head. The appendix contains a small rod or thread-like column of fæces. Below the intussusception vascularity and softening of the mucous tissues, with some pasty, yellow and greenish fæcal matter were noticed ; the large intestine from the valve to the anus is enormously distended with fæces, the greater portion of which is natural ; at the cæcum and at the great arch of the colon and in the lower portion of the rectum, there are the same changes of the mucous tissues as in the pyloric half of the stomach. The mesentery and its glands dark and injected ; the glands some-what enlarged ; a few traces of chyle were seen in dividing the lacteals ; bladder contracted, injected, contained three or four ounces of turbid urine, with sedimentary branny matter. Kidneys engorged, but of natural consistence, as are the spleen and pancreas. The liver is rather pale on its convex surface ; brittle, but somewhat supple ; its convex surface for one or two lines in depth, is dyed of an iron color (this is often seen, and is really a curious change of color whether morbid or not); the gall bladder distended, its coats thickened and permeated or dyed with bile, which, though very thick, dark, and abundant (two or three ounces,) had began to exude and dye the contiguous tissues ; the bile ducts pervious ; the solitary glands of the large intestine enlarged, and of a dark hue.

:I:.

J. H., born in France, aged 57, laborer, resident six years ; sick five days before admission into the hospital, on the 7th of February, 1848. During the last stage he was treated with castor oil, carb.

ammon., etc. He was comatose, insensible ; had laborious, noisy respiration ; quick pulse ; eyes and mouth partially open ; no cutaneons eruption, or subsultus, except in the muscles of the face, which twitched ; skin hot. Continued in this condition until he died, at 1, P. M., February 10th.

Autopsy, February 11th, 10, A. M.—Medium size ; moderate emaciation ; abdomen concave ; a few purplish patches, apparently from cadaveric hyperæmia ; rigidity; animal heat natural, except in the extremities, which were cool ; muscles and adipose tissue natural.

Head.—Dura mater extensively adherent upon the superior portions of the hemispheres for half an inch on each side of the falciform process, requiring dissection or tearing of the inferior envelopes. The union or consolidation is owing to bloodvessels and dense, semi-transparent bands and false membranes, lymphy matter ; increased vascularity of the dura mater. The falx contained some small, irregular bones. Arachnoid serosity 1 to $1\frac{1}{2}$ oz.; sub-arachnoid and ventricular effusion about as much ; excessive vascularity, turgescence, and dilatation of the sub-arachnoid net-work, or pia mater, chiefly venous ; choroid plexuses and cerebral substance injected ; increased tenacity, with opacity of the cerebral membranes, one lobe of brain was lifted by a band of the arachnoid and pia mater about half an inch wide ; cerebral substance natural in consistence.

Chest.—The tracheo-bronchial membrane red and injected, particularly the bronchiæ of right side ; the pulmonary and costal pleura on that side had formed recent or red engorged adhesions, and $2\frac{1}{2}$ to 3 oz. of blood were effused on this side in the pleural sack ; both lungs crepitant, completely filling the chest, being loaded with blood, especially in their central and posterior parts, being, perhaps, five times heavier than is usual with healthy lungs; the parenchyma somewhat brittle ; blood dark and fluid.

Heart large and thin ; left ventricle indurated and thickened, the systemic aörta double size, the arch three or four times larger than usual ; the abdominal aörta considerably enlarged, but otherwise not altered ; a polypous concretion in the left ventricle ; a little fluid, black blood in the heart. The cavas yielded considerable fluid blood, which did not coagulate, except a few shreds.

Abdomen.—Omenta attenuated ; the left lobe of the liver thinned out, or rather formed a supplemental lobe covering the stomach, etc.;

liver of a natural appearance, inclining to paleness and friability; gall-bladder collapsed, small, attenuated, containing a few drops of thin liquid of a gamboge color ; the spleen, which is *transposed to the right side,* is enlarged, puffy, crepitant ; its envelopes thickened, strong, having attached to their inner aspect a dense, bony plate, two inches long, one inch wide, and from two to three lines thick ; though thinning towards its margins, the parenchyma or body of the spleen disorganized into a pulpy mass as soft as lard, though nearly without odor. The ureters and adjacent tissues engorged. Right kidney *transposed to the left side* of the spine, one occupying the place of the absent spleen, the other in its usual position. The bladder contracted, injected, containing about an ounce of dirty liquid, having a sediment ; pancreas natural.

The œsophagus, towards its lower end, and the pyloric half of the stomach, had similar lesions with the last-mentioned case, though more intense ; stomach collapsed, small, and extremely thin in such portions as are denuded of the mucous tissue, leaving the injected bloodvessels in arborized, foliated, or leaflet figures ; intestines injected, thinned by the softening and removal of the mucous membrane ; the caliber of the bowels narrowed or collapsed ; no elliptical or peyerian plates developed ; the mesentery engorged ; its glands natural in size and consistence ; natural fæces from the cæcum throughout the colon and rectum.

Other organs were natural, excepting the chest, which presented an abnormity, doubtlessly congenital, namely : the chest corresponding with the diaphragm, and just above the termination of the ensiform cartilage, was compressed on both sides, forming a deep concavity of several inches.

III.

W. J. F., born in Maryland, aged 22, steamboatman, last from Natchez, resident in New Orleans two weeks, sick seven days before admission into the hospital (Jan. 24, 1848). The principal symptom which accompanied his fever in the early stage was that of diarrhœa ; the latter stage was characterized by delirium, requiring, during the last two days, physical restraint.

The treatment consisted of opiates, sod. chlorin., brandy, sinapisms, blister on the nape.

He died February 15, at 1, P. M. In fifteen minutes afterwards the experiments and observations began. The temperature of the axilla, in a trial of 10 minutes, 103°; 5 m., 103°; 5 m., 103½°, stationary ; 2½, P. M., after having been laid out an hour in the deadhouse, axilla 100°, and falling. Muscular nisus, upon percussion, without flexion of the arms. No eruptions ; no cadaveric injection or discoloration ; no rigidity, except in the neck and jaws. At 2, P. M., body on an inclined plane, the head highest, resting as usual on the occiput, the left eye was extirpated for microscopic purposes; the blood ran freely from the eye socket, until 3, P. M. (when the dissection began), amounting to sixteen or twenty ounces, though the eye was the highest portion of the body except the frontal sinus and forehead. The blood coagulated moderately, not firmly. But little adipose tissue ; muscles firm, natural ; scratching them caused contractile ridges. Abdomen concave ; body of medium size, rather emaciated and pale ; no venous fulness externally.

Autopsy two hours after death. Venous and capillary system of all the cavities highly congested, the blood appeared to be moving rapidly, if one might judge by the distension and bleedings upon the most elevated portions of the heart, omentum, bowels, mesentery ; the slightest wounds of the minutest vessel bleed, as might be expected in the living state ; the venous congestion of the most elevated portions of the stomach as seen through the serous coat, is like a blue net work of veins ; the mesentery when elevated and drawn out artificially was, and continued to be, turgescent in the extreme ; the exterior of nearly every organ, except the liver, appeared to be injected ; nearly the whole blood of the body appeared to be in the cavities ; the eye had already discharged at least a pint; the heart and lungs perhaps two pints, the mesentery, cavas, porta, etc., still more. Nothing could be imagined more striking than the general venous congestion ; the coronary and other veins of the heart were everywhere full and bled from the smallest orifice ; the interior of the hollow organs were in the same congested state generally, but in different degrees.

Head.—Serosity in the arachnoidal sac about one ounce ; in the ventricles nearly as much ; subarachnoid vascularity and turgescence ; the substance of the brain and the choroid plexuses injected; the substance of the brain slightly diminished in consistence ; the arachnoid increased in cohesion or tenacity, being milky.

Chest.—Trachea slightly injected ; left lung universally adherent to the costal pleura by a white, bloodless network ; lungs healthy ; heart a little diminished in cohesion.

Abdomen, etc.—Tongue, tumid, short, dark red, especially on its dorsum, coated with a brown fur ; fauces dark red ; lower portion of the gullet had its epithelium brittle, white, thickened longtitudinal portions or strips were gone. About half of the interior of the stomach next the cardia denuded of its mucous tissues, leaving large trunks of blood vessels with leaflet injections and red gelatinous bloody exudations at their terminations ; the stomach contains three or four ounces of a yellowish, chymous matter, has general injection of the submucous tissues ; the ileum in some places denuded of its mucous coat; half a yard above the valve of the cæcum a few elliptical plates were noticed as large as the nail ; at the valve, and a few inches above, several plates about two and a half inches long and one inch wide arose internally with very acute perpendicular or rather projecting salient edges, very firm, almost scirrhous, at least the one-sixth of an inch thick, though a little depressed in the central part ; ulcerations of the glands in the cæcum ; apparently all the solitary glands of the large intestine are developed, red or even black, sometimes ulcerated and softened, generally elevated in solid crusts or scabs, some depressed in the centre or excavated, being nearly as large as grains of maize ; some resembled small boils or furunculi in various states of firmness. Bladder generally injected, enormously distended with urine, one and a half pounds ; kidneys engorged; spleen enlarged three times, of good consistence ; liver enlarged, good consistence, rather purplish ; coats of the gall bladder infiltrated, contained a gamboge-colored mucosity, about two ounces. Mesenteric glands enormously developed, being darkened from engorgement and injection ; some half the size of a hen's egg; none had suppurated, but some were soft or brittle ; their weight probably ten times increased.

IV.

J. H., born in Buffalo, State of New York, aged 38 ; carpenter ; resident six months ; duration of his fever eighteen days ; treated in the last stage with brandy, carb. ammon ; delirious ; for two days before death tied down in bed; vomits; thin, yellow involuntary stools; a little thirsty ; delirium declined during the last day of his life; took gruel freely, etc.

Died at 11 o'clock, A. M., Feb. 25, 1848 ; one hour afterward the body flexible ; stout and muscular; no eruption; a few minute vesicles (sudaminia) upon the skin; a bed sore as large as the hand over the base of the sacrum; the skin of dependent parts roseate with dark discolorations; on turning the body over on the face, the same colors took place on its other or lower aspect in five minutes, but receded on pressure ; heat of the body about 100°, but declining.

A blow on the left arm, over its flexors, caused the forearm to ascend nearly to the perpendicular; three or four blows and flexions at short intervals, exhausted the contractile force for a time, but it returned repeatedly after a rest of a few minutes, and with increased energy during half an hour, after which, only a few feeble motions were excited. The right arm was now manipulated; its flexions were much more complete, lasting and vigorous, though insufficient to carry the hand to the breast through the vertical, before reaching which it was deflected either towards the side of the head or abdomen; the death-stiffness of the left arm (the first manipulated) had taken place before the contractility of the right had been exhausted.

Autopsy.—Adipose and muscular tissues natural. The trunk and centres nearly as warm as in health. The blood dark, fluid, abundant, clotting feebly after having been discharged.

Head.—The left hemisphere of the brain had a coagulum of blood as large as the palm over it, partly organized, having two whitish membraniform surfaces, the one towards the brain and the other towards the dura mater, and a partly organized coagulum resting upon and adherent to the superior central portion of the hemisphere reaching back towards the posterior lobe, amounting to about two ounces, with an equal quantity of dark fluid blood surrounding the same, all of which being removed, a subarachnoid button-shaped or pyramidal coagulum as a large as a cent, with a salient apex, was discovered ; this apex was surrounded by what seemed to be the open mouth of a minute artery about the size of a large bristle. The subarachnoid effusion was firmly coagulated—was probably the first deposit of the ruptured artery, but having been confined in the meshes of the arachnoid and pia mater ruptured these membranes at the point where the ruptured artery appeared, pouring out at least four ounces of blood above the central arachnoid or in the arachnoidal sac. The false membranes around this point adhering to the central envelopes, resembled certain recent aneurismal sacs which I have met with in operating for false aneurism. The arterial system of the brain was comparatively, if not completely empty ; the veins greatly developed, especially upon the cerebral surface, forming a network of a close texture. There was at least three ounces of serosity, chiefly in the base of the brain and ventricles. The consistence of the brain good.

Chest.—Trachea natural; right lung adherent generally along its base, red vascular adhesions; the lower half of the lung red, vascular dense, nearly as much so as in recent hepatization ; several portions of clotted blood were found in its parenchyma; it discharged great quantities of blood from every cut; half of the left lung loaded densely with blood; pericardium natural; heart large, loaded with fat ; the right auricle enormously distended. Both sides of the heart contained fibrinous concretions partly white and partly red ; cavas distended. Diaphragm on both surfaces on the right side vascular.

Abdomen, etc.—Tongue retracted, that is, shortened, tumid, or rather indurated, clean, red, cracked; fauces and gullet natural ; the mucous tissue very white. The salivary and some of the lymphatic glands red and tumid. The pyloric half of the stomach had its mucous tissues softened, pulpy, red, vascular and thinned ; the duodenum and jejunum contained much green or bilious matter, which appeared to have dyed the mucous tissue. The ileum, in many places, much altered, its mucous tissue softened, or pulpy, or dissolved, intensely vascular ; a few oblong pustular plates, the tissue being brittle, and in and about the plates non-vascular. The large intestine, in some places, enormously dilated, in others much contracted ; the cæcum dilated, being as large as the stomach ; the mucous tissue often softened, its glands developed, or pustulated. The large intestine contained semi-fluid and solid fæces, a part of which was of the most healthy kind, in the rectum. The greater and lesser omenta, with the mesentery, highly vascular; the pancreas, mesenteric glands, the left kidney and the bladder natural ; the latter completely empty and contracted. The spleen enlarged about six times ; its cohesion greatly diminished, readily breaking into a semi-pulp; a supplemental spleen unconnected with the large one was found, as big as a crab apple; right kidney red, engorged, vascular; liver enlarged nearly twice, had a strong, red, vascular, adhesion to the abdomino-diaphragmatic walls near the spine, where the parenchyma was loaded with blood and had a darkish red hue ; gall bladder distended with green ropy bile, three ounces, which had begun to exude, staining the tissues ; great quantities of similar bile variegated with mucous and chylous matters prevailed in the small intestines.

Experiment.—After opening the brain and the chest, the heart was found still greatly distended on the right side. The veins of the heart proper were distended also ; this organ was raised out of its pericardium, its apex elevated and the veins of its surface emptied by pressing their contents downwards ; still, after many trials, the blood was forced upwards against gravity towards the apex, distending the vessels strongly. The cavas were not emptied by these experiments, but remained distended until severed. I cut down to and half severed one of the carotids, and on compressing the heart with the hand, in imitation of its systolic action, the blood jetted from the artery several times responsive to the action of the hand, until the organ appeared to be nearly or quite empty. But in a few minutes the heart appeared to be as full as ever, which was proved by repeatedly compressing it, thereby causing the arterial jets as before. These experiments were repeated with like results a number of times, the heart refilling as often. All this while the large blood vessels had not been cut except in the brain and one carotid, as already mentioned. The quantity of blood discharged from the heart by these experiments must have been about ten or twelve ounces. Whether this blood reached the left side of the heart by arterial regurgitations, or suction, or by the capillaries and veins of the lungs may be matter of conjecture ; but the rapidity of its accumulation indicates both agencies as probable.

Art. V.—*Contributions to the Pathological Anatomy and Natural History of Yellow Fever :* By BENNET DOWLER, M. D.

NUMBER ONE.

I.

1848 ; Sept. 15 and 16. R. D., male ; born in Manchester, England; aged 21 ; resident three years ; sick three days ; muscular ; well proportioned ; skin variegated with yellow, cyanosed, marbled with dark, dirty, dusky red discolorations ; eyes prominent, injected and yellow; pupils natural ; tongue tumid, retracted, completely smooth, dry, and of a pale cherry red ; abdomen and epigastrium concave ; respiration easy, 36 ; pulse, 88, natural ; hand, 96°; bend of the arm 97½°; axilla 99°; quiet delirium, with glimpses of intelligence especially when interrogated ; in the midst of his incoherency is much annoyed when flies and mosquitoes alight on his person. His delirium augmenting, he was tied down in bed. Swears, and some- times for an hour cries out " O dear, O dad." Deep coma succeeded with loud stertorous respiration. He was untied. Threw up black vomit and expired about the middle of the night of the 17th of Sep- tember.

Treatment.—Sinapisms ; pills of quinine and blue mass in moder- ate doses ; spts. nitre ; lemonade ; epistast. to epigast.; iced drinks.

Dissection nine and a half hours after death. Body rigid, except the neck ; skin, eyes, and fat, moderately yellow ; neck, face, and dependent parts darkish red ; black vomit running from the mouth without fermentation ; abdomen concave ; the blistered surface red, firm, dry ; the internal surface of the skin, the cellular and other tissues, as the peritoneal, unaltered opposite the blister. Muscles massive, firm, and red ; no gases or other indications of putrefactive action ; body cool externally ; about 100 deg. in the centres. The air was not only dry, but cool, having descended during the night to 67 deg., but had reached 80 deg. at the time of the examination.

. *Head.*—Universal vascularity and injection of the brain and its envelopes ; the arachnoid and pia mater opaque, and tenacious ; a band an inch wide suspended half of the brain without breaking.

Chest.—Mucous tissues red ; both lungs distended and highly en- · gorged, particularly the left, which was five or six times increased in weight ; the chest of that side contained eight to ten ounces of effused blood and serosity ; the pericardium injected externally, the valves of the heart yellow ; incipient polypi in both ventricles.

Mouth.—Fauces, pharynx and glands red, papillæ at the base of the tongue hypertrophied ; tongue clean, swollen, its muscular tissue firm, and comparatively dry, discharging no blood ; the œsophagus and its cellular annexæ much injected, the lower two-thirds of the submucous tissue marked with numerous longitudinal black striæ, (black vomit petechial infiltration)—these shone through the trans- parent mucous tissue which was of the natural consistence—the latter it was found necessary to scrape completely away, before reaching the melanoid stratum or infiltration. The stripes which had no tinge of blood were coal black in the middle, but faded towards their margins ; the tissue appeared colored as well as infil-trated with the black fluid. The cardiac orifice red and vascular ; this tube loaded with black vomit matter, which latter was also abundant in the stomach, duodenum, also in a portion of the jejunum (where chylous paste, faintly yellow, was found); the lower half of the ileum, and the entire cæcum contained nothing else ; the ascend-ing and transverse arch of the colon contained the same ; portions of solid black vomit had descended into the rectum, forming, with the pale solid fæces, a striking contrast, scybalæ being in some instances formed with one part or side black and the other whitish or gray ; the omental tissues injected ; the liver of good consist-ence, but pale or cork-colored ; bile dark, but yellowish on dilution ; the urinary bladder injected and distended ; much of the lower part of the ileum red, vascular and injected, with softening and thinning of the mucous tissue ; on the left side of the spine from the diaphragm to the lower end of the kidney injection, vascularity, thickening, fibrinous, red, and yellow infiltration prevailed in the subserous and cellular tissues ; the peritoneum thickened ; the kid-ney enlarged, engorged, discharging much blood from incision ; the spleen softened, grayish-red ; the lymphatic glands enlarged and injected ; the submucous tissue of the duodenum infiltrated with pink-colored blood ; the cellular tissue abundant in connection with the duodenum also injected ; more than half of the mucous tissues of the stomach commencing with the cardiac, to a great extent, gelatinous, consisting of red, yellow, black and grayish matter, flakes, shreds, resting on an immense number of blood-vessels greatly enlarged, as if varicose, the smaller arborizations in blood-like leaflets ; this portion of the membrane presented no rugosities, being thin, flaccid, and like a worn out wet rag ; the residue of the stomach thick, pale, rugous, resilient, perhaps natural ; the line be-tween the disorganized and healthy portion elevated, very regular, and as well defined as that noticed when mortification is arrested by healthy reaction. The great veins of the abdomen, the cavas, porta, etc., enlarged or at least distended greatly with coagula and with fluid blood of an unusually black hue.

It is difficult to determine the order, or succession, the primary or secondary nature of these lesions, and the more so as contiguity of organs rather than identity of tissues often serves to connect them. The greatest alteration was midway between the greater curvature of the stomach and the left kidney in the serous cellular and lymphatic tissues. Did the inflammatory radii extend from this as a common centre, involving the stomach, duodenum, spleen and kidney ? It appears that this man vomited but three times, though much of his stomach was disorganized.

II.

R. R., Irishman, large and muscular ; aged thirty ; last from St. Louis, resident six days ; sick one day ; admitted Oct. 9th, 1842 ; the same day was bled from the arm, cupped over the stomach, where he was also poulticed ; he had a footbath, and was cupped again during the day, behind the ears. Oct. 10th ; seidlitz ; footbath. The next day he had a mustard plaster over his stomach. During his treatment he vomited often, and had delirium at night, but was quiet until the night before his death, when, becoming unmanageable, was tied down in bed. He died at three o'clock, A. M., on the 13th, after a sickness of four days and three hours' duration.

Dissection, eight hours after death : *Body* warm, extremities cool; skin, eyes, and fat, *yellow;* muscles, firm and red ; fingers and toes strongly *contracted ;* no emaciation ; skin of natural elasticity ; external tissues along the back unaffected by cadaveric infiltration.

Head.—Serosity, chiefly, without the cerebral arachnoid, seven to eight ounces ; brain, of good consistence ; pia mater, vascular, and was, with the arachnoid, so strong, that a strip two inches wide, suspended half of the brain without breaking.

Spinal Marrow.—Natural.

Mouth.—The tongue covered with a white, thin fur ; its muscles pale ; velum, elongated and tumid ; posterior fauces, reddish. The gullet had its epithelium white like paper. The mucous membrane of the trachea, pale, but became red in the bronchial tubes.

Chest.—Lungs natural, though extensively adherent by a bloodless, non-vascular tissue ; heart, of normal size and color, was somewhat brittle in texture ; the pleuræ, yellowish ; other thoracic organs, natural.

Abdomen.—Peritoneal tissue, yellowish. The stomach contained *a dark liquid ;* its size moderate ; its mucous tissue had a slight *reddish tinge,* without any concentration of color, at any one point ; it peeled well ; being free from puffiness, though slightly softened, with arborizations and some turgescence in the outer portion of the submucous tissue ; the duodenum and small intestines, natural, contained a small quantity of a pasty mucosity, gray, lead-colored, odorless, without bile, fæces, etc ; this liquid became somewhat thicker in the lower portions of the bowels. The large intestine was contracted to the size of the thumb, but otherwise natural. Several folds of the small intestine in the lowest situations injected. Bladder, contracted to the size of a *hen's* egg, injected, empty. In the scrotum, around each testicle, about one ounce of yellow liquid was effused. Liver, enlarged about one-third, of a gingerbread color, diminished in cohesion, every where brittle, except at its edges ; its parenchyma exsanguineous ; its large vessels white ; its membranes diminished in their adhesions to the parenchyma ; the gall-bladder, thickened, contained a teaspoonful of gamboge-colored serosity. Other organs natural.

Are not the injection and other slight changes in the stomach and small intestine to be attributed to cadaveric gravitation alone ?

III.

R. H., female ; born in Germany ; aged twenty-three ; last from the city of Bremen ; for ten months resident in New Orleans ; sick two days ; admitted August 22d ; the next day was cupped ; took but little medicine, and expired at one o'clock, P. M., upon the fifth day of her malady. During her illness, she complained chiefly of pains in the head and back.

Dissection, five to ten minutes after death. *Body* everywhere hot, as in fever, and free from emaciation ; considerable adipose tissue which had a pale orange tinge ; eyes and skin, yellow ; muscles, natural ; incisions discharged blood of a good color ; neither rigidity nor abdominal distension. The abdomen and chest were instantly opened. The omenta, mesentery, the linings of the cavities, etc., in elevated, as well as depressed situations, had their arterial and venous tissues gently distended with blood, apparently in motion ; the smallest vessels of parts the most elevated, discharged blood on being punctured. The subclavian veins discharged, in a few minutes, about three pounds of good-colored blood, which coagulated in the ordinary time.

Head (opened last).—Dura mater dotted with blood ; venous vascularity of the pia mater excessive ; tenacity of the arachnoid ; the choroid web (plexus) in each of the lateral ventricles, resembled a bunch of grapes, the main artery being like a stem which was every-where surrounded with *cysts* (some nearly an inch in circumference); these contained a pelucid liquid, nearly as thick as albumen, with surrounding vascularity and injection.

Chest.—A slight *red adhesion* of the pleuræ, as large as the hand, in the left side ; other organs natural.

Abdomen.—The stomach contained about twenty ounces of thin, claret-colored liquid, with a heavy, black vomit sediment ; the mucous coat pink-colored, thickened, wrinkled, rough, with bark-like granulations, intersected with fissures, rounded, and elevated two or three lines (mammillated), but free from softening or brittleness, peeled well ; the duodenum resembled the stomach, with respect to its inner coat ; the small intestines contained, in some places, black vomit, in others, blood, with several lumbricoid worms and consolidated portions of black vomit ; the lower portion of the ileum, and the whole of the large intestine, were contracted to a cord, except in the latter, where a few balls of inodorous fæces, nearly dry, were found. The gullet and intestines were generally blanched, but otherwise everywhere natural.

The liver had a mottled, milky brown color ; its substance had red granules, which did not bleed ; size natural ; consistence, brittle in the center ; its coats diminished in adhesion ; the gall-bladder enlarged ; its coats infiltrated with button-shaped extravasations of blood ; the bile thin, greenish yellow. Several watery cysts in the broad ligaments of the uterus, near the ovaries. Other organs natural.

IV.

August 31. M. B., female; born in Ireland; aged twenty-two; married ; throwing up black vomit ; brain oppressed ; intelligence extinguished ; copious hæmorrhage from leech-bites upon the epigastrium, which her physician arrested with difficulty by the application of lunar caustic. Died September 1.

Dissection two and a half hours after death. Air of the dead-house at its maximum, 85° ; calorification for forty-five minutes ; axilla 100° ; vagina 104½° ; epigastrium 103° ; left chest 102½° ; vagina 103¾° ; contractility ; a blow with the edge of the hand caused the right arm to rise slowly nearly to the perpendicular ; half an hour after, the other arm was completely flexed, the hand was carried within half an inch of the ribs, below the mamma, where it remained without touching or falling back until rigidity set in ; neck moderately rigid ; jaws fixed ; legs moderately rigid ; abdomen concave ; skin yellow, positional injection along the back ; adipose tissue abundant, and orange-colored ; muscles natural ; body of medium size, and symmetrical ; features calm ; cicatrized lines, indicative of child-bearing.

Head.—The envelopes and substance of the brain natural in cohesion ; the former vascular and injected to the utmost extent, chiefly venous.

Chest.—The mucous membrane of the trachea, and all its bronchial ramifications, injected, uniformly red, bathed in fluid blood ; in both lungs blood was effused or extravasated into their parenchyma, the anterior portions, particularly of the right, appeared through the pulmonary pleura to consist chiefly of densely-impacted blood ; the lungs were five to six times heavier than natural ; there was scarcely the one-tenth part of the parenchyma not densely congested, though not solid, as in hepatization ; the lungs natural in texture, excepting the apparently recent infiltration ; a general hæmorrhage appears to have taken place in the pulmonary tissue, and wholly within the pulmonary pleuræ, none into the pleural cavity ; the blood being intimately blended with the lung-substance ; heart on both sides contained a little dark coagulated blood.

Mouth.—The salivary glands enlarged ; the posterior fauces dark red ; pappilæ at the base of the tongue strongly developed ; surface of the tongue nearly clean ; tumidity of that organ with redness, increasing towards the center of its body.

Œsophagus, injected and vascular, particularly near its lower end.

Abdomen.—Omenta and mesentery congested ; the glands of the latter enlarged considerably ; the cavæ and porta distended with blood, being larger in calibre than several portions of the ileum. The great nerves, pancreas, lymphatics, spleen, and bladder, natural. The whole venous system of this cavity from the largest to the smallest vessel was distended with dark blood ; the stomach pale, of good consistence, and moderately vascular in the sub-mucous tissue of the cardia, being distended, with nearly a pint of homogeneous, intensely-colored black vomit, a little of which was found in the duodenum ; a great portion of the bowels, viewed externally, was black and vascular to the utmost degree ; the jejunum had a strong, tumid, injected intussusception, two inches of the bowel had descended into the inferior portion ; several tracts of pasty chyle were met with ; the lower third of the small intestine contained a dark water ; the bowel, inside and out, was black, attenuated, and vascular in branches and leaflets, forming a close netting ; the mucous tissue of the large, and nearly half of that of the small, intestine, dotted over with very salient, firm, round, isolated points, larger than mustard seed (glandulæ solitariæ); a dime would cover perhaps a dozen.   The large intestine contained some mucus and water, but no fæces ; the rectum had a little gruel-like liquid ; kidneys engorged ; liver pale ; gall-bladder half an ounce of thick, greenish bile, but yellow when spread thin.   The uterus contained a vascular or shaggy web, confined to its fundus ; the ovaries were engorged ; had a number of ova or vesicles, some being peripheral, round, and prominent ; when cut open, several corpora lentea were found, having sacks of various sizes, some contained yellow, corrugated, membranous projections or duplications ; others had thick, brittle walls ; all without a central nucleus.   The os tincæ and vagina engorged and red.

v.

1848. M. L., born in Ireland ; aged thirty-three ; resident six years ; last from Boston ; laborer ; has coma, stertor, and black vomit. Died September 7, at half-past 8, A. M., on the fourth day of his disease.

Dissection two and a half hours after death. Body stout ; free from emaciation and rigidity; six feet two inches in height ; eyes, skin, and fat yellow; belly concave ; positional injection upon the limbs and trunk moderate ; contractility good in the arms for an hour, flexing the extended arm horizontally to the sides.

From the tip of the nose to the inside of the foot below the maleölus, both points being marked with an incision, the distance was five feet eight inches ; in half an hour the distance was lessened nearly three-quarters of an inch. Was this not owing to contraction, as the heat was declining ? Axilla 96 deg.; rectum 100½ deg.; left of the epigastrium 99¾ deg.; to the right 100 deg.; left chest 97½ deg.; right 97 deg.; in all places falling. Dead-house 84½ deg. The jaw, neck, and limbs became rigid during dissection.

Head.—Brain firm, meninges opaque and tenacious ; pia mater infiltrated, injected ; serosity four to five ounces in the arachnoidean sack.

Chest.—Left lung natural, completely collapsed, not filling the one-fourth of the cavity ; the right lung about ten times heavier, partially adherent ; sub-pleuræ red and vascular ; parenchyma loaded with fluid blood, which streams from every incision (doubtless a hæmorrhagic exudation into the cells); heart natural, but loaded with yellow fat.

Abdomen.—The omenta and mesentery injected and bled freely (like wounds in the living body), in the most elevated, as well as in the lowest, situations ; the lymphatic, particularly the mesenteric glands, reddish and somewhat enlarged ; urinary bladder contracted into a solid mass, and nearly empty ; spleen hypertrophied, double size, its coats opaque, as if from a former hyperæmia, its parenchyma brittle and soft, discharging a bloody, pasty, thick liquid ; liver enlarged ; coats readily peeled ; exterior a little pale, tinged with yellow, its parenchyma nearly normal in color, its large vessels much engorged with fluid blood ; in the gall-bladder about two ounces of dark, green bile.

Stomach small ; contained two or three ounces of tenacious, bloody paste or mucosity, in which a little flakey black vomit was found ; the sub-mucous tissue had several longitudinal red stripes ; black vomit in the duodenum ; the jejunum natural in cohesion, contained chylous paste ; the ileum loaded with black vomit, and towards its lower end with pasty, dark red, bloody liquid ; this bowel, generally attenuated, had a few dilatations ; nearly everywhere black ; its sub-mucous tissue presented a net-work of vascularity, nearly naked ; the cæcum red ; contained the same kind of paste, which increased in consistence throughout the colon. The rectum and other organs natural.

VI.

F. P., female ; born in Georgia, aged 33, widow ; resident six months, Sept., 6; comatose; *in articulo mortis;* extensively blistered over the abdomen ; died next morning about 4, A. M.

Dissection eight hours after death. Neck becoming limber; extremities rigid ; fingers and toes flexed strongly and irregularly, disfiguring the hands and feet ; skin yellow, and dotted on exposed parts (the face, neck, breast, legs, arms and most of all the hands) with mosquito-petechiæ of a dark red, inclining to blue, not receding on pressure, as during life; much dark red discoloration of dependent parts, particularly of the neck and sides of the face ; eyes and adipose tissue yellow ; abdomen concave ; body stout, and rather muscular, with moderate development of adipose tissue ; muscles natural ; extensive cantharidian vesications covering nearly half of the abdomen.

Temperature.—Axilla 94 deg.; vagina 100½ deg.; left hypochondrium 99 deg.; right 100 deg.; left chest 99 deg.; right 99 deg.; center of the thigh 98 deg.; under the liver 100 deg. Dead-house 87 deg.

Brain.—Excessive vascularity of the pia mater, and injection; with tenacity, opacity of the arachnoid and pia mater ; albumen-like sub-arachnoidal infiltration.

Chest.—Natural.

Abdomen.— Œsophagus, pancreas, kidneys, bladder, natural ; omenta, mesentery, and glands injected ; spleen diminutive, a little softened, discharging reddish, pasty liquid ; liver pale, supple, enlarged one-third, its parenchyma bloodless, its great vessels enlarged, varicose, contained much clotted blood ; gall-bladder, which was thickened, white, contained half an ounce of dark green bile ; the sub-serous tissue around the connections of the gall-bladder infiltrated ; the stomach displaced, or forced downwards, so that its great arch encroached upon the upper boundary of the pelvis ; the stomach contained a pound or more of intensely-colored, flakey black vomit ; the cardiac half of the mucous tissue softened ; the duodenum and upper part of the jejunum contained black vomit, like that in the stomach ; a little chylous paste found in the middle of the small intestine ; its lower half attenuated, as it were, wilted, non-elastic, brittle, nearly black, vascular to the utmost degree ; the vessels generally denuded of their mucous tissue ; a little bloody, adhesive mucosity prevailed to the cæcum and throughout the arch of the colon. From the descending arch to the anus the intestine was strongly contracted, was pale, had a little tenacious gray paste, alternating with enormous masses of nearly inodorous, solid, natural fæces*. The cæcum and arch of the colon contained nearly a pint of bloody mucosity, the mucous tissue being of a logwood hue, and thickened.

The uterus was pretty firmly fixed ; its direction diagonal, the os tincæ directed to the sacro-iliac junction ; the ovaria enlarged, had several sacks, one of which contained blood, the cavity being

---

* These fæcal masses had probably accumulated before the attack, which is often preceded by constipation.

as large as a hazelnut ; some were red, others white, others yellow ;
from the middle of the body of the uterus arose a scirrhous mass,
apparently identified with or planted in the substance of that organ,
and expanding into a kind of second uterus, its distal end resembling
the fundus ; the membranous coverings, and a little of the exterior
of the tumor, were of a grayish color ; the great mass consisted of
solid, white, fibrous matter, colored like the medullary matter of the
brain, exceedingly tenacious, cutting with difficulty; the scirrhous
tumor was homogeneous with a portion of the fundus ; uterine cavity
extremely small. The womb, when the scirrhous portion was excised, was of the normal size; the os tineæ had escaped the scirrhous
degeneration.

The mammæ were not scirrhous. The kidneys were firm, perhaps not morbid.

The uterine tumor was free from surrounding redness, but the adjacent membranes, etc., were much thickened.

The death of this patient, probably, was not in any degree influenced or accelerated by this scirrhous deposit. It may be presumed
that the tumor had long remained dormant, awaiting some exciting
cause or contingent change, which, about the period of the disappearance of the menses, is apt to develop cancerous ulceration, ending in a death incomparably more painful and terrible than that from
yellow fever.

VII.

G. W., born in France ; last from Havre ; blacksmith ; aged
nineteen ; resident eighteen months. During the last two days of
his illness he was often delirious ; was tied in bed ; his skin hot ;
he vomited but once, throwing up a mouthful or two of dirty liquid,
supposed not to be black vomit ; his strength was good, got up and
down unassisted, until a few hours before his death.

Treatment.—Lemonade ; epispastic to the abdomen ; cold to the
head ; six pills of quinine. Died September 10, at 9, A. M.

Experiments began an hour and a quarter after death. Axilla,
10 m., 102½ deg.; 5 m., 102¾ deg.; rectum, 5 m., 103 deg.; two
hours and a half after death, axilla 100½ deg.; rectum 102¾ deg.;
left hypochondrium 101 deg.; right 100 deg.; left chest 101 deg.;
right 101½ deg.; thigh 99 deg. Dead-house 85 deg.

Dissection two hours and a half after death. Body large, muscular, fat, rigid ; eyes, adipose tissue, and skin yellow, the latter

discolored from positional or cadaveric injection ; abdomen flat ; a slight prick of the lancet on the tip of the nose discharged about half an ounce of blood, which soon separated into a clot and serum, the quantity supposed to be as great as a similar wound would discharge in health ; muscles firm, natural, except a high degree of redness, which increased on exposure to the air.

Head.—Pia mater vascular, injected, turgid with blood ; arachnoid opaque from reddish, albuminoid infiltration of the sub-arachnoid tissue.

Chest.—Bloody mucosity in the air passages ; sub-pleural infiltration of the periphery of the left lung ; bloody exudations in patches, with congestion of the parenchyma ; the heart and right lung natural.

Abdomen.—Omenta, sub-peritoneal tissue, and mesentery execssively injected ; the sub-serous cellular tissues around and near both orifices of the stomach, the duodenum, the pancreas, gall-bladder, kidneys, particularly along the left side of the spine, much thickened, minutely injected, and largely infiltrated with a yellow, albuminous or lymphy liquid ; the liver of natural consistence, uniformly of a cork-color, its large vessels contained much clotted blood ; the gall-bladder thickened, injected, infiltrated, being of a dull white, variegated with purplish hues—contained a yellowish, watery mucus, with some concrete lumpy matter, the lymphatic, particularly the mesenteric glands, enlarged and red ; spleen and bladder natural ; kidneys and pancreas somewhat indurated ; the stomach, which was less pale than natural, contained half a pint or more of black vomit, which latter prevailed in the duodenum, jejunum, and in a portion of the ileum ; the large intestine loaded with fluid blood of a dark claret hue, having comparatively but little odor ; the middle portion of the small intestine contained a little adhesive chylous matter ; the ileum, much of which was impacted within the pelvis, was collapsed, thickened, dark ; its mucous tissues intensely vascular, injected, reddened, and coated with a dense bloody exudation or jelly; the glandulæ solitariæ, near the valve, were salient ; the lower half of the jejunum contained, at short intervals, four firmly-impacted intussusceptions, from three to four inches of the bowel in each case having descended into the contiguous portion ; each presented a conical appearance, the apex being the downward end ; the enclosed portion being compressed and bloodless ; the outer being thickened and darkish from congestion and tumefaction. The pelvis contained several ounces of serosity.

The central venous system contained much fluid blood, which coagulated in due time. The viscera of the abdomen having been removed, and consequently the great cœlic artery cut, it was observed that on pressing the left ventricle of the heart a free stream of blood was projected directly upward one inch high ; this was often repeated for about a quarter of an hour, discharging from eight to ten ounces, the supply continuing.

After the excision and removal of the heart, its great coronary and other external veins were found to be still distended with blood ; the heart was suspended, its apex being downward ; its veins, particularly some of its long superficial ones, which pass upward to the base of the organ, were emptied by pressure, and by repeatedly passing the finger-nail over them, so as to empty them, yet they were as often refilled by capillary or other motion contrary to gravity.

VIII.

J. Z., born in Germany; aged twenty-two; last from Havre; wheelwright ; resident five months. Died of yellow fever September 10, at half-past 10, A. M.

Dead half an hour. Axilla, 5 m., $99\frac{1}{2}$ deg.; in half an hour 100 deg., and stationary ; the body muscular, and free from emaciation ; well proportioned ; yellow, mottled with livid and black ; blood oozing from scarifications on the nape of the neck, as in the living body, being fluid at first, and clotting afterwards ; the entire body flexible ; abdomen without distention ; the skin, where blisters had been applied, is red and raw ; on turning the body on the face or side, the skin of the under surface became quickly livid or black.

Experiments on contractility for one hour, that is, an hour and a half after death, at which time the contractility, though apparently good, was interfered with by incipient rigidity. The arm having been extended so as to form a right angle with the trunk, the biceps was struck repeatedly, at intervals, either with the edge or with the palm of the hand ; the flexions were as complete as possible, unless when the intervals were not sufficiently prolonged ; for example, two complete flexions following each other quickly, were followed by a demi-flexion, the arm not quite reaching the perpendicular ; after the arm fell back, another blow immediately given produced scarcely any effect beyond the twisting of the hand ; but subsequently, that is after rest, the muscular contractility returned.   Extensions (not to mention pronations, etc.) were performed in various ways.   Thus, the right arm was flexed upon the breast, the palm resting on the opposite shoulder, so that the arm could not fall back by gravity; the extensors were then percussed, the arm was extended, the hand was lifted from the left shoulder and carried to the opposite side, extending the limb completely, though at various angles with respect to the trunk.   The thigh was raised perpendicularly to the trunk and horizon, the leg hanging down ; a blow on the extensors caused the leg and foot to arise several inches from its original position ; the body was made to rest on the right side ; the left arm was made to rest on the side, the elbow being near the hip, the fore-arm was bent so that the hand touched the left jaw ; a blow caused the fore-arm to extend itself so that the hand was carried to the thigh, the fore-arm forming a straight line with the body.   The experiment was varied—the arm was placed in a right line with the body, the fore-arm was flexed to a right angle, that is, directly across the abdomen, the hand hanging down on the opposite (the right) side ; a blow caused the fore-arm to extend, dragging the arm and hand over the abdomen, throwing the entire limb not only to a line with the body, but beyond it, behind the back.   These experiments upon the extensors become the more striking from the fact that I have not found any convenient method to avoid the great loss of force from friction, in dragging, etc.

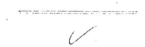

Art. VI.—*Medication ? or non-Medication ? That is the Question:* By Bennet Dowler, M. D.

" In regard to the employment of the experimental method, we stand much upon the same point as that upon which chemical experiment stood in the times of phlogiston, or even of alchemy ; and as the phlogiston hypothesis so long stood in the way of every more exact investigation, so *our* attempts have been impeded by the old hypotheses of an ' archæus' or a ' pneuma,' and by the more modern ones, of a vital force, a typical or healing force, and, lastly, by the so-called ontological conception of diseases as special entities, no less than by the belief in mystical medicinal forces."—F. Oesterlen, M. D.   *Med. Logic,* p. 262.

The recent unexpected and much lamented death of Dr. Todd, of London, just as he had completed his new book on " *Clinical Lectures on Acute Diseases,*" seems to have drawn much attention to this work as the last will and testament of a man whose previous career of authorship had been alike useful and illustrious. Although there may be but little merit in praising a dead competitor, yet, it is but just to say, that the living not less than the dead Dr. Todd seems to have been highly appreciated at home as well as in this Republic. It is, however, difficult to account for the special eulogy and sanction awarded to his last work by practitioners, teachers and reviewers, seeing that it utterly denies the existence of acute inflammations, acute diseases, and sthenia, and interdicts antiphlogistics altogether. Dr. Todd is not, however, a strict non-medicationist ; he has a remedy, if not a panacea. It is, O, Sons of Temperance ! rejoice O, ghost of John Brown of Edinburgh, it is alcohol, brandy, wine. Leave the rest to Nature. The poet but followed the faculty of former days in his anathema :

> "To those whom fever burns, the smell
> Of vigorous wine is death and hell."

Of Dr. Todd's book, which is devoid of novelty, originality and sound logic, it is not intended to make any special mention, further than that it seems to have given an almost epidemic impetus to skepticism. It is easy to see, that its chief eulogists are delighted with, and emboldened by its authority. In this defection, it is asserted many of the younger members of the profession are included. Doubtlessly, the great majority will never join in the revolt, but imitate Milton's

> "Abdiel, faithful found
> Among the faithless—
> Among innumerable false, unmoved,
> Unshaken, unseduced, unterrified,
> His loyalty he kept, his love, his zeal ;
> Nor number nor example, with him wrought
> To swerve from truth, or change his constant mind "

In making a few unpremeditated and unsystematic remarks upon the existing skepticism in regard to medicinal treatment, doubtlessly the strict logician may discover some errors and inconclusive arguments ; but if the leading postulates be on the whole sustained with more or less probability—if there be no undue biases in favor of untenable theories, or over estimates of the valid claims of therapeutics—no malice towards those who wholly repudiate these claims, the reader will, it is hoped, excuse the attempt to defend the truth, though it may not be in all respects successful.

Dr. Todd's rejection, *in toto*, of the doctrines of sthenia and antiphlogistics, is received with acclaim by the skeptics. These terms may or may not be pathologically correct. Sthenia and asthenia, though convenient and useful words, are of hypothetical import in pathology if literally applied. The very excess of sthenia is often the parent of asthenia. It is, however, impossible to provide accurate terms for that which is but imperfectly known. Even active and passive hæmorrhages differ, not in their nature, but degrees. Active medication has no antithesis which can be conceived, much less practised as being medication at all.

The old doctrine of phlogiston has given impetus to the hypothesis that there is a fundamental class of medicines which are antiphlogistics and constitute a method of cure, namely, the antiphlogistic method or system—which, as all know, a few years ago reigned with unrelenting despotism. The medicinal agents which were given under this name in diseases called phlegmasial, phlogistic or inflammatory, because of their real or supposed efficacy in removing inflammation by acting antiphlogistically, became a class, and every cure thus achieved was supposed to prove the correctness of this classification; thus doctrine, language and therapy mutually confirmed each other, and a mere hypothesis was regarded as the deduction from rigid science. What has been gained in therapy by labored arguments for and against the antiphlogistical character of quinine, mercury, opium, etc. The using this word either to designate a class of medicines or a method of treatment may be convenient, rather than correct. If brandy in certain cases of fever or inflammation should, as it may, lessen the disease, it would be entitled to the character of antiphlogistic as well as venesection ; and so of other remedies among stimulants and tonics and diet.

After writing this last paragraph, the following *jeux d'esprit*, half argument, half irony, by M. Forget, was met with in the *Med. Times and Gaz.*, of last June, and will be subjoined, although its import is little favorable to drugs and druggists, and their prescribing patrons the doctors :

"Dr. Forget on Antiphlogistic Treatment.—Broussais invented

inflammation and bleeding it seems. Hippocrates, Celsus, Galen, never suspected the existence of inflammation. MM. Andral and Gavarret are only the satraps of the reformer ; and as for bleeding, this same Galen, and Sydenham, Botal, Guy-Patin, Chirac, Sylva, Hecquet, Bosquillon, and *tuti quanti*, never used the lancet. Hence, then,

> " Si nous saignons sans succès,
> C'est la faute de Broussais."

Unable to destroy inflammation, we have begun to calumniate it ; it has completely changed its nature we are told. For three thousand years it has been considered as an *exaggeration* of the vital forces, but we have it now demonstrated as a *depression* of the nervous system. For three thousand years bleeding has been used as the most natural means of disgorging the inflamed tissues, and now it is irrefragibly proved, that bleeding aggravates and produces inflammation. We have not only theoretical proofs of the fact, but we have practical proofs, which no one will refuse—clinical experiment. Thus English, German, and French practitioners have taken it into their heads to lay the bridle on the neck of the phlegmsiæ of pneumonia, and erysipelas, for example; some of them have the courage even to treat them with alcohol, by the aid of which their patients do admirably. Ah! you will say, that does not surprise me at all ; we have had expectant doctors, like Hippocrates ; and busy doctors, like Asclepiades; and debilitating doctors, like Sydenham and Broussais ; and stimulating doctors, like Morton and Brown. At all times there have been empirics and methodists who have, turn by turn, ruled the medical world. Broussais dethroned Brown, and now behold Brown revenging himself on Broussais. Science, like representative government is a system of balancing. The truth of to-day is the error of the morrow. All which proves that there is no constancy in Nature, as Bichat has said, and proves also that Nature is stronger than physic and physicians, for if she were the slave of systems, the world would soon be a desert. But statistics? you will say. Statistics are always on the side of the party who invokes their aid ; they are kindly handmaids, at the service of the first comer. The value of statistics is the value of the observer. Science, good sense, and honesty are of more worth than figures."

It appears from an interesting and finely illustrated memoir, for which the Academy of Sciences lately awarded M. Forget a prize (a memoir kindly sent to the *N. O. Med. and Surg. Jour.*), that while M. Forget says, "I am a partisan, pathogenically of the doctrine of naturism," yet the very first case reported in his work, he calls an "ulcerous inflammation," and the treatment first adopted is called antiphlogistic. He says: "In November, 1854, a violent inflammation occurred. Antiphlogistic treatment was employed, two applications of leeches were made, and the inflammatory symptoms decreased." (*Dental Anomalies and their Influence.* Pp. 7, 8, 28.)

Sthenia and antiphlogistics, I may further remark, are innocent and legitimate babes, compared with numerous phrases and terms in use, which, however, serve admirably to conceal our ignorance of certain pathological and therapeutical topics, as nervous, reflex, dynamic, etc., among which is one now becoming axiomatic, as if it were as clear as that a part is less than the whole—namely: that pathology is nothing but diseased or deranged physiology; symptoms, pathological anatomy, all quantitative, qualitative, all dynamical and material aberrations and changes being purely physiological. But if it were expedient to look very closely into this seemingly lucid explanation, it would soon appear that there is more darkness than light in it. One might as well define falsehood by deranged truth, insanity by deranged sanity, vice by deranged virtue; all of which are antitheses, being neither analogous nor identical. Whatsoever is morbid is a constant recession from and incompatible with physiological function. Sickness is not health. Whether we rely upon what we observe in the ordinary maladies of people, or produce, artificially, that is, by experiment, diseased conditions, it will be seen that every morbid symptom or change is just so far a departure from the normal physiological actions which constitute health. Physiological sickness and physiological venesection, or drugs, as opiates, quinine, blisters, etc., do not, at least, appear to be very happy examples of medical nomenclature. The same remark may be applied to those writers who mention that sensation is sometimes not perceived or felt. Now, any sensation which is not felt, is not. The feeling of a sensation is the whole of it, and essential to its very nature. Hearing, seeing, smelling, tasting, pain, anger, which produce no sensation, have no reality for the individual, neither for the judge nor jury, and could not be received as evidence in any court.

According to the new, or rather according to the old sect now revived, "nature healeth our diseases:" what may this goddess be? Is she material or immaterial? mind? or matter? or both? The German pantheists believe that there is no God other than the universe, the whole of matter and mind. Pope's idea is, that

" All are but parts of one stupendous whole,
Whose body Nature is, and God the soul."

One philosopher maintains that phenomenal Nature is a self-revelation of the Deity, while another announces that Nature conceals God !

Mr. Stallo, in his work on the *Philosophy of Nature* (or one might call it the Philosophy of Germany), gives the following exposition of Nature and her laws : " The teleological system, or the doctrine of *causæ finales*, with its laws, for which, on account of their formal generality, it was impossible to give any empirical [experimental] warrant [are]: the *lex parsimoniæ*, that Nature attains her ends by the shortest possible route and by the fewest possible means ; the *lex continui*, that Nature never proceeds *per saltum*, either in the succession or the coärrangement of her products ; the *lex subsumptionis*, that Nature's variety reduces itself to a few principles."

The student of history, from its earliest records to the present day, will have found that there have been all sorts of gods and goddesses relied on or appealed to in the science and art of healing, as demons, astrologes, conjurers, witches, and in our day homœopathists, spiritual table-turning doctors, and many other sects.

The revival of non-medication (if a negation may be revived), and the re-discovery of Nature, and that she alone can heal the sick, without drugs—or, as others affirm, with the aid of alcohol, full diet, etc., are doctrines which have been avowed by not a few men of learning and moral excellence.   Have these men received a revelation from Nature or any other goddess ?   This they neither can nor do avow.   But they virtually claim to know the intentions and conduct of Nature better than the great mass of medical professors and practitioners of all nations and of all ages, not to mention the non-professional world, not one in a thousand of whom doubts the efficacy of medication.   Now, all of these classes have derived their opinions from the same Nature and Art in disease which the skeptics themselves rely upon to prove the mischievous effects of the medication, however skillful.   Now, this overwhelming majority who attest the efficacy of medication have at least an equal opportunity of knowing all the facts necessary to the formation of an enlightened opinion, and of drawing rational deductions from both personal observations and experience, and the experience of all ages, times, and places.

There never was a time in the history of legitimate medicine when either the physicians or the people generally supposed that medicinal agents, judiciously applied, were always injurious or wholly inefficacious in relieving from suffering or in removing disease and preventing untimely death. Now, the speculative opinions of the few cannot overthrow the speculative opinions of the many, in matters where all are equally qualified to judge, having equal opportunities to observe. Under these circumstances, in a matter purely experimental, the opinion of one man cannot outweigh the opinion and experience of a million, especially when fortified by all traditional and historical testimony. That emetics, cathartics, stimulants, opiates, etc., have been valuable remedial agents when given with ordinary judgment and skill, all history testifies.

We have no evidence but that of the skeptics themselves showing that they have peculiar and indisputable claims to interpret the purposes, plans, and powers of Nature, nor that they alone have a knowledge of what she can and will do.

That Nature, or, as some have it, God, is a doctor, has not any foundation in revelation.

The very first book of Sacred History, Genesis, recognizes doctors : "Joseph commanded his servants, the physicians, etc." Throughout the whole series of Sacred writings, no reference is made to a metaphysical abstraction or myth as being the only doctor, called Nature—the most ambiguous word known in human vocabularies ; while, on the other hand, physicians and their vocation are often mentioned. Pious and rational doctors of modern times, who say "God healeth our diseases," intended to say that the means of cure, or the functions of the physician, were also implied or enjoined in the process just as much as industrial means are implied in producing corn, clothing, printing, gunpowder, telegraphs, railroads, etc.

The learned Dr. Renouard, of Paris, in his recent work, the *History of Medicine* (translated by Prof. Comegys), makes the following quotation from the Ecclesiasticus, a book indubitably very ancient, and held to be canonical by the Catholic Church, and generally bound in the protestant version of the Bible, between the Old and New Testaments. I have added from the same chapter referred to by Dr. R., several additional passages :

" Honor a physician with the honor due to him, for the uses which you may have of him. For of the most High cometh healing, and he shall receive honor of the king. The skill of the physician shall lift up his head ; and in the fight of the great men he shall be in admiration. The Lord hath created medicines out of the earth ; and he that is wise will not abhor them." (xxxviii, 1, 2, 3, 4.)

The following, from the same sacred record, is a true exposition of the manner in which the "Lord healeth :" "He hath given men skill, that he might be honored in his marvelous works. With such doth he heal men, and taketh away their pains. Then give place to the physician, for the Lord hath created him ; let him not go from thee, for thou hast need of him. There is a time when in their hands there is good success." (v. 6, 7, 12, 13.)

In the eighth verse, the apothecary and his pharmaceutical preparations are alluded to : "Of such doth the apothecary make a confection," etc. Whether this confection was like any of the numerous formulæ of the American Dispensatory, as the *confectio opii*, c. *scammonii*, c. *sennæ*, etc., does not appear in the record ; but, at all events, Israel, when sick, was sometimes drugged, which is contrary to the growing science of non-medication.

Medicine, or rather therapy, is not an absolutely exact science, but one of reasonable cumulative probability. It does not rest on the dictum of any one, but is founded on experience and observation. It is more reasonable to suppose that the general experience and observation upon which therapy rests, are less likely to deceive than the opinion, contrariwise, of a single or a few individuals. The testimony of the former must preponderate, other things being equal.

Therapy in no case can claim as its foundation a necessary truth ; indeed, experience cannot prove a necessary truth, but probability only. It is not a pure science, like mathematics, astronomy, etc. Its materials, though consisting of facts, are related to and blended with vitality, or life, or antecedents,- the nature of which have hitherto transcended experimental research. Those who deny the laws of vitality because they cannot define its cause, might deny as well many things altogether true. The nature of life, of mind, and even of matter, remain unknown. Physiologists have been no more puzzled to define life, than physicists to define matter. Hegel says that "a thing is nothing more nor less than the complex of its relations to other things. These relations are called its qualities ; hence, the whole existence of a thing is *qualitative* ; it is not primitive, mere *quantitative* being to which qualities are subsequently imparted." Now, on the contrary, "it is a fundamental proposition in the philosophy of Schelling, that all difference is *quantitative.*" Some of the greatest philosophers, including Bishop Berkeley, maintain that the existence of matter has never been, nor can it be proven.

The efficacy of medication—active medication (for all medication is more or less active)—can in no way be invalidated by the improper and unnecessary administration of drugs, as to their kinds, doses, times, cases, etc. A man sinking from hæmorrhage should not be bled, nor one collapsed from cholera be purged ; nor should another, who has already eaten too much, for that reason eat still more. All arguments against the use derived from the abuse of drugs are fallacions and irrelevant. The true question is this : Is the skillful use of quinine or any other drug less likely to arrest and remove a disease, an intermittent fever, for example, than non-medication or Nature ; or, to use the language of common sense, can the malady be sooner or more certainly or completely cured by letting it run its course without any interference ? The question, then, at issue, is not whether medication is required in all cases, as no enlightened practitioner will hesitate to admit that it is not. Whether unskillful treatment is not more dangerous than the omission of all treatment— whether antiphlogistic or stimulant treatment should be preferred— are all foreign to the issue involved, which may be thus put : Cannot a physician who is thoroughly acquainted with the existing medical sciences, as well as with the observation and experience of the past—one who during his education has witnessed and studied the effects of therapeutic treatment, as now practised at the bedside—cannot he apply remedial agents, so as in all probability to cure a greater percentage of the sick than would be in all human probability cured by abandoning them to the natural course and tendency of their diseases ; such, for instance, as intermittent fever, pleurisy, pneumonia, cholera morbus, scurvy, diarrhœa, dysentery, itch, syphilis, gonorrhœa, etc.

If it were possible for an educated physician to be wholly ignorant of the therapeutical history of past experience, when called to treat his first case, he might not be able, upon the recovery of his patient, to say whether the treatment, even in a case of actual cure, had or had not contributed to the recovery. The testimony of the past and a comparison with the present, together with daily experience in such cases, will enable him to arrive at probability, if not absolute

certainty, even in individual cases, and this probability is strength-
ened in proportion to the number of observations, and in many cases
he may attain to a reasonable certainty, such as in most departments
of science and business is deemed reliable for human belief and conduct.

In no isolated case, from Hippocrates to the present, can it be
demonstrated beyond the possibility of a doubt, that a cure has ever
been effected by any mode of medicinal treatment. Nor can it be
demonstrated that the sun will rise to-morrow, and that some person
will die during that day. Nevertheless, the evidence of analogy, or
past experience and observation, give the utmost probability that
both events will happen. That Cæsar, Napoleon I, or Washington
lived, is less probable than that either of these anticipated events mentioned will fail. History has often been falsified, as experience has
shown, but the rising of the sun has failed neither during our own
experience nor that of our predecessors in all the historical period.

The efficacy of the medical treatment of disease is founded neither
upon any certain knowledge of the nature of vitality nor upon the
mode of action by which a remedial agent removes pain and arrests the
march of a malady. All that is known in the premises is empirical,
that is, experimental. The same is true of the whole circle of the
experimental sciences, with, however, this great difference, that
throughout the whole realm of inorganic nature, there is a fixity or
uniformity unknown to the vital or organic world. It may be, nay,
it is probable, that uniformity reigns in the latter equally with the
former, but unfortunately the antecedents, functions, and nature of
the living economy are, in relation to our senses and modes of cog-
nition, neither known nor fixed with the certainty which appertains
to inorganic or non-vital matter.

Observation and experience, however extensive these may be, are
not knowledge. The latter is the act of a sound, comprehensive understanding, together with rational deduction from facts. Therapeutical facts are peculiarly liable to misinterpretation. A gentleman, a few days since, took the trouble to relate to me the great
success of a deceased doctor (of this city) in curing hydrophobia.
" Now it has been ascertained," says Dr. Oesterlen, " by the exact
observation of hundreds of dogs which had been inoculated with the
poison, or bitten by others which were mad, that even under the
circumstances most favorable for the production of the disease, that

is, where no means, or so-called preservatives of any kind had been employed, scarcely sixty or seventy per cent. of the animals became rabid." Now, if these sixty or seventy cases in the hundred, had been treated by any remedy, that remedy alone would obtain the credit of so great a success.

If the physician possessed any certain means of knowing that particular cases would eventuate in recovery without any advantages from treatment, a vast amount of medication would thereby be prevented. But neither the believers nor skeptics in physic can predict with absolute certainty such a result, in any case whatever. Prophets there are none. Probabilities there may be for or against the occurrence of one of the only two possible events in a given case.

The theoretical stand-points from which therapeutical methods are viewed and the consequent contrarieties, real or apparent, in practice, afford skeptics with plausible if not logical arguments against medication. In illustration of this and some kindred positions, I beg eave to introduce a few paragraphs from Dr. Oesterlin's work on *Medical Logic* (Sydenham edit., p. 238, *et seq.*).

"If we bring to the bedside of the same patient a disciple of Brown or of Broussais, an empiric of the old, or one of the modern stamp, an adherent of the so-called Vienna anatomical, or of the Giessen chemical school, a nerve-pathologist or a blood-pathologist, each will recognize a different state of things. The opinion which each forms of fever, for instance, and similar aggregates of symptoms, of their casual connection and dependence upon various local or general changes and conditions, and of these in their relations to each other, will be different from that of the others. Each of them, if he reflects upon it at all, will form a different notion of all that he has been able to observe; he will arrange and combine the various phenomena in the patient after his own manner—*i. e.*, in accordance with his own point of view; and, if the same remedy be administered in a given case, the assertions and opinions of each concerning its effects will equally differ. For each has expected from it different services and modes of operation in accordance to his previously formed theory; he will, therefore, interpret what he has observed in the manner which best corresponds to his own views, and in the remedy employed will acknowledge only such effects as it has been his aim to produce.

"So long as Brown's system prevailed, many believed that digitalis produced an excitement of the heart and circulation. According to their view the pulse was first accelerated and rendered fuller before it could become weaker and slower, and they asserted that the subsequent depression depended upon the previous excitement (Saunders, Hutchinson, and others). If another, a disciple of Broussais,

for instance, had observed exactly the same thing, his interpretation
of it would have been entirely different, because he would not attach
the same signification, or an equal importance to such excitement of
the circulation, etc. In like manner, at the period when the simple,
non-mercurial treatment of syphilis prevailed, patients were believed
to be injured by mercury in a degree never observed before or since.
A homœopathist of the old school, and a modern disciple of Rademacher, will equally claim for themselves, and for the influence and
mode of operation of their remedies, credit for much which the impartial, and, perhaps, correctly reasoning physician, regards simply
as dependent upon the natural course of the disease. The ordinary
practitioner will scarcely hesitate to assert that he has obviated
various diseases or abnormal conditions ·by means· of some remedy
or mode of treatment. He willingly regards the changes which
take place in the state of his patients after the employment of them,
as their effects, when those changes are favorable—*i. e.*, as the results' of his practice, while, if the changes are unfavorable, he
attributes them to the natural course of the disease, or to various
other influences and circumstances. He will further interpret the
effects of his remedies in exact accordance with his own theories
and views. Because, for instance, in persons submitted to the influence of anæsthetic agents, intelligence and consciousness, in the
first place, then sensation, motion, and respiration, are successively
suspended, ether and chloroform are said to act first upon the cerebrum, then upon the cerebellum, next upon the posterior, and, lastly,
upon the anterior pyramids of the spinal cord and their nerves.
And when their action is extended to the medulla oblongata, life is
said to hang by a single thread. A Flourens, a Baudens, and others
take this view of their mode of operation, because it happens to
correspond with their theories of the functions of those portions of
the nervous system.

"In relation to the accuracy and scientific value of our conclusions,
there is scarcely any difference to be found between the ordinary
practitioner, or even the homœopath or disciple of Rademacher, and
the modern physiological physician ; for the endeavor of the latter
towards a more scientific advance and judgment is still far from
complete, and seldom to any great extent feasible. His interpretation of what he observes, though it may approach nearer to the
actual state of things than theirs does, will not be less uncertain
and arbitrary. Just so will the physicist interpret the same phenomena and processes in the living body, and even in the inorganic
world—*e. g.*, in the air, water, or the soil, with their action upon each
other, upon vegetation, man, and animals—very differently from the
chemist, and both again differently from the professed physiologist
or ordinary practitioner.

"In all that has been already advanced, many may, doubtless, if
they are so inclined, find sufficient grounds of discouragement, and
feel justified in mistrusting even the first and most indispensable
methods of comprehension in medical science. Yet, to perceive difficulties does not necessitate that we should allow them to overcome
us, and in the case of observation, especially in such a science as

medicine, it has already been shown that it is by no means such a simple and intelligible thing as might be at first believed, and that Fontenelle was quite right when he said 'l'art d'observer, qui n'est que le fondement de la science, est lui-même une très-grande science.'

"If we compare, for instance, our present methods of observation and investigation in the whole field of vital phenomena, and even at the bedside, with those employed but a few decennia ago, we cannot fail to recognize a great improvement in them. Not only have we acquired, by the recognition of various anatomical relations and chemico-physical processes, better starting points for our observations, but, by the employment of such aids, the general value of our observations is advanced far beyond that of earlier periods. In illustration of this it may be sufficient here to mention the more frequent and efficient employment of various auxiliary means, such as the thermometer, scales, etc."

The ethical question involved in medication or in non-medication is in numerous points of view of grave import. If opium, quinine, calomel, blistering, bleeding, etc., can either directly or indirectly remove disease, or even lessen pain, teachers, writers and practitioners who deny the efficacy and withhold the application of remedial agents might seem to plain people, not altogether guiltless of hypocrisy, the omission of duty, and the propagation of fatal errors. Is it not hypocrisy to assume the office of a physician, which both virtually and openly holds forth to the public a belief in the efficacy of remedial agents, while at the same time, the practitioner who receives compensation from patients for services wholly worthless, according to his own showing? does he not obtain money under false pretenses? Would he, in any case, be employed, if he candidly told the patient that all medicine is not only useless but injurious, and that Nature only, not the doctor, is competent either to relieve or cure the sick? Can an honest man hold such opinions, and at the same time continue to practise his profession? Are not his principles and his conduct the antithesis of the true and the good? the concentration of the false and immoral? If sincere in his belief, should he renounce practice altogether? His opinion, in opposition to that of a vast majority of his contemporaries and predecessors, who have had an experience in therapy to which his own is as a drop to the ocean, may in all reason be disturbed; at least, until further discovery he can never be certain that science and art can do nothing to arrest disease and prolong life.

If he can do nothing himself, how can he be certain that others cannot do something to arrest disease? Can he fix the limits of the possible ? Is he entitled to teach, write, or say anything more than that for himself, he knows of no remedy which can in any case be useful for the sick, although others equally able to judge in the premises may know how to apply medicinal agents so as to cure, and, therefore, he cannot, from his own negative knowledge, infer that the positive knowledge of all others is to be rejected as useless, and, therefore, he cannot conscientiously propagate, by lectures, writings, or otherwise, a mere personal negative which might endanger the lives of millions, should medicinal agents, after all, be efficacious or curative.

Homœopathy, under the cloak of medication, when really carried into effect, is strictly non-medication. All its cures, if any, are effected by practising directly the reverse of its theory, of its infinitissimal doses, dilutions, and attenuations. The expectant method of cure, a pleasant phrase or refinement in language, which means skepticism or non-medication—no more, no less, the practice of which (if the practice of nothing were a possibility at all conceivable) is but a deception as far as the public is concerned, and would not be considered otherwise if candidly avowed at the bedside. Can any sane man suppose that a planter of Louisiana would send at midnight, in a rain, storm, and thunder, over rivers and bayous, through canebrakes, morasses, and among crocodiles, for a physician to visit his family, or his negro, if the sender knew that the doctor would not in any case administer any medicine, but leave the case wholly to what is fancifully called Nature. If the doctor mean by Nature, God, and that God is the medical attendant, he must be competent, even though he may not have a sheepskin diploma. Would it not be presumptuous in such presence to prescribe pills, syrups, and distilled waters, which the prescriber himself acknowledges to be wholly inert and intended only to deceive ?

PROGRESS OF MEDICINE.

Art. I.—*Notes of Selected Cases from the Wards of the Charity Hospital, at New Orleans:* By T. G. Richardson, M. D., one of the Attending Surgeons, and Professor of Anatomy in the Medical Department of the University of Louisiana.

Dislocation of the Head of the Femur into the Thyroid Foramen, of eight days standing, reduced by Manipulation.—W. S., aged twenty-six, a very stout, athletic man, was admitted into the hospital on the first of November, 1859, having been injured eight days previously by falling from the side of a schooner into a skiff. Attention being directed to the left hip, only a very slight examination sufficed to determine the nature of the accident. The patient lying upon his back, the leg was found to be flexed to a right angle at the knee-joint, the thigh strongly abducted and everted, and the limb lengthened about an inch and a half ; in fine, all the signs of dislocation of the head of the femur into the thyroid foramen were well marked.

Determined to attempt reduction by manipulation, I had the man carried into the amphitheatre before the class and brought fully under the influence of chloroform. Complete insensibility and muscular relaxation having been effected, I seized the limb just above the ankle, flexed the leg still further at the knee-joint and the thigh upon the pelvis, bearing the latter down upon the left side of the abdomen, then carried the knee over to the middle line of the abdomen, and rapidly extended the limb, drawing it at the same time obliquely underneath its opposite fellow. Just before the extension, which required the exertion of a good deal of force, was completed, the limb suddenly yielded and fell into its natural position, but a single manipulation having been employed. The usual after-treatment was instituted, and in ten days time the patient, being able to walk with little or no difficulty, left the hospital.

Notwithstanding the readiness and comparative ease by which reduction was accomplished in this case, I am not prepared to recommend manipulation as a substitute in all cases for the old method of extension by the means of pulleys. It is, without doubt, a great improvement in the surgical art, but when abused as it oftentimes is, it is liable to do great mischief to the soft parts around the joint. We read of practitioners who, in their efforts to accomplish reduction in this manner, have thrown the head of the bone from one position to another ; say, from the dorsum of the ilium into the sciatic notch, from the latter into the thyroid hole, and then back again upon the ilium. When this happens, great laceration and bruising of the soft parts must, of course, be produced, and hence the necessity for an accurate knowledge of the mechanism of the procedure and unusual care in its application. In reduction by the pulleys, the force being applied only in the direction of the displacement, no such accident can be produced. When the knowledge referred to is not possessed by the operator, I would advise adherence to the old method.

Concussion, with Laceration of the Brain, and slight Extravasation of Blood ; Death ; Autopsy.—An Irishman, name unknown, aged about thirty, was brought into the hospital on the afternoon of Oct. 11, 1859, in a state of complete insensibility from an injury to the head received an hour previously. The history of the case, as gathered from those who witnessed the accident, was substantially as follows : The man was standing on the levee near the river's edge when a spar, extending from an adjacent boat to the shore, suddenly gave way, flew up, and struck him under the jaw with such force as to raise him entirely from the ground and throw him several feet distant. He was picked up in an apparently lifeless condition and conveyed immediately to the hospital, where I saw him the following morning.

Upon making inquiries of the student of the ward, I ascertained that the man was completely insensible when admitted, and that his vital powers were so much prostrated that the house surgeon deemed it advisable to administer brandy and water, which was gotten down only with great difficulty. Partial reaction followed the use of the stimulant, but up to the time of my visit, about twenty hours after the accident, there was no evidence of returning consciousness. Upon examination, I discovered the mark of the blow just below the lower jaw on the left side, but the skin was not lacerated nor the bone broken. His intellectual functions were completely suspended, nor could he be in the least aroused, or even made to open his eyes, by forcible shaking or by hollowing in his ears. His breathing was natural, pulse a little accelerated, and extremities warm. He had not vomited since his admission, but passed his urine involuntarily. The pupil of the left eye was slightly dilated, but the right was of its natural size, and responded readily to the influence of light.

While making this examination, I noticed that he was continually moving the left leg and arm, but that only now and then did he lift the right leg from the bed or move the fingers of the right hand ; and upon directing my attention more particularly to these symptoms, I found that a partial paralysis of sensibility existed throughout the whole of the right half of the body, and that the muscles of the right arm, with the exception of those going to the fingers, were in a state of *rigid contraction;* so much so indeed that the limb could be bent at the elbow only by using considerable force. The sensibility of the arm was manifestly not entirely destroyed, for pinching the skin excited an effort to move the limb, as evinced by the contraction of the muscles of the corresponding shoulder. The right leg was relaxed, but when pinched or pricked was now and then feebly raised from the bed.

No fracture of the skull could be detected. Reaction having been in a measure established, as indicated by the character of the pulse, temperature of the surface, and other signs, I did not consider it necessary to repeat the stimulant which had been given the previous evening, but simply ordered cloths wrung out of cold water to be applied to the head, and the bed to be surrounded by curtains to shut out light and noise.

On the following morning I found the temperature of the skin, both of the extremities and trunk, quite hot but moist; pulse 120, soft and compressible ; respiration somewhat hurried but easy; the bladder still emptying itself involuntarily without any discernible accumulation. I also learned that a large semi-liquid evacuation from the bowels had occurred during the night. There was, however, no reäction in the mental faculties, and the partial loss of sensibility in the right side, and the rigidity of the muscles of the right arm continued.

The directions of the day before repeated, with the addition of a large blister to the inner side of each thigh. The patient died, however, during the ensuing evening, fifty-three hours after the accident.

Autopsy.—The body was opened fourteen hours after death, the examination being limited to the head, as it was evident from the history of the case that this was the only part injured.

Upon lifting the brain, surrounded by the greater part of the dura mater, from its place, attention was first directed to the bones of the cranium, but no sign of fracture or other injury could be found, nor was there any effusion of blood between the dura mater, and the bony surfaces. Removing the dura mater from the brain, the first abnormal appearance that I observed was a slight congestion of the veins of the pia mater, but no extravasation. Proceeding next to slice the brain carefully, commencing above, I could detect no unusual fullness of the vessels of the organ; but situated near the centre of the anterior lobe of the left hemisphere was a very small longitudinal rent containing a tolerably firm clot of blood about the size and very nearly the shape of a large pea. The clot was easily lifted from its bed, and, what was singular, the surrounding parts were scarcely stained by the effusion and not in the least congested. Continuing the dissection, I came upon a similar clot, but not larger than a No. 4 shot, in the posterior lobe of the right hemisphere, just beneath the gray layer.

Remarks.—The value of this case, both in a diagnostic and pathological point of view, will be readily appreciated. With the exception of the partial paralysis of the right side of the body, the symptoms were those of a pure but severe case of concussion. The exception in question was, however, sufficient to induce a strong suspicion of grave and probably fatal lesion to the central substance, and I so expressed myself from the time that I first saw the patient. As to the complete and protracted suspension of the intellectual powers, this is not unfrequently witnessed in cases of simple concussion, and, except when it continues for some time after entire reäction of the circulatory and secreting functions is not a very alarming symptom.

The post-mortem appearances account sufficiently, according to our present notions of the relations of the cerebral hemispheres to the two sides of the body, for the partial paralysis of the right arm and leg ; but how is the rigidity of the right arm to be explained ?

This was a puzzling symptom to me, and is worthy the attention of physiologists.

Concussion; Suspension of Intellectual Faculties for Four Days; Recovery.—J. W., aged fourteen, was admitted into the hospital, October 8th, 1859, having been injured a few hours previously by being thrown upon the sod from the back of a mule. It could not be ascertained what portion of the body struck the ground first. The symptoms were those of an uncomplicated but severe case of concussion ; heart's action feeble, and pulse correspondingly weak but slow, beating only sixty per minute ; countenance pale, and features pinched ; respiration natural ; pupils unaltered and contracting promptly under the influence of light ; vomiting and involuntary passage of urine. The intellectual faculties, as is usual in such cases, were not completely suspended ; for when the body was forcibly shaken, a muttering complaint could be elicited, but no intelligent answer to the simplest question could be obtained, however loudly spoken in his ears.

Dr. Dirmeyer, who attended the case for two days before it fell into my hands, employed none of the ordinary means to bring about reaction, except the administration of a little brandy and water, which, being vomited, was followed by only partial success. At the time of my first visit, forty-eight hours after the accident, all the symptoms above mentioned were present except the paleness of the countenance, contraction of the features, and coldness of the extremities. As the functions of the body generally seemed to be in a tolerably good condition, and the symptoms not alarming, I did not consider it prudent to repeat the stimulants, but ordered the head to be placed low, perfect quiet, and the regular administration of milk and beef-tea every three or four hours.

On the following day the color of the face was decidedly better ; extremities warm ; pulse somewhat increased in force, but no improvement in the cerebral symptoms. Ordered blisters to the thighs, and continuance of regimen.

On the morning of the twelfth, four days from the receipt of the injury, the patient opened his eyes as though awaking from an ordinary sleep, looked around evidently in perfect ignorance of his situation, and being told where he was, tried to get out of bed in order to go home. Upon being questioned, he could give no account whatever of the accident, but remembered only having been upon the mule's back. By gentle confinement to bed, low regimen, and slight purgation added to the counter-irritation which had already been made by the blisters, inflammation of the brain was prevented, and in four days more the boy was allowed to be taken home, with directions to continue the treatment a few days longer.

Remarks.—The object in reporting the above case is to show the good effects of a more negative course of treatment than is usually pursued in such cases. It is true that the patient had taken brandy, but this had been ejected very soon after, and he subsequently took nothing whatever except milk and beef-tea. The great advantage which such a plan possesses is the security which it affords against inflammation of the brain. It is only where the prostration is excessive that a resort to stimulants is, in my opinion, at all justifiable, and I am convinced that if the majority of cases were let alone, we should have fewer deaths from subsequent inflammation.

Compound Fracture of the Skull, with Depression of Bone and no Symptoms of Compression; Remarks upon the General Treatment of such Cases.—During the month of February, 1860, three cases of compound fracture of the cranium, with depression of bone and no symptoms of depression, were admitted into my wards at the Charity Hospital. Of these, one was what Mr. Erichsen terms a "longitudinal punctured fracture," made with the edge of a hatchet ; the second, an extensive compound comminuted fracture, with laceration of the brain, produced by a blow from a hammer ; and the third, a compound fracture, with angular depression of bone, inflicted by a stone or brick. In the first case, the wound was closed by the house surgeon, by means of stitches, and the parts kept constantly cool and moist by the application of cloths wrung out of water. The patient recovered without a bad symptom. In the second case, inflammation of the brain, induced by the injury which the organ received at the time of the accident, supervened upon the third day, and death resulted at the end of a week. The third case is here reported in full for the purpose of illustrating the treatment which I usually pursue under such circumstances, in opposition to that of a large majority of American and British surgeons.

J. C., a large, well-built, hearty-looking Irishman, about thirty years of age, was struck upon the forehead by a stone or brick, he did not know which, on the night of the first of February. He fell to the ground in a state of insensibility, but soon recovering his consciousness, got up, and was led by his friends to the hospital, where he was put to bed, and cloths wrung out of cold water applied by the student of the ward. Examining the next morning, I found a contused, lacerated wound of the forehead, situated a little to the left of the median line, and an inch and a half above the orbital arch. The wound was sufficiently large to admit the end of the forefinger, upon introducing which, and also by exposing the parts to the light, I readily ascertained that there existed a fracture of the skull, with angular depression. Two irregular pieces of bone, each about as large as a ten-cent piece, had been driven in obliquely upon the brain, and were so firmly impacted as to be immovable by any ordinary force made with the finger or forceps. The depth of the depression at its lowest point below the level of the surrounding bone was nearly eight lines. There were also a few small splinters or chips of bone lying loose in the wound.

As already intimated, the man had no symptoms of compression, and, at the time of my visit, expressed himself as entirely comfortable, save a very slight headache. Under these circumstances, and as it was impossible to remove or even raise the depressed fragments without recourse to the trephine, I contented myself with simply picking out the loose bits, and directed the cold cloths to be continued, a rigid antiphlogistic diet, perfect quietude, and the administration of a dose of compound cathartic pills. Under this treatment,

which, with the exception of the purgation, was continued from day to
day, the wound gradually filled up from the bottom with healthy granulations, and in less than three weeks was entirely healed, the patient
not having had a single untoward symptom. It is now four months
since the accident, and although I have not seen the man since he
left the hospital, as he has not sent for me nor applied again for admission, I have good reason to believe that he remains perfectly well.

Remarks.—My object in reporting this case, and in mentioning the
other two in connection with it, is to show, in the first place, that
compound depressed fractures of the skull without symptoms of
compression are not very rare, Mr. Erichsen to the contrary, notwithstanding ; and, secondly, to furnish evidence in favor of modifying a generally received surgical dogma concerning their treatment.
In regard to the latter question, if the reader will take the trouble
to refer to the standard surgical works, published in this country
and in Great Britain within the past half century, he will find that
the trephine or the elevator is directed to be employed in all cases
of compound fracture with depression, whether symptoms of compression exist or not. Take, for example, the recently published
"System of Surgery," by Professor Gross, pronounced by Professor
Simpson, of Edinburgh, to be the most complete treatise on surgery
in the English language. The following is his language : "the proper treatment in compound fracture is to elevate the depressed bone
and remove any loose or partially detached pieces, this plan being
adopted whether there be any compression or not. The case being
a compound one cannot be aggravated by operation, though it is not
to be forgotten that this should be executed with the greatest care
and gentleness." Mr. Erichsen is equally positive ; and if we go
back a few years to the great modern lights, such as Sir Astley
Cooper and Mr. Abernethy, we find this same doctrine laid down as
a law not to be questioned. Accustomed as the Anglo-Saxon race
has been for so many centuries to obedience to law, departing from
it only by slow degrees, as circumstances seem gradually to require,
or breaking suddenly away from it only under the pressure of great
emergencies, it is not strange that a doctrine backed up by such
authority, and reäffirmed by nearly all subsequent teachers, should
have all the force of an enactment of the Medes and Persians, which,
we are told, altereth not. Now, with all due defference to the opinions and decrees of those who have established or perpetuated this rule,
and without partaking in any manner whatever of the spirit or temper
of the party who pleasantly style themselves "Young Physic," I am
disposed to object to the wide range which has been given to this
dogmatic precept. I have no objection to picking out pieces of bone
which are completely detached from their connections with the dura
mater and pericranium, or so nearly so that their little vitality must
be inevitably lost in the subsequent reäction ; nor would I hesitate
to remove a jagged or splintered fragment that might be sticking
through the dura mater into the brain ; but I cannot understand the
necessity of removing the bone simply because it is found resting upon
the dura mater. To elevate it to its place, when this can be accomplished without further injury to the cranium, would be all right

enough, but it is rarely feasible, the great majority of cases demanding for this purpose the use of the trephine.

If I understand the matter, the practice is grounded upon the fact that the depressed bone is necessarily a cause of irritation which will subsequently develop inflammation of the brain or its membranes, whether these structures be wounded or not. Upon this subject I have two suggestions to make.

In the first place, those who take this ground also advocate non-intervention in simple depressed fracture without symptoms of compression. Now if the depressed bone be a cause of inflammation of the encephalon in compound fracture, it is not less so in simple fracture. Indeed, this unfortunate result, according to these premises, would be more likely to occur in the latter than in the former, in consequence of the additional pressure exerted by the extravasated blood and the products of the subsequent inflammation of the sub-cutaneous structures. And this, I think, will be found to hold good in practice ; that is to say, that inflammation of the brain and its membranes oftener occurs in simple fracture with depression than in compound, the same expectant treatment being employed in both.

Secondly, it is not true that pressure upon the brain induces inflammation of the organ, and in proof of this I need only refer to the fact that apoplectic effusions are seldom if ever followed by such an occurrence. The cause of inflammation of the brain after fracture I conceive to be the bruising, laceration, or jarring to which the organ has been subjected ; and if such be the fact, the removal of the depressed bone will in no degree serve to prevent this much-dreaded result, except in those cases in which the fragments have penetrated the dura mater. I might even go still further and state, as has been suggested to me by my distinguished colleague, Professor Stone, that it is not altogether improbable that the removal or elevation of the depressed bone, independently of the injury done by the trephine, may even contribute to the establishment of inflammation by permitting the entrance of a greater amount of blood into the bruised part when reaction takes place than could occur if the pressure were allowed to continue.

In regard to the statement made by many writers, that the use of the trephine does not in any manner complicate a case of compound depressed fracture, I would simply ask whether that exposure of the dura mater which is what they so much fear in simple fracture as to advise against the use of the trephine, is not largely increased by the application of the instrument in compound fracture, to say nothing of the further injury to the bone? It is true that in times long gone by, and it is to be hoped never to return, when a perfect mania for trepanning prevailed among surgeons, large portions of the cranium are said to have been removed with evident advantage to the patient ;* but this by no means proves the innocuousness of the operation.

---

* It is mentioned, in John Bell's " Principles of Surgery," that Godifredus, chief surgeon to the States of Holland, was accustomed to boast that his friend Henry Chadborn, chirurgion, during King William's wars on Philip, Count of Nassau, trepanned the skull of the Count *twenty-seven* times, and substantiated the fact by the most indisputable authority, for he made the said Count of Nassau, after he was recovered, on the 12th of August, 1664, write the following curious certificate : " I, the under-written Philip, Count of Nassau, hereby declare and testify that Mr. Henry Chadborn did trepan me in the skull twenty-seven times, and after that did cure me well and soundly."

Lastly, I would state, without fear of contradiction, that the number of persons who recover after compound fracture with depression, in whom the trephine is not employed, is far greater than of those who have been subjected to the operation. Common observation proves this beyond any doubt; but as additional evidence, I would refer the reader to the statistics of Mr. Lawrie and Mr. King, in Cormack's *Monthly Journal*, 1844, where it will be found that of 77 cases reported of compound fracture, there were 29 cures and 48 deaths; 26 of these 77 cases were not trephined, and of these 18 were cured and 8 died ; 51 of the 77 cases were trephined, and of these 11 were cured and 40 died.†

The only question that remains to be considered in this connection is, the liability to epilepsy after depressed fracture when the fragment of bone is allowed to remain in its unnatural position. The number of cases of epilepsy directly ascribable to this cause, compared with the total number of cases in which depressed bone is permitted to remain below the level of the surrounding surface, is acknowledged by all to be very small, and does not therefore usually enter into the discussion of the subject. But according to the views here enunciated concerning the propriety of using the trephine in the class of cases under consideration, the question becomes, in my opinion, of considerable importance. In the absence, however, of sufficient data, I am compelled to leave it for further investigation.

Subnitrate of Bismuth, in the Treatment of Burns and Scalds.—To the thousand and one local remedies resorted to by medical men, as well as non-medical persons of both sexes, in the treatment of burns and scalds, I have the temerity to add another, if, indeed, I have not been anticipated by some one else. The substance referred to is the subnitrate of bismuth, which I employed during the past winter with remarkable success in the wards of the Charity Hospital. Heretofore I was in the habit of using the white lead and linseed oil, as recommended first by Professor Gross, in the March number of Dr. John Bell's *Medical Bulletin*, for 1844, and, although I consider it far superior to any other application in common use, I am now convinced by ample experience that the bismuth is better. I was induced to give it a trial from a consideration of its well known effect in calming irritation, and even actual inflammation occuring in mucous membranes, the condition of these structures under such circumstances bearing a very close analogy to that of the skin after a burn of the first or second degree.

When I first began its use, I combined it with linseed oil in such proportions as to form a consistent paint, but subsequently substituted glycerin for the oil, and I am now inclined to think that the combination can never be surpassed, since by it every local indication is fully met. To prepare it, it is only necessary to rub the bismuth in a mortar with a sufficient amount of glycerin to form a paste or thick paint, which should be applied to the affected surface by means of a camel's hair pencil or a mop made of soft linen. Previously, however, to making the application, the parts should, if

† Mott's Velpeau, vol ii, p. 942.

possible, be thoroughly dried, and for this purpose it is necessary to prick with a needle or other fine instrument any blisters that may exist, and carefully wipe the surface, by gently pressing upon it a a piece of dry lint or charpie. A thick coating having then been put on, the parts should be protected from the pressure or friction of the bed clothes by covering it with a sheet of clean carded cotton or a layer of cotton batting, which may be confined, if necessary, by a thin bandage lightly applied. In burns of the first degree, one such application will often suffice, but in those of the second degree, it may be necessary to repeat it, in part at least, from day to day, in consequence of its disturbance and the wetting of the cotton by the subjacent discharges. The great object is to keep the denuded and tender surface entirely protected from atmospheric contact, which is especially important in the wards of hospitals where the air is always more or less loaded with noxious gases.

In slight burns of the first degree in which there is only an erythematous inflammation without any vesication, the glycerin may be conveniently dispensed with and the dry bismuth dusted thick over the surface, in which case the watery exudations from the skin will form with it a pasty coating sufficiently protective. But still the glycerin, possessing of itself properties powerfully soothing in their influence, should always be combined with it, unless there be some reasonable objection to its use.

The carded cotton or cotton battery I look upon as a most valuable adjuvant, and is superior to anything with which I am acquainted for warding off pressure.*—*The North American Medico-Chirurgical Review*, July, 1860.

ART. II.—*The Arsenic-Eaters of Styria:* By CHARLES HEISCH, Lecturer on Chemistry at the Middlesex Hospital.

AT the last meeting of the Manchester Philosophical Society, I observe that Dr. Roscoe called attention to the arsenic-eaters of Styria. Having for the last two years been in communication with the medical men and other residents in the district where this practice prevails, I shall feel obliged if you will allow me through your journal to make known the facts I have at present collected. The information is derived mainly from Dr. Lorenz, Imperial Professor of Natural History, formerly of Salzburg ; from Dr. Carle Arbele, Professor of Anatomy in Salzburg ; and Dr. Kottowitz, of Neuhaus, besides several non-medical friends. If human testimony be worth anything,

----

* Since writing the above, Dr. W. C. Nichols, the highly accomplished House Surgeon of the Charity Hospital, has informed me that he has given the bismuth and glycerin a fair trial in a number of cases of burns under his charge, and freely accords to it all the praise which my experience elicited in its behalf.

the fact of the existence of arsenic-eaters is placed beyond a doubt. Dr. Lorenz, to whom questions were first addressed, at once stated that he was aware of the practice, but added, that it is generally difficult to get hold of individual cases, as the obtaining of arsenic without a doctor's certificate is contrary to law, and those who do so are very anxious to conceal the fact, particularly from medical men and priests. Dr. Lorenz was, however, well acquainted with one gentleman, an arsenic-eater, with whom he kindly put me in communication, and to whom I shall refer again more particularly. He also says that he knows arsenic is commonly taken by the peasants in Styria, the Tyrol, and the Salzkammergut, principally by huntsmen and woodcutters, to improve their wind and prevent fatigue. He gives the following particulars :

The arsenic is taken pure, in some warm liquid, as coffee, fasting, beginning with a bit the size of a pin's head, and increasing to that of a pea. The complexion and general appearance are much improved, and the parties using it seldom look so old as they really are ; but he has never heard of any case in which it was used to improve personal beauty, though he cannot say that it never is so used. The first dose is always followed by symptoms of poisoning, such as burning pain in the stomach, and sickness, but not very severe.

Once begun, it can only be left off by very gradually diminishing the daily dose, as a sudden cessation causes sickness, burning pains in the stomach, and other symptoms of poisoning, very speedily followed by death.

As a rule, arsenic-eaters are very long lived, and are peculiarly exempt from infectious diseases, fevers, etc.; but unless they gradually give up the practice, invariably die suddenly at last.

In some arsenic works near Salzburg, with which he is acquainted, he says the only men who can stand the work for any time are those who swallow daily doses of arsenic, the fumes, etc., soon killing the others. The director of these works, the gentleman before alluded to, sent me the following particulars of his own case. (This gentleman's name I suppress, as he writes that he does not wish the only thing known about him in England to be the fact that he is an arsenic-eater ; but if any judicial inquiry should arise which might render positive evidence of arsenic-eating necessary, his name and testimony will be forthcoming.)

"At seventeen years of age, while studying assaying, I had much to do with arsenic, and was advised by my teacher, M. Bönsch, Professor of Chemistry and Mineralogy at Eisleben, to begin the habit of arsenic-eating. I quote the precise words he addressed to me : ' If you wish to continue the study of assaying, and become hereafter superintendent of a factory, more especially of an arsenic factory, in which position there are so few, and which is abandoned by so many, and to preserve yourself from the fumes which injure the lungs of most, if not of all, and to continue to enjoy your customary health and spirits, and to attain a tolerably advanced age, I advise you—nay, it is absolutely necessary, that besides strictly abstaining from spirituous liquors, you should learn to take arsenic ; but do not forget, when you have attained the age of fifty years, gradually to decrease your dose, till from the dose to which you have become accustomed, you return to that with which you began, or even less.' I have made trial of my preceptor's prescriptions till now, the forty-fifth year of my age. The dose with which I began, and that which I take at present, I enclose ; they are taken once a day, early, in any warm liquid, such as coffee, but not in any spirituous liquors." The doses sent were, No. 1, original dose, three grains ; No. 2, present dose, twenty-three grains of pure white arsenic, in coarse powder. Dr. Arbele says this gentleman's daily dose has been weighed there also, and found as above. Mr. —— continues : "About an hour after taking my first dose (I took the same quantity daily for three months), there followed slight perspiration, with griping pains in the bowels, and after three or four hours a loose evacuation ; this was followed by a keen appetite, and a feeling of excitement. With the exception of the pain, the same symptoms follow every increase of the dose. I subjoin as a caution, that it is not advisable to begin arsenic-eating before the age of twelve, or after thirty years." In reply to my question, if any harm results from either interrupting, or altogether discontinuing the practice, he replies : " Evil consequences only ensue from a long-continued interruption. From circumstances I am often obliged to leave it off for two or three days, and I feel only slight languor and loss of appetite, and I resume taking the arsenic in somewhat smaller doses. On two occasions, at the earnest solicitations of my friends, I attempted entirely to leave off the arsenic. The second time was in January, 1855. I was induced to try it a second time, from a belief that my first illness might have arisen from some other cause. On the third day of the second week after leaving off the dose, I was attacked with faintness, depression of spirits, mental weakness, and a total loss of the little appetite I still had ; sleep also entirely deserted me. On the fourth day I had violent palpitation of the heart, accompanied by profuse perspiration. Inflammation of the lungs followed, and I was laid up for nine weeks, the same as on the first occasion of leaving off the arsenic. Had I not been bled, I should most likely have died of apoplexy. As a restorative, I resumed the arsenic-eating in smaller doses, and with a firm determination never again to be seduced into leaving it off, except as originally directed by my preceptor. The results on both occasions were precisely the same, and death would certainly have ensued had I not resumed arsenic-eating." One of the most remarkable points in this narrative is, that this gentleman *began* with a dose which we should consider poisonous. This is the only case of which I have been able to obtain such full particulars, but several others have been mentioned to me by those who knew the parties and can vouch for their truth, which I will briefly relate.

One gentleman, besides stating that he is well aware of the existence of the practice, says he is well acquainted with a brewer, in Klagenfurth, who has taken daily doses of arsenic for many years. He is now past middle life, but astonishes every one by his fresh, juvenile appearance ; he is always exhorting other people to follow his example, and says : " See how strong and fresh I am, and what an advantage I have over you all ! In times of epidemic fever or cholera, what a fright you are in, while I feel sure of never taking infection."

Dr. Arbele writes : " Mr. Curator Kursinger (I presume curator of some museum at Salzburg), notwithstanding his long professional work at Lungau and Binzgau, knew only two arsenic-eaters—one the gentleman whose case has just been related, the other the ranger of the hunting district in Grossarl, named Trauner. This man was, at the advanced age of eighty-one, still a keen chamois hunter, and an active climber of mountains ; he met his death by a fall from a mountain height, while engaged in his occupation. Mr. Kursinger says he always seemed very healthy, and every evening regularly, after remaining a little too long over his glass, he took a dose of arsenic, which enabled him to get up the next morning perfectly sober and quite bright. Professor Fenzl, of Vienna, was acquainted with this man, and made a statement before some learned society concerning him, a notice of which Mr. Kursinger saw in the *Wiener Zeitung*, but I have not been able to find the statement itself. Mr. Krum, the pharmaceutist here, tells me that there is in Sturzburg a well-known arsenic-eater, Mr. Schmid, who now takes daily twelve and sometimes fifteen grains of arsenic. He began taking arsenic from curiosity, and appears very healthy, but always becomes sickly and falls away if he attempts to leave it off. The director of the arsenic factory before alluded to is also said to be very healthy, and not to look so old as forty-five, which he really is.

As a proof how much secrecy is observed by those who practise arsenic-eating, I may mention that Dr. Arbele says he inquired of four medical men, well acquainted with the people of the districts in question, both in the towns and country, and they could not tell him of any individual case, but knew of the custom only by report.

Two criminal cases have been mentioned to me, in which the known habit of arsenic-eating was successfully pleaded in favor of the accused. The first by Dr. Kottowitz, of Neuhaus, was that of a girl taken up in that neighborhood on strong suspicion of having poisoned one or more people with arsenic, and though circumstances were strongly against her, yet the systematic arsenic-eating in the district was pleaded so successfully in her favor that she was acquitted, and still lives near Neuhaus, but is believed by every one to be guilty. The other case was mentioned by Dr. Lorenz. A woman was accused of poisoning her husband, but brought such clear proof that he was an arsenic-eater, as fully to account for arsenic being found in the body. She was, of course, acquitted.

One fact mentioned to me by some friends is well worthy of note. They say: "In this part of the world, when a graveyard is full, it is shut up for about twelve years, when all the graves which are not private property by purchase are dug up, the bones collected in the charnel-house, the ground plowed over, and burying begins again. On these occasions the bodies of arsenic-eaters are found almost unchanged, and recognizable by their friends. Many people suppose that the finding of their bodies is the origin of the story of the vampire." In the *Medicinischer Jahrbuch des Oster: Kaiserstaates*, 1822, *neuest Folge*, there is a report by Professor Schallgruber, of the Imperial Lyceum at Grätz, of an investigation undertaken by order of government in various cases of poisoning by arsenic. After giving details of six *post-mortem* examinations, he says : " The reason of the frequency of these sad cases appears to me to be the familiarity with arsenic which exists in our country, particularly the higher parts. There is hardly a district in Upper Styria where you will not find arsenic in at least one house, under the name of hydrach. They use it for the complaints of domestic animals, to kill vermin, and as a stomachic to excite an appetite. I saw one peasant show another on the point of a knife how much arsenic he took daily, without which, he said, he could not live ; the quantity I should estimate at two grains. It is said, but this I will not answer for, that in that part of the country this poison is used in making cheese; and, in fact, several cases of poisoning by cheese have occurred in Upper Styria, one not long since. The above-mentioned peasant states, I believe truly, that they buy the arsenic from the Tyrolese, who bring into the country spirits and other medicines, and so are the cause of much mischief." This report is, I believe, mentioned in Orfila's *Toxicology*, and one or two other works, but I have not seen it quoted myself ; it is interesting, as being early and official evidence of arsenic-eating. Since I received the above information, a gentleman who was studying at this hospital, told me that, when an assistant in Lincolnshire, he knew a man who began taking arsenic for some skin disease, and gradually increased the dose to five grains daily. He said he himself supplied him with this dose daily for a long time. He wrote to the medical man with whom he was assistant, and I have been for a long time promised full particulars of the case ; but beyond the fact that he took five grains of arsenic, in the form of Fowler's solution, daily, for about six years, and could never leave it off without inconvenience, and a return of his old complaint, I have as yet not received them. I have delayed publishing these facts for some time, hoping to get information on some other points, for which I have written to my friends abroad ; but as considerable delay takes place in all communications with them, I have thought it better to publish at once the information I have already received. All the parties spoken of are people on whom the fullest reliance can be placed, and who have taken much pains to ascertain the foregoing particulars. The questions which still remain unanswered are these :

1st. Can any official report be obtained of the trials of the two people mentioned by Drs. Kottowitz and Lorenz?

2d. Do medical men in these districts, when using arsenic medicinally, find the same cumulative effects as we experience here ? Or is there anything in the air or mode of living which prevents it ?

3d. Can any evidence be obtained as to how much of the arsenic taken is excreted ? To show whether the body gradually becomes capable of enduring its presence, or whether it acquires the power of throwing it off.

I have proposed to the gentleman who furnished me with the particulars of his own case, either to make an estimate of the arsenic contained in his own urine and fæces during twenty-four hours, or to collect the same and forward them to me, that I may do so; but as yet have received no answer.—*Pharmaceutical Journal. Edinburgh Medical Journal.*

Art. III.—*Absorption of Arsenic by Plants.*

Dublin, June 6, 1860.—At the last evening meeting of the Royal Dublin Society, held May 25, Dr. E. W. Davy communicated the results of some further experiments he had instituted on the subject of the absorption of arsenic by plants, both when that substance was directly applied to their roots by watering the soil with a solution of arsenious acid, as well as when different artificial manures containing that substance (as they frequently do) were used in the ordinary manner as fertilizing agents.

Dr. Davy first referred to the numerous attacks which had been made on his former experiments on this subject, which appeared in the *Pharmaceutical Journal, Gardener's Chronicle,* and other scientific periodicals. Thus, one gentleman, Mr. B. S. Kensington, of Dartmouth (see *Pharmaceutical Journal* for November, 1859), states, from his experiments, that he doubts that plants are capable of absorbing arsenic at all ; whereas, Dr. Davy not only detected the presence of that substance in plants which had been watered with a solution of arsenious acid, but in several instances determined the amount which had been taken up or absorbed. Again, Mr. Ogston, of London, in the *Pharmaceutical Journal,* for March, 1860, states that in plants which he had similarly treated, he found arsenic only in the portion of the stem close to the roots, but that in no case could he discover in the leaves, or in the stem at more than five inches from the ground.

Dr. Davy, on the other hand, detected it in the leaves, and in every portion which he examined, of the different plants which had been watered with a solution of arsenious acid ; and he accounted for Mr. Ogston's failing to detect it in the leaves, where probably it existed in a smaller quantity, by his using Marsh's method, which, as Professor Odling has recently shown, is not applicable for the detection of minute quantities of arsenic where much organic matter is present.

Again, Mr. Sibson, of the Royal Agricultural College, Cirencester, asserts in the *Gardener's Chronicle,* for September, 1859, that the occurrence of arsenic in superphosphates is rare, and its quantity when present is generally exceedingly small ; and he gives the results of some experiments which would appear to indicate the same.

Dr. Davy's experience, however, is diametrically opposed to the results of Mr. Sibson, for he found arsenic in almost every sample of superphosphate which he examined, as well as in different other artificial manures, in the preparation of which, sulphuric acid had been employed ; and, as this acid, which is used in large quantities, frequently contains, he finds, several pounds weight of arsenic in the ton of acid, the amount of that substance in superphosphate and other artificial manures, cannot be so very inconsiderable as Mr. Sibson would have us believe. Dr. Davy also noticed some interesting experiments which Mr. Horsley, of Cheltenham, had made and communicated to him, on the same subject of the absorption of arsenic by vegetables, which confirmed, in the most satisfactory manner, his former statements, and showed that plants, under different circumstances, were capable of taking up that substance ; from which he (Mr. Horsley) has come to the conclusion that arsenic applied to the roots of plants, under any form, is taken up by them, some perhaps, absorbing it more readily than others. Finally, Dr. Davy stated that he had succeeded in detecting the presence of arsenic in different crops, as for example, in turnips, mangold wurzel, etc., which had been grown with superphosphate in the ordinary way, and though the amount present was very minute, and as this manure was usually applied, it could only be very small; yet circumstances might occur in which from unequal distribution of the manure, and from other causes, plants might be placed within reach of a greater quantity of arsenicated manure, and, under these circumstances, imbibe such a quantity of arsenic as might render those vegetables unwholsome and unfit for food. He, therfore, maintained what he had before asserted, that a substance containing such a quantity of arsenic as pyritic sulphuric acid usually does, should not be used in the preparation of artificial manures which are intended to be applied as fertilizing agents to our plants which are grown for food.—*Med. Times and Gaz.*

ART. IV.—*The Reproduction of Bone.*

DURING the last two years, a series of interesting experiments has been carried on by M. Leopold Ollier, on the function of the periosteum as a producer and regenerator of osseous tissue. The subject is of some importance in a surgical as well as in a physiological point of view ; and we propose to give a full abstract of M. Ollier's papers, combining with them such other notices as we have been able to find in the Journals. The following are the sources from which we derive our information ; the principal being the essays of M. Ollier in *Journal de la Physiologie.*

1. Berruti, M. Experiments on the Transplantation of Periosteum. *Giornale delle Scienze Mediche della Reale Academia de Torino ; and Gazette Hebdomadaire,* July 1, 1859.

2. Flourens, M. On the Dura Mater or Internal Periosteum of the Skull. *Gaz. Méd. de Paris*, August 20, 1859.—On the Osteoplastic Properties of the Dura Mater, and on Cerebral Osteophytes. *Gaz. Hebd.*, September 9.

3. Larghi, Dr. Contributions to the History of Subperiosteal and Subcapsular Operations. *Gaz. Méd. de Paris*, Jan. 29, Feb. 19, May 21, July 23 and 30, Aug. 27, and Dec. 10, 1859.

4. Ollier, M. Leopold. Experimental Researches on the Artificial Production of Bone by Transplantation of Periosteum; and on the Regeneration of Bone, after complete Resection and Removal. *Journal de la Physiologie*, January and April, 1859. Experimental Researches on the Grafting of Bone. *Ibid.*, January, 1860. The same subjects. *Gazette Médicale de Paris*, April 2 and 9, 1859. Experiments on the Transplantation of the Dura Mater, showing that this Membrane may be regarded as the Internal Periosteum of the Skull. *Ibid.*, September 10, 1859, and *Gaz. Hebdomadaire*, August 12. Case of Superiosteal Resection of the Elbow-joint followed by Reproduction of the Bone. *Ibid.*, December 3, 1859, and *Gaz. Hebd.*, December 2. On the Reality of the Reproduction of Bone after Superiosteal Resection. *Gaz. Méd. de Paris*, January 28, 1860. On the Transplantation of Bones taken from Animals which have been dead some time. *Ibid.*, same date, and March 24.

5. Paravicini, M. Superiosteal Resection and Disarticulation of the Lower Jaw. *Annali Universali di Medicina;* and *Gaz. Méd. de Paris*, July 16.

6. Rouget, M. Charles. The Skeleton of Vertebrate Animals, in Relation to the Morphology of the Locomotive Apparatus.—*Jour. de la Phys.*, January, 1860.

7. Sédillot, M. On Regeneration of Joints after Resection. *Gaz. Méd. de Paris*, November 12, 1859. On Subperiosteal Resection. *Ibid.*, December, 31 ; and *Gaz. Hebd.*, Dec. 30.

Taking as a groundwork M. Ollier's papers, we find him first describing the results of his experiments on the

ARTIFICIAL PRODUCTION OF BONE BY TRANSPLANTATION OF THE PERIOSTEUM.

The experiments were performed on rabbits of various ages. A marked difference was observed in the results, according to the hygienic condition of the animals. In healthy rabbits, operated on in the country, union most frequently commenced at once, and in four or five days the secretion of ossifiable blastema could be felt through the skin. In animals, on the contrary, kept in Paris in cages or boxes, death frequently followed the operation. After operation, the animals were kept in a cage during two or three days ; after which they were allowed more freedom. A good supply of food is necessary; otherwise the work of reparation is arrested. In proof of this, M. Ollier removed the radius and the second metatarsal bone of a rabbit, and placed the animal for three weeks in a small unhealthy place, with scanty food. Although the periosteum had been preserved, reparation had scarcely commenced at the end of the time. The operation was then repeated on the opposite side; and the rabbit was placed in an airy situation, and well supplied with food. At the end of six weeks, the bones removed by the second operation were found to be more completely restored than those which had been taken away at the first. The experiments of M. Ollier are divisible into three series : 1. Those in which a slip of periosteum was partially removed, but left more or less adherent to the bone ; in these the slip was grafted among the muscles or under the skin, but still received some vessels from the bone. 2. Those in which the periosteum was separated from its final attachment to the bone from three to five days after the operation. 3. Those in which a portion of the periosteum was entirely removed at once, and transplanted to another part.

1. *Transplantation of a Flap of Periosteum, left adhering to the Bone, by one end.*—The part operated on was the tibia. An incision having been made along the crest of the bone, the muscles were carefully turned aside, so as to denude the periosteum. The part to be detached was then marked out by a scalpel, and was dissected up, leaving one end attached; it was there introduced into a channel made for it under the skin or among the muscles, and the free end was fastened by a suture, to prevent it from becoming twisted. In three or four days, in young healthy rabbits, the piece acquired a cartilaginous consistence, and sometimes became almost as thick as the tibia itself ; but, whether this was from infiltration from the surrounding tissues, or from the blastema intended for the formation of bone, it soon diminished, and gradually became more distinct and osseous. In almost all the experiments there was a small nucleus of bone developed in the end of the periosteum beyond the suture. If the flap of the periosteum escaped from the suture, it took the form of a spur, which projected more or less under the skin. In old rabbits, the result was different ; the wounds secreted a serous pus, and there was, at the end of a month or six weeks, little or no trace of ossification. This shows that, as age advances, the osteogenetic power is diminished, though not entirely abolished.

To meet the objection that periosteum merely conveyed the blastema from the bone, M. Ollier calls attention to the formation of an osseous nucleus beyond the point where the periosteum was strangled by the suture. He also, having detached a flap of periosteum, twisted it several times on itself, and fastened the end by suture, as in the other experiments ; the result was the formation, not of a perfect ring of bone, but of a circle formed of several separate movable osseous deposits, like a string of beads.

2. *Excision of the Pedicle of Communication three or four days after Operation.*—In these experiments, the ossific process continued; in one instance, the newly formed bone became reunited to the tibia, but, in another, where a large portion of the attached end was removed, the new bone was found to be joined to the tibia only by some fibrous deposit.

3. *Complete Removal of a Portion of Periosteum, and Transplantation into neighboring or distant parts.*—M. Ollier dissected a piece of periosteum from the tibia of a rabbit eleven months old, leaving it attached by a few filaments of the extensor muscle of the great toe. Six weeks afterwards, the piece had ossified, and was entirely inde-

pendent of and movable on the tibia. In other experiments, he transplanted portions of periosteum from the tibia under the skin of the groin, the back, and the popliteal space ; in these cases, also, bone was formed. The new bone was not equal in size to the removed portion of .periosteum, from the shrinking which the latter had undergone.

The osteogenetic property does not reside alike in the periosteum of all bones. M. Ollier dissected up a portion of the pericranium of a rabbit three months old,· leaving it attached .at one end, and fastened it by suture under the skin, so that the deep surface was turned outwards. At the end of six weeks, there was but very slight trace of ossification, except along the edge of the slip where it still adhered to the bone. This result is in conformity with the demonstration of Heine, that the pericranium is not of itself sufficient for the reparation of bone.

At a meeting of the Société de Biologie in July, 1859, M. Ollier exhibited some specimens bearing on the question whether the dura mater performs the functions of a periosteal membrane. He transplanted portions of the dura mater of young rabbits under the skin in various parts of other animals of the same kind ; at the end of five or six weeks, portions of bone were found to be formed. The osteogenetic property of the dura mater he found to diminish with the age of the animal ; and this, he thinks, explains why bone is so often not reproduced after the operation of trephining. Bone was not formed from the parts of the dura mater not in direct contact with the skull—the falx cerebri, for instance ; pathological ossification, however, takes place very frequently in this situation. Ossification was more abundant in portions taken from the base than from the concavity of the skull.

M. Berruti has performed some experiments, which confirm those of M. Ollier. In dogs, he has raised flaps of periosteum, leaving them attached at one end, and has laid them with their inner surface in contact with a muscle ; a plate has been formed, having all the histological characters of bone. In another instance he removed a flap of periosteum from the radius of a young dog, and fixed it to the muscle of one of the thighs of the same animal. The wound in the skin united without suppuration. On examination, after some time, the muscle was found to have a bony plate deposited on it. In another similar experiment, the transformation into bone was observed to be in progress. M. Berruti did not find any trace of cartilage in the tissue undergoing the osseous transformation.

External Characters and Structure of the Bone formed by Transplantation of Periosteum.—The heterotopic bone presents all the characters of normal bone. [M. Ollier uses the term *heterotopique* (from ἕτερος, another, and τόπος, a place) to denote development in abnormal or extraordinary situations. We retain it in an English form, as being convenient and expressive.] Externally, it is covered by periosteum ; internally, it contains medullary spaces, which unite in a tolerably large canal. At the periphery there is a layer of compact tissue. When the periosteum has been allowed to remain partly connected, the heterotopic bone contains a medullary canal perfectly distinct from that of the original bone. The canal is formed gradually, by thinning of the osseous tissue, the development of vacuoles or spaces, and the removal of the trabeculæ which separate them. Bones formed from transplanted periosteum are generally smaller than the piece of membrane, probably because of the necessity for the formation of a new vascular organization, and from the contraction of the piece of periosteum ; but they also present a tendeney to the formation of a medullary canal in their interior.

On examining thin slices of heterotopic bones under the microscope, they are found to contain osseous corpuscles, arranged in the compact substance in distinct layers round vascular or Haversian canals, not, however, so regularly as in normal bone ; but the specimens examined by M. Ollier were, it must be noticed, not more than eight or ten weeks old. The Haversian canals are generally parallel to the axis of the bone. The medullary canal contains (a) free nuclei, and small cells with a distinct round nucleus ; (b) patches of numerous nuclei, generally infiltrated with fatty granulations, and containing several nuclei analogous to the free nuclei ; (c) fat ; (d) fibro-plastic elements, and fibrils of connective tissues ; (e) bloodvessels. The vessels enter through one or more nutritive foramina.

The heterotopic bone frequently presents a longitudinal groove on the whole length of one of its surfaces. It is always observed on the side where the edges have been turned on themselves, towards the internal surface of the periosteum, and indicates an inequality in the secretion of the blastema. The furrow is generally noticed, also, on bones reproduced after subperiosteal resection ; it here corresponds to the incision in the membrane, through which the bone has been removed.

At their commencement, at least, the heterotopic bone is more or less adherent to the neighbouring parts ; the external surface of the periosteum is less distinct from the surrounding cellular tissue than the periosteum of normal bone. When developed round the leg, the bone adheres to the sheaths of the muscles, so as to impede the action of these organs. At first, the tendons also are more or less completely fixed to the bone ; but gradually motion is allowed, by means of a loose cellular tissue, which would, perhaps, at last form a serous bursa.

Mode of Development of Heterotopic Bones.—From the first there is an effusion of lymph, at first serous, afterwards more consistent, infiltrating the slip of periosteum and the adjacent tissues. The periosteum then becomes turgescent, and its capillaries are filled with blood ; on its internal face there is produced an exudation, which at first sight resembles that furnished by the external surface and the neighboring tissues, but which is soon distinguishable by its greater density; it goes on increasing, while the other becomes absorbed. In four or five days, or thereabouts, there is an accumulation of transparent or slightly yellowish-gray firm matter under the periosteum, or rather in it (for the edges are glued together so as to form a complete sheath). This blastema is chondroid rather than cartilaginous. At about the seventh or eighth day, the deposition of earthy matter commences. It is not necessarily preceded by true cartilage ; but sometimes there is a hard elastic substance, having the external characters of this tissue. Ossification commences at the center, and advances rapidly to the periphery ; and, when the whole mass is permeated, the process goes on while the periosteum deposits new layers of blastema. Although the deposit of earthy matter is general, the bone remains flexible for some time, and might be considered as still cartilaginous until laid bare and examined, when it is found to be friable and finely granular. It gradually acquires the appearance and consistence of normal bone. The process here described indicates that the production of heterotopic bone is not necessarily preceded by the formation of cartilage ; and this might be expected, inasmuch as cartilage is not normally formed under the periosteum.

By scraping the internal face of the periosteum at the commencement, a layer of blastema is detached. On placing this under the microscope, it is found to consist of a large number of nuclei, and of cells analogous to those which are found in the embryonic tissues. The free nuclei, which form the predominant element, lie in the midst of a more or less granular amorphous substance. Here and there some fusiform cells are found, as well as very fine fibres—the latter being more apparent if some force has been used in scraping the periosteum. There are also cells, some with one nucleus, others larger, with several nuclei. These large cells are often very regular in outline. The younger the animal, the more abundant is the blastema. In this blastema, the process of ossification goes on, in the same manner as has been described, with regard to the formation of normal bone beneath the periosteum, by Virchow, Sharpey, Kölliker, Robin, and Rouget.

When cartilage is met with, it is rare to find cavities containing many cells ; and there is nowhere the regular arrangement observed in ossific cartilage.

Do the heterotopic bones continue to increase in size ? M. Ollier observes that, to answer this question, a period of several years would be required ; but, in the meantime, reasoning from analogy, it is fair to infer that they would at least increase in thickness, like normal bones, since the periosteum exists in both cases.

Nature of the process which takes place on the Internal Surface of the Periosteum—Immediate Origin of the New Bone.—If, after detaching a portion of the periosteum, one-half of it is gently scraped on the internal surface, the osseous tissue will be formed from the part only which has not been so treated. M. Ollier dissected up a flap of periosteum, leaving it attached at one end, and scraped the part nearest to its attachment to the bone. At the end of ten days this portion was merely fibrous, although traversed by numerous vessels; the part which had not been scraped presented a partly ossified deposit. Hence he concludes that neither vessels nor the external part of the periosteum are sufficient for the production of bone. The production of bone may also be prevented by touching the internal surface of the periosteum with a caustic.

In order to determine more closely the action of the sub-periosteal blastema, M. Ollier proceeded to transplant it alone to distant parts. Having gently scraped some from a flap of periosteum, he inserted it under the skin of the axilla of one animal. In a week there were found small masses of a yellowish substance, having the external appearance of fat, but which, under the microscope, were found to contain nuclei of sub-periosteal blastema, mixed with fragments of a granular fibroid substance, in which the presence of carbonate of lime was detected by hydrochloric acid. These masses, when treated with acid, presented elongated nuclei with more or less irregular outline.

M. Ollier makes some comments on the doctrines advanced a century ago by Duhamel, with reference to the function of the periosteum in the formation of bone. At first Duhamel regarded the bone as increased by the ossification of layers of the periosteum ; but he subsequently modified this view; and, in 1757, he thus expressed the analogy between the formation of wood and that of bone : " Wood increases by the addition of fine layers deposited between the wood and the bark. Bones increase in size by the formation of layers between the periosteum and the bone." He could not, M. Ollier observes, be more explicit at a period when the knowledge of the production of tissues was very imperfect.

Transplantation of Periosteum after Death.—In his experiments, M. Ollier took care to operate rapidly, lest the properties of the periosteum should be destroyed by the least amount of cooling and desiccation. He finds, however, that, though rapidity in operation is most important to the production of regular and abundant ossification, the osteogenetic property is not at once lost. In January, 1859, he transplanted a piece of periosteum, which had lain on his table seven or eight minutes, and had been washed with cold water; it became adherent, and granules of bone were formed in it. In other cases he has succeeded with pieces which had been removed from fifteen to twenty minutes ; and, in periosteum removed from animals even as late as an hour and a half after death, the osteogenetic property was not entirely lost. He believes, moreover, that this limit may be carried still further under favorable conditions of temperature, etc., and according to the mode of death.

Transplantation of the Periosteum of an Animal to another of a Different Species.—In the experiments already referred to, the periosteum was transplanted to animals of the same species ; but M. Ollier has further tried the effects of introducing portions of periosteum under the skin of animals of different species from those from which the membrane was taken. He has thus experimented on the dog, cat, rabbit, guinea-pig, calf, goat, sheep, and hen, with the following general results : 1. The flap transplanted is entirely absorbed in a longer or shorter time. At first the wound heals ; and for some time a small hard nucleus is felt, which, however, gradually diminishes and disappears, so that no trace can be found on *post-mortem* examination. 2. The flap sloughs, and is thrown off by suppuration ; this result was most frequently observed in rabbits on which periosteum from the dog had been engrafted. 3. The flap becomes encysted, without suppuration. At first the experiment appears to have succeeded ; the flap is retained in its place by plastic lymph ; but this lymph soon becomes organized into a cyst, and the periosteum undergoes fatty change. Sometimes the cyst contains thickened pus. This latter result was observed chiefly in rabbits ; the former in experiments with the combs of cocks. 4. The periosteum becomes adherent to the neighboring tissues ; vessels are formed in it, and it continues to live, as a fibrous membrane ; but no bone is produced. This was observed several times in cases where periosteum was transplanted from the dog to the rabbit, and from the rabbit to the hen. 5. The periosteum not only forms a fibrovascular adhesion to the neighboring tissues, but produces osseous tissue. This result, however, is very rare, even in animals of closely allied species.

Modifications which Bone undergoes when denuded ; Regeneration of the Periosteum.—It has long been known that a bone deprived of periosteum is not of necessity condemned to necrosis. Tenon proved this by experiment ; and Macdonald, in 1799, showed that periosteum was reproduced after being destroyed. At a later period this opinion has been supported by Cruveilhier and Flourens. In none of his experiments has M. Ollier observed a sequestrum at the part where the bone has been denuded. Immediate union takes place, or the wound suppurates.

In the first case the following phenomena are observed : In a short time after the bone is denuded it becomes covered by a thin, soft, transparent layer, which soon becomes distinct from the effused plastic lymph. Towards the eighth day it resembles a coat of varnish spread over the bone. It unites with the edges of the old periosteum. At first it is without vessels ; but, three or four days later, these appear at the edges, being furnished by the periosteum ; and in the center, where they are supplied by the bone. The old periosteum is puffed up and thickened all around ; and small tufts of vessels are seen advancing from the circumference to the center of the denuded portion, so as to cover the varnish-like layer of blastema. In the meantime cellular and fibrous elements are developed, and form a fibrous membrane analogous to periosteum.

To ascertain whether the new membrane thus formed is really periosteum, M. Ollier, in two instances, removed and transplanted it ; but the experiment failed, probably from being performed at too early a stage (three weeks). He subsequently performed other experiments, taking care to allow six or seven weeks for the formation of the new periosteum. In an instance related in the *Journal de la Physiologie* for July, 1859, he removed the newly-formed periosteum forty-three days after the first operation ; it was thicker than the normal membrane, and was easily isolated. He then inserted it among the muscles of the leg ; and, at the end of twelve days, bone was found to be formed. Periosteum was again commencing to be formed in the bone which had been thus twice denuded.

M. Ollier differs from the opinion of M. Flourens, that the periosteum is capable of being reproduced indefinitely. He allows that periosteum may be removed and reproduced again and again ; but this, he says, can occur only when the bone which it covered has not also been taken away.

Bone, when denuded, becomes slightly roughened while the new periosteum is being formed ; it loses its whiteness, and becomes reddish, and presents punctiform vascularity on its surface.   When, however, the new periosteum is formed, the bone continues to grow regularly ; and in rabbits, at the end of two months it has regained its normal appearance.

When the wound is the seat of prolonged suppuration, the bone remains denuded for several days ; then fleshy granulations appear on its surface, and the superficial layer is gradually absorbed. When cicatrization is perfect, the surface of the bone is unequal ; round the denuded part, at the limits of the old periosteum, there are projections, sometimes large; while more or less deep depressions are seen in the part which has been the seat of exfoliation. These inequalities tend to disappear gradually.   While this work is going on, the bone is covered with a fibrous layer ; but this new membrane is always more or less confounded with the cicatrix outside it, so that it is not certain whether it is a true periosteum.— *British Medical Journal.*

ART. V.—*Practical Observations upon the Nature and Treatment of Prostatorrhœa.*   Read before the Medical Society of the State of Pennsylvania, in June, 1860 : By S. D. GROSS, M. D., Professor of Surgery in the Jefferson Medical College of Philadelphia.

THE disease which I am about to describe has not, so far as is known to me, received any attention either from specialists or from the authors of general treatises on surgery.   The term by which it is here designated appears, it is true, in M. Nélaton's *"Elémens de Pathologie Chirurgicale,"* but altogether in an incidental manner, and evidently without any definite idea on the part of that distinguished writer as to the true nature of the affection in question.

Prostatorrhœa is, as the term implies, a discharge from the prostate gland, generally of a thin mucous character, dependent upon irritation, if not actual inflammation, of the component tissues of that organ.   The reason why the disease has not hitherto received any specific name or place in surgical nomenclature, is simply because it has always been confounded with other lesions, as gleet, or chronic urethritis, seminal losses, and cystorrhœa, or chronic inflammation of the mucous membrane of the bladder; from which, in fact, it is often difficult to distinguish it.   As for myself, I have long been familiar with the affection, and latterly have described it in my lectures at the college.

I have not met with prostatorrhœa in children or very young subjects, probably because all kinds of diseases of the prostate are so very rare at that period of life. That it may occur, however, even at a very tender age, is altogether likely, especially in children laboring under stone in the bladder, prolapse of the bowel, or worms in the rectum, causing the organ to suffer from reflected irritation. After the twentieth year the disease is sufficiently common, and instances are occasionally met with even in very old persons. As long as the prostate gland remains small and inactive, or is not brought fully under the influence of the sexual organs, with which it is so intimately associated, it is comparatively infrequent.

I am not able to say, from my experience, what classes of persons are most liable to suffer from this affection ; but it has seemed to me that it is most frequent in those of a sanguineo-nervous temperament, with strong sexual propensities, leading to the frequent indulgence of the venereal appetite, if not to positive venereal excesses, either in the natural manner or by masturbation. An irritation would thus seem to be established in the prostate gland, attended with more or less discharge of its peculiar secretion, either in a normal or abnormal state. Single and married men are, apparently, equally prone to it. Once established, it is probable that certain occupations may serve to keep it up; and it is also likely that there are certain employments which may predispose to it, although it would require a much longer experience than what is possessed by any one individual to point them out in a definite or satisfactory manner. Intemperance in eating and drinking, frequent horseback exercise, sexual abuse, and disease of the bladder, anus, and rectum, may all be regarded as contributing to such a result.

The exciting *causes* of prostatorrhœa are not always very evident. In most of the cases that have fallen under my observation, the affection was traceable, either directly or indirectly, to venereal excesses, chronic inflammation of the neck of the bladder, stricture of the urethra, or disease of some kind or other of this canal. In some cases it has its origin in disorder of the lower bowel, as hemorrhoids, prolapse, fissure, fistule, ascarides, or the lodgment of some foreign body. It is easy to conceive how reflected irritation might induce this disease. The connection between the prostate gland and ano-rectal region is very close and intimate, and, hence, whatever affects the one will almost be sure, in time, to implicate the other, either in consequence of proximity of structure, or as an effect of the laws of sympathy. However this may be, no judicious surgeon ever omits to examine these parts most thoroughly in the event of any serious disease of any of them, before he attempts a course of treatment. Temporary prostatorrhœa is occasionally excited by the exhibition of internal remedies, as drastic cathartics, cantharides, and spirits of turpentine; or, in short, whatever has a tendency to invite a preternatural afflux of blood to the prostate gland and neck of the bladder, or to the posterior portion of the urethra. Another cause of the disease, and, according to my experience, a very common one, especially in young men, is masturbation or self-pollution. Many of the most obstinate and perplexing cases of it that have come under my notice were the direct result of this detestable practice.

The *symptoms* of prostatorrhœa are sufficiently characteristic. The most prominent, as already stated, is a discharge of mucus, generally perfectly clear and transparent, more or less ropy, and of varying quantity, from a few drops to a drachm and upwards, in the twenty-four hours. It is seldom that it is puriform, and still more rare that it is purulent. When considerable, the flow keeps up almost a constant moisture at the orifice of the urethra, and may even make a decided impression upon the patient's linen, leaving it wet and stained, somewhat in the same manner as in gleet or gonorrhœa, though in a much less marked degree. The most copious evacuations of this kind generally occur while the patient is at the water-closet, engaged in straining, especially if the bowels are constipated, or the fæcal matter is uncommonly hard, or greatly distends the rectum, so as to exert an unusual amount of pressure upon the prostate gland.

The discharge, whether small or large, is often attended with a peculiar tickling sensation, referred by the patient to the prostate gland, from which it frequently extends along the whole length of the urethra, and even to the head of the penis. In some cases, indeed in many, the feeling is of a lascivious, voluptuous, or pleasurable nature, not unlike that which accompanies the earlier stages of sexual intercourse. Not a few patients experience what they call a "dropping sensation," as if the fluid fell from the prostate gland into the urethra. Other anomalous symptoms often present themselves, such as a feeling of weight and fatigue in the region of the prostate, the anus and rectum, or along the perineum, with, perhaps, more or less uneasiness in voiding urine, and a frequent desire to empty the bladder; some patients are troubled with morbid erections, and their sleep is interrupted with lascivious dreams.

It is astonishing how much the patient's mind often suffers in this affection. The discharge, even if ever so insignificant, occasions him the greatest possible disquietude; for at one time he imagines that it is a source of much bodily debility, or that it is productive of weakness and soreness in the dorso-lumbar region, especially if these symptoms happen to coëxist ; at another, that he is about to become impotent, under the delusive idea that the flow is one of a seminal character; an idea which not unfrequently haunts him day and night, and from which hardly anything can, perhaps, even temporarily divert his attention. His mind, in short, is poisoned, and the consequence is that he is incessantly engaged in trying to obtain relief, running from one practitioner to another, distrusting all, and affording none an opportunity of doing him any good. In the worst forms of the affection, his business habits are destroyed, he becomes morose and dyspeptic, and he literally spends his time in watching for the discharge which is the source and cause of his terrible suffering.

The affections with which prostatorrhœa may be confounded are the various forms of urethritis, especially gleet or gonorrhœa, discharges of semen, and chronic inflammation of the bladder.

From urethritis, whether common or specific, it is generally easily distinguished by the history of the case, the nature of the discharge, and the attendant local phenomena. In most cases the affection comes on gradually, not suddenly, as in gonorrhœa or simple inflammation, and without impure connection ; the discharge is white or grayish, translucent, and ropy, not purulent, opaque, and yellowish; and there is ordinarily no burning or scalding in micturition. Moreover, there is seldom any evidence of inflammation in the urethra or penis. In gleet or chronic urethritis the signs of distinction are sometimes more difficult ; but even here a satisfactory conclusion may generally be reached by a careful consideration of the history of the case, and a proper examination of the discharge, which is nearly always more or less puriform, as well as more abundant than in prostatorrhœa. When the discharge of the urethra is kept up by the presence of a stricture, the diagnosis can be determined only by a thorough exploration with the bougie.

Very many patients confound this discharge with a flow of semen; an idea in which they are often encouraged by their attendants, in consequence of their ignorance of the nature of the affection. Much has been said and written respecting diurnal spermatic emissions ; but, according to my experience, these evacuations are among the rarest occurrences met with in practice. We are often told that they take place at the water-closet, during efforts at straining, and this is, no doubt, occasionally the case; but more commonly it will be found that these discharges are of a strictly prostatic character, the fluid being forced out of its appropriate receptacles into the urethra, along which it is presently discharged. This delusion will be more likely to take hold of the mind if the escape of the fluid be accompanied by a sort of pleasurable sensation, somewhat similar to that which follows a feeble emission. Persons affected with prostatorrhœa will often tell us that they have quite a number of such evacuations—perhaps as many as six or eight—during the twenty-four hours, especially if they are troubled with disease of the ano-rectal region, leading to frequent visits to the water-closet, or if they are much in female society, engaged in exciting reading, or addicted to the pleasures of the table, or to inordinate sexual intercourse, eventuating in general and local debility. Should the history of the case fail to afford the requisite light, it may be promptly supplied by a microscopic examination of the suspected fluid, semen always revealing distinct spermatozoa, whereas the prostatic and urethral secretions never afford any such indications. This will be the case whether the discharge be taken fresh from the orifice of the urethra or from the stiffened spots left upon the patient's linen.

The characteristic symptom of cystorrhœa, or chronic inflammation of the bladder, is an inordinate secretion of mucus, associated, in nearly all cases, with an altered condition of the urine, frequent and difficult micturition, pain in the region of the affected organ, as well as in the surrounding parts, and more or less constitutional disturbance. In prostatorrhœa there may also be more or less uneasiness low down in the pelvis, with trouble in voiding urine, especially where the prostate is much enlarged, so as to cause constant vesical irritation ; but the two disorders are so widely different as to render it impossible to confound them.

The *pathology* of this affection consists in some disorder of the prostate gland, especially of its follicular apparatus, leading to an inordinate secretion of its peculiar fluid, and to a discharge of this fluid along the urethra, at longer or shorter intervals, and in greater or less quantity. That this disorder is, at times, of a real inflammatory nature, would seem extremely probable from the character of the concomitant phenomena, and also from the fact that this organ is frequently, if, indeed, not generally, found to be more or less enlarged and indurated. Nevertheless, there are cases, and these are by no means uncommon, in which it is, to all appearance, either entirely healthy, or so nearly so as to render it impracticable, by the most careful exploration, to discover any departure from the normal standard. The discharge under such circumstances seems to be the result solely of a heightened functional activity, probably connected with, if not directly dependent upon, disorder of the seminal vesicles, the urethra, neck of the bladder, or recto-anal structures; in other words, upon reflected irritation, or, as our professional forefathers would have denominated it, sympathetic disturbance.

The *prognosis* of the prostatorrhœa is generally favorable; for it does not, in itself, present anything grave, being, as just stated, not a disease, but merely a symptom of a disease, usually slight, and, therefore, easily removable. Its obstinacy, however, is often very great, and hence the surgeon should always be guarded in the expression of his opinion respecting a rapid cure. When the mind deeply sympathizes with the local affection, as is so frequently the case, especially in young men of a nervous, irritable temperament, there is no disease which, according to my experience, is more difficult of management, or more likely to result in vexation and disappointment.

In the *treatment* of this affection, one of the first and most important objects is to inquire into the nature of the exciting cause, and, if possible, to remove it. To set about it in any other way would be the climax of absurdity; for here, as everywhere else, our therapeutic measures must be based upon a rational pathology, or a full appreciation of the nature and seat of the disease. The points which should more especially claim attention are; first, the condition of the prostate and its associate organs, and, secondly, the habits and state of health of the patient.

The first of these indications is best fulfilled by a thorough exploration of the genito-urinary apparatus and of the anus and rectum. For this purpose a catheter is employed, with a view of ascertaining the condition of the urethra, the prostate, and the bladder, aided by the finger in the bowel, previously emptied by an enema. In this manner the surgeon becomes at once apprised of the existence or non-existence of stricture of the urethra, and of the presence or absence of morbid sensibility of its mucous membrane; the size and consistence of the prostate, and the state of the urinary reservoir, particularly as to whether there is inflammation, stone, hypertrophy, or other lesion. The finger in the rectum will be of great service, not only in detecting disease in the prostate and bladder, but also in this tube itself and in the anus. Indeed, without this aid no ex-

ploration of these organs could be at all satisfactory. If disease of
the seminal vesicles exist, it will usually be evinced by tenderness
on pressure through the wall of the bowel, provided the finger is
sufficiently long or the prostate is not too voluminous.

The habits of the patient should be particularly inquired into. In
many of this class of persons they are decidedly lascivious, or marked
by excessive sexual indulgence, either naturally or in the form of
masturbation, the prostate gland, seminal vesicles and adjoining
structures being thus kept in a state of continual excitement, highly
favorable to the production of prostatorrhœa. The nature of the
patient's diet, his temperament, the state of his health, and his mode
of life as it regards sleep and exercise, both of mind and body, also
deserve special consideration.

Having ascertained the above facts, or, in other words, having
made himself perfectly familiar with the local and general condition
of the patient, the surgeon will be able, in most cases, to institute
something like a rational mode of treatment. This should be directed, as a general rule, partly to the system at large, partly to the
suffering structures.

In many of the cases the patient is weak, or deficient in muscular
and digestive power, indicating a necessity for tonics, as iron and
quinine, a nutritious diet, with a glass of generous wine, and gentle
exercise in the open air, either on foot or in an easy carriage ; riding
on horseback being scrupulously avoided as likely to keep up undue
excitement in the parts.   One of the best preparations of iron is the
tincture of the chloride, in union with tincture of nux vomica, in the
proportion of twenty drops of the former to ten of the latter, four
times a day. If the patient be plethoric, he may use with great advantage small doses of tartar emetic in the form of the antimonial
and saline mixture, care being taken not to nauseate.   In either case
it is of paramount importance to correct the secretions and to maintain a soluble condition of the bowels. Drastic purgatives are of
course avoided, as they would only tend to perpetuate the mischief.
Unless the patient is actually debilitated, he should rigorously ab-
stain from condiments and high-seasoned dishes.

Among the more important topical remedies are, first, moderate
sexual indulgence, as a means of allaying undue excitement of the
prostate and its associate organs ; secondly, cooling and anodyne
injections, or weak solutions of nitrate of silver and laudanum, or,
what I generally prefer, Goulard's extract with wine of opium, in the
proportion of from one to two drachms of each to ten ounces of
water, thrown up forcibly with a large syringe three times a day,
and retained three or four minutes in the passage. In obstinate
cases, cauterization of the prostatic portion of the urethra, or even
of the entire length of this tube, may be necessary, the operation
being repeated once a week. The cold hip-bath should be used twice
in the twenty-four hours ; the lower bowel should be kept cool and
empty; and if the disease do not gradually yield, leeches should be
applied to the perineum and around the anus.

Such, in a few words, is a brief outline of the treatment which I
have found most efficacious in this affection. Whatever plan may be

employed, perseverance and an occasional change of prescription are indispensable to success. When there is deep mental involvement, hardly anything will effect a cure; or, more correctly speaking, it is almost impossible to induce the patient to believe that he is well, or that nothing serious is the matter with him. Under such circumstances our chief dependence must be upon traveling and an entire change of scene and occupation. If the patient be single, matrimony should be enjoined.—*The North American Medico-Chirurgical Review*, July, 1860.

ART. VI.—*Experimental Pathology :* By M. CLAUDE BERNARD, Member of the French Institute ; Professor of General Physiology at the Faculty of Sciences.

IN examining the various tissues which enter into the composition of the living frame, it is easily ascertained that peculiar and distinct properties are separately enjoyed by each of them ; and that, in this manner, they are enabled to fulfill the various functions which devolve upon them. At the same time we discover that certain general systems exist, which by their distribution are brought into constant communication with all the various elementary tissues of the body; you have already named the vascular and nervous systems. The blood, as you are well aware, is brought through the capillaries to every part of the body, and its presence being indispensable to the physiological existence of all living tissues, they rapidly perish when accidentally deprived of this all important and vivifying fluid. The blood, therefore, must be looked upon as the medium in which all our tissues have their being ; it brings them in contact with an immense number of substances, derived from various sources, some of them drawn from the atmosphere through the process of respiration, others contained in the animal's food, and assimilated by the digestive organs ; others again introduced into the economy through various absorbent surfaces, and all of them equally necessary to the continuance of the physiological conditions of life.

Such, however, are not the only bodies which the circulating fluid brings into contact with the primitive elements of which our organs are composed ; the blood is, at the same time, the vehicle through which medicinal agents, intended to modify their properties, are conveyed into living tissues, and penetrate into their substance. We must, in consequence, consider medicines as physiological agents of an unusual nature ; introduced into the system through the same channel as the bodies with which it is naturally supplied, they reveal their presence exactly in the same manner, viz.: by giving birth to a series of phenomena peculiar to each substance, and widely different from those which exist in the physiological state. But another question now presents itself ; *how* are these foreign substances enabled to act upon our tissues ? Not through their physico-chemical properties, as has been sufficiently proved in our last lecture ; a *physiological* property must therefore be had recourse to, as in the case of all the powers which support life. When oxygen, for instance, is brought into contact with elementary, nervous, or muscular fibres, it quickens their activity, and keeps alive all their properties within them; and, when deprived of so powerful a stimulus, both nervous and muscular fibres quickly die. Similar actions are, no doubt, in their intimate essence, of a physical or chemical nature; but in the present state of our knowledge, the observer can only point to a physiological agency.

Histological elements, as we have already shown, are in every case endowed with special properties ; and the wider is the difference which separates one tissue from another, the higher is the animal's rank in the scale; in the nobler species peculiar organs are adapted to each individual function ; and in no other animal is their number so great as in man. We are, therefore, justified in supposing that the primitive muscular fibre, for instance, is widely different in every respect, from the nervous filament and the glandular cell ; and, in consequence, that agents entirely powerless as regards all other tissues, may be found to exercise, over the muscles, an almost unbounded influence.

Among the innumerable agents which possess the power of destroying life, there exist an immense number, which the medical philosopher cannot, by any means, consider as diseases ; no one, for instance, would think for a moment of giving that name to the bullet which slays the soldier in the battle, or the thunderbolt which strikes the ploughman dead in the fields ; the same, of course, might be said of all the various causes of violent death; now, reasoning by analogy, might we not place a large number of so-called diseases in the same class ? A tumor which, by its situation, compresses the windpipe, and gradually increasing in size, superinduces suffocation at last ; a stricture of the œsophagus, which prevents the passage of food into the stomach, and ultimately starves the patient to death ; are not these mechanical obstructions, which, acting as impediments to some of the more important functions of life, gradually bring on death, by a slow, but inevitable process? It would, of course, be superfluous to adduce other instances to the same purpose, but we are supported by the authority of Professors Trousseau and Pidoux, in assimilating to such cases those valvular affections of the heart, which, by constantly opposing the natural course of the blood, sooner or later produce a complete stasis of the circulation.

The word disease, must, therefore, be understood to signify disorders of a more extensive nature, the existence of which is revealed by phenomena of an entirely general character. Such, however, are frequently the results of local affections ; the fact is established by daily experience ; and we need only allude to the well known effects of wounds and sores, in order to convince you that local causes frequently become the starting point of general diseases. The results of our physiological experiments are, in this respect, perfectly in accordance with clinical observation ; let, for instance, a poison be introduced under an animal's skin ; its action, during the first few moments is entirely confined to a single point, but within a given space of time, its effects are felt throughout the living frame ; in what manner can similar facts be best explained ? Such is the problem, the solution of which we are about to seek ; the difficulty, as you perceive, has been distinctly stated.

That poisonous substances cannot act upon the tissues which compose the body, without having previously been absorbed, is perfectly clear ; but when, under their influence, general phenomena are produced, the vessels or nerves must evidently have been called into play; the vascular and nervous systems alone, as you are well aware, are distributed throughout the body in one unbroken chain ; and physiology, in this case, abundantly confirms the inferences drawn from our knowledge of anatomy.   The well known experiments of Magendie have shown that after injecting into the arteries of a limb any given toxic substance, its ordinary effects may be indefinitely suspended, by tying the veins which connect the diseased part with the remainder of the economy.   The animal's life might, in this manner, be almost indefinitely prolonged ; but as soon as the vessels are untied, the poison flows into the torrent of circulation, and gives rise, as usual, to a series of phenomena which end in death. The fact is well known to the inhabitants of tropical countries, who, when bitten by venemous serpents, immediately apply a close ligature over the limb, in order to prevent the passage of the venom into the blood until proper remedies have been applied.

But the vessels which convey into the depth of our tissues both poisonous substances and the ordinary elements of nutrition, belong, as you are perfectly aware, to the arterial system ; on the other hand, all foreign bodies which pass into the blood through the process of absorption, are conveyed into the arterial circulation by the veins; we thus discover that when general symptoms have been produced in this manner, the two great divisions of the vascular system have both been called into play.   It sometimes occurs, however, that the noxious principle which circulates in the veins is eliminated during its passage; such, for instance, is the case with sulphuretted hydrogen, one of the most dangerous substances we are acquainted with ; when injected into the veins, it escapes from the lungs, and is, in this manner, prevented from passing into the arterial current ; and the animal, in consequence, does not experience the slightest injury from the operation, the poison having been expelled before it could reach the tissues, which its contact would have disorganized.   The venous, or absorbent system, is, therefore, that part of the vascular network which contributes to the production of general phenomena, when deleterious agents are introduced into the economy; nor do the arteries begin to play their part before the veins have accomplished theirs.   But, as we have just stated, the poison is sometimes expelled before reaching the left side of the heart ; and this elimination takes place on various points ; but the pulmonary apparatus is the ordinary seat of the process.   For this very reason the inner coat of the lungs is, perhaps, the most powerful of all absorbent surfaces ; and poisons, when directly brought to bear upon it, produce a more instantaneous effect than when deposited upon any other point ; introduced, as it were, into the very center of the arterial system, they pass at once into the circulation without any possibility of being expelled. Thus sulphuretted hydrogen, when introduced into the lungs, extinguishes life within a few seconds ; while the same gas exists, to a considerable amount, in various parts of the intestinal tube, and even circulates in the veins, without producing the 'slightest inconvenience. It must, of course, be understood that the presence of poisons within the animal economy is perfectly inocuous as long as they are not collected together in sufficiently large quantities at a given moment. Small doses of the most dangerous substances may be successively poured into the vessels, at distant intervals, with perfect impunity. In estimating the noxious power of toxic bodies, the amount actually contained within the blood must alone be taken into consideration.— *Medical Times and Gazette.*

ART. VII.—*Investigation of Trichina Spiralis :* By R. LEUCKART. ·

PROFESSOR LEUCKART has communicated the following results of his investigation of trichina spiralis to the Royal Academy of Sciences of Göttingen :

1. Trichina spiralis is the young state of a hitherto unknown, small, nematode worm (of 1.5–2.8 mill. in length), for which the generic name of trichina must be retained.

` 2. It inhabits the intestinal canal of numerous warm-blooded animals, not only mammalia (dogs, cats, pigs, sheep, rabbits, and mice; also, undoubtedly, man), but also birds (the common fowl), and, indeed, always in large quantity.

3. The intestinal trichina attains its full sexual maturity as early as two days after its immigration.

4. The eggs of the female are developed in the vagina into minute filaria-like embryos, which are extruded without egg-shells (from the sixth day onwards).

5. The new-born young immediately set about their migration. They penetrate the wall of the intestine, and pass through the cavity of the abdomen directly into the muscular envelope of their host.

6. The course upon which they advance is indicated beforehand by the intermuscular masses of cellular tissue.

7. The majority of the migrating embryos remain in the groups of muscles immediately enclosing the cavity of the body (the abdominal and thoracic cavities), especially the smaller ones, and those containing most cellular tissue.

8. The embryos penetrate into the interior of the individual muscular fasciculi, and here attain, within fourteen days, the size and organization of the well-known trichina spiralis.

9. The infected muscular fasciculus loses its previous structure immediately after the penetration, the fibrillæ becoming broken up into a finely granular substance, and the muscular' corpuscles acquiring the form of oval nucleated cells.

10. Up to the full development of the trichina spiralis, the infected muscular fasciculus still retains its original tubular form ; whilst subsequently its sarcolemma thickens and it becomes gradually shriveled from the extremities.

11. The spot occupied by the parasite persists, in the form of a spindle-shaped enlargement, in which the well-known lemon-shaped or globular calcareous shell is afterwards deposited (although only after a long time).

12. The migration and development of the embryos take place also after the transference of pregnant trichinæ into the intestine of another (suitable) host.

13. The further development of the trichina spiralis into the sexually mature animal is quite independent of the formation of this calcareous shell, and takes place as soon as the young state is fully developed.

14. The male and female individuals are distinguishable even in the young state (trichina spiralis).

15. The immigration of the brood of trichina in large quantities causes very serious symptoms ; namely: peritonitis, in consequence of the penetration of the wall of the intestine by the embryos; and lameness, in consequence of the destruction of the infected muscular fasciculi.

16. Feeding upon flesh containing trichinæ is also followed by more or less dangerous symptoms, according to the quantity of the imported parasites; namely: an enteritis, often causing death, accompanied by bloody *(crupòser)* exudations, which are sometimes thrown down in ragged clots and evacuated (rabbit), and sometimes converted into psorospermia (dog), or pus-corpuscles (cat, mouse).—*Göttinger Nachrichten*, April 30, 1860, p. 135. *The Annals and Magazine Natural History*, June, 1860.

BERLIN, May 16, 1860. ·

The microscopical preparation which I have the pleasure to forward to you, has not only a serious pathological importance, but, I may venture to say, with regard to the discovery of the new and alarming disease it tends to illustrate, is invested with a truly historical interest. It is a minute portion of the pectoral muscle of a rabbit, which died under symptoms of progressive muscular paralysis, after being fed with the flesh of another animal of the same species, which died under similar symptoms from the same cause ; for it likewise had been fed with a piece of muscle taken from a rabbit which had perished from the immigration of myriads of trichinæ into its muscular system, about a month after a piece of human muscle, in which a number of these parasites were imbedded, had

been introduced into its stomach. The piece of human muscle, however, was taken from the body of the first patient whose death was
ascertained to have been due to trichinatous disease.

From the remarks made by Professor Virchow in the opening lecture of his most excellent course of pathological demonstrations for
the present session, and from a series of papers by that eminent
pathologist, and by Professor Zenker, of Dresden, I have compiled
the following sketch, which will serve to illustrate for the information of your readers the salient points of this most important
subject.

Trichina spiralis, known formerly only in a capsulated state, was
considered more as a zoölogical curiosity than as a subject of pathological interest. No symptoms were known to betray its presence ;
and it was, perhaps, more frequently discovered in the dissecting-
room of the students than at the post-mortems conducted by the
pathologist. Since its discovery by Owen, numerous conjectures
have been formed relative to the nature, origin, and propagation of
this singular parasite. Herbst believed it to be identical with
filaria, Meissner and Davaine regarded it as a larva of trichosoma,
and Küchenmeister considered it to represent an undeveloped, juvenile stage of tricocephalus dispar. The latter idea seemed to be
confirmed by some experiments of Leuckart, who found trichinæ in
the muscles of an animal fed with tricocephali ; these experiments
could, however, not be considered as conclusive, as the examination
of the muscles before the experiment was commenced had been
neglected. Herbst was the first to institute feeding experiments
with trichinatous muscles. He found trichinæ in the muscles of the
animals experimented upon ; but the connective links between the
parasites introduced into the stomach and those found in the muscles
being deficient, no perfect light was thrown on the subject by these
observations. The first experiments of Virchow, instituted last
summer, tended materially to supply these deficiencies. In the
intestinal canal of an animal fed with trichinatous muscle, he found
the villi crowded with psorospermia; and free in the intestinal mucus
numerous thread-like worms, of the form of trichinæ, of both sexes,
the sexual utricle of the male filled with sperm-cells, that of
the female densely stocked with ovules. Trichinæ were thus proved
to be bi-sexual. Their non-identity with tricocephali was also placed
beyond doubt. The numerous points still requiring elucidation
were being reserved for further inquiry, when in January of the
present year, the following case was observed by Prof. Zenker, of
Dresden, which, in conjunction with the experiments to which it
gave the impetus, and for which it supplied the material, not only
served to bring about a final settlement of the zoölogical part of the
question, but disclosed the startling and alarming pathological fact,
that trichina spiralis, hitherto considered to be an innocent parasite,
is in reality the most terrible and dangerous of its kind—that it can
actually kill a healthy adult in a few weeks, under the most distressing symptoms

On January 12, 1860, a robust maid-servant, twenty-four years of
age, was admitted into the Dresden Hospital. She had been indis-

posed since Christmas, and confined to bed since New Year's day; complaining of depression, lassitude, sleeplessness, loss of appetite, heat, and thirst. These symptoms persisted on her admission ; there was considerable pyrexia ; the abdomen painful and tympanitic ; and although neither splenic tumor nor roseola were present, the case was put down as one of typhoid fever. A remarkable affection of the whole muscular system now rapidly supervened, consisting in extreme painfulness of the extremities, with contractions of knee and elbow joints, and œdematous swelling, particularly of the legs. The pain was so severe that the patient was continually moaning. Pneumonic symptoms supervened, and death took place on the 27th inst., preceded for twenty-four hours by an apathetic condition. The post-mortem examination showed in the internal organs merely an atelectatic condition of the left lung, with numerous small lobular infiltrations, bronchitis and hyperæmia of the mucous lining of the ileum. The muscles, however, which showed a grayish-red color and a slightly freckled appearance, were found, on a microscopic examination, to harbor vast numbers of non-capsulated trichinæ. The parasites were living, some coiled in spirals, others with extended bodies ; and all (as Prof. Virchow was the first to show, in a fragment of muscle which was forwarded to him for examination) living within the sarcolemma of the primitive fibrils. They showed various stages of development ; they were diffused over all the striated muscles of the body, with exception of the heart, and that in such vast numbers, that under a small magnifying power as many as twenty were in the field of vision simultaneously. The muscular substance was otherwise fragile, homogeneous, non-striated, and showed numerous transverse fissures. The intestinal mucus was found to be swarming with mature trichinæ of both sexes ; and the remarkable fact was elucidated, that female trichinæ are viviparous ; the central portion of the bodies being observed to be full of well-developed embryos.

Inquiry being directed to the probable source of the trichinatous infection, it was ascertained that on December 21, four days before the patient was taken ill, two pigs and an ox had been slaughtered in the establishment of her master. Some smoked ham and sausage, prepared from the meat of one of the pigs, were fortunately obtained, and on examination proved to be full of trichinæ. The parasites had a shrunken appearance ; otherwise unchanged ; resumed a normal appearance on the addition of water, but showed no signs of vitality. It is particularly worthy of remark, that to the naked eye the ham appeared perfectly healthy. It is very likely that the deceased had partaken of some of the raw meat. The butcher of the establishment (butchers notoriously indulge in raw meat) had also been taken seriously ill a short time afterwards, and was confined to his bed for three weeks with severe muscular pains, his whole body being semi-paralytic, etc. This complaint was ascribed to rheumatism at the time, but Prof. Zenker correctly surmises that an immigration of trichinæ, not sufficiently extensive to prove fatal, may have been the cause of the attack ; and that capsulated trichinæ would very likely be discoverable in his muscle. Professor

88

Virchow immediately commenced a series of feeding experiments with the pieces of human muscle forwarded to him by Professor Zenker.

The following is a brief statement of the results, as published in the last number of *Virchow's Archiv.*:

Rabbits fed with trichinæ die in about a month under symptoms of general muscular paralysis.

The trichinæ, which, as long as they reside in muscle, have no perfect sexual organs, become perfectly developed in the ileum. They are found free in the duodenum, about six hours after a piece of trichinatous muscle has been introduced into the stomach. In about a month they attain a length of four lines, and during that period not only mature eggs and sperm-cells, but numerous embryos, resembling small filariæ, are developed, which leave the maternal body through the anterior sexual orifice, are found in the mesenteric glands, and rapidly invade the whole muscular system, dwelling within the sarcolemma, and feeding upon the contractile substance of the muscular fibres. They are found in all the striated muscles of the body, with the exception of the heart (Zenker states that he found a few in the heart of a rabbit fed with trichinæ); liver, lungs, kidneys, etc., are free. In case the immigration is not sufficiently extensive to cause a fatal result, the trichinæ become enclosed in a capsule, which consists originally merely in a thickening of the sarcolemma, and this is the only condition in which they were formerly known. The trichina now shows the highest development it is able to attain within the muscle, into which it originally penetrated in an embryonic stage. It still retains its vitality, and quietly waits for an opportunity to find its way back into the intestinal canal, where, as Virchow's observations have shown, the two sexes attain the stage of puberty, and a wonderful productiveness, so pernicious to the individual who is unfortunate enough to harbor such terrible guests, is displayed.

The same applies to the non-capsulated trichinæ, which the enclosed preparations will make you acquainted with. The flesh of the rabbit had to the naked eye a perfectly normal appearance. The trichinæ are not near as numerous in this case as they were on former occasions. The intestinal mucus contained mature trichinæ of both sexes.

Professor Zenker made a feeding experiment with a piece of the ham. No trichinæ were found in the rabbit a week after. These experiments will, no doubt, be repeated, as the time elapsed was far too short to enable a definite conclusion to be formed.—*Med. Times and Gaz.*

Art. VIII.—*Bloodletting in Fever.*

[Practitioners who "have made up and expressed an opinion" (to use a judicial phrase) that bloodletting is wholly inadmissible as a remedial measure, will, of course, read with incredulity statistical statements such as the following. The numerical, in common with all other methods, may fail to eliminate certainty, and the more so in cases wherein the various or peculiar conditions and circumstances under which numerical facts actually occur, cannot be accurately appreciated, or are not mentioned in the numerical history. The most hopeful phlebotomist could hardly expect that forty individuals "affected with fever of a typhoid nature," taken at random in the varied conditions of civil society, would, "in every case" be cured by "a quantity of blood drawn from each patient ranging from sixty to near two hundred ounces in the space of two or three days."

B. D.]

Sir—I herewith beg to send you for the *British Medical Journal*, a copy of a letter which I addressed, forty-five years ago, to the late John Burns, Professor of Surgery in the University of Glasgow, thinking its contents may be acceptable to many of our associates.
I am, etc.,   J. B.

GLASGOW, December 4th, 1815.

Sir—In your inculcating this morning the decided utility of blood-letting in fevers, even of a partial typhoid nature, whether in this country or in hot climates, some facts naturally recurred to my mind (in complete apposition, I thought, to the doctrine under your re-view), ·namely, the extent and phenomena of bloodletting I had occasion to observe last summer in the West Indies ; and I humbly hope that the desire to communicate them, though not very import-ant of themselves, will serve as some apology for intruding them on your leisure.

During the months of April and May last, upwards of forty men of the ship I belonged to, while on the Leeward Island station, were successively attacked with the endemic remittent of the country, and venesection was carried to a very great extent, the quantity of blood drawn in each patient ranging from sixty to near two hundred ounces in the space of two or three days ; the consequence of which depleting plan was recovery in every case.

On the first attack, thirty ounces were immediately taken away, or the patient was generally bled to syncope, and the bleedings were repeated, often from the same orifice, in a few hours afterwards, or from incisions in the opposite arm, in frequency and extent as the symptoms of vascular action arose and indicated. The pulse, before the insertion of a lancet, was generally small, wiry, or hard ; some-times quick and tremulous, with much depression of the nervous system, and with sensations of much debility, irregular chills and heats ; but it became fuller and rose in strength, in a pretty direct ratio with the extent of the bleeding, and the system seemed to gain fresh action, a more phlogistic circulation, and as if it had been let at liberty from some oppressive power.

Being an early subject of an attack, I had not the opportunity of witnessing the incipient features of many of the cases, but when they arrived at the hospital, after copious bleedings on board, the fever still assumed, in the majority of cases, its bold obvious character—exhibiting a strong vascular over-action, as violent headache, pains about the region of the stomach, painful suffused eyes, florid blushing countenances, and hot unperspiring skins ; but, after renewed venesection, the system recovered its equilibrium, the appetite in a few days became keen, and very little or no emaciation followed the severest attacks.

The few observations these cases gave rise to in my mind were :

1. That the sensations and symptoms of debility in the attack were fallacious, and the greater or less extent of nervous depression and mental despondence were followed by a corresponding degree of arterial action.

2. That bleeding during a period of chilliness, sickness, or vasenlar depression, increased the nervous sensibility and weakness, and was less efficacious than when an evolution of heat and action took place ; and I thought that venesection then was even somewhat hurtful, and laid the foundation for a more formidable reaction when this again took place.

3. That the system seemed, as it were, to generate blood in preternatural quickness, as if venesection was a stimulus to sanguification ; or that the lancet had let loose a latent reservoir of blood, so little did the patients seem to feel the loss of a great quantity.

4. That the tepid bath elicited the type and paroxysm of the fever, and allowed a fresh quantity of blood to be withdrawn, as opening a vein in its imperfect or irregular formation was followed by syncope, or a trifling flow of blood.

5. That the blood drawn did not exhibit any extraordinary inflammatory crust, or that this tended much to concavity on its upper surface ; and that doses of a scruple of calomel and half a drachm of jalap scarcely produced any desired effect before the violence of the disease was subdued by the lancet the "sheet-anchor," as it was termed, of the patient's life.

This curtailed statement of the above simple facts can add little corroboration to a practice generally adopted, in the navy at least ; but as isolated examples of the successful issue of copious bloodletting in fevers, they are respectfully laid before you, and

I am, sir, your most obedient humble servant,

J. B.

To John Burns, Esq., Professor of Surgery.

Art. IX.—*On the Treatment of Inflammation:* By Dr. Lawson, Professor of the Theory and Practice of Medicine in the Medical College, Ohio, Cincinnati.*

Dr. Lawson's paper is an elaborate and very able criticism of the well-known views of Dr. Bennett, of Edinburgh. Of the ability of this criticism, sufficient proof may, we think, be found in the remarks upon the value of statistics as a guide in the treatment of disease, and upon the fallacy of supposing that the type of disease is fixed, and that a treatment which is right to-day will also be right to-morrow.

"It becomes an important question for the practitioner to decide, *how far confidence can be placed in medical statistics,* especially such as bear on this subject, and to what extent such evidence can be made a guide in the treatment of disease? An examination of the statistics of pneumonia, which occupy so important a position in Dr. Bennett's theory, will reaveal results so variable and contradictory as to deprive them of the slightest claim to authority. Thus, without depletion, Dr. Bennett's statistics show a mortality of 1 in $21\frac{1}{4}$; Deitl's, 1 in 13; the homœopathic, 1 in 6; and the non-bleeding plan in Vienna, in 1856, in 1 in 4. With antimony, bleeding, etc., Grisolle lost 1 in 8; Dr. Bell, 1 in 77.7; Trousseau, 1 in 26; Burkart, 1 in 60; Wossildo, none in 76. Pneumonia treated by inhalation of chloroform furnishes the following mortality: in the hands of Baumgärter, 1 in 10; Varrentrapp, 1 in 23; Wucherer, 1 in 90 ! In the Royal Infirmary, Edinburgh, former statistics show a mortality of 1 in 3; and this constitutes, mainly, the foundation for Dr. Bennett's denunciation of depletory treatment.

"In addition to this, Kissel treated 112 cases with a mortality of 5—1 in $22\frac{1}{5}$. When the urine was alkaline he gave iron ; when it was acid he gave copper.

"Here is exhibited a very wide range of figures. The non-bleeding plan varies from 1 in 4 to 1 in $21\frac{1}{2}$; the antiphlogistic from 1 in 3 to 1 in 90. Are not these results too variable to constitute any sound basis of practice ? If we take Dr. Bennett's statistics, we would certainly not deplete; if we take Wossildo's results as the guide, we will as certainly resort to bloodletting ; but if we chance to adopt the tables of Wucherer, then we will administer chloroform ! or iron and copper, if we depend on Kissel. Each partisan will find his theory fully sustained by these figures ; but the judicious praetitioner will perceive that some unseen agency has modified the results, and that the mere figures are but so many fallacies. It is evident, therefore, that the statistics of pneumonia, as a whole, are utterly worthless and unreliable as practical guides.

"If we seek an explanation of these contradictory results in the

---

* In a letter dated at Cincinnati, July 18, 1860, I learn from Professor Lawson that he has been appointed Professor of Clinical Medicine in the University of Louisiana, and will remove to New Orleans before the opening of the course of Lectures in autumn. As a pathologist and clinical teacher, he is highly distinguished, and will doubtlessly do credit to the Institution and the cause of science.

B. D

treatment of pneumonia, it will be found in the numerous qualifying conditions connected with age, season, climate, epidemic and endemic influences, early treatment, stage, extent, and complications of the disease. And to these conditions we must add, in a general sense, the *individuality* of each case ; indeed, so great are the differences in constitutions, that no two examples will exhibit the same characteristics throughout, nor will they admit of precisely the same method of treatment. And it is a due appreciation of these more minute shades of differences, as well as the broad distinctions observed in the varying *forms* of the disease, that constitutes the truly skillful physician, and which enables him to meet the emergencies of each case, instead of relying on conclusions drawn from *groups* of cases.

"Viewing nationalities in a somewhat prejudiced light, a critical writer intimates that the English think more of some other case than the one under treatment, while the French think more of the disease than of the patient ; hence the former individualize the disease, the latter generalize the patient ; but the true course is that indicated by Hufeland, to *generalize the disease and individualize the patient.* It is quite immaterial to our present purposes, whether these distinctions exist among French, Germans, and English, or not, but we cannot fail to observe their strong development in individual writers. Statisticians rob each case of its individuality, and cast it upen the sea of uncertainties pertaining to others of a different character. Thus one series will all be bled, another will receive tartar emetic, and a third left to the chances of nature. In the first class, some are bled who should have been stimulated ; in the second, tartar emetic is administered when bleeding would have been preferable ; and in the third class, some are permitted to die from mere over-action. In this blundering, if not criminal procedure, individuality is ignored, and the practitioner prescribes for a mere *name*, leaving the patient to the mercies of chance or fate.

"It is evident, therefore, that a rational treatment must secure to each case its own individuality; and as the shades of differences, and the corresponding modifications of treatment, cannot be expressed in *groups*, statistics, in this sense, become simply an impossibility. For example, bleeding, antimony, mercury, and blisters may be demanded in one case; quinine, opium, and wine in the next ; a third may require but little interference, except a well-regulated diet, with moderate stimulants ; and so on, *ad infinitum.* The treatment of pneumonia demands not a single but many agents ; and he who would attempt to develop results by statistics will be required to make each group a *unit.* It is the proper *combination* of remedies, and not a single agent or mode of practice, which is capable of securing the best results in the treatment of disease.

* * * * * * * *

"The variation of inflammatory affections may be clearly observed, on a limited scale, in what occurs during the different seasons of a single year. Thus, it is well known that inflammatory diseases bear and require more antiphlogistic treatment during winter than summer. But still more distinctly are these variations observable in different years ; indeed, every practitioner must have remarked that the same classes of disease manifest a much higher grade of action, and require more depletion, during some years than others. And, if this is true of seasons and years, there is no obvious reason why the same influences may not extend through longer periods or cycles of time. In our own country we have numerous illustrations bearing on this question of the change of the type and character of disease. Thus, it is well known that, since the prevalence of Asiatic cholera in 1832, there has been manifested a greater degree of irritability of the alimentary canal, and consequently diminished tolerance of cathartic medicine. Purgatives have fallen into disuse since the days of Hamilton, even to a greater extent than has bloodletting since the days of Cullen and Gregory. And it may be safely affirmed that the change of practice in this respect cannot be ascribed to an improved pathology, but to a broad and enlightened experience growing out of an obvious change in the *type* of disease.

"In the western and southern portions of the United States, another and even more striking change has occurred. The endemic fevers of this vast region were originally of the periodical type ; but as early as 1842 we were invaded by a well-defined (typhoid) fever, which in many localities superseded the periodical fevers. The continued type predominated in many localities for a period of ten years, since which time it has gradually diminished, while periodical fever again becomes more common. I do not assert that these changes were radical and complete in every district, but the predominance of the two types occurred, as I have stated, in many regions of country, and the typhoid element seems to have permanently impressed most of the diseases incident to the climate. And this important modification of disease demanded at once a radical change of treatment. The preparations of bark and mercury, together with bloodletting, were no longer efficient ; but, instead of these, the employment of stimulants and nutrients became the leading agents. Quinine, so efficacious in periodical fevers, was not only inefficient in the new form of disease, but was often found positively pernicious ; mercury was seldom required, and frequently wholly inadmissible. This great change of treatment was not due to an improved pathology, but it arose from the introduction of a new form of disease, and experience soon indicated the necessary changes of treatment.

"But still another modification in the type of disease has occurred here and elsewhere. Practitioners have observed, for some years past, a *nervous* type, with often a decided tendency to prostration, so much so, indeed, that depletion must be resorted to cautiously, or entirely interdicted

Now, it is evident, from the concurrent statements of writers in Europe and America, that these changes are general and common to both countries ; and that a corresponding modification of treatment has occurred, coëxtensive with the changes in the type of disease. Typhoid fever has of late years spread over England, and has been fully recognized by the practitioners generally. In 1845, the writer of these remarks observed cases of typhoid fever in the London

Fever Hospital, but they were limited in number, and, perhaps, not well defined, for Dr. Tweedie remarked that the disease had not been recognized, and that they made no distinction between the typhus and typhoid forms. Soon, however, typhoid fever multiplied, and its existence was fully recognized by Dr. Jenner and other observers.

"I may also mention here, as evidence of the change which the *type* of fever undergoes, that Dr. Tweedie's report for the year 1845 shows the low form of disease by the large quantity of stimulants demanded. He states that, in the epidemic of 1843, when 1100 patients were admitted, the quantity of wine administered was about 1800 ounces, and 60 of brandy; while the next year, although not half the number were admitted, they consumed 14,000 ounces of wine and 760 of brandy, besides gin and porter ! No fact could be more striking and conclusive than this.

" It ceases, therefore, to be a matter of surprise or doubt that these zymotic causes, with others probably unknown, should modify the *type* of disease and require treatment greatly changed in character. The choleraic and typhous poisons, to say nothing of the causes which have so extensively modified the nervous system, must be regarded as fully competent to effect these important changes.

" It is contended, however, by Dr. Bennett, that *inflammation* is always essentially the same, and hence there has been no change in the *type* of disease. It is very true, indeed, that the elementary actions characteristic of inflammation must necessarily remain unchanged ; that is, the adhesion of the corpuscles, distension of vessels, stagnation of blood, and, finally, the exudation of lymph, are the same in the days of Bennett that they were in those of Cullen. But this does not embrace the main question, for it is not the local changes occurring in an inflamed tissue which are supposed to have undergone changes, but it is the condition of the *general system*—of innervation, circulation, and all the vital functions. These become, from general causes, depressed ; and although there may be no change in the microscopic appearances of inflammation, nevertheless the *reäction* is less intense, the tendency is to depression, and depletion is less demanded. Hence the *type* of disease may change, while the minute process of inflammation remains unaltered.

" It is not contended, however, that this change of type will be observed in every example of disease ; on the contrary we still witness the old division of sthenic and asthenic inflammations. The former, however, have diminished, until, finally, the latter predominate; or what would, perhaps, be more correct, there is a general lowering of the grade of action, which requires less depletion than did the same classes of disease in former years.

" At the same time, I am strongly inclined to believe that the great outcry against bleeding has driven us to the opposite extreme, and we now deplete less than the interests of our patients frequently require. With the prevailing aversion to bleeding, cases are liable to be overlooked, and depletion neglected from sheer habit. Dr. Christison clearly proves, within his own personal experience, that the synocha of Cullen has several times recurred, and each time demanding depletion. But he who would regard that form of fever as a *myth*, would not recognize its new introduction, and, therefore, would fail to meet its exigencies."

Dr. Lawson concludes his paper with this *argumentum ad hominem*. Dr. Bennett himself has been attacked by inflammation, and, lo ! his case *demands bloodletting !* His colleague, Dr. Miller, moreover, informs us that his sthenic constitution nobly sustained depletion. Alas for theory ! — *The Half-Yearly Abstract of the Medical Sciences*, June, 1860.

ART. X.—*On Fermented and Aërated Bread, and their Comparative Dietetic Value:* By J. DAUGLISH, M. D.

SINCE the new process of preparing bread has been introduced—a process which effects the raising of bread wholly by mechanical means, imparting to it the most perfect vesicular structure, while it leaves the constituents of the flour wholly unchanged and uncontaminated—there has not been wanting those who doubt whether the process of fermentation, by which bread has been hitherto prepared, is not really beneficial in other respects than that of imparting the vesicular structure to it; whether, in fact, the changes which the constituents of the flour—especially the starch—undergo, are not essential to healthy digestion in the stomach.

Although I believe there are few members of the medical profession who will be prepared to maintain that fermentation is beneficial, still, as some do hold such an opinion, and have asserted likewise that starch which has not undergone the fermentive process is wholly unfit for human food, I am desirous of stating what I believe are good reasons for rejecting the process of fermentation for the new one which I have introduced.

In order to dispose of the assertion that starch requires to be disposed of by the fermentive changes to render it fit for human food, it is but necessary to remark, that the proportion which the inhabitants of the earth, who thus prepare their starchy food, bear to those who do not, is quite insignificant. Indeed, it would appear that the practice of fermenting the flour or meal of the cereal grains is followed chiefly by those nations who use a mixed animal and vegetable diet, while those who are wholly fed on the products of the vegetable kingdom reject the process of fermentation entirely. Thus, the millions of India and China, who feed chiefly on rice, take it for the most part simply boiled ; and that large portion of the human race who feed on maize, prepare it in many ways, but they never ferment it. The same is true with the potato-eater of Ireland, and with the oatmeal-eater of Scotland. Nor do we find that even wheat is always subjected to fermentation; but the peculiar physical properties of this grain appear to have tasked man's ingenuity more than any other, to devise methods of preparing from it food which shall be both palatable and digestible. In the less civilized states, a favorite mode of dressing wheat grain has been, by first roasting and then grinding it. On the borders of the Mediterranean it is prepared in the form of maccaroni and vermicelli, while in the East it is made into hard thin cakes for the more delicate, and for the hardworking and robust into thicker and more dense masses of baked flour and water. Even in our own nurseries wheaten flour is baked before it is prepared with milk for infant's food. The necessity of subjecting wheaten grain to these manipulations arises from its richness in gluten, and from the peculiar properties of that gluten. If a few wheaten grains are taken whole and thoroughly masticated, the starchy portions will be easily separated, mixed with the saliva and swallowed, whilst nearly the whole of the gluten will remain in the mouth in the form of a tough tenaceous pellet, on which scarcely any impression can be made. A similar state of things will follow the mastication of flour. In this condition the gluten is extremely indigestible, since it cannot be penetrated by the digestive solvents, and they can only act upon its small external surface; hence the necessity to prepare food from wheat in such a manner as shall counteract this tendency to cohere and form tenaceous masses. This is the object of baking the grain and the flour as before mentioned, of making it into maccaroni, and of raising it into soft spongy bread ; by which latter means the gluten assumes a form somewhat analogous to the texture of the lungs, so that an enormous surface is secured for the action of the digestive juices ; and this I believe is the sole object to be sought in the preparation of bread from wheaten flour.

Wheat is said to be the type of adult human food. It supplies, in just proportions, every element essential to the perfect nutrition of the human organism. And yet in practice, we find that the food which we prepare from it, and furnish to the inhabitants of our large towns and cities, is quite incapable alone of sustaining the health and strength of any individual. This is the more remarkable, since in Scotland we find that the food prepared from the oat, a grain possessing the same elements of nutrition as wheat, though in a coarser form—furnishes almost the exclusive diet of a very large number of the hardiest and finest portion of the population.

In the large towns of France wheaten bread certainly forms a very large proportion of the diet of the laboring classes, but not so large as oatmeal does in Scotland. And yet it has been remarked by contractors for public works on the Continent, that the chief reason why the Englishman is capable of accomplishing double the work of a Frenchman is, that the one consumes a very large proportion of meat, while the diet of the other is chiefly bread. In Scotland, however, the laboring man is capable of sustaining immense fatigue upon the nourishment afforded by oatmeal porridge.

The deficiency of wheaten bread in affording the nourishment due to the constituents of the grain, is to be attributed solely to the mode of preparing the flour, and the process followed for making that flour into porous bread.

The great object sought after both by the miller and the baker, is the production of a white and a light loaf. Experience has taught the miller that the flour which makes the whitest loaf is obtained from the centre of the grain ; -but that the flour which is the most economical, and contains the largest proportion of sound gluten, is that which is obtained from the external portions of the grain. But while he endeavors to secure both these portions for his flour, he takes the greatest care to avoid, as much as possible, by fine dressing, etc., the mixture with them of any part of the true external coat which forms the bran, knowing that it will cause a most serious deficiency in the color of the bread after fermentation.

It is generally supposed that the dark color of brown bread—that is from bread made from whole wheaten meal—is attributable to the colored particles of the husk or outer covering of the grain. · But such is not really the case. The colored particles of the bran are of themselves only capable of imparting a somewhat orange color to bread, which is shown to be the fact when whole wheaten meal is made into bread by a process where no fermentation or any chemical changes whatever are allowed to take place. Some few years since a process was invented in America for removing the outer seed coat of the wheat grain without injuring the grain itself, by which it was proposed to save that highly nutritious portion which is torn away, adhering to the bran in the ordinary process of grinding, and lost to human consumption. The invention was brought under the notice of the French Emperor, who caused some experiments to be made in one of the Government bakeries to test its value. The experiments were perfectly satisfactory so far as the making of an extra quantity of white flour was concerned, but when this flour was subjected to the ordinary process of fermentation and made into bread, much to the astonishment of the parties conducting the experiments, and of the inventor himself, the bread was brown instead of white. The consequence, of course, has been that the invention has never been brought into practical observation.

It has been estimated that as much as ten or twelve per cent. of nutritious matter is separated adhering to the bran, which is torn away in the process of grinding, and until very lately this matter has been considered by chemists to be gluten. It has, however, been shown by M. Mège Mouriès to be chiefly a vegetable ferment, or metamorphic nitrogenous body, which he has named cerealin, and another body, vegetable caseine.

Cerealin is soluble in water, and insoluble in alcohol. It may be obtained by washing bran, as procured from the miller, with cold water, in which it dissolves, and it may be precipitated from the aqueous solution by means of alcohol ; but, like pepsine, when thus precipitated it loses its activity as a solvent or ferment.

In its native state or in aqueous solution, it acts as the most energetic ferment on starch, dextrine and glucose, producing the lactic and even the butyric changes, but not the alcoholic.

It acts remarkably on gluten, especially when in presence of starch, dextrine or glucose. The gluten is slightly decomposed at first, giving ammonia, a brown matter, and another production which causes the lactic acid change to take place in the starch and glucose. . The lactic acid thus produced immediately combines its activity with that of the cerealin and the gluten is rapidly reduced to solution.

The activity of the cerealin is destroyed at a temperature of 140° Fah., according to M. Mouriès, but my own experiments show that it is simply suspended even by the heat required to cook bread thoroughly; thus bread made without fermentation, of whole wheaten meal or of flour in which there is a large proportion of cerealin, will, if kept at a temperature of about 75° to 85° Fah., pass rapidly into a state of solution, if the smallest exciting cause be present, such as ptyalin or pepsin, or even that very small amount of organic matter which is found in impure water—while the same material, when it has been subjected to the alcoholic fermentation, will not be affected in a like manner.

The activity of cerealin is very easily destroyed by most acids, also by the presence of alum ; and while it is the most active agent known in producing the earlier changes in the constituents of the the flour, it cannot produce the alcoholic, but so soon as the alcoholic is superinduced the cerealin becomes neutralized and ceases to act any longer as a solvent. M. Mouriès, taking advantage of this effect of the alcoholic fermentation, has adopted a process by which he is enabled to separate ·from the bran all the cerealin and casein which are attached to it. He subjects the bran to active alcoholic fermentation, which neutralizes the activity of the cerealin, and at the same time separates the nutritious matter; and then having strained this through a fine seive, he adds it to the white flour in the preparation of white bread, by which an economy of ten per cent. is effected, and the color of the bread is not injured.

The peculiar action of cerealin as a special digestive solvent of the constituents of the flour—gluten and starch—has been practically tested by Mr. Stephen Darby, of Leadenhall street, in a series of careful experiments. He found that when two grains of dry cerealin were added to 500 grains of white flour, and the whole digested in half an ounce of water at a temperature of 90° for several hours, ten per cent. more of the gluten, and about five per cent. more of the starch, were dissolved than when the same quantity of flour was subjected to digestion without the addition of the cerealin, but in which of course there was the small amount of cerealin that is present in all flours. The action of cerealin upon the gluten of wheat is precisely similar to that of pepsin on the fibrine of meat. Pepsin acting alone on fibrine dissolves it, but very slowly, but if lactic acid be added solution takes place very rapidly. In like manner the starch present with the gluten of wheat is acted upon by the cerealin, and produces the necessary lactic acid to assist in the solution of the gluten by cerealin.

With the knowledge thus obtained of the properties of this substance, cerealin, it is not difficult to understand why the administration of bran-tea with the food of badly-nourished children, produces the remarkable results attributed to it by men both experienced and eminent in the medical profession ; and why, also, bread made from whole wheaten meal, which contains all the cerealin of the grain should prove so beneficial in some forms of mal-assimilation, notwith-standing the presence of the peculiarly indigestible and irritating substance forming the outer covering of the grain.

It will be seen that in all the methods of bread-making hitherto adopted, the peculiar solvent properties of this body, cerealin has been sought to be neutralized simply because it destroys the white color of the bread during the earlier stages of panary fermentation. It is by thus destroying the activity of the special digestive ferment which Nature has supplied for the due assimilation by the economy of the constituents of the wheaten grain, that wheaten bread is ren-dered incapable of affording that sustenance to the laboring man which the Scotchman obtains from his oatmeal porridge. Although the new bread has been as yet but little more than experimentally introduced to public consumption, I have already received from members of my own profession, who have recommended it in their practice, as well as from non-professional persons, accounts of the really astonishing results that have followed its use in cases of de-ranged digestion and assimilation. Private gentlemen have sought interviews with me to record the history of their recovery to health, after years of suffering and misery, by the simple use of the bread as a diet. Children that have been liable to convulsive attacks from an irritable condition of the alimentary canal and nervous system, have been perfectly free from them immediately the new bread was substituted for fermented bread. And cases are now numerous that have been communicated to me by medical men of position, in which certain distressing forms of dyspepsia, which had remained intractable under every kind of treatment, have yielded as if by magic almost immediately after adopting the use of the aërated bread.

The delicate flavor of the new bread renders it peculiarly grateful to the stomachs of invalids and children, as well as of those whose tastes have not become vitiated by the habitual use of baker's bread, which is slightly sour, and tastes of yeast. The new bread was sup-plied to two wards in Guy's Hospital, in place of the ordinary bread (which is of a very fine quality, made on the premises), for two months, and in no case were there any piece, left in the wards uncen-sumed, while of the fermented bread large quantities of scraps are collected daily, for the consumption of which the appetites of the patients have been deficient.

That persons who have been long used to the strong yeasty-flavored bakers' bread should consider the new bread tasteless at first is not to be wondered at, since the delicate sense of taste is of all other senses the most easily lost by rough usage. Hence the argument put forth in defence of adulteration by some London tradesmen, es-pecially the beer-sellers, that the public will not buy the pure article, as it is wanting in the flavor to which they have been accustomed; and hence, also, the dislike of the Viennese of the fresh oysters sup-plied to them when the railway was completed, as they deemed them insipid, after the habitual use of oysters slightly decomposed, with which they had been supplied when it required a lengthened period to transport them from the sea.

I am disposed to attribute the beneficial effects of the new bread

to two causes. The one to the *absence* of the prejudicial matters imparted to ordinary bread by the process of, fermentation, and the
other to the *presence* in the bread, unchanged, of that most essential
agent of digestion and assimilation, cerealin.

I believe the prejudicial matters imparted to bread by fermentation
to be chiefly two—acetic acid and the yeast-plant. The first is produced in large quantities, especially in hot weather, by the oxyda-
tion, by atmospheric contact, of the alcohol produced. The second
is added when the baker forms his sponge, and is also rapidly propagated during the alcoholic fermentation, and cannot of course be
afterwards separated from the other materials in the manner that
the yeast and the other *débris* of fermentation separate themselves
from wine and beer by precipitation in the process of fining. Nor is
the life of the yeast-plant generally destroyed in baking, because it
requires to be retained at the boiling point for some time before it is
thoroughly destroyed ; and bread is generally withdrawn from the
oven, for economical reasons, even before the centre of the loaf has
reached the temperature of 212°. It is not difficult to understand
how the most painful and distressing symptoms and derangements
may follow the use of bread in which the yeast-plant is not thoroughly
destroyed previous to ingestion, in those cases of impaired function
in which the peculiar antiseptic influence of the stomachal secretions
is deficient, and is incapable of preventing the development of the
yeast-plant in the stomach, and the setting up of the alcoholic fermentation to derange the whole process of digestion and assimilation.

The presence of cerealin in bread is as beneficial as that of acetic
acid and the yeast-plant is prejudicial. Digestion, or the reduction
of food, is evidently essentially dependent on the action of a class
of substances which chemists, for the want of a better term, have
called ferments—to these substances belong pepsin, ptyaline, emulsion, diastase, and cerealin ; these are evidently types of a very
numerous class, which act by producing those molecular changes in
organic substances in which digestion consists ; and since the purpose of digestion or solution is to prepare from heterogeneous substances taken as food, a chyle, which shall not only when absorbed
present all the elements of healthy blood, but shall, previous to
absorption, possess the properties which will constitute it the proper
stimulus to the functional activity of the lacteals, it would appear
to be necessary that each distinct substance taken as food should be
furnished, not with its simple chemical solvent, but with that peculiar form of solvent or ferment which alone can carry it through
those molecular changes which shall terminate in the production of
healthy chyle. Hence we should infer that a substance is digestible
or indigestible, just in proportion to the provision that is made for
its reduction to the standard of healthy chyle, and that substances
which have hitherto been incapable of affording any nutrition whatever, may at some future day be rendered highly nutritious, simply
by adding to them suitable ferments, artificially obtained or otherwise, that shall secure their passing through the proper molecular
changes. Indeed, I think this subject opens up to us that very wide
field of inquiry, as to whether the cause and prevention of disease,

and the beneficial administration of remedies may not, for the most part, if not entirely, be dependent on the action of substances analogous to such bodies as ptyaline, pepsin, cerealin, etc., acting in concord with, or retarding and opposing the vital functions of tissues ; and that by more profound inquiry in the field of research, the physiologist and the pathologist may not at a future day lay the foundation of true scientific medicine.—*Medical Times and Gazette.*

Tunbridge Wells.

ART. XI.—*On the Pathology of Lead-Colic :* By WILLOUGHBY F. WADE, M. B., Physician to the Queen's Hospital and to the General Dispensary ; Professor of the Practice of Physic in the Queen's College, Birmingham.

THE received opinion that this painful disorder depends upon some perverted action of the colon, as its name implies, has already had its antagonists. When we come to inquire a little more closely what this perverted action is, we find that no satisfactory answer can be given. Some contend for an empty and contracted condition of the gut, others for a distension by gas or fæces.

Dr. Copland says that in his cases distension was as frequent as retraction, owing evidently to inflation and fæcal engorgement of the colon, the course of which could be distinctly traced under the abdominal parietes. De Haen and Merat found contraction of the colon and cæcum in all the cases they examined. But, as Dr. Watson judiciously remarks, " with regard to the contraction of the large intestine in these cases, we must not be too ready to attribute it to spasm, for the bowel, when empty, is apt to be contracted." Andral details six cases in which no such contractions were found. Indeed Andral, Louis, and Sir George Baker, concur in describing the intestines as being normal throughout their whole extent. I doubt very much whether an unopposed contraction of a hollow muscular canal can be attended with pain. It is the vain endeavor to shorten the muscular tissue, and the resistance offered by an incompressible material, that causes the pain in biliary calculus and ordinary crapulous or flatulent colic. An empty intestine might, I think, go on contracting till its calibre was obliterated before it produced pain. The after-pains of labor do not offer any necessary objection to this view ;· for the contraction of one layer of fibres can be well resisted by the large mass of inactive ones. Besides, they often depend on the presence of clots. On the other hand, did the pain of lead-colic depend upon the presence of flatus, I cannot conceive how it is that this should not, in such cases, be readily removed, for a time at least, by opiates and carminatives, as happens in ordinary flatulence. If, again, it depended upon retained fæces, the removal of them should remove the pain. But the operation of the bowels is by no means necessarily followed· by this relief. It is, indeed, true that the two often coincide, but this is quite as easily explicable in another way, as we shall see directly. The retraction of the abdominal parietes, so constantly noticed in this form of the complaint, is by no means so constantly observed in other varieties of colic.

The pathology of lead-colic is then, I submit, unsatisfactory and vague as at present taught.

Various pathologists of distinction have been disposed to refer the symptoms to cramp of the external abdominal muscles, instead of to the intestines at all. Giacomini first broached this notion, and M. Briquet of La Charité has more lately revived this view, which he supports with skill and vigor. The existence of cramp in these muscles has been recognized by those who are entirely committed to the generally accepted pathology. Thus Dr. Copland says, "the voluntary muscles often become so sore that they cannot bear the slightest pressure ; and the pain frequently alternates between the stomach and bowels and the external muscles." Besides the spasmodic contraction of the abdominal muscles, which he has observed more particularly in the severe cases, Grisolle says that three-fourths of these patients suffer from cramps, or a feeling of numbness, or from lancinating and tearing pains in the muscles of the lower extremities ; half of them have similar affections of the muscles of the upper extremities, and a third in the lumbar muscles.

The fact that in the most severe cases the abdomen was found to be retracted is important ; for there was evidently a spasm of all the abdominal muscles. Hence, on Briquet's theory, the acuteness of the pain ; whereas in the slighter cases there would be only a moderate spasm or perhaps affection of one or two muscles only, which would not produce retraction, and which might be readily overlooked unless attention were specially directed to it.

There can be no question that this condition is more than sufficient to produce any amount of pain—even the excruciating agony of lead-colic. To any one who has suffered from cramp in the leg or any other part of the body, further proof of this point is quite superfluous. That it is the actual cause of the suffering M. Briquet shows by the following arguments :

Muscles which are thus affected may be excited to more energetic action by rubbing them with the point of the finger or with any rigid, bluntly pointed instrument, such, for example, as a penholder. They can also be reëxcited if they have previously become quiescent. We can thus reproduce or exacerbate the pains of lead-colic, and this artificial excitement cannot be distinguished by the patient from the natural exacerbations so common in this complaint.

Some little time ago I had an opportunity of proving the truth of M. Briquet's assertions.

A boy, aged 13, who was engaged in polishing black glass brooches with a powder containing lead, and whose gums were marked with the blue line, was brought in great suffering to the Dispensary, in

October 1858. The pain was constant, with paroxysmal exacerbations; it was referred to the upper part of the abdomen; the bowels had been open two days before, but for a week had been very costive. The pain also was of a week's duration. The upper half of each rectus abdominis was tonically contracted, and the spasm evidently increased during each exacerbation. The spasm might be artificially excited by manipulation with the finger, as described by Briquet. This produced just as much pain as occurred during the inartificial exacerbations, and this pain was just of the same character as that which came on spontaneously. In this case the bowels were moved, not before, but after the pain had ceased. In another less severe case, in a girl, the pain ceased twenty-four hours *before* the bowels were opened.

There can be, I think, no difficulty in understanding that the pains of lead-colic, and the retraction of the abdomen, may be completely explained by the existence of tonic and clonic spasm of the abdominal muscular parietes. The question then which remains to be answered is, whether it is possible for the constipation to depend upon this spasm. It appears to me that this question may be safely answered in the affirmative.

In ordinary defecation these muscles take an active part. "The act of defecatiou (as of urination)," says Dr. Carpenter, "chiefly depends upon the combined contraction of the abdominal muscles, similar to that which is concerned in the expiratory movement; but the glottis being closed, so as to prevent the upward motion of the diaphragm, their force acts only on the contents of the abdominal cavity; and so long as the sphincter of the cardia remains closed, it must press downwards upon the walls of the rectum and bladder, the contents of the one or the other of these cavities, or of both, being expelled according to the condition of their respective sphincters; these actions being doubtless assited by the contraction of the walls of the rectum and bladder themselves."

The muscles, then, of the abdomen being already firmly contracted without closure of the glottis, the diaphragm is unable to descend, and pressure upon the rectum becomes impossible. This, combined with the heardened state of the fæces and the contraction of the sphincter ani, both of which are, according to the best authorities, *common* occurrences in lead-colic, are undoubtedly sufficient to explain the constipation which characterises this disorder. The bladder requiring a less sustained voluntary effect, is emptied; this applies also to the stomach. This theory explains also why micturition is sometimes painful; and the connections of the cremaster account for its spasmodic contraction, and the consequent painful retraction of the testis. And we can also comprehend why the action of the bowels, and cessation of the pain, should be so commonly contemporaneous, and why, as in the cases I have cited, the pain should cease before the bowels are moved.

It now remains to consider in what relation·the lead-poisoning stands to this spasm; and what relation there is between this latter and the disorder of the abdominal organs, which is certainly a com-

90

mon feature of the complaint, such as the slight icterus, the hardened fæces, the vomiting, loss of appetite, and so on.

I presume that the members of this Association are acquainted with the papers which have been published from time to time in our Journal, by our ingenious *confrère* Dr. Inman of Liverpool. In these and in a volume which he has published separately, Dr. Inman has contended that the symptoms which have been grouped together under the title of "Spinal Irritation," arise from the irregular contraction of muscles which have been enfeebled from any cause ; as, for instance, from over-exertion, or malnutrition. He points out, too, that the term over-exertion is a relative one ; that whereas one person might walk fifty miles or lift enormous weights, others might evidently be overtasked did they accomplish a tenth part of such labors. Muscles so affected present, generally perhaps in a minor degree, those appearances and phenomena which are found in the abdominal muscles of patients with lead colic.

Now, we know, from examination, that muscles impregnated with lead lose their color, and become enfeebled in various degrees, even to the extent of actual paralysis. The malnutrition, if extreme, ends in fatty degeneration so complete that all the proper functions of the muscle are rendered impossible. It is especially, if not exclusively, the voluntary muscles upon which lead exerts its morbid influence. I cannot assert that the abdominal muscles are impregnated with lead in these cases, because sufficient time has not elapsed since attention has been directed to this view to permit of the necessary investigations being completed. But if this be made an objection, I answer that it applies equally to the intestinal involuntary muscles, which have not been shown to suffer disorganisation, but which, on the contrary, have been stated by independent observers to be apparently healthy. Besides, the frequency with which spasm does attack the external muscles has been admitted by the same observers.

Whether the absorption or ingestion of lead produces any direct effect upon the abdominal viscera, I am also unable to state ; if not, we must attribute their disorder to general causes, such, for instance, as intemperance in men, a vice to which painters are much addicted, and which we have the authority of Dr. Copland for stating aggravates and reproduces the effects of lead on the system. Induration of the fæces has a direct influence upon the production of parietal spasm, by necessary unwonted activity of the muscles during the act of defæcation. The occupation of many of these people involves considerable exertion.

In a case of so-called spinal irritation, with costiveness, in a young girl, not a lead-worker, the act of defæcation was always attended with pain in the abdominal muscles, and a subsequent soreness in the upper portions of the recti abdominis. This ceased in a great degree when the bowels were rendered more soluble by medicine, and this long before there was any or much amelioration of the other muscles which were liable to these painful contractions.

Congestion of the liver, irritability of the stomach, and irritation of the colon, from Scybala, may tend in another way to produce this spasmodic affection. It is not uncommon to find the muscles contracted where they overlie an internal organ which is in an abnormal state; indeed, Dr. Copland explains this contraction by supposing that it is involuntarily instituted for the purpose of compressing the distended colon.

In conclusion, let me ask, why should we seek to offer an explanation of lead-colic which cannot be substantiated, when we can find another one which is not only supported by admitted facts, but which is capable of adequately explaining not merely the colicky pain and the constipation, but also of embracing those, as they have been held, minor and accidental features, the existence of which must, on tne old theory, have been explained in the very way which I now seek to extend, so as to embrace and harmonize all the phenomena of the disorder. Whether lead-colic, using the term in its strict acceptation, ever exists is, I think, extremely doubtful; but that many cases reputed to be such are to be referred to a totally different category rests upon evidence which cannot, I think, be controverted. It therefore behoves those who are prepared to admit, as I think all must, the occasional simulation of lead-colic (in the strict sense) by a spasm of the external muscles; it behooves them, I say, to distinguish carefully in each case its exact nature, both with the view of ascertaining the real pathalogy of these two disorders, and of regulating their treatment by this, and not merely by the name, under which they have been hitherto confounded.—*Brit. Med. Journal.*

ART. XII.—*Physiological Discoveries claimed* by Prof. PAINE, A. M., M. D., LL.D. (From his work on *The Institutes of Medicine.**)

[BEFORE proceeding to give the author's summary of his researches, a casual glance at the work is sufficient to show that it is a numerical curiosity. It probably contains, independently of foot notes, one million of references to the work itself or to other works by Dr. Paine, though the primary sections of *The Institutes* number only 1,090. Thus, section 892 is by means of Arabian numerals, vulgar fractions, and alphabetical lettering and duplications, not to name formal paragraphs sub-divided into 76 sub-numbers before reaching the next normal or whole figure, that is 893, or one of the 1,090 §. Now, this single sectional figure has 285 references to the author,

* *The Institutes of Medicine :* By MARTYN PAINE, A. M., M. D., LL.D., Professor of the Institutes of Medicine and Materia Medica in the University of the City of New York ; Corresponding Member of the Royal Verein für Heilkunde in Preussen ; Corresponding Member of the Gesellschaft für Natur und Heilkunde zu Dresden ; Member of the Medical Society of Leipsic ; of the Medical Society of Sweden ; of the Montreal Natural History of Society ; and of many other Learned Societies ; 5th edition. Pp. 1109, 8vo. New York : Harper & Brothers. 1859.

regularly noted with the figures and the symbol §. Although this is a long section, yet it has not, perhaps, one-tenth as many references, paragraph for paragraph, as some others. Now, if one section gives 76 sub-sections, 1,090, at this rate, give 82,540 §, or sub-sections, with references to Dr. Paine's work, amounting to 1,390,650, provided 892 be taken as an example, the only one counted. But deducting about four hundred thousand, a million, more or less, remains! Although Dr. Paine professes to have made but 39 original discoveries, yet 999,961 arguments, laws, opinions or references, in the premises, must be difficult to retain in the memory, and moreover, they show that scientific discoveries may be very complex. From the history of previous discoveries, however, it appears that when known, their simplicity is so great, almost every person wonders how they should have remained unknown so long ; such as the circulation, vaccination, the identity of lightning and electricity, the steam engine, telegraph, anæsthesia, the cure of aneurism by ligature, or by digital compression, etc.

As it is probable that this work cannot be reviewed in the present number of this Journal, it is proposed to give the learned author's summary in his own words, commencing at page 912, and ending at 920, omitting only such passages, or figures, controvesies, etc., as are least important, in order to bring Dr. Paine's manifesto within the necessary limits of journalism.　　　　　B. D.]

Of his "rights" as a discoverer, Professor Paine says : The Author of these Institutes (and it will soon appear that he acted wisely) has sometimes thought it expedient to assert his claim of originality, in advance, to many doctrines promulgated in the work ; as for example, all that is most essential in the application of the nervous power, or reflex action of the nervous system to pathology and therapeutics, and to much of what is most important in the natural state of the functions. This may be readily seen by consulting, p. 106, § 222 b, etc., where all the subjects relate to the reflex action of the nervous system, and present the nervous power as an important vital agent in the various processes of organic and animal life, in the production of disease, in the operation of remedies, in all the results of bloodletting, in the changes which take place in the secreted and excreted products ; the same doctrines are at the foundation of the author's *Medical and Physiological Commentaries*, published in 1840. * * *

When the foregoing works were first published, it was in the midst of a universal prevalence of the chemical and physical doctrines of life and disease, and the author stood alone in the field of vital physiology, and in the application of the reflex action of the nervous system in resolving the great problems in physiology, pathology and therapeutics. * * * But the author has lately seen so great an indisposition, in certain quarters, to allow him any credit for his labors.

The author represents, also, the reflex action as variously *alterative* in organic life, and this imputed attribute pervades the author's writings. He enforces, everywhere, the doctrine that the reflex action of the nervous power is the modifying cause through which all the changes are effected by morbific and remedial agents in parts that are not immediately connected with the direct seat of their action ; and, farther, that the principle is precisely the same when the nervous power is brought into operation by *direct* influences upon the nervous centres (as in the case of their diseases, or when the passions operate, or as the will determines voluntary motion), as it is when it is brought into operation in that indirect manner known as reflex action. Indeed, every one of the foregoing doctrines, in all their particularities, as quoted from the American Claimant, are taught, at great extent.

The whole of this doctrine of reflex nervous action, and of the operation of the nervous power as an *alterative*, an *excitant of the secretions* and of vascular action (both direct and reflex), a *depressant* and *sedative* (according to the nature of exciting causes), and the *great immediate cause of diseases and their cure*—variously modifying organic actions—was set forth extensively and circumstantially in an "*Essay on the Modus Operandi of Remedies*," in 1842, of which the author distributed, at that time, a large number of copies in London, and addressed four thousand copies to physicians throughout the United States. The author not only sent a copy of the work to Dr. Hall, but dedicated it to him (along with Prof. J. Müller and Dr. A. P. W. Philip).

In 1848 the author applied the doctrine of reflex nervous action to a physiological demonstration of the substantive existence of the soul and instinctive principle.

* * * Nor can the reader fail of the conclusion that, were Dr. Hall's "adjudication," and Dr. Allen's after-thought, founded in any justice, and were not the claimants themselves the obnoxious parties, the present writer would have been long ago convicted by them and by others of arrogant assurance and the grossest plagiarisms. Nevertheless the author is most happy to find that his solitary position is becoming relieved, and that a practical direction has been given to his labors by others which cannot fail of carrying forward the great doctrines at which he has toiled, and against manifold obstacles, during his professional life.

The author regards it as a duty to himself and to the cause of that Philosophy in Physiology and other branches of Medicine which he has labored to introduce, that he should set forth the principal details of what he considers himself the unquestionable author. Following, therefore, the foregoing admonitory examples, he proceeds to assert his claim of originality to—

1. All that is relative, in principle, to *Reflex Action of the Nervous System* in Pathology and Therapeutics, including the application of

antecedent experiments to determine the "Laws of Sympathy" and of the Vital Functions," as they respect the natural conditions, to all the great problems in those branches of Medicine, so far as the Nervous Influence is involved as a modifying cause ; and a systematic *generalization* of the whole subject.

2. The doctrine of *Modification of the Nervous Power* by the Causes which bring it into action, and according to the nature of each Cause, whether mental or physical, remedial or morbific, external and internal, and through which its *Alterative* influences are exerted in conformity with its various modifications, respectively—regarding, therefore, the Nervous Power as a *Vital Alterative Agent* and susceptible of an endless variety of changes in *kind* from the influence of exciting causes ; being thus rendered, in its extremes of change, either a vital *stimulant* or *sedative*, exerting *alterative* effects, with corresponding results in both the solids and fluids.   The application of this philosophy equally to the cure and production of diseases in all their gradations.   (Index I and II.)

3. The doctrine and demonstration of the operation of *Remedial Agents* and *Morbific Causes* by *Reflex Action of the Nervous System*, as, also, through the foregoing *modification* of the Nervous Power (No. 2), and all that is relative to the same action in Pathology and Therapeutics.

4. A distinct exposition of the modus operandi of *Counter-Irritants* through *Reflex Action of the Nervous System*, and their associate *local influences ;* exemplifying, also, by these agents, the modus operandi of all other agents applied to the skin when they produce constitutional, or any internal effects, whether remedial or morbific —as in the case of cold, mercury, etc.   (Index II, *Counter-Irritants ; Causes, Morbific ;* and *Remedies*)

5. A distinct exposition of the modus operandi of the *Seton* through *Reflex Nervous Action and local organic influences*, as exemplifying all the essential philosophy that is ever concerned in the operation of all remedial and morbific agents, as set forth in the author's essay on the Modus Operandi of Remedies (1842), and in these Institutes (p. 679—681, § 905 *a*)—being, however, only parallel with the author's demonstration of the operation of Blisters and other Counter-Irritants through the same causations.

6. The operation of *Anæsthetics* through *Reflex Nervous Action*, as contained in this work.

7. Distinction between the agencies of *Reflex Nervous Action* in the modus operandi of the author's group of *Alteratives* and among other denominations of Remedies (Index I and II)—an important consideration, by which the *gradual* operation of remedies through *Reflex Nervous Action* is rendered clearly intelligible, as in the progressive influences of small and frequently repeated doses of tartarized antimony, mercury, etc. (p. 344–345, § 516 *d*, No. 6, p. 568–569, § 889, *m, mm*).   And so, slso, of the progressive operation of Morbific Causes, either physical or mental—as in hydrophobia, sympathethic diseases, etc. (p. 421–422, § 657 *a, b*, p. 465–466, § 715, p. 661–663, § 894–896).   The example of the *Seton* illustrates the principle (No. 5).

8. All embraced in this work, and in the Medical and Physiological Commentaries '(vol. i, p. 124–384) upon the *Influences and Modus Operandi of* LOSS OF BLOOD (whether in General Bloodletting or Leeching) which are interpreted by the Author upon purely Physiological Laws, and mainly through *Reflex Action of the Nervous System.*

9. The LAW OF ADAPTATION, operating through *Reflex Nervous Action* (INDEX I).

10. The philosophy of the natural operation of the *Will* and *Mental Emotions* through the *direct* development and action of the *Nervous Power*, and its effects as an *Alterative* agent when the latter operates in the cure or production of disease, as embraced in this work.

11. Demonstration of the *direct* development and propagation of the *Nervous Power* as an *Alterative* agent, or a simple *Stimulant* or *Depressant*, in diseases of the nervous centres, etc., and as concerned in Loss of Blood along with *Reflex Action*, etc.

12. What is relative, in this work, to peculiarities of *Structure* in its Vital constitution in different parts (p. 50–73, etc.), and their important bearings upon Physiological, Pathological, and Therapeutical doctrines, as it relates both to the direct action of remedial and morbific causes, and their operation through *Reflex Action of the Nervous System.*

13. The proof and reasoning embraced in these Institutes, and in the Medical and Physiological Commentaries, and other works, in behalf of VITAL SOLIDISM, as applied to Physiology, Pathology, and Therapeutics, and in opposition to the Chemical hypotheses.

14. Special deduction of *Vital Principle*, and peculiar Laws of Organic Beings, from their *Composition*, as embraced in this work (p. 23–49).

15. Special deductions from *Nitrogen Gas*, as contra-distinguishing the Organic from the Inorganic Kingdom, as contained in the Essay on the Philosophy of Vitality (1842), and briefly in this work (p. 34–36, § 62 a–k).

16. Special deduction of the principles of *Vital Solidism*, Physiological and Pathological, from the development of the incubated *Egg* and the physiology of *Generation*, as contained in the Essay on the Philosophy of Vitality, and in these Institutes (p. 36–49, § 63–81).

17. Analysis and elaboration of the *Properties of Life*, as contained in this work (p. 73–125).

18. The proof adduced in this work, and in the Medical and Physiological Commentaries (vol. i, p. 1–119), of the existence and office of the *Vital Powers* or *Vital Properties*, with a disproof in the latter work of the supposed identity of the Nervous Power and Galvanism, with the variety of proof herein contained of the wonderful attributes of the Nervous Power, as one of the properties of the Vital Principle of Animals.

19. Exposition of Law of *Vital Habit* (p. 363–370, § 535–537).

20. All embraced in these Institutes and the Medical and Physiological Commentaries in disproof of the Chemical and Physical hypotheses as applied to Physiology, Pathology, and Therapeutics.

' 21. All herein and in the Medical and Physiological Commentaries (vol. i, p. 385–712), in refutation of the *Humoral Pathology.*

22. Demonstration of the dependence of *Digestion* upon Vital Laws, and to the exclusion of the Chemical, as contained in this work and in the Medical and Physiological Commentaries (vol. ii, p. 79-122).

23. Demonstration embraced in these Institutes, and in the Medical and Physiological Commentaries (vol. ii, p. 1-78), of the dependence of *Vegetable* and *Animal Heat* upon Vital Laws, and against the Chemical hypotheses.

24. Experiments relative to the *Circulation in the Brain*, showing that the organ is depleted in Bloodletting (p. 824-828).

25. Demonstration of the dependence of *Absorption* and *Circulation* in Plants and Animals upon Vital Laws (p. 817-824, § 1053-1055, and *passim*).

26. Much of what herein relates to the Powers which circulate the Blood, and in the Medical and Physiological Commentaries (vol. ii, p. 398-426).

27. The distinction between *Inflammation* and *Fever*, and what is most essential in proving an active condition of the immediate instruments of Inflammation, and the dependence of its different stages, and of all its phases and products upon Vital Laws, as embraced in these Institutes, and in the Medical and Physiological Commentaries (vol. ii, p. 141-214).

28. All herein relative to the philosophy of *Venous Congestion* and *Varix*, and in Medical and Physiological Commentaries (showing that *venous inflammation* is the pathological condition), and the proof of the dependence of *Tubercle* and *Scrofula* upon Inflammation, and *Cold* as a cause of Congestion, etc., in the several Appendixes to Venous Congestion in Commentaries (vol. ii, p. 215-640).

29. Much of the Physiological bearing of organic changes incident to different periods of Life upon practical medicine (p. 373-383, § 570-584).

30. The uses and abuses of *Morbid Anatomy* as contained in this work and in Medical and Physiological Commentaries (vol. ii, p. 641-677).

31. A generalization of the *mutability of the Properties of Life*, as lying at the foundation of disease and of its cure, and of many natural changes of organization at the different stages of life, of gestation, lactation, etc. Also, of the doctrine of *substitution of pathological conditions* by Remedial Agents, through *reflex nervous action*, more favorable to the law of recuperation than such as had been impressed by the truly morbific causes, and their progressive nature; and the *physiological distinction* which the author has drawn between remedial and morbific agents.—See *Index* I, Vital Properties.—*Index* II, Remedies ; Causes, Morbific ; Therapeutics.

32. The demonstration of the operation of *Astringents* upon Vital Principles, and through *reflex action of the nervous system* (p. 370-378).

33. The demonstration of the operation of *Tonics* upon Vital Principles, and through *reflex action of the nervous system* (p. 579-583, § 890½, p. 676-679, § 904 c. d.).

34. Attempted refutation of *Theoretical Geology* and of *Spontaneity of Being*, to which there are references at p. 908, § 1079 b, p. 910-911, § 1083.

35. A critical exposure of the fallacies of the Medical Doctrines embraced in the WRITINGS of P. CH. A. LOUIS, in Medical and Physiological commentaries (vol ii, p. 679–815, and *passim*).

36. A critical exposure of the fallacies contained in the WRITINGS of LIEBIG, so far as he has applied Organic Chemistry to Physiology, Pathology, and Therapeutics (p. 147–178, p. 234–279, and *passim*).

37. A *Therapeutical Arrangement of the Materia Medica* upon Physiological principles, and in the order of the relative therapeutical value of the different substances, and as applied to particular forms of disease.

38. All that is relative to the Substantive Existence and Physiology of the SOUL and INSTINCTIVE PRINCIPLE, as embraced in this work, and in the former Essay upon those subjects. (See INDEX II.)

39. Opinion that the *Will* exercises a controlling influence upon the *Intestine* in Defecation, and as evincing a remarkable instance of Creative Design, p. 325, § 500, *e*.

ART. XIII.—*Pharmaceutical Memoranda.* (From the *Am. Jour. of Pharmacy*, for July, 1860.)

i. *On Liquor Ferri Peracetatis :* By WILLIAM PROCTER, Jr.

A tincture of acetate of iron has long been known as an officinal of the Dublin Pharmacopœia, made by double decomposition, between alcoholic solutions of the ter-sulphate of iron and of acetate of potassa.

Recently Dr. W. R. Basham, of Westminster Hospital, London, in Lancet, Jan. 28th, 1860, has suggested a new form of acetate of iron, which he has found to answer remarkably in many cases where other preparations of iron have disagreed with the patient or have excited disgust. This solution is made from the officinal tincture of the chloride of iron and solution of acetate of ammonia, and was brought to my notice by Dr. John F. Meigs, who has frequently prescribed it.

Take of Tinct. of chloride of iron, (U. S. P.) three fluid drachms.
Solution of acetate of ammonia, three fluid ounces.
Syrup of orange peel (or other syrup) a fluid ounce.
Acetic acid, ten minums. Mix.

Of this solution the dose is a dessert-spoonful three or four times a day.

. The chemical affinities result in the formation of peracetate of iron, and muriate of ammonia, with an excess of acetate of ammonia. Its impression on the palate, though astringent, is but slightly ferruginous, and has none of the inky taste of the chloride. When made without the free acetic acid, the solution undergoes change much sooner than with it. The preparation has the deep ruby red color of·

a solution of acetate of iron, and has a tendency to change by keeping. To give greater permanency, and a more agreeable taste, I
have, after a variety of experiments, adopted the following formula
as worthy of acceptance :

Liquor Ferri Peracetatis.

Take of Acetic acid, five fluid ounces.
        Carbonate of ammonia (pure), a sufficient quantity.
        Tincture of chloride of iron (U. S. P.), four fluid ounces.
        Curaçao, four fluid ounces.
        Ginger syrup, a pint.

Reserve a fluid drachm of the acetic acid, and saturate the remainder with the carbonate of ammonia, then add the acetic acid
and tincture of chloride of iron, and mix them. Lastly, add the
other ingredients.

This solution is about one-third stronger than the other solution,
and may be given in the dose of a tea-spoonful to a dessert-spoonful,
mixed with a little water, three times a day, for an adult, after meals.

The proportion of sesquioxide of iron contained in this solution, is
three-quarters of a grain to the teaspoonful, or six grains to the fluid
ounce; a dessert-spoonful is equal to sixteen minims of the tincture
of chloride of iron, as regards its iron strength. The curaçao cordial may be substituted by any other suitable flavoring, except such
as contain astringents, which of course will blacken the preparation.
A sweetened tincture of recent orange peel, slightly aromatized with
canella and oil of coriander or caraway, may be used.

This preparation has proved to be a valuable tonic and diuretic.
Dr. Basham recommends it very highly in renal dropsy. Dr. John F.
Meigs has found it particularly serviceable in cases of children requiring a ferruginous tonic. The presence of the muriate of ammonia, no doubt, has a modifying influence, as well also as the small
excess of acetate of ammonia. Dr. Keating has derived valuable
diuretic effects from it in cases of albuminuria. In a case of dropsical effusion attendant on heart disease, with great debility, its tonic
action was decidedly efficient, proving acceptable to the stomach
when other preparations had occasioned disgust.

PHILADELPHIA, June 25, 1860.

ii. Use and Properties of Perchloride of Iron.

The solution of this persalt is now almost universally employed to
arrest arterial or venous hæmorrhage, resulting either from accident,
or as a consequence of surgical operations. It has also been found
useful in intestinal hæmorrhage; in one case in particular. M.
Demarquay, of Paris, administered, morning and evening, enemata
of seven ounces of fluid, with twenty drops of the concentrated solution of perchloride of iron, and a teaspoonful of the perchloride
syrup (five or six drops to the tablespoonful), where the hæmorrhage
from the bowels was considerable, and had resisted the ordinary
remedies. The result was extremely satisfactory. The same surgeon relates a second case of extensive abscess of the shoulder,
where an injection of iodine caused severe hæmorrhage. This was

arrested by throwing into the sac a lotion composed of seven ounces of water and ten drops of the perchloride.

In gonorrhœa, and leucorrhœa, injections of the perchloride have been tried with success in weak and lympathic subjects, the proportion of the perchloride being twenty drops to three ounces and a half of water.

As a *Hæmostatic.*—1. As a local or external hæmostatic, 3 to 5 parts chloride of iron to 100 parts of distilled water. Lint soaked in this mixture is to be applied with more or less pressure on the seat of hæmorrhage. 2. As an internal hæmostatic, 1 part of chloride of iron to 500 of distilled water, sweetened to taste. One table-spoonful to be given every hour, or oftener, if necessary. This formula suffices to check the fiercest hæmorrhage within twenty-four hours. The same formula, without sugar, forms a useful uterine injection or astringent lavement in cholera or colliquative diarrhœa. 3. A hæmostatic ointment is composed of 4 to 15 parts of chloride of iron to 30 of axunge.

In a letter in the *Medical Gazette*, August 27th, Mr. J. Zachariah Laurence states that having, a few months ago, drawn the attention of the profession to the powerful local styptic properties of the *solid* perchloride of iron, he has since that time found a superior method of employing it. "If the solid perchloride of iron be kept in a bottle, a small portion of it after a time deliquesces into a thick brown fluid, which is constantly kept in a state of super-saturation by the unde-liquesced portions of the salt. This liquid, applied by means of a spun-glass brush to a bleeding surface, arrests the bleeding almost instantaneously. This mode of application is particularly valuable in applying the styptic to such cases as excision of the tonsils, bleeding from the deeper-seated gums, etc."—*Pharmaceutical Journal*, October, 1859.

iii.—*Pyrophosphate of Iron:* By Mr. ROBBINS.

One of the most recently introduced curative agents is (the so-called) pyrophosphate of iron, a salt more beautiful in appearance than the ammonio-citrate, or any other of the scaled salts before introduced. Its color varies according to the manufacture ; may be made from a decided green to a greenish hue, yellow, or more or less of a reddish tint. Water dissolves it readily. In taste it has nothing to indicate its ferruginous character, but is rather that of a pleasant saline, so that the youngest children, or the most fastidious in palate of a larger growth, cannot object to its use. With regard to its efficacy as a tonic, when compared with other preparations of iron, that, of course, can only be decided by medical men.

The name given to the above is decidedly objectionable. The science of chemistry, within the last few years, has made such rapid progress that there is scarcely a day but some new compound is an-nounced to the scientific world, some of which compounds have such long and formidable names that it requires more courage than many possess to attempt even to pronounce them ; others are more simple, yet, from their immense number, but few memories can command them at pleasure. I think it, therefore, a pity, when a new preparation is introduced of rather an indefinite composition, to increase the necessary difficulties already existing by giving it the name of a definite chemical compound well known. The salt in question physically bears no relation to pyrophosphate of iron, and all that can be said chemically is, that the latter is one of its constituents.

Pyrophosphate, or bibasic phosphate of iron, is obtained by adding a solution of persulphate or perchloride of iron to a solution of bibasic or pyrophosphate of soda. A white precipitate is thrown down, quite insoluble in water and dilute acids. Pyrophosphate of soda is obtained by simply igniting to redness in a crucible the the bibasic or ordinary phosphate of soda. The two are best distinguished by nitrate of silver, which gives with the former a white, and with the latter a yellow, precipitate.

Recently precipitated pyrophosphate of iron, obtained as above, is readily dissolved by the pyrophosphate of soda and the alkaline citrates, viz : potash, soda, and ammonia.

When pyrophosphate of soda is used as the solvent, and the solution allowed to evaporate spontaneously in shallow vessels in a warm place, a nice-looking, transparent salt is obtained, which, however, is now nearly insoluble in water, evidently from some change that has taken place during desiccation.

Citrates of soda, potash, and ammonia dissolve freely pyrophosphate of iron, yielding salts readily dissolved by water ; but the soda citrate I find to give the most satisfactory result. With it an elegant preparation may be made, easily scaled, readily dissolved by water, and which, when exposed to the air, retains its brilliancy for a much longer time than when prepared with citrate of potash or ammonia.

To prepare the citro-pyrophosphate of iron (perhaps the best name we can give it), take citrate of soda in solution, or dissolve citric acid and neutralize it with carbonate of soda, and, with the assistance of heat, dissolve in it as much recently precipitated pyrophosphate of iron as it will take up. Filter and evaporate to the consistence of a syrup. Lastly, spread on glass plates to dry, when beautiful scales of a greenish-yellow color will be obtained.

One part of dry citrate of soda is required to dissolve the pyrophosphate precipitated from one part of pyrophosphate of soda, free from water of crystallization.

As it may be considered desirable to introduce as much bibasic phosphoric acid into this preparation as possible, the following formula may be preferred :

> Take of pyrophosphate of soda, 1 part ;
> "   syrupy citrate of ammonia, 1 part ;
> "   citrate of soda, 2 parts.

Dissolve in it as much recently precipitated pyrophosphate of iron as possible, and proceed as before.

The salt formed by this process is also a very elegant one, having a greenish hue, and is perfectly soluble. If a reddish tint be desired, that can be easily attained by the smallest addition of ammonio-citrate of iron, after being reduced to a syrupy consistence.

One of the chief points of success in scaling the above preparations, is to take care that the glass plates be not subjected to a heat much above summer temperature.—*London Phar. Jour.*, April, 1860.

iv.—*Kamela (Rottlera Tinctoria); its History, Properties, Medical Uses, Doses, etc.*

History.—This plant was known to the Hindoos from the remotest antiquity, the fruit of which was employed by them as a remedy for worms, and also in certain skin diseases. They likewise used it for dying and printing silks, etc., but for this purpose it underwent a chemical process, viz: an alkaline solution was mixed with the powder of the fruit, which yielded a beautiful orange-brown color. But its properties have only recently been demonstrated by Drs. Anderson and Mackinnon, who first introduced it into England. Kamela belongs to the natural order of *Euphorbiacea*. It grows abundantly on the hilly districts of India, Burmah, the Philippine Islands, and the north-east portions of Australia. Its fruit ripens in February and March, when it is gathered, and the powder, which appears as an excrescence, is carefully brushed off and preserved for use.

Properties.—The powder of kamela is of a red brick color, with little or no odor and flavor, and like lycopodium, it is difficultly miscible with water. Ether extracts a quantity of its resinous components, and if the solution be allowed to stand for a few days, a precipitate of granular crystals is formed, which, when purified, is seen to consist of small scales of a yellowish color and satiny lustre, and named by Dr. Anderson rottlerine. Alcohol extracts its medicinal constituents most perfectly, and the tincture made with rectified spirit is found to be very suitable for administration.

Medical Uses.—Kamela has been successfully given in cases of tænia, and Dr. Mackinnon considers it of much greater value in those cases than either kousso or turpentine. Dr. Anderson describes "ninety-five cases of tænia, in ninety-three of which the worms were expelled after the third or fourth dose." It has been used also with very great success for tapeworm and ascarides, by Dr. Arthur Leared, of the Great Northern Hospital, and by Dr. William Moore, of Dublin. The *Lancet*, of May 15th, 1858, records six cases of cure of tapeworm by Dr. Ramskill, of the Royal Free Hospital. In some instances sickness, headache, and purging are produced by it, but generally its administration is attended by no unpleasant result.

Dose.—In powder, the dose of this remedy is from one to three drachms early in a morning, fasting. The tincture* may be given in doses of from one to two drachms, night and morning, on lump sugar.—*Chemist and Druggist*, London, March 19, 1860.

v. *On some Failures of Marsh's Process for the Detection of Arsenic.*

At the last meeting of the British Association, Dr. Odling read a paper, which has been since published in *Guy's Hospital Reports*, showing that the presence of certain organic and saline substances prevents the formation of arseniuretted hydrogen, and consequently

---

* Tincture of kamela is made by macerating half a pound of powder of kamela for fourteen days in a pint of rectified spirits of wine.

destroys the action of Marsh's test. The author had occasion to examine a soil which contained 0·07 of arsenious acid. Ready indication of the presence of the arsenic was obtained by Reinsch's process, but, most unexpectedly, when the dilute hydrochloric or sulphuric decoction was tested in Marsh's apparatus, no result could be obtained. Thus, 100 grains of the dried soil, boiled with half an ounce of muriatic acid and three ounces of water, yielded a solution in which no arsenic could be detected by Marsh's test, yet the liquid poured out of the apparatus and boiled with copper foil gave a metallic deposit from which crystals of arsenious acid were obtained. Another acid decoction prepared in the same manner, was distilled to dryness, and the distillate transferred to Marsh's apparatus, when characteristic stains were observed with the greatest facility. Also, when the 100 grains of soil were heated with strong oil of vitriol, so as to thoroughly char the organic matter, then diluted with water, and the filtered solution tested by Marsh's process, a satisfactory reaction was obtained. One-fifteenth of a grain of arsenious acid was then added to ordinary non-arsenical soil, and precisely the same results obtained—that is to say, the simple dilute acid decoction gave no evidence with Marsh's test.

Two different specimens of grass that had been grown upon arsenical soil, and also some hay to which one-fifth of a grain of arsenious acid had been added, were examined ; the acid decoctions tested by Reinsch's process readily furnished arsenical deposits, but afforded no evidence in Marsh's apparatus. Two quantities of human stomach, each weighing two ounces, were boiled for an hour, one with dilute muriatic, the other with dilute sulphuric acid, and the decoctions filtered off and mixed with from a fourth to a third of their bulk of rectified spirit. To about three ounces of each decoction 0·01 of arsenious acid was added, and the liquids then tested in Marsh's apparatus, but no arsenical stains could be procured; whereas, ordinarily, the one-hundredth of a grain of arsenious acid in three ounces of dilute muriatic or sulphuric acid, affords characteristic arsenical stains with the greatest facility.

From these results it appears that Marsh's process cannot be relied upon to detect minute quantities of arsenic in the presence of organic matter, that is, under conditions in which it can be most satisfactorily detected by Reinsch's process. The plan recommended by Dr. Odling for extracting the arsenic from an animal tissue, in a state suitable for testing, is as follows : About a quarter of a pound of the tissue, cut or broken up, is placed in a beaker glass with an ounce and a half of water, and half an ounce of muriatic acid. The beaker, with its contents, covered by a glass plate, is then stood upon a sand bath, and maintained at an almost boiling temperature, for half an hour. There is no fear of any arsenic being lost during this digestion, for even the first half of the distillate from such a liquid does not carry off a trace thereof, unless, indeed, a very large proportion be present. The decoction when cold is filtered, and a clear liquid obtained, holding dissolved all the arsenic originally present, even when a great portion of it existed in the state of tersulphide, from the action of sulphuretted products of decomposition.

This solution is then in a suitable condition for being tested by Reinsch's process, but to fit it for Marsh's apparatus it is distilled to dryness, or almost to dryness. There is no frothing or any other difficulty until the liquid has nearly all passed over, when it is necessary to be careful. To the residue, another half ounce of strong muriatic acid is added, and the distillation continued. On first applying heat after this addition, there is usually considerable frothing, lasting, however, for a few minutes only, after which the distillation can be carried to dryness without any difficulty. In this way, a colorless acid liquid, well fitted for testing in Marsh's apparatus is obtained, and a small *caput mortuum* entirely free from arsenic. This residue may be dissolved or oxidized by the usual methods, and examined for other metals. The distillate, instead of being tested in Marsh's apparatus, may be treated with sulphuretted hydrogen gas, when the yellow sulphide of arsenic, in a well characterized condition, is precipitated and may be collected and weighed. The arsenic present in the soil before referred to was estimated by this process, the precipitated sulphide being dissolved in ammonia, the solution evaporated to dryness, and the residue weighed. The residue remaining in the retort did not contain a trace of arsenic.

This process also serves for the detection of arsenic in the presence of certain metallic compounds which interfere with the action of Marsh's process, such as the salts of copper and mercury, in the presence of which no arseniuretted hydrogen is formed. The author states that the presence of bismuth does not at all detract from the delicacy of Marsh's test.

When oxidizing salts, such as chlorate or nitrate of potash, are present, which impede the action of this test, the author recommends their reduction by means of bisulphite of soda, the excess of sulphurous acid being afterwards driven off by heat.—*London Pharmaceutical Journal*, Jan. 1860.

vi. *Legislation on the Sale of Poisons.*

The apothecaries were recently taken by surprise by the announcement in the newspapers of the passage, during the late session of the Legislature of Pennsylvania, of a law on this subject, which rendered them liable to being fined for selling certain poisons unless with specified precautions. From the Druggists' Circular we learn that the New York Legislature also passed a law more stringent and applying to a larger number of poisonous articles than that of this State. The following is the Pennsylvania law, viz :

" No apothecary, druggist, or other person shall sell or dispose of by retail, any morphia, strychnine, arsenic, prussic acid, or corrosive sublimate, except upon the prescription of a physician, or on the personal application of some respectable inhabitant, of full age, of the town or place in which such sale shall be made. In all cases of such sale, the word *Poison* shall be carefully and legibly marked or placed upon the label, package, bottle, or other vessel or thing in which such poison is contained ; and when sold or disposed of otherwise than under the prescription of a physician, the apothecary, druggist, or other person selling or disposing of the same, shall note in a register kept for that purpose, the name and residence of the person to whom such sale was made, the quantity sold, and the date of such sale. Any person offending herein shall be guilty of a misdemeanor, and on conviction be sentenced to pay a fine not exceeding fifty dollars."

The general effect of this law will no doubt be useful, if its provisions are carried out by apothecaries and druggists, and all should endeavor to do so as strictly as possible, at least in spirit if not in letter. There are, however, some points arising out of its application which need attention. After setting forth to what class of persons only the apothecary and druggist shall dispose of poisons, viz.: those presenting a physician's prescription, and those considered to be "respectable inhabitants of full age," etc., the law says, "in all cases of such sale, the word *Poison* shall be carefully and legibly attached," etc. Now if we understand the tenor of the law, it means that when a physician prescribes either of the five poisons named in the law, the apothecary is bound to mark the vial or package with the word *poison*. Will physicians submit to this ? Is the apothecary justified in construing the law as applying to unprofessional demands only ? If not, must it apply to every case where the poison is diluted or associated in mixtures with other drugs, equally with those cases where sold pure and unmixed ? In a word, must the Liq. Morphiæ Sulphatis of the Pharmacopœia, and a solution of a grain or two of corrosive sublimate in a pint of syrup of sarsaparilla, be marked *Poison ?*

In our private opinion the law was framed to meet a particular class of cases, where these poisons are sold in a pure and concentrated form, and better adapted to be used maliciously, or with evil intent, and hence only those more commonly used for that purpose are named. If it were not so, why were not the long list of narcotic and irritant poisons named in the law, as opium and its preparations, aconite, veratria, tartar emetic, belladonna, croton oil, elaterium, etc. ? And if. the poisons of the law were intended to be marked "poison" when prescribed by the physician, why was not the same requirement extended to those other poisons which are more frequently prescribed ?

In regard to that part of the law requiring registration, it is all right and proper, and apothecaries and druggists should carry it out conscientiously for their own sakes and for the public good ; yet there is one case of frequent occurence which will cause trouble if literally construed. We mean where the head of a family sends a servant for corrosive sublimate for vermin—a very frequent occurrence. In such case can the apothecary consider the servant or messenger as a "respectable inhabitant" in the view of the law ? If not, will a note from the "head of the family," by the servant known to be such, be a sufficient guarantee ? if not, and the head of the family has to come and make "personal application," it will create great difficulty.

Before leaving the subject, it may be interesting to give a sketch of the requirements of the New York law, which we take from the Druggists' Circular of June, 1860.

"The New York law, as reported in this paper, requires that persons who sell poisons shall register the names and residences of parties purchasing, unless in cases of a physician's prescription. The labelling must be attended to properly. The poisons here referred to, are arsenic and its preparations, oxalic acid, corrosive sublimate, chloroform, sugar of lead, tartar emetic, opium and its preparations, oil of bitter almonds, the cyanides, deadly nightshade, and poison hemlock."

"The sale of the following poisons by retail is prohibited, except by the written order of a regularly authorized practising physician, whose name and residence shall be attached to such order : prussic acid, aconite, and its preparations, atropia and its salts, cantharides, croton oil, daturia and its salts, delphinia and its salts, digitalis and its preparations, nux vomica and its preparations, elaterium, ergot and its preparations, veratria and its salts, and cannabis indica and its preparations. A fine of one hundred dollars may be recovered for a violation of these restrictions."

This law, if literally carried out, will occasion much trouble to the apothecaries, and in practice it will be found nearly impossible, from the fact that various of the articles named are already in common legitimate family use, and for every demand the law requires a physician's prescription.

ART. XIV.—*Therapeutic Employment of Arsenic.*

DR. CHARLES ISNARD concludes a series of papers in *L'Union Médicale* with the following summary : Arsenic is an agent of the Materia Medica at once the most constant and certain in its effects, being altogether harmless in the hands of the skillful physician who knows how to administer it so as to be tolerated by, and advantageous to the sick. Equal to quinine in efficacy as a febrifuge, its cheapness brings it within the reach of the poorest patient. In simple intermittants it may be employed quite as successfully as the former, being useful even at the febrile access of both intermittents and remittents even when they are attended with symptoms of organic lesion, as for example, tubercular softening. Possessing as it does equal power with quinine, it should be nevertheless, for a time, interdected in the access of pernicious fever, as in this stage, the motive for its employment is not altogether evident, and, moreover, this fever is less rapidly supressed by it than by quinine ; its employment, however, should be reserved for exceptional cases of this fever, whether administered alone, or in combination with quinine. For relapses of intermittents which have resisted quinquina, arsenic is a heroic remedy. It appears, also, to be destined to play an important part in the treatment of nervous affections, as the great neuroses, particularly those whose therapy remains uncertain, as chorea, hysteria, epilepsy, asthma, and other nervous affections of the respiratory apparatus which are favorably influenced by this remedial agent ; while from the great facility with which it may be administered, it is preferable to the repulsion and excessively bitter preparations of quinine. It should, above all, be held in reserve for children. (" *Il doit être réservé principalement pour la médecine des enfants."*) During the infantile age, its employment is so easily instituted, that it deserves to be the general method in all those cases in which febrifuge medication is indicated, even in pernicious fevers. B. D.

ORIGINAL COMMUNICATIONS.

Continued from page 662.

ART. VII.—*Inguinal Aneurism Cured by Digital Compression:* Reported by W. C. NICHOLS, M. D.

HAVING a wish, during the past winter, to observe the treatment adopted by Dr. Warren Stone in various surgical affections, I frequently visited the wards in his charge at the Charity Hospital. Entering one of these on the 15th of February, ultimo, my attention was directed to a nurse who was attempting to adjust a compress to the groin of a patient in bed.

This patient informed me that his leg grew painful, and began to swell in January of the present year, and that a diversity of applications had been made to the tumid member by persons ignorant of his condition.

On the 2d of February, 1860, he consulted Dr. Andrew Smyth, at that time Assistant Surgeon of the Charity Hospital, who readily appreciating the cause of his malady, referred him to Dr. Stone for treatment.

I found, on examination, a pulsating tumor, about the size of a goose's egg, situated in the right groin above Poupart's ligament. The hand applied over the course of the external iliac artery received an impulse and a thrill characteristic of arterial tumors, whilst auscultation recognized a distinct aneurismal murmur. In point of fact, as each contraction of the heart sent a wave of blood along the artery, the heaving pulsation of the tumor was evident to inspection. The patient complained of great pain in the tumor when the blood rushed freely into it, and apprehensive of torture, he was eager to break the force of the current by digital or instrumental compression. By thrusting a thumb or finger deeply into the iliac region along the course of the artery, the painful mass could be circumscribed, and the flow of blood into the sac could be easily arrested. The superficial vessels of the corresponding leg and thigh, owing to the pressure of the aneurism, were tortuous, whilst the member was swollen and of a livid color. Satisfied that all pulsation in the tumor could be checked by pressing the thumb on the course of the artery, I felt assured that by securing competent assistants, the flow of blood into the aneurism could be moderated a sufficient length of time to promote the fibrination of its contents and effect a cure.

With the permission of Dr. Stone, I undertook the treatment of this case by digital compression. The rapidity of this cure must be attributed, in great part, to the intelligence of the gentlemen, both physicians and students, who kindly afforded assistance; for imbued with enthusiasm in their profession, they were ever vigilant in adopting such measures as would facilitate recovery and conduce to the comfort of the patient. I subjoin their names: Drs. Roberts and Fournier ; Messrs. Murphy, Tate, Turner, Shields, Robertson, Ford, Richardson, Parker, Jackson, McGregor, Lewis, Jones, Campbell, Denman, Collins, Moody, Profilet, Stickney, Sawyer, Haynes, Duffel, and Burke.

This patient, named Patrick Gilday, a native of Ireland, aged 28, was admitted to the Charity Hospital on the second of February, 1860.

Digital compression was begun in this case at five minutes after five o'clock, P. M., on Friday, February 17th, 1860. The treatment was begun by thrusting the thumb directly against the neck of the sac, so that all pulsation was speedily arrested. We at first found much difficulty in accomplishing our purpose ; for the tenderness of the parts produced spasm and rigidity of the abdominal muscles, and this condition, conjoined with the alternate elevation and depression of the abdominal walls, rendered doubtful our ultimate success. The indication was to benumb the sensibility of the patient, and a draught containing half a grain of morphia was administered. The benign influence of this potion rendered compression tolerable, and we entered upon our night watch with hopes of success.

On Saturday morning, February 18th, the tumor had diminished in size, and the pulsations were less forcible. The most flattering indications of recovery were presented during the day; for the patient, buoyed with hopes of relief, and calmed by the opiates, submitted without a murmur to the treatment. During the afternoon, when each assistant gave place to his successor, we discovered that pulsation would be arrested for several seconds ; and at eleven, P. M., pulsation entirely disappeared. We continued pressure during the remainder of Saturday night, and on Sunday morning, February 19th, at nine o'clock, A. M., during Dr. Stone's customary visit to the ward, he pronounced the cure effectual, and advised the withdrawal of pressure. Surprised at the rapidity with which this sac was obliterated, and fearful of untoward accidents, I requested the students to remain with the patient during the day. They continued their watch till eleven, P. M., only giving occasional pressure, and then retired, confident of a triumph in conservative surgery.

Thus, after making pressure for *thirty hours*, all pulsation ceased ; and within *forty hours* the cure was announced as successful, and within *fifty-four hours* our watch over the patient was withheld.

The patient was not permitted to leave his bed for several days ; yet, excepting a bandage applied to his leg to counteract œdema, no further treatment was directed. This patient left the Hospital on the 29th of February, 1860. He has returned on two occasions, submitting himself to inspection ; and on May 3d, he came, by request, to the Hospital, exhibiting a leg free from enlargement, yet presenting about the ankle a more livid hue than the opposite member. The aneurismal tumor had contracted to a firm nucleus about the size of a walnut. The patient informed me that since his departure from the Hospital, he has continued to work at a cotton press, around which every laborer is required to undergo great muscular exertion. It is a matter of surprise that no ill consequences have ensued.

In glancing over the records of surgery, I am unable to find a parallel instance of success in treating inguinal aneurism by digital compression. The cases reported by Broca, Michoux, Vanzetti, Gross, and others, were confined to the extremities ; and I am not aware that any surgeon has hitherto succeeded in controlling an aneurism by digital compression applied so near the great centre of the circulation. Dr. Gross, in his treatise on Surgery (1859), estimating the value of digital compression as compared with other modes of treatment, remarks : " It is to aneurisms of the extremities that this procedure is mainly, if not exclusively applicable, as the compression must be made to bear upon some point of the principal artery of the limb." And he adds : " The external iliac has been subjected to the same procedure in two cases of inguinal aneurism ; in one, the pressure was unbearable, and in the other, the assistants became so fatigued that it was discontinued. Moreover, it is very difficult in this situation to keep up the pressure, and such cases should, therefore, be excluded."

Satisfied, from the knowledge acquired in the treatment of this aneurism, that digital compression should be more frequently resorted to by surgeons, and hoping to invite attention to this mode of managing such maladies, I willingly submit this report for publication. Should failure ensue with this procedure in some cases of aneurism, its use prior to more serious operations, must necessarily protect the patient against many untoward accidents conseqent on the sudden arrest of the nutritive current to an important organ.

ART. VIII.—*Observations on Toxicology :* * By BENNET DOWLER, M. D.

ARSENIC, among poisons, is the principal agent used for both suici-

---

* This article has been suggested by the Articles II and III (in the Progress of Medicine), on Arsenic-Eating and on the Absorption of Arsenic by Plants, in the present number of this Journal. See page 671, *et seq*.

dal and homicidal purposes. The symptomatic evidence of poisoning by this mineral is most fallacious. Medical witnesses, courts, and juries should in no case consign an individual to the dungeon or hangman upon evidence solely of this character. Although this proposition is indisputable, yet there is reason to fear that the evidence of the symptoms supposed to be incidental to, or characteristic of, individual poisons, has been greatly overrated. Every experienced physician has encountered cases in which no poison had been taken, and yet the symptoms so closely resembled those produced by poisoning by narcotics, strychnine, arsenic, etc., that he has not been able to pronounce the difference with absolute certainty.

The chemical evidence of poisoning, though far more reliable, has been, and still is, received, to a great extent, as absolutely certain. Christison, one of the best of toxicologists, says, in his elaborate work on Poisons, that "the chemical evidence in charges of poisoning is generally, and with justice, considered as the most decisive. It is accounted most valid when it detects the poison in the general textures of the body, or in the blood, or in the stomach, etc. When poison is detected in any of these quarters, more especially in the stomach and intestines, it is seldom that *any farther proof is needed to establish the fact of poisoning*" (P. 54).

Authority, rather than direct personal observation and experience, governs the opinions of many. Even in chemistry this is true. The analytic chemist tells the world that certain reäctionary tests are the infallible indicants of certain poisons. But does any chemist hold in his experimental grasp a perfect synthesis of the infinite possibilities and potentialities of the whole, in virtue of his knowledge of a little part? What can analysis claim? Universality? Never. So far as I have experimented, this test is reliable. But am I certain that I have exhausted all the possible elements and combinations? May not some other poison, or even a substance not poisonous, afford a similar reäction? Accordingly, certain reägents, once deemed infallible as tests of certain poisons which cannot be reduced to their primitive state by art, have, in the course of experimental research, proved illusory, seeing that they give results common to different elements or combinations. Thus, the chemist, when unable to reproduce a poison in its primitive, sensuous, or concrete form, has recourse to various tests, seldom satisfied with one. The chemist is not in possession of a single necessary or universal truth, in the strict, absolute sense of those terms. His truths are conditioned, experimental, not being intuitions, the antitheses of which are not only absurd, but inconceivable, impossible. His utmost universality is soon told, namely: so far no exception to this rule is known, though this does not prove the impossibility of exceptions.

A professed toxicologist, who is a mere compiler, cannot be considered the best authority. However destitute he may be in originality, he may, by repeatedly verifying the experiments of others, be far more reliable than the busy practitioners of medicine usually are. The latter seldom, if ever, see a sufficient number of cases of poisoning to enable any single individual, either from symptoms or autopsies, not to mention chemical analysis, to testify positively in all cases. It is lamentable to hear or read the testimony on this subject in many cases, as given before courts of justice, by physicians and toxicologists. Inconsistency follows inconsistency—contradiction, contradiction—theory, theory. The accused at the bar is quite as likely to be honorably acquitted as a medical witness who is afraid to acknowledge that his knowledge is not universal ; that his experience is too limited, and that the state of science is too imperfect for him to answer categorically and positively, under oath, a tithe of the questions which the greatest sciolist at the bar may easily propound.

With regard to the quantity of arsenic which will prove mortal, there is little unanimity among writers.* Dr. Taylor, the latest authority in Medical Jurisprudence, says " a medical witness will be justified in stating that, under circumstances favorable to its operation, the fatal dose of this poison, in an adult, is from *two to three grains.*" Christison regards four and a half grains the smallest fatal dose on record. A quantity thus minute, diffused throughout the whole body, much of which is probably very quickly excreted, must be exceedingly small in any one part, or even all parts of the body at death. But suppose a trace, or even a notable quantity is found— what then ? Do not some of the very ablest chemists testify that arsenic is found in the human body as one of its normal products or elements ? Professor Lehmann, in his Physiological Chemistry, says:

---

* It will be seen (p. 673) in this Journal that arsenic-eaters begin with three and increase the dose to twenty-three grains ! How, then, can a medical witness swear that " from two to three grains " will kill ? Here, as in many other cases, it were better to " swear not at all."

"Devergie* and Orfila believed that they had found arsenic in all animal bones, and hence that it should be regarded as an integral constituent of the animal organism. Subsequent investigations have, however, shown that there must have been some fallacy in the method of analysis pursued by these chemists, and that this view is altogether erroneous." (i, 401.) Now, without affirming that Devergie and Orfila were right, it may be affirmed that higher adverse authority has not been cited by Prof. Lehmann. · Perreira (*Mat. Med.* i, 52) says : "Orfila asserts that arsenic exists in the bones of man and several other animals. But the experiments of Dr. G. O. Rees, MM. Danger and Flandin, and of the commissioners appointed by the French Academy of Sciences *(Jour. de Pharm.*, 1841) to report on Marsh's† apparatus, have failed to corroborate his statements." Is this impotent negation an infallible test ?

Those who read the second and third articles of the Progress of Medicine in this Journal, on Arsenic-Eating and on Arsenic in Vegetables, and accept them as authentic, must admit that forensic medicine, in relation to poisoning with this substance, can, upon the strongest chemical ground—namely: its reduction—arrive at little more than an "impotent conclusion." For, allowing that arsenic is not a normal constituent of the human economy, its secret use as a diet—the use of vegetables containing it—not to name utensils that may possibly sometimes be contaminated with its presence, and especially the two former facts, if facts they be, will, to a great extent, nullify the chemical evidence, *per se*, of criminality.

---

* Ann. d'Hygiène, Oct., 1830. *Ib.* July, 1840.

† It is now asserted by analytical chemists, that " Marsh's method is not applicable for the detection of minute quantities of arsenic, where much organic matter is present." This information comes too late for courts and juries whose verdicts .and sentences have led to the execution of many persons accused of poisoning.

REVIEW.

Review of a part of Professor PAINE'S *Institutes of Medicine:* By BENNET DOWLER, M. D.

IN discovery or originality, No. 14 (see Progress of Medicine in this Journal), Dr. Paine claims to have made the "special deduction of a *vital* principle," which he reïterates often as peculiar to his works at the æra of their advent : "When the foregoing works were first published," says he, "it was in the midst of a universal prevalence of the chemical and physical doctrines of life, and disease, and the author stood alone in the field of vital physiology." 913. In page 100, he says : "Sensibility, which is peculiar to the vital principle of animals, resides exclusively in the nervous system."

Without allowing that Dr. Paine ever stood alone or now stands alone on the vital platform—without conceding that his "deduction" or that of any other, has brought to light and demonstrated a vital *ens*, having attributes—*substantia et accidens*, nevertheless, a vital principle always was, now is, and perhaps will ever be admissible as a strong probability, although, as yet, neither its synthesis nor analysis has been discovered. Its "deduction" *per se*, from anatomy, chemistry, and physics has not been achieved, although its phenomenal history is very ancient.

The exact date of its discovery from this point of view, is not known ; but it is reasonable to infer, that it was anterior to the death of Abel. Adam and Eve must have studied its phenomenal history with intense interest (the only mode of investigation yet known, its *ens* being wholly undiscovered).

Although they were not professional anatomists, nor physiologists, they must have witnessed the death of birds and beasts—nay, they must have practised a little anatomy in killing animals for food, or for sacrificial offerings. Their son Abel was a "keeper of sheep," and was in the habit of slaying and offering as sacrifices, "the first-lings of his flock and of the fat thereof ;" and when Cain slew Abel, his sorrowing parents must have studied *Life and Death* as deeply as Bichât himself, whom M. Gigon, calls *the divine young man (le divin jeune homme)*, Hippocrates being "the divine old man."

At the present moment, the vital principle is the cause of a violent

93

war in Paris, concerning which, M. le Dr. AMÉDÉE LATOUR's Bulletins,
as reported in his able Journal, *L'Union Médicale*, will compare with
Ossian's : " Loud, rough, dark—chief mixes his strokes with chief—
steel clanging sounds on steel—helments are cleft." This may be
called the long war. With the first dawn of medicine, many a glittering sword leaped from its scabbard, and formidable fortifications
of logic were erected in defence of vitalism. M. Renouard, in his
History of Medicine, says of the Hippocratic æra, that " Physiologists
gave themselves up to transcendental speculations on the nature of
the principle of life." 95.

This quarrel, however, unlike the civil and religious quarrels
(about opinions) which have desolated the world, is for the most
part, a good one, and tends to renewed researches; and although the
nature of and formula for producing vitality will never be discovered
as a material or immaterial *ens*, yet the investigations which have
been made, and are now in progress (instance that on spontaneous
generation), must advance the science of biology, just as the search
after the philosopher's stone led to the ultimate establishment of
scientific chemistry. If the chemico-organical physiologists could
only succeed in combining the organic elements of a baby, so that
vitality would be the result, what a preventive of the pangs of childbirth there would be ! By keeping the elements *in equilibrio*, according to a given formula, death would never occur as long as chemical
knowledge and the supply of the elements abounded. This would
be infinitely preferable to spontaneous generation, which gives no
protection against death spontaneous.

Physiologists have assigned the vital principle to various tissues ·
of the economy as its seat. The Jewish lawgiver defines the vital
principle as follows : " *For the life of all ?flesh is the blood thereof.*"
(Leviticus, xvii, 14.) Harvey assigned the special seat of the vital
principle to the blood ; Hunter maintained the vital principle of the
blood ; Dr. Brown-Séquard says, that all the nervous and contractile
tissues in the brain, the spinal cord, nerves, muscles, etc., may, after
having lost their vital properties, their life, recover those properties
again, and in some respects be resuscitated by injecting fresh oxidated blood into the arteries, both in men and animals recently dead;
all of which he has established by actual experiments. Professor
Carpenter says, that the " physical, chemical, and other relations of
the blood, are quite subordinate to its *vital* reactions"—" its vital en-

dowment," being the "life of the body generally." In fact modern physiology is drifting rapidly towards, or rather is anchored with that of Israel's lawgiver.

Vitalists ought, however, to be prudent, since they cannot be positive in their definitions and demonstrations concerning the nature and seat of the vital principle. Let the *onus probandi* of disproving the vital principle, or of proving it a merely physical one, be as much as possible thrown upon the mechanical and chemical organicists. These latter philosophers cannot produce the analysis, and still less the synthesis of any kind of matter in which the vital principle is a necessary element or result, whether brain, sensation, understanding, will, stomach, womb, heart, eye, ear, etc. They cannot make similar structures and functions, like those inherent in the living economy; their finest crystals cannot think, nor their most elaborate compounds feel, nor their most perfect machines perform voluntary motion. Their most perfect combinations of the organic elements are as dead as the nails in a coffin, without the superadded, coöperating or antecedent force, essence, principle, or something else, known by its phenomenal history, not anywhere recognizable in mechanics or chemistry, being known by its fruits only.

The chemico-physiologist charges the vitalist with being an ontologist, and construes the vital principle as a veritable *ens* or entity. But the same logic applies with double force against the chemist. For, while he professes to reject unknown entities, he straightway substitutes one, namely, an unknown chemical entity or force no where found in the mere chemical or physical world of matter—a position far worse than that of the vitalist. The subjective evidence or the consciousness of possessing a vital principle, as a primary endowment, an essential element in his *ego* or personality, though no more explicable than understanding, will, and reason, is no insignificant evidence—but is a kind of evidence, not an iota of which is found in the materials and forces with which the mere chemist pretends to be conversant. Passion, health, pain, sickness, and with rare exceptions, medicinal action, cannot be accountable for, or attributed to, chemistry or physics.

Upon the whole that Adam and Eve must have understood the vital principle just as Dr. Paine understands it, may be inferred from the *Institutes*, page 73 : "It [the vital principle] is, in all but the vulgar acceptation, synonymous with the term *life.*"

Dr. Paine says, " All that we can know of the nature of any substance, material or immaterial, is by the phenomena it manifests " (117).

" Sensibility" says the author, " is peculiar to the vital principle of animals and resides *exclusively in the nervous system*. That which gives rise to *true* sensation is *mainly* limited to the cerebro-spinal system" (100). " *True* sensation is *mainly* limited to the cerebro-spinal system." What may be the meaning of *true* sensation ? can any sensation be *false?*

" The impressions transmitted by common sensibility are received by the brain alone, or its equivalent. The spinal cord is only a medium of communication" (100). Sensation is first ascribed to the brain and cord or " cerebro-spinal system," next to " the brain alone " or its equivalent !" What is this equivalent? certainly, not the cord, because " the spinal cord is *only* a medium of communication." " Impressions transmitted by sensibility." This new theory, is contrary to that which this book advocates, namely, " impressions are transmitted by the nerves exclusively to the brain alone ; the spinal cord is only a medium of communication." This cord, with the brain is, nevertheless, the seat of " true sensation." " Impressions transmit sensibility !" The book teaches that impressions are transmitted to, and received by, the brain alone ; but here the sensibility is first transmitted. The transmission of the impression and the sensibility both, is incomprehensible, superfluous and contradictory. If this review may be allowed to extend beyond the page 100, which at first was not intended, it will be seen that Dr. Paine announces as a law, that " sensitive impressions received by the sympathetic nerve, although conveyed to the cerebro-spinal axis, may *not be perceived by the sensorium !*" (350). This is a contradiction; for, " all sensitive impressions " not perceived, are not. It is impossible to conceive that a sensation can be such unless it be perceived or felt as such, all other impressions being insensible. Sensibility or feeling is not an objective or external entity, but is wholly subjective or internal, and is altogether restricted to individual sentient beings. Love not felt ! pain not perceived, are not. Here

> " Nothing is
> But what is not."

" The nervous power is an agent" (117). " The *attributes* of the nervous *power*" (91). "The nervous power with all its attributes" (116). Power is an attribute, not a substance. But here a power or attribute, has attributes, that is, attributes of attributes! White is an attribute of snow—ponderosity of gold. Has each of these attributes other inherent attributes? "Motion does not depend on the nerves" (127). "It is an assumption to say that the nerves have any generating effect upon the secreted products" (289). "Perception is necessary to sensation" (282). "The foundation [of medicine] is laid in the *principle of life, and its various attributes*" (405). "One principle, namely: *a vital principle, with various elements or properties*" (411). "The nervous power is superadded to the vital principle" (116). [A power added to a principle!] "The nervous power possesses the remarkable characteristic of being a vital agent to the property of irritability" (107). [The power is an agent!] "The nervous power does not generate motion either in animal or organic life" (110). [The power and the agent are motionless, powerless!] "It is important that the hypothetical words *motor* and *sensitve*, and *senso-motory*, do not betray us into the belief that the nerves are the causes of motion, or that there is any sensation connected with the organic phenomena of sympathy" (294). [The nerves cause no sensation! no motion! Yet, "sensation resides exclusively in the nervous system" p. 100]. According to page 100, the spinal cord, as an agent, is an entire negation, a perfect nonentity, an absolute antithesis of all sensation—yet, with the brain it is the seat of "true sensation," "the brain alone" is the seat of sensation, the cord is nothing but a conductor to the latter! propositions which logicians cannot reconcile.

Upon page 100 it is affirmed that "the nerves are the *organs of sensibility,* and the brain and spinal cord the *recipients* of impressions *transmitted by this property* through the medium of the nerves." Is not every part of this statement, so far as it is comprehensible, contradicted by every other part of it? The nerves are called the exclusive organs of sensibility, and at the same time nothing but the media by which impressions are transmitted to the brain and spinal cord where these impressions are received, after having been already sensationalized by the said organs of sensibility. If the nerves be the organs of sensibility—if they transmit this property and impressions also to the brain and spinal cord, the latter being mere receivers, must play but a secondary part, like the echo of the kiss mentioned in *Taming of the Shrew.*

"The impressions transmitted by common and specific sensibility are received by the brain alone, or its equivalent." Passing by this "equivalent," which is most equivocal, and omitting to notice the repetition that both sensibility and impressions are antecedent to their reception by the brain, it may be affirmed that the postulate implied that the hand cannot feel but the brain alone, or the latter and the cord, is a proposition contrary to the consciousness and intuition of every sane person—contrary to the writers' postulate already quoted, namely, "sensibility, which is peculiar to the vital principle of animals."

In the most literal manner impressions are said to be transmitted, sometimes to the brain alone, and sometimes to the latter and the spinal cord, while the nerves and even the cord are mere insensible conductors, conveying certain things to other things or places, called "their recipients." Neither vital nor moral principles are known to be transmitted to or by nerves and spinal cords, especially such as are wholly insensible. These runners which go along a material nerve, and are received by their material recipients, at a material place, must be material themselves, but as no one has discovered them microscopically or otherwise, their is no proof that they really exist. They are myths, or worse. The ancient mythology can be conceived as possible, but it is contrary to intuition or self-consciousness to affirm that the hand cannot feel as well as the head, that a burnt finger has no sensibility, etc.; and if the greatest physiologist in the land were to depose, in open court, to this as a fact, he would, as a witness, be set aside as *non compos mentis.*

"All of the modifications of sensibility are designed for the transmission of impressions from the circumference to the nervous centres" (100). Here the suface or periphery is not only the seat but the modifier of sensibility, a veritable sensorium which transmits these sensiferous impressions to the centres, which is contrary to the orthodox doctrine as received by the writer, and is withal an unnecessary circumlocution; for the *ego* or individual is conscious of these modified sensibilities or sensations upon the periphery, or sometimes in the centres; he can feel all over, all through. A burn on the surface can be felt there without taking the trouble to go to the centre, just as well as a colicky pain or a headache, can be felt in the centres without going to the outside to establish its status and obtain recognition.

While the brain subserves, or rather rules as lord paramount the intellectual faculties and the essential conditions of life, the periphery is its rival in acuteness of sensibility, as in seeing, hearing, tasting, smelling, and touch ; these are its antennæ or feelers thrown out for sensational purposes—a view which anatomy, as well as the testimony of the vulgar confirms—a view which even the book builders always advocate when they happen to forget, as they often do, their theory of the unknown sensorial spot in the brain. Thus Professor Carpenter, in his Principles of Comparative Physiology, says : " By the sense of touch is usually understood that modification of the common sensibility of the body, *of which the surface of the skin is the especial seat*, but which exists also in some of its internal reflexions. In some animals, as in man, nearly the *whole exterior of the body is endowed with it,* in no inconsiderable degree, being greatest in the fingers and lips," etc. That a stomach, heart, or brain, is necessary to the normal condition and perpetuation of life, does not disprove that the burnt nerves of a finger possess no sensibility whatever, but serve only as insensible conductors.

Great is common sense even in the text book theories of neurology. Although the nerves are divided into four distinct and separate kinds, and some say into six, the sensori-volitional, the excito-motory, the secretory and excito-secretory systems, yet only one kind is known to the anatomist and microscopist. All of these imaginary nerves, and the one set known to exist, are said to be mere insensible conductors of impressions to one or more unknown centres or spots, which do all the work of sensation. But when this theory is finished and testified to by every text-book—every lecturer, and every clinical teacher, is forced by intuition and common sense not only to ignore but flatly contradict the entire theory. He afterwards tells you that sensation prevails everywhere except in a few tissues, as the hair, nails, etc. Carpenter says, " where no nerves exist there is an entire absence of sensibility, as in the epidermis, hair, nails, cartilage, and bony substances of the teeth. The most sensible of all parts of the body is the skin," and so on from Alpha to Omega, all of which contradicts his theory and that of the orthodox text-books, namely, that all sensations have their seat in an unknown spot in the brain.

Suppose one of these system builders, with these views, to enter the great New Orleans Charity Hospital filled with patients, attended by a class of students seeking clinical instruction : the professor asks each patient where is the seat of your pain ? One answers, in the knee. Here, says the professor, is a case of articular rheumatism (writes pain in the brain). Another answers, the pain is in my finger—Whitlow (writes ditto)—Urethritis (ditto)—Ophthalmia (ditto)—Dysentery (ditto)—Abscess (ditto)—Burn (ditto). Thus the teacher goes on throughout M. de Sauvage's three hundred genera, not to mention his countless species of disease, writing down and referring all aches, as well as head-aches to the brain alone. He might, in this way be consistent, but he would be deemed insane. A theorist when sick himself never describes his colic pains or those from inflamed corns as being in the brain. Molière however, mentions a doctor who referred every symptom of disease to the lungs alone.

The Institutes is a book of commentaries upon the Physiological Commentaries and other works of the author, abounding with heterogeneous clippings from journals and books. The style is involved, obscure, tautological, and sometimes hardly grammatical; its rhetoric is as faulty as its logic often is ; all of which could be shown by a literary analysis of, and quotations from, the work, were such an undertaking likely to be either useful or consistent with the brevity of life and the narrow limits of journalism. The only originality characteristic of the book is in its infinitesimal numerals and references, nearly all of which centre in the author, together with laborious attempts to prove a number of self-evident truths.

Of those who do not assent to the laws of sympathy, Dr. Paine kindly says : " These they have yet to study and learn ; but it may be well objected that their ignorance shall prove an obstacle to the progress of knowledge. He, indeed, must have been an imperfect spectator of human events, who anticipates the acquiescence of ignorance or prejudice, or the ready concurrence of inferior minds, in the intricate problems which relate to the laws of the vital functions " (112). " Is there a scientific effect of morbific and remedial agents, operating through the nervous systems, which cannot be clearly, perfectly, explained by the doctrines which I have propounded in relation to the nervous power ? Can a like affirmation be made of any other thing ? " (314). Several parallel statements were made by Paracelsus. " We have already compassed the general philosophy of life, of disease, and of medicine" (411). At last! Celsus considered the art of medicine conjectural ("*ars conjecturalis*") and experience itself as in the same category, which it virtually is, not in itself, but owing to our imperfect interpretation of its apparent anomalies—a view fully sanctioned by all his successors whose opinions are entitled to respect. The progress of scientific medicine is a progress in probability—a cumulative certainty, characterized by an abandonment of systems, or, " general philosophies of life and of disease."

" He [the physician] knows as much of the properties of life as of the remedial agent. He knows them far better; and that he admits their existence and specific nature is manifest from his deliberate action. Whoever prescribes for disease upon any other ground is a mere charlatan " (119). Physicians prescribe quinine for intermittents and analogous diseases, not from a knowledge of "the specific nature " of the vital principle—not from a "specific" knowledge of the nature, *modus operandi* and adaptation of this remedial agent in the cure of the disease, but from an abundant experimental evidence, showing that quinine is an efficacious remedy; and so all other cases in practice. For anything known of the "specific nature of the vital principle," quinine should cause—not cure intermittents.

"By no artificial means can the diseased properties and functions of life be converted into their healthy state. The most efficient remedial agents institute their favorable effects by establishing new pathological conditions ; which farther shows that it is nature alone which cures, and through the foregoing principle " (122); that is, medicines can't cure, but they make new diseases which can cure. Does like cure like ? or contraries, contraries ? Has the vital principle or "the new pathological conditions instituted in it by medicines," any anatomical characters discoverable upon post-mortem examination? According to a prevalent anecdote, a certain doctor gave notice that he could not cure a fever, but would change it into fits, and that he was death on fits. This is a complete parallelism with the doctrine quoted. "Connected with the foregoing law is another not less fundamental, which shows the fallacy of reasoning from the effects of remedial agents upon healthy to morbid conditions" (*Ib.*). If this be true, experimental pathology must be false.

The science of therapeutics is based on this principle and analogical reasoning.

"Those who have regarded it [morbid anatomy] of paramount importance have entertained but very limited views in physiology, or of the laws of disease. The multitude lost sight of disease in its vital aspects, and undertook a system of pathology out of the last wrecks of disease * * * when I undertook their systematic examination" (456). "Morbid anatomy, as taught by the materialist school, has precluded all regard for those pathological conditions upon which the lesions of structure and physical products truly depend, and about which the art of medicine is mainly interested. Morbid anatomy has not, in an original sense, ever given us a solitary clue to the pathology of disease, any more than healthy anatomy to the natural organic functions" (458). The intelligent physician needs no argument in refutation of these dogmas.

Professor Paine says of the homœopathist, that " his doctrines in pathology and therapeutics are a thousandfold better, more rational, more consistent, more conducive to health and life, than any or all the tenets of the chemical and physical schools" (558).

"There is no objection to admitting that all remedial and morbific agents find their way, very scantily into the circulations, excepting as it regards the matter of fact. No conclusions can be formed from the effects of injections into the circulation" (677). Sympathy and reflex action can do almost everything in "his philosophy."

"The laws of life and the laws of chemistry are as wide as the poles from each other" (419). If this be endorsed "by his own country with great unanimity," the said country must, like the Professor, "stand alone." Simon's big book, *Animal Chemistry on the Physiology and Pathology of Man;* Lehmann's voluminous work, *Physiological Chemistry;* and Lowig's *Physiological Chemistry,* and many other elaborate works of a kindred character now in the hands of medical students, " are falsifications and perversions of his [Prof. Paine's] statements and opinions " (see preface), and, therefore, false guides and enemies to science. Is no chemical law (nearer than the poles) concerned either in the fluids, as the blood, urine, etc., or in the solid tissues, both in their normal and diseased states ?

At every successive application of remedial agents, the new pathological conditions should form the ground of the new prescriptions" (428). Now, as the first prescription, according to the author, must be for the purpose of producing "*a new pathological condition,*" and all subsequent ones must have the same effect. Hence, it is to be feared, that the medication would be perpetual, as the last prescription would always create a "new pathological condition" or cause for the next, and so on *ad infinitum.* There is only one way to avoid this logical conclusion, namely, to deny the premise and to affirm that, with rare exceptions, a prescription is intended, not to create a new pathological condition but to destroy an existing one, and, this being accomplished the medication might "surcease," which would be an advantage to the patient, if not to the doctor and apothecary.

In his preface, Dr. Paine avers that all of his critics who do not commend his books, are falsifiers and perverters. He says : "The author feels it his right to say that, in *all* the critical reviews which have fallen under his observation, whose *objects* have been to affect his writings *injuriously, such* reviews have consisted *altogether of falsifications and perversions* of his statements and opinions." The author does not fail to show the other side of the picture, namely: "Another preface enables him, also, to express his sense of obligation for the generous opinions which have recently appeared in the Medical Press of *his various professional writings.* It is especially gratifying that this *tribute* has been rendered with *great unanimity* in his own country, and he desires no greater reward for his toil and anxiety." (The Italics have been added.)

Neither Dr. Paine nor any other doctor is of sufficient importance to be an "object" of "injurious" attacks by "all the critical reviews" which dissent from him ; nor has Dr. Paine "the right" to charge "*all*" their "reviews" as being "*altogether* falsifications and perversions." With rare exceptions, far other objects impel the reviewers of medical books. The interests of science and of truth are paramount. Neither friendship for author nor publisher, should bias critical reviewers. Praise unworthily bestowed is robbery of the worthy. Readers have a "right" (for which they pay) to an honest editorial opinion "without fear, favor or affection," and for reasons which might be readily imagined indiscriminate praise, rather than malicious censure is the weak point of editors in reviewing authors. Reviewers may be mistaken, or they may be "falsifiers ;" but that "*all* the reviewers" which dissent from what Dr. Paine in the first page of his work announces as the "difficult achievement," namely, his purpose to establish the "laws that shall stamp the whole as the *Philosophy of Medicine*," have originated " altogether in falsification and perversion," is a gratuitous statement, and by no means charitable. These .dissenters (some whom the writer of this paper knows and believes to be men of ability and moral excellence) doubtlessly felt it to be a duty to advise their readers that Dr. Paine's philosophy and medical philosophy were not identical, and, that the former ought to be prevented from rising into credit, for fear that it might displace the latter. Dr. Paine's book is what is called a success. It has reached the fifth edition (the *Principia* reached a second edition in thirty years), and its praise has been sounded, according to Dr. Paine, " with great unanimity," which is presumptive, though not demonstrative proof, that "stamps the *whole as the Philosophy of Medicine*," and which he naïvely says " is especially gratifying."

MISCELLANEA.

A PHILOSOPHER'S ACCOOUNT OF HIS OWN CASE OF PALSY.—A PHYSICIAN'S
ACCOUNT OF THE PROGRESS OF HIS* DEATH.

Varnhagen, the confidential friend and correspondent of Humboldt, in his diary of Feb. 27, 1857, says : "M. Hermann Grimm called, coming from Humboldt's apartments, where he had conversed with Seiffert, the valet. It is not a cold that has befallen Humboldt, but a far more serious attack, a paralytic stroke. After the court ball on Tuesday evening, he felt unwell; in the night he left his bed to drink some water—wished to avoid disturbing the servant—and fell upon the floor. Seiffert awoke with the noise, and found his master speechless and unconscious ; it was some time before he revived. Privy Councillor Schœnlein is not sanguine ; he had not a very good night."

Humboldt (March 19, 1857), who gives an account of his own case, in a letter to Varnhagen, says : " What my nervous affection

was, which produced a paralysis of such short duration, with the
functions of the brain remaining entirely free, with pulse unchanged,
with preservation of sight, and of all motion of the extremeties
subject to will, I cannot divine. There are magnetic storms (the
polar light), electric storms in the clouds, nervous storms in man,
heavy and light ones—perhaps, also sheet lightning, *foreboding* the
others. I had serious thoughts of death, *comme un homme qui part,
ayant encore beaucoup de lettres à écrire.*" (*Humboldt's Letters*, 1860.
Pp. 357-8, 360-1.)

The late Professor Retzius, of Stockholm (born 1796 — died
April, 1860), is reported (in the medical and literary journals) to
have speculated upon the progress of his own death thus : This
struggle of death is hard, he said to those about him ; but it is of
the highest interest to note this wrestle between life and death ; now
the legs are dead, now the muscles of the bowels cease their function, the last struggle must be heavy, but for all that it is highly
interesting. These were his last words.

[This eminent Swedish physician had gained for himself a solid
reputation, not only throughout the medical world, but also throughout the world of science. In a letter which I received (before Prof.
Retzius's death) from Prof. Rafn, Councillor of the State of Denmark,
the most honorable mention is made of Prof. Retzius as a man of
science. B. D.]

HORA HARVEIANA :

An Address delivered at the Annual Meeting of the Harveian Society, Edinburgh,
April 13, 1860: By JAMES MILIER, F.R.S.E., P.R.C.S.E., etc., late President
of the Harveian Society, Prof. of Surgery in the University of Edinburgh, etc.

[THE following extracts from an article of twelve pages are copied
from the *Edinburgh Medical Journal.*]

Harvey was not gifted profusely by Nature.—" In person," we are
told, " he was not tall, but of the lowest stature; round-faced ; oli-
vaster (like wainscot) complexion ; little eye, round, very black,
full of spirit ; his hair dark as a raven." Yet, notwithstanding
these bodily defects, he grew to be a *great* man—somehow—a very
" giant in those days."
Neither does he seem to have had any surpassing gift of natural
talent ; his mental stature, at first, bulks no larger than that of
other men. We look in vain for any sign or proof of those flashings
of early genius which, in others, have more or less plainly foretold
the coming might of the coming man. And yet, step by step, he

trod the steep and slippery path of renown, until at length he rested
securely on its very topmost ledge.

He was of noble descent, however ; *he had a good mother.* On her
tombstone her qualities are thus described : " A godly, harmless
woman ; a chaste, loving wife ; a charitable, quiet neighbor ; a
comfortable, friendly matron ; a provident, diligent housewife ; a
careful, tender-hearted mother ; dear to her husband, reverenced of
her children, beloved of her neighbors, elected of God ; whose soul
rests in heaven, her body in this grave—to her, a happy advantage ;
to hers, an unhappy loss." An American writer has quaintly said,
that "it is far more noble to be born of those who have been born
of God, than to be grandchildren of the devil," however illustrious,
in some respects, these latter may be, or have been. "Far more
noble ?" Ay, and far more profitable too. It is a goodly inheritance, the sonship of a good mother. The virtues by her side of the
house descend, and are, in a sense, hereditary. "She may drop into
the grave ; but she has left behind her influences that will work for
her. The bow is broken ; but the arrow is sped, and will do its
office." The "mother wit" often proves the best patrimony. For
gifts are better than gold, and a good name more precious than
rubies.

He had a liberal education.—Grounded in elementary knowledge
at the grammar school of Canterbury, he "studied classics, dialec-
tics, and physics," at Cambridge ; and, leaving that university at
the end of four years, with the degree of B. A., he spent five years
more at Padua, in mental training of a more professional kind, under
Fabricius ab Aquapendente, graduating at the age of twenty-four.
This was good capital to start in business with ; and such like it is
in the power of all to give, besides the inheritance of an honest
name, to their descendants.

Harvey married early, securing a helpmeet for his working, and
that in good time. Graduated at 24, he wived at 26, and *then*
launched fairly into practice. This is at variance with the principles
of some—directly and rightly at variance. To initiate exertion is
not so difficult as to sustain it.

But it is not in mortals to command success. At the most, we can
but deserve it. Harvey's wife was childless.

The atmosphere of a Royal Court is not supposed to be usually
very favorable to professional study and scientific progress ; but in
the case of Harvey it proved no bar to either. When first appointed
Extraordinary Physician to King James, he had already mooted his
views in regard to the circulation ; and his patient inquiries on that
subject seem to have been steadily prosecuted during the reign both
of that monarch and of his successor, Charles, until, in 1628, they
culminated in the production of his celebrated Treatise on the
"Motion of the Heart and Blood." In the society of Vandyke and
Rubens, the delights of their art could not beguile him from the love
of his own ; and the frivolous fascinations of the courtier-throng
seem to have but given him a fresh zest and quickened appetite for
his own peculiar pursuits.

Upright conduct on the part of Harvey, the Court physician, was not without its reward. Not only did it secure the respect, and even love, of his royal master, who took quite a personal interest in the prosecution of the physiological inquiry ; but in the end came the perfecting of the discovery which rendered the name of Harvey immortal.

Then, however, stepped in envy and detraction ; and the proverb was to be realized, that "a prophet is not without honor, save in his own country." The physiologist could be no physician, forsooth ! Now, at the ripe age of 50, it was suddenly discovered that he was "cracked-brained." "He fell mightily in his practice," says Aubrey, "and all the physicians were against him." Giving him every credit as an excellent anatomist, they could not "admire his therapeutique way ;" they turned up their noses at his "bills," or prescriptions, and vowed that they could not tell what he therein aimed at. Wise and disinterested creatures ! Was it the knowledge they had gained from Harvey that so cleared their eyes and understandings as to enable them to see the failings of their master, to which they had before been blind ? or was it but the fruit of moral jaundice come upon them, casting the eye, so that it

' Sees strains upon the flowers most chaste,
And hates all goodness (greatness), for it shares it not ?''

But though patients forsook Harvey, patience did not. Ais aim was, not practice, but progress ; the voice that he regarded was not that of the multitude, but the still, small voice within himself. Confident in the truth and strength of his own position, he could afford to let the lesser things pass by—much too honest, through any compromise of truth, to higgle for a following. Galileo, threatened with loss of life, is said to have retracted the assertion of his great discovery : Harvey, less pressed indeed, yet facing the loss, if not of life, at least of living, wavers nothing ; but stands upon his ground, upright, like a man ; and, ready for all comers, offers fair and honest fight, assail him who so may.

Originally, he was of a most choleric disposition ; and "in his younger days," says Aubrey, "he wore a dagger, as the fashion then was, which he would be apt to draw out on every occasion." But, as the philosopher grew and ripened in his knowledge of outward things, the man grew and ripened in knowledge of himself, attaining ultimately to such self-command as kept him from all strife and contention with his enemies—content to reason quietly with those amenable to reason, and leaving the rest, unheeded, to bark and bite as they chose. To the wordy Primerose he deigned no reply. But with Caspar Hofman, "a foeman worthy of his steel," he argues patiently in his native Nuremberg, with scalpel in hand demonstrating the truth of his averments ; and when at length all present are convinced, save the obdurate Caspar, Harvey, without a word, lays down the knife and walks away. The choleric youth, dagger in hand, had grown into the calm and cool philosopher ; yet, not wanting in dignity and self-respect, ready to assert his rights and privileges becomingly. For we find him testifying to "the very excellent John Nardi," that he "makes no case of the opinions and criticisms of our pretenders to scholarship, who have nothing but levity in their judgments, and indeed are wont to praise none but their own productions; while, with the unbelieving Hofman he remonstrates thus, epistolarily : "Do not vilipend the industry of others, or charge it them as a crime; do not derogate from the faith of an honest man, not altogether foolish or insane, who has had experience of such matters for a long series of years. Farewell! and *beware!* and act by me as I have done by you."

And in the end comes the reward. Harvey *lives* down all scoffs and scepticisms as to his own merits. Real worth needs no aid from angry words. And he lives, too, to see his discovery triumphant over all opposition, openly established and acknowledged in the schools. Truth asks no help from the strife of tongues. Do we not well to remember this in all our contendings for it?—never sacrificing one atom of truth for peace, and never invoking war for anything short of truth. "Peace is so precious a jewel," said one, "that I will give anything in purchase of it save truth." "First pure, *then* peaceable," is the axiom, infallible and inflexible. Contend for truth, assuredly, and seek that first ; but let all our contendings be largely tinctured with that "softness of answer" that "turneth away wrath ;" and, discarding the personal quite, let us so shine that, while in opinions on *things* we may be at open and prolonged war, we shall, notwithstanding, " if it be possible, as much as lieth in us, live peaceably with all *men*."

In taking a side, too, it may be well to have a preliminary combat with oneself, not only to bring into wind and condition for fighting, but also to make sure that we are right as to place and cause on and for which we propose to fight ; and this all the more as we grow in what ought to bring wisdom—years. It is a portentous fact that no man believed in Harvey's discovery, at the time, who numbered more years than forty. And so, let those of us who may have turned that intellectual climacteric, beware of doggedness and dogmatism in any cause which at the first sight may seem either false or offensive ; making sure, as far as we may, that, ere we close in combat with our opponent, we have conquered all bigotry and prejudice within ourselves.

To ensure this self-command, this εγκρατεια, Harvey no doubt lived by rule, and temperately. Yet, I fear we cannot lay claim to him as an absolute Nephalist, inasmuch as we learn that *gout* laid hold of him in his latter years—not very severe, however, and not connected with organic disease, else he had not found his simple treatment either so safe or so successful. "He would sit with his legs bare, though it were frost, on the leads of Cockaine House, put them into a pail of water till he was almost dead with cold, and betake himself to his stove—and so 'twas gone." So aqueous in his tendencies for the outer man, we incline to think he must have used wine most sparingly for the inner ; all the more, as we know for certain how devoted he was to the coffee-cup, ere that grew much in fashion, bequeathing his favorite "coffey-pot" as a special legacy to his well-beloved niece, Mary West. The discoverer, not only of the circulation of the blood, but also of the muscular mótive power of the heart, may well be supposed to have known that the normal action of that organ, and the normal distribution of that fluid, ordinarily needed no fierce and fiery stimulant.

His own calm circulation brought sweetness and sociality of disposition with it. The quarrelsome young bantam had grown into the most amiable of roosters. The dagger—fit token of heat and anger—had long been laid aside ; and Harvey, in his mature age, is said to have "possessed, in a remarkable degree, the power of persuading and conciliating those with whom he came in contact. In the whole course of a long life we hear nothing either of personal enemies or of personal enmities." " Man," he says himself, naturally taking a physiological view of the matter, "comes into the world naked and unarmed, as if nature had destined him for a social creature, and ordained that he should live under equitable laws, and in peace." And, indeed, he seems to have ultimately acquired an absolute distaste for war, even in its most attractive and exciting form. Moving with the army, he attended his royal master at the battle of Edgehill ; and "during the fight the Prince and Duke of York were committed to his care. He told me," says Aubrey, "that he withdrew with them under a hedge, and took out of his pocket a book and read ; but he had not read very long before a bullet of a great gun grazed on the ground near him, which made him remove his station." Fighting suited neither his business nor his inclination ; and so engrossing was his devotion to the main pursuit of his life, that even in the din and bustle of a battle he could find time for carrying it on, all but undisturbed, save by the occasional and random grazing of a "bullet from a great gun."

Harvey, in his old age, made himself master of Oughtred's " Clavis Mathematica," according to Aubrey, who found him "perusing it, and working problems, not long before he died." Himself tells us— "Did I not find solace in my studies, and a balm of my spirit in the memory of my observations of former years, I should feel little desire for longer life." And in a letter to his friend Nardi, in reference to physiological and psychological researches, he says : "I myself, though verging on my 80th year, and sorely failed in bodily strength, nevertheless feel my mind still vigorous, so that I continue to give myself up with the greatest pleasure to studies of this kind." And in another place he refers to the promised appearance of Nardi's " Noctes Geniales " thus—"I am used to solace my declining years, and to refresh my understanding, jaded with the trifles of every-day life, by reading the *best* works of this description."

So he passed calmly on—pleasantly to himself, usefully to others —adding one thing more to all we have already spoken of, *the* " one thing needful ;" not deferring that till now, at the last, but having taken it with him all the way—as a bright thread of gold intertwining the entire web of life ; at length able to say these grave and good words at parting, "I do most humbly render my soul to Him that gave it, and to my blessed Lord and Saviour Christ Jesus."

95

THE great bulk of our readers are necessarily men of literary tastes, and we are proud too to know that we secure the attention of that portion of the Profession whose habits are also literary, and who have the ear and the respect of the public. All are more or less interested in the question of International Copyright. This we brought forward in a somewhat practical tone a few weeks ago. There has now been time for an echo to reach us from the other side of the water, and the surge and boom of it are thoroughly Trans-atlantic. England has a great literature; America "has authors second to none." England has disclosed many noble truths of science; "the greatest scientific discoveries of the last twenty years have been made in America." England demands an interna-tional copyright on the wide, open ground of justice and the good of all; "America does not propose to discuss this question in the abstract," but calculate some of the benefits to American literature which would result from an international copyright. These are the grand reverberations which beat upon us. Much better this big, young talk, than mere stagnation; and we can afford to listen placidly, and to smile hopefully. But let us also catch up and exam-ine some few of the fainter utterings which the subject prompts an American editor to say. He would altogether repudiate and abjure sympathy with "international stealing," "the larcenies committed by some of our American journalists," "common plundering," and "scissoring." He acknowledges "piracy to be a crime," and spurns the flimsy fallacies about "cosmopolitan philanthropy," "the univer-sal character of science," and the "hardship of the lets and hindrances of legal enactments." The whole American system of reprinting is admittedly bad, and it is not worth while spinning fine webs of sentiment about it to conceal its deformities, or wasting grand language in trying to defend it. Let it go; and let America have the advantage of an international copyright. After all, it is better to look at the matter in its practical bearings, for *(aside)* if we have not a national Medical literature, we have a good share of American Medical vanity; and there is something to be said about that. The real truth is, that foreign and especially English books, are not reprinted on account of their superiority, or, at any rate, on account of their superiority to what might be done in America. It is cheaper to reprint than to pay authors; and it lies in human nature to buy cheap reprints, provided they are not much worse than the original works which there are American writers always ready to produce if circumstances permitted. The system starves the foreign author, and represses native talent. The English book-maker would write better if he had American remuneration; and the Americans do not write at all because the bookseller will not pay them. The literary labor of England and the literary "labor" of America, may be declared the highest and hardest work that man is capable of performing, and both should have a pecuniary reward. Pay both, and we should soon see where one would be.

Then, again, the respectability of American authorship is an im-portant consideration. The "social evil" of American literature is the "American editor." Trains have their conductors, Atlantic steamers have their harbor pilots, Washington's nurse and Jenny Lind had their Barnum, and it seems to be a settled point in the American constitution, that every English book is to have its "American editor." An American editor equivalent to a Barnum and a social evil ! what are we to understand by this questionable title ? Simply, we are informed that in the great majority of of cases it means nothing more nor less than the "proof reader," bestowing cheap literary honor and repute, frequently where it least belongs, and in other cases humbling those who are fully competent to produce as good an original work as the one which they edit to the position of proof readers and American editors, because it pays better to the publisher to reprint than to *risk* an original work." Now, this is quite wrong, and there are all sorts of American reasons why the evil should be suppressed by an international copyright. Honesty, equity, the advancement of science, are all good reasons ; and the liberation of original research and scientific "labor" from the oppression of the yearly inundation of reprints in every branch of science is imperative. America need not be dependent any longer on foreign discoverers. Why should the young country always have to be reading accounts of what the old ones have done and are doing, instead of cutting out a career and immortality for itself ? Let American booksellers be made to pay, and let American authors and original researchers flourish ! So say we also. There are good hearts and sound minds, steady observers and eloquent writers, in that land of our children ; and we wish for nothing more than that they should have fair play in the race, and speedily outstrip their fathers, if they can, in the work of doing good to mankind.—*Med. Times and Gaz.*

SINGULAR DEATH FROM INHALING CHLOROFORM, ETC.

Sir—An anomalous or unusual death from chloroform, probably from asphyxia rather than syncope, has occurred at Doncaster. As the case is suggestive, showing the danger of accumulative doses of this anæsthetic, or (however we are to explain it) the danger of single small doses, the facts are deserving of being placed on record.

The lady (Mrs. M.) had originally chloroform given her about four years ago, I am informed by Mr. Moore, her medical attendant, for violent attacks of hysteria, amounting at times to temporary mania. Chloroform, he states, *at once* (all other means having failed) relieved all the symptoms; and, in doing so, produced such a feeling of abiding relief, that the poor lady continued for more than four years to take it at very frequent though uncertain intervals. Repeated expostulation with herself personally, and with the druggists of the town, failed to prevent her getting large quantities of chloroform. She has been known to consume or purchase as much as ten or eleven ounces in a day (one chemist says fifteen), and has, I believe, seldom passed a month without procuring some similar doses of her suicidal anodyne.

The point in the case I think most remarkable is the evidence given at the inquest by a little girl ten years of age, who was in the habit, poor child ! of sprinkling the chloroform on a handkerchief for her mamma, and was so engaged the day of the fatal accident, when it seems Mrs. M. happened to suffer more than usual from her hysteric pains, and went to bed three several times, to have chloroform three several times administered, about an ounce each time ! The first ounce was taken before breakfast. Mrs. M. then got up quite well, and went out about her ordinary household duties. She then had another dose in the middle of the same day, which also did not seem to produce any unusual effect. She then got up, and we find her again going to bed in the evening (a third time), and taking with her an ounce and a half bottle of chloroform ; the same little girl and the children playing about her bed ; so that the skill of this little girl, which answered twice the same day already, and on hundreds of opportunities before for the administration, now failed. Nay, we find this little girl saying that at nine o'clock the chloroform was " taking " very well ; but, in about an hour after, the children suspected something was wrong; *"the cloth was over mamma's face."* Their mamma was dark-colored, and had been snoring. She was, in fact, some time cold and dead at ten o'clock !

I am inclined to think this lady took no food this day, and that she was very much exhausted from pain and want of food. The death was probably from simple suffocation or asphyxia. The post-mortem examination, though very carefully made, tells us nothing; it is, however, in its details, very like four other post-mortem examinations of this sort that I have seen. We have, too, the old and curious contradiction—a patient taking one day fifteen ounces with impunity, and sinking under about an ounce another day l

I am, etc., CHARLES KIDD.
Sackville street, Picadilly, June 12th, 1860.
British Medical Journal.

STEARATE OF IRON.

Dr. Calvi, states, in the *Union Médicale*, for May 5th, that M. Ricord has successfully employed a plaster of stearate of iron as a dressing for phagadænic ulcers of the thighs in a syphilitic patient, which had resisted all previous treatment. . A comparative trial was made with this preparation and coal-tar ; and the former was found to be by far the most efficacious.

Stearate of iron is made in the following way : Take of sulphate of iron one part ; soap, two parts. Dissolve the sulphate of iron and the soap in water separately. On adding the solutions to each other, a greenish white precipitate is obtained ; this is dried, and melted at a temperature of from 175° to 190°; essence of lavender (40 per cent.) is then added, and the whole is stirred until it cools. A plaster can be formed by gently melting it and spreading it on linen.

IODIDE OF AMMONIUM.

M. Gamberini of Bologna has, from an experience of fourteen

cases, arrived at the following conclusions regarding the use of iodide of ammonium in constitutional syphilis.

Iodide of ammonium is indicated in all cases where the iodides of potassium and sodium are employed, and produces a rapid cure. In syphilitic cases the following results were obtained: five were cured in a fortnight, three in three weeks, five in a month, and one in five weeks. In the last case, the medicine was not well tolerated, and had to be given in small doses.

The dose is from two to sixteen grains daily; the last named quantity is but rarely required. Intolerance is an exceptional occurrence. Externally, iodide of ammonium has been usefully employed in frictions (three grains to an ounce of olive oil), in cases of nocturnal syphilitic pains of the muscles or joints.

Intolerance of the medicine is denoted by a burning sensation in the throat and heat in the stomach; these rapidly cease when the medicine is suspended for a day or two.

M. Gamberini states that he has removed, by means of iodide of ammonium, the indurations following the cicatrisation of chancre, and the enlargements of inguinal glands. The other syphilitic affections in which he has employed it successfully are, astralgia, rheumatic pains, periostoses, and enlargement of the cervical glands.

M. Gamberini states that iodide of ammonium possesses the following advantages over the analogous salt of sodium: 1. Its action in attaining the same therapeutic object is more rapid. 2. A much smaller dose is required. (*Bulletino delle Scienze Mediche;* and *Gazette Hebdomadaire,* June 1st, 1860.)

The conclusions at which M. Gamberini has arrived with respect to the iodide of ammonium agree very closely with those stated by Dr. Richardson in a communication to the Medical Society of London, reported in the Journal for the present year.—*Ib.*

ANIMAL GRAFTING. (Translation.)

A Case of Animal Engraftment. (Observation de Greffe Animale) communicated to the *Journal de Médecine de Bordeaux,* for July, 1860, by M. Azam, is of great interest. He reports, that on the 5th of May, 1860, Jean Desplats, of Talence, near Bordeaux, while dressing a piece of wood with a very sharp hatchet, from a badly directed blow cut off about three *centimètres* of the index finger of the left hand, in an oblique direction cutting the nail in two, and shaving the phalangette laterally, including the almost entire ball of the finger. The pain and loss of blood caused complete syncope. A neighbor who was present, directed his first care to the assistance of the patient; after which, the happy thought occured to him to replace the separated portion, which he did, about ten minutes after the accident, covering the part with copaiva. Three hours afterward, the paitent came to my ward for advice. The resident adjunct, M. Vergely, who was in attendance, found that the part had been completely separated. It was bandaged.

Three days later, Desplats attended the ward, at the time of my visit, and again, three or four days afterward. A stylet passed through the bandages to the ball of the finger, proved that the part was perfectly sensible. The engrafting was certain and perfect ; the color, however, being black, caused some fears of mortification.

On the fourteenth day the bandages were all removed. The black portion mentioned was found to be nothing more than a clot effused beneath the cuticle ; the latter only was mortified.

The line of the cicatrix indicated in the most evident manner, that the fragment had been completely separated, affording an indelible proof that the attempt (which in parallel cases ought to be imitated) was altogether successful.—B. D.

THE EXPENSES OF THE LAST SICKNESS BEFORE DEATH, AND ALSO BEFORE INSOLVENCY.

It appears from the *Gazette des Hôpitaux* (July 10, 1860), that the Commercial Court of Montargis has interpreted the Napoleon Code (Art. 2101) in relation to the expenses of the last sickness in an enlarged sense and in a liberal manner highly interesting to the medical profession of France, and consequently interesting as a matter of medical jurisprudence and legislation in all countries, particularly in Louisiana, where the civil code has been not only virtually annulled, but replaced by the most eccentric and unwarrantable legislation, as may be noted in the sequel, or upon some other occasion.

The Napoleon Code provides that the costs of justice (courts), of funerals, and of the last sickness, shall be privileged debts. Ought this reserved privilege to be restricted to the disease which caused the decease ? may it not include that malady which immediately preceded the events by which an insolvent debtor makes a declaration of insolvency, and distributes his effects ? and, finally, may not the privilege, in the case of this insolvent, apply equally in favor of the costs of attendance upon his sick children ?

Upon these points the tribunal of commerce of Montargis, has decided that the *honorarium* of the physician for medical attendance on a bankrupt during the year preceding bankruptcy, is privileged, and this privileged debt applies in like manner, during the same period, for services to his sick children.

This judgment, *in extenso,* is too long for the space which can be allowed in this Journal. · B. D.

TOADS LIVING WHEN SHUT UP IN PLASTER FOR YEARS...

M. Seguin, wishing to ascertain what amount of truth there is in the marvellous tales told of batrachians being found living within the substance of stones, has undertaken some experiments upon the matter. He enclosed some toads very firmly in plaster, and left them for years in the middle of these blocks of factitious stone. At various intervals he has broken some of these blocks, and has found a certain number of the toads alive. One of the animals had remained thus deprived of air during ten years, another twelve, and a third fifteen years. Two still continue enclosed, and as M. Seguin is very old, and fears that these two blocks may be lost to the purposes of science, he offers them to the Academy of Sciences in order that it may hereafter test the truth of the phenomenon. M. Flourens announces on the part of the Academy its willingness to accept them, intending after a verification of the dates of sequestration to have the plaster broken in presence of a commission *ad hoc.—Med. Times and Gaz.,* 1860.

PROFESSOR JEITELLES, of Olmütz, has taken up the dispute about the true discoverer of the reflex movements. He gives the whole credit to Prochaska, who anticipated both Dr. Marshall Hall, and Müller, and Sir C. Bell. He gives quotations from Prochaska's work and says of them: "These quotations are enough to show that Prochaska established in all essential points the doctrine of reflex motion ; and it will be remarked that he makes use of the expressions sensitive and motor nerves, although the experiments of Sir C. Bell were only made twenty-seven years afterwards (1811)."—*Ib.*

[Abundant evidence to the same effect was given in the *N. O. Med. and Surg. Journal,* many years ago.]

IN criticising a work of Dr. Edwin Lee, the *Gaz. Médicale* observes : "The state of moral degradation in which the Medical Profession in England languishes, has been for some years the constant consideration, and the source of the legitimate complaints of the most eminent men of the country. Political journals, literary reviews, the scientific press, all these have echoed their complaints, and have propagated the idea of the necessity of a reform. Meetings, commissions, associations, have been formed for the purpose of investigating and proposing to the Ministry legislative measures. All sorts of plans for reform have been recommended, but they have always turned out impracticable. . . . The perusal of the two memoirs of M. Lee, shows us what a long path English Medicine has yet to follow out, in respect of its institutions and professional conditions, before it can attain the height and social dignity that it occupies in our country (!!!). We hope, however, that better days are in store for it. We have the guarantee in the zeal and talents of men who, like M. Lee, labor at its regeneration."—*Ib.*

PRESERVATION OF BODIES FOR ANATOMICAL PURPOSES.

Professor Budge has found that bodies may be admirably preserved for a long period of time, whether for anatomical purposes, or for courses of operative surgery, by injecting into the carotid a preservative fluid composed of pyroligneous acid and sulphate of zinc, of each from eight to twelve drachms to seven pounds of water. Bodies thus injected have kept well during eight weeks of intense summer heat, without giving rise to any putrefactive smell, the muscles retaining their red color, and though a little softened, admitting of good dissection. The injection does not prevent the subsequent injection of colored matters ; and the knives used in dissection scarcely suffer at all.

PENCILS OF TANNIN FOR AFFECTION OF THE UTERUS.

Becquerel has recommended the following mode of applying tannin in certain affections of the uterus, in which cases it has been found very useful :—Take of

Tannin, 4 parts.
Gum Tragacanth, 1 part.
Crumb of Bread,

sufficient to give the required consistency for forming pencils, which are made about one inch in length, and one-fifth of an inch in diameter.—*London Med. Review, July,* 1860.

Mortality Statistics of New Orleans, from June, 1860, to Aug. 12, 1860, compiled from the Weekly Reports politely furnished by Dr. Dirmeyer, Secretary of the Board of Health.

Time.	Total Deaths.	Children under 2 yrs.	Under 20.	U. States.
June (5 weeks)	927	379	503	435
July (4 weeks)	789	210	304	255
August (2 weeks)	306	77	132	106

Principal Diseases.	April (5 weeks).	May (4 weeks).	June (2 weeks).
Apoplexy	22	62	8
Cholera Infantum	44	16	2
Congestion of Brain	16	29	6
Consumption	63	51	28
Convulsions, Infantile	61	44	21
Croup	6	4	4
Diarrhœa	60	34	12
Dysentery	30	27	18
Diphtheria	11	5	2
Dropsy	3	11	0
Bronchitis	8	8	1
Fever, Miasmatic	41	40	27
" Scarlet	29	12	8
" Typhoid	11	13	4
" Yellow	0	3	7
Gastro-Enteritis	13	10	9
Whooping-Cough	19	11	3
Inflammation of Liver	5	3	0
Inflammation of Brain	7	1	1
Inflammation of Lungs	18	9	0
Marasmus, Infantile	29	18	4
Measles	20	5	0
Pleurisy	2	0	1
Still-born	37	18	16
Sun Stroke	20	57	5
Teething	45	25	6
Tetanus	7	15	6
Trismus Nascentium	8	1	2

THE

NEW ORLEANS

MEDICAL AND SURGICAL JOURNAL.

NOVEMBER, 1860.

ORIGINAL COMMUNICATIONS.

Art. I.—*Letter from* Stanford E. Chaillé, M. D., *on Experimental Physiology, etc., etc.*

Paris, August 10, 1860.

To Dr. Bennet Dowler, *Managing Editor N. O. Med. and Surg. Jour.*

Dear Doctor: Among physiologists the question has been much disputed whether the muscular fibre possesses in itself the power to contract ; or is this power due to its connection with the nervous elements which penetrate it? This question has occupied your attention, and from experiments and observations on post-mortem contractility, and the rigor mortis, you arrived at Haller's conclusion, that contractility was a power inherent in the muscular fibre itself. Such is the doctrine now inculcated in our text books, and in its favor might be adduced the authority of many names illustrious in physiological researches. I have been a witness to some experiments in support of this view, which to my mind are conclusive ; and since they are not only instructive, but may be readily repeated, I am induced to record them in our pages.

Bernard, seeking to analyze the effects of poisons on the system, and their *modus operandi* in producing death, has established, that if either strychnine, curare (woorara), or sulphocyanide of potas-

96

sium be introduced into the circulation of an animal, death results in each case from paralysis, but in each case the paralysis has a different cause. Strychnine produces it by destroying the functions of the nerves of sensation, curare the nerves of motion, and sulphocyanide of potassium the contractility of the muscular system. If a frog be poisoned with curare, there is no stimulus which, applied to a nerve, will excite the slightest motion, but stimulants applied directly to a muscle, causes it to contract instantly. The nerve has been killed by the poison, the muscle left intact.

If the animal be poisoned with sulphocyanide of potassium, contraction does not respond to any stimulants applied to the muscles. But if the posterior extremities of the same animal be protected from the poison by ligating all the parts at the level of the sacrum, the lumbar nerves alone being excluded, then it will be found that an excitant applied to the skin or nerves of the anterior portion of the animal (the only portion poisoned), excites no motion in this part, while reflex movements are excited in the posterior extremities. Thus proving that the nerves have remained intact, while the contractility of the muscular fibres has been destroyed.

These experiments of M. Bernard, though but recently seen by me, are by no means new ; for the scientific world has been rendered familiar with them through his published treatise upon " *Les Effets des Substances Toxiques*." However conclusive they may be, I introduced this subject of muscular contractility not to detail these which are well known, but others which are still simpler, equally as conclusive, and I believe as yet unpublished in America.

A German friend, W. Kühne, who, though but twenty-four years of age, has already made a name for himself, has written an essay (untranslated from the German) on this subject of muscular contractility, and has fortified his conclusions with many original experiments. Some of these he has demonstrated to me, and any one who is at all skeptical, may repeat them in a very few moments, if he has a few frogs, a little chlorohydric acid, and some sugar. The principle of these experiments is simply this: Kühne discovered that chlorohydric acid, applied locally, is an excitant to muscular fibre, and has no action when applied to a nerve ; whereas, a concentrated solution of sugar or glycerin produces the reverse effect, excites the nerve to action ; but as a muscular irritant, is inert. The principle given, the following experiments were performed:

The sartorius muscle was dissected with its tibial tendon, from the thigh of a frog, the tendon fastened to a small stand, left the muscle pendent, its pelvic extremity being cut off with the scissors close to its attachment. This smooth cut extremity was then gently dipped in a dilute solution of chlorohydric acid, when strong muscular contractions followed. A leg was now·removed with an inch or more of the sciatic nerve attached, the nerve was then dipped in the same solution without producing the slightest effect ; although any nervous irritant would, when applied to the nerve, produce violent muscular contractions.

The second experiment was as follows : A leg with its nerve attached was prepared as before, the cut extremity of the nerve was dipped in a concentrated solution of sugar, when well marked and persistent contractions of the muscles to which the nerve is distributed, followed. These contractions do not, generally, begin instantaneously with the introduction of the nerve in the solution, but in a few moments thereafter, as if it were necessary that the fluid should have time to permeate and saturate the nervous structure. Continuing the experiment with sugar solution (this excitant of the nerves, but *not* of the muscles), the sartorius was prepared as before, and dipped in the solution without causing the slightest muscular contraction. But when this same muscle was severed about its middle or lower third, and *this* extremity was dipped in the same fluid, contraction of the muscular fibres did follow. This latter result would seem to invalidate the experiment, but in reality confirms it, for nerves are distributed to the sartorius about its middle, but no fibres can be traced into·the extremities of this muscle. Hence the solution of sugar did not excite contractions in the first extremity of the muscle, because in that extremity no nerve-fibres are mingled with the muscular ; whereas, when the muscle was shortened by removing its lower third, and this extremity containing nerve-fibres was dipped in the solution, contractions ensued. In performing this latter experiment, a difficulty is often encountered, and to it an objection may be made. The difficulty is this, that on separating the muscle from the body, spontaneous contractions often persist, so that on dipping it into the fluid, it is impossible to prove that *no* contractions result from such application. In the experiment performed, three frogs were sacrificed before a sartorius was found which was perfectly tranquil, and suitable for the purpose, With it ensued the result as stated. The objection which may be made to the experiment is this : it is not proved that the extremities of the sartorius are unsupplied with nerve-fibres. The microscope gives no evidence of them, which is only negative evidence, since nerve filaments might exist which the microscope could not demonstrate. More conclusive proof is derived from the fact, that if you destroy the function of the nerve with curare, it will be found that the whole muscle has become like its extremity, viz unexcitable on its application to a solution of sugar, while excitable to all muscular stimulants. Farther, if you suspend the function of the nerve, which may be done by transmitting through it a *constant* galvanic current, the same result ensues which followed the destruction of the nerve by curare. Here, then, we have a part of a muscle in which no nerve-fibres are *supposed* to exist, and other parts in which they are *known* to be present ; in these latter the nerves are destroyed, when it is found that the muscular fibres supplied with nerves have become subject to the same laws and give rise to the same phenomena, as those prevailing in that portion of the muscle where no nerve-fibres were supposed to exist. This identity of condition can only be explained by the fact, that the extremities of the muscle contain no nervous tissue.

In previous experiments upon this subject, the difficulty has been, that all the galvanic, chemical and mechanical stimuli which act on the nerves, also excite the muscles to action ; whereas, we have now acquired the knowledge of simple and delicate tests for each tissue separately. Touch a muscular fibre with a dilute solution of chlorohydric acid, and it will contract forthwith ; whereas, the nerve which supplies this same fibre may be bathed in the solution without producing the slightest contraction. Change the nerve from the preceding solution, place it in a concentrated solution of sugar, and the tranquil muscle responds to the excited nerve ; but kill the nerve, and then your sugared solution will produce not the slightest effect, whether it be applied to the nerve alone, the muscle alone, or both combined. And yet, the muscle is notdead—apply the solution of chlorohydric acid, and its contractions will prove it. In conclusion, these experiments have a most commendable virtue, they may be performed in half the time it has taken me to describe them.

For the past four months I have attended, assiduously, Bernard's lectures, and been present at his experiments, whether in the laboratory or lecture room. The more I see him, the higher is my opinion of his ability. I can bear witness to his honesty of purpose, and having assisted in recording many of his experiments, can testify to the care with which he excludes every source of error, and how faithfully he practises his oft-repeated precept, "observe the *fact*, and record it as it exists, explanations and theories after." I have heard him allude to the sneers which experimental physiology often excites, and the ridicule aimed at deductions from a bull-frog to a man.

He contends that the same laws govern identical tissues in all animals. That if certain phenomena are found to exist in the mus-- cular, nervous, or other tissues of one animal, the same phenomena will, in *like* conditions, be found to exist in the same tissues of other animals; and where the observations have been extended through, and verified upon each of the great divisions of the animal kingdom, the evidence accumulates until it becomes indisputable. Farther, that contradictory phenomena are only *apparently* so, resulting sometimes from the difficulty or impossibility of having all the con- ditions of the experiment identically the same; and often from a difference in *degree*, but not in the essential *nature* of the thing itself.

In illustration : many contradictory phenomena have been reported in reference to the action of poisons ; that the bite of a venomous snake has no effect upon the hog. Is it because the hog is an ex- ceptional and peculiar animal, whose tissues are exempt from the laws governing the same tissues in other animals ? or is it because his skin is so tough, and the adipose tissue beneath so thick, that the poison is not absorbed into his system ? He who desires to *see* a reply, may take this venom before inert and inject it into the same animal's circulation, and may rest assured the response will be a *dead hog.* Some years ago, a French savant discovered that sheep could eat enormous quantities of arsenic with impunity, and his pub- lications on the subject gave rise to so much discussion, that the skeptical Magendie, with Bernard (then his assistant), introduced into his lecture room four of these innocent animals. To three of these, kept fasting sufficiently long to *empty* their stomachs, an ordinary dose of the innocuous (?) arsenic was administered. The result was that M. Magendie eat the fourth, which no man who valued his life would care to have done with the three dead sheep experimented on.

Still more recently, an eminent physiologist, M. Vulpian, published the result of many interesting experiments upon the venom of the toad, which he found was a poison for all animals except for the toad itself. Repeated experiments by himself and others gave the same result. Bernard, consistent with his doctrine, came to the conclusion that *if* the venom of the toad was a poison for other animals, but not for the toad itself, then physiology was not worth studying, and that it would be well for him to resign his chair. This, fortunately, is not likely to take place, since I have seen him kill a number of toads with their own venom, notwithstanding M. Vulpian. The latter's experiments would force the conclusion, that there was something in the *nature* of the toad different from other animals, which is not true, although there is a difference in degree, for the toad does require a much larger proportionate quantity of its own venom to kill it, than other animals.

Pardon me, if I attempt to illustrate still farther this subject of contradictory phenomena. Charles Bell, or Alexander Walker, as you please, first taught that the spinal nerves are compound, the posterior roots supplying filaments of sensation, the anterior filaments of motion. Magendie, experimenting to confirm this result, found that on irritating the anterior root, the animal often gave unmistakable evidences of suffering. Hence, he concluded that the anterior root was not composed exclusively of filaments of motion. However, subsequent experiments failed to reproduce the phenomena he had several times observed, and after many fruitless attempts to produce pain by exciting the anterior roots, he was convinced he had erred, yielded his former position, and concluded that irritation of the anterior root of a spinal nerve caused motion only, and no manifestations of sensation.

In this case Magendie had observed a contradictory phenomenon. One year pain could be excited in a nerve, another year a similar nerve gave not the least evidence of sensation. Although Magendie conceded his previous convictions in consequence of his failure to produce the results he had observed, M. Bernard who had assisted in his experiments, and had *seen* evidences of pain on irritation of the anterior root, was not convinced by any theories that he had *not* seen it. Deeming the positive evidence stronger than the negative, he concluded that the *fact* had, and probably still existed; and that if the phenemenon had disappeared, it was probably because the conditions of the experiment were not identical. After various trials he at length succeeded in proving that irritation of the anterior roots does cause pain, and in establishing the conditions necessary to the success of the experiment, and the reasons why Magendie, after observing the phenomenon, had failed in his attempts to reproduce it. Now, I and hundreds of others have seen, over and over again, what Magendie denied, and few of our text books teach, that the anterior roots do give unmistakable evidence of containing filaments of sensation. M. Bernard, seeking the source of this sensation, severed the posterior root, fellow to the anterior root experimented on, and found that all trace of sensation had disappeared from the latter ; and thence concluded that the anterior derives its sensation from the posterior root. Seeking still farther to discover from what portion of the nerve of sensation the motor root derived its sensory fibres, he found that in many cases the section of the compound nerve as near its distribution as it could be followed, produced the same effect as action of the posterior root, and destroyed quite as effectually all evidence of sensation in the anterior. From this result he concluded that the nerves of sensation at their *periphery* send back to the nerves of motion as far as the spinal cord some of its sensory fibres, and from the fibres thus derived it is that the motor root gives rise on irritation to manifestations of pain. In relating these experiments, I have no desire to go any farther than the experimenter himself, who does not give his conclusions as unquestionably established, but as the most reasonable to account for the phenomena observed ; and who is more anxious to record the facts which are undeniable, than the theories thereon, which may be disputed. I did propose to detail to you the requisite conditions for performing these experiments successfully, and the very simple (when known) reasons why Magendie and others failed in theirs, but I have too great a fear of wearying a large class of our readers who are constantly demanding something *practical*, and are obstreperous for remedies to cure disease, and make a fortune with. Dear souls, I wish I could help them, and forward to order a panacea. But, alas ! I have seen nothing so far to induce me to believe that Europe is any nearer this discovery than America, or that the treatment of disease is a whit more scientific or successful at the Charity of Paris, than the Charity of New Orleans. No one has succeeded in abbreviating the road to knowledge, which here, as elsewhere, and now, as heretofore, must be trod long, laboriously, and patiently. When I have done all this let my suffering readers expect the *practical* results of my experience!

However, speaking of things practical, you, of course, know all about syphilitic inoculations, syphilization, etc.; but did you know, what I did not until recently, that there are physicians here in Europe who treat chancres exclusively with *chancres*, never administering a particle of medicine either internally or externally? A man comes with a chancre, they give him another from the original, then another from the second, and so on until the poison loses its power, or the patient gets well, or some other striking result occurs which renders farther treatment unnecessary.

With this practical episode, I return to some other experiments, and promise with them to conclude this *experimental* letter. Bernard and others have long since established that division of the sympathetic nerve is accompanied by an elevation of temperature in the parts supplied by the nerve. On its destruction, the vessels are distended with an increased amount of blood, which flows with greater rapidity. Galvanize the cut end of the sympathetic, and the distended vessels contract, their contained blood flows less rapidly and in less quantity, and the temperature of the part lowered. I have witnessed the action of the sympathetic in the neck several times, as also the results given ; but the point to which I desire to attract attention is this, that when the temperature of the part is augmented as stated, the veins which conduct the blood from this part contain *red arterial* blood ; while if the temperature be lowered in the manner described, it will be found that the veins contain black, very black blood. Neither Lavoisier's theory of animal heat, nor Liebig's modification of it, help us to any explanation of this phenomenon ; so far from it, the phenomenon disproves the theory, which so long prevailed, and which you have often and well combatted.

The presence of red blood in the veins is by no means infrequent or exceptional. The experiments which I have seen have convinced me of the truth of Bernard's conclusions, that whenever a *gland* is in action, performing its function of secretion, the veins leading from it *always* contain *red* blood. Hence the renal vein, which appertains to a gland which has no repose, but is constantly eliminating the urine, never contains the black blood which is supposed to be a necessary characteristic of the venous circulation. Open any animal quickly, the quicker the better, expose the renal vein, and you may *see* the correctness of my statement.

A more forcible illustration of the same fact may be produced by cutting the branch of the sympathetic which supplies the sub-maxillary gland, then with an electric current stimulate the branch of the chorda tympani which supplies the same gland and you will have before you the following phenomena, a flow of blood augmented in quantity and rapidity; an elevation of temperature in the part; an increased secretion from it; and its vein has gained two striking attributes of an artery, its blood is as red as the arterial, and its walls pulsate with such vigor that if a small incision be made, the blood spirts out for a foot or more in rhythmical jets. I regard facts like these as an acquisition to our physiological knowledge, however incapable we may be of explaining them. It takes many bricks to make a house, but every brick must be made separately before the house can be completed. However, the phenomena above cited admit an explanation which is good as far as it goes. The sympathetic is a vaso-motor nerve which in action causes the vessels it supplies to contract; paralyzed by division, the vessels are *passively* dilated by the blood flowing through them. On the other hand, the function of the branches of the chorda tympani which supply the vessels of the sub-maxillary gland would seem to be *active* dilatation of those vessels. That the sympathetic is the contractor, and the chorda tympani the dilator, the following proofs are offered: Irritate the sympathetic, the flow of blood in the part is diminished; sever the same nerve, and the flow of blood is increased. Irritate the chorda tympani, the flow of blood is increased; sever it, and the quantity of blood is diminished. The action of the one is just the reverse of the other. Now, perform the experiment above cited, viz: cut the sympathetic, thereby increasing the circulation, and, at the same time, irritate the chorda tympani, which also has the effect of augmenting the flow of blood, and by this simultaneous action on the two nerves, the greatest possible dilatation of the vessels is produced, and, as consequences of this dilatation, we have the results detailed, viz: augmented circulation, temperature, and secretion, with the blood coursing so rapidly through the dilated vessels that the pulsation is transmitted even to the veins. But why the venous blood remains red is but imperfectly explained. One would be disposed to explain it by supposing that the blood coursed too rapidly through its capillaries to admit of its deoxydation, and yet one important duty of the capillaries is performed, the function of the gland (its secretion) is augmented. Still farther, it is found that though the circulation is increased in a muscle when in action, as well as in a gland, yet the venous blood flowing from such muscle is truly venous or black, and, therefore, unlike the red arterial condition of the venous blood coming from a gland in action. In the case of the muscle, the temperature is also found augmented, which is in accordance with Liebig's theory of calorification.

In giving a *résumé* of the result of these experiments, it may be stated : That when glands are in action the venous blood flowing from them is red, when the glands are in repose the venous blood is black. For the muscles, the reverse is true ; whereas, the temperature is augmented, as also the circulation, in both muscles and glands when these latter are performing their functions.

M. Leconte, our able organic chemist, and M. Bernard's asssistant, has analyzed the blood in the several conditions referred to, and his analyses often repeated prove that the chemical condition of the blood is such as its physical appearance would indicate. His analyses were directed simply to the relative proportions of carbonic acid and oxygen, and he found that the blood taken from the

Artery of a Muscle	Vein of Muscle in repose.		Vein of Muscle in action.	
gave of acid carbonic, ...0.00	2.01	N. B. red.	3.21	N. B. bl'k
" oxygen,.........9.31	8.21		3.31	

whereas the blood taken from the

Artery of submaxillary gland.	Vein of the Gland in repose.		Vein of the Gland in action.	
gave of acid carbonic, ...0.98	2.94	N. B. bl'k	2.10	N. B. red
" oxygen,.,. 9.80	3.92		6.31	

You will perceive that the red or black appearance of the blood corresponds as was to be expected with the relative proportion of the two gases, and that these analyses confirm what has already been stated. You will also observe that M. Leconte gives. a much smaller quantity of carbonic acid in arterial blood than is given in the many analyses quoted in our books. If this is an objection, his reply is that he gives what he found, and that he believes that the analyses differing from his own were not conducted with the same precautions, nor was the blood analyzed guarded as carefully as were his specimens from all atmospheric contact.

I leave Paris in a few days, and shall spend the next four weeks in Switzerland, Austria and Prussia. · I shall remain several days in Vienna, and in Berlin—both of them medical centres—which I find are preferred to Paris, by those students who have had an opportunity of judging. Should I be enabled to pick up any professional information likely to prove interesting, I will be probably taken with another attack of scribbling, the results of which would be forwarded for our January number. Should I find nothing better I think I could write a letter which would be serviceable and interesting to those of our students or medical men, who contemplate spending some time in Europe in the study of their profession. Before leaving New Orleans I was most anxious to procure information in regard to expenses, college and hospital regulations, dissecting, and so on, which was furnished to me meagerly and unsatisfactorily. I feel sure that many of our subscribers would pardon the introduction of a few pages on these topics in one of our numbers.

I am now corresponding with a physician in London, and hope to engage him as a regular correspondent of our journal from that place ; if so, you will soon have something from him ; and if not I shall do all in my power to obtain some one else. Dr. Nichols and myself had determined to engage correspondents from both Paris and London, and anticipated no difficulty in finding them. But I have been disappointed, and have found that medical men have great reluctance to labor, even when well paid, for an American periodical, since their publications would not be as well known as if published in their own journals, nor their reputation increased at home, where a reputation is valuable to them.

As to exchanges I find the course adopted by us is decidedly the best to procure them through their agents in New York.

Rely upon it I shall study the interest of our journal, and strive to make it deserving of the patronage it enjoys. For all its readers and yourself, I remain their and your humble servant.

STANFORD E. CHAILLÉ.

ART. II.—*Contributions to Comparative Anatomy and Physiology.—*
(Crocodilus Mississippiensis): By BENNET DOWLER, M. D.

NUMBER TWO.

" All our science is but an investigation of the mode in which the Creator acts."
PROF. CARPENTER, COMP. PHYS.—726.

"It is very true, as Cuvier said, in the last Lecture he delivered, 'If we were agreed as to the crocodile's head we should be so as to that of other animals; because the crocodile is intermediate between mammals, birds and fishes.'"—(*The principal forms of the skeleton and Teeth:* By PROF. R. OWEN.)

"Buffon has well remarked in the introduction to his great work on Natural History: 'It is only by comparing that we can judge, and our knowledge turns entirely on the relations that things bear to those which resemble them, and to those which differ from them; so, if there were no animals the nature of man would be far more incomprehensible than it is.'"—(*Ibid.*)

DURING the present generation a great and beneficent change of opinion in favor of the propriety and utility of experimental physiology, pathology and surgery, has taken place. Experiment artificially planned has greatly enlarged the boundaries of the organic sciences, and much of the knowledge thus gained has been more or less available in the practice of the philosophical physician and surgeon. The prejudice against the vivisection and other experiments on the inferior animals as being cruel or immoral, has nearly, if not quite ceased. While the carnivorous animals not only devour each other, but sometimes kill for mere wantonness, or the love of killing, and man himself not only "slays and eats," but even kills for sport, the medical man kills for the benevolent purpose of learning the laws of the human economy, in order that he may regulate and sustain them, and remove whatsoever may obstruct or derange their healthful action.

The great advances recently made in the organic sciences in the rational classification of the animal kingdom, chiefly by fixed anatomical criteria, by homological identities, by analogies, by differentiæ, by the eternal unities of type or of plan, by infinite diversities of execution throughout the four great branches of living organisms, the *vertebrata, mollusca, articulata,* and *radiata*—the great progress recently made in deducing the principles of philosophical anatomy, are mainly owing to zealous researches into comparative anatomy and comparative experimental physiology.

In view of these undeniable facts it is believed that the readers of this journal will not disapprove the attempt to illustrate the natural history of the great saurian of Louisiana, and the more so because the text books of the most eminent comparative physiologists and anatomists, whose works, though generally excellent, abound with errors in regard to this animal—inadvertant errors which these writers, as lovers of truth must desire to see corrected, however humble the historian may be. Such investigations so far from being foreign to the studies of the physician are of great advantage to him, and constitute a part of the regular education of the medical man in some countries where professorships have been established for this purpose. A few years ago, according to the foreign journals, fifteen professors and as many assistants, were employed in the Museum of Natural History of Paris, in lecturing upon Natural and Physical Science.

It appears from the programmes för the examaination of applicants for admission into the medical service of the British Government, that candidates are always examined upon Natural History. The course of examination for medical degrees in the University of Edinburgh, at present, is " both in writing and *vivâ voce:* First, on chemistry, botany, and natural history ; secondly, on anatomy, institutes of medicine and surgery ; and thirdly, on materia medica, pathology, practice of medicine, clinical medicine, clinical surgery, midwifery, and medical jurisprudence. The examinations on anatomy, chemistry, institutes of medicine, botany, and natural history, shall be conducted, as far as possible, by demonstrations of objects placed before the candidates ; and those on medicine and surgery, in part by clinical observations in the hospital."

Without attempting to give a description of the cranial bones of the alligator, and much less a treatise upon this animal, I may take the liberty to remark, in a general way, that the fundamental ideas of philosophical anatomy in relation to morphology, type, unity of composition or plan, etc., advanced by Gœthe, in 1784, and subsequently, though long repudiated with scorn and contempt by his cotemporaries, as being innovations by a poet (not perceiving that he was also a profound naturalist) were finally adopted by the most eminent anatomists and physiologists in nearly the whole of Europe, as Oken, Meckel, Geoffroy St. Hiliare, Carus, R. Owen and some others ; but probably the great majority of medical men have either not studied these views or think them too abstruse—perhaps not always well founded in Nature ! Gœthe's views of the unity of the various forms of the skeleton and of the resolution of the cranial bones into six vertebræ seem to have given origin to Oken's researches upon the vertebral theory of the skulls of animals, which he assumed to consist of four vertebræ—a theory which Professor Owen has investigated with great learning and ability, with numerous diagrams, and many neologisms requiring a new dictionary for their explanation. The vertebral theory of the cranium of the crocodile (Prof. Owen's most perfect realization of this theory) appears scarcely tenable if all of the bones, which are extremely numerous, be considered. When, however, great anatomists agree it may be most prudent not to differ from them.

The mouth of the Alligator never completely closed against either air or water, owing to the absence of lips, presents on each side double curves or gently undulating lines of the jaws, the general bearings of which rise above the horizon considerably from the tip of the muzzle to the posterior angles of the mouth.

The teeth, variable in size and length, are conical or of the canine type, a portion being somewhat blunt, especially posteriorly, but none adapted to grinding. They are more formidable in appearance than in reality, being hollow shells and easily fractured, even by biting hard substances.

In an animal from ten to twelve feet long, the largest tooth is less than a quarter or the third of an inch in diameter, while a vast majority are much smaller. The teeth are inserted into distinct sockets, except about one-fourth, which enter a trough or gutter, forming the posterior angles of the mouth.

Anatomical adaptation, as well as actual observations, show that the teeth are designed to seize, hold fast, pierce, and kill their prey. Alligators find much difficulty in preparing their prey, when the latter are too large to pass the unyielding bony strait of the jaws and palate. To facilitate this preparation for deglutition, they bend their heads laterally so as to bring the mass within the reach of one of the forelegs, in order to tear the food to pieces. The limb and claws however, are feeble aids for this purpose, being comparatively small. In fact they appear to be generally unable to divide solid bodies which are too large to be swallowed whole, as will more fully appear in the sequel.

From the curves of the jaws, the variable size, length, and non-opposition of the teeth, and from the position which the teeth of the under jaw take within the dental arch of the upper, and from the fact that the under teeth enter into shallow holes, or a kind of sockets, in the soft parts or alveolar gums of the roof of the mouth, as well as from the acute, almost needle-pointed shape of the teeth, especially the longer ones, it is evident that the dental apparatus can have no horizontal motion forward, backward, or laterally, and that they act only perpendicularly to the plain of the jaws, penetrating, but never masticating by grinding ; nor can they divide by incising their food or prey, if solid, resisting, and coherent. The reader will recollect that, from the days of Aristotle to the present century, it has been generally asserted that the upper jaw opens without moving the head. Even Denon (born 1747, died 1825) of the French Egyptian Expedition, is quoted as authority for this anatomical myth (*Voy.* i, 185). St. Hilaire, naturalist to the same expedition, embarrassed by the classics (Aristotle, Herodotus, and Pliny), does not [fully deny their statements in this behalf. The missionary Labat (born 1663, died 1738), a voluminous and instructive writer of travels in the West Indies, including the Natural History of these islands, maintained, according to ancient authority, that the crocodile's upper jaw only is movable (T. ii, p. 344, *Nouvelle Ed.* 1742).

The number of the teeth, though little variable, has been generally estimated by writers so contradictorially as to show that their accounts are little reliable, even in the osteology of this animal, though less so in the dental apparatus than in some others.

Cuvier says crocodiles have twenty-seven teeth above and twenty-five below. He subsequently says they have nineteen above and fifteen below. (*Anatomie Comparée*, T. ii, p. 517.) Of the American crocodile, he says, it has nineteen teeth above and nineteen below, on each side (*dix-neuf en haut et dix-neuf en bas, de chaque côte. Ib.*). Again, in his *Ossemens Fossiles*, he says of living crocodiles, that the alligator has at least nineteen, and sometimes twenty-two teeth on each side of the under jaw, and at least nineteen, but often twenty, on each side of the upper one ; of the Nilotic crocodiles, that they have fifteen below and nineteen above, on each side. St. Hilaire's enumeration differs from the preceding, being $36+30=66$.

Mr. Gore, the translator of the first edition of Carus's Comparative Anatomy, quotes from Cuvier as follows : "The cayman [alligator] has nineteen teeth on each side, both in the upper and lower jaw ; in the crocodile there are nineteen above and only fifteen below " (ii, 50). By the way, Carns's plate (xi, figs. 10 and 11), purporting to represent the head of the Nilotic crocodile, is highly erroneous in regard to the teeth ; and as it regards the representation of the viscera, the plate (xii, fig. 19) is almost wholly incorrect, for the alligator, and equally so, it is believed, for the crocodile of the Nile.

In his *Personal Narrative of Travels* (vol. vii, 294), Humboldt says: " Crocodiles have 38 teeth in the upper jaw, and 30 in the lower= 68; the fourth tooth *touches* freely the upper jaw. The fourth tooth of the alligator *enters* the upper jaw." This is an error, noticed in another part of this paper.

Cuvier, in describing crocodiles and alligators, distinguishes the latter from the former by the teeth, a distinction almost wholly without a difference ; for example, one, he says, has "unequal," the other "uneven teeth," etc. The only important difference to which he alleges is an error of fact as it regards the alligator, namely: that the alligator has " the fourth tooth below entering into cavities in the upper jaw, and not the interstices of the upper teeth, as in the crocodile." (*An. King.*) Now, the fourth tooth does not enter into the upper jaw at all, though it and many others enter slightly into the dense, thick membrane of the vault of the mouth.

In his splendid work on *Odontography*, Mr. Richard Owen (plate 75 A, fig 1, vol. ii) represents all of the teeth as conical, except five or six on each side of each jaw, posteriorly, which have the appearance of grinders. One anterior tooth near the tip of the muzzle, on each side of the inferior jaw, is represented as passing quite through, rising considerably above the superior jaw. He describes, in the text, one on each side as penetrating the upper jaw, whereas, in the alligator, at least, none even enter, much less pass through the superior maxillary bone. More than half of the teeth of the lower jaw enter more or less into the dense, semi-cartilaginous membrane of the upper. In the bone there are shallow depressions, with slightly separate and very faint indentations, corresponding more or less to about a dozen of the front teeth of the lower jaw; about four or five on each side, the farthest back, rest in indentations, which, however, are barely perceptible ; the next three or four are a little more developed. The deepest of these cannot be called holes, much less sockets, being superficial, ill-defined fossæ or depressions within the alveolar arch of both the young and adult.

I will here add some personal provings of the teeth, without, however, adopting any principle of selection, except size : In an alligator six inches long, I counted 40+38—that is, 40 above and 38 below=78 ; in another, sixteen and three-quarter inches long, 38+38=76 ; another 38+40=78 ; one two feet five inches long, 40+38=78 ; one of two feet four inches, 34+34=68 ; one of four feet 38+34=72; one of four feet five inches, 40+40=80; one of ten feet, 40+40=80 ; one eleven feet, 40+40=80, etc. Other enumerations might be added, were it necessary. It will be seen that the maximum is 80, the minimum 68, the mean of eight animals 76·25.

In a perfect specimen of the mummied crocodile from Egypt, measuring four feet eight inches, the jaws being immovably closed, I counted thirty-six teeth in the upper and thirty-two in the lower— sixty-eight. Although these only were visible, yet, from the anatomical conformation, others were doubtlessly concealed by the closed position of the jaws, the dried skin, and the bituminous and other matters used in the mummification. Beginning in the middle of the anterior portion of the under jaw, the first tooth penetrates through the upper jaw. The fourth tooth, the longest of all, does not penetrate the bone of the upper jaw, but compresses or indents it, entering outside of the same, forming a notch, the very thing which some writers have erroneously supposed to characterize the Mississippi crocodile. The transverse diameter from notch to notch is one and five-eighths inches. The diameter of the muzzle, just before this notch, is greater than that through the notch itself, by one-quarter of an inch. In the living animal, the notch doubtlessly appears as a kind of socket in the skin or semi-cartilaginous alveolar gum or membrane. At this point, as also forward and backward, the under teeth retire within the line of those of the upper jaw, never being opposite or in any respect like grinders, as some erroneously represent them.

The most salient difference between the Nilotic and the Mississippian crocodiles is this slight, but by no means fundamental one, in the teeth, and, strangely enough, the descriptions usually met with intended to fix this differentiation is erroneous in regard to the alligator, as explained elsewhere. "Nothing," say MM. Duméril and Bribon, "better distinguishes the crocodiles from the alligators than the narrowness of the muzzle behind the nostrils ; a narrow-

98

ness which is produced by the deep notch on each side of the upper mandible, serving for the passage of the fourth lower tooth."

Of numerous measurements of the head, etc., I will here give only a few, more or less illustrative of the muzzle : No. 1 is a mummied Nilotic crocodile, four feet eight inches in length ; No. 2 the skeleton of a Mississippi crocodile, four feet five inches long, being three inches shorter than the other, and without either dried flesh or skin ; No. 1, from the tip of the muzzle to the posterior angles of the orbits, eight and a half inches ; No. 2, from ditto to ditto, six and a half inches ; No. 1, from tip of the muzzle to the posterior angle of the mouth, nine inches ; No. 2, from same to same, seven and three-quarter inches ; No. 1, from the angle of jaw to the opposite, over the orbits, five and three-quarter inches ; No. 2, from same to same, four and three-quarter inches ; No. 1, circumference of head just behind the orbits, fourteen and a half inches ; No. 2, from same to same, twelve inches ; No. 1, circumference just before the orbits, eleven and a half inches ; No. 2, same place, ten inches ; No. 1, circumference at the nostrils, five and three-quarter inches ; No. 2, same place, five inches. I believe that these measurements differ more than elsewhere in the skeleton.

The teeth enclose a series of smaller ones, which, it is reasonable to assume, successively replace the outer when the latter are shed, or broken, as they often are, by accident.

Buffon, who viewed (at a distance) the crocodile and alligator as terrible animals, says, " that travelers, rather than Nature, have made a distinction between them ; for, in the general outline and in the nature of these two animals, they are entirely the same." He alludes to and admits a difference in the teeth : " The fourth on each side of the lower jaw of the alligator enters a hole in the upper when the mouth is closed." (*Nat. Hist.*, Eng. ed., vol. iv, p. 60.)

Mr. Owen says that crocodilians " have three and sometimes four generations of teeth, sheathed one within the other, in the same socket." In a number of specimens which I have examined, from the youngest to the adult ages, I have never found more than two well-developed and one rudimentary one in the skeleton. Mr. Owen, in a later work (*On the Skeleton, etc.*), says, that the processes of succession and displacement are carried on uninterruptedly through the long life of these cold-blooded, carniverous reptiles." The man who bought a hawk in order to settle the disputed question, whether its natural term of life reached one hundred years, must have forgot the brevity of his own life. It must be exceedingly difficult, in man's short life, even were crocodiles daily under his observation, to determine how many generations of teeth take place during crocodilian life, which is generally supposed to be very protracted, extending through centuries.

In an alligator four feet long, which I had vivisected, a large number of the teeth were broken, some had probably been shed, at least, they were missing, so that I was obliged to interpolate or guess at the number, as follows: $38+34=72$. I attempted to draw several of the longer teeth with forceps, but failed—the teeth being hollow shells, were crushed to pieces, not having sufficient solidity to permit extraction. I might mention other examples of broken teeth. It is evident that, as the longer teeth are the most finely pointed, and show no marks of having been worn, their use is restricted to prehension and piercing and crushing soft bodies, as fishes, being powerless in grinding down the bony skeletons, heads, limbs, and pelves of large animals so as to fit them for deglutition.

The tongue, white at its apex, becomes faintly roseate underneath and on its sides, towards the middle and backward ; it constantly augments in size, from its tip to its base, where it is massive ; its dorsum is studded with very large, white papillæ, chiefly on its anterior half, but declining from the outer third to the base. On both sides, and on a level with the under surface of the anterior third of the tongue, are several folds of loose white membrane. The entire bucal membrane, together with the tongue, is nearly dry, being but little more moist, when not immersed, than the skin, and wholly destitute of mucus, and of mucous follicles or salivary glands.

The *Museum of Animated Nature* describes the crocodilidæ as having "the space between the two branches of the lower jaw covered internally with a yellow skin, full of glands, whence oozes a viscid saliva. This part represents the tongue, if, indeed, we may not say that this organ is wanting" (ii, 79). In his Comparative Anatomy, Carus says : "There is a musky secretion produced by *a gland* on the lower jaw of the crocodile" (ii, 123); whereas, there are always *two* musk glands on the outside and underneath the jaw, in a kind of valved pocket in the skin.

The epithelium of the tongue and mouth is very dense and thick, like the sole of the human foot, or the laborer's palm. The tongue is soldered down to the central floor of the mouth, a large triangular area, extending from one side of the lower jaw to the opposite. Between the inferior surface of the tongue and skin, there is a little dense, areölar tissue, the whole forming rather a thin flooring, and but a slight protection to the tongue, the skin being destitute of osseous plates below. The frænum (if such it may be called) is not altogether under the center of the tongue, but also on its sides, and may be regarded as a kind of double or broad frænum, holding the tongue down firmly, and preventing its protrusion altogether, but permitting a little upward and backward action. The base of the tongue is so massive that it may, with very little motion, exercise an upward pressure against the roof of the mouth.

Mr. Broderip, a pleasing writer, who quotes authorities to show (and what writer does not?) that crocodiles swallow man and beast, ox, mule, and horse, says, in writing about reptiles : "Take the head of a crocodile. A more solid, bony mass you could hardly see. Now, turn to that of a boa. The skull, you see, is made up of a considerable number of pieces, all admirably fitted and joined together, but with such an adaptation as easily to admit of separation. Why is this? The long head and widely-extended jaws of the crocodile enable it to secure and take into the stomach a comparatively large prey. But the serpent frequently has to master and swallow an animal utterly disproportioned to the usual gape of the mouth ; the skull is, therefore, so framed as easily to admit of partial dislocation, so that it may aid the dilatation of the jaws and throat, and facilitate deglutition" (Note Book, 79). Now, "the solid, bony mass of the crocodile's head," when measured, will convince any one that solids larger than the entrance between the jaws and palatine bones, cannot pass, any more "than a camel through the eye of a needle."

The palatine bone, firmly set at its base, stretching across the isthmus of the posterior fauces, and descending nearly to the middle of the base of the tongue, and much lower laterally, is a barrier to the deglutition of bodies of considerable size. In swallowing, the base of the tongue is necessarily depressed so as to allow a large mass of food to pass under this depressed arch or door way, so that, making every allowance for the depression of the base of the tongue, the segment of a circle within the condyles of the lower jaw, limiting the vertical diameter, makes it smaller than the inter-maxillary horizontal diameter at the isthmus of the posterior fauces. Hence no

✳ solid substance larger than this latter diameter can possibly be swallowed. Now, this diameter, in the skeleton of an animal five feet long, after the removal of all the soft parts, is, from the interior of one ramus or condyle to the other, but two and a half inches.

In view, therefore, of the anatomical structure of the osteological passage to the gullet and stomach, what becomes of such statements as the following, not to mention others more extravagant, but less reliable. In the fourth volume of the English edition of Buffon's Natural History, Mr. Audubon, the distinguished ornithologist (a native of Louisiana), is quoted as follows : " The drivers of cattle from Opelousas, and those of mules from Mexico, on reaching a lagoon or creek, send several of their party into the water, armed merely each with a club, for the purpose of driving away the alligators from the cattle ; and you may then see men, mules, and those monsters all swimming together, the men striking the alligators, that would otherwise *attack the cattle, of which they are very fond. They will swim swiftly after a dog, deer, or horse.*"

" It [the alligator] is found in the Mississippi, in the lakes and rivers of Louisiana, and of Carolina, and specimens have been brought from Savannah and New Orleans. According to Bartram, these formidable reptiles may be seen in troops, in creeks and bays of the river, where fish abound ; and he states that he saw in Florida vast numbers of alligators, as well as fish, in a mineral spring, near the Mosquito river, though the water at its exit from the earth was nearly at the boiling point, and strongly impregnated with copper and vitriol. They attack both quadrupeds and men." (*Mus. Animated Nature*, ii, 82.)

Humboldt and his companions, during all their sojourn in the equinoctial regions of America, saw no instance of ferocity in, or danger from, the crocodiles of the Madelena, Oronoco, Amazon, and other rivers, although the party sometimes slept in houses infested by these animals. (See his Narrative, 7 vols.)

In Lacépède's celebrated French work on Natural History, there is a frightful engraving representing an alligator in the act of carrying away in its mouth a bleeding negro. Cuvier (*Oss. Fos.*) quotes authority to show that the alligator prefers negroes to whites for food. " *Il préfère la chair de nègre à cette de blanc.*"

It is remarkable that the wonderful, but still classical tales of alligators devouring oxen, horses, and negroes (especially the latter,

as being their favorite food), were told chiefly by the earlier writers
on Louisiana, South Carolina and Florida. The negroes, credulous
enough, would be amused at such statements, as well as with the
killing of alligators. It is the negro who eats the alligator, or at
least a part of the tail, as I have been informed.*

The Nilotic crocodile, according to the late George Gliddon, U. S.
Consul in Egypt, long resident in that country, is one of the most
timid and retiring animals, and the least willing to encounter the
presence of man.†

Humboldt, in his *Aspects of Nature* (1849, p. 39), says that the
South American horses and oxen are attacked by crocodiles.

. The Rev. Wm. Kirby, author of the *Bridgewater Treatise on Animals*,
who was, as he truly says, "*officially* engaged to prove the great
truths of Natural Religion from the instincts of the animal creation"
(and for which he got a heavy golden consideration), affirms that
" were it not for the number of their enemies, the crocodiles would
drive man from the vicinity of the great rivers of the torrid zone."
Natural Religion founded on such official statements ! He also says :
"Crocodiles send forth lowings almost as loud as those of an ox.
They respond to each other by hundreds, especially in the evening,
which makes in the swampy forest a frightful and thundering din—
cries that may be heard from a great distance, which seem as if they
issued from the ground." (17.)

Bory de Saint Vincent, chief editor of the French Dictionary of
Natural History, quotes authors, as Michaux, Catesby, and Bartram,
to show that the Mississippi, Carolina and Florida alligators attack
and devour dogs, hogs, beeves, oxen, bulls, cows (bœufs), and
negroes, and, when the latter cannot be had, white people.

Sir Charles Leyell, the eminent geologist, in his *Second Visit to
the United States* (i. 251, *anno* 1845), having seen an alligator about
nine feet long, takes occasion to make the following statements :
" When I first read Bartram's account of alligators more than twenty
feet long, and how they attacked his boat and bellowed like bulls,

---

* The negroes find little difficulty, either in killing or capturing alligators. A few years ago several
negroes, who had captured and carted to my door enormous live alligators, were sorely disappointed at
my refusal to purchase such unwieldy animals, one of which must have been about seven feet in
circumference.

† Mr. Gliddon, some years before his death, addressed to me an interesting communication, still
unpublished, concerning the crocodile of the Nile, in answer to some interrogatories which I had
addressed to him.

and made a sound liked istant thunder, I suspected him of exaggeration ; but all my inquiries here [in Georgia] and in Louisiana convinced me that he may be depended upon."* A few years ago a venerable negro, formerly of Savannah, having related to me in the most serious manner, an alligator story still more extraordinary than that vouched for by the geological traveler, was evidently chagrined at my incredulity as to his veracity : he knew as well as the geologist, that "alligators swallowed cows," but he knew more, for he had "seen small trees growing from the backs of large alligators."

Mr. Brooke, an Englishman, the Rajah of Sarawak, though not known as a naturalist, is doubtless a writer of veracity. He gives the following statement in his Journal (vol. ii, p. 70 *et seq*, Lond., 1848) : During one of his expeditions against the pirates of Borneo, he relates that "a crocodile was caught (Nov. 25, 1845) measuring fifteen feet four inches. It is astonishing how *quiescent* these animals are when taken, allowing their feet to be fastened over their back, and a strong lashing to be put round the mouth *without any resistance*, and then brought down, floated between two small canoes. When dragged out of the water to be killed, the monster only moved his tail *gently* backwads and forward. * * * The bones of a poor fellow were found in his stomach. The thigh and the leg bones of the Malay were perfect, and the feet had some portions of the flesh adhering to them, and were crushed into a roundish form, whilst the head was found separated at the joinings or processes. The poor man's jacket and trousers were also found, which enabled the relatives to recognize his remains, and, from his having been a fisherman, it is probable he was attacked whilst occupied with his lines. A Dyak of Sarambo, who was with him, must have been carried off at the same time." Now the Dyak story is, of course, mere conjecture. The fisherman was doubtlessly drowned accidentally, and after having been greatly softened and decomposed, the animal seizing the head and the leg in succession, detached them by jerkings and scratchings—with the head the jacket, with the limb the trousers. The shirt, arms, ribs, spine, breast-bone, hips, and some two hundred bones of the normal skeleton, were not found in the stomach. Hence, it appears that the whole body was not swal-

* Sir Charles made a curious discovery at New Madrid, namely, a German who was so poor that he had " not even a negro boy or girl." Perhaps a majority of Sir C.'s countrymen at home are too poor to be able to pay £500 for " a boy " or £400 for " a girl."

lowed. Now the account, as given by the Rajah, concerning the complete torpidity of this unresisting, helpless monster, which gave no signs of pain while being killed, except a "gentle motion of the tail," shows that this crocodile was captured, dragged through the river and upon land, and was killed, during hibernation. Although the climate of Borneo is altogether tropical, yet the alligator has a hibernating sleep, which occurs, as Humboldt and others affirm, in the hottest and driest season of the year, in the intertropical regions of America at least.

Rajah Brooke's report (which is reproduced because it is deemed *true*), bears date November 25th, when the alligator had probably fallen into its annual sleep. Mr. Audubon, the ornithologist, says : " So truly gentle are alligators at this season of the year (beginning of autumn), that I have waded through the lakes, merely holding a stick in one hand to drive them off. If you go towards the head there is no danger, and you may safely strike it with a club four feet long, merely watching the operations of the tail." (Quoted in Buffon's Nat. Hist., Eng. ed.)

The Eastern is, if possible, more inoffensive than the Western crocodile, according to the most reliable writers. Miss Harriet Martineau, who, a few years ago, " traveled from end to end of Egypt," represents the crocodile as altogether harmless : " Our crew seemed to have no fear of these creatures, plunging and wading in the river without hesitation. Crocodiles abounded. We never witnessed any sign of fear of crocodiles, or heard of any disasters by them." (*Eastern Life*, p. 51, 157.) She mentions that the party in the vessel in which she voyaged, passed near many of these animals, killing some of them.

In a Description of the Province of South Carolina, bearing date at Charleston, Sept., 1731, and reprinted in Mr. Force's *Tracts*, the following account is given, namely : " There are also some crocodiles in the rivers [of Carolina], but the people fear them no more than if they were so many fishes, since it was never known that they have hurt any person whatsoever."

The alligator, after passing the hibernating season, so far from being voracious and ready to devour every thing alimentary, negroes and bullocks, seems to have no appetite for food for weeks, and swallows his first meal, which is a very small one, with great difficulty, after many fruitless efforts. With the increase of the atmospheric heat, there is not only a greater power to swallow, but a gradual gain of appetite, which, however, recedes, if cool weather supervene. Their digestion is at all times very slow, and, if the weather be cool, nearly or quite null.

I may here refer to some experiments illustrative of these subjects. The air for several weeks before the 31st of March, had ranged at sunrise from 50° to 64°. Several alligators had been recently offered food ; the offer was renewed to-day, but all refused to eat, as heretofore. The mouth of one animal (measuring eleven feet) was opened by a lever, and a piece of a hog's spine, including the adherent fleshy portions, around which a rope was tied, was forcibly placed in the mouth, but the mass was not swallowed as long as it was observed. On returning half an hour after, the whole had disappeared but the end of the rope. Fifteen hours afterward, I drew the rope with force ; it slipped off from the mass, bringing away, however, a portion of the hog's flesh, quite unchanged, together with a mass of mucus ; the latter was thick, transparent like the white of an egg ; neither the meat nor the mucus had any perceptible odor. The mucus, tested with litmus, gave neither an alkaline nor acid reaction.

April 3, noon : air 68°. A strip of pork, including the skin, two feet long and as wide as the finger, was doubled together, having a small cord firmly tied around these duplications ; the mass was placed in the mouth of a large alligator, but not having been swallowed, was forced down the gullet by a rod, leaving the end of the cord out. The next day, twenty-five hours after the introduction of the pork into the stomach, the mass was drawn up by pulling at the free end of the cord. The food was unchanged in cohesion, size, and general appearance, excepting, perhaps, a little blanching ; a good deal of mucus had been deposited in the coils of the long strip of meat and skin. The whole was free from odor ; the mucus, which was tasteless, caused no effervescence in a solution of the carbonate of soda ; it caused very little change of litmus paper, except a very faint tinge of redness.

In the month of October, a piece of meat, tied with twine having blue and white strans, was swallowed by an alligator, which, a few days after, was vivisected. The meat had disappeared, but the colors of the twine had not changed in the least.

Dr. Carpenter attempts to account for the long fast of reptilians thus : "It is to be borne in mind, however, that a large supply of food is frequently ingested at once by these animals ; and that, owing to the slowness of their digestive powers, the introduction of the aliment into the system is protracted over a very long period— as is seen, for example, in the case of the *Boa Constrictor*, which occupies a month in the digestion of a single meal." *(Prin. Comp. Phys.* 178.)

At no season of the year will alligators eat often, and if food be forced down their throats in comparatively cool weather, no digestion takes place ; as already said, digestion is slow in even the hot season. Mr. Audubon says : " In those I have killed (and I have killed a great many), when opened to see the contents of the stomach, or to *take out the fish* " * * (Eng. edit. of Buffon). The idea of killing of alligators " to take out the fish" for diet, is calculated to produce nausea, though it is indicative of a preservative power of the animal's stomach. Dr. John Davy kept a torpedo many days ; when it died, a fish was found in its stomach, much in the same state as when it was swallowed ; no portion of it had been dissolved. (i, 17.)

It may be allowable, in this place, to pause a moment in order to examine several current errors, alike discreditable to crocodiles and the received text-books on natural history, comparative anatomy, and physiology. These errors are, however, of little importance, compared with others which may be noticed hereafter.

Of these animals, Cuvier says : " Their habit is to drown their prey, and then place it in some hole beneath the surface, where they leave it to putrefy before they devour it." *(Règne Animale.)* This statement stands unimpeached and uncontroverted in the fine, new edition* of Cuvier's *Animal Kingdom*, edited by Professor W. B. Carpenter, aided by Messrs. Westwood, Blythe, Mudie, and Dr. G. Johnston. Now, without relating in detail various experiments from year to year, with different kinds of meat, fresh and stale, it is sufficient to say, that alligators always prefer the best, never eating that which is putrid. Inferior pieces of beef or other meat, for example, are rejected for those which are more palatable ; if the latter be insufficient, they may return to the inferior pieces, not otherwise. They prefer the bones of fowls which they can crack, to larger bones

---

* London : 1851. The plate in this work, intended to represent the crocodile, is inaccurate in the head, body, tail, etc.

which they cannot break—fleshy to gristly and bony—fresh to salt— muscle to skin—lean to fat, and so on. The larger animals take the lion's share ; the smaller, what is left, or what they can slyly get without interfering with their more powerful, august masters. If, after being satisfied, any food be left until it becomes in any degree putrid, they will not eat it, while at the same time fresh food will be taken quickly if offered. They will not eat a dead rat, especially if putrid.

It has been already stated that the great ornithologist of Louisiana, Mr. Audubon, was in the habit of killing, according to his own ac- count, a great many alligators, for the purpose of taking the fish out of their stomachs, instead of fishing with hook, line, and rod. If, however, these fish were buried until putrid before they were swallowed, they must have been worse than worthless afterward.

The distinguished naturalist of London, Prof. R. Owen, in his recent work *On the Principal Forms of the Skeleton and Teeth*, says : " In the cold-blooded ferocious crocodile, the cavity for the brain, in a skull three feet long, will scarcely contain a man's thumb. Almost all the skull is made up of instruments for gratifying an insatiable propensity to slay and devour : it is the material symbol of the lowest animal passion " (222-3). "This is a hard saying ;" but it is not punishable under the law against cruelty to animals : it is, nevertheles, a cruel injustice. For the crocodile is one of the most peaceable—one of the most temperate and abstemious of animals. It fasts for half the year, and during the other half, seldom eats more than once or twice in a week, even during the four hotter months. During the latter part of spring, and in mid-autumn, it eats little or none, unless the temperature be near that of summer. It kills nothing wantonly, but for food only—attacks nothing, unless in self-defence, nor even then, if it can escape. Its appetite is easily satisfied ; and, for the quantity of food supplied, yields more fat, perhaps, than almost any animal. Hence an alligator pen, in domestic economy, might be profitable, for the purpose of fattening alligators, the internal fat of which is very beautiful and abundant, being deposited upon the internal parietes of the abdomen, not in the omenta, for this animal has neither the greater nor lesser omentum, though writers say the contrary.

Aug. 7 : Fed a number of alligators. They all eat moderately. Threw them fresh food on the 10th ; this, which they refused, remained the following day, and soon become putrid. On the 16th of August, they all eat fresh beef, having fasted nine days. Sept. 6 : These animals eat heartily ten days ago—since which, food has been repeatedly offered them, but not taken ; they look full and well. Sept. 10 : Some bacon and putrid meat lie in their pen. To-day they eat freely of fresh beef. They eat in like manner on the 19th and 26th of September. They would not eat again until the 14th of October, which was their last meal for the season. The hibernating sleep now set in.

Now, if an alligator, in the hot season, is satisfied with a moderate meal once a week, more or less, why should it be characterized by naturalists as the most voracious of animals ? Do not these authors eat more than twenty meals a week, not to mention luncheons ?

Writers who disparage the alligator on account of the smallness of the brain, and the absence of the numerous convolutions or protuberances on the cerebral surfaces, fancifully assumed to be so many distinct, special and independent organs or faculties, might correct their statements by rigidly comparing the numerous facts adverse to their theory, presented by comparative anatomy and physiology.

Dr. Roget (in the *Encyc. Brit.*, Art. *Anat.*) says that "the cranium of a crocodile measuring from thirteen to fourteen feet is scarcely capacious enough to admit the thumb" ! Without stopping to examine the exactitude of this statement, I may mention, that in the skeleton of a very young alligator now before me, the head of which is but $1\frac{3}{4}$ inches long, there is an inter-cranial transverse diameter of five lines. This, though shorter, of course, than the longitudinal diameter, is nearly one-fourth of the length of the head.

Nevertheless, the crocodile "has the wisdom of the serpent," and, compared with most reptilians, "the harmlessness of the dove," too, notwithstanding the smallness of its brain. That "it is the material symbol of the lowest animal passion," is no more reasonable than its deification in the days of the Pharaohs. As some compensation for its lack of brains, I could relate some remarkable examples of its sagacity in action under peculiar and unusual circumstances. If reason can be inferred from rapid contrivance or the adaptation of means to ends, the alligator reasons.

It is easy to announce, but difficult to apply, theories to the facts of comparative anatomy and physiology. For example, Dr. Carpenter reasons thus : " The tiger is furnished with a cranial cavity of considerable dimensions, in order that the size of the brain may correspond with the degree of intellect which the habits of the animal require.   The face is short, so that the power of the muscles which move the head may be advantageously applied," etc. (*Comp.* *Phys.*) Now the carniverous alligator has not " a short face " nor a large " cranial cavity," but its " degree of intellect " is probably in no wise inferior to that of the tiger.

Without now entering upon the anatomy of the alligator's brain, it may be proper to allude to Cuvier's estimates of this organ (*Anat.* *Comp.*, ii, 71, *et seq.*), which, in man, he says, from infancy to old age, is to the whole body as 1 to 22, 1 to 25, 1 to 35.   In many animals the brain is in a much higher ratio, according to him : as the little American monkey (*saïmiri*), 1 to 22; monkey of Guiana, 1 to 28; field-mouse, 1 to 31; blue-headed tomtit, 1 to 12; great titmouse, 1 to 16; sparrow, 1 to 25; canary, 1 to 14; linnet, 1 to 24; jay, 1 to 28; cock, 1 to 25, etc.   The cerebellum is to the brain proper, as 1 to 9 in man and the ox ; in the dog 1 to 8; in the baboon, monkey, wild boar, and horse, 1 to 7; beaver 1 to 3; rat 1 to $3\frac{1}{4}$; mouse, 1 to 2; sheep, 1 to 5, etc.

Alligators can in various ways take their diet, but in none so readily as in water.   When they become somewhat tame, they will sometimes open their mouths and catch the food thrown to them, as a dog often will.   If the food fall on the ground, which is not a convenient position, they turn the jaws so as to take it up, not at the tip of the muzzle, but laterally or sidewise, and by a backward muscular action of the tongue, bring it to the palate or isthmus of the fauces.   When the food is thrown in the water, they seize it with the utmost facility, and then elevating the head out of the water, the mass falls back by its gravity, and aided by the tongue, they swallow it at once, if not too large.

I have not seen them swallow under water.   But from the action of a remarkable valve not yet described, it is apparently possible, though not altogether probable, for this to occur without the ingress of water.   The constant action of this valve prevents water from passing into the posterior fauces and the glottidian aperture, and the more the mouth opens the more actively is this valve forced up before the partially cleft palate.   As the nostrils can be closed, which is apparently their usual condition, unless when voluntarily opened, water, which always enters the mouth during immersion, seems to be completely excluded from the posterior fauces, trachea, and gullet. Neither in nor out of the water does respiration occur in the ordinary sense of the term. A large supply of air is taken into the capacious lungs, consisting of innumerable air-sacks, and this serves, as it seems, for a long time, perhaps for days, while the carbonated or deteriorated portion is probably discharged into the water, if the animal should be long immersed. I have watched from year to year without noticing regular respirations.

While immersed, air-bubbles, supposed to be carbonic acid, have been sometimes noticed arising through the water, yet judging from the apparent absence of respiratory motion when the animal is in repose, and not irritated, it would seem that neither inspiration nor expiration is rythmical or regular. Is air, like food, taken in only at long intervals? or is the air taken in and expelled without apparent respiratory movements? · Kirby, in his *Bridgewater Treatise on the History of Animals*, asserts that "the crocodile cannot remain under water more than ten minutes" (418), which is quite erroneous, as it sometimes remains quietly for hours or days altogether immersed, especially when sudden changes of weather occur. Experiment shows that the most direct and rapid method of killing an alligator is to tie its windpipe, or to introduce water into its lungs. How, then, can the animal remain long under water, seeing that during submersion it cannot inspire? The most probable answer to this question that occurs to me, is this, namely: that while inspiration is only occasional, expiration, though little perceptible, is constantly required to eliminate carbonic acid.

June 13, 1853. An alligator, nearly two feet in length, was taken to the Medical College, with a view of ascertaining by experiment how long it would live in carbonic acid gas. Mr. Riddell, an accomplished chemist (now Prof. Riddell, M. D., of Texas), conducted the experiment. The animal was placed in a box, into which carbonic acid gas was introduced. The box or receiver, it should be mentioned, was not perfectly air-tight ; but, on testing the air of the box repeatedly, it was found that lighted matches were always speedily extinguished in it. The supply of gas was continued for nearly three hours, without either killing or greatly annoying the animal, which, however, at the close of the experiment, kept its mouth open or rather gaping, although its strength and spitefulness were undiminished. After having repeatedly tied the tracheæ of alligators, I am inclined to think (for I speak not by the watch) that not one so treated lived half an hour, and that the majority died in half of that time ; that is, the usual phenomena of life ceased, but they could be reproduced by inflating the lungs artificially. Now, decapitation leaves the head and the body alive for a long but variable time.

Now, if there were no defects in the experiment, is it not probable that the animal did not inhale the gas, but lived through the experiment on its previous stock of air, expelling, in the meantime, the carbonic acid generated in its own lungs ?

1851, June 13, 14. Two alligators have been lying completely submerged for several days, without any apparent respiration, being in a deep sleep, the nictitating membranes only covering the eyes ; these animals, in the meantime, were closely and often observed. It is scarcely among possibilities that at night, or at any other time, they could have risen to the surface to respire, and afterwards have placed their bodies at the bottom of a large tub, in precisely the same attitudes as at first. The temperature of the air of the place at sunrise for the two weeks preceding, had ranged from $67\frac{1}{2}°$ to 77°. Other similar observations were made before and since these dates, and often with the same negative results in regard to regular respiration. The vast, but greatly underrated capacity of the lungs, enables the alligator to take in a large quantity of air, which it probably appropriates very slowly. Hence, it is probable that, in tying the trachea, death takes place not so much for want of air or inspiration as from inability to expire that already contaminated. This provisional explanation, though unsatisfactory, is submitted with the hope that a better one may be given.

It has been said by several writers that "alligators roar like a thousand mad bulls engaged in fight." The aligator makes generally no noise, except that of hissing like a goose when angry. Young ones, on being vivisected, have, in very rare instances, uttered a sound which may be spelled oupe ! or houpe ! the English of which may be, help ! This sound is, however, very uncommon. On one occasion, an alligator having been wholly defeated after a prolonged fight, in retreating to a corner, uttered a plaintive moan, not loud, but sorrowful.

I will here glance at, without anticipating, the anatomical description of the manner in which the alligator hisses. This is not accomplished by expelling the air directly from the glottidian aperture, but from the posterior fauces and funnel-shaped pharynx. (The latter should, I venture to think, be regarded as the cheeks of the alligator.) The air first accumulated in the lungs in great quantity, is expelled through the glottis into the posterior fauces and pharynx, which become largely inflated, the upward action of the thyroidian valve, which is of great size, preventing the air from escaping, while this cavity is being blown up like a bladder ; then, at the will of the animal, the muscles of the throat contract, expelling the air over the anterior margin of the great thyroidian plate, through the cleft palate above, and at the base of the tongue below.

ART. III.—*Vesico-Vaginal Fistula—Improvement on the Common Yoke Speculum of Prof. Sims.—Improvement in the Introduction of Sutures.* By H. ESTES, M. D., Edwards' Depôt, Hinds county, Mississippi.

I WOULD respectfully submit the following report of an operation for the closure of a vesico-vaginal fistula : The patient, a negress, æt. 21 years, the property of Mr. J. W. Ratliff, of Hinds county, was first seen by me on the 26th of December, 1858, being at that time in labor with her third child. The fistula was first observed immediately after her first delivery. Prior to the time of my seeing her, she had been operated on twice for closure of the fistula, but without success.

The fistula was of circular shape, five-eighths of an inch in diameter, and belonged to the fourth class of Dr. Bozeman. Before I could procure certain instruments which I deemed requisite to the performance of a successful operation, the patient again became pregnant, thus (as I then thought) necessitating a postponement of the operation.

On the 8th of May, 1860, having procured the desired instruments, and the patient having been delivered about two months before of her fourth child, I proceeded to operate, the patient being placed in the usual position, viz : on her elbows and knees, upon a table presenting to a side window. Present : Drs. McKay, Rice, Kirby, and

Robinett. Chloroform was administered *by the stomach*, not to the extent, however, of producing complete anæsthesia.

The steps of the operation were—1st, The removal of a strip of vaginal surface, three-eighths of an inch in width, from the entire circumference of the fistula. 2d, The introduction, antero-posteriorly, of six silver sutures, No. 29. 3d, The application, after the manner of Dr. W. L. Atlee, of Philadelphia, of the button or splint of Dr. Bozeman, as modified by Dr. Atlee (for an account of which, see *American Journal of Medical Sciences* for January, 1860).

The after treatment was not worthy of note. The suture apparatus was allowed to remain ten days, and was then removed in the presence of Drs. Rice, Kirby, Robinett, Williamson, and Wydown, when I had the satisfaction of finding an entire union. The patient was then permitted to walk about in accordance with her strength and inclination; and finding that she had full control over her urine, the catheter, which she had worn since the performance of the operation, was removed, and not reintroduced. An examination a few days afterwards displayed a firm cicatrix with perfect closure of the fistula. In a few days more the patient went about her ordinary avocation.

I have been induced to offer this report, with the following remarks, for publication, from the fact that surgeons, in accordance with their skill, or the lack of it, in the use of instruments, find little or much difficulty in the performance of operations for the cure of this affection. Every one acquainted with the nature of such cases is aware that, *cæteris paribus*, there is but one obstacle to success— that obstacle, inaccessibility. The difficulties in satisfactorily paring the margins of the fistula, and in introducing the sutures—difficulties which have taxed the inventive ingenuity of both surgeons and instrument makers no little—are both dependent on this inaccessibility. They are dependent, too, to some extent, on the flaccidity of the parts to be denuded, and through which the sutures are to be passed.

When I first examined the patient mentioned in this report, I used the common yoke speculum of Professor Sims, which displayed the fistula—its posterior or upper margin overhung by a prominence caused by a partial uterine prolapsus. I saw at once that, on this account, there would be much difficulty in paring this margin; in fact, that I could scarcely hope to be able to do more than scarify it with the point of the knife. I found also, that I could not so use the

100

speculum as to level this prominence. But these were not my only difficulties, for on elevating the rectum with the speculum, the lateral walls of the vagina collapsed to such an extent as to interfere materially with easy and free access to the fistula ; and not only so, but by their collapse they converted the floor of the vagina into an irregularly acute angle, thus ill-adapting it for a successful operation. These same difficulties, yet not in such degree, are attendant also on the single broad-blade speculum of Prof. Sims. To rid myself of these difficulties, I invented an attachment, consisting of two lateral blades, one inch in width, for the common yoke speculum, as represented in the following cuts. (They were made and attached for me, by Messrs. Otto and Reynders, 58 Chatham street, New York.)

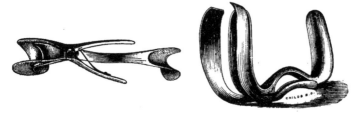

The patient being placed in position, the speculum, its blades closed, was introduced with perfect ease. The blades were then gradually expanded until their extent of separation measured from $2\frac{1}{4}$ inches to $2\frac{3}{4}$ inches. The vertical space measured from $1\frac{1}{2}$ inches to 2 inches, in accordance with the position given the speculum. It will be seen at once that these measurements are such as admit of perfect freedom of access to the parts immediately concerned, thus reducing this difficult operation to one perfectly simple, and that may be performed successfully by even the unskillful.

But there are other advantages gained by the use of this particular form of speculum, which are not gained by the use of any other. They are—1st, That it reduces the floor of the vagina, on which the operation is to be performed, to a plane surface in its whole extent, thus, in the case herewith reported, leveling the prominence overhanging the posterior margin of the fistula. 2d, That the blades, by their expansion, put the floor upon the stretch, thus rendering the paring easier, as also, the introduction of the sutures, and admirably adapting the surface to the easy and accurate application of the button or splint.

For the introduction of the sutures, I used a very small trochar and canula, smaller than Prof. Simpson's tubular needle by one-fourth of the diameter of the needle, and suggested instead of the same, and furnished me by Dr. Rice. The trochar and canula being introduced, the trochar was withdrawn and the suture introduced instead, which, as soon as it was passed sufficiently far, was grasped with a pair of forceps and drawn through to the extent required, being drawn over the fork invented by Dr. Bozeman, which, by being passed beyond the extremity of the canula, prevented injury to its very delicate edge. Thus the sutures were passed with an ease and rapidity which elicited commendation from all present.

In connection with the case herewith reported, it has lately become necessary to add the following : In a few weeks after the patient was discharged, she became pregnant again, and about the middle of August, having lifted a heavy stick of wood and walked a short distance with it, she found that she could not retain her urine. On examination, I found a fistula which would barely admit a pocket-case probe, and situated at the left extremity of the cicatrix of the former operation. In accounting for this, it is necessary that I mention (which I omitted for the sake of brevity in my report), that I cut two small arteries very near together, and in left extremity of the pared surface. The hæmorrhage from them was considerable at the time, interfering materially with the remaining steps of the operation, and continuing to bleed slowly for some time after the patient was put to bed. The result was the formation of a clot partially keeping assunder the pared surfaces, and thus rendering the new vesico-vaginal septum thinner at this point than at any other in the line of union.

On the 5th of September, although the patient was two and a half months advanced in pregnancy, I again operated, assisted by my friend, Dr. J. E. Slicer, late of Richmond, Virginia. On the 14th, I removed the sutures, three in number. The operation proved a successful ,one, and was unattended by even the least threatening of abortion.

In conclusion, I would beg leave to say that this is the second time that I have operated successfully for closure of vesico-vaginal fistula, with the help of only one assistant, thus demonstrating the utility of the speculum to which I have called attention, as a labor-saving instrument, in addition to its other self-recommending properties.

SEPTEMBER, 1860.

Art. IV.—*Some account of the Hot Springs of Arkansas*: Communicated in a letter from A. J. Wright, Esq., to Dr. Samuel A. Cartwright, asking for information.

[Dr. Cartwright says that he has been in the habit of requesting intelligent patients, willing to take the trouble, whom he sends to the various watering places, to communicate to him an account of the effects of the water upon them, and whatever other truths they may extort from Nature by their own experience and observation, with a view of adding something to the general stock of medical knowledge, which is very deficient in regard to American medicinal springs. He thinks this letter of Mr. Wright contains more useful information in regard to the Hot Springs of Arkansas than any account heretofore published. Ed.]

Hot Springs, Arkansas.

Dr. Samuel Cartwright, New Orleans, Louisiana:

Dear Sir—The trip to this place, except in midsummer, is not an unpleasant one. There are tri-weekly first-class packets running to Napoleon, and comfortable little boats thence to Little Rock, whence extra coaches may at all times be had to transport passengers by easy journeys, at reasonable prices, over good roads to the Springs.

In giving you so much of the information asked for as I may be able, excuse me if I insert matters with which you are already familiar.

On many of the old maps two ranges of mountains are marked, running east and west, parallel and distant from each other eighty to one hundred miles, but the whole western and north-western part of the State is so thickly studded with numerous hills as to resemble one vast mountainous tract or group of mountains, of which no geological survey has ever been made. The whole abounds in minerals, and especially in mineral springs. No doubt is entertained but that the deep shafts, crumbled furnaces, and mining implements found among them are the traces of DeSoto and his followers. (*See Remarks.*)

You strike these hills soon after leaving the Arkansas river at Little Rock, after which you do not leave them. The Hot Springs are situated about six miles from the Ouachita,* near the point where that river emerges from the range of mountains in which it

---

* This orthography is likely to become obsolete, as Washita is rising into favor.—Ed.

rises. Thereabout, the hills, from 400 to 700 feet above the level of the valleys, are composed almost entirely of silicious rocks of various colors, greenish, red, etc., but chiefly white. The streams, which are numerous, including Hot Springs Creek and the Ouachita, here about 250 yards wide, all run on beds of slate stone—somewhat irregular and broken, and often protruding near the margins in thick shelving masses very precipitous ; their sides, and all that portion of the valleys not washed out by the torrents, being covered with broken quartz rocks, of all sizes, which the elements have been crumbling down for ages. The soil is thin and flinty, supporting, however, a growth of pines and some varieties of oak. At the summits, the quartz is piled in huge irregular sharp-edged blocks, forming, often, perpendicular precipices, but without any trace of volcanic action. It seems that in the disturbance which protruded these vast masses of quartz through the slate, the disturbing or central fire did not reach the surface here. Bits of mineral heavy with iron, and apparently cooled on the surface into beautiful globules, found about half a mile from the Spring mountain, were often shown in proof of an extinct volcano, but they are well known by geologists, and indicate the reverse, being, in fact, the substance commonly called bloodstone. Iron ore is found scattered among these hills, and one or two large masses of it on the Spring mountain, which, like the others, is almost wholly composed of flint, freestone, and quartz of all sizes.

But its Westerly side, to the height of 80 or 90 feet, is covered with, or is apparently composed of calcareous tufa from out of and over which the springs run. This tufa, blackened and made porous by the weather—heated in some places by the overrunning water and lying in rounded shape, as if cooled in rolling down—is regarded by the vulgar as another proof of igneous origin ; the undoubted fact being, that the springs ordinarily deposit this very substance in gutters and in excavations made for the purpose, to the extent, in most cases, of about one-eighth of an inch annually—a few days sufficing to obtain a coating of it in an excavation—and that the whole hillside is "a deposit from the springs, having assumed, in the course of ages, just the rounded or cascade-like form we might expect from their action. (See Remarks.)

Hot Springs Creek rises in the valley of Horse-Shoe Mountain, about a mile and three quarters from the Hot Springs. Its source consists of springs, and it is in fine weather a rivulet over which you can step with ease. Passing through a deep gorge or valley not much more than one hundred yards in width, it here laves the base of the Hot Springs Mountain on the east and the "Cold Mountain" on the west, each near five hundred feet above its level ; and into its waters, by cascades and *jets d'eau,* fall the healing ones of the Hot Springs.

It is worthy of notice that on the opposite side of the same mountain, and not three-fourths of a mile from it, there is a plentiful chalybeate spring, gushing from an immense quartz rock, of which the waters are so cold as to be drunk with difficulty.

The considerations which go to prove that these waters derive their heat from a great depth, are too obvious to require mention ; nor is there any thing improbable, to my mind, in the supposition that it is derived from the central heat of the earth.

Of the Hot Springs, there are some fifty-four distinctly recognizable, besides a considerable number in the bed of the creek. With one exception, their temperature ranges from 120° to 148° of F., and their composition is nearly the same. The exception is a warm spring (temperature 100°) discovered a year ago on the bank of the creek beneath the others. It has a strong odor and taste of sulphur, and is believed to have considerable virtues. *(See Remarks.)*

The quantity of water discharged by the various hot springs is estimated at 350 gallons per minute (one spring affording 60 gallons), or, say about 500,000 *gallons per diem.*

The analysis of the water is as follows (by Prof. Owen, State Geologist, Arkansas) :

1½ (one and a half) gallons of water contain—

Of Silica, with Sulphate of Lime	1.04 grains.
Carb. of Lime, 1.68, and with Bi-Carb. of Lime...	2.04 "
Carbonate of Magnesia	0.326 "
Bi-Carb. of Magnesia	0.05 "
Sulph. of Lime, dissolved in water	0.35 "
Chloride of Potass	0.05 "
Chloride of Sodium	2.18 "
Oxide of Iron, with a little Alumina	0.133 "
Dry Powder (insol.)	1.16 "

The average attendance of visiters this spring and summer has been about four hundred, chiefly of persons afflicted with rheumatism, neuralgia, paralysis, dyspepsia, mercurial affections, and syphilis. Rheumatism is the most frequent of these.

The baths are taken according to the custom of the place, without immediate medical supervision. Small wooden bath-houses are fitted over the creek, and close to the precipitous edge of the hill. Wooden reservoirs retain the water which they receive through wooden troughs, until it is sufficiently cooled to be borne : it is then dropped in a stream of about an inch in diameter, from a height of nine or ten feet, upon the affected part, or the body generally (the time, according to the patient's power of endurance), and is received into a large wooden tub used for the plunge bath. A small chamber adjoining receives the steam from the constant flow of the water, through wooden strips on which he stands, and drinking copious draughts of "hot and hot" in the meanwhile, the patient endures the vapor for five or ten minutes without any apparatus for breathing of fresh air, an occasional protrusion of the nose at the door being necessary : After which, more drinking of "hot and hot," and to bed to sweat profusely under blankets from half an hour to two. This, once or twice a day, and the frequent drinking fresh hot during the day, other medicines being laid aside. This is what custom prescribes.

As a first effect of this treatment, rheumatics generally experience a return of pain to all parts previously attacked, and frequently in parts not previously affected, and throughout the body, the pains being frequent and often severe. I myself had been for some weeks free from pain, except in one ankle ; but, after a single bath, began to have the aches and pains peculiar to rheumatism in nearly all the joints and muscles. They continued with me for about two weeks (from one to three weeks is their common duration), a relief from them being experienced for an hour or two after the bath. Their gradual disappearance is regarded as indicating a cure. There are, however, well authenticated cases where they have continued during a stay of two months or more, and soon after leaving the springs the patient has found them to disappear and a permanent cure to have been established. *(See Remarks.)*

Another common effect is an active salivation in such as have used mercury—the soreness and spitting often continuing two to four weeks ; and on recovery from this, some disease dependent on it, supposed perhaps to be neuralgia, rheumatism or ophthalmia, disappeared. This I have seen repeatedly.

A number ·resort here· for the cure of gout, not generally with success.

The curative effects are not generally perceptible to the patient, many complaining of being worse, or no better, who ultimately go away cured.

Drinking the fresh hot water seems to have a very soothing effect on irritable conditions of the stomach—acts, I guess, on the mucous membrane. No nausea attends its first or its frequent use, and it is drank in large quantities with relish and relief before and soon after meals.

Its first effect on the bowels vary much, and frequently cause a temporary derangement, constipation, or the reverse, which disappears during the first fortnight.

Paralytic cases, stiffness in the joints, contractions of the muscles, swellings on the bones, are relieved slowly in general, sometimes quickly, sometimes not at all, though the cases are few in which some relief is not experienced. They are treated with overdoses of douche. Some three or four, I saw come, unable to walk, or moving slowly with assistance of others, and crutches. They seemed to improve in general health, and to gain a little freedom of motion daily, without seeming aware of the improvement themselves. Hands that were knotted up gradually relaxed, and rheumatic swellings disappeared without other previous indications of a cure than improved appetite and regular perspiration. The swelling you may recollect on my left hand, disappeared in about a month. I saw one young lady arrive, walking with great difficulty on crutches. She had had fever, and as a result of it, an affection apparently paralytic in her ankles. In about a fortnight she was conspicuous in the ball room for her graceful dancing. There seemed to be no doubt about the cure, but some opined that Cupid had lent her his wings, which accounted for the lightness of her carriage. My *vis-à-vis* at the table, was a lady who had one knee and one hip useless from old rheumatism, and who could not get to her meals except with assistance of her husband and a crutch. Although very delicate, she took the douche for a half hour or so twice a day. Her health improved daily, and at the end of two months she walked slowly by herself. My own impression was very strong that a continuance of the treatment would have cured her.

The improvement of the appetite, after the first week, was almost universal. Coarse food becomes palatable.

Palpitation of the heart was a symptom frequently caused by immoderate or ill-timed use of the bath, as were also headache and nervousness, and, occasionally, the victim of chill and fever to such as had had it (other baths, of similar temperature, are said on high authority to have the latter effect uniformly) ; but in this region, the chill and fever yields promptly to the proper treatment, at least it did in my case, and in every one which I saw.

The presence of a good physician to superintend the bathing and record its effects, would be a great thing for patients and for the science of medicine. The only physician practising there, Dr. Hammond, died shortly after our arrival. For want of advice, or for excess of it from everybody, the injudicious use of the baths has doubtless proved fatal in a number of cases to persons who came here extremely ill.

There is one disease, in the cure of which these waters have no rival : I mean syphilis in its advanced stages, and especially where it has been unsuccessfully treated with mercurials. From what I have seen, I believe they have no rival in the cure of this affection.

When spacious hotels, built of stone, which is so plentiful here, and abounding in numerous comfortable bath-rooms, shall fill this valley, so admirably adapted to their construction—and when a railroad now building shall bring passengers from nearly all the great travel lines of the Union converging at Memphis—from what island in the Pacific or Indian Ocean will not the afflicted seek these healing fountains, and what number of thousands shall be the limit of the concourse ! For I do not hesitate to say that buildings could be so constructed as to accommodate with the waters from 8,000 to 10,000 visitors.

There are numerous other springs in the neighborhood, as sulphur, chalybeate, etc.; but one eight miles distant, and called the Sulphur Spring, seems worthy of notice, as it is said to contain *an excess of nitrate of potash*, some bi-carb. of soda, sulphur, chloride of sodium, magnesia, iron, alumina, and iodine (?). I have seen its use produce the happiest effects in rheumatic cases.

You ask me for some observations on the *modus operandi* of the waters. I can give you none. Their mode of action seems to be of the kind called insensible. My own opinion is that the chief virtue lies in the following things : Pure, dry mountain air (the valley is fifteen hundred feet above the sea level), and an abundant supply of

101

pure hot water, free from every taint of cooking utensil or hurtful metallic substance. These conditions any where fulfilled would have the same result. I believe, too, the water drunk acts by soothing irritation of the stomach, improving digestion, and that the baths act as powerful stimulants, and at the same time, in conjunction with the drinking, cause constant uniform perspiration. And it is my opinion that good digestion and healthful perspiration, with exercise and pure dry air, will leave only one cure out of a thousand for the doctors to perform.

The chief disadvantage of a residence here results from the insufficiency of the accommodations. The parties to the protracted litigation for the ownership of the springs are unwilling to expend money for their improvement until the suits are decided. The houses are old and rickety, and but one room in many cases is allotted to four persons, in some to five. The discomfort and danger to health from these causes are better imagined than described.

Yours very respectfully,   A. J. WRIGHT.

AUGUST 25, 1859.

REMARKS BY DR. CARTWRIGHT.

In 1804 and 1805, Wm. Dunbar, Esq., of Natchez, and Dr. Hunter, at the instance of President Jefferson, explored the Washita as far the Hot Springs. In his report to the President of the United States (see Medical Repository, vol. 9, p. 305, etc.), Mr. Dunbar, speaking of the Hot Springs, says : "The water is palatable, and very good to drink, having but little foreign impregnation. The body of the mountain from which it issues, is silicious, partly flint and partly freestone ; but the superficial parts which have been overflowed by the effusions from the Springs, are incrusted with a stratum of calcareous matter, that, in the course of time has been deposited from this water. A trifling portion of iron is contained in it, too, and precipitated with the lime. In the hot water of these springs a green plant vegetated, which seemed to be a species of the *conferva*, probably the *fontinalis*. But what is more remarkable, a bivalve testaceous animal adhered to the plant and lived in such a high temperature too."

"This country," continues Mr. Dunbar, "was colonized early by the French. They projected and began extensive settlements on the Washita ; but the general massacre planned, and executed in part, by the Indians against the French, put an end to their undertakings, and they were never resumed under the French government." He mentions a silicious composition resembling oil-stone or Turkey-stone, and also mineralized wood and carbonated wood found in the vicinity of the springs, but found no lava, pumice, or other volcanic matter.

A very interesting account of the Hot Springs of Arkansas is contained in a letter from Dr. Joseph Macrery, of Natchez, published in the Medical Repository, vol. 9, p. 47–50. New York : 1806. We learn from this letter, that several persons of Natchez, and the Mississippi territory, visited the Hot Springs in 1804, a little prior to the exploration of W. Dunbar, Esq. This letter states that the spring mountain or hills consist mostly of silex in its various combinations, and schistus or slate. The exploring party discovered antimony, mineralized by sulphur, of a bluish grey metallic appearance with radiated crystalization, composed of slender hexahedral prisms ; zinc, mineralized by sulphur, forming the ore called blende; feldspar, of a white, inclining to a red color, granulated texture, the surface covered with crystal, of a rectangular form, and very brilliant ; black schorl, with pieces of quartz intermixed." They analyzed the mineral substances met with in search of gold and silver, but found none. They analyzed the water and found it to contain less mineral impregnation than common spring water usually does. A little carbonic acid was detected in it, a slight trace of iron, a small quantity of calcareous matter, and a little muriate of soda. They tried it by the various reägents commonly used to detect minerals, viz : Muriate of barytes, spirits of ammoniac, caustic potash, acetate of lead, nitrate of mercury, the sulphuric and muriatic acids ; but these reägents produced no effect upon the water. The party learned that the Hot Spring mountain had, from time immemorial, been called by the Indians *the Land of Peace,* and that hostile tribes, while there, remain in harmony with one another. They learned that the aborigines resorted to these Springs on account of their medicinal virtues, and that the white people in the nearest settlements "testified to their efficacy in curing or relieving chronic pains, paralytic affections, and inability to motion generally.

"Many of the white hunters, who are very liable to disease from exposure to the vicissitudes of climate and season, have been restored by the use of these Springs from a state of entire inability of motion to complete health and activity.

"The water is soft and limpid, without smell. The taste is agreeable. It is used in preference to the cold springs in the vicinity. In July, 1804, it was very dry ; the degree of heat was so great that persons could not expose themselves to the vapor, which is the usual mode adopted by those who visit them on account of their health. Meat was boiled in the water in a shorter time than could be accomplished by a culinary fire ; it was made use of to prepare both tea and coffee. The temperature of the water is [not] influenced by the season."

REMARKS BY SAMUEL A. CARTWRIGHT, M. D.

[*Explanatory Note by the Managing Editor.*—The delay in publishing Mr. Wright's paper, which in itself is acceptable, was caused by the inability of the editor (under which he still labors) to reconcile the analysis, which Mr. Wright quotes from Prof. Owen, with the remarks which Dr. Cartwright attached to the original paper. This explanation is necessary, in order that the reader may understand the purpose of this second series of remarks by Dr. Cartwright. It will be seen, according to Prof. Owen, State Geologist, that twelve pints of the waters of the Hot Springs contain but 7.219 grains of foreign ingredients, divided among very numerous substances, so that there is, of this compound, but little over half a grain in one pint. How such a water, which by various accounts contains enormous quantities of mineral matter, and which turns to stone, can be almost wholly pure, is the question which the learned writer has undertaken to solve. *Audi alteram partem.*]

I visited the Arkansas Hot Springs two years ago, and remained there several weeks. I am sure the water is charged with something which has not been mentioned in these analyses. I think it is electrified oxygen or azone. I noticed the green plant mentioned by Mr. Dunbar, as a species of *conferva,* and by Prof. Bell and others regarded as a deposit from the water. I could arrive at nothing satisfactory in regard to it. It is not a deposit from the water, as is generally supposed ; nor do I think it a *conferva.* If it were a deposit, it would occupy some fixed place in the stream of hot water, at the bottom, top or sides ; but it is found in all these places. I put some of it in my ears, and in a few days had great difficulty in getting it out. It had turned to a gritty substance, like stone. It was soft and unctious, yet it soon hardened into a calcareous looking substance like that which covers the hill side from whence the hot springs issue. I take it to be, not a vegetable, but a mineral animal, or stony polyp, a jelly-like animal—the *coral rag*. Information is needed in regard to it. I am sure it will prove to be a species of *coral*, bearing the same relation to hot mineral water that the coral bears to sea water. It is so abundant in the hot water as to lead me to the conclusion that the upper crust of the Hot Spring Mountain, or calcareous matter, mentioned by Dunbar and other explorers, is entirely formed from it, and not from any deposit in the water itself. The water itself is proved, by direct and repeated experiments, to deposit nothing whatever.

"Consider how many and how different distempers are cured by the use of the hot baths and medicated waters." "There is observed in all those medicated waters, a certain spirituous principle, very volatile, which renders them easily movable through all the vessels of the body, and makes them that they can be drank in *much greater quantity* than even the purest common water. In some medicated waters, that volatile principle is so very subtle, that they ought to be drunk at fountain head. But as soon as they are deprived of their volatile principle, they taste perfectly vapid. Some of these waters contain nothing else besides that volatile principle and pure water, at least nothing can be obtained from them by any chemical experiments." [See vol. 10, page 244, Van Swieten's Commentaries on Boerhaave.]

There is a spirituous principle in the water of the Hot Springs of Arkansas. It may be electrified oxygen or ozone. There is another principle in them, which causes a little salt and pepper to convert them into a very *palatable soup*, or, at least, a liquid tasting like soup. It is, perhaps, the basis of gelatin. But will the fact be believed that a little salt and pepper thrown into water, almost chemically pure, will convert it into a palatable soup, or a liquid tasting like soup made from the flesh of animals? Shall the fact be suppressed on that account, is the question? It may be asked, if there be gluten in the water why does it not show itself by gelatinizing when the water cools? Researches in animal chemistry have proved, that long boiling *destroys* the property of gluten to gelatinize, and hence the substance, which forms at least a third of the tissues of man, and is the basis of his bony structure, eludes all the senses, when boiled in water, except the sense of taste. The sense of taste detects it in the Hot Springs of Arkansas, when a little salt and pepper are added to the water containing it. Leucine and glycine can be produced from gluten by boiling with caustic potash. Leucine may also be obtained the same way from the protein compounds. Shall the fact be ignored or suppressed, that a large proportion of the human body is composed of gelatinous substances, because no chemist has ever yet been able to detect gelatin in the blood, or in any healthy fluid of the body? There is surely glue in the bones and all those tissues, whose functions are mechanical, although the chemist cannot detect it in the blood or other healthy fluids of the body. How did it get into the tissues, and why is the glue from the skin and bones of old animals more tenacious and cohesive than from younger animals, are questions more difficult to explain, than the question why salt and pepper will convert the almost chemically pure water of the Arkansas Hot Springs into a beverage like soup? If all facts which cannot be satisfactorily explained were suppressed, the sciences would be half demolished. But when facts apparently conflict with one another, does the cause of truth and science require that one or the other be suppressed? Surely not if they are ascertained to be facts cognizable to one or more of the senses. They may be antagonistic facts only in appearance, artificially and not naturally antagonistic, made so by antagonistic explanations of them. Thus, Wm. Dunbar, of Natchez, long known to the scientific world, attributes the calcareous upper stratum of the Hot Spring Mountain as deposited by the water of the Hot Springs itself. The conflicting fact is the almost chemical purity of the water. How can it be pure, and contain so much calcareous matter to encrust a mountain? How can it be pure, and filled with a green gelatinous substance, which he calls conferva? How can it be pure, if a stick or twig left in it a short time becomes encrusted with a calcareous substance like the upper stratum of the mountain? Are we to deny the existence of these facts, or deny the purity of the water? The antagonism is in the theory of explanation—not in the facts themselves. The calcareous matter is there on the mountain in and around the springs. A similar calcareous matter, in the shape of shoals and islands, is found in the ocean. It is admitted that these shoals and islands are not formed by vegetable growth, by sea-drift, or by depositions from sea water, as their first discoverers may have supposed, but are built up by the exuviæ of little animals, called *polypiers*, inhabiting the waters where the shoals and islands are found. These animals are found to consist of a gelatinous substance and the salts of lime. The latter, being a stony substance is indestructible, and accumulates with every generation of these animals. Suppose, before science could satisfactorily account for their formation, the makers of the charts for mariners had said to the discoverers, we will not put down your shoals and islands on our charts, because you contradict yourselves: "you say that the sea water, where these shoals and islands exist, does not differ perceptibly from the common water of the ocean ; we cannot swallow the contradiction that there is no extra sediment in the water beyond other sea water, and yet believe that the shoals and islands you pretend to have discovered have any existence, and we will not insert them on the charts ; we could not do so without involving you in contradictions ; we have more respect for you and ourselves than to make liars out of you." Nature is true to herself: she does not lie. Those who faithfully report the phenomena of Nature, as witnessed by their senses, may not be able to explain them, but their statement of the facts cognizable to their senses, may involve apparent contradictions ; but the lie or contradiction is imaginary, not real : it is in the brain of the theorizer, whose theories weave it into a contradiction, and not in Nature or the observer of Nature. The brain of the individual who has got the theory in his head that the upper crust of the Hot Springs Mountain is deposited by the water, and that the green gelatinous substance in it is also deposited by the same fluid, will not permit him to believe in the fact that the water is purer than common spring water usually is. But his belief does not add a particle of impurity to the water, or take away a particle of the calcareous matter forming the upper crust of the side of the mountain from which the Hot Springs issue. His belief in regard to the green slime found in the water, does not alter its character : it turns to stone when dried, whether he believes it or not. All polypiers, when dead, leave behind them an indestructible substance resembling stone. The green substance in the Hot Springs water of Arkansas cannot be any thing lse than polypiers. The upper crust of the mountain consists of their dead bodies. While living, they attract lime from water. "Enfin, on croit que les polypiers absorbent la part calcaire de l'eau, et qu'ils la purifient." *(Dic. du Science Méd.*, vol. 44, p. 262.) " La forme extérieure des polypiers, qui est souvent celle de certaine plantes, les a longtemps fait regarde comme des véritables végétaux. Les naturalistes ayant reconnu des animaux dans plusieurs d'entre caux." (Page 161, vol. 44). * * * Mr. Dunbar discovered animals of a bivalvular form in the green substance in the Hot Springs water. He took that green substance to be a conferva, but Dunbar's theory does not alter the facts.

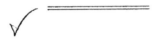

ART. V.—*Remarks on Medical Hydrology and Mineral Waters, includ-ing the Hot Springs of Arkansas:* By BENNET DOWLER, M. D.

ALTHOUGH the number of letters which I have received from the readers of this Journal, making inquiry concerning the medicinal properties of mineral waters, particularly those of Arkansas,* may to some extent excuse, if not wholly justify some general remarks upon these topics, without my having had the advantages of a large experience in, or much opportunity for personal observation on medical hydrology, yet, I hope by calling attention to this subject to induce the friends of science to contribute such information in the premises as they may possess, particularly in reference to the medicinal waters of the South, so that an interchange of facts and opinions may be of mutual advantage, and at the same time supply a want long felt in the conduction of this Journal. Many physicians, during the summer season, find their clientship greatly reduced by absentees to Northern watering places, while, perhaps, waters equally good or better, but not equally known, abound nearer home. The nature, and uses, both internal and external of the mineral and thermal waters of the whole country should be objects of medical study as well as the preparations of the Pharmacopœia.

At the present time, medical hydrology, or hydrotherapy, is attract-ing great attention, not only on the part of the profession, but is becoming an object of imperial legislation, particularly in France,

---

* STEEP CREEK, P. O., LOUNDES CO., ALA., May 4, 1860.

DR. B. DOWLER, *Editor N. O. Med. and Surg. Journal*—Will you be so kind as to give the readers of your Journal your views of the virtues of the Hot Springs of Arkansas, in the treatment of rheuma-tism; judging from the many failures to cure this very painful disease, I am confident your views upon this subject will prove acceptable to many of your readers.

Yours, etc.,   D. S. N****, M. D.

wherein a decree of great length, including thirty-six articles, was, on the 28th of January, 1860, issued in that country, establishing medical inspectorships and regulations for all the mineral springs and establishments of the empire. Legislation regulating the medicinal uses of the mineral waters of France date many years ago, the rehabilitation, extension, and improvement of which, are contemplated in the recent law. The revenues and fees of proprietors and inspectors, and the gratuitous attendance on the indigent sick, and the free use of the waters, are comprehended in the civil and medical administration created by this decree, which must in its practical operations be very complex—a wheel in a wheel. In Europe, special treatises, societies, and periodicals,* are devoted to these investigations, which, however, must not be confounded with the charlatanries of hydropathy,† the pretended universal water-cure for all maladies.

Opinions seldom clash with or contradict each other so much upon any other topic as they do in regard to the curative property of various mineral waters. Both professional and non-professional persons are apt to be biased in favor of the reputed medicinal springs which are situated in their vicinity. The therapeutic universality ascribed to these waters, which are often highly charged with medicinal agents of apparently opposite or different qualities, seems, theoretically speaking, hard to reconcile with the well defined indications which are supposed to characterize the skillful prescriber. Alkaline, acid, or neutral ; tonic, purgative, or astringent ; stimulant, antiphlogistic, or sedative ; or whatsoever other qualities these medicinal waters may possess, they are by many supposed to be curative, if not panaceas, in almost all diseases. A vast deal of limestone, in the form of sulphates and carbonates, are swallowed, together with

---

* The French Journals, as the *Gazette des Eaux; Annales des Maladies Chroniques (Medecine et Chirurgie) et de L'Hydrologie Medicale, Revue d'Hydrologie Med;* as also numerous published documents, official reports, pamphlets, and special treatises, upon mineral springs, both in and outside of France, show that in this country at least, these waters are deemed of very great importance for prophylactic and curative purposes.

† HYDROPATHY. Water-cure, or the method of curing diseases by means of water ; introduced by Vincent Priessnitz, of Silesia. (Worcester's Dict., 1860) This definition omits one fundamental particular of this system, namely : the water must be pure, cold, etc. " It is not sufficient," says Weiss, " that the water should be cold, but it must also be fresh." Dr. Dunglison's definition affords nothing very satisfactory, thus : " HYDROPATHY, hydrosudotherapeia." This latter word, he says, " expresses the mode of treating diseases systematically by cold water, sweating, etc." " Hydro-therapeia " he defines with one word, that is, " bydrosudotherapeia." Hydropathy is appropriated to a sect, with which hydrotherapy or medical hydrology should not be confounded, from merely etymological reasons.

the salts of soda, as glauber salts and table salt—the salts of magnesia, particularly epsom salts—also salts and other combinations of iron, alumina, sulphur, and the like, the purpose of which is not always evident.

If the patient need a ferruginous preparation, he has generally to swallow much which he does not need, as vast quanties of water, chloride of soda, sulphate of magnesia, carbonate of lime, and many other similar and dissimilar substances, held either in solution or suspension. This complexity of mineral springs is so great, that a chemical, physiological or therapeutic classification of them is provisional rather than rigorously correct; for whether called ferruginous, sulphureous, saline, alkaline, or acid, other and different properties are often present, and may neutralize each other, or constitute polypharmacy, as well as more or less incompatibility. Where, however, a predominating quality is found, as in the alkaline water of Bladon (Alabama), or in the saline purgative property of the Bedford water (Pennsylvania), a clear indication is afforded, and theory and practice verify each other.

In excessive acidity, an alkaline water would, doubtlessly, at least for a time, be useful, even though it might not, as it probably would not, cure the original malady or morbid alteration from which the acidity proceeded. But, according to the received doctrines, the introduction into the economy of alkaline agents might be injurious or beneficial, according to the condition of the sick, as is the case with all medicines. In perfect health they would be only detrimental, and the same may be affirmed as to some maladies. Prof. Wood regards the alkalies as antiphlogistic in their action. He further says : "When in excess in the stomach and bowels, the alkalies act as irritants, and, very largely given, or in a concentrated state, may cause severe inflammation, and even corrosion. Their abuse is apt to induce want of appetite, gastric uneasiness, and other symptoms of dyspepsia. A certain excess of alkali in the blood is essential to the continued solubility of the albumen and fibrin, and possibly for other purposes; but, beyond the normal amount, it produces effects, dependent probably on a direct alteration in the condition of the organized constituents of that fluid. The coagulability of the febrin is probably impaired, and, under a very powerful influence, the blood corpuscles themselves, to a certain extent, broken up and dissolved," and, as he thinks, a tendency to the formation of calculi may be thus promoted. (*Therap. and Pharm.*, i, 845–6.)

Now, from this exposition, which applies chiefly to the carbonate of soda, the best and most generally used of the alkalies, it is difficult to understand how the Vichy Springs of France, and their analogue, the Bladon Vichy Spring of Alabama, the best perhaps of their kind, deriving their fundamental character from the carbonate of soda, can be safely used by all sorts of people, sick and well, in all varieties of disease, and especially in such as dyspepsia, stone, and a multitude of asthenic or non-inflammatory and chronic maladies. It is remarkable that such waters should be recommended by medical hydrologists, as common beverages.

Some writers, however, disdain to take refuge in mineral mystery and occult history. Dr. Durand Fardel says : " Medical hydrologists, those more particularly who belong to certain spas, admit still, and with great complacency, the antiquated doctrine that each mineral watering-place is endowed with occult and specific virtues, that render it suitable to certain distinct maladies; whereas, the real state of the question is, not to ascertain whether such a water be specific against gout or rheumatism, or a uterine disease, or a complaint of the kidneys, but under what conditions of a certain given case of disease a certain mineral water is sure to be useful. Thermal medicine is a matter of appreciation and tact. A mineral water has no other value than that which a skillful physician knows how to elicit from it. To consider it as a medicament, prepared and supplied by nature for a single special object, is an error. Mineral waters are simple instruments in the hands of the physician, from which it is for him to obtain the most advantageous results."

The same author quotes from Dr. Barthez's account of the physiological and therapeutic action of the Vichy waters, which the *Br. and For. Med. Chir. Rev.*, July, 1860, sums up as follows (the latter portion of which, concerning the prolonged use of the waters, confirming Dr. Wood's statement) : " In quantities of twelve or fifteen glasses a day, and continued during thirty days or so, the Vichy waters have no very sensible influence upon the circulation ; if any thing, it is somewhat lessened. Sometimes a desire to sleep is induced ; at times a slight feeling of excitement or species of intoxication. The appetite is usually increased and digestion improved ; slight constipation rather than relaxation is apt to be induced. The urine is generally rendered alkaline in less than an hour after drinking the water, and remains clear and free from sediment of uric acid or urates. It is usually rendered in smaller quantities than the amount of water drank, which is accounted for by an increased action of the cutaneous function. The generative organs are commonly somewhat excited, especially at the commencement of the course. If the waters be continued even in moderation beyond a certain time—say three weeks—atonic dyspepsia is often induced, with diminution of muscnlar strength, at the same time diarrhœa is apt to supervene, and other signs of irritation of the abdominal organs. The action of the Vichy waters is evidently due to the large amount of bi-carbonate of soda contained in them, which, when introduced into the system, renders the blood more than normally alkaline—a condition which diminishes the plasticity of the several constituents of that fluid, alters the characters of the various secretions and excretions derived from it, and likewise stimulates the different glands."

Mineral waters, however, of a complex character, in which numerous substances are chemically combined, are therapeutically and even analytically of very uncertain import, being compounds of compounds, the general characters of which may or may not be represented in the analysis of the members of the group. The chemistry and the common effects of this unity may elude research, or be changed by artificial methods, so that a predominating ingredient of the analysis may be but a subordinate one in the natural or original chemical combination.

Rational therapy, whether theoretical or practical, appears, therefore, no where more equivocal and faulty, than at mineral springs, if the rôle assigned to them by writers be considered impartial. A dyspeptic patient is, perhaps, directed to drink, before breakfast, from a quart to a gallon of water differing little from sea water or a strong brine of common salt ; another patient, with chronic diarrhœa, is advised to a similar dose of a water, the fundamental element of which is epsom salts. Thus, the Bedford waters of Pennsylvania (admirable as an aperient as I know from the experience of one season) are highly recommended in diarrhœa, whereas, they are chemically and practically purgative, forming an elegant prescription in place of the usual bitter solution of epsom salts, having a little lime variously combined, a sprinkling of table-salt, and a little touch of iron, which, with carbonic acid gas, disguise the taste without impeding the action of the sulphate of magnesia ; and yet, plethoric people, appoplectics and the like, have been cautioned against the risk of taking these tonic waters—a barrel of which might be safely taken at one draught without any risk from the iron tonic in the same. Of the carbonate of iron, Wood and Bache say, " No nicety need be observed in the dose. The usual dose is from five to thirty grains three times a day." A barrel of this water which does not contain 100 grains of the carbonate of iron, holds in solution 2,560 grains of epsom salts, which latter give it a value, simplicity, and consistency rarely met with in mineral springs.

Neither a spring nor a prescription should generally be sought which is based upon a mixture of stimulant and contra-stimulant, tonic and debilitating, astringent and purgative agents, which, according to the principles of pharmacology, are either incompatible with each other, or of doubtful therapeutic import, owing to their complexity and their possible reäctions as influenced by the physiological chemistry of the economy.

The most frequented springs in the United States appear to be those of Saratoga, in New York, the celebrated congress water of which contains, as analists report, abundance of common salt, amounting to about two-thirds of its solid contents ; the remaining third is nearly equally divided between the carbonates of lime and magnesia, the carbonate of iron being almost nothing—not one per cent. This brine, not so strong as that of the Red Sea, in doses from three to eight pints, will doubtlessly purge many people. Dr. Steel, who wrote a book on these waters, says, " some invalids drink thirty and even'forty tumblers full of congress water, in the morning, without much apparent inconvenience" (118) ; such a dose would contain about 2,000 grains of salt ; *his* dose is *three pints*, which, according to his analysis, contain 144.36 grains of salt. Than this, perhaps no mineral water is more generally used, not only at its source, but in distant places. Salt, lime, magnesia, in purgative doses, as in these waters, may be useful in a limited number of cases, but not as an universal remedy. Among the fifteen thousand visitors to these springs during this season, considering the quantity of water required for a dose, it is difficult to understand how all could be supplied, as Dr. Steel says that this famous congress spring " issues at the rate of something less than a gallon per minute !" Many celebrated waters contain medicinal agents of opposite tendencies to each other, or substances which are either inert or injurious, all of which the therapeutist tries to eliminate or avoid in practice.

Fatal eases, often the most instructive, are seldom reported by physicians and surgeons, and especially such cases as have been blunderingly or unjustifiably treated, and the same remark applies in medical hydrology. It is unreasonable to suppose that any medicinal spring is adapted to the cure of all maladies and conditions whatsoever. How discriminating soever may be the choice of a spring, as being adapted to a special case, still the enormous quantity of liquid usually taken at once or in quick succession, whereby the stomach is suddenly distended, seems, upon mere mechanical principles, not altogether free from risk. Reasoning from analogy, injurious effects might be anticipated from using many of the fashionable waters, which, for the most part, are contaminated with enormous quantities of heterogeneous substances. The water-cures and the water-failures, and even the maladies which these waters may cause, should be alike considered. The former might be increased and the latter diminished by making mineral waters, as well as drugs, a part of regular study and education in all the medical colleges. Whether wise or otherwise, there is every summer a great and increasing number of visitors to the mineral springs, and, consequently, it is desirable that the physician should be able to advise his clientship understandingly in the premises, so that they may not be misled and deceived by interested parties, who are ready with certificates, advertisements and documents, to prove that at their springs a cure is almost certain.

However, the opinion long entertained in favor of the curative action of mineral waters, whether well or ill founded, appears to be extending in the medical profession, or at least beyond its pale among a considerable portion of the public. During the hot season, many whose pecuniary resources are not restricted, travel to "the watering places" for the purpose of regaining or preserving health, and, it may be, for other purposes. Without taking into view the auxiliary influences of change of air, travel, new scenery, novelty, relaxation from care and business, there can be little doubt as to the curative effects of some mineral waters in several chronic maladies, as rheumatism, nervous affections, diseases of the serous, mucous and cutaneous membranes, scrofulous and syphilitic diseases, ulcers, and swellings and stiffness of the joints, etc.

There is as much need of medical advice in using medicinal waters as there is in using other medicines. The internal and external uses of these waters, whether for antiphlogistic, tonic, resolutive, depurative, alterative, or revulsive purposes, which must be learned from experience, analysis and analogy, require judgment that few can be expected to possess, as this branch of medical education is neglected, and the compound character of these medicinal agents renders their therapeutic value difficult to appreciate and apply, and the more so, because few physicians have practical knowledge, derived from a prolonged residence at mineral springs, to guide them in giving advice, and have, therefore, to depend on interested persons for that necessary kind of information.

Upon one salient point of hydrology there is no room for differences of opinion, namely, temperature ; and with respect to the therapeutic applications and uses of temperature, there is more unanimity than is usually found in regard to a majority of the agents employed for remedial purposes. The physical distinction between cold and hot, and the pathological distinction between sthenic diseases having a high temperature, and asthenic diseases having a lower one, present physical and physiological parallelisms of great significancy for the practitioner of medicine, the discussion of which is not intended on this occasion. Admitting, what indeed few will question, that a considerable number of asthenic chronic diseases may be advantageously treated by thermal waters, it may be questioned whether any thermal springs extant equal those of Washita, in Arkansas—whether any afford quantities so copious—springs so numerous—temperatures so varied—elevations so convenient for bath-houses—in a climate so mild (34° 31' N. lat.)—where so much is done by Nature, and so little by art ? Tne efficacy of these waters, when used internally and externally, has been greatly extolled both by physieiaus and patients ; but visitors have been so few, and verbal accounts so general and indefinite, that in the absence of rigorous medical statistics and authentic reports, very little is positively known, particularly in reference to the medicinal effects of the water when taken internally. When consulted as to the internal use of these waters, I have not been able, after considerable inquiry, to give any satisfactory opinion, seeing that, according to the analyses which have been announced from time to time, these must be the purest of all waters except distilled, and at the same time the most impure, being loaded with minerals which are held in solution or suspension, and which, on reaching the air, solidify !

Nevertheless, if these springs are not mineralized, but are purer than almost any others yet analyzed, as has been affirmed by some persons, it follows that no physiological or therapeutical value beyond that possessed by any other water equally warm, can be attributed to them. A hot bath at home, and a hot bath abroad, must be similar in curative action, while it is easy to determine which is the more economical and convenient to an invalid. To leave home, family, and comforts, and to travel a thousand miles simply to get a hot bath, merely because blind routine or rumor requires it, is unreasonoble, if not fanatical.

For the physician, clinical experience and observation constitute the complemental finality of the thermal and chemical history of all waters whatsoever. But this complemental result is, in regard to these hot springs, involved in more uncertainty than in most other remedial waters.

Viewed from a therapeutical stand-point, no active mineral water, especially such as are purgative or debilitating, should be taken daily for indefinite periods, and for a multitude of diseases fundamentally differing in their nature and indications. All medication should cease when the object for which a medicine was given is attained. Analogy would teach that active mineral waters, like other medicines, might, if improperly taken, cause disease. The taking of some quarts of strong mineral waters regularly every morning, is a routine medication similar to that recently alledged (in the newspapers) as prevailing in a Canadian town, namely, " at Dunville, where the bell rings at noon each day for the inhabitants to take quinine." The charlataries at the mineral springs, and in essays and advertisements upon their virtues, would have afforded Molière good subjects for ridicule. The following satire on "The Fashionable Watering Places," from the *Southern Literary Messenger*, is as replete with hygienic and medical suggestions as some grave but unreliable and interested representations in which neither satire nor irony is intended :

HOW TO ENJOY THE SPRINGS AND STAY AT HOME.

WHITE SULPHUR.—Tie a roll of brimstone under your nose, and drink freely of thick warm water. Break some doubtful eggs in your pocket, and run round till you are exhausted. Procure a second-hand diabetes, change your linen six times a day, and strut loftily under a tree.

OLD SWEET.—Get a large tub, and put some white pebbles in the bottom. Sit down in it and blow soap-bubbles. Dress your best, and don't know any body.

RED SWEET.—Obtain some iron filings, paint 'em red, put 'em in a tin-pan or pitcher, and look at 'em in solitary silence. Eat much mutton, and go to bed early. Whisky julep eight times a day.

SALT SULPHUR.—Call yourself a South Carolinian, and take things easy. Live well. Stay in one place a long time. Tincture of brimstone occasionally.

MONTGOMERY WHITE.—Wear a loose sack coat and look at mulattoes frequently. Eat a great variety of raw meats and undone vegetables. Play at faro and draw-poker.

YELLOW SULPHUR.—Get good living on the top of a hill, where you can't see anything whatever. Dominos, draughts and backgammon.

ALLEGHANY.—Sit down in a hard chair, in a deep, hot hole, and drink citrate of magnesia and Epsom salts. Gamble some with dyspeptics.

ROCKBRIDGE ALUM.—Select some cases of cancer on the face, with a few necks scrofulously raw, and dine with them daily on indifferent victuals. Then catch the drippings from the eaves of a very old house, in a tin cup with a long handle, thicken the drippings with powdered nutgalls, and drink three times a day.

ALL-HEALING SPRINGS.—Throw a green blanket in a shallow pond, and wallow on it. Cut off a strip of blanket and clap it to your ribs. Read old novels, and talk to old ladies about chronic diseases of the digestive tube.

WARM SPRINGS.—Diet yourself on the unadulterated juice of the tea-kettle.

HOT SPRINGS.—Wear a full suit of mustard plasters, and walk about in the sunshine at noonday, swearing you have got the rheumatism.

BERKELEY SPRIGNS.—Keep your shin clear, and know nothing but Baltimore ten-pins.

PEAKS OF OTTER.—Climb a high pole on a cold day at sunrise. Shut your eyes and whistle.

WEIR'S CAVE.—Go into the cellar at midnight—feel the edges of things, and skin your shins against the coal-scuttle. Sit down on a pile of anthracite, with a tallow candle, and wonder.

OLD POINT COMFORT.—Build a hog-pen in a mud-puddle ; fill it with cockle-burrs and thistles, and call it surf-bathing. Drink bad brandy. Don't sleep. Lie down with your windows wide open, and no clothing on. Come home with a fish-bone in your throat, and oyster-shell in your head, a pain in your stomach, and ten thousand musquito bites in your body.

CAPE MAY.—Penetrate an immense crowd of male and female rowdies. Drop some salt water in both eyes. Shoot pistols. Eat some ice cream and claret, and send up one sky-rocket every night. Have yourself insulted often by niggers. At mid-day smell of an oven with a dead pig in it. Fill your pockets with cut glass broken into minute fragments.

YANKEE WATERING PLACES GENERALLY.--Keep a stale codfish under each arm ; live on onions and pumpkins ; go in strong for the Union and freesoil ; and dance the round dances in big breeches.

If the reader does not relish these levities, let him pass on to what the late Dr. Drake says in his elaborate work on *The Diseases of the Valley of the Mississippi*, namely: "Near the base of the south-eastern slope of the Ozark Mountains, about six miles north of the Washita river, lie the celebrated Hot Springs. According to Nicollet, their elevation is 718 feet above the level of the Gulf of Mexico ; the altitudes of several neighboring ridges being 997, 1162, and 1406. The springs are about seventy in number, and burst out near each other in the same valley. In temperature they range from 92° to 151° of Fahrenheit. They are limpid, emit no bubbles of gas, and have no particular taste. Like many other hot springs, they hold silex in solution ; for they deposit a tufa which is composed of that earth, with lime and oxide of iron. The surrounding rocks manifest more or less of a volcanic character, as I am informed by Dr. Warder, who has specimens in his cabinet ; and according to Col. Long, many of them are in strata highly inclined to the horizon. The scenery of this region has an aspect of wildness and grandeur, and its summer and autumnal salubrity is unquestionable. For the people of the far South, the Washita Springs might be made an interesting summer resort, as this is their nearest mountain locality ; and to invalids of the southern part of the interior valley whose diseases require a resort to the hot springs, those of the Washita are far more conve-nient than the hot springs of Virginia. If our physicians would turn the attention of their patients to this locality, the only objec-tion--a want of comfortable accommodations--would soon be obvi-ated" (i, 162-3).

In his Gazetteer (1845), Darby says of the region in which these springs arise, that "the water is pure and the air elastic, affording a most delicious retreat from the summer and autumnal temperature of Louisiana and southern Arkansas. The Washita is navigable with steamboats within thirty miles of the springs."

G. W. Featherstonhaugh, U. S. Geologist, in his Geological Re-port published by Congress (1835), alludes to the large deposits of travertine by the Hot Springs of Washita, in Arkansas, which he had examined in 1834. (P. 21.)

It may be acceptable to the readers of this Journal, to give a sketch of Mr. F.'s observations upon the geological formation and characteristics of the Hot Springs, and the more because his official report is not only little known, but is at variance with other authorities upon these subjects, as the readers of the present number of this Journal will have seen. These discrepancies constitute a sufficient apology for the large space devoted to these topics, as well as reasons for further researches.

Mr. Featherstonhaugh says :

On leaving the town [Little Rock], I soon got once more upon the old red sandstone, reposing on the grauwacke, and, indeed never left it, with one exception, until I drew nigh the little Missouri river, south of 34° north latitude.

Of the streams crossed on his way from Little Rock to the Springs, he says :

I invariably found, upon a minute investigation of their beds, the same tertiary deposit of marine shells* which I had seen at Little Rock. In the bed of the Saline, I found, at a depth of not more than a foot under the surface, a regular calcareous rock, enclosing immense quantities of oyster shells, the rocky part being evidently formed from the broken down exuviæ of marine animals, disintegrated in long periods of time. The settlers in the neighborhood, whose chimneys are built of mud, which had to be replaced annually, were extremely well pleased with the discovery of a mineral so useful to them for domestic purposes.† At thirty-five miles from Little Rock, the country is covered with ferruginous conglomerate of the old red sandstone. Wherever this latter rock is found, the pine‡ prevails, as is usually the case in silicious countries ; but, about forty-eight miles from Little Rock, I observed an approaching change in the timber, the pine having entirely disappeared, and being replaced by deciduous trees.

Where this change commenced, I found a total change of mineral structure ; the old red sandstone had given place to an ancient greenstone, containing great quantities of crystalized hornblende. The rocks rose here about one hundred and fifty feet, and having reached the top, I saw I was upon the brim of what—in the western part of Virginia, near the Clinch Mountain, where I have seen several, as well as in the neighborhood of Sequatchee valley, in Tennessee—is called a cove ; this cove, which is not quite circular, but rather affecting the form of a gourd, has an interior basin, which slopes pleasingly down, and contains, probably, one thousand five hundred acres of very excellent soil. In various parts of the bottom, I found large masses of decomposing felspar, studded with black tourma-

---

* Of the Eocene period of Mr. Lyell.

† These deposits evidently belong to the period when the ancient littoral shore was washed by the ocean.

‡ Pinus Australis, Mich.

lines, some of which were in long prisms, whilst others formed a stellated figure of beautifully delicate acicular rays. Some of the felspathic rocks were filled with amorphous masses of white sulphuret of iron, believed by many persons · to be silver. In other parts of the cove I found masses of coarse-grained syenite, consisting of red felspar, hornblende, mica, and some quartz. But what will always give celebrity to this remarkable locality, now called Magnet Cove, is the magnetic iron which abounds there. There is an extensive mound of it covered with pebbles of magnetic iron, from an ounce to four pounds weight. From some examinations I made by digging, I am certain these loose pebbles, like those of the vein of iron in Missouri, overlie masses of the metal of prodigious extent. Some of the specimens I obtained possess a surprising magnetic power ; and such is the influence of the mass in place, that Colonel Conway, the Surveyor General, informed me he had been unable to survey the country, as the needle will not traverse on approaching this locality. From a careful examination of the different portions of this most interesting cove, I came to the conclusion that the whole structure of this elevation, as far as its exterior, as well as its interior slopes were concerned, was an old greenstone belonging to the intrusive rocks, and occupying, for a limited space, a place amidst the old red sandstone. That as far as the greenstone extends, all the trees are deciduous, and without its limit all the trees are evergreens and pines. It is impossible to look at this quasi-circular brim, and the cove below, and take into consideration, at the same time, all the minerals and metals found there, without being impressed with the opinion that it is the result of a very remote volcanic action, and is, perhaps, one of those extremely ancient craters that may have preceded those of which basalt and lava are the products.

The distance from Magnet Cove to the Hot Springs of the Washita is about sixteen miles, keeping always upon the old red sandstone, and no change in the mineral, except one vein of greenstone, with small plates of brown mica, which crops out at about half the distance. At length, nearing a considerable ridge, and turning into a small valley about fifty yards broad, I saw, from the appearance of things, that I had reached the Hot Springs of the Washita, so great an object of curiosity to men of science, and so little known to the rest of the world.

This valley which runs about north and south, and divides two lofty ridges of old red sandstone, extends about eight hundred yards, and then deflects to the west. At the foot of the eastern ridge, which is about five hundred feet high, flows a lively stream, which rises in the hills to the northeast ; this ridge has, towards the top, a dense growth of pine and oak trees, amongst which are strewed fragments of the rock, often very ferruginous, and pieces of a strong band of ironstone, which traverses the ridge in the direction of N. N. E. and S. S. W., and dipping S. E. with the sandstone, at an angle of about 45°. There is, also, some conglomerate on this hill, held together by ferruginous cement. The stream, for a considerable distance, runs upon the grauwacke slate, upon which the sandstone rests. I had entered the valley but a short distance before I saw, on the flank of the east ridge, a rock of a totally different character from that constituting the ridge, impending, like a curtain, down to the stream, and .I at once recognized it for a travertin deposited by the mineral waters. The curtain, with some intervals, extends along the stream for about four hundred yards from the slope of the ridge, presenting sometimes abrupt escarpments of from fifteen to twenty-five feet, and at other times showing itself in points and coves advancing into and receding from the stream. This travertin extends back east from the stream about one hundred and fifty yards, leaning upon the aclivity of the old red sandstone, to where several powerful springs are now situated. Some of the springs rise in the bed of the stream ; one very fine spring rises in its west bank, and numerous others, of which perhaps thirty rather copious ones are found at various heights on the ridge, rising through the old red sandstone rock. Of springs of feebler force there are a great many. Sometimes one or more of these are said to disappear, and it is certain that new ones are frequently breaking out. Some of them issue from the rock at an elevation of at least one hundred feet from the valley where the present log cabins are built, and where a flourishing village will no doubt exist ere long. A more beautiful and singularly convenient situation for a town cannot be imagined ; for, by the aid of the simplest frames to support spouts, the hot water may be conveyed to the houses in great profusion, for baths and medical purposes, as well as for domestic uses. Upon repeated trials with my register thermometers, I found the water of some of the principal springs to be 146° of Fahrenheit, and I never found it higher, although I should not doubt that, during very dry weather, when the mineral springs are not attenuated by the atmospheric waters, they would mark a few degrees more. But, during my stay, I always found the water hot enough to make my tea without any further boiling, as well as to wash my clothes. Indeed, in this locality, the hot water is so abundant that I found it often troublesome to procure that which was cold, for the Hot Springs occupying a breadth equal to four hundred yards of the base of the ridge, all the hot water was discharged into the creek, which in many parts was of a temperature just fitted for a warm bath ; and what further assists to keep up its temperature, is the great number of hot springs rising through the slate at the bottom of the brook. This can be seen at almost a hundred places ; and although the water does not scald the hand there, still, upon insinnating my fingers a few inches below the ground at the edge of the stream, I was obliged to retire them instantly, having more than once burnt them in that way. If this stream were turned; it is incredible the quantity of water, of a temperature perhaps always equal to 145° Fahrenheit, which might be obtained. During the summer drouths, when the stream is low, no fish are ever seen in it, the water being too hot ; but when the season arrives for the cold waters to enter the stream in considerable quantities, then trout, perch, and other fish are taken in all parts of it. I was told, however, that at other portions of the summer, when the whole volume of the stream was not so much heated, the fish would sometimes come up the brook in those parts where no springs came through the slate, but always swam at a particular depth ; when crumbs of bread were dropped in to them, they rose to them, but stopped when they reached the stratum of hot water, which, being rarified, was at the top. Frogs and snakes, when forced into the hot water, or falling in inadvertently, immediately stretch themselves out and die. These mineral hot waters, except one or two of the springs, which are slight chalybeates, are tasteless, having not the least saline trace. A person totally unacquainted with mineralogy, and not aware of any difference between travertino and old red sandstone, might suppose the mineral structure of all the rocks to be homogeneous, and that the waters, not differing in their taste from ordinary warm water, were without any mineral constituent, as the hot waters of the Washita have been reported to be ; but these immense deposits of carbonate of lime attest the contrary. On digging about twenty-five feet above the level of the brook, I went through a foot of the carbonate, with traces of sulphate of lime, and then through a dark red oxide, with reniform masses of nodular iron, with botroidal faces. The sulphate was deposited in layers in acicular form. I then came to masses of ferruginous sandstone belonging to the ridge. These seemed to have been loose, and to have been recemented by the deposits from the water, which had filled up all their interstices. I took out one large mass of iron, the walls of which were, in some places, two and a half inches thick, of rich hematite ore, the inside of the nodule containing gypsum and a deep red oxide. These masses almost led me to suppose that they had been deposited by the springs, and that the iron had thus been aggregated by molecular attraction. It is not improbable that the ferruginous matter has been carried to them during the immense periods of time which have elapsed since these springs first appeared, by atmospheric waters trickling amidst the ferruginous materials of the ridge ; the iron certainly appears to be accidentally there. I observed, also, that where these great quantities of the oxide of iron were, it was evident a stream of hot water had passed for a long period of time, and beneath the superincumbent deposit of carbonate of lime, which, as these hot waters have frequently changed, their direction, might very well be. I perceived one considerable underground stream of hot water issuing from a cavity near the bank of the brook, and, upon examining it, found the process going on, iron depositing on the sides, and soft seams of sulphate of lime already established. Under these circumstances, I would not pronounce any of these waters to be natural chalybeates. It is probable that a great many mineral waters acquire some of their properties in transitu. I have supposed this to be the case in some sulphuretted springs I have seen, that rise through beds of slate and coal, loaded with sulphuret of iron, much of which may reasonably be thought, at particular depths, to be in a state of decomposition. For the carbonate of lime contained in these hot waters, we may infer a different origin ; nor can we consistently assign to the prodigious quantity of caloric which has probably for such immense periods of time raised the temperature of these springs, any source short of those depths from whence the intrusive rocks, the veins of iron, and various other mineral phenomena of the vicinity, have sprung.

These thermal waters rise in a very limpid state, but as soon as they get into motion, and their parts become exposed to the atmosphere, a mineral deposit commences, attaching itself to dead leaves, to sticks, to anything that serves for a point of adhesion ; upon this deposit a brilliant green enameled looking substance presents itself, which increases and thickens, in favorable situations, until it takes the thickness of half an inch. When this can be detached from the calcareous matter it covers, it has a vitreo-gelatinous appearance, somewhat of the consistency of those glairy substances produced in stagnant water in very hot weather. As long as the water runs over it, it continues to thicken and look green ; but when the deposit has dammed up the course of the water, and another course is formed, which is constantly doing, then this green substance, being forsaken by the water, dries up, and crisps on the surface of the ground, like dead lichens. This dead stuff I examined with a powerful glass, and found that it was a mineral substance of a whitish gray color ; on the under side it preserved still a deadish green appearance. In the course of time it undergoes a change, and changes to a deep black calcareous mould, on the surface of which I found, as is frequently done in decomposing travertins, an immense number of individuals of various species of helix.   *   *   *

That these waters annually perform very admirable cures of chronic complaints incident to southern climates, is well known there ; and that their efficacy, and the beauty and salubrity of the country, will soon cause the place to be resorted to from far and near, as soon as proper accommodations for visitors can be prepared, is very obvious. They seem providentially placed there for the use of the inhabitants of the low lands in the vicinity of Red River, and their value deserves to be made extensively known.

About six years ago, the late Judge Watts, who was distinguished for his intelligence, and who had experienced in his own person the effects of the Hot Springs, wrote, agreeably to my request, an account of these springs. The MS. I transmitted to the learned Dr. John Bell, of Philadelphia, who published a part of it in his work on Mineral Springs, a portion of which will close this paper, already very long:

They [the Hot Springs] are about thirty or forty in number, and some of them are very copious in their discharge, rushing out from under the rocks in a volume three feet in width by five or six inches in depth. The temperature of the springs varies from 140° to 145° (Fah.), and is sufficiently hot to scald a hog or a chicken ; and the water is constantly used for these purposes.

The mode of using the waters, most generally, is by taking a steam bath. For this purpose a small building, fifteen feet long by five feet wide, is erected. One half of it is used for an ante-room, in which to dress and undress—the other half is the bath-room. The floor of the bathing room consists of slats which are two inches wide and two inches apart, and is placed over one of these large springs, which issue from the rock. The water throws off the steam, which rises between the slats. For the first three or four minutes the body is dry, but afterwards a profuse perspiration breaks out, which runs from every pore. The temperature of the steam-room is about 116° F. This occasions no inconvenience, but for persons who apprehend a congestion of the vessels of the head, a hole is made in the roof through which a person can breathe the external air, the body being immersed in steam. The patient usually remains thirty to forty minutes in the bathing room, and when he comes out, it is not uncommon for two or three buckets of cold water to be thrown over him in the dressing room. There is no danger of taking cold if the most ordinary precaution is used. It is not unusual to take a steam bath in the forenoon, and a water bath in the afternoon. The water bath is frequently taken in a creek, into which all the hot springs run. After a spell of dry weather, it is necessary to go half a mile, and sometimes three-quarters of a mile below where the hot springs run into the creek, before the water is of a temperature to bathe in. If the water is carried from the spring to a bathing tub, it must stand about four hours before it can be used. * * * * There have been some attempts to analyze the water, but I have no faith in any of them. The water is much impregnated with lime and magnesia, and the deposit of these substances is very great on the mountain, and in the channels in which the water runs, and leaves and sticks are continually petrified into a kind of rotten stone, composed of lime and magnesia.

The water may be drank without nausea as soon as the throat can bear it, and if a little salt be put into it, it could not be distinguished from chicken broth. The best season for the use of the water is late in the fall, and in the winter and spring. Every species of chronic disease is cured by these waters, to wit: rheumatism, gout, scrofula, venereal, mercurial, erysipelas, consequences of measles, of scarlet fever, and of whooping cough, and all diseases occasioned by obstructions.

Three miles from the Hot Springs is a very fine chalybeate spring, and at the distance of forty miles, at a place called Irons, is a spring of highly exhilarating properties, so much so as to produce a species of intoxication.

The Brocken of the Hartz Mountains, where the Spectre of the Brocken and even witches are said to be seen, can scarcely rival the representations which some give of the scenery of the Hot Springs as to picturesqueness. "The Hot Mountain," says Dr. Bell, "is covered with the most luxuriant growth of vines. There is a solitary spring seventy feet higher than the others, on the side of the mountain, but it is, also, of an equal temperature, and differs in no respect from those below. A dense fog continually hangs over the springs, and upon the side of a hill, which, at a distance, looks like a number of furnaces in blast. It is probably the condensation of this vapor which produces such a rank growth of vines on the side of the mountain."

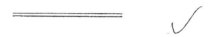

ART. VI.—*Partial Deficiency of the Vagina, with a Rudimentary Condition of the Uterus, and Probable Defect of the Fallopian Tubes: Remarks, etc.,* by Nathan Bozeman M. D., of New Orleans :

MISS F., aged 21, of light hair and complexion, stout, heavily built, and, to all appearances, enjoying good health, was sent to consult me last fall, by a medical gentleman of Auburn, Alabama, under the supposition that there was an abnormal development of the genital organs. His advice had been sought in the case in consequence of the non-appearance of the menstrual flow.

I learned from the lady, herself, that ever since she was twelve or fourteen years old, she had experienced monthly pain in the back, soreness in the lower part of the abdomen, and a light feeling of the head, though never had any discharge from the vagina until within the last few years ; then it was even so scanty and light-colored as to leave scarcely any stain on her linen. Now, at these periods she has great oppression in breathing, and suffers from severe pain in the head, which latter sometimes continues varying in intensity, from one period to another. Occasionally she is relieved to some extent by bleeding from the nose.

Upon examination, I found her well formed. The pudenda presented nothing of an unusual appearance. The mons veneris had its usual covering of hair, and the mammæ indicated nothing out of the way in their development.

But when I came to introduce my finger into the vagina to determine its condition, I found that it could not be passed further than just beyond the meatus urinarius. The obstacle encountered here I at first took to be a firmly developed hymen ; but by opening the vulva and making a close inspection of the parts, I found that such was not the case. If there ever existed a perfect hymen, it had in some way been destroyed. There were to be seen the carunculæ

104

myrtiformes, indicating its usual place. The obstruction my finger met with was just about three-quarters of an inch above this point, which now proved to be the termination of the vagina. The urethra appeared to be of the proper length, with the external orifice in the proper place, though considerably thickened.

At the bottom of the *cul de sac* in which the vagina terminated, I discovered a very small opening, around which the parts felt firm, and yielded but slightly to pressure. Upon introducing a small probe at this point and passing it up, I found that it took pretty much the same course as that of a normal vagina, and at a distance of something over two inches, it was arrested by what appeared to be the end of the canal. By no manipulation or justifiable force could the probe be carried any further. The index finger of the right hand being now introduced into the rectum and brought against the anterior wall, the whole distance which the probe had passed was found to be occupied by a cylindrical body, nearly the size of the little finger. It was hard and somewhat unyielding, and could be readily traced to its upper extremity. Here the point of the finger was made to sweep over it, and off on either side, upon what appeared to be well defined borders of the broad ligaments. A metallic bougie, No. 6, was next introduced into the bladder, and its extremity brought against the tip of the finger. This was done in the measial line, and upon either side as far as the bowel would allow of the finger being carried.

After withdrawing the probe and bougie, the finger being still in the bowel, I made an attempt to discover the ovaries, but in this I utterly failed, not being able to feel any thing that indicated either their existence or that of the Fallopian tubes. Next I introduced the same bougie, that had been used, into the canal leading out of the vagina, to determine more definitely its size. The instrument was passed to the same depth that the probe had been, though it required considerable force, thus indicating the full extent of capacity.

Remarks.—The above case is one that must be regarded as possessing no little interest. A consideration of this, and the fact of having been spoken to a few weeks since by a medical friend of this city in relation to a case somewhat similar, I would offer as an excuse for the following remarks :

My friend's case, judging from the account given me, differs from mine in these respects, namely; that the vagina terminates in the urethra, and the woman is married—the latter step having been taken, I should observe, contrary to his advice.

Now, the deplorable condition of such unfortunate creatures, especially when they have unadvisedly entered into a matrimonial alliance, is calculated to arouse the tenderest sympathies of almost any one; but it is to the medical man that the appeal is made for advice. It becomes his duty, although his skill may promise but little aid, to investigate, as a careful physiologist and pathologist, the nature of such cases, that he may be well prepared to give the proper advice to all parties interested; for an error in his decision might not only involve the happiness of an entire family, but would place the unfortunate victim of matrimonial responsibility in a position to become an object of the deepest commisseration for life, as must sooner or later take place in the case related by my friend. Here coitus can only be effected through the urethra, and the result of this will be an extensive and permanent dilatation of the passage, followed by incontinence of urine. Burggraëve relates a similar case, which was followed by the above result after marriage.

Although such an occurrence would not likely take place in the case I have described, for the reason that the vagina terminates in a *cul de sac* sufficiently far beyond to preclude the possibility of injury to the urethra; nevertheless, the act of coition, under such circumstances, could not be effected otherwise than imperfectly and with more or less pain.

As to the precise state and relation of the parts in this case, I could not at first satisfactorily determine. My first impression was that there was an entire absence of the uterus and the Fallopian tubes, and that the small canal leading from the bottom of the vagina was a part of the latter congenitally contracted. But the firmness indicated around the orifice of this canal and throughout its entire course, as felt through the coats of the bowel, as well as a kind of grating sensation imparted to the probe, as when introduced into the cavity of a normal uterus, I was induced to think that I was mistaken, and what I took to be a contracted state of the vagina, was nothing more nor less than the uterus in a rudimentary state. I believed that the ovaries existed, from the fact that there were present the normal development of the mammæ and the pudenda, and the periodical prodromes of menstruation.

It was and is still a question in my mind, whether the Fallopian tubes exist or not ; and if they do, what is their relation to the uterus ; whether they communicate by open mouths with the canal we traced with our probe, or do they terminate as blind ducts in the vicinity of the organ. The presumption is that they do not com- municate with the cavity of the rudimentary uterus, or we would have some show of a menstrual discharge. Now, with these doubts and uncertainties weighing on my mind, I was led to examine what authors I could lay my hands upon for an analogous case. Wri- ters, especially in our own country and Great Britain, say but little about such abnormities of the genital organs. By reference, however, to Rokitansky's Pathological Anatomy, I find that he is very elabo- rate and explicit upon this subject, and certainly there is no one whose opinion is entitled to more credit. It seems that he and sev- eral other writers, to whom I shall presently allude, take the ground that complete absence of the uterus is exceedingly rare ; that there had been instances in which it was supposed to be wanting during life, but it turned out that, in a *post mortem* inspection of these cases, the organ was found to exist in a rudimentary state. Here is what he says : " The most common case of arrest, which is generally considered as absence of the uterus, is that in which the fold of the peritoneum, which is destined for the reception of the internal sexual organs, contains, on one or both sides, posteriorly to the bladder, one or two small flattened, solid masses, or larger hollow bodies, with a cavity of the size of a pea or a lentil, which is lined with mucous membrane. They are to be viewed as rudiments of the reterine horns, and the Fallopian tubes bear an exact relation to their devel- opment. These may either be totally deficient, or terminate in the vicinity of the uterus in the peritoneum as blind ducts, or they may communicate with the uterus with or without an open passage.

" This formation of the uterus, and especially the existence of two lateral, hollow, elongated and rounded uterine rudiments, each of which is connected with a corresponding Fallopian tube and ovary, constitutes what Mayer terms the uterus bipartitus. From each of the uterine rudiments, a flattened, round cord of uterine tissue, ascends within the fold of the peritoneum, and the two from each side coalesce. *The place of the uterus is occupied by cellular tissue, in which a few uterine fibres, derived from the just-mentioned cord, may be traced ; it presents the general outline of a uterus, and, reaching downwards, rests upon the arch of a short vaginal cul de sac. The external sexual organs and the mammary glands, as well as the general sexual character of the individual, attain a normal development."*

The italics here are mine, and I call attention to these lines particularly, as suiting very well the description of our case, excepting that it is not stated whether the body occupying the place of the uterus ever has a cavity or not. Such we found to be the case ; and however much doubt there may be as to the true relation of the Fallopian tubes and ovaries to this cavity, it certainly presents an interesting feature, as showing the organ itself complete in every essential particular, though in a rudimentary state.

Vidal (de Cassis), in speaking of the anomalies and deformities of the uterus, thus expresses himself as to the rarity of its absence : " L'absence complète est l'anomalie sans contredit la plus rare de toutes ; suivant quelques auteurs, elle est même sans exemple. On oppose, en effet, avec quelque apparence de raison, aux faits rapportés par Colombus, par Théden, et surtout à ceux beaucoup plus douteux de Richerand, de Lemettrie, de Baudelocque, etc., cette remarque très juste, que les recherches anatomiques modernes, faites avec plus de rigueur qu'on n'en mettait autrefois, n'ont pas encore permis de constater l'absence complète de l'utérus, dont il existe toujours quelques rudiments."†

Dr. G. S. Crawford, of Chicago, relates a case of absence of the uterus, in the *North-Western Med. and Surg. Journal,* for Nov., 1850.

Dr. Warren also reports a case, which we find among the " Extracts from the Records of the Boston Society for Medical Improvement," published in the *Boston Med. and Surg. Journal,* of June 14th of the present year. Both of these subjects were living ; and as it is only by a *post mortem* inspection that the existence or non-existence of the uterus can be determined with certainty, they may be put down as doubtful. This is what Scanzoni says on this point, as translated into French from the German, by Drs. Dor and Socin : " Nous ne croyons pas qu'il soit possible de diagnostiquer avec certitude l'absence complète de l'utérus. On ne pourra que la soupçonner, lorsqu'il n'existera que des rudiments du vagin et des parties externes, lorsque acun des symptòmes qui caractérisent la rétention du sang menstruel dans la cavité de la matrice ne pourra être perçu ; enfin, lorsqu'une sonde introduite dans la vessie, et la doigt dans le rectum, celui-ci

---

* Op. Cit., vol. ii, p. 206.

† Pathologie Externe, Tom. v, p. 346.

aura la sensation du rapport immédiat de ces deux organes. Nous répétons que tous ces phénomènes n'excluent pas absolument la présence d'un utérus rudimentaire." *

Notwithstanding now the difficulty which must be admitted in the diagnosis of absence of .the uterus, still we cannot enter. tain the same doubts upon the subject as some of the authors we have mentioned, especially the latter, who, in the whole course of his extensive practice, never met with a single instance of this abnormity. There are cases on record, well substantiated. Dr. Ziehil gives us the example of a woman fifty-seven years old, who, dying of phthisis, became the subject of his observation. He says : " On examination, not the slightest trace of a uterus could be found. The external organs were well developed. The vagina was so contracted as scarcely to admit the index finger, and terminated at the extent of an inch in a *cul de sac*. The Fallopian tubes were in the broad ligaments ; the fimbriated extremities were normal ; the abdominal opening of the tubes was open ; there was no uterine opening. The ovaries were firm and dry, puckered on their surface, and containing in their interior small and compact protuberances." †

There is also another example recorded by R. Boyd, M. D., Resident Physician to St. Marylebone Infirmary. The subject of his case was seventy-two years old, and died of disease of the brain and lungs. In the autopsy he found both kidneys out of their proper place, and supplied by arteries from abnormal sources. "The situation of the left ovary," he says, " was occupied by a fibrous tumor of an irregular globular shape, connected by a round ligament smaller than that on the right side, but which took a similar course to the bladder. The Fallopian tubes were not present. There was a slight projection of the peritoneum, behind the bladder, from cellular tissue beneath it. A careful examination of the parts in their recent state was made by Dr. R. Lee, also by Mr. Kiernan, afterwards by Mr. Perry. No vestige of the uterus could be discovered.

" The external parts of generation presented no unusual appearance ; the mons veneris but thinly covered with hair ; a *cul de sac*, about half an inch deep, beneath the orifice of the urethra, is all that exists of a vagina. The mammæ were well developed for so old a person." *

---

* Traité Pratique des Maladies des Organes Sexuels de la Femme, p. 46.

† Am. Jour. of the Med. Sciences. vol. xxii. Taken from Gaz. Méd. de Paris, June 4th, 1851.

* Med. Chirurgical Review, vol. 36 ; 1842 ; p. 41.

ART. VII.—*Albuminuria Gravidarum. Report of a case of, with remarks:* By HUMPHREY PEAKE, M. D., of Yazoo City, Mississippi.

ON the 7th of July inst., I was called to see Mrs. L. G. of the age of twenty years. She resides fifteen miles in the country. I found her presenting an extremely anasarcous condition—the upper and lower extremities greatly swollen, and pitting deeply under pressure, and her breathing very much oppressed. She had been unable to assume the recumbent position for nearly two weeks, and the little sleep she was able to get was by being propped up almost vertically in bed. On assuming the recumbent position, suffocation seemed imminent. The infiltration of the lower extremities was to an extent which precluded the possibility of walking, and looked as if almost ready to burst: I could not satisfy myself of the existence of fluid in the peritoneal cavity, for the abdominal walls partook of the general infiltration, but I much feared, from the greatly labored breathing, that a collection was going on in the thorax. Owing to the extremely swollen condition of the arms, I was utterly unable to perceive the pulse at the wrist. She suffered a good deal from headache and a painful sensation in the left breast, shoulder, and arm. She was losing some blood daily, from a uterine hæmorrhage. This had continued for three or four weeks. The bowels were constipated, for which she had been taking, by direction of a physician, rhubarb pills. She is married, and six weeks before my visit had miscarried in her first pregnancy, at about the sixth month. Her lower extremities began swelling two months before this time. With her anasarcous appearance is blended an extremely exsanguineous hue.

I had some of the urine sent to my office, and on examination found it highly charged with albumen. I then put her upon the following treatment, which has been continued, with the exception of the saccharum saturni, ever since. The saturnini solution was only continued for a week, the hæmorrhage, for which it was partly given having given way in a very few days. The improvement has been so rapid and regular as to give every reason to expect a rapid and perfect recovery. Indeed, within ten days from beginning of treatment, her condition was so much improved that she was able to walk a distance of some hundred yards. In the language of her husband, it seems hardly possible that a person could have improved more rapidly.

℞. Sacchari Saturni, ℨi.
 Syrupi Simplicis, ℨiv.
 Aquæ,   ℥xii. M.

S. A teaspoonful every night.

℞. Magnesiæ Sulphatis.
 Potassæ Bi-Tartratis.
 Potassæ Acetatis, aa℥i.
 Aquæ Cinnamonii ℥iv.
 Aquæ,   ℥xii. M.

S. A wine-glassful three times a day.

℞. Quiniæ Disulphatis, ℨi.
 Pulveris Ferri, ℨij.
 Strychniæ,   grs. ii.
 Mucilaginis q. s.   M.
 Make 60 pills.

S. One to be given three times a day.

A wine-glassful of the purgative and diuretic mixture having been found to operate a little too much upon the bowels, the dose was accordingly lessened.

One week after commencement of treatment, the urine was again examined, and found to have had its albumen considerably diminished.

Remarks.—The above case is one of a kind with several of which I have met in the course of my practice. These cases are classed in most of the systematic works in use with us, as cases of *anæmia gravidarum*, but we are of opinion that had he who proposed this name been acquainted at the time with the albuminous condition of the urine not unfrequently found in pregnant women, and more particularly in primaparæ, and its connection with anasarca, a distinction, based upon this particular condition, would have been made.

It is generally stated by writers on this subject, that the anasarca is caused by the pressure of the enlarged uterus upon the veins returning the blood from its lower extremities, and that as soon as delivery shall have taken place, this condition will disappear. So I was at one time of opinion, and imbued with the teachings of the justly esteemed Dr. Meigs, I was always ready, and never failed, in these cases, to predict a speedy recovery after the delivery should be accomplished. It generally happened that my predictions were justified by the result, but I have an unpleasant recollection of several cases in which this favorable termination did not occur. In some cases weeks, and in others months, elapsed without any return to health, and it was only after a treatment similar to that adopted in the case reported above, that the health was reëstablished.

While, according to the best authorities, albuminuria of the pregnant female may be present without an accompanying anasarcous condition, yet we believe that, in the great majority of cases of powerful anasarca, when the anasarca is *general*, there will be found an albuminous condition of the urine, while there may be very great œdema of the lower extremeties, without any such accompanying condition.

The question has been settled, we believe, that an albuminous condition of the urine does not necessarily indicate that the pathological condition of the kidney known as characteristic of morbus brightii ; but while this is so, many contend that albuminous urine always precedes this pathological change in the organ, and that it is a stage of the disease. We favor this opinion, and, should it be correct, the importance of paying strict attention to the urine of women affected with puerperal anasarca, or even œdema of the lower extremeties during pregnancy, becomes at once apparent.

The plan of treatment pursued in the case reported, is not claimed as *par excellance* the best. Any one having a fair knowledge of the profession will be able to discern the indications it was intended to fulfill.

JULY 28, 1860.

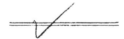

ART. VIII.—*Antigalactic Property of Belladonna.*

LIBERTY, Mississippi, August 13, 1860.

DR. DOWLER—As it is a subject which has been attracting considerable attention lately, I beg leave, through your Journal, to report that I have lately tried, *with perfect success*, belladonna as an antigalactic. Patient was a well-grown negro woman, primipara ; labor natural ; child well-formed and at full term ; but (as the midwife in attendance informed me) born with animation suspended, and could not be revived.

Three or four days after confinement the breasts were tumid and hard, and patient presented the symptoms of an attack of milk fever. The preparation of belladonna used was the ordinary *extract* found in drug stores, not diluted or mixed with anything. Directed it to be applied for two or three inches around the nipple.

Three applications were made, about twelve hours apart, when the tumidity, hardness, and heat had disappeared from the mammæ, and no constitutional symptoms of fever remained.

Respectfully,   S. C. Young.

ART. IX.—*Obstetrical Reflections, Suggested by passages in the First Chapter of Exodus.*

THE verses in this chapter which have suggested the following reflections, extend from 15th to 19th inclusive, and read as follow :

"15. And the King of Egypt spake to the Hebrew midwives, of which the name of the one was Shiphrah, and the name of the other Puah :

"16. And he said, when ye do the office of a midwife to the Hebrew women, and see them upon the stools, if it be a son, then ye shall kill him ; but if it be a daughter, then she shall live.

"17. But the midwives feared God, and did not as the King of Egypt commanded them, but saved the men-children alive.

"18. And the King of Egypt called for the midwives, and said, unto them, why have ye done this thing, and have saved the men-children alive ?

"19. And the midwives said unto Pharaoh, because the Hebrew women are not as the Egyptian women ; for they are lively, and are delivered ere the midwives come in unto them."

It appears to me that the following thoughts are naturally suggested by the reading of these verses :

1. That there were in Egypt at that time persons whose business it was to assist women in childbirth.

2. That these obstetricians were women.

3. That the women were delivered in a sitting posture.

4. That these midwives feared God, and regarded the interests of their patients more than the threats of their king.

5. That these midwives were in the habit of attending both the Hebrew and Egyptian women in childbirth, or, at least, were familiar with the processes of labor in both classes.

6. That the Hebrew women were more easily delivered than the Egyptian women were.

1. The first proposition, I think, seems evident, from the mere reading of the context. The writer refers to the "Hebrew mid-wives" as persons whose office was well understood, as it doubtless was. Indeed, it is to be presumed that midwives, or persons who assisted women in childbirth, have been needed since the earliest ages, almost from the time God said to Eve, "thou shalt bring forth children in great pain." Their art was rudimentary in the beginning, but improved as the opportunities for practising it increased, and necessities demanded, until, at the time this was written, it seems to have been a regular profession or employment, and to have made considerable progress. The rapidity with which the Hebrews increased and multiplied, must have made very frequent demands for their services ; and it is but natural to suppose that, with such constant practice, they would soon become familiar with the processes of labor, both normal and abnormal, and would after a while make out a rude classification of the various positions and presentations, and, indeed, of all the phenomena of labor. Their answer to the king proves their familiarity with one very important phenomenon ; and since they had observed enough to know this, they doubtless knew many others.

2. These obstetricians were *women.* This is proved by the facts, that the Hebrew word has been translated *midwives* throughout the whole connection, and the names given of two of them (Shiphrah and Puah) are the names of women. The translators were well aware of the original meaning of this word, and would not have translated it midwives so often, unless they had been thoroughly convinced that this was its true meaning, although Mr. Bush affirms that the Hebrew word means "one who causes to bring forth," without regard to the gender of the one performing this service. Admitting, then, that the translation, "midwives," is correct, it is evident that these obstetricians were *women,* for midwife means a *woman* who assists other women in childbirth, and can never be correctly applied to a man, though he performs the same service. Indeed, woman enters into the very composition of the word midwife, *mid* with, and

wif a woman ; and this is true of the analogous word in several other languages, as Danish, Swedish, Spanish, etc. (see Webster's Dict.). This proposition is confirmed by the fact that both of the names of these persons here given are *feminine* nouns, and the names of women ; and further, by the fact that Plutarch informs us that, about this time, there were, among some nations, schools for the instruction of *women* in midwifery. I think, then, it is plain to every unbiased mind, that these persons who assisted in childbirth were *women*.

Though far from being one of those who think that all that is good in medicine comes to us wrapped in mystery, from ancient times, or uncultivated nations, yet I think we might learn a useful lesson from this, viz : to *educate* women, more than we do, for the practice of obstetrics. As tending to this, I hail with pleasure the successful establishment of a Female Medical College in Philadelphia. I am aware that it has been said by its enemies that many of those who have attended this school are turning their professional knowledge to a very bad purpose, that of procuring *abortions* for those of their sex who have been so *unfortunate* as to reap the just reward of their departures from the paths of virtue, and become pregnant ; but this, even if true, which I doubt, is the fault, not of the cause, but of its representatives, or rather *mis*-representatives, and is no argument against it. Indeed, every *good* cause has been misrepresented and abused. Again, it has been said that women have not intellect or application sufficient to master the complications of the science of obstetrics ; but this is a slander on the sex that cannot be proved. As instances that women have sometimes, in spite of the opposition and success of their lords, attained eminent and enviable notoriety in the prosecution of the medical sciences, I need only refer to Mrs. Preston, of Philadelphia, and Madame Boivin, of France. Away, then, with such frivolous reasoning. I, for one, will rejoice to see the time when more intelligent, well-educated women will be found prosecuting the study of medical sciences, especially obstetrics, and when the practice of obstetrics will be intrusted entirely to them.

3. These Hebrew women were delivered in a *sitting* posture. I am aware that some commentators have contended that the word here translated "stool," sometimes means a stone trough in which new-born infants were washed previous to being dressed, and that *them* in the context refers to the infants, not the mothers ; but this

position, I think, is altogether untenable ; and it is evident, from observing the language and punctuation of the passage, that the " stools " here referred to were some kind of seats on which women were placed for delivery. Although most obstetricians of modern times have selected more appropriate positions for women during parturition, yet the practice of placing them in a sitting posture still prevails in some country provinces. (See article in a late num-ber of this Journal, by the editor.)

4. These Hebrew midwives feared God, and regarded the interests of their patients more than the threats of their king. In the present state of religious intelligence, the obligation of every one to "fear God and keep his commandments," is a proposition which no longer need be argued ; it is universally admitted. Yet, when we reflect upon the absolute powers of the king, and the risks which these women were running in disobeying his cruel order, their conduct presents a commendable instance of piety, worthy the imitation of all, and is a sovereign rebuke to the blasphemous oaths which we *occasionally* hear from our eminent lecturers on obstetrics.

5. These midwives were in the habit of attending both Hebrew and Egyptian women in childbirth; or, at least, were familiar with the processes of labor in both. If not, how could they say to the king, " the Hebrew women are not as the Egyptian women ; for they are lively, and are delivered ere the midwives come in unto them ? " Would not he have instantly detected their falsehood ? and severely punished them for disobeying his order ? But, on the contrary, it appears that their tale, though false, was sufficiently probable for him to believe without questioning it. This is a proof that the science of medicine, even in this barbarous and tyrannical age, was free, and not commingled with or fettered by diversities of national, political, or religious opinions. Such should be the case at all times.

6. The Hebrew women were delivered easier and quicker than the Egyptian women. This, though resorted to for the purpose of de-ceiving the king, and not really the reason of the midwives for saving the male children, was doubtless true. If this had not been a fact, the king would have suspected them. Besides, the ease with which women accustomed to labor (as the Hebrews were) give birth, compared with those effeminately and luxuriously raised (as the Egyptians were), is evident to the most careless observer.

Such are some of the reflections suggested by the reading of the passages quoted at the beginning of this article ; an attentive consideration of which (passages), I think, affords one of the many proofs of the vast amount and diversity of knowledge contained in the Bible, which I consider one of the evidences of its divine origin.

S. C. YOUNG.

LIBERTY, Mississippi, September 4th, 1860.

ART X.—*Medical Intelligence.* [From the London Correspondent of the New Orleans Medical and Surgical Journal.]

LONDON is at a stand-still ! Professional and general news are alike silent. The court, the aristocracy, all who have time and means, have taken flight ; and after the fatigues of a weary season of pleasure, of excitement, of toil, and business, have fled from the bustle and turmoil of the great city, to seek rest and regeneration in the balmy air of some country retreat. The moors of Scotland, the relaxing airs of the sunny south, the watering places, the continent, all have their votaries ; but London, the great metropolis of the world, is left deserted, to such alone as are bound to her by stern necessity. Even our professional brethren, who of all men are most tied to the scenes of their labors, have been swept along by the common tide, and for a brief space are at rest. Now are assistant surgeons in the ascendant, their seniors absent ; they flesh their maiden scalpels, and for a while rule predominant in the wards of our hospitals.

The medical societies, lately so active, are closed, and the question of their amalgamation under one grand head, a question the issue of which must be interesting to all, is deferred until next session ; and even scandal, which unfortunately amongst us is far from silent, has been for a while hushed in most desirable repose. Hence, I repeat that London, as regards news, is at a stand-still ! and you will at once perceive that little of interest can be afloat, beyond such as we may extract from those unfailing mines of information, the hospitals. Here, indeed, we may always look with certainty for instruction, as Death and Disease little heed the seasons mapped out by custom for the convenience of the wealthy and the great !

I shall confine myself almost entirely, in my first letter, to the notices of some interesting cases which have occurred within the last few weeks at one of these noble institutions.

At St. Bartholomew's, at St. Mary's, and elsewhere, several cases of calculus vesicæ have presented themselves, exemplifying the ever-changing variety in this disease, and the various modes of procedure adopted for its cure.

At St. Mary's Hospital, Mr. Ure has attempted the destruction of a stone by the application of the lithotrite, assisted by solutions of carbonate of lithia, under the exhibition of this solvent of uric acid. The stone apparently became friable, and broke down with great ease under the gentle application of the instrument. The case, however, is unsatisfactory, inasmuch as, when to all appearance advancing so steadily towards its cure, the patient suddenly became depressed, and sunk without any apparent cause, excepting the presence of a second stone in the bladder, which was discovered after death.

At St. Bartholomew's, the veteran Mr. Lawrence performed lithotomy upon a man of forty-five years of age, and extracted a lithic acid stone—three days sufficing for the recovery of the natural functions of the bladder, and the discharge of urine through its proper channel.

Mr. Skey had some very successful cases of lithotrity, from which I select the following, as exemplifying the ease and rapidity with which this operation often effects its end. John Barry, æt. thirty-five—suffered from every symptom of calculus visicæ, for twelve months, accompanied by those of chronic inflammation of that organ, namely, frequent and painful micturition with great straining, spasm of the bladder, and pain referred to the extremity of the penis ; his water, upon standing, became stringy and tenacious. The stone was readily detected with the sound, and appeared, as it afterwards proved to be, of about the size of a walnut. Lithotrity was per-formed five days after admission, without chloroform—the stone seized and broken once across, according to an invariable rule of Mr. Skey's at a first operation ; after this, several small fragments of lithic acid culculus were voided with the urine, and the vesical symptoms subsided to a remarkable extent.

It is worthy of notice, how almost invariably severe symptoms of irritation, etc., of the bladder, yield under the *first* application of the lithotrite. The operation was repeated at the end of a week; the stone being crushed several times, and fragments sufficient to fill an ordinary sized pill-box, were the result. Pain diminished. The next operation took place three days subsequently; and after two more " sittings," at intervals of three days, no stone could be detected by the sound.

Thus, in five operations, neither of which occupied beyond four minutes, rarely beyond three, within three weeks, completed the cure. Mr. Skey possesses the art of seizing the stone by means of a slight shake of the lithotrite, with singular tact. As quickly as the upper blade is withdrawn, it is screwed home upon a fragment.

At the same hospital, Mr. Wormald extracted a curious hour-glass shaped stone, lodged partly in the bladder and partly in the urethra of a child, six years of age. It being impossible to carry the staff beyond the neck of the bladder, by reason of the presence of the calculus in that region, the surgeon made a transverse incision between the rami of the bones, down to the point of the staff, as it lay in contact with the stone, in the first portion of the urethra; he then divided the remainder of the urethra and the neck of the bladder, employing the calculus as a director, and extracted the stone, which proved, upon section, to consist of triple phosphate, and to be developed from two distinct nuclei.

Mr. Edward Atkinson, surgeon to the English Hospital for the Jews at Jerusalem, has removed a stone of great size from the bladder of a Jewess, aged fifty-four. A straight staff having been introduced along the urethra into the bladder, with its groove facing downwards and outwards to the left; a probe-pointed bistoury was passed along it into that viscus, and the wound enlarged externally during the withdrawal of the knife; the calculus, however, proved so considerable in size, that it became necessary to repeat the incision upon the opposite side, avoiding, however, the " strong fibrous ring around the neck of the bladder," as described by the operator. After this, a stone was removed with great difficulty, the circumference of which proved to measure, in its shorter axis, four and a half inches—in its longer, six inches; its weighed nineteen drachms. Her recovery was rapid and complete.

An interesting case of axillary aneurism is at present under treatment by Mr. Paget, in the St. Bartholomew's Hospital. A fine healthy man, of fifty-four years of age, presented himself at this institution, with a well defined pulsating tumor, evident to the touch, both above the clavicle and in the axilla upon the right side. All the usual symptoms of aneurism of the main artery of this region were present ;. and had, with the exception of the swelling which he had only perceived a few days previous to admission, been remarked by the patient himself for some months. On June 26th, after the attempt had been made to treat the case by pressure, the subclavian was tied, and the man progressed favorably until the commencement of the third week, when the lint with which the wound was dressed was found bloody. However, he appeared well ; and it was not until the morning of the 14th July, nineteen days after the operation, that a severe rigor set in, lasting nearly twenty minutes, on account of which, brandy, with twenty minims of tinct. opii, were administered. He perspired profusely for the remainder of the day. This was the first constitutional symptom which had presented itself ; and Mr. Paget, believing it to be the result of pyæmia, ordered him brandy ℥viij daily, with large doses of quinine every two hours. Under this treatment his pulse, which in the morning had reached 144, fell before evening to 124. On the 16th, the ligature came away with the dressing. Perspires a great deal, and is a little tremulous, but otherwise as well as could be expected. Continues quinine every *two* hours ! He now complained of severe pain in his left shoulder, followed at an interval of three days by a similar pain in the right elbow joint, which was rather distended, and for which was ordered unguent. hydrarg. c. pulv. opii ; the quinine every *four* hours. Pressure in the axilla caused healthy pus to flow from the wound in the neck, although suppuration had occurred around the sac. On August 6th, hæmorrhage came on from the wound, and in a few minutes the patient lost above twenty ounces of blood. This reduced him very much. The same evening an abscess was opened at the elbow, with considerable relief ; and on the following day, fœtid bloody serum appeared from the wound in the neck. On examination of the elbow, the lower end of the humerus was discovered to be bare. Pulse 108. A few days later, a small opening was made in the axilla, as the swelling in that region appeared to be approaching the surface ; but nothing but blood presented, which flowed freely from both wounds, and was stopped with difficulty. Mr. Paget believed that he had punctured the aneurismal sac. Pulse very feeble ; perspires profusely. On the 10th, at about one o'clock, r.

106

M., he suffered a second rigor of about twenty minutes' duration, during which about an ounce of very fœtid bloody fluid welled up from the upper wound. The patient improved gradually until the 17th, when hæmorrhage again occurred to the extent of ten or twelve ounces ; and on the same evening he suffered another rigor of about twenty minutes' duration, during which a small quantity more of blood escaped. The patient remained in this precarious condition, vibrating between hope and fear, now suffering a rigor, now losing a small quantity of blood, and now improving in spite of the heavy drain upon his vital powers, until about the 24th, when a more steady amendment seemed to set in.

In my next communication, I hope to give your readers the final notes of this interesting case, if any thing further occurs in the course of it worthy of notice.

Some interest was attached to the following case of secondary traumatic aneurism of the ulnar artery. A woman, aged thirty years, sustained a wound on the front aspect of the right wrist. The division of the parts, which was effected by a piece of glass, was considerable, but apparently no large vessel was wounded. The wound having healed, she left the hospital at the end of three weeks; shortly after which, a tumor appeared on the ulnar side of the palm of the hand, and she returned to the hospital at the end of the week ; the swelling had reached the size of two-thirds of a pigeon's egg, and pulsated distinctly. Pressure upon the ulnar artery arrested the pulsation, and the tumor became flaccid. Mr. Skey tied the radial and ulnar arteries, from one to two inches above the wrist—the external incisions being made over the arteries at an angle of about thirty-five degrees with the line of the vessels, on grounds advocated in his own work upon Operative Surgery. Mr. Skey deemed the operation essential to recovery from a traumatic aneurismal tumor of the ulnar artery ; but added, that in the case of a simple wound of the vessel in the palm, he should resort to local pressure, and the flexed position of the fore-arm at the elbow joint, by which the circulation in both radial and ulnar arteries is almost entirely arrested. The recovery was complete.

A rather curious case of extravasation of urine in the person of a little boy twenty months old, occurred in the practice of Mr. Holden. The mother had observed nothing peculiar in the child until the day of admission, when he had not made water for twenty-four hours, and evidently suffered greatly from the difficulty in evacuating the bladder. Upon examination by the house surgeon, it was discovered that a small stone had passed along the urethra, and had become impacted between the prepuce and the glans penis, effectually barring the passage of water through the orifice of the prepuce—in fact, acting as a sort of ball valve. Extravasation had taken place to a considerable extent, from before backwards—that is to say, the urine had passed from the urethra, and, unable to escape from the prepuce, had made its way backwards through an opening in the fossa corona glandis, and under the integument of the organ into the scrotum and perineum. The stone was removed without difficulty. Two or three incisions relieved the infiltrated parts, and the child is about to leave the hospital recovered. It is now fourteen days since admission.

A case of traumatic tetanus, the result of a crushed finger, was treated, in London, the other day, by cold baths, with beneficial, but only temporary effect. The patient died.

"*Vesico-Vaginal Fistula treated with Nitrate of Silver*"!—A ricketty little woman was admitted into "Lucas" ward, St. Bartholomew's Hospital, under the care of Mr. Skey. She was confined five months ago, when it was found necessary to complete a very lingering labor by the aid of instruments ; since which time she has been utterly unable to contain her urine, which constantly flowed from her per vaginam. On examination, a large rent was found close to the os uteri, in the anterior vaginal wall, through which the fore-finger readily passed into the bladder. By means of a speculum, the solid stick of nitrate of silver was applied to the edge of the wound, about every five or six days. After six such applications, she was enabled to hold her water for a full hour at a time, and some of it passed by the natural channel. The fissure will now admit no more than the tip of the finger. She continues to improve, and will probably leave the hospital in a few weeks, perfectly well. It is a question whether the nitrate of silver might not in many cases supersede the use of the knife. It is a remedy easily applied, and leaving the patient, in case of its failure, in certainly no worse predicament for the performance of the usual operation for vesico-vaginal fistula. It seems to be one of those means of cure, which should at all events be attempted in most cases, before the long and painful operation of paring the edges of the wound, and bringing them together by means of silk, silver wire, or other sutures, is entered upon—an operation fraught with so much difficulty, and attended by such doubtful success.

In no disease has treatment undergone a more marked change in England, than in that of that most common and depressing malady, " Influenza." Purgatives and salines are no longer deemed available for good ; and in their place mulled port wine, in considerable and frequent doses, is a favorite and successful substitute. A medical practitioner of considerable experience informed me that during a recent epidemic of this disease, he had ordered the following, with most happy results :

R : Ammon. sesquicarb........................ℨss.
Ætheris Chlor. .... ℨi.
Tinct. Cardam. Comp....................... ℨi.
Mist. Camph. ad........................ . ℨvj.

Ft. Mist. partem quartam 4tis horis.

This prescription, or slight variations of it, I have myself prescribed in several cases, with complete success.

And now, in conclusion, let me add one word upon a subject which must be more or less interesting to our brethren in every quarter of the globe where scientific surgery is recognized.

The health of Sir Benjamin Brodie continues to be the source of much anxiety to his friends, and the profession. He is the leading spirit of progress among us—not alone as a man of a high order of mind, which, coupled with great industry, has achieved, during a period of a quarter of a century, an unrivaled eminence as a surgeon, but as President of the Royal Society he stands foremost in the paths of general science of Great Britain. For six or eight months past Sir Benjamin's sight has become more and more impaired, and about two months ago he consulted two of our leading ophthalmic surgeons, between whom, however, some slight difference of opinion prevailed as to the precise nature of his disease, which was deemed glaucoma, with the doubtful existence of incipient cataract of the right eye. The operation for glaucoma, first suggested by Graefe, which your readers will remember as consisting of the removal of a small section of the iris, and the ciliary muscle, was performed on both eyes, but without the beneficial result which is said by its advocates generally to follow it. At the expiration of three weeks from this date, Sir Benjamin left town for his seat, Betchworth Park, near Dorking, little, if at all, benefited by the operation. During the last month cataract has developed itself in the right eye, which presents a hope of improved vision for the future, when it has become sufficiently matured in its condition to sanction the operation of extraction. At the present date the sight of the left eye is slightly improved, objects being perceptible in the direction of the outer canthus, although to a limited extent. It is impossible even to glance at the services rendered to the cause of scientific surgery by this great surgeon, without deploring the compulsory cessation of labors fraught with so much benefit to the world ; for, although of a good advanced age, the activity of his mind and the energy of his pursuit of knowledge have been, up to the period of his illness, almost unimpaired. Large and numerous as have been Sir Benjamin Brodie's contributions to surgical literature—and every work he has published is full of knowledge—he is not less remarkable as a philosophic thinker, and of him it may truly be said on every subject he has handled, "nihil tetigit quod non ornavit."

To the familiarity with surgical facts, surpassed neither by our own countryman, Sir Astly Cooper, nor by the great French surgeon, Baron Dupuytren, Sir Benjamin Brodie superadds a more reflective and reasoning faculty than either. His practical familiarity with almost every variety of surgical disease, has probably never been surpassed, while his opinions upon the subject of their treatment, founded upon a thorough knowledge of the vital powers, have been notoriously successful throughout his long and eminently successful career.

LONDON, September 1st, 1860.

PROGRESS OF MEDICINE.

ART. I.—*Goitre—The Whey Cure—Iodism.*

i.—*Goitre.*—Prof. F. H Hamilton, of Buffalo, New York, in his tour of Europe a few years ago, mentions that in Valais canton, two-thirds of the inhabitants are goitrous, and that the absence of the usual appendage is considered as a deformity ! Dr. H. C. Lombard,

of the Geneva Hospital, considers that to effect a cure it is necessary to remove from the valleys to the mountains, and then use
iodine. Dr. Blakie, of Edinburgh, now Professor of Botany in the
University of Nashville, in a memoir on Goitre, published a few
years ago, gives a very interesting account of this deplorable disease, which has so greatly deteriorated the minds and bodies of the
Swiss and others.

Its prevalence in Mexico and some other American countries, in
climates very different from those of the Alpine and some other regions of the old world, shows that the usual explanations of its
causes are altogether unsatisfactory ; such as the use of snow-
water, deficient solar light, the humidity of the deep valleys, etc.

In a book of travels (1846), by A. Gilliam, Esq., formerly United
States Consul to California, the author gives accounts showing the
prevalence of goitre rivaling that of the Alpine regions ; as, for example, at Canales. He says : " The climate of Canales is spring
and summer. The trees are perpetually green ; for as fast as the
leaves fade and fall, others are fresh and expanding ; added to which
the golden harvests of the orange are ever beautiful " (314). Yet
he says one-half of the population is diseased with these tumors ;
he saw some of these which were of great size, requiring a handkerchief or bandage by which to suspend them (316). "Children born
of goitred parents are certain to be idiots, or deaf and dumb; in
some instances feeble and rickety" (316). He says that it does
" not originate from the water."

To what extent this malady prevails in the Southern regions of
the United States, I am unable to determine, having seen only one
case of it in Louisiana. If one may judge by the silence of the
medical journals, it must be an exceedingly rare affection in the
South.

The following extracts are from the August (1860) number of the
Edinburgh Medical Journal, written by A. Mercer Adam, M. D., .
Edinburgh, late Physician to the Dumfries and Galloway Royal Infirmary (No. VII of " Medical Notes from the Continent). These
notes, for the most part, are not strictly professional, but they are
quite interesting to the medical reader and traveler.   B. D.

On in the evening to Berchtesgaden—a most picturesque little
town in a lovely valley, lying at the foot of the lofty Watzmann
mountain. Here we rest for the night. This is the summer retreat

of the King of Bavaria. His *schloss*—a plain-looking country house—is close by the town. Before leaving Berchtesgaden we visit the celebrated Königsee—the wildest of all the Salzkammergut lakes—lying in the hollow of lofty mountains, which rise so abruptly from the water-edge that no pathway for human feet can be found along their precipitous sides. Deep green are its waters ; deeper and darker in their hue from reflection of the sombre pine forests which clothe the hills on every side up to their glacier-crowned summits. Here and there bold rocks rear their rugged but picturesque forms from out the depths of the thick leafage. No sounds of life are heard in this scene of savage grandeur, save the faint tinkle of the cattle bells, or the scream of some eagle. We are rowed along the lake by two good-looking Tyrolese girls, who break the dead silence by singing us their native Jödeln. As their sweet voices carol the air, and the notes are thrilled out with a peculiar guttural intonation, the strange wild melody seems well to accord with the native majesty of the lonely lake.

But let not the reader think that everything is romantic in these charming regions. The inhabitants of these valleys are fearfully afflicted by cretinism ; and the two fair rowers of our boat, despite their sweet voices and pretty faces, are disfigured by enormous goitres. There is little wonder that cretinism is common here, because we find that all the physical causes which conduce to its development are in existence in the deep solitudes of many of these mountain valleys. Take, for example, Hallstadt, one of the places where I was most struck by the prevalence of cretinism. This is a village on the shores of the romantic Hallstadt-See. This large lake lies between lofty mountains, which give a wild and gloomy character to the scenery, and prevent all access to the wind, except when blowing in certain directions. The village is built on the side of one of these mountains, which descends so abruptly to the lake that the houses seem to cling to the steep hillside, "like swallows' nests against a wall." The situation is, therefore, damp and ill-ventilated ; it is, moreover, gloomy for want of sufficient light, as the sun never shows his face to the poor inhabitants from the 17th November to the 2d February, and often, at other times, is very niggardly of his beams. Hallstadt is, therefore, a perfect focus of cretinism ; and as I climbed up the long flights of stairs which constitute its streets, I was followed by a rabble of idiots, with enormous goitres, dwarfish bodies, and unmistakable cretin physiognomies—all jabbering clamorously for alms.*

A few years ago Professor Virchow† published some interesting papers on the subject of cretinism in the Bavarian Highlands ; and, as regards the ætiology of this disorder, he believes that there exists, in certain districts, a certain diffusible agency (arising from the soil), or *specific miasma*, which occasions goitre in adults, and which affects the fœtus in utero, and young children still more seriously—producing in them, not only enlargements of the thyroid glands, but

---

* The word *Fex* has long been used in this district to designate these unhappy beings. Some people think it a corruption of " Vir vexabilis."

† Ueber den Cretinismus, u. s. w.; *Ges. Abhand. zur wissensch. Med.* 1855–56.

also morbid changes in the development of the central nervous apparatus and its envelopes. This diffusible miasmatic element mixes with the air, and impregnates the water of the region producing it ; and thus it is received into the human system by means of respiration, or by absorption through the mucous membranes of the skin. This poison may be communicated by a mother to her child, during its fœtal life, without any manifestation of the disease in herself; so that a cretinous child may be born of parents apparently healthy, in districts where the miasm is prevalent. A curious illustration of this has been observed at Reichenhall, by Dr. Schierlinger. The Government officials sent thither to be employed at the great salt mines of which I have spoken, have been known to beget goitrous and cretinous infants during their residence at Reichenhall, although they had always previously had healthy offspring ; and, on their being removed from this place to some other locality, where the miasma was not prevalent, the infants born to them were strong and healthy as before. Virchow believes that the amount of cretinism, like that of other epidemic diseases, undergoes periodical fluctuations. In certain districts it begins to decline, and eventually to disappear ; while in others it makes its appearance, and spreads quickly, Virchow says, in the neighborhood of the Spessart Forest*, where cretinism was very prevalent from 1822 to 1832, the disease seems now to have become extinct, because in 1851 no single instance of its reäppearance could be elicited by the most careful inquiries. The cretinism miasma is only communicable to man ; for animals in Alpine regions are not found to have goitre†. Certain races appear to be more affected by it than others ; thus, in Styria, cretinism occurs among the Germans in the proportion of 1 in 113, and among the Sclavonic population only as 1 in 513‡. Females also seem more liable to it than males. Köstl tells us that of every 1000 cretins in Styria, 803 are females§.

ii. *The Whey Cure.*

I may say a few words on this system of treatment, which is carried out to a great extent at Ischl. "We give whey," says Beneke, in his well-known work¶ on the subject, "in those cases where we wish to diminish the nitrogenous elements of the blood, without altering the quality and quantity of the various inorganic compounds which are essential to the proper nutrition of the body." In other words, whey is given in cases where we wish to reduce plethoric conditions, and to correct deranged action of the liver and bowels, without perceptibly lowering the vital powers. As used at Ischl, and other Alpine villages where there are institutions for treatment by this remedy, the medicinal whey is not only a bland nutrient agent, but is a gentle yet efficacious laxative and diuretic. It is prepared by the Tyrolese from the milk of their sheep, cows, and

---

* See "Concerning Bavaria!" by the author, in *Edinburgh Medical Journal,* January, 1859.

† Fabré, *Traite du Goître et du Cretinisme.* Paris, 1858.

‡ Kostl, *Der endemische Cretinismus als Gegenstand der öffentliche Fursorge.* Vienna, 1855.

§ Ibid.

¶ *Die Rationalität der Molkenkuren,* 1853.

goats, which browse on the wild herbage of the mountains. It has an opalescent appearance, a pale yellowish-green color, and a sweet aromatic taste. It contains all the nutritive elements of the milk, separated from the casein or nitrogenous part. The watery constituents of the whey act on the kidneys, and gently favor the metamorphosis of tissue, while its sugar of milk, if not too quickly absorbed, acts as a mild laxative. Goats' whey is more' efficacious than the others as an aperient, on account of its containing a larger proportion of sugar of milk. When a slightly purgative effect is desired, the whey is taken about one or two hours after breakfast, instead of on an empty stomach, when it would be too rapidly absorbed. In all other cases, however, it is drunk fasting, before breakfast, and a brisk walk is taken between each glassful. The quantity taken varies from one to four small tumblerfuls; and mineral waters of various kinds, e. g., those of Kreuznach, Kissengen, Selters, Vichy, etc., are mixed with it when ordered by the physician. The use of whey is highly recommended in cases of abdominal plethora, in hyperæmia of the liver and spleen, in threatened phthisis, in scrofulous affections generally, in chronic dyspepsia and constipation, and in cases of impaired nervous energy, where the circulation is languid and the extremities are constantly cold. I fancy that it gets the credit of many cures which are effected by change of scene, fresh mountain air, plenty of open air exercise, and the cheerful society of a watering-place. But it is a pleasant depurative agent, if it does not possess all the virtues which enthusiastic German physicians ascribe to it ; and if the reader goes to Ischl, let him drain off the crystal gobletful, handed him by a buxom Tyrolienne, with faith and thankfulness.

In conclusion, there are few places more attractive than Ischl for pleasant situation and romantic scenery. And those of my hard-worked professional brethren, who can spare time for a "physician's holiday," will never regret spending part of their vacation amid the charming lakes and valleys of the Salzkammergut.

iii. *On Iodism :* By M. RILLIET.

In this paper M. Rilliet, of Geneva, takes a review of the recent discussion upon this subject which has taken place in the French Academy. This originated in a paper by M. Boinet, in which he maintained the power of iodized alimentation to effect all the good derivable from iodine administered medicinally, as also its absolute innocuity. This produced a note from M. Rilliet, in which he stated that the absorption of small doses of iodine during a long period of time, sometimes gives rise to a cachectic condition which he terms "iodism," and he related three cases in which this state had been brought on by the consumption of iodized salt during several weeks. M. Boinet having flatly denied the accuracy of the statement, M. Rilliet set himself to work, with the aid of other Swiss practitioners, to produce a full memoir upon the subject, containing accounts of sixteen cases, thirteen of them occurring in persons the subject of goitre, and three in those who were not goitrous. This memoir was

107

made the subject of an able but adverse report by Prof. Trousseau, and thereupon a lively discussion ensued.

M. Rilliet did not confine himself to his own personal experience. But found that this was corroborated by the testimony of various authors who had written on iodine, from Coindet downwards. However, his facts were disputed by M. Pierry, and his explanation of them by M. Trousseau. With regard to the facts, he is contented to leave them undefended, observed, as they were, with care, consciousness, and professional publicity. M. Trousseau well knew the amount of reliance to be placed upon the powers of observation of the celebrated author of the *Traité des Maladies des Enfants ;* and, therefore, while admitting in the cases observed the emaciation, bulimia, palpitations, enervation, and agitation described, denies that iodine has been the cause of such persistent, and sometimes such grave, functional disturbances. He is disposed to attribute these symptoms to the so called exophthalmic cachexia. He said he had met with cases of anæmic exophthalmia, which presented every analogy with the cases described by M. Rilliet. But the latter declares that in none of his cases was this condition of the eye present. The patients before taking the iodine exhibited no signs of any cachectic condition, the cachexia appearing in different degrees, only after taking it for a more or less long period, and not recurring unless the drug was again administered. While, too, many instances of iodism were observed at Geneva in 1820, six months after Coindet's discovery, and have been seen frequently since, none of the practitioners of the town have met with an instance of cachectic exophthalmia. On the other hand, it is very possible that some of the reported cases of exophthalmic cachexia observed elsewhere were in fact examples of iodism. In fact, this so-called cachexia does not always seem to have exhibited well-defined characters. As has been well observed by Stokes, the exophthalmia and the thyroid enlargement are both epiphenomena, resulting from active or passive sanguineous congestion. There are also notable differences between the two cachexiæ. In the exophthalmic cachexia the derangement of the health usually precedes the appearance of the exophthalmia and the goitre, the cachectic symptoms attain their maximum at the period of the greatest development of the protrusion of the eyes, and of the enlargement of the thyroid, and it is a disease of continuous progress, accompanied by frequent exacerbations, during which every symptom becomes aggravated. In the iodic cachexia, although the patients may have their thyroid glands enlarged, the general health has been good, it is just at the period when the goitre diminishes that the iodism manifests itself, and once cured, it does not recur unless iodine is again administered. The one is a disease of years, the other, at most, of a few months ; the gravity of the two affections being also markedly different. Even the individual symptoms are not alike in the two cases ; for not only is the exophthalmia wanting in the iodism, but there is not in it the same vascular development in the thyroid. On the other hand, emaciation and bulimia are not always observed in the exophthalmic cachexia, and the nervous symptoms are not alike in the two affections. As, however, persons of a nervo-sanguineous temperament are especially those who are liable to iodism, it is no wise surprising that a morbid condition like exophthalmic cachexia, which is only an exaggeration of such temperament, should sometimes act as a predisponent to it; and, in fact, iodine has several times acted with disastrous effect in exophthalmic cachexia.

In answer to M. Trousseau's objection, that cases of iodism are of rare occurrence, M. Rilliet admits the fact, though not to the extent stated by the reporter. Slight cases exhibiting iodic susceptibility, are of constant occurrence at Geneva, and many of these would proceed to confirmed iodism if the use of iodine were persisted in. Even with this limitation, the author has been enabled to collect in two months in Geneva, a town of 30,000 inhabitants, accounts of sixteen well-marked cases, being a very small portion of those observed since the time of Coindet; while M. Charcot, who has collected all the observations on exophthalmic cachexia contained in medical literature, has not been enabled to get together more than forty cases. Again, when it is objected that the small doses of iodine exhibited at Geneva are not competent to produce this slowly poisonous effect, it is replied that if doses of the iodide of potassium varying from 1-18th to 1-36th of a grain are competent—of which there can be no doubt—to cure goitre at Geneva, why should they not, in certain predisposed subjects, induce this cachectic condition termed by M. Rilliet "chronic iodism."—*Gaz. Méd.*—*Med. Times and Gazette.*

Art. II.—*Parisian Medical Intelligence.* [From the Correspondent of *The Lancet.*]

Goître; removal by the écraseur.—M. Chassaignac, of the Hôpital Lariboisière, some years ago drew the attention of the profession to certain enlargements of the thyroid body, which, although apparently insignificant from their smallness of volume, yet, from their unyielding density of texture and prolongation along the trachea into the chest, not unfrequently proved the cause of a degree of disturbance in the respiratory function amounting at times to suffocation. To this variety of goitre M. Chassaignac assigned the epithet of "constricteur," recommending in all cases, when feasible, the immediate removal by operation of the tumor.

In one case, especially dwelt upon by this surgeon, so considerable had been the pressure exercised by the enlarged gland, that the pneumogastric nerve had been flattened out through several inches of its course, like a piece of tape. In this patient, the dyspnœa, added to the constant recurrence of a violent form of neuralgia, made existence intolerable; and not until the autopsy (for death occurred suddenly) had revealed the condition of the pneumogastric trunk, were the symptoms, inexplicable during life, ever referred to the compressive action of the small and seemingly innocuous goitre. The enucleation of the whole of the thyroid body is a most grave affair ; the hæmorrhage from the large blood-vessels, divided so close to their origin from the main trunk is something fearful, and most difficult to control—such attempts having on more than one occasion necessitated the ligature of both common carotids.

· An example of the "goitre constricteur" presented itself last week in the wards of M. Chassaignac, and this surgeon resolved on using the écraseur to effect the extirpation. The patient was a lad of six-teen ; the tumor was small, apparently as big as a full-sized walnut, but peculiarly firm and low down in the neck, near the sternum. Much distress was complained of, and very slight pressure caused the breathing to assume a spasmodic, gasping character. Chloroform having been administered, the boy lying on his back with a narrow bolster under his shoulders and the head well thrown back, an incision was made with the écraseur through the skin and successive layers of cellular tissue and fascia down to the surface of the enlarged gland. The isolation from surrounding tissues was effected by the finger, and the chain of the écraseur passed round the base of the tumor, so as to include all its fibrous and vascular connections. The handle of the instrument was worked at the rate of one notch per half minute, and in about twenty minutes the whole of the thyroid body came away. The size was that of a small orange ; in density and texture it much resembled a fowl's gizzard, and was traversed in all directions by large vessels, some of them exceeding a goose-quill in calibre. There was a little oozing, which was controlled by a small bladder of ice ; and the patient shortly afterwards awoke from his chloroformal lethargy, highly delighted at feeling his throat freed from the preëxisting constriction.

It struck me, during the operation, that the écraseur might be employed with advantage in craniotomy on children. The trachea might with this instrument be reached and laid bare in five minutes by a bloodless incision ; and I feel sure all who have tried the operation on a child will fully appreciate such a benefit. With regard to the écraseur, I think Mr. Chassaignac is becoming a little more discriminating in its employment ; he has had the good sense to stop short of that narrow frontier which divides the honorable practitioner and the valuable medicament from the charlatan and his panacea, and has thus avoided the danger he would otherwise have incurred by "riding the willing nag to death," and bringing into discredit one of the most useful additions to modern surgery.

There is much summer diarrhœa in the hospitals just now ; the weather is changeable, and fruit abundant, so that we have both the catarrhal and dyspeptic forms of this complaint. M. Trousseau, in his wards of the Hôtel Dieu, is treating both classes of diarrhœa with ipecacuanha, in large doses, and says he is most successful in his cures, which are more rapid than those obtained by any other means he has hitherto attempted. He says that ipecacuanha is as much of a specific in catarrhal or irritative hypersecretion of the mucous membrane as is colchicum in gout.

It is impossible for an Englishman, in going through the hospitals here, not to be struck by the capricious and experimental nature of the practice now in vogue. At home, the routine of treatment adopted in one hospital differs little from that in another. What is ascertained to be good by one is copied very readily by the rest, without recourse to academical arbitration or without giving rise to discussion about priority. This never-ending struggle for priority is, at the present moment, one of the greatest stumbling-blocks to scientific research. Men are led to seek novelty irrespectively of utility. The rich vein of ore is often abandoned simply because others have already worked and enriched science from that source. I believe that this competitive system in hospital practice, if tested by statistical calculation, will be found to exercise a most baneful influence upon the main object of this branch of charitable relief—namely, the preservation of human life. This great object is not sufficiently borne in mind in France, and many great and really good men are, I think, carried away by the current, which, as a body, they would certainly have the power, but lack the courage, to stem.

PARIS, JULY 30, 1860.

* * * * * * * * * *

Treatment of Gleet.—Every one knows how tiresome and difficult to cure a gleet may become, and how weary of each other both patient and surgeon occasionally grow in consequence. A little "dodge," which may not yet have crossed the Channel, and which I have seen succeed here, when the whole armament of balsamics, injections, and derivaties have failed, is the following : Take a moderate sized wax bougie (the common yellow wax ones are the best), warm it slightly, and then roll it for a few seconds in well-powdered alum ; when thoroughly whitened with the salt, roll it between the hands so as to press the alum well into the wax, and the instrument is ready for use. Make the patient micturate previously, and then pass your bougie, without the assistance of oil or cerate, as far as may be deemed advisable, cutting it off to within an inch of the orifice of the meatus, where it may be tied or not, and then left one hour each day. In this way a tiresome and refractory old gleet may be cured in ten days.

Paris Practice: New Style.—One of the drawbacks to such a system of practice as that followed by M. Trousseau—namely, novelty hunting—is the impatience with which any return to old-fashioned modes of medication is tolerated by the circle of admiring copyists, the volunteer *claquers* of the performance. In going round with M. Trousseau a day or two back, we came upon a case of lead colic, newly admitted ; and M. Trousseau dictated the prescription as follows : an emetic of ipecacuanha, an enema of nut oil, a dose of bolus theriacalis in the evening, and low diet. "But that is as old as the hills," murmured out one recalcitrant follower, the Aaron of the company—a truth which the Professor was forced to admit. This trifling remark, however, reminds one of the fact that M. Trousseau has saddled himself with an unpleasant and thankless task—namely, that of having indefinitely to cater novelties and original modes of treatment for the fast-palling tastes of his numerous audience.

Another of the Paris practitioners who has struck out much in the same manner, though rarely in the same direction, as M. Trousseau, is Dr. Beau, of the Charité. Although not very happy in some of his therapeutic innovations (the employment of carbonate of lead in phthisis for example, the virtues of which consist in anticipating by medicine what nature generally effects by disease), this physician possesses many of the qualities of a good clinical teacher. He has much originality of conception, and great happiness and facility of expression. M. Beau's practice is always decided, and undertaken with a definite purpose. His clinical remarks are particularly interesting and suggestive. Some of the favorite modes of treatment are the following : In typhoid fever, continued purgation to the amount of ten or twelve stools daily ; he uses castor oil, croton oil, seidlitz water, tartar emetic, etc., varying the drug each time the effect is to be produced. In acute rheumatism, he begins with antimonial emetics *(ad plenum vomitum,* to last a day at least), and then gives large doses of sulphate of quinine. Ascites, if without grave complications, he taps and treats with injections of iodine as readily as a case of hydrocele. I have merely jotted down the above as specimens, and I strongly recommend any countryman about to visit Paris to note down Dr. Beau's service at the Charité as one of the indispensable " memoranda and agenda."

PARIS, AUGUST 6, 1860.

———

At the Imperial Academy of Medicine, on the 24th ult., M. Malgaigne ascended the tribune, and amid a profound silence delivered the most eloquent address I ever had the good fortune to hear within the walls of the Academy. In spite of a disagreeable southern accent, a nasal tone, and a total lack of " presence," M. Malgaigne's charm and power as an orator are undeniable. His wit, quickness of perception, brilliant illustration, and happy citations, added to great rhetorical skill and knowledge of effect, make him a most potent advocate, or most formidable opponent, in any medical question. It is unfortunate, however, that none of these qualities can be conveyed in an epitomized *compte-rendû,* and your readers must be contented with the raw material, bereft of its fashioning, and consequently as much like the original as would be a heap of pulverized marble to the statue it may formerly have composed. M. Malgaigne began by rallying the head of the chemical school, M. Poggiale, on the subject of his antipathy to the word *chimiatre.* " Remain, then," said he, " in your chemical province, and be simply a chemist ; but encroach one foot upon our domain of medicine, you will incur the penalty, and we shall ruthlessly brand you a *chimiatre.* Chemistry has done much for medicine ; she has been a faithful handmaid, but like all handmaids must be taught her proper place, and be kept there : her powers are limited, and this she must not forget." M. Poggiale had expressed a hope that more ample justice would be rendered by the future to chemistry and her services to medical science than the present seemed inclined to accord. M. Malgaigne would remind the learned Professor that the future is often a more impartial judge than the present, and that although it often raises a

throne for the great genius, yet as often does it dig the grave of the
dreamer. M. Poggiale had boasted of the power possessed by
chemistry of forming, by synthesis, one or more of the principles
produced in the human body, and would thence, by analogy, argue
that chemical agency is alone competent to the formation of the rest.
" I grant you," continued M. Malgaigne, "that a few of the crystalli-
zable products of the human laboratory may be mimicked by chemical aid, but there are other materials in the body besides chemical
products, and when we come to the formation of tissue, more than
crystallization is needed. We want for the organization of tissue,
the touch of the weaver; we want the warp and woof. Can chemistry furnish these? No, she cannot, in spite of all the boastful
encomiums of her devotees. There is still, and ever will be, between
the operations of nature and those of chemistry an unfathomable
gulf which no effort of man will ever succeed in sounding. The
chemists generally are too fond of calculation, and too little of experiment, and from this fault even M. Lavoisier was not free. Take
their many years of fruitless search after the source of animal heat
as an illustration. In this they remind me forcibly of the story told
of the hydrographers of Frederick the Great, who, when consulted
by his majesty on the subject of a well he wished to sink at Sans
Souci, and requested to point out a likely spot for the finding of a
spring, fell to calculating. They took into account the nature of the
soil, and its geological conformation; the possible interference of
chance disarrangements, and all the other contingencies, from the
probable to the impossible, were allowed for, the calculations were
made, and a site was indicated. A pit was dug, and no water was
found. Fresh calculations, and similar results. At last Frederick,
a positive man, got tired of the philosophers, and sent for a little
pump-maker in the adjoining village. The illiterate fool, with no
knowledge of geology, mathematics, or the doctrine of chances,
pointed out a spot; a well was sunk, and water obtained in abundance. M. Malgaigne seemed to wish that modern chemists had a
little more of the pump-maker in them than they have. " M. Poggiale
does not admit the existence of a vital force in the economy; and
yet he speaks of life and its presidence over the functions. This
surely was more than a half-vitalist admission." M. Malgaigne then
reverted to the works of one of the leading organicians of the day,
M. Rostan. "Here," he observed, "the theory of vital property is
rejected, and the doctrinal datum of organs endowed with 'disposition to function' maintained; a healthy organ implying a healthy
function, an unhealthy organ a deranged function. How does this
theory explain death, when no change of structure, no organic lesion
can be detected; or how, that of two grains of wheat taken from a
mummy-case, neither distinguishable from the other in appearance
or structure, both organically the same when planted, one will die
and the other grow and fructify. Thanks to the organicians and
their infamous treatment of pneumonia by bleeding and leeching—
thanks to their sacrifice of human life thereby, we have seen the day
when the statistics of homoeopathy have been laid by the side of our
own, and the results have not been what they had a right to be."

"It is a falsehood!" roars out M. Barth, of Beaujon Hospital, "and the statistics were untrue."

"So I trusted and so I believe," went on M. Malgaigne; "but the insult has been offered to the profession through you, and the credulous, unenlightened section of the public does not stay to sift facts; and the report, untrue as it is, will have already borne its fruits. The vitalists, on the other hand, cure pneumonia perfectly well without bleeding, and lose an infinitely smaller proportion of cases."

An interruption by M. Bouillaud—"That is inexact; and were you attacked to-day with severe pneumonia, and not bled, I think we should not have the pleasure of hearing you speak again in the Academy."

"That I should be very sorry for myself also," replied the orator; "nevertheless I have not always been of the same opinion regarding blood-letting. In my days I have bled, cupped and leeched with the best of my contemporaries. I began as Broussais' *chef de clinique*. I continued the system through part of my hospital career; but I am proud to say I know better now. I have hardly used even leeches for the last six years, and I am well satisfied with my change of opinion. I believe that your organism, carried to the bed-side, blinds the physician, making him neglect the more important general indications in order to attend to the more trifling local manifestation."

After citing two cases illustrative of the superior value of the general vital indications over the local organic condition in the formation of a prognosis, M. Malgaigne terminated his brilliant speech by a short consideration of the character of vital force. "Its alliance," he said, "with caloric and electricity is indisputable. It is, like them, a special agent, possessing both affinity and attraction for matter, but independent of it and separable from it; the dead body differing from the living man as the uncharged Leyden jar differs from the charged one."

The meeting broke-up considerably later than usual. There will probably be no discussion next week, as a new member is to be elected, and this ceremony is performed with closed doors.

A Russian, of the name of Lukomski, some months ago requested permission of the head surgeons of the two great venereal hospitals here, the Midi and Lourcine, to continue in their wards a method of treatment which he declared had succeeded in Russia, and especially in an hospital at Simpheropol, where he had been allowed to experiment. The plan was based on the hypothesis of the incompatibility in the system of the venereal and vaccine virus, and the primary object of the treatment was stated to be the accumulation of the latter in the blood—this to be effected by repeated vaccinations, to the extent of nine or ten consecutively. A committee, consisting of MM. Cullerier, Folin, and Alphonse Guérin, was named some weeks back by the Society of Surgery, for the purpose of examining the results obtained, and the report was presented on Wednesday last. I am informed by the reporter, M. Guérin, in whose wards at the Lourcine part of this investigation was conducted, that the failure of M. Lukomski's experiments has been complete, and that the "anti-syphilitic power of vaccine" has been proved to be a myth. The idea is not a new one, and was, years ago, worked threadbare by Sigmond, in Germany.

PARIS, AUGUST 6, 1860.

Erysipelas has been raging in the central Paris hospitals for some weeks past, and at the Clinique more especially. At this latter nearly all the operations have been followed by this most distressing complication, and M. Nelaton has deemed it prudent to postpone treatment in several cases in consequence. The Hôpital Beaujon and the Lariboisière enjoy a perfect immunity from this scourge, thanks, no doubt, to their excellent hygienic arrangements, airy situation, and more spacious distribution. I believe we shall some day find out the mistake of planting great depôts for the sick in the centre of our cities, and, reversing the plan of centralization, retain simply receiving houses in town for the registration of patients, who will immediately, as on the field of battle, be conveyed by a sort of civil ambulance corps to the destined hospital, itself placed in the most healthy situation procurable, and at easy railway distance.

Taken by themselves, the Clinique, the Charité, and even the Hôtel Dieu, are hospitals of which a casual observer would augur favorably. The buildings are large, almost *grandiose;* the wards are lofty, well-lighted, and scrupulously clean: the first two institutions have gardens full of green trees and flowers, and a far greater air of comfort than is usually seen in such establishments elsewhere, and yet they are rarely free from some one or other of the manifestations of atmospheric impurity. Why is this? In the case of the Clinique the question is not difficult to answer. The hospital, though it has an open square of about an acre in extent within its walls, is yet built in with old houses, the veteran architecture of the classic "quartier Latin." One end of the building juts into the Court of the École Pratique, the dissecting school of the Faculty of Medicine ; and the opposite side, as the ground rises towards the Rue de Monsieur, is much below the street level, and receives, no doubt, a due contribution from the house-drains of that thoroughfare. The Charité stands in the damp soil of the Pré aux Clercs, the old Battersea-fields of Paris, in which so many duels were fought in days of yore. The Hôtel Dieu is as old as the hills, and never was regularly built, but, like Paddy's shoes, "only patched;" the ventilation is very ill contrived, and it overlooks the Seine, a river bidding fair some day to rival, in its powers of evolving ammoniacal and sulphureous perfumes, the great model, Father Thames. I know that many will think I am exaggerating ; to such I say, "Come and smell for yourselves."

A work, entitled "Les Cures de Petit Lait et de Raisin," from the pen of Dr. Edward Carrière, has just appeared in Paris, and has been courteously received by some of the medical reviews. A full-sized octavo volume is devoted to a pæan in praise of the healing virtues of milk-whey and the juice of the grape (unfermented, be it understood). It appears from this book that Germany and Switzerland alone rejoice in the possession of several hundreds of establishments, where health and whey, salubrity and grape-juice, are dispensed with a lavish and ungrudging hand. The two panaceas are apparently all-powerful, and universal in their adaptations. The over-fed gourmand, oppressed with fat, and the emaciated victim of tuberculosis, are both equally benefited by a course of these much vaunted remedies. As the culture of the vine in England is a very artificial process, and as grapes hardly ever ripen in our foggy climate without the assistance of a greater or less degree of forcing, it may be difficult to establish a comparison in this particular respect ; but surely, unless indeed M. Carrière's partiality for the Teutonic cow and its Helvetian sister has led him into exaggeration, that animal must be endowed with some special quality denied to the less fortunate bovine, or rather vaccine, race in our island. Or is it that milk-whey in the Swiss mountain districts, and grapes from " the vine-terraced hills of the Rhine " are possessed of properties as wonderful as that lately attributed at Geneva by M. Rilliet to iodine—a special *ism* resulting from their prolonged use ? The Academy of Medicine pondered over these wonderful cases of iodism for several weeks with an air of stupefaction and astonishment (analogous to that of a child reading the "Adventures of Baron Munchausen"), and returned the cautious verdict of "curious if true." Some such kindred feeling it was, I confess, that took possession of my mind during the perusal of this carefully written and perfectly readable book of M. Carrière. It is very evident that the author, in extolling the merits of his therapeutical hobbies, and in attributing to their exclusive agency the numberless cures referred to, has forgotten to take into account the pure air of the mountains, the regular habit, the wholesome diet, the bodily exercise, and mental relaxation or distraction, which, though apparently, and according to his showing, only accessories, are in reality the essential conditions of the benefits accruing from the salutary *régime* he has treated of in his work.

Paris, August 13, 1860.

———

Academy of Sciences.—At a meeting of this Academy, on the 6th instant, an essay by M. Fasoli, on the Employment of the Sulphuret and Sesquioxide of iron as antidotes in cases of Poisoning by Arsenous Acid, was read. Nineteen dogs, it appeared by this paper, were experimented on and dosed with arsenic : to five out of the number no counter-poison was administered—they were left to their fate, and all died ; out of the fourteen others, to whom considerable doses of hydrated sesquioxide and sulphuret of iron were given, only two died—a result which powerfully upholds the already good reputation enjoyed by these two salts as arsenical counter-agents.

Academy of Medicine.—The discussion on the perchloride of iron continued : M. Devergie again addressed the Academy, and urged very strongly upon his hearers some of the facts which are daily occurring to prove the efficacy of this preparation in the treatment of purpura hæmorrhagica, reports of eleven well-authenticated cures by the perchloride, in very severe types of this disease, having been received by the Academy since the discussion commenced ; which fact alone the speaker considered as condemnatory of M. Trousseau's contemptuous rejection of this remedial agent, which it will be remembered that he qualified as the least beneficial, when administered internally, of all the salts of iron—threatening those who should adopt its employment with an *avenir de déceptions.* M. Devergie again reverted to the experiment quoted from M. Claude Bernard, proving that carbonate of soda, when introduced into a dog's stomach through a fistulous opening, will render the secretion more acid than before, instead of neutralizing this reaction ; and, also, that this secretion of acid increases in proportion to the amount of alkali introduced. " It is curious," said he, "that both MM. Trousseau and Poggiale, in their several speeches, should have used the very same weapons for attacking each other ; and I dare say it will be found still more curious that I should take up the same arms to assail them both. I refer to the cure of acid dyspepsia by alkalies, and the abduction of M. Claude Bernard's experiment by M. Trousseau in support of his own views. I believe that this gentleman has misapprehended the effects of carbonate of soda when used, as by M. Bernard, in concentrated solution upon the mucous coat of the stomach. He forgets that a small portion only of the alkali is neutralized by the acid actually present in the stomach, and that the rest, during the interval preceding the moment when saturation is effected, acts as a direct irritant, and provokes the increase of secretion, which irritant action, and consequent outpouring of secretion, can be repeated and reproduced as often as the operator desires. But to compare such a process to our treatment of acid dyspepsia, is to establish a very false analogy, one of the main conditions of that treatment being, if we desire to ensure success, the copious dilution of the remedial agent—as in Vichy water, for example, and in the artificial preparations of the same nature. Neither can I admit, with M. Poggiale, that in acid dyspepsia the curative action of alkalies on the malady is one of a purely chemical nature ; my own opinion being, that such remedies operate in the same way that absorbents act in certain cutaneous affections—that is, by removing or nullifying and rendering inert a product of morbid secretion, the presence of which was detrimental to healthy action ; and the obstacle thus removed, nature is able again to take the reins into her own hands." In terminating, M. Devergie requested a vote on the adeption of the conclusions of his report ; this was agreed to, and the conclusions were carried. Consequently, the perchloride of iron, in spite of M. Trousseau's very powerful opposition, may be said to have achieved a great victory, and to have taken a high place amongst the quasi-specifics of the Pharmacopœia. The discussion, however, is not ended, as M. Piorry has given notice of his intention to speak next Tuesday in answer to M. Malgaigne.

Functional Spasm.—M. Duchenne (de Boulogne), well known by his indefatigable researches on the subject of nervous disorders, has lately described, under the double name of *functional spasm* and *functional muscular paralysis,* an affection which, though often noticed in a vague way by most clinical observers, had never been seriously studied by pathologists. The conditions which are implied in the name of this disorder are not permanent, or, at all events, are not permanently prominent, requiring for their reproduction or manifestation the exercise of some special function, of which they then impede the progress. The commonest form of this affection is that called the "scrivener's cramp," and the seat of the spasm or paralysis is in one or more of the fingers, which either curl up, or may become so powerless as to cause the writer to drop his pen—this condition being often observable after a few strokes of this implement, and consequently wholly unconnected with fatigue or nervous sur-excitation. Other muscles besides those of the hand and arm are also found to be liable to this affection—*e. g.*, the sterno mastoids, the abdominal muscles, and also those of the shoulder. It is, according to M. Duchenne's observation and experience, generally incurable, and out of thirty-five cases treated by cutaneous Faradization, only two were benefited, and no amelioration whatever was noticed in the remaining thirty-three.

August 20, 1860.

* * *

Academy of Sciences.—At the last meeting, M. Bourguet presented a paper on the reparation of long bones, as occurring after extensive resections of their shafts. This essay, which possesses considerable merit, and the materials of which are drawn from the inexhaustible mine of clinical observation, tends to establish the following : The new bone formed after removal of part of the shaft of a long bone, is shorter and thicker than the old. The presence of the periosteum in its integrity is *desirable*, but *not indispensable* to the reproduction of osseous tissues ; as the surrounding textures, such as vessels, muscles, fibrous and areolar tissues, are sufficient of themselves, in the absence of the periosteum, to do the work of regeneration. This last conclusion is, so far as I know, a new view of things, and will require further confirmation before it can be accepted.

An excellent *compte-rendù* appeared lately in the *Moniteur Scientifique*, due (as I understand) to M. Gratiolet, one of the curators of the Museum of the Jardin des Plantes, well known by his important work on the "Brain and Nervous System." This *résumé* goes over all the evidence, experimental and rational, for and against the doctrine of spontaneous generation, primitive generation, heterogeny, or whatever it may be termed, revived since 1858, by Prof. Pouchet, and communicated to the Academy in his note "On the Protoorganisms, both Vegetable and Animal, produced spontaneously in Artificial Air and in Oxygen Gas." Without passing a definite verdict, M. Gratiolet's mode of summing up the evidence would imply that he is himself in nowise a partisan of the opinions expressed by M. Pouchet ; but still that he is desirous that the refutation of the doctrine should be arrived at by scientific research and experiment, and this, to use his own words, "in common, without passion or prejudice ; and that, for once, at least, the noble and touching example of Schröder van der Kolk and Vrolik should be imitated," namely : that of two philosophers working out the truth or falsity of a question on which they differ, in harmonious coöperation, each lending his light to the other, and receiving back assistance when needed. Whether, however, Messrs. Fouchet and Pasteur are likely to follow the suggestion, does not at present appear. M. Fouchet's pretension of being able to invoke a special creative power by the mere juxtaposition of certain natural conditions, seems, to say the least of it, somewhat presumptuous ; and the seriousness with which his views are propounded only confirms the fact that science, as well as history, has its share in the domain of fable and romance, and that M. Fouchet's revelations are only a recent chapter of the philosophic *contes des fées*.

PARIS, August 27, 1860.

ART III.—*Discussion on the Therapeutic value of Perchloride of Iron before the Imperial Academy of Medicine.*

[THE discussion (*debate*, it might be termed) on the perchloride of iron, in the French Academy of Medicine, protracted from week to week, from month to month, is, from its prolixity (not to say personality), little adapted to the narrow limits of a bi-monthly journal. The following fragment of this debate, from the *Maryland and Virginia Medical Journal*, defines M. Trousseau's position on the iron platform.]

M. Devergie, in the name of the committee, of which he was a member with Messrs. Bouchardat and Bouillaud, reported on a memoir by M. Pize, a medical practitioner of Montélemart (Department of La Drôme), and entitled : *De l'emploi de perchlorure de fer dans le traitement du purpura hemorrhagica et de son action sédative sur le cœur* (On the use of sesqui-chloride of iron in the treatment of *purpura hæmorrhagica*, and its sedative action on the heart). This paper is divided into two entirely distinct parts—one relating to the exposition of practical facts, the other to the mode of action of sesqui-chloride of iron on the system in disease.

The following are the obvious inferences from the cases relating to *purpura hæmorrhagica* :

1. Sesqui-chloride of iron is preëminently the agent for the cure of the disease ; it arrests the hæmorrhagic tendency in the space of twenty-four or forty-eight hours, and, continued for a few days, rapidly brings about the convalescence of the patient.

2. This medicine produces an immediate diminution in the rapidity of the circulation, decreases the quickness of the pulse in twenty-four hours from 110 to 80 pulsations, and may, therefore, fairly be considered as a direct sedative of the action of the heart.

M. Trousseau addressed himself to both the questions of fact and of theory. The four cases, which form the basis of M. Devergie's report, although relative to very serious instances of *purpura hæmorrhagica*, seemed to him insufficient to justify inferences so exclusive as those brought forward by M. Pize. In this respect M. Trousseau participated in the opinion expressed in committee by M. Bouillaud. This reserve and these doubts are more especially conceivable, as sequi-chloride of iron failed in M. Devergie's hands in two cases of febrile *purpura* with successive eruptions. The lowering of the pulse after four or five days is usual in the natural course of febrile *purpura hæmorrhagica*. The diminished activity of the vascular system is, therefore, a spontaneous phenomenon, of which sesqui-chloride of iron does not deserve the credit. If, however, this remedial agent were a vascular sedative equal to digitalis and aconite, it would, like these substances, display this peculiar power in healthy subjects, a circumstance which occurs neither in man nor in animals.

M. Trousseau was of opinion that M. Devergie was wrong in dividing physicians into two camps, as to the interpretation of the therapeutic action of medicines. For most remedies, all are agreed ; thus, none pretend to explain the efficacy of opium, belladonna, nux vomica, etc., on chemical grounds. If differences of opinion still exist with regard to a small number of substances, iron, in particular, it is unnecessary to make a distinction between vitalists, on the one hand, and dynamists on the other.

Is sesqui-chloride of iron a hemostatic ? It is and it is not. It is a *direct* hemostatic, and one of the most energetic ; Pravaz's experiments, and the daily experience of medical practitioners, abundantly prove it.

But is it an indirect hemostatic ? The Professor did not think so; he argued that in uterine hæmorrhage, for instance, it was inadmissible to suppose that sequi-chloride of iron would successively traverse the capillaries of the alimentary duct, of the liver, of the lungs, etc., and pass through the greater part of the vascular system without coagulating one drop of blood, without producing the least hemostatic effect, and precisely exercise all its astringent and coagulating power on the capillaries of the womb ! It is difficult to understand so strange a phenomenon ! M. Trousseau did not, however, contest it ; but he feared that it would be received with incredulity, even by the warmest friends of chemistry among his colleagues.

The restorative action of sesqui-chloride of iron has been also much exaggerated. M. Trousseau estimates that this salt, in this respect, is very inferior to other ferruginous preparations ; it has, in addition, the disadvantage of not being easily managed, and of being tolerated in general with difficulty.

Here the learned Academician raised the difficult and still very obscure question of the mode of action of iron as a restorative. It had been long believed and taught that iron, as an ingredient of the blood, was much decreased in quantity in chlorotic subjects. Recent experiments, instituted by Messrs. Favre and Reveil, have demonstrated that the contrary is the ease. Thus, these skillful chemists have found that in the chlorotic, the amount of globules of the blood being represented by 40, the proportion in weight of normal iron is equal to that of a non-chlorotic subject, in whom the figure of the globules rises to 120 or 130, according to the investigations of Messrs. Andral and Gavarret. If, therefore, for the same quantity of blood the same proportions of iron are found in chlorosis, and when that disease does not exist, although the blood in the latter case contains three times more globules than in the former, it must be admitted that the iron is condensed in the globules of the blood of chlorotic subjects.

M. Trousseau admits the passage of iron into the blood, but hence it does not by any means follow that it remains in that fluid, and that it becomes assimilated to the system. No substance is assimilated by force. If albumen be injected into the blood of an animal, it is eliminated by the kidneys. Sugar given in excess, or injected into the vessels, also, instead of being assimilated, passes into the urine.

Thus, iron penetrates into the blood, but does not sojourn there; the quantity absorbed is inappreciable, according to the experiments of M. Natalis Guillot, who has constantly detected in the fæces almost all the iron ingested into the stomach.

Therefore, although iron is of incontrovertible utility in the treatment of chlorosis, the mode of action of this medicine has not yet been discovered any more than that of the other agents of the materia medica.

Two illustrious chemists, Leibig and Dumas, have attributed to chemistry an exaggerated part in therapeutics. Chemistry must not direct, but merely enlighten medicine. And yet, God knows if it is so! M. Garrod publishes a work on gout, in which he professes that this disease depends on an excess of urate of soda in the blood. Hence the chemical treatment so well known; hence those innumerable drugs, colchicum, Boubee's syrup, Lartigue's pills, Laville's remedy, etc., which have killed as many gouty subjects as the waters of Carlsbad and Vichy.

In this respect, the orator observed that the waters the most highly extolled for the lithic diathesis, Vichy, Carlsbad, Pougues, Contrexéville, produce effects varying in inverse proportion to their alkalinity. Nothing is, however, more common than cures obtained by waters containing different mineralizing ingredients, or even containing none whatever, such as, for instance, those of Plombières and Bagnères-de-Bigorre, which are scarcely more mineralized than river water. How can a purely chemical theory account for the fact that a patient, after a season at Vichy or at Pougues, remains a year without ejecting any calculi? Will it be argued that the lithic acid has been neutralized by the alkaline virtues of these waters? But obviously this alkali has long been expelled from the blood! If oncretions ceased to be formed, it is merely because the constitution has been replaced in a more healthy condition.

Dyspepsia, attended with acidity, is cured by the use of the alkaline waters of Vichy, Carlsbad, Vals. But when patients find it more convenient to repair to Bagnères or Plombères, they at times recover quite as rapidly, or even more so. Here, again, therefore, if the alkaline medication is beneficial, it is not from its *alkalinity*. Moreover, M. Claude Bernard has demonstrated that, if an alkaline salt is given to a dog, bearing a fistulous opening in the stomach, the salt, it is true, instantly neutralizes the gastric juice ; but at the same time a more abundant secretion of that juice takes place, so that the surest means of filling the stomach with acid fluids would, perhaps, be to exhibit an alkaline preparation.

Why is uterine hæmorrhage checked by cold affusions ? Why are the catamenia suppressed after a glass of cold water has been taken into the stomach ? We know not. Can we say we possess more accurate information on the subject of the unquestionable efficacy of the water cure, or do we know why metallic armatures, applied to a limb, increase ten-fold its muscular power in the space of half a minute ? Why the irritation produced on the gastric mucous membrane by the contact of ipecacuanha, of tartar emetic, or of sulphate of copper, throws into convulsion all the respiratory muscles, and induces emesis ? Can chemistry supply us with an explanation of these phenomena ? Why is it that waltzing, swinging, or the rolling of a ship bring on vomiting and vertigo ? Why protracted tickling of the soles of the feet may cause death ? Any physical or chemical explanations of these phenomena are untenable : far better is it to confess our ignorance.

I am reproached, said M. Trousseau, with always demolishing and never constructing. Granted ; but I declare my utter inability to supply the required explanations.

I am asked whether I am a vitalist or an organist. I do not know; I am, perhaps, both. Instead of discussing these grave and insoluble questions, we should act more wisely were we to attach ourselves, in the first place, to ascertaining facts. In therapeutics, experiment must be the starting-post ; systematization follows. Disease was first empirically cured ; this has been the origin of the most active medications, and of those reputed the most rational. Before establishing the substitutive medication, irritant collyria were empirically introduced into the inflamed eye ; before goitre and tertiary syphilis were treated by iodide of potassium, they were empirically cured with burnt sponge. Let us not be more ambitious, and our therapeutics will be sound.

I recapitulate and say: therapeutics will be nearer to the truth in proportion to the candor with which we shall agree to confess our ignorance as to the intimate mode of action of remedies ; in proportion as we shall study more specially each medicine, and more closely apply ourselves to experiment. This does not exclude spontaneity or the primitive direction of experiments, which we should conduct and not permit to conduct us ; nor does it exclude sagacity in research or philosophical deduction.

ART. IV.—*Properties of Erythroxylon Coca.*

i. · *On the Dietetic and Medicinal Properties of Erythroxylon Coca :*
By DR. MANTEGAZZA. (Prize Essay. Pamphlet. Milan, 1859.) .

THE erythroxylon coca, a plant which grows in moist and woody regions on the eastern slopes of the Andes, is highly valued by the inhabitants of Peru, Chili, and Bolivia, not only as a medicine, but also as an article of food ; and serves with them as a substitute for the tea, coffee, betel, tobacco, haschisch, and opium, used by other nations. Its culture, upon which, since the time of Pizarro's conquest, much care has been bestowed, has recently increased to such a degree that, in the year 1856, the revenue of the Republic of Bolivia, from the sale of this herb, amounted to thirteen millions of francs—a very large sum, if compared with the small number of consumers (800,000). According to the account of M. Pöppig and of other well-known travelers, the natives use the dried leaves of the coca plant either by themselves or in combination with a highly alkaline substance called *llipta*, which is prepared from roasted potatoes and the ashes of different other plants ; they masticate them like the Malays and the inhabitants of the Indian Archipelago do the calcined leaves of the clavica betle. The use of this masticatory, which is considered a great delicacy, is not, however, confined to the rich ; on the contrary, it is particularly among the hard-working Indians that the coca enjoys a high reputation as a nutriment and restorative, and its use is considered absolutely essential for the endurance of fatigue and exertion, so that a laborer, in making his contract, has a view not only to wages, but to the amount of coca to be furnished. The Inca, who lives at a height of seven to fifteen thousand feet above the level of the sea, and whose meagre fare consists principally of maize, some dried meat, and potatoes of bad quality, believes that he can sustain his strength solely by the use of coca ; the porter who carries the mail, and accompanies the traveler over the roughest roads at the quick pace of the mule, invigorates and strengthens himself by chewing coca ; the Indian who works half naked in the silver and quicksilver mines, looks upon this plant as an ambrosia capable of imparting new life, and of stimulating to new exertions. It is not surprising, under such circumstances, that this article should be very much abused, and that the evil of intemperance in the use of coca, known as coquear, should be quite as prevailing among the natives of those districts, as intemperance in the use of tobacco, alcoholic liquors, and opium is among other nations. They often intoxicate themselves for several weeks, hide in the deepest forests, in order not to be disturbed in their enjoyment, and not rarely return home to their family suffering from delirium or decided idiocy.

The child and the feeble old man seize with equal eagerness the leaves of the wonderful herb, and find in it indemnification for all suffering and misery. Be it that the praised efficacy of the plant is merely the effect of fancy or tradition, or that the plant really contains a powerful principle unknown to science, the solution of this mystery is certainly a worthy theme for scientific inquiry, and the

investigations of Dr. Mantegazza deserve, therefore, our full atten
tion.

Dr. Mantegazza observed that the chewing of a drachm of the
leaves of the coca increased salivation, giving at first a somewhat
bitter, and afterwards an aromatic taste in the mouth, and a feeling
of comfort in the stomach, as after a frugal meal eaten with a good
appetite. After a second and third dose, a slight burning sensation
in the mouth and pharynx, and an increase of thirst, were noticed ;
digestion seemed to be more rapidly performed, and the fæces lost
their stercoraceous smell, the peculiar odor of the juice of the coca
becoming perceptible in them. On using the coca for several days,
the author observed on himself, as well as on other individuals, a
circumscribed erythema, an eruption around the eyelids resembling
pityriasis ; from time to time a not unpleasant pricking and itching
of the skin was felt. An infusion of the leaves, taken internally,
was found to increase the frequency of the pulse in a considerable
degree. In making observations on the frequency of the pulse, the
author was very careful to consider all the conditions which might
influence it ; he found that the temperature of the air being the
same, and the liquids being heated to an equal degree, an infusion of
coca will increase the action of the heart four times its normal
standard, while cocoa, tea, coffee, and warm water only double it.
By taking an infusion prepared from three drachms of the leaves, a
feverish condition was produced, with increased heat of the skin,
palpitation of the heart, seeing of flashes, headache, and vertigo ; the
pulse rose from seventy to one hundred and thirty-four. A peculiar
roaring noise in the ear, a desire to run about at large, and an apparent enlargement of the intellectual horizon indicated that the specific
influence upon the brain had commenced. A peculiar, hardly de-
scribable feeling of increased strength, agility, and impulse to exertion follows ; it is the first symptom of the intoxication, which is,
however, quite different from the exaltation produced by alcoholics.
While the latter manifests itself by increased but irregular action
of the muscles, the individual intoxicated by coca feels but a gradually augmented vigor, and a desire to spend his newly-acquired
strength in active labor. After some time the intellectual sphere
participates in this general exaltation, while the sensibility seems to
be hardly influenced ; the effect is thus quite different from that produced by coffee, and resembles in some degree that of opium. Dr.
Mantegazza could, in this excited condition, write with ease and regularity. After he had taken four drachms, he was seized with the
peculiar feeling of being isolated from the external world, and with
an irresistible inclination to gymnastic exercise, so that he who in
his normal condition carefully avoided the latter, jumped with ease
upon the writing-table without breaking the lamp or other objects
upon it. After this a state of torpidity came on, accompanied by a
feeling of intense comfort—consciousness being all the time perfectly clear—and by an instinctive wish not to move a limb during
the whole day, not even a finger. During this sensation sleep sets
in, attended by odd and rapidly changing dreams ; it may last a
whole day without leaving a feeling of debility or indisposition of

any kind. The author increased the dose to eighteen drachms in one day; his pulse rose in consequence of it to one hundred and thirty-four, and in the moment when delirium was most intense, he described his feelings to several of his colleagues, who observed him, in the following written words : "*lddio é ingiusto perche ho fatto l'uomo incapace di poter vivere sempre cocheando*" (this is the expression for intoxication by coca). "*lo preferiscta una vitta di 10 anni con coca che un di 1,000,000 secoli senza coca.*" After three hours of sleep, Dr. Mantegazza recovered completely from this intoxication, and could immediately follow his daily occupation without the least indisposition—on the contrary, even with unusual facility. He had abstained for forty hours without food of any kind, and the meals then taken were very well digested. From this fact, the author finds it explainable that the Indians employed as carriers of the mail are able to do without food for three or four days, provided they are sufficiently supplied with coca.

From these experiments, made repeatedly on himself, and on other individuals, Dr. Mantegazza draws the following conclusions :

1. The leaves of the coca, chewed or taken in a weak infusion, have a stimulating effect upon the nerves of the stomach, and thereby facilitate digestion very much. 2. In a large dose coca increases the animal heat and augments the frequency of the pulse, and consequently of respiration. 3. In a medium dose, three to four drachms, it excites the nervous system in such a manner that the movements of the muscles are made with greater ease—then it produces a calming effect. 4. Used in a large dose it causes delirium, hallucinations, and finally congestion of the brain.

The most prominent property of coca, which is hardly to be found in any other remedy, consists in the exalting effect it produces, calling out the power of the organism without leaving afterwards any sign of debility. The coca is, in this respect, one of the most powerful nervines and analeptics. These experiments, as well as the circumstance that the natives have used the coca from the earliest period as a remedy in dyspepsia, flatulency, and colic, have induced Dr. Mantegazza, and several of his colleagues in South America and Europe, to employ the leaves of the coca in a variety of cases, partly as masticatory, partly in powder, as infusion, as alcoholico-aqueous extract in the dose of ten to fifteen grains in pills, and as a clyster. Dr. Mantegazza has used coca with most excellent results in dyspepsia, gastralgia and entralgia ; he employed it not less frequently in cases of great debility following typhus fever, scurvy, anæmic conditions, etc., and in hysteria and hypochondriasis, even if the latter had increased to weariness of life. The coca might also be employed with great benefit in mental diseases, where some physicians prescribe opium. Of its sedative effect in spinal irritation, idiopathic convulsions, nervous erethism, the author has fully convinced himself. He proposes its use in the highest dose in cases of hydrophobia and tetanus. It is a popular opinion that the coca is a reliable aphrodisiac ; the author has, however, observed only two cases in which a decided influence upon the sexual system was perceived.

Dr. Mantegazza, finally, recommends this remarkable plant, which could be easily introduced into trade, to the profession for further physiological and therapeutical experiments, and adds the full history of eighteen cases by which the medicinal virtues of the remedy are proved to satisfaction.—*London Pharm. Jour.*, June, 1860, *from Oesterreichische Zeitschrift für Praktische Heilkunde,* November 4, 1859—*American Jour. Pharm.*, September, 1860.

ii. *A New Alkaloid in Coca.*

Coca is the name under which the leaves of several species of erythroxylon are and have been known in Peru from time immemorial, and which, especially among the Indians, are used for chewing, mixed with a little unslacked lime or wood ashes. Numerous and somewhat fabulous accounts are given of their physiological action, as, for instance, in "Tschudi's Travels in Peru." A moderate use is said to produce excitement of the functions, to enable the chewer to remain some time without food, and to bear the greatest bodily exertions ; while an immoderate chewing of coca, like that of opium, frequently becomes an habitual vice, producing all the deleterious symptoms and consequences of narcotics, such as a state of half intoxication, half of drowsiness, with visionary dreams, premature decay, complete apathy, and idiocy. These peculiar symptoms rendered the presence of a narcotic principle very probable, and have induced Prof. Wœhler and Dr. Niemann, of Goettingen, to undertake the investigation of the substance. The material was furnished by Dr. Scherzer, the naturalist of the exploring expedition in the Austrian frigate Novara. The examination has so far succeeded, by the usual method for the separation of alkaloids, in eliminating a crystalizable base, *cocaine,* crystalizing in small prisms, devoid of color or odor, slightly soluble in water, more readily in alcohol, and very easily in ether. It possesses a strongly-marked alkaline reaction, and a bitter taste; and acts in so far peculiarly, as it transiently benumbs, or almost paralyzes the part of the tongue which it touches. It bears some resemblance to atropine in its chemical relations, and forms perfect salts with the acids. It is, however, without action on the eye, and its compound with the chloride of gold is remarkable for forming benzoic acid in large proportion upon being heated. Further experiments will throw light on its physiological properties. —*Druggists' Circular,* August, 1860.—*Am. Jour. Pharm.*

Art. V.—*Iodide of Potassium in Large Doses.* To the Editor of The Lancet :

Sir—I think the profession and the public at large are much indebted to the gentlemen who volunteer to test the powers of drugs in heroic doses upon their own persons ; and the letter of Dr. Sisson in The Lancet, detailing experiments, tried upon himself, with iodide of potassium, does credit to his courage, and entitles him to thanks for his experimental inquiry ; at the same time I feel assured that larger experience will satisfy him that the salt in question ought in all cases to be prescribed with due caution. True it is that a large proportion of patients can take it, even in large doses, with impunity; but, judging from my own experience, there are many to whom it cannot be given, without inconvenience, even in small doses. I confess I was staggered on reading of the iodide having been given by our continental brethren to the extent of an ounce per diem ; still, I know that some constitutions will tolerate almost any dose of powerful drugs when gradually augmented. Calomel may be given to some persons to an almost unlimited extent without producing any of its ordinary effects upon the system ; whilst in another individual a single grain will excite ptyalism. Thus it is with the iodide of potassium ; one patient may possibly take an ounce per diem with impunity and perhaps benefit ; and another will be half killed by a grain or two. I gave to a middle-aged gentleman a mixture containing iodide of potassium—a dose, containing three grains, to be taken three times a day. He took one dose at night ; I saw him in the morning, when his sister informed me he had been, to use her own expression as near as I can recollect, half mad all night, and she dared not give another dose of the medicine. He was getting better, but had ferrety eyes, when I saw him. He took no more. The party had suffered from some head affection, resulting in partial paralysis of the lower extremities some years before I knew him, and the iodide was prescribed for chronic enlargement of the testis. The same dose was given to another middle-aged person affected in a like manner, but otherwise healthy. He took a dose at night, and in the morning I found him in bed with his head wrapped up in a flannel night-cap ; he had got a desperate cold, somehow, the day before, with which he woke up, but was getting better. He took no more iodide, and was free from his desperate cold the next day.

I gave the same dose recently to a lady, the subject of ovarian dropsy. A few doses made the head very uncomfortable, and brought out blotches on the face and other parts of the body. Its use was discontinued, and afterwards resumed with the same results.

To the daughter of the same lady, eight years old, it was given in one-grain doses. On the second day I found the patient with a shade on ; she had caught cold in the eyes and could not bear the light. The iodide was discontinued, and the eyes were well in twenty-four hours.

A lady suffered from neuralgia of the face, for which the iodide had been prescribed on a former occasion—she told me in one-grain doses ; it cured the neuralgia, but deprived her of voice for a long time. I doubted her report as to dose, so the prescription was looked up, and it proved to be a five-grain dose. She was anxious to try it again, if its inconveniences could be obviated. I directed a few drops of laudanum to be added to each dose, which proved effectual.

I took the iodide myself, some time back, for a rheumatic affection of the acromio-clavicular joint. The dose I began with was three grains, thrice daily. This was taken three or four days, when a grain per dose was added. Finding no inconvenience or advantage, another grain was added in a day or two. The effects of the medicine now began to show themselves. I awoke the morning after the five-grain dose had been taken with an uneasy feeling of the left eye. On applying the hand, I found the edge of the orbit, at the external part, tender on pressure, and on inspection the eyelids were found swollen and infiltrated on that side. The following morning the right side was similarly affected : the tenderness was evidently seated in the periosteum of the orbit, and exclusively at the outer part. On the following day, a strange sensation was felt : it appeared like a pain extending in a direct line from the external border of one orbit to that of the other at the same spot ; the sensation was very peculiar and difficult to describe—it was pain and something more, which made me decide at once it was better to have rheumatism than that, for to-morrow, perhaps, the dura mater may be quarreling with the iodide in a like manner to that manifested by the periosteum of the orbit to-day, and so I gave up my remedy.

The foregoing, amongst similar cases that might be adduced, will suffice to show that iodide is not a medicine that may be prescribed at random in heroic doses in all cases. Like opium and other medicines, iodide may be safely administered in large doses to some individuals, and with advantage ; at the same time, common prudence requires that the drug should be prescribed with caution in all cases, seeing that no one can tell beforehand whether the individual for whom it is prescribed can tolerate its action or not. I have seen an ounce of the ordinary tincture of opium taken at once as an agreeable cordial, and known a half-grain dose of opium, given to an adult, followed by all the urgent symptoms of poisoning by that drug. The iodide of potassium appears to act specifically on mucous membranes, as shown by its action upon the bowels, causing much irritation in some cases, irritable bladder in others ; affections of the conjunctiva, fauces, nasal cavities, and larynx, together with the integument ; and also on fibrous structures, as periosteum, and capsular ligaments of joints, etc.

I am, sir, yours, etc.,   H. C. Roons, M. D.

Art. VI.—*Note on Fluid Extract of Wild Cherry Bark:* By William Procter, Jr.

The recipe for this preparation, published at page 108, vol. 28th (1856), has been received with such general favor that it may be looked upon as an established formula, and probably is, in substance, the one to be adopted in the revised edition of the United States Pharmacopœia. In a paper on fluid extracts read before the American Pharmaceutical Association, last year, and published in the November (1859) number of this Journal, I included a process for this fluid extract of double the original strength, so as to be in the proportion of an ounce to the fluid ounce in accordance with the general strength adopted in that paper ; but at the same time it was doubted whether the bark could be properly extracted and condenssd in so small a bulk without the loss of a portion of its valuable qualities. As the strength of eight ounces to the pint gives the dose a teaspoonful, the Committee of the College of Physicians of Philadelphia adopted the formula as originally proposed, in preference to the stronger preparation.

The object of this note is to offer a few hints in regard to the details of the process, which have been suggested by considerable practical experience with the manipulations required.

Wild cherry bark contains amygdalin, a bitter principle not yet isolated, tannic acid, resin and fixed oil, besides other less important matters. It is desirable to get all the amygdalin and the bitter principle and a part of the tannic acid in the fluid extract, whilst the remainder of the tannic acid and all of the resin and fixed oil should be excluded. In order to render these comments intelligible to the reader who may not have the volume for 1856 at hand, I will recapitulate an outline of the formula, with the quantities altered for a gallon of the fluid extract.

Take of Wild Cherry Bark (Cerasus serotina)..................64 ounces Troy.
Sweet Almonds .... 8 "   "
Granulated Sugar (pure)...........................96 "   "
Alcohol (U. S. P.)
Water, each a sufficient quantity.

Macerate the bark (powdered and passed through a No. 60 seive) moistened with two pints of alcohol, for two hours, pack it firmly in a cylindrical percolator, and gradually pour on alcohol until twelve pints have slowly passed. If the powder has not been carefully prepared as directed, the passage of the liquid must be regulated by a cork or stop cock. The tincture is then poured in a still, and ten pints of alcohol drawn over by distillation, the residue is evaporated to a syrupy consistence, and, while hot, mixed with two pints of cold water. Separate the resinous and oily matter which precipitates, and evaporate the liquid again till all traces of alcohol are removed. The almonds, without blanching, are now to be thoroughly beaten, with a little water, until reduced to a smooth paste. (This part of the operation is most effectually performed in an iron mortar with a flat-faced pestle.) They are then rubbed down with sufficient water to make the emulsion measure four pints, without straining it. This is then incorporated with the syrupy extract of the bark in a bottle, securely closed, and agitated from time to time for twenty-four hours, at least, and unless the weather be very warm forty-eight hours will be better, as on prolonged contact of the almonds with the amygdalin of the bark, depends the development of the hydrocyanic acid and volatile oil. The liquor is now thrown on a cloth, rapidly and forcibly expressed, to remove the solid residue, which is reserved, and the liquor filtered through paper into a gallon bottle containing sugar. If the liquid, thus obtained, is not sufficient to dissolve the sugar by agitation and make the measure of a gallon, pour water on the dregs in the cloth, express and filter until sufficient liquid is obtained to make that measure, and strain.   The most annoying part of this process is frequently experienced in the extreme slowness with which the liquid passes the filter (owing to the fixed oil and fine particles of the almond paste), and the consequent tendency to loss of strength by the prolonged exposure. After many experiments, with gelatin, etc., and various filters, I have found the most satisfaction from the following plan : For the quantities mentioned take half a pound of prepared chalk, triturate it in a mortar with some of the turbid liquid, add it to the remainder, and shake the mixture well several times. It may now be poured at once on a muslin filter supported in a large funnel with ribs, when the liquid, which at first is cloudy, soon becomes transparent and passes with considerable facility.   When the liquid ceases to pass, pour on water carefully to displace the portion retained in the chalky sediment. The chalk in no respect injures the preparation, having no reaction with any of the principles present that are medicinally important.— *Am. Jour. Pharmacy.*

ART. VII.—*On the Employment of Chloride of Zinc in Diseases of the Skin.* By Dr. VEIEL, of Canstätt. (Zeitschrift der Gesellchaft der Aerzte zu Wien, February 20th, 1860.)

DR. VEIEL has employed the chloride of zinc for the last nine years as a caustic whenever it was requisite to destroy morbid growths in the areolar tissue, or to remove abnormal secretions, as happens in different forms of lupus. He therefore employed it for a long time only in the cure of lupus and some allied diseases, such as lepra vulgaris, elephantiasis, and small circumscribed forms of scirrhus ; but latterly he has also used it for the purpose of altering the condition of suppurating surfaces, and in chronic ulcers of the legs, chronic eczema and sycosis.   Three forms of this are in use, namely, the alcoholic solution, the aqueous solution, and the solid cylindrical form.   The first consists of equal parts of rectified spirit and chloride of zinc ; the second of ten parts of the chloride, ten of hydrochloric acid, and five hundred of water ; and the third is prepared by fusing the chloride, and pouring it into moulds, as in the case of caustic potash. Dr. Veiel selects the solid form when his object is to penetrate as deeply as possible in order to destroy hypertrophic secretions, as happens in inveterate cases of lupus, in which the stick of chloride is used in the same way as caustic potash.   The chloride was thus employed with the best results in thirteen well-marked cases of lupus, one of alæ nasi, six of the upper lip, four on the cheek, and two on the ear. The proceeding is as follows : when there are scabs or thick scales, which have already destroyed the epidermis, poultices are used to remove them ; but when the epidermis is preserved, it is dissolved by blistering plaster or spirits of ammonia. Then the solid chloride, fixed in a quill and pointed, is pressed deep into the hypertrophied and tuberculous tissue and the structures for two or three lines around it, until the salt has penetrated all the morbid growths in different directions. Immediately after this operation, the honeycomb-like and perforated surface discharges a dark bloody fluid, succeeded by a brighter colored serum, which after a few hours hardens to a smooth and firm scurf. On the third or fourth day, a thin pus is formed on the edge of the scurf, and the removal of this fluid by puncture generally relieves tension. On the sixth or eighth day, the scurf is loosened at the edges, and it may be entirely removed by poultices continued for several days. It is seldom necessary to use the solid chloride more than three times, but in cases where the diseased structures are very thick, it must be employed much oftener. When the large ulcer is at last free from all swollen prominences, and on a level with the surrounding healthy parts, it should be poulticed for several days, then lightly touched with the alcoholic solution of the chloride every three or four days, and afterwards, when the edges begin to contract, with the watery solution, until a complete cure is effected, which seldom requires more than three or four months.

Besides lupus, there are a great number of skin diseases which are relieved by chloride of zinc. In obstinate eczema, occurring on the limits of the skin and mucous membrane, as on the eyelids, the lips, the labia, and the anus, the spirituous solution affords great relief. In eczema solare and impetiginodes, the daily employment of the aqueous solution is sometimes the only cure. In psoriasis, some indurations are occasionally left, after the cure of the complaint, on the elbows, back, and thigh, but they are easily removed by the alcoholic solution of the chloride, although the scales must first be removed. There is also a form of psoriasis palmaris, with painful watery indurations, which yield to no other means than the solid chloride, after they have been previously raised from their source by a blister. In sycosis and favus, after the beard or hairs are removed, the watery solution is very useful, partly in dissolving the swelling and infiltration of the follicles, partly in removing fungous growths. It is also useful in certain forms of acne, and in a great number of warty, circumscribed scirrhous growths on the nose, the cheeks, and the lips.

Dr. Veiel considers that chloride of zinc is especially useful as a caustic, on the following grounds : 1. It enters into combination with all the elements with which it comes into contact, particularly with the proteinaceous matters, which again occasion a caustic effect upon the deep structures, whereby the parts in the immediate vicinity of the cauterized matter contract, and thus the diseased portion is diminished, and the edges of the sound parts approximate. 2. Because the irritation thus excited causes a more rapid formation of pus and dissolution of the scurf, whereby the cure is more rapidly accomplished, and the raw surfaces form better granulations. 3. Be-

cause the cicatrization following the peculiar contraction, the attendant destruction of the disease is more complete ; and 4. Because the
pain of the application, although severe, lasts only a short time, and
may be easily moderated by chloroform. Dr. Veicl considers, for various reasons, that the chloride of zinc is preferable to the strong
acids, caustic potash, nitrate of silver, the preparations of iodine,
the chloride of gold, and other caustics. It should be mentioned
that as the chloride of zinc in the solid form is remarkably prone to
attract moisture, it ought to be kept for use in a well-stepped glass
vessel.—*Br. and For. Med. Chir. Rev.*

Art. VIII.—*Alcoholism—Typhoid—West Indian Fevers—Typhoid
and Typhus in Dublin.*

i.　*On the Treatment of Alcoholism :* By Dr. Smirnoff.

Dr. Smirnoff states that he has become convinced by repeated trials,
that the *asarum Europœum* well deserves the reputation it has obtained in Russia, of being an excellent remedy for the effects of
drinking. The influence of a.continuous abuse of alcoholic drinks,
is first exerted locally, but afterwards dyspepsia is produced ; and
the nutrition and functions of the entire economy, especially of the
central portions of the nervous system, becoming interfered with,
the blood itself being loaded with an injurious foreign material, the
dyscrasia potatorum is at last completely established. The asarum
fulfills various indications, acting beneficially on the alimentary canal
in those cases in which the digestive powers are so much at fault.
Its aromatic principle confers upon it a stomachic power, and regulates the condition of the intestinal discharges, producing vomiting
and purging when given in large doses. Its most beneficial action,
however, is manifested on the defective appetite, and by its counteracting the invincible longing for alcohol. The horrible sensations
with which the drinker awakes in the morning, and which impel him
to seek temporary and delusive relief from renewed libations, are
much blunted and mitigated by means of a glass of strong infusion
of asarum and some other nervine—*e. g.*, valerian. Its immediate
effect is often to produce vomiting, and sometimes purging ; but the
painful sensations at the epigastrium undergo relief, and the appetite becomes invigorated. Persons who have been long habituated
to alcoholic drinks cannot, however, have these suddenly suppressed
with impunity; and in such cases the author gives the asarum in
brandy, applying at the same time a blister or an issue to the pit of
the stomach. By this means the normal activity of the stomach becomes excited, and the longing for alcohol diminished. The author,
however, cannot agree with those who would still allow a small

quantity of spirits to habitual drinkers, even when the morbid desire for it has become appeased. The continuous use of a decoction of asarum, even when it does not succeed in extinguishing the desire for alcohol, always supports the powers of the patient; and it is remarkable in some cases, in which the individuals have been long accustomed to periodical intervals of drunkenness, ending in delirium tremens, how much longer these intervals will become, and how much less likely delirium tremens is to recur. The patients themselves are sometimes surprised at the comparative impunity with which they can continue their drinking. The author prescribes three or four glasses a day of an infusion made with ℥iij of asarum root, ℥j of valerian root, and ℥½ of orange peel, but he does not state the quantity of water employed. In cases of drunkenness, another formula is composed of decoction of asarum (made by boiling from ℥½ to ℥j of the root) ℥vj, tinct. valerian ʒij to ʒiij, Sydenham's laudanum gtt. xij, syrup of orange peel ℥½. A tablespoonful of this is taken every two hours. He finds from two to five grains of bismuth, taken four times a day, a valuable adjunct. He has also found the following popular Russian remedy of service in cases of drunkenness: R. Ammon. carb. ℥½, aceti vini ℔j, oxymel scill. ℥½. Two tablespoonfuls every two hours.—*Med. Zeit. Russland*, 1859, No. 8.—*Medical Times and Gazette.*

ii. *Emetics in Typhoid Fever:* By Dr. BRINTON. (From the *Lancet*.)

1. Emetics, early in fever, are most advantageous; with proper precautions, always harmless; in most instances, extremely beneficial; in some cases, positively cutting short the malady by a speedy cure.

2. They ought only to be given in an early stage, for which we may generally find an arbitrary limit in the first four days from that of the inaugural rigors, but which is practically better defined by the access and duration of the nausea or vomiting of this epoch.

3. Later than this period, they seem to have much less influence. Indeed, in many cases, it may be doubted whether they have any effect at all. While, on the other hand, the purging they often cause—a purging itself also decidedly useful in the outset of the malady — obscures the symptoms subsequently requiring to be recognized and treated, by its resemblance to that diarrhœa (of intestinal lesion) which systematically occurs in typhoid fever, and to that diarrhœa incidental to typhus.

4. Ipecacuanha seems, on all grounds, the best emetic; and the wine, in ounce or two-ounce doses, the best preparation. Warm water should be plentifully taken to facilitate its action.

5. Once or twice a day, for three or four days, is the greatest number and frequency of vomitings I have found it advisable to induce.

iii. *Observations on the Intermittent Fevers of the West Indies, and on the action of Quinia as a Specific in their Treatment:* By Mr. HUGH CROSKERY.

The object of the author in this communication was to point out

the necessity of a sedative treatment during the hot stage, and fre[e
purgation before the administration of the specific. The mixture h[e
had found most beneficial was composed as follows : Solution d [f
acetate of ammonia, two ounces ; spirit of nitrous ether and spir[it
of juniper, of each half an ounce ; potassio-tartrate of antimon.y,
four grains ; tincture of hyoscyamus, two drachms ; tincture [Of
opium, one drachm ; to twelve ounces of camphor mixture. Of th,is
a tablespoonful is given to an adult every half hour until diaphoresis
comes on. The mixture may be either preceded or followed by ten
grains of calomel, with a saline aperient a few hours later. He considered that the action of the mercurial purgative tended to assist
the subsequent action of the quinia. He condemned the administration of quinine in large doses, and stated that he had obtained the
most satisfactory results from its employment in small doses at
repeated intervals. He believed that to administer it in any form
during the paroxysm was injurious, and that the exhibition of large
doses at this period of the disease was fraught with the greatest
danger. The formula adopted by the author for its administration
is the following : Disulphate of quinia, forty grains ; tincture of
oranges, half an ounce ; dilute sulphuric acid, one drachm ; to ten
ounces of water. Of this mixture he gives to an adult a tablespoonful every hour during the intermission, until singing in the ears or
the presence of headache shows that the system is saturated by the
remedy, when it is to be repeated at longer intervals, and even con-
tinned in small quantity for some days, so long as any unpleasant
feelings are experienced at the time when the paroxysm ought to
occur. He has found that in this manner from forty to sixty grains
may be given before the recurrence of the attack, and that in the
majority of instances the next paroxysm is either entirely prevented
or is very much modified. One large dose of the salt very often
produces disagreeable head symptoms, which prevent its repetition
so as to get the system saturated with the remedy sufficiently early
to obviate the return of the hot stage. In cases of severe quotidian
he had occasionally given with benefit ten grains of quinine at once,
along with the calomel ; this, however, he considered rather as the
exception. The paper concluded with the narration of five cases
illustrative of the author's method of treatment. Of these cases,
four were adults, and one a child nine years of age. In most of
these the attack was quite recent, but in one case it had continued
six weeks. The author remarked that in such circumstances the
prolonged use of quinine during convalescence was essential to ultimate recovery.—*Medical Times and Gazette.*

iv. *Typhus and Typhoid in Dublin.*

Dr. Henry Kennedy's article on Typhus and Typhoid Fevers, as
seen in Dublin (published in the September number, 1860, of the
Edinburgh Medical Journal), maintains the following propositions :

1. That typhus and typhoid fevers exist in Paris, London, Sweden,
parts of America, and Dublin ; and relapsing fever in Great Britain
and Ireland. 2. That in Dublin other types of fever exist, equally

distinct from any of these; of which gastric, remarkable for its great duration, the congestive typhus of Armstrong, the febris nervosa of Huxham, and in summer the inflammatory fevers may be adduced as examples. 3. That these may exist in the same family, and at the same time. 4. That when a whole family is attacked at once, some may exhibit spots and others not. 5. That two crops of eruption, as observed long since by Grant, are not uncommon in the typhus of Dublin; and either may precede the other. 6. That one of these may be a bright red, and the other of a much darker hue; and that they often coëxist. 7. That patechiæ may exist with typhoid fever; and bright lenticular spots without this fever. 8. That bright lenticular spots may be followed by petechiæ. 9. That it would seem as if typhus and typhoid fever could exist in the same patient, and at the same time. 10. That whilst in London intestinal hæmorrhage is common in typhoid fever, it is much rarer in Paris and Dublin. 11. That in Dublin the same hæmorrhage is not uncommon in typhus. 12. That cerebral complication is more common to typhoid fever than is usually taught.

Dr. Kennedy says that the Dublin physicians follow the stimulant plan of treating typhoid fever : But then there is this difference between us in Dublin and what has been lately advocated ; we do not use stimulants because we have fever to treat, but because the particular case requires them. We know that fever is a depressing disease (few, indeed, are not), and that it has a tendency to lower the powers of life ; but we also know that a certain lowering is essential to nature's cure ; and from the way that she points out we are very slow to depart. Hence we do not use stimulants so generally, or so much as a matter of course, as has been advocated elsewhere. This much I may say, however, that in particular cases I have known a very large quantity of them given, and this many years ago—as much as two bottles of wine and half a pint of brandy in the twenty-four hours, and with the best results. * * * I do not hesitate to treat the symptoms as they arise. If there be pain in the right iliac fossa, a few leeches are directed—care being taken they do not bleed too long. If these be not required, a blister is applied, and after it a warm poultice ; nor have I the slightest doubt in my mind, that, used with common prudence, these measures are most beneficial. The internal medicine which I now use, by much the most frequently, is the dilute sulphuric acid. It appears to me to be far superior to any others in common use ; and I have tried largely lead, gallic acid, opium, etc. But I have not used the phosphoric acid so strongly recommended by Huss. The mixture I myself am in the habit of ordering has from one to three drachms of dilute sulphuric acid in the eight ounces, with from two to five drops of laudanum in each ounce. Of this an ounce is given at intervals proportioned to the urgency of the case. One remark is, however, to be made of this medicine. It may act too powerfully—I mean as an astringent ; for I am sure that a gradual lessening of the diarrhœa is much the best plan to pursue, and that if it be suddenly checked, mischief will be very apt to follow in the chest or head. If this caution, then, be only kept in view, I repeat that this acid has, in my hands, proved the most useful means of treating the diarrhœa of typhoid fever.

In this particular fever there still remains one point of treatment to notice. Cases like those just spoken of occur naturally ; that is, without any means used to check the diarrhœa, it will suddenly cease, and the chest or brain become engaged, often very seriously; and then, again, when the chest symptoms moderate, those of the abdomen recur. All such are, in my experience, most critical cases, and too often fatal ; and latterly I have been in the habit of adopting the expedient of keeping a blistered surface open for some days. This was commonly done on the chest, and, as I believe, with very beneficial results. It seemed to have the effect of ridding the system of the poison ; for, in the course of two or three days, all went on smoothly. The idea is probably worthy of being kept in mind.

ART. IX.—*On the Treatment of Hæmorrhoids :* By MM. NÉLATON and HEYFELDER. *(Gazette des Hôpitaux,* 1860, No. 23.)

IN a recent clinical lecture, M. Nélaton made the following remarks : I was some time since a great partizan of the actual cautery in hæmorrhoids, at least since it could be employed under conditions formerly impossible. In fact, nothing can be more painful than its application. I have seen cauterization employed many times by Dupuytren, who first excised the tumor and then cauterized ; but so terrible were the sufferings of the patients, that I could scarcely have made up my mind to have recourse to it, had not the means of preventing pain by chloroform been discovered. I have since then frequently had recourse to cauterization, with the best results ; and if I do not employ it now, it is because we have at our disposition another operative procedure, which is just as good, and which is not painful, either during or after its application. I mean *écrasement linéaire.* It is usually unattended with hæmorrhage, and when, as is sometimes the case, there is a certain amount of bleeding, this may at once be arrested by means of a powerful hæmostatic, the perchloride of iron. The union of these two means, then, constitutes an excellent method for the ablation of hæmorrhoids.

One word about ligatures. All surgeons, at the end of last century and the beginning of the present, were very fearful of applying them, owing to an instance of fatal hæmorrhage which occurred after the application of the ligature by J. L. Petit. I believe I am right in affirming, guided by the cases related by Amussat, and by those which have occurred in my own practice, that these surgeons entertained the most erroneous notions concerning the results of the ligature employed for hæmorrhoids. It is an excellent operation, by means of which patients may be cured in eight or ten days, without any accident ; and, indeed, I may place it on the same line with *écrasement linéaire.* The latter has, however, the indubitable advantage of causing the fall of the tumor within a few minutes, although perhaps it offers somewhat less security against hæmorrhage.

There is one thing to be well borne in mind, viz: that all these operations practised in the vicinity of the anus, however simple they may be in appearance, may terminate in a fatal manner. This is a powerful motive for insisting, as long as possible, on palliative treatment, only performing an operation as a last resort. Quite recently one of our leading surgeons applied a small portion of Vienna caustic to a hæmorrhoidal tumor, and the patient was dead next day ; while, in another case, an incision made into a fistula scarcely a centimetre in length, was followed in a few days by fatal purulent infection. I was myself consulted some years since by a man who, having acquired great wealth, complained bitterly of not being able to enjoy it in consequence of a hæmorrhoidal tumor. I advised him to bear with it, but some time after, abundant hæmorrhage having come on, he entreated its removal.. He manifested all the signs of complete anæmia. He was put under the influence of chloroform, and the actual cautery was employed. He did not suffer during the operation, but scarcely had he recovered consciousness when he complained exceedingly. I appeased the pain, and all seemed doing well, when on the sixteenth day violent shivering ushered in purulent infection, and he died. The conclusion to be drawn from all this is, that you should never operate except when you cannot possibly avoid doing so, since when you least expect it you may meet with sinister events similar to those just adverted to.

One more word with respect to *écrasement linéaire.* This operation has during some time been frequently resorted to; and it is for this description of tumor it is, perhaps, best adapted. But I ought to inform you that in most cases the operation is badly executed. For a short time after its performance, the patients are delighted, and the surgeon believes that he has attained a splendid result ; but in the course of a few months the cicatricial tissue contracts, and the patient suffers from an anal stricture. During about a twelvemonth I have had a great number of patients, who have come to me in order to undergo an operation for the relief of this unfortunate consequence of removal of hæmorrhoidal tumors—the stricture sometimes scarcely admitting the passage of a quill. It has arisen because not only the mucous projection, which alone constitutes the disease, has been removed, but also a more or less considerable portion of the skin of the orifice of the anus.

[Professor Heyfelder, of St. Petersburg, commenting upon the above article (*Deutsche Klinik*, No. 20); adds some corroborative instances of fatal results speedily following apparently trifling operations in the anal region. He is inclined to regard such cases as examples of irritation of the nervous system, somewhat analogous in nature to the *delirium nervosum* or *traumaticum* met with after injuries ; and this the more so, as such excitement is often manifested in persons suffering from hæmorrhoids, owing, doubtless, to some extent, to their want of rest.]—*Brit. and For. Med. Chir. Review.*

ART. X.—*Emphysema of the Lungs. Drowning.*

i. *Observations on the Morbid Anatomy, Pathology, and determining cause of Emphysema of the Lungs:* A paper communicated to the Royal Medical and Chirurgical Society, by Mr. A. T. H. WATERS.

ALTHOUGH much has been written on the subject of pulmonary emphysema, there are yet many points in connection with it which require investigation. There is perhaps no disease the symptoms and physical signs of which are so readily explicable, from a knowledge of the structural changes by which it is accompanied, as this particular affection, and hence an acquaintance with the minute anatomy of the healthy lung-tissue becomes of the utmost importance, in order fully to appreciate the morbid changes which take place. (Here follows a brief description of the arrangement of the "ultimate pulmonary tissue.") Pulmonary emphysema is of two kinds—1. Interlobular emphysema. 2. Vesicular emphysema. The second, or vesicular, is by far the most important, and will be alone considered. It exists in three forms, differing only in the extent to which they involve the lung. 1. *Partial Lobular Emphysema,* involving a few air-sacs, or at most only a single lobulette. This is not often seen as an independent affection, but in lungs which are the seat of the second form it occasionally exists in small patches along the margins of the lobes. These patches resemble small vesicles, and when numerous have somewhat the appearance of a row of beads. 2. *Lobular Emphysema.* This is the form most frequently met with. It involves one or more lobules in different parts of the lung, and is especially found along the margins of the base, the anterior border, and at the apex. It frequently exists in connection with phthisis, and occasionally with pneumonia. In this form it is easy to trace the divisions of the lung ; the boundary walls of the lobules have not usually given way, and generally no interlobular emphysema exists. The air-sacs of a lobule are not necessarily all equally dilated, those at the circumference being most so. The emphysematous lobules may be seen projecting above the level of the lung, and in some instances they become developed into "appendages." 3. *Lobar Emphysema.* This form involves the whole of a lobe or an entire lung, or very frequently both lungs. It constitutes a very formidable affection, and often destroys life at an' early period. The lung is much increased in size. The outlines of the lobules frequently cannot be distinctly seen, in consequence of the rupture of their boundary walls, and the production of interlobular emphysema. In investigating the morbid anatomy of emphysematous lungs, the same methods of preparation were used by the author as had been previously employed in the examination of the healthy organ—viz : injection, inflation, and desiccation. With regard to the structural changes which take place in the disease, we recognize, in the early stages, a simple dilatation of the air-sacs, and a diminution in the height of the alveolar partitions. A further dilatation takes place, with more or less complete obliteration of the alveolar septa. This distension produces a divergence of the elastic fibres of the air-sacs, and is soon followed by a perforation of the walls themselves, so as to give in the advanced stage a perfectly cribriform appearance to the membrane of which the walls are formed. This is followed by rupture of the elastic fibres, a further distension of the air-sacs, with a general breaking down of their walls, so that in the most advanced stages of the disease large cavities are found, traversed in all directions by membranous shreds or fibrous cords. The inner surface of the emphysematous lung-tissue presents the same microscopic appearances as that of the healthy tissue. In some lungs in which lobular emphysema existed, the air-sacs were found much distended, but no perforations existed ; while in others, and especially where the disease was of the lobar kind, extensive perforations were found, with not more, and in some instances less, dilatation than in the former. This would seem to indicate some degeneration of tissue in the one case, which might be absent in the other. The condition of the blood-vessels explains the anæmic appearance of the emphysematous lung. In the earlier stages the capillaries of the pulmonary plexus are wider apart than in health ; and as the walls of the air-sacs are perforated, and the latter more distended, the capillaries become ruptured and absorbed. The vascularity of the lung, in a condition of advanced emphysema, is very slight. The bronchial tubes are usually dilated in old-standing cases of emphysema, their mucous membrane is pale, and there is increased development of the circular muscular fibres. An important question in connection with the emphysema is, whether the disease is preceded by, or attended with, any degeneration of tissue. With regard to the existence of fatty matter in the emphysematous lung, a considerable number of specimens were examined with great care ; and although in one or two instances indications of its presence were found, as a rule it was entirely absent. Dr. Jenner has stated that a fibrous degeneration frequently exists. A number of specimens were examined to ascertain whether any alteration of this kind could be observed in the elastic fibres as compared with those of the healthy lung. The results arrived at on this point were imperfect, and the question is left for future investigation. Some kind of degeneration is believed in many cases to exist. With reference to the determining cause of pulmonary emphysema, the view that the disease is produced by expiratory efforts appears to the author most tenable. Serious objections seem to present themselves to the theory advocated by Dr. Gairdner, that the disease results from increased distension, during inspiration, of one part of the lung, in order to fill the space previously occupied by a collapsed portion. During inspiration, the chest expands to make room for the dilating lung ; air is drawn equally to all parts of the lung, and is not driven by any external force to one part more than to another. It is difficult, therefore, to understand how an excessive quantity of air should find its way to any particular portion. If the chest must reach a certain expansion, it would rather appear that the entire lung would be every where slightly dilated, except where collapsed ; or else that those parts nearest the collapsed portions would be most distended. Such parts, however, are not the most frequent seats of emphysema. Further, the lungs can undergo very considerable distension without suffering any injury. Although the lungs undergo equable pressure during ordinary expiration, this by no means proves that such is the case during acts of coughing ; in fact, the contrary is true, as has been shown by Dr. Jenner. The conformation of the walls of the chest, and of the lungs, seems to render it necessary that the latter should undergo unequal compression during violent expiratory efforts with a partially closed glottis, and that air should be driven first to those parts of the lungs where the walls are least resisting, and secondly to those portions which contain the least volume of air. The least resisting part of the thoracic walls is that which covers the apex of the lung ; it consists of membranous expansion, and plays no active part in the expiratory process. As a fact, we find, in coughing, that the lung bulges into the lower part of the neck. The parts of the lung which contain the least volume of air are the margins. These are out of the direct line of pressure which the lung undergoes in violent expiratory efforts, which are chiefly effected by the abdominal muscles, especially the recti. The contraction of these latter muscles, forcing upwards the abdominal viscera and the diaphragm, produces the greatest amount of compression at the base of each lung ; the air is driven upwards in a strong current, which overcomes the current from the other portions, and these, instead of becoming emptied, remain forcibly distended. The phenomena witnessed in M. Groux, probably seen by many of the Fellows present, may be adduced in support of the view that during coughing the lungs become distended in any part where the walls of the chest offer but little resistance. Lastly, the cases recorded in a paper written by M. Guillot—in which what he describes as sub-pleural emphysema was found after death, preceded by long-continued and violent spasmodic cough—may be cited in favor of the expiratory theory of the production of the disease, a theory to which anatomical arrangement and physiological phenomena seem to point.—*Med. Times and Gaz.*

ii. *The Cause of Death in Drowning.* By M. BEAU.

Death in cases of drowning has been attributed to various causes—the introduction of air into the stomach, into the bronchial tubes, closure of the epiglottis, syncope, and asphyxia. M. Beau believes that the cause of death is asphyxia from want of respirable air ; but that the small quantity of water which enters the bronchial tubes requires to be explained. Is it that, in drowning, there is an arrest of the respiratory movements ? To the solution of this question, M. Beau has applied himself, and has performed the following classes of experiments, which are recorded in the *Archives Générales de Médecine* for July, 1860.

CLASS I.—A dog is plunged rapidly into a vessel of clear water, and held there on its back. At the first moment, on its surprise, it makes a more or less complete inspiration ; this is immediately followed by a jerking expiration, during which a tolerably large quantity of air escapes in bubbles to the surface of the liquid from the mouth and nose. After this, there are no further expiratory movements. The animal struggles, and there is energetic action of its trunks and limbs ; but no more inspiration or expiration. The lips remain convulsively closed. In about two minutes, the movements cease completely ; but the animal is not dead, and, if now withdrawn from the water, it may recover. Death does not take place until two or three more minutes have elapsed. On *post mortem* examination, the lips are found to be firmly closed ; the glottis is also closed. There is a variable quantity of frothy water in the small bronchial ramifications, the trachea, and frequently the large bronchial tubes. There is also a little water in the stomach, and some emphysema of the lungs.

CLASS II.—A dog is plunged into water in the same way, and removed at the end of two minutes, when he had ceased to struggle, and had lost consciousness without being really dead. He soon performs some respiratory movements, and opens his eyes ; presently he rises on his feet ; and gradually, without cough or symptoms of suffocation, he recovers rapidly and completely. If the animal be killed by pithing while he is recovering, and the chest be opened immediately, frothy water will be found in the air-passages, as in the first class of experiments.

CLASS III.—The trachea of a dog is opened, and a canula is introduced. The animal is immediately plunged into water, and held under it on his back. Scarcely has submersion taken place, when air enters the chest by an inspiration, probably through the glottis and the canula ; this is immediately followed by a jerking expiration or cough, during which bubbles of air escape from the mouth and through the canula. After this, the course of the symptoms, and the *post mortem* appearances, are the same as in the first class.

CLASS IV.—The trachea of a dog is opened, and a canula is introduced as in the first class of experiments. The animal is held under water, with his head free, but so that the opening of the canula is under the surface of the fluid. Immediately on this complete submersion taking place, water is drawn by an inspiration through the canula, and is partly rejected by cough by the same passage, with a certain quantity of air which escapes in the form of bubbles. The respiratory movements now cease, and the animal becomes restless ; but, in a few secods, respiration returns, and the animal makes regular inspirations and expirations, bubbles of air escaping at each expiration through the canula, and forming a froth on the surface of the water. As the inspiration of water goes on, and the interchange between the water and the air from the bronchi becomes complete, the quantity of bubbles diminishes at each expiration, until at last nothing but water passes through the canula. At last all movements cease, and the animal dies in the course of five minutes. On examination, the trachea and bronchi are found to be literally filled with water, which is not frothy. The lips and glottis are not convulsively closed as in the former experiments.

CLASS V.—This is a modification of the second class of experiments, introduced to show that the mere withdrawal of the muzzle from the water, so as to leave the respiratory orifices free, while the rest of the body remains submerged, is sufficient to bring about recovery.

CLASS VI.—When the trachea of an animal is constricted by a ligature. so that no air can pass, the animal struggles as if drowning ; for about two minutes, he opens his lips and nostrils as if to admit air. In five minutes, death occurs ; and, on examination, nothing is found in the bronchi, but the lungs are congested and emphysematous.

These experiments are held to show that death takes place in drowning from an irresistible horror of the water inducing an arrest of the movements of respiration and closure of the respiratory orifices ; and that this takes place irrespectively of the actual introduction of a small quantity of water into the air-tubes at the moment of submersion. There is then, in the words of M. Beau, a *hydrophobia of inspiration* in the drowning, analogous to the *hydrophobia of injection* in persons bitten by rabid animals. The last class of experiments shows that death in these cases is comparable to that which arises from strangulation.—*Gaz. Hebdom.*—*Brit. Med. Jour.*, August 25, 1860.

ART. XI.—*On Epidemic Dysentery :* By Prof. TROUSSEAU.

THE year 1859 was remarkable in France for the prevalence of a terrible epidemic of dysentery. While in former years the affection has been observed only in circumscribed localities, it prevailed during the past year almost universally. Paris, too, which has, perhaps, been exempted from epidemic dysentery for a century, has had, on the present occasion, to pay a large tribute. Commencing towards the end of July, the epidemic attained its maximum in September, undergoing a notable diminution in intensity towards the end of October. Of all epidemic diseases, dysentery is the most murderous, typhoid fever, cholera, diphtheria, variola, and scarlatina being but as child's play compared with it. These affections prevail only accidentally, while dysentery decimates whole populations, returning at certain fixed epochs, as every three years, for example. Desgenettes declared that it killed more soldiers than the enemy's cannon did between the years 1792 and 1815. The etiological circumstances of the invasion of an epidemic may be quite inappreciable. Thus, at Tours, there are two barracks placed in identical hygienic conditions, and yet, during thirty years, it has always been the cavalry barracks in which dysentery has prevailed epidemically. The reputed effects of the excessive use of fruits in generating the disease, is very doubtful, seeing that it sometimes rages when fruits are very scarce, as in 1859, while it may not be met with when they are in excessive abundance, as in 1858.

Passing by M. Trousseau's description of the disease, we come to his account of the treatment. His right to speak with some authority upon this point, is derived from the fact of his having witnessed four epidemics of the disease at Tours, Versailles, and Paris, during which the victims were either young and vigorous soldiers, aged men and women, or young children. Moreover, as Reporter on Epidemies to the Academy, he has to peruse the accounts of the various epidemics which appear throughout France. Some thirty or forty years since the traditions of the former age were abandoned, Broussais sweeping away the whole of the empirical modes of treatment in favor of his doctrines. In fact, with an inflammation so violent in view, it was then difficult not to 'give in to them ; and the antiphlogistic treatment was put freely into force, and when unsuccessful, this was believed to be because it had not been carried far enough. In 1823 or 1824, however, M. Bretonneau, imbued with the medical doctrines of Stahl and Sydenham, set on foot a reaction against the doctrines of Broussais, by resorting to a substitutive mode of treatment. He gave an ounce of the sulphate of soda internally, and administered the same dose in a very copious enema, once or twice a day, continuing the practice as long as the stools remained bloody. As soon as they became bilious and serous, the sulphate was only given once a day, then every other day, and afterwards at still rarer intervals. In 1828 or 1829, M. Trousseau published an account of an epidemic treated with success in this manner. In 1842, an epidemic occurring in the garrison at Versailles was similarly treated, but with less marked success ; however, at all events, the military surgeons in attendance—almost all pupils of Broussais—agreed that the sulphate of soda was preferable to bloodletting. Unanimity in favor of neutral salts, of one kind or another, has also nearly prevailed in the reports addressed to the Academy from all parts of France. Frequent failures have undoubtedly occurred, but, in general, when advice is sought early, considerable and extremely rapid success is the result. Induced by the success of the calomel treatment employed by the English at Gibraltar, M. Trousseau has several times put it into force, and frequently with good effect in severe cases of dysentery, occurring, however, sporadically. He still resorts to it when the weather is very hot, but in cold and wet seasons he has found salivation and other ill consequences result from its employment. In children, too, who can only be got to take the sulphate of soda with the greatest difficulty, he prefers giving calomel. Ipecacuanha, which was so much in vogue during the last century, is now seldom employed. Opium is one of the sovereign resources of the *materia medica*, and is, perhaps, the pharmaceutical substance with which most harm may be effected. It is in incessant use, and is strangely used, being, in M. Pidoux's happy phrase the "knout of the therapeutist." With it every patient who complains or suffers is fustigated. In vain may you try the rational procedures consecrated by usage, and in vain do you appeal to your intelligence and your experience—all goes for nothing—pain is present, and the indication which dominates all others is to assuage such pain, for which opium must be prescribed. With such logic as this we make but a bad business of it, or may engage in a very perilous work. A distribution of opiates with easy compliance is the mark of an impatient and ignorant practitioner. It is a very convenient procedure, and one to which every capacity is competent, which consists in "drying up the intestinal canal" by laudanum in a case of diarrhœa, and in roughly imposing silence upon the symptom pain in a case of dysentery attended with horrible tormina. "I do not pretend to say that, after having put into force the evacuant treatment, we must never, when the patient is suffering cruelly, temper his pains by a few drops of laudanum, but I entirely object to the practitioner at once drying up the intestinal canal (for this is the aim) in a case of diarrhœa or dysentery. Let him not meddle with opium except with cautious reserve, or he will be the cause of the typhoid symptoms, which will soon make their appearance." After passing in review the various other means of treatment, to which he does not seem to attach much importance, M. Trousseau adds, that all these means will be of little avail if not adopted prior to the occurrence of important pathological changes. Otherwise, every effort will be paralyzed, and no means will avail against the horrible ravages of an epidemic. In conclusion, above all things, let the condition of the diet be attended to, for this is of vital consequence. Insist that two, three, or even four quantities of soup *(potage)* be taken daily, and prescribe feculent drinks, as barley and rice waters. In all the comparative trials which have been made of treating dysentery by rigorous abstinence, or by allowing aliment in wise moderation, advantage has attended the latter procedure.—*Gazette des Hôp.—Med. Times and Gaz.*

ART. XII.—*On Hereditary Syphilis:* By M. NOTTA.

IN a paper published in the fourth volume of the *Memoires de la Société de Chirurgie*, by M. Cullerier,* its author endeavored to demonstrate that the hereditary transmission of syphilis is due only to maternal influence—the male parent exerting none. The transmission may take place at any age of fœtal life, and at all periods of the maternal infection—during the existence of the chancre, during the course of secondary or tertiary symptoms, and in the interval of these constitutional manifestations, although the mother may present every appearance of a flourishing state of health. The chief objection to M. Cullerier's views was, that they were based only upon two carefully observed cases; and it is in answer to his appeal for a further investigation into the subject that M. Notta, Surgeon of the Lisieux Hospital, now adduces several cases since observed by himself, with great care and circumspection, uninfluenced by any preconceived opinion upon the subject. These cases are completely confirmatory of M. Cullerier's views. Eleven in number, they really comprise eighteen observations, since, in two of them, observation was extended to two births, and in one to six

* *Vide British and Foreign Medico-Chirurgical Review*, January, 1857, vol. xix, p. 156.

births. In twelve of these eighteen instances the fathers, at the time of conception, had syphilitic symptoms, the mothers being healthy, and the children were born healthy. In two instances the fathers had no syphilitic symptoms, although heretofore they had suffered from the disease, and here, too, healthy children were born. In one instance the father neither had, nor ever had had any syphilis, but the mother was formerly syphilitic, and the child was born syphilitic ; and in three instances, father, mother, and offspring were all syphilitic. Thus, whenever the mother was healthy and never suffered from syphilis, the child was always exempt, whatever might be the condition of the father in this respect ; while, whenever the mother has or has had syphilis, although all manifestations may have disappeared, there is a great chance that the child will not reach its full time, or will be born with a congenital syphilis. M. Follin also has informed the author that he has never met with a case of congenital syphilis, without the mother herself being syphilitic. It is not meant to be stated that whenever a woman has had syphilis, she must always give birth to syphilitic infants. The hereditariness, although frequent, is not invariable. The objection, which the partisans of the hereditary transmission by the father may advance, that in some of the author's instances the women may have played false to their husbands, so as to leave the true paternity of the children in doubt, is anticipated by the author ; and he states that he has taken the most scrupulous care to establish his convictions upon this point—a matter of much easier accomplishment in the provincial town where his observations have been made, than it would be in the capital. These cases, then, scrupulously observed, corroborate M. Cullerier's views, and besides their scientific interest, they are of importance in reässuring fathers whose early lives may have been attended with syphilitic manifestations that these will not be entailed on their offspring in after years.—*Archives Gén.*, 1860, tome i, pp. 272-284.—*Med. Times and Gaz.*

The same journal, of September 1, 1860, announces the following recent medico-legal decision :

An action for transmission of congenital syphilis has just been tried in France. The infant of a couple named D—— was placed at nurse with the wife of a couple named R——. When about three months old, it became the subject of a syphilitic eruption, and five days afterwards its nurse, the mother of a family, up to that period in good health, and of an excellent moral character, presented on her breast ulcerations and pustules, the venereal character of which was indubitable. The husband became in his turn infected, and his wife, who had before borne three fine, vigorous children, aborted. In spite of the efforts of the counsel, who invoked the facts showing the non-transmissibility of secondary syphilis, the couple D—— were condemned by the Civil Tribunal of the Seine to pay 3000 francs damages. The medical attendant of the latter, also charged with negligence, was acquitted.

ART. XIII.—*Experimental Pathology:* By M. CLAUDE BERNARD, Member of the French Institute, Professor of General Physiology at the Faculty of Sciences, Paris.

[THE following extracts, taken from the original department of the *Medical Times and Gazette,* of July and September, are but mere specimens from a rich mine.]

If we examine some of the diseases which most frequently produce death, we shall equally be obliged to have recourse to general effects, in order to explain the mechanism through which the ultimate result is attained ; numberless patients die of peritonitis, and in a very short space of time, too; how does this take place ? for peritonitis, at first sight, does not seem to interfere with any of the higher functions of life. Inflammation of the lungs, or pleura, frequently proves mortal in a few days ; and in such diseases the respiratory functions are of course impeded ; yet mere asphyxia is evidently not the cause of death in acute cases of pneumonia ; and, in affections which rapidly prove fatal, the animal, although deprived of food, cannot evidently be supposed to die from mere inanition in so short a space of time. It therefore becomes necessary to proceed to a rational investigation of *all* the diseased tissues, in order to ascertain the mechanism through which death has been produced ; both nerves, muscles, glands, and other tissues ; both the solids and liquids of the body require to be examined. If, for instance, the substance of the liver is submitted to chemical analysis, it is found to contain no more glycogenic principles ; the total disappearance of which is, in our opinion, one of the most ordinary causes of death ; for animals kept fasting for several days together, still retain a certain amount of sugar in the blood. It therefore seems that life may be extinguished in two different ways : firstly, by the introduction of deleterious principles into the blood ; and, secondly, by the total absence of indispensable elements in that fluid. From such instances it is hardly difficult to judge what degree of scientific accuracy we may expect to find in ordinary post-mortem examinations ; local lesions are exclusively sought for, while the general disturbance passes unperceived ; and, even supposing its existence to have been suspected during life, how difficult it becomes, in the human subject, to ascertain the fact after death ! Twenty-four hours must have elapsed before we are allowed to touch the corpse ; now, although in animals recently slain the natural properties of healthy tissues persist, during a certain space of time, we are perfectly aware that, after a few hours, they are no longer to be found ; such, for instance, is the case with respect to the galvanic excitability of muscles and nerves in birds and mammiferous animals. If, therefore, the effects of woorara, digitalis, and other poisons, which act upon these very tissues, had been exclusively studied in the human species, we should never have been able to ascertain by comparison the precise nature of the injury.

It is, therefore, altogether indispensable to combine experimenta researches with clinical observation ; to create artificial disease by known means in living animals, and proceed, immediately after death, to a rational post-mortem examination ; all the tissues must successively be compared to those in a normal condition, but the state of the blood more especially deserves our attention. Towards this subject the energies of all physiologists ought to be mainly directed. Organic chemistry, however, is unfortunately not in an advanced state, especially as regards the constituent principles of the animal organization ; and chemical analysis must, therefore, be in a great measure left aside when the properties of the blood are the subject of investigation ; in other terms, a physiological analysis is in this respect far preferable. Let the vital properties of the nervous system be brought into play, and modifications of the very highest importance will be discovered, which neither morbid anatomy nor the known methods of analysis would have been able to render apparent. The same is the case with muscles—when poisoned by certain substances, they lose their contractile power, but no modification whatever is to be discovered in their chemical constitution. The blood, therefore, may naturally be expected, in various states of health and disease, to present changes which none but the physiologist can appreciate ; thus, when oxyde of carbon has been inhaled, the blood-globule is deprived of its characteristic property of absorbing oxygen in exchange for carbonic acid ; the fact is ascertained by physiological experiments, but ordinary analysis gives no clue whatever to the solution of the problem. Far be it from me to disapprove the chemical researches of which the blood has been made the subject ; on the contrary, they deserve to be carried out on a more extensive scale than ever ; but if performed apart from experiments on the living animal, their results will never contribute to the real progress of science.

The study of morbid principles can, therefore, alone enable us to discover the means of curing the disorders to which they give rise ; and for this purpose two different systems might be adopted ; firstly, to neutralize the morbid agents ; and, secondly, to eliminate them from the body. In the present state of our knowledge, we possess no means whatever of neutralizing their actions ; as in the case of poisons, they must be expelled before they cease to act. To this result do all the efforts of nature tend, and to this result also must all the physician's endeavors be devoted.

From the earliest period to which our knowledge extends, it has been a favorite object with medical philosophers to connect, as far as possible, the symptoms exhibited by patients during life, with the morbid alterations discovered in the various organs after death. In many instances these laudable efforts have been fully crowned with success ; and the light thrown on this branch of the medical sciences, since the commencement of the present century, has in no slight degree contributed to the progress of the healing art. But, although in the majority of cases the results of post-mortem examinations enable us to ascertain the direct and immediate causes of death, our expectations are too often deceived in this respect ; the most attentive survey leads sometimes, as you are well aware, to no satisfactory conclusion whatever ; all the organs appear as

th   112

sound as in the healthy state, and it becomes altogether impossible to account for the cessation of life. On the other hand, how frequently are extensive lesions discovered within the body after death, the existence of which had been previously revealed by no corresponding symptoms! All physicians whose attention has been devoted to the diseases of old age, have met with numerous instances of this kind. I remember myself having, more than once, witnessed similar cases, at the time when I was attached as an *interne* to the Salpêtrière.* On one occasion I discovered a large tumor in the immediate vicinity of the pons Varolii, the presence of which had not been attended with symptoms of paralysis, notwithstanding the pressure exerted on so important a portion of the brain.

Morbid anatomy must not, therefore, be considered as a key to all the phenomena of disease ; viewed by itself, it is utterly incapable of pointing out the hidden sources from which they spring ; and mere anatomical investigations, however minute, are altogether insufficient in this respect. In making experiments upon the abdominal nerves, I have frequently seen animals die, before any symptoms of inflammation had made their appearance ; and Chossat's interesting researches on the effects of starvation equally affords instances of sudden death under similar circumstances. Thus, in animals entirely deprived of food, a given period usually elapses before life is altogether extinct ; but, when the process is already far advanced, the slightest shock is sufficient to destroy life at once. A pigeon, which has been kept fasting for a considerable length of time, falls down, and instantaneously dies, when its claws are nipped ; while, if not interfered with, the animal's life is usually prolonged for several days. It would, of course, be quite unnecessary to state, that, in making the autopsy, no alterations besides those which ordinarily result from inanition are met with. In what manner, therefore, is death to be accounted for in such cases ? Chossat attributes it to syncope ; an opinion which our own experiments tend to corroborate. In fact, the heart's motion (as we have elsewhere stated) is momentarily arrested when a sensitive nerve is painfully excited ; it would, therefore, be quite possible that in animals reduced to a state of great debility, a slight sensation of pain should immediately produce death. There also exist, in such cases, other conditions, which the mere anatomist is unable to appreciate. The temperature of the medium in which the animals are kept during the process of starvation, has a considerable influence upon the duration of life ; for cold accelerates and warmth opposes the destructive process ; and, in experiments in which circulation has been arrested in some of the larger vessels, we also find this to be the case. When the vena porta, for instance, has been tied, the animal is soon deprived of its natural heat, and rapidly dies, if the temperature of the body is not maintained in a proper state by artificial means ; but when this precaution has been taken, the results of the operation seldom prove fatal.

It would not be difficult to accumulate a still larger amount of

---

* An Asylum for aged women, which contains upwards of five thousand inmates. ◆

evidence upon this point, but you have no doubt been fully convinced, by the facts to which we have just drawn your attention, that nothing beyond the mere mechanical causes of death is explained by morbid anatomy, and that other and more comprehensive modes of investigation are indispensable to those who wish to acquire a deeper insight into the secrets of living nature. To fill up this void as far as possible, is the chief purpose of our present researches, but in pursuing this object we must never lose sight of the example left us by those illustrious observers to whom the biological sciences are indebted for all the progress they have accomplished in moderations. The concatenation of natural phenomena, their mode of precession, and the laws according to which they are produced, must alone become the subject of our studies ; as to the intimate nature of things, it lies entirely beyond the reach of human knowledge. It would not, for instance, be sufficient to state that certain poisons act upon the nerves, others upon the muscles or the blood ; but when the peculiar mode of action of such bodies upon our tissues and the mechanism through which life is extinguished, have been thoroughly ascertained in each case, we can go no further ; to explain the mysterious properties which enable a given poison to disorganize a given tissue, is not within the power of science. You remember, no doubt, the effects produced by oxyde of carbon upon the blood-globules, you are aware that a chemical combination takes place between these two bodies, which opposes the absorption of oxygen, and brings on a peculiar kind of asphyxia ; the mechanical process of respiration still continues, but is no longer attended with the revivification of the blood in the lungs. Here, then, we have a satisfactory explanation of the deleterious influence exerted by this substance ; but if we were asked *why* the combination takes place, we should, of course, be unable to answer the question. The affinity of oxyde of carbon for the blood-cells is evidently superior to that of oxygen, but the primitive reason of this difference lies beyond the limits of our scientific knowledge.

The physiologist must, therefore, be contented with tracing back the effects produced by disease to some primitive cause, the discovery of which puts an end to his inquiries ; and the influence exerted by toxic agents upon the organs of the living body, will, in this respect, be found to exhibit a striking analogy with that of morbid causes. In what manner is the agency of poisons to be conceived ? Ought their effects to be viewed in the light of chemical combinations, which supersede the physiological changes that support life ? Such is, in fact, the explanation we have adopted as regards the action exerted by oxyde of carbon upon the blood-globules ; but would it be proper to extend these views to all the different poisons with which we are at present acquainted ? Are we to suppose that woorara is chemically combined with the substance itself of the motor nerves, so as to impede the progress of the nervous fluid ? A similar hypothesis would evidently not be in accordance with facts ; we find that when life has been protracted by artificial means, the deleterious agent is gradually expelled from the economy; now, if a permanent impression had been produced upon the nerves, we should not find this to be the case.

It therefore appears that toxic agents exert different modes of action upon the fundamental conditions of life ; in some instances they seem to be chemically combined with the histological elements of the disorganized tissues ; such, according to Liebig, is the case with respect to metallic salts. Other poisons, on the contrary, circulate freely with the blood, and destroy, for the time being, its vital properties ; now, the blood, as we have already stated, is the common medium in which all the tissues exist ; if, therefore, a deep change occurs in its physiological properties, both muscles, glands, nerves, and other organs, are liable to experience a total derangement in their usual functions. The well-known experiments of Bichat upon the injection of venous blood into the arteries, afford a striking example of this ; and it can scarcely be questioned, that such is the mode of action exerted by woorara, strychnia, and all the other substances which are speedily eliminated from the body, when death has not been almost immediately the result of their presence.

It would, therefore, appear that poisons might, in this respect, be divided into two principal classes ; some of them give rise to stable and definite chemical compounds, are retained within the economy, and may be discovered by the process of analysis after death ; others are speedily expelled from the body, and leave no visible marks of their passage. In the first case, permanent and incurable effects are produced ; in the second, a transitory action is alone exerted, and when the patient recovers, the noxious principle has entirely disappeared. In short, we find, in all respects, a perfect resemblance between the effects of poison and those of ordinary diseases.

The experimental method, to which the physical sciences are wholly indebted for the progress they have hitherto realized, has rendered equally important services to physiology ; it has taught us to consider the various phenomena exhibited by animated beings as the result of properties enjoyed by matters in the living state, instead of referring them to the mysterious agency of a power entirely independent of the animal organization, but controlling all its internal changes, and which, in the language of ancient physicians, received the name of *vis vitæ*, or vital force.

A similar revolution is no less indispensable in pathology ; and the actual bias of science is rapidly leading us to this desirable result. A great number of our cotemporaries, however, still adhere to the notions of the old classical school, and consider the rejection of their favorite views as a proof of materialism ; an assertion altogether unfounded, and which must not arrest us in the course of our present investigations. The experimental method is equally applicable to all the sciences. Why, therefore, should we endeavor to establish, with respect to pathology, a distinction as erroneous in theory as it is injurious in practice, to the progress of our art ? No medical philosopher who truly deserves that name will dissent from us on this point.

What is disease ? A question which evidently must be the first that presents itself to the physician's mind, but which none of the definitions laid down up to the present time has satisfactorily answered ; in fact, these definitions having in almost every case been established à *priori*, are of no value whatever in the actual state of our knowledge. Synthetical reasoning is, of course, the starting-point of all sciences ; they arrive by degrees at the analytical process of inquiry, and are thus at length enabled to reconstruct their principles on solid foundations ; a progress which has already been realized in the case of physiology, while pathology still lingers behind in that state of uncertainty from which our present endeavors are intended to release it. The existence of essential diseases, as opposed to symptomatic disorders, has, for instance, been long a subject of discussion among medical men ; but the precise meaning of these terms must be accurately determined before we can possibly come to an understanding on this subject. If, by the words " an essential disease," it is implied that certain disorders exist without corresponding material lesions, a similar hypothesis cannot be too strongly condemned ; for an organic apparatus can never cease to accomplish its physiological functions, as long as all the parts of which it is composed remain in perfect order ; to suppose the contrary would be to deny the necessary connection between cause and effect. But if, on the other hand, the expression is intended to convey no other meaning, than that our actual methods of investigation are not capable of revealing the existence of certain lesions, and that we must be contented with registering the fact, without attempting for the present to explain it, no objection whatever can be raised against this latter view, which is perfectly in accordance with facts. Notwithstanding the progress of microscopical anatomy, our knowledge is still very imperfect in this sense, and we constantly meet with difficulties the solution of which will reward, no doubt, the labors of a future generation. Let us not, however, be discouraged, nor abandon the research es undertaken for this purpose ; for science, after all, entirely cons sts in the study of the relations of natural phenomena with their material causes. If, therefore, the existence of affections altogether independent of physical .changes were admitted as a positive fact, the whole fabric of our knowledge would fall to the ground at once.

Experimental pathology (according to our view) is, therefore, the application of the analytical method to the study of disease. A given series of disorders, all belonging to the same nosological tribe, having been selected, we shall proceed to inquire into their causes, symptoms and development, by means of direct experiments—that is to say, by artificially creating similar disorders in animals whose organization closely resembles our own ; and we shall, in this manner, successively review the great natural divisions of pathology. We might, for instance, direct our attention to inflammations in the first place ; and, after exhausting the subject, proceed to the study of fevers ; and the whole field of scientific nosology will thus be brought by degrees within the pale of our investigations.

We now meet with one of those difficulties with which all scientific classifications are encumbered : ought the effects of poison to be viewed in the light of ordinary affections, or to set apart as belonging to an entirely different science ? The latter is the opinion of many an eminent toxicologist; we are far, however, from partaking of these views. There exists, on the contrary, so remarkable an analogy between the symptoms of legitimate diseases, and the disorders which result from the introduction of toxic agents into the economy, that the effect of poisons may, up to a certain point, be considered as the most perfect specimen of morbid actions which can possibly be selected as a type. You are, no doubt, already prepared for this assertion, the preceding lectures having been mainly devoted to this subject; we shall now endeavor to complete the demonstration of the fact.

When we examine the lesions which result from the injection of toxic substances, we invariably discover that one peculiar histological element, one given tissue has been invaded in all the parts which compose the animal economy; and the direct consequence of such modifications is a total derangement of the physiological functions which, in the healthy state, devolve upon the injured elements. A general disturbance, therefore, arises from the suppression of their vital properties; and in this respect, the action of poisons is strictly parallel to that of internal diseases. Nor is this all; you are fully aware that the characteristic symptoms which attend the introduction of each particular substance into the system, enable the physician to establish as precise a diagnosis as in the case of any affection. Are not the effects of arsenic, or those produced by the salts of lead, as easily distinguished from those of other poisons, as typhus fever or pneumonia from all other diseases? Now this is a property which has at all times been viewed as an essential characteristic of well-defined diseases; we give, in fact, this name to a definite succession of morbid phenomena, which, arising from a given anatomical modification of tissue, undergoes a regular evolution, and terminates either in death, when the more important phenomena of life have been suspended, or in the patient's recovery when they have resumed their natural course.

But a highly plausible objection might now be raised against us; the effects of poison, it may be said, can be reproduced at all times upon a healthy subject; while morbid agents are entirely beyond our control. Our reply to this argument is, that a variety of diseases may be created by artificial means, especially when a peculiar virus exists; the inoculation of small-pox and of venereal diseases sufficiently prove this; and we have previously shown that mere surgical lesions frequently enable us to create at pleasure in sound animals, a series of well-known disorders.

The astonishing rapidity with which the symptoms of poisoning often succeed the introduction of the toxic agent into the body, ought not to prevent us from assimilating them to the ordinary effects of disease; for the duration of the morbid series entirely depends upon the nature of the poison, and the state of concentration in which it is employed: if prussic acid, when pure, produces instant death, its destructive powers may be reduced by successive dilutions to the very lowest degree; and a large number of other poisons (metallic salts, for instance) act with comparative slowness, and may be assimilated to chronic affections, when taken in small doses.

The absence of all visible lesions after death, which not unfrequently occurs in cases where poison has been administered ; and the possibility of an entire recovery, when the noxious substance has been completely expelled, may be adduced as additional proofs in favor of our views ; and lastly, as a further resemblance to certain diseases, an incubation to a certain extent often takes place. The deleterious agent does not always exhibit at once its destructive properties, but remains during a certain lapse of time in a latent state (so to speak) within the economy. In short, the phenomena of life, whether viewed in connection with physiology, pathology, or toxicology, obey the same natural laws, and ought not to be studied apart from each other. But in the case of poisons, the observer is placed in the most favorable conditions that can possibly be imagined ; he administers definite substances in given quantities ; he notes the effects produced from the very commencement of the consecutive disorder—a condition which can never be realized in clinical practice ; and lastly, he selects according to his convenience, the age, size, constitution, and species of the animal on which the experiment is performed : he therefore enjoys every possible security for the perfect success of the operation.

It is a well-known tendency of the human mind, never to rest satisfied with the mere observations of facts without seeking to know their primitive causes ; in this respect an absolute parity exists between the medical observer and the experimental physiologist ; they both endeavor to combine facts in such a manner as will enable them to arrive at general conclusions. It has been stated that scientific observation consists in remarking the effects produced by the unassisted efforts of Nature : while experiments, according to the well-known definition of Laplace, consist in disturbing the natural evolution of phenomena by direct interference, so that observation is the only method available in certain sciences ; for as long as the phenomena which attract our attention do not lie within our reach, their natural evolution cannot be modified for scientific purposes, and the experimental method is no longer applicable. Such, for instance, is the case with astronomy ; the motions of the celestial bodies lie open to our observation, but cannot possibly be diverted from their course.

We have no objection to make against these definitions, viewed in a general sense ; but when applied to the medical sciences, it would not be safe to place an entire reliance upon them. Clinical observation is perpetually disturbed by medical treatment ; and experimental physiology is frequently reduced to mere observation ; when, for instance, a fistulous opening has been formed in an animal's stomach, in order to examine as closely as possible the digestive process, all interference with the natural course of the function is cautiously avoided by the scientific observer ; we are, however, entitled to call the operation a physiological experiment ; and, on the other hand, in the practice of medicine, a vast number of experiments are daily made under the name of " clinical observations ;" when the physician administers to his patient a substance, the action of which is as yet unknown, when he notes down its effects, and publishes the result of his inquiries, has he not been actually making an experiment? We therefore believe that no positive distinction could be safely established between these two modes of investigation, and that in all cases in which the process of analysis has been introduced into the study of facts, and logical inductions have been drawn from the results of observation, an experiment has been made.

ART. XIV.—*Case of supposed Congenital Absence of Uterus, and Occlusion of Vagina.* (Sheffield General Infirmary, under the care of Mr. BARBER. Notes of the case by Mr. H. J. KNIGHT, House-Surgeon.)

H. E., a healthy, good-looking girl, aged twenty-one, applied at this hospital last month for advice under the following circumstances: She stated " that she had been married nine months, during the last two only, however, she had cohabited with her husband ; that the marriage had never been properly consummated, and she thought 'there must be something wrong with her.'" She had always enjoyed good health, though she had never menstruated. When about the age of fourteen, she had fits of an epileptic character, which have recurred at irregular periods, sometimes with an interval of six months. She had never suffered from lumbar or abdominal pains.

An examination was accordingly made externally. The external parts presented a perfectly natural appearance. On separating the labia pudendi, the nymphæ were found to be well formed, but there was no meatus urinarius, or any communication with the bladder external to or above the vagina. A small caruncle of mucous membrane, about the size of a pea, and having on its upper surface a preputial membrane, represented the clitoris. The finger passed into the vagina revealed the following state of parts : That passage, instead of leading to the uterus, terminated in a cul-de-sac about two inches from its commencement ; the mucous membrane moved freely on the subjacent tissues, and there was no fullness or tension in any part. Just within the vagina was a septum or mucous fold, formed by its anterior wall, in front of which the finger passed forwards through a passage of about an inch in length, grasped by a sphincter muscle, into a large cavity, from which, on introducing a catheter, urine was drawn. She was examined also per rectum, and by means of a catheter passed into the bladder through the urethral opening in the vagina, but no hard body or sign of an uterus could be detected, nor was there any fullness in or about the rectum or lower part of the abdomen. The diameter of the outlet of the pelvis was rather more contracted than natural, and the perineum was about half an inch in length. The mammæ were well developed ;

but she asserted that she had never experienced sexual desire or feeling, either prior to or since her marriage, though micturition was always excited by coitus. At a consultation held on the case, it was considered undesirable to attempt any exploratory operative proceeding, and she therefore left the hospital in a few days.

The evidence in the above case as to the absence, or rather the non-development of the uterus, may be classed under three heads : 1st. The non-occurrence of menstruation. 2d. The state of the parts as ascertained by tactile examination. 3d. The asserted absence of sexual desire. The latter point is one of course to which little or no weight can be attached ; since, apart from the doubt which must be felt as to a woman's statement on such a subjcet, it is probable that the instinct in question has more to do with the ovaries than the uterus. In a case recorded by M. Depaul (*L'Union Méd.*, No. lxxix, 1851), a young woman, aged twenty-two, whose sexual organs were in almost exactly the same state as those of the Sheffield patient, had well developed breasts, and had displayed marked venereal desire. M. Depaul, in this instance, believed that he detected the right ovary. Every month the woman had all the symptoms of menstruation except the flux. In place of the vaginal opening was a simple depression.

The absence of menstruation in a well-grown and healthy woman of upwards of twenty, when it has been complete, and without any indication of retained secretion as afforded by the presence of a tumor in the pelvis, is a very significant fact as regards the absence of the uterus. It is, however, far from a conclusive one, and must only be relied on in connection with others bearing on the same point.

Dr. Meigs, of Philadelphia, in his translation of Colombat's work on Diseases of Women, mentions a case which had come under his own notice, in which "a handsome woman," aged twenty-two, had never menstruated. Although two years married, satisfactory coitus had never been accomplished. On examination, the vagina was found to be a cul-de-sac two inches in length; and, as far as could be ascertained, the uterus was wholly wanting. The reviewer of Dr. Meigs's translation, in the *Medico-Chirurgical Review*, mentions, without giving any details, that a similar case had lately fallen under his own notice and adds : "When proceedings were instituted to obtain a nullity of marriage, no precedent was discovered in the records of the court."

Thus, it is probable that entire absence of the uterine function is more frequent than that of all trace of its structure. It is with such an arrest of development as involves total inability to take on functional activity that the practical physician and medical jurist have to deal. It does not affect their conclusions to know that in these cases the absence of all rudiment is rarely entire. The pathological fact to which the Professor's remark points is nevertheless an important one. It would seem that these instances of absent uterus and closed vagina are examples of local arrest of development only, and approach but little towards those more general malformations (often with excess of parts) grouped together under the head of

113

hermaphrodites. In all the cases which we have mentioned above, the women possessed well formed external genitals, and had probably no reason, prior to marriage, apart from the emansio mensium, to suspect that they were in any way differently constituted to others. This fact increases the practical importance of the non-occurrence of menstruation very greatly. It is clear that a medical examination ought to precede marriage in all cases in which the intended wife has never menstruated.

Dr. Taylor adverts to "the remarkable circumstance," that suits for divorce on account of alleged impediment to intercourse or procreation, are almost always by the female against the male, and explains it by reference to the much greater difficulty in establishing sterility against a woman than impotence against a man. There can be little doubt, however, but that in such cases as those quoted above, very couclusive medical evidence might be given in a court of law. Although these malformations may but rarely give occasion to suits for divorce, yet the amount of mutual unhappiness caused by them is probably very great.

It is a curious fact, that two murdered women have been proved to be subjects of absence of the uterus, one case being that of Hannah Brown, murdered by Greenacre, and the second that of a woman whose mutilated remains were found in the streets of a London suburb some years ago, and the mystery concerning whose death was, we believe, never unraveled.—*Medical Times and Gazette*, July 14, 1860.

━━━━━━━━

ART. XV.—*Wound of the Carotid in a Child—Abscesses of the Brain.* Care of Mr. LLOYD. (St. Bartholomew's Hospital Reported by Mr. F. LLOYD.)

THE danger after ligature of the common carotid, that the patient may die of abscess in the brain on the side from which the supply of blood has been cut off, is well known. In the following case the internal carotid trunk had become obliterated as the result of a punctured wound, and the child died a month after the accident with abscesses in the brain. It might have been expected, *à priori*, that young children would have been less liable to this occurrence than adults ; but there are very few facts on record bearing on this question. For obvious reasons, the operation of ligature of the carotid has been very rarely performed in children. The subjoined case has, however, several other features of interest distinct from the one alluded to. It gives an instance of Nature's cure of a wound of the large trunk, namely: obliteration. The hæmorrhage had been wholly arrested, and had the vessel involved been any other than the internal carotid, in all probability the patient would have recovered.

He died of a secondary, not of the primary, lesion. It is remarkable, also, in respect to the cause of the accident, the age of the patient, and the recurrent attacks of hæmorrhage.

Arthur A., aged four, was admitted into St. Bartholomew's Hospital on April 14th last, in consequence of a wound in his neck, from which it was said he had lost a very large quantity of blood. The bleeding had then ceased. His appearance, when admitted, was that of a remarkably fine and fat boy, with an unusually large head. His face and the whole of his body was blanched and of a waxen hue ; his lips and tongue were very anæmic ; his eyes glassy and half closed ; his pulse at the wrist was scarcely perceptible and slow. In fact, he was in a state of syncope. The wound, which was about the size of a large pea, was situated on the right side of the neck, about an inch below and anterior to the angle of the jaw. It had been caused by his falling on the point of a stick, which he was holding in his hand. A probe gently introduced into the wound passed inwards and very slightly backwards for an inch and a half. As the bleeding at this time had entirely ceased, he was merely put into bed, and a piece of wet lint applied to the wound. On April 16th, however, hæmorrhage again took place, but was easily stopped by means of a pledget of lint strapped over the wound. The blood was of a dark venous color, and did not come in a rapid jet, but merely in a continuous stream, so that, altogether, he did not lose more than an ounce or so of blood. At this time he seemed to have recovered from the first loss of blood to a great degree, his face was flushed, and his skin generelly had lost the blanched appearance it presented on admission. His pulse was sharp and quick, and of moderate volume. As his bowels had not been open for days, an aperient was given, and quinine was ordered three times a day.

On the 21st, as he was very restless, and seemed to suffer a good deal of uneasiness from the wound, which at this time was discharging a healthy pus, he was ordered (in addition to the quinine and acid draught) ten-minim doses of the compound tincture of camphor. On the 22d there was again some hæmorrhage, to about the same extent as before, and of the same character. It was, however, easily stopped by a compress of lint.

On the 29th, in the middle of the day, the wound bled again, and in rather larger quantity ; and the same night he had some kind of fit, after which the left side of his body was completely paralyzed. He was ordered three grains of mercury, with chalk, immediately, and every six hours, with nitrate of potash in almond and manna mixture. From this time he gradually sank, without any marked symptoms supervening, or any fresh hæmorrhage, and he died on May 9th.

Autopsy, Twenty-four Hours after Death.—The neck was the first part examined, and on dissection the wound was found to pass through the skin, superficial fascia, platysma, and deep fascia, between the external carotid artery and the internal jugular vein, and finally to terminate in a lymphatic gland lying on the rectus capitis anticus major. The wound was, in fact, a deep sinus, with thickened indurated walls, and implicated in the posterior wall was the internal carotid artery, which was quite impervious. On opening the skull and removing the dura mater, which was healthy, the right hemisphere of the cerebrum appeared much softened, and in it were found three circumscribed abscesses, two in the middle lobe and one in the posterior. The rest of the brain was healthy.—*Med. Times and Gaz.,* September 8, 1860.

ART. XVI.—*Two Cases of Resection of the Hip-Joint.* (King's College Hospital, under the care of Mr. FERGUSSON and Mr. BOWMAN.)

FOR the notes of the two following cases we are indebted to Mr. William Wickham, the present House-Surgeon of King's College Hospital

CASE 1.—*Abstract of Case—Disease of the Hip-Joint in a Young Girl—Profuse Discharge, Emaciation, and Hectic—Resection—Head of Bone found Necrosed and Loose—Recovery.*—Mary A. K., aged six, was admitted into King's College Hospital, under the care of Mr. Bowman, on February 4, 1860, with disease of the hip-joint. From the history of the case, it appears that fourteen months previous to this date, she had slipped down an area, and injured the left hip, so that she could not stand, and suffered a great deal of pain. She was admitted into the Hospital for Children, in Great Ormond street, where she remained four months ; during this time two abscesses formed in connection with the joint, one pointing behind and the other below the great trochanter. These were opened, and have continued to discharge ever since. On admission, the patient presented a pale and very emaciated appearance. The diseased hip presented an appearance as if dislocated, the left leg being considerably shorter than the right, and much drawn over towards the right side, the trochanter major very prominent and near to the crest of the ilium. There was some motion in the joint, which gave very little pain. There were two wounds, discharging freely, one behind and the other below the great trochanter (the same as previously noticed); these did not communicate with one another, but a probe passed through either of them to the joint. By measurement, the limb was three-quarters of an inch shorter than the right. The pelvis was very much tilted. The liver was found to be very large, and the abdomen full and tense, the surface being much marked by veins. Ordered ol. morrhuæ and syr. ferri iodidi aa ʒj quotidie. This treatment was continued for five or six weeks, with rest in bed, and the child's general health improved, but the hip continued to discharge very freely, and excision of the joint was therefore decided upon.

May 19th. Chloroform having been administered, a vertical incision was made through the posterior opening, and another at right angles to this, for an inch backwards. The outline of the trochanter major was then exposed, in the posterior part of which was a deficiency, through which the finger could enter the cavity of the joint. The head and neck of the bone were found to be necrosed and loose ; in an excavation on the inner surface of the trochanter major, which was sawn off just above the trochanter minor. The acetabulum had partly disappeared, the outline of the socket not being recognizable ; the disease did not extend beyond this, and from the surface of it some small loose fragments were removed. Scarcely any blood was lost during the operation. The limb was placed on a long interrupted splint.

20th. The patient slept well, and complains of no pain ; healthy discharge from the wound.

28th. Has continued to progress most favorably. The discharge, which, before the operation, was so great, is now moderate and healthy. The limb in very good position, and the patient's health has much improved.

July 5. The splint was removed to-day, and the limb placed between sand bags. The wound has nearly healed, the discharge being very slight. She is quite free from pain, and able to move herself easily in bed. There is considerable freedom of motion in the joint. Her health is now very good, and she is very much fatter than on her admission, or previous to the operation. She was discharged cured, on August 2, 1860.

CASE 2.—*Abstract of Case—Disease of the Hip-Joint in a Little Boy—Profuse Discharge—Resection—Partial Dislocation and Absorption of the Head of the Bone—Recovery.*—William K., a strumous-looking child, aged four years, was admitted into King's College Hospital, under the care of Mr. Fergusson, in February, 1860, with disease of the right hip. From his previous history, it appeared that in May, 1859, he fell down some steps, and injured his right hip. This was followed by a great deal of pain, and he could not support the weight of the body on the leg ; he underwent treatment, but without deriving any benefit. He was admitted into the hospital on February 28, 1860. At this time there was some considerable fullness about the joint, and any attempt at moving the limb caused the child a great deal of pain. The limb was placed on the body, and drawn over to the opposite side. After he had been in the hospital three weeks, some deep fluctuation was perceptible over the outer part of the joint, and an abscess finally pointed behind the great trochanter, which was opened. On passing the finger through this opening, extensive disorgization of the joint was found to exist. After this, the child's health improved, and the pain in the joint much diminished. He was discharged on May 19, to go into the country, and return to the hospital in six weeks' time.

On readmission, July 4, the child's general health was pretty good, but the disease of the joint was more advanced. The opening behind the great trochanter still discharged freely, and there was more shortening and distortion of the limb than when discharged in May. There was great fullness of the tissues around the joint, and any motion in the joint was attended with much pain.

7th. Chloroform having been administered, an incision, about three inches in length, was made over the 'great trochanter, and, on examination, the head of the bone, a great portion of which had disappeared, was found to be partially dislocated; this, with a few touches of the knife, was readily detached from the surrounding tissues, and made to project through the wound. It was then sawn off through at the base of the trochanter major, which latter was slightly diseased. The acetabulum was found to be perfectly healthy. Scarcely any blood was lost during the operation. On examination of the portion of bone which was removed, it was found that the cartilage was destroyed, and a large portion of the osseous structure beneath it absorbed. The patient was then removed to bed, and an interrupted side splint applied.

9th. Patient doing very well; has had very little pain; wound looking healthy, and discharging freely; appetite good; sleeps well.

18th. The splint was reapplied this morning, and the whole body placed between heavy sand bags, extension being made by means of a weight hanging over the end of the bed. The wound is healing rapidly, and the discharge very slight. There is considerable motion in the joint, unaccompanied by pain.

August 7. The splint was left off to-day. The wound is nearly healed, and there is no discharge.

16th. The child is now quite well, and can move the limb of his own accord. Since the splint was left off, the leg is somewhat shortened, on account of the tilting of the pelvis. Extension is therefore being continued for a short time, by means of the weight over the end of the bed.—*Med. Times and Gaz.*, September 1, 1860.

ART. XVII.—*Inquiry into the Treatment of Congenital Imperfections of the Rectum by Operation; Founded on an Analysis of One Hundred Cases, Nine of which occurred in the Practice of the Author:* By. T. B. CURLING, Esq., F. R. S. (Royal Medical and Chirurgical Society. Tuesday, June 26th, 1860. F. C. SKEY, Esq., F. R. S., President, in the Chair.)

WITH the view of ascertaining and estimating the results of the operations which have been resorted to in the different forms of congenital imperfections of the rectum, either for the preservation of life or its future comfort, and of assisting to establish the best modes of proceeding in these cases, Mr. Curling had collected and tabulated one hundred cases in which operations have been performed by himself and other surgeons. Of these cases, sixty-eight were males and thirty-two females. He classed the congenital malformations of the rectum as follows : 1. *Imperforate anus, the rectum being partially or wholly deficient.* Of this form the table furnished 26 instances—21 males and 5 females. 2. *Anus opening into a cul-de-sac, the rectum being partially or wholly deficient.* Of this the table included 31 cases—17 males and 14 females. 3. *Imperforate anus in the male, the rectum being partially or wholly deficient, and communicating with the urethra or neck of the bladder.* Of this the table contained 26 cases. 4. *Imperforate anus in the female, the rectum being partially deficient, and communicating with the vagina.* Of this the table furnished 11 cases. 5. *Imperforate anus, the rectum being partially deficient, and opening externally, in an abnormal situation, by a narrow outlet.* Of this form the table contained 6 cases.

A few other congenital deviations had been observed, but they were of very rare occurrence ; and the five forms enumerated above were alone included in the table. The author briefly related a case of fæcal fistula, passing from the back of the sacrum to the rectum, which fell under his own observation.

After reviewing the causes of these malformations, and showing that, though in most instances consequent on an arrest of development, they sometimes result from a pathological change, due probably to inflammation occurring during intra-uterine life, the author noticed the relations of the peritoneum to the bowel in the different forms of atresia, as having an important bearing on the operations performed in the perineal region ; and stated that, in several instances in the table, the fatal result was due to the opening made in the serous sac. He also called attention to an imperfect development of the pelvis in those cases in which the rectum is wholly deficient.

1. The 26 cases in the table of the first form furnished the following results : In 14 cases the gut was opened in the anal region, and in 12 the operator failed to reach it ; of the former, 9 ended fatally, and 5 proved successful ; of the 12 cases in which the gut was not reached, 2 ended fatally without anything further being done ; in 7, colotomy was performed in the groin—1 only proved fatal ; in 3 the colon was opened in the lumbar region—1 recovered and 2 died. The author gave some particulars of the five successful cases, and noticed that there was only one of complete success in which the rectum was wholly wanting. In three of the cases in which the bowel was simply incised, more or less difficulty was experienced afterwards in maintaining a free passage for the fæces ; but, in two of the cases, subsequent contraction was prevented by drawing the bowel down to the anal region.

2. In 16 of the 31 cases of the second form, the gut was reached and opened. In 11 the operator failed in finding it. Of the former, 6 were fatal, and 10 recovered. Of the 11 cases in which the gut was not reached, 6 ended fatally without any further operation. In 2, colotomy was performed in the groin, with a fatal result. In 3 instances, the colon was opened in the loin ; 2 were fatal and 1 recovered. In 4 cases, colotomy was performed without any previous subpubic operation, three times in the groin with successful results, and once in the loin with a fatal termination. In analyzing the ten

cases of success after a subpubic operation, the author observed that in several cases in which the septum was slight, the passage was readily established ; that in others, where a space of some extent intervened between the two ends of the bowel, great difficulty was experienced in preventing contraction, unless the bowel was drawn down and attached to the skin ; and he gave the particulars of a case treated by himself in this way with complete success.

3. The author adduced some cases of the third form, in which, the communication between the rectum and the urethra being more free than usual, life has been preserved for many months, the fæces escaping entirely by the urethra, until the passage becoming at length blocked up, death has ensued. Of the 26 cases in the table, the gut was reached in 15 ; in 9 the operator failed to find it. Of the former, 9 recovered and 6 proved fatal. Of the 9 cases in which the gut was not reached, 7 ended fatally without any further operation. In 1 colotomy was performed in the groin, in the other in the loin ; both ended fatally. In two cases no attempt was made to reach the bowel from the parinæum, but the colon was opened in the loin. One did well, the other died. In 7 of the successful cases treated by incision, more or less difficulty was experienced afterwards in maintaining the passage. In the only case in which the bowel was drawn down and secured to the skin, no contraction took place, and the boy was well and thriving at five years of age. After the establishment of a passage at the anus, the escape of fæces by the urethra did not always cease, and several instances are given in which serious inconvenience resulted from non-closure of the abnormal communication.

4. The author, after alluding to instances of persons born with imperforate anus, the rectum opening into the vagina, who had passed through life submitting to the annoyances consequent upon it, stated that the recto-vaginal communication is not always sufficient, and that obstinate constipation sometimes ensues. As the rectum descends low in the pelvis in this form, the operator cannot well fail to reach the bowel. In all the 11 instances in the table the gut was opened, and only 1 ended fatally, from over distension of the rectum, consequent on the operation having been delayed too long ; 8 of the 10 remaining cases were reported as successful, and 2 as unsuccessful, owing to the tendency to contraction and neglect by the parents of the means recommended to maintain the passage. In one of the successful cases the bowel was drawn down and secured to the skin. The author gave the particulars of two cases which came under his own notice—one successful, the other unsuccessful. In this malformation the establishment of a new passage at the natural site is not all that is required ; the abnormal communication with the vagina must also be closed. A case in which this opening is reported to have closed spontaneously, is the only one of complete success in the table. The author was unacquainted with a single case in which, after the formation of an artificial anus, a successful operation had been performed for the closure of the recto-vaginal aperture.

5. Of the fifth form there were 6 cases in the table—4 males and

2 females. In the males the abnormal outlet was in the perinæum, just behind the scrotum, in 2; in 1 in the scrotal raphé; and in 1 anterior to the scrotum. In the females the opening was in the perinæum, close to the vagina, or at the posterior commissure of the vulva. In all the cases the vent was insufficient, and defecation more or less difficult. In this form, as in the last, the rectum could be easily reached, and it was opened in all 6 cases. Two different operations have been practised to remedy this imperfection; 1, the enlargement of the original outlet, which was done in two instances; and 2, the establishment of a new anus at the natural site, which was performed in the four other cases. The author, after giving a detailed account of one of the cases in which he had recourse to the latter operation, contrasted the advantages of the two methods.

In cases of imperforate anus in which a passage is successfully established, the retentive functions of the bowel generally exist in sufficient force. Evidence on this point was furnished by several of the cases in the table, and the existence of an external sphincter had been frequently recognized in dissection.

The author, after noticing that in cases of imperforation unreme died by operation, death is sometimes caused by extreme distension and rupture of the colon or the terminal pouch, remarked that the most common causes of death after operation are peritonitis and diffuse inflammation of the areölar tissue. The former is generally produced by a wound of the serous membrane, the latter by the passage of fæcal matter through the tissues of the pelvis, both being chiefly due to faulty methods of operating. He condemned the use of a trocar as a most unsafe instrument, and advocated the plan of drawing down the bowel and attaching it by sutures to the margins of the wound in the skin—an operation first performed by Amussat, in 1835, and since described and recommended by Dieffenbach. The important advantage obtained by it is the securing a lining of mucous membrane for the passage traversed by the fæces. By this means not only are the tendency to contraction, with its consequent miseries and dangers, guarded against, but the early risks of inflammation and fæcal absorption are avoided.

In some instances troubles in defecation have continued after a sufficient passage for the fæces has been fully established, owing to an organic change in the bowel, consequent upon an obstruction of long continuance subsisting after removal of the cause. The author gave an account of some dissections in which the muscular coat of the rectum was found remarkably hypertrophied and its mucous follicles enlarged, and stated that when the vent for the fæces has long remained insufficient, and the bowel has undergone these changes, its expulsive functious become seriously impaired and weakened, and the infant consequently suffers in the same way as adults laboring under stricture of the rectum.

Having investigated the results of the operations performed in the perinæum, the author proceeded to inquire into the degree of success which had followed the operation for opening the colon in the groin and in the loin, to ascertain the inconveniences consequent. upon an anus in these regions, and to estimate the comparative value of the two operations. Colotomy was performed in 21 of the cases in the table—in 14 by the inguinal operation, and in 7 by the lumbar. In 9 of the former an unsuccessful attempt had been made to reach the gut from the perinæum—4 proved fatal and 5 recovered. Of 5 cases in which no previous operation had been performed, 1 only proved fatal and 4 recovered. Of the 9 recoveries after inguinal colotomy, 1 survived only a month, 2 died of cholera within fourteen months, and a fourth was doing well at seventeen months ; a fifth survived three years, and a sixth was doing well at thirteen years of age. M. Rochard had recently given an authentic report of the remaining three ; one died at the age of forty-three ; the two others are alive and well—one at forty-six years of age, the other at forty-three. Of the seven cases in which colotomy was performed in the left loin, attempts had previously been made to open the bowel from the perinæum in five, of which three were fatal. In another fatal case an attempt was made after the lumbar operation. The author related the particulars of a case operated on by himself, in which death was caused by injuries inflicted in the perineal operation before the infant came under his care. Of the two recoveries after lumbar colotomy, one infant lived to the age of seven years, and of the other there was no report more recent than seven weeks, and the child is supposed not to have long survived.

The author considered the two operations in reference chiefly to three questions—the difficulties of the operation, its dangers, and the condition and convenience of the artificial anus. The operation was admitted to be one of greater difficulty in the loin than in the groin ; and after remarking on some of the causes of this, the author noticed the irregularities in the disposition of the colon, which render it impossible to open the bowel in the left loin without wounding the peritoneum, and which prevent the operator finding the colon in the left groin. The author practised both operations on the bodies of twenty infants, and in two he was unable to open the colon in the left groin, in consequence of the colon making a sharp curve and passing over to the right side before reaching the pelvis. In six subjects lumbar colotomy was impossible witnout opening the peritoneum, owing to the colon being attached by a distinct mesentery, and being loose in the abdomen. This serious impediment once occurred to the author in performing lumbar colotomy in a case of imperforate anus. In respect to the dangers of the two operations, the results of the cases in the table were much in favor of colotomy in the groin. The author quoted the description given by Rochard of the condition of the anus in the groin in two patients, who had been operated on many years previously. Both were in good health, and suffered very little inconvenience. One had married and borne children. In all the patients observed by Rochard, prolapsus had taken place from the lower part of the bowel, but it was easily restrained. The author also gave a particular description of a case, which had recently come under his own notice, of an artificial anus in the loin in a boy eight years of age, born with an imperforate anus, the rectum opening into the urethra. The anus was sufficient, but fæces escaped occasionally into the lower part of the bowel, and caused difficulty in micturition. To obviate this difficulty, he had suggested the lodgment of a sponge-plug in the lower opening. The author saw very little to justify a preference for either operation on the ground of the position of the anus ; but the greater difficulties and dangers of lumbar colotomy would induce him in future to select the inguinal operation.

The author controverted the views recently advanced by Huguier in favor of the performance of colotomy in the right groin in preference to the left, and showed by several examinations of the infant subjects that the passage of the colon from the left iliac fossa to the right iliac fossa is not so constant as he states.

In conclusion, he gave particular directions for conducting the operative treatment of imperfections of the rectum, based on the results of this inquiry.—*Brit. Med. Jour.*, September, 1860.

ART. XVIII.—*Wound of the Humeral Artery Cured by Digital Compression.*

IN the *Union Médicale*, of September 18, 1860, a case of wound of the humeral artery, which was cured in forty-eight hours by digital compression, is reported. The wound was inflicted on the 17th of June, and various means were adopted to arrest the hæmorrhage, but without success, before and after entrance into the hospital. On the 22d of June, the limb being threatened with gangrene, amputation was at first thought to be the only remedy; but fortunately the idea of digital compression occurred, and was carried into effect by the *interne* and four sisters of the hospital, each attending for one hour, and alternately relieving one another.

On the 31st of July the patient was discharged from the hospital, cured.

The case was under the care of Dr. Bury, of Saumur (Maine-et-Loire), and was communicated by him, through M. Boinet, to the Society of Surgery, at Paris. In this case, owing to secondary hæmorrhages, the inflammation, and the infiltration of the surrounding tissues with blood and pus, it was deemed impossible to find and tie the wounded artery.   B. D.

MISCELLANEA.

FEMALE PHYSICIANS, MEDICAL COLLEGES, AND MEDICAL ETHICS.

It appears from the *Transactions of the Medical Society of the State of Pennsylvania*, held in Philadelphia, June, 1860, recently published, that the Medical Society of Montgomery county, in the State of Pennsylvania, made a protest against the action of the Philadelphia County Medical Society, and also against the action of the State Society, at its previous annual session, in approving the course of the Philadelphia County Society, in relation to female physicians and colleges The preamble of the Montgomery County Society, as addressed to the State Society, will be given entire, without its appended resolutions, which are too much extended for the space of the Journal ; and for the same reason, the resolutions offered on this topic in the State Society will be omitted, with the exception of the final and sole resolution, " which was unanimously adopted."

" At a meeting of the Montgomery County Medical Society, held in Norristown, May 26, 1860, the following preamble and resolutions were adopted :

"*Whereas*, The Philadelphia County Medical Society has passed a resolution forbidding the members to consult with the Faculties of Female Medical Colleges, the graduates of those institutions, and female practitioners generally; and

"*Whereas*, The Board of Censors of said Philadelphia County Medical Society caused these resolutions to be presented to the State Medical Society at its last meeting—whereupon a committee was appointed to consider them and report thereon, which committee reported that they believed the course pointed out by these resolutions is a consistent one, and such as deserves the sanction of this Society, and they would urge its observance by all the County Societies throughout the State ; therefore, *Resolved*," etc.

On the following day, the State Society, after having considered several resolutions, " unanimously adopted" the following: "*Resolved*, That it is the sense of this Society, that members of the regular profession cannot, consistently with sound medical ethics, consult or hold professional intercourse with the professors or graduates of female medical colleges as at present constituted, inasmuch as some of the professors are irregular practitioners, and all of those colleges are ineligible to representation in the American Medical Association."

As there is no sex in science, so there is no ethical code by which competent female physicians must be excluded from the pale of the profession solely on account of their gender. It is, as a general rule (be that rule right or wrong), inexpedient and contrary to pub-lic opinion for women to enter upon the study and practice of physic. But in what way are the duties of the profession incom-patible with purity of motive, moral excellence, and usefulness of female practitioners, apart from expediency? But what is ethics, medical ethics? Is a violation of æsthetics, *ipso facto*, a violation of ethics?

In his Moral Philosophy, Paley defines ethics as "*that science which teaches men their duty, and the reasons of it.*" Medical ethics is, therefore, that science which teaches medical men their duty, and the reasons of it. In the next place, what is æsthetics?

"Æsthetics. The science which treats of the beautiful, or of the principles of taste." (*Worcester, Quarto Dict.*, 1860.)

Ethical and æsthetical principles, so far from being identical, may be, in some instances which might be named, antithetical. Although a female physician, having an equal education and ability with a male physician, stands equally on the same ethical platform, yet the sanctioned principles of æsthetics, arbitrary though they be, virtu-ally repel her and attract him, when medical aid is asked.

But when a competent female physician, who has been already in attendance, asks, in conformity with the wish of the patient, for a consultation with a male physician, and is refused because he and all his associates are forbidden officially to consult with any one of her sex, a very serious ethical complication arises, hazardous alike to the wellfare of the patient and the dignity, wisdom, and morality of the members of the medical societies. Here advisory, not co-ercive, measures—a judicious discretion, not an unconditional pro-hibition—would seem expedient, just, benevolent. To give univer-sality to a non-consultation rule, as if it were a self-evident principle of morality—as if an exception were impossible—is to deprive a member of his freedom and judgment, while it exposes him to charges for violating a rule, which may lead to his expulsion and disgrace. If what all the world and the American Medical Asso-ciation say concerning the incompetency of the male graduates in medicine, be true, is it not possible that some of the female grad-uates may have, not only equal, but superior qualifications to many of the former? and would it be a violation of any moral principle in the former to consult with such as possessed greater skill than them-selves?

The Code of Ethics of the American Medical Association declares neither the ineligibility of females to membership in that Society, nor forbids consultation with female physicians. The Code says : " No one can be considered a regular practitioner, or a fit associate in consultation, whose practice is based on an exclusive dogma, to the rejection of the accumulated experience of the profession, and of the aids actually furnished by anatomy, physiology, pathology, and organic chemistry."

The isolated fact that female physicians are not members of the American Medical Association, is neither a sin of omission nor commission. If membership in that society be required by medical ethics, to qualify a practitioner for consultations, perhaps forty in every fifty physicians and professors in the Republic would be disqualified, not being members. Many physicians are not members of any medical society; those who are members, cannot be members of the American Medical Association unless they be the elected delegates sent by the medical societies as their representatives in the Association, the number being limited by an act of the Association, which fixes the numerical ratio of representation. Hence no physicians are eligible to membership but the small number of the delegates. Many medical societies are not represented at the annual meetings of the Association. It does not appear that female medical colleges have ever sent delegates to the Association, nor that delegates from such institutions are ineligible. The Code of Ethics is silent on this subject. The enactment of an ethical rule by a local society, forbidding its members to consult with the professors of female colleges (some of whom are males), is an assumption of power which it is difficult to reconcile with the freedom and duty of the physician, or to the rights of chartered female colleges and their graduates, whose education and modes of practice are based on legitimate bases, organized in the same manner, and teaching the same branches and principles as those colleges in which male practitioners graduate. If " some of the professors are irregular practitioners," ought not an exception be made in favor of such as are regular, skillful, and worthy ?

The question is not whether it be culpable to consult with Thompsonians, homœopathists, hydropathists, mesmerists, spiritual-rappers and the like, but whether the practitioner may, in any case, be allowed to consult with an individual having all the evidences of qualification in medicine equally with himself, gender excepted, without being amenable to rebuke, or liable to expulsion from a medical society ? At the least, ought not this question to be left wholly to his own judgment, discretion, and conscience for solution according to the merits of individual cases ? Is not the rule forbidding consultation with all females, regardless of their qualifications and merits, an unnecessary restriction ? an aggression ? an injustice which will react injuriously upon the profession, and give rise to well-grounded charges of prejudice and persecution ? Silence on the part of the faculty and the force of public opinion, will *probably* teach the female doctor sufficiently well the inexpediency of entering upon the duties and difficulties of medical practice, though her motives may be as disinterested as Miss Nightingale's, and her learning as great as that of Madame Boivin, and other authoresses of high authority, particularly in obstetrical medicine.

If, contrary to all expectation, female physicians should obtain the approbation of the public, and consequently a large and lucrative practice, would not the enactment of the rule against consultations with them be quickly rescinded ? Is ethics unstable as the winds ? Is it but the echo of æsthetics ? While the well-wishers of woman should discourage her from entering into the perils of the medical profession, any coersive measures for this purpose will create public sympathy in her behalf, and precipitate movements in the contrary direction, which, there is reason to fear, would promote neither her well being nor that of society.   B. DOWLER.

They do not always "manage these things better in France." We some weeks ago referred to the work of M. Topinard on English Surgery. M. Topinard's countrymen—some of them at least—do not admit the much greater mortality after amputations in Paris than in London. M. Topinard answers by saying that in England he had not the slightest difficulty in collecting the history of 3000 cases of amputation. "All the hospitals of London," he says, "have registers, which are kept by one of the students, or by the *Director*, who is generally a medical man   Many of them print annually a summary of patients treated, etc. The *Medical Times and Gazette* gives a trimestrial *resumé* of all the operations practised in London and in the country. The benefits of this custom and labor are immense. But what opposition I have met with here !   The Administration of Public Charity has refused to allow me to consult its registers, although I was furnished with the best recommendations.   All I have met with is one single statistical account of any importance, by M. Malgaigne, eighteen years old."

We often hear it said, What a pity that we never hear or enjoy in our Medical Societies the brilliant discourses which adorn the French Academy ! This is what a French critic thinks of those elocutional performances : " A strife of words kept up by a confusion of principles ; entire absence of conviction in one party, and extreme narrowness of views in another ; fighting in empty space ; reasonings in a circle ; and false conclusions."

Hydrotherapeutics is all the fashion just now in France. " Here is an ordinary bathing-house, with the device on its doors—'*Traitement hydrothérapique complet*.' There we find a retired tailor ambitious of playing the character of Priessnitz. Then, again, we have a widow who, to make the best use of her park, founds an establishment, which she carries on with the aid of a clientess *Officier de Santé*. Then a thermal establishment, which, after having boasted of the wonderful efficacy of its waters in all diseases—known or unknown— considers it necessary to recommend a new cold spring for douches and lotions to satisfy the taste of all. Besides this, we have an inventor who recommends those about to travel to take with them in their carpet-bag his portative apparatus, complete for all hydrotherapeutie treatment."—*Med. Times and Gaz.*

Mortality Statistics of New Orleans, from August, 1860, to October 14, 1860, compiled from the Weekly Reports politely furnished by Dr. Dirmeyer, Secretary of the Board of Health.

Time.	Total Deaths.	Children under 2 yrs.	Under 20.	U. States.
August (5 weeks)	704	184	298	250
September (4 weeks)	612	157	247	233
October (2 weeks)	254	55	95	92

Principal Diseases.	August (5 weeks).	September (4 weeks).	October (2 weeks)
Apoplexy	14	18	3
Cholera Infantum	5	6	2
Congestion of the Brain	21	8	3
Consumption	74	55	40
Convulsions, Infantile	46	45	22
Croup	7	4	0
Diarrhœa	31	24	11
Dysentery	27	16	7
Diphtheria	7	9	6
Dropsy	6	8	4
Bronchitis	5	9	2
Fever, Miasmatic	70	61	21
" Scarlet	23	9	2
" Typhoid	12	16	6
" Yellow	11	5	0
Gastro-Enteritis	18	11	5
Whooping-Cough	8	7	3
Inflammation of Liver	0	4	3
Inflammation of Brain	4	3	2
Inflammation of Lungs	11	0	2
Marasmus, Infantile	11	12	5
Measles	1	0	0
Pleurisy	1	0	0
Still-born	36	29	21
Sun Stroke	5	2	0
Teething	14	12	5
Tetanus	17	18	7
Trismus Nascentium	4	5	5

To our Subscribers, Correspondents and Contributors.

All payments should be made, and business letters addressed to Drs. CHAILLÉ and NICHOLS, proprietors; and *not* to the publishers; all literary contributions to Dr. BENNET DOWLER.

Office of the Journal at the University Buildings, on Common street, near Baronne street.

Office hour, from 11 to 12 o'clock.

Copies of the Journal may be purchased, and the Journal subscribed for, at J. C. MORGAN & Co.'s, Exchange Place, at BLOOMFIELD, STEEL & Co's Book Store, No. 60 Camp street, and at T. L. WHITE'S, 105 Canal street.

This Journal will be published bi-monthly, each number to contain 152 pages.

The Journal will be sent a second time to those who have not received it one month after the time for its appearance, if the subscriber write that he has not received it.

Those once ordering the Journal to be sent to them, will be considered subscribers until they order its discontinuance, which should be at least two months before they wish it discontinued.

No subscription discontinued unless at the option of the proprietors, until all arrears are paid up.

Numbers of the Journal sent as specimens to gentlemen who are not subscribers, will not be continued, unless a written order to continue it is forwarded, with $5 enclosed for the first year.

Payments should be made to those only who bear the written authorization of one of the proprietors. When sent by mail it will be at the proprietor's risk, if registered as a valuable letter.

No personal matters, unless of general interest to the profession, will be published, except as advertisements, and as such must be paid for.

All communications for publication must bear the signature of the writer.

Original articles should be sent two months in advance, should be written on only *one side of the paper*, and those which are short and practical will be preferred.

Postmasters and Booksellers are requested to act as agents both in collecting debts, and procuring new subscribers. To collect debts a written authority will be forwarded upon their application, and they will be allowed to deduct a liberal percentage on any payments passing through their hands.

The contributors to this Journal can have forwarded, to their address, at small expense, 100 copies or more of their articles, in pamphlet form, provided the order to this effect accompany their articles.

TERMS OF THE JOURNAL—Five Dollars per annum, in advance.

TERMS OF ADVERTISEMENTS—always in advance—

     One page, per annum, $50; one insertion, $10.
     Half page   "   30; "   "   5.
     Quarter page, "   15; "   "   3·

Special arrangements will be made for inserting a few lines, cards, etc.

EDITOR'S OFFICE.—NOTICES.

[Managing Editor's Office and Residence, 89 Constance, between Melpomene and Thalia streets; box 106 D, Post Office; box of the Journal at Mr. Morgan's book store, same place where communications, etc., may be received.]

MARCH, 1860.

NEW MEDICAL JOURNAL.

Louisville Medical Journal: Edited by Thomas W. Colescott, M. D.: John R. Timberlake, M. D., publisher and proprietor. No. 1, Vol. I. Feb., 1860.

BOOKS AND PAMPHLETS RECEIVED.

Observations on some of the Physical, Chemical, Physiological and Pathological Phenomena of Malarial Fever: By Joseph Jones, A. M., M. D., Professor of Medical Chemistry in the Medical College of Georgia, at Augusta. Extracted from the Transactions of the American Medical Association. Pp. 419. 8vo. Philadelphia: 1859. From the Author.

The Retrospect of Practical Medicine and Surgery, being a half-yearly Journal, containing a Retrospective View of every Discovery and Practical Improvement in the Medical Sciences: Edited by W. Braithwaite, Lecturer on Obstetric Medicine at the Leeds School of Medicine, etc. Part XL, for January, 1860. Uniform American Edition. New York: W. A. Townsend & Co.

The Diagnosis, Pathology and Treatment of the Diseases of the Chest: By W. W. Gerhard, M. D., one of the Physicians to the Pennsylvania Hospital; Fellow of the College of Physicians of Philadelphia; Member of the American Philosophical Society, etc. Fourth Edition, Revised and Enlarged. Pp. 448. 8vo. Philadelphia: J. B. Lippincott & Co., 1860. From Messrs. J. C. Morgan & Co., booksellers, Exchange Place, New Orleans. Price $3.

The Obstetric Catechism, containing 2347 questions and answers on Obstetrics Proper: By Joseph Warrington, M. D. One hundred and fifty illustrations. Pp. 445. 12mo. Philadelphia: J. B. Lippincott & Co., 1860. From Messrs. J. C. Morgan & Co., booksellers, Exchange Place, New Orleans. Price $1 50.

Lobelia-ism—Its Prospects and Policy: By J. Dickson Smith, M. D., Macon, Georgia. Pp. 16, 1859.

Elements of Medical Jurisprudence: By Theodore Romeyn Beck, M. D., LL. D., etc., and John B. Beck, M. D, etc. Eleventh Edition, with notes by an association of the friends of Drs. Beck; the whole revised by C. R. Gilman, M. D., Professor of Medical Jurisprudence in the College of Physicians and Surgeons of New York. Vol. 11. Pp. 884 and 1003. 8vo. Philadelphia: J. B. Lippincott & Co., 1860. From Messrs. J. C. Morgan & Co., booksellers, Exchange Place, New Orleans. Price $10.

The Medical Profession and its Claims: By James Bryan, A. M., M. D., Professor of Anatomy. Pp. 25. New York, 1859. From the Author.

Report Eastern Lunatic Asylum. Pp. 39. Frankfort, Kentucky, 1858-9.

Selections from a Report on Ovariotomy: Read before the Kentucky State Medical Society, at its Annual Meeting at Louisville, April, 1857: By J. Taylor Bradford, M. D., Augusta, Kentucky. Pp. 58. 1859.

Report of the Superintendent of the Lunatic Asylum of the State of Texas: Printed by order of the Eighth Legislature. Pp. 12. Austin, 1859.

The Influence of Surroundings: By John T. Hodgen, M. D., Professor of Anatomy and Physiology. Pp. 20. St. Louis, 1859.

Transactions of the Medical Society of the State of Pennsylvania, at its Eleventh Annual Session, held in Philadelphia, June, 1859. New Series—Part IV. Published by the Society. Pp. 120. Philadelphia, 1859.

Annual Report of the Board of Health to the Legislature of the State of Louisiana. January, 1860. Baton Rouge, 1860. From the Board.

First Report of Progress of the Geological and Agricultural Survey of Texas: By B. F. Shumard, State Geologist. Printed by order of the Eighth Legislature. Pp. 17. Austin, 1859. From Dr. W. P. Riddell.

On the Effect of Pressure upon Ulcerated Vertebræ, and in Morbus Coxarius, and the Relief afforded by Mechanical Remedies, with Cases: By H. G. Davis, M. D., No. 67 Union Place, New York. Pp. 8. Reprinted from the New York Journal of Medicine, for November, 1859. New York, 1859.

Inaugural Address delivered at the Opening of Lind University: By N. S. Davis, M. D. Pp. 26. Chicago, 1859.

Minutes of the Tenth Annual Meeting of the Medical Society of the State of North Carolina, held at Statesville, North Carolina, May, 1859. Pp. 28. Wilmington, North Carolina, 1859.

Botany as an Ally of Medicine: By George S. Blackie, M. D., A. M., F. B. S. E., Member of the Medico-Chirurgical Society of Edinburgh, etc. etc. etc., Professor of Botany and Natural History in the University of Nashville, and Assistant Editor of the Nashville Journal of Medicine and Surgery. Pp. 24. Nashville, 1859. From the Author.

On Criminal Abortion in America: By Horatio R. Storer, M. D., of Boston, Member of the American Medical Association. From the North American Medico-Chirurgical Review, January to November, 1859. Pp. 107. Philadelphia: J. B. Lippincott & Co., 1860.

The Half-Yearly Abstract of Medical Sciences: Being a Practical and Analytical Digest of the Contents of the Principal British and Continental Medical Works Published in the preceding Six Months, together with a Series of Critical Reports on the Progress of Medicine and the Collateral Sciences during the same Period: Edited by W. H. Ranking, M. D., Cantab., Physician to the Norfolk and Norwich Hospital; and C. B. Radcliffe, M. D., London, Fellow of the Royal College of Physicians in London, Physician to the Westminster Hospital, and Lecturer on Materia Medica at the Westminster School of Medicine. *Apparatu nobis opus est, et rebus exquisitis undique et collectis, arcessitis, comportatis.*—CICERO. No. 30, from July to December, 1859. Pp. 303. 8vo. Philadelphia: Lindsay & Blakiston, No. 25 South Sixth street, 1860.

Introductory Lectures and Addresses on Medical Subjects, delivered chiefly before the Medical Classes of the University of Pennsylvania: By George B. Wood, M. D., LL. D., President of the American Philosophical Society, President of the College of Physicians of Philadelphia, Professor of the Theory and Practice of Medicine in the University of Pennsylvania, etc. Pp. 460. 8vo. Philadelphia: J. B. Lippincott & Co., 1859. From Messrs. Morgan & Co., booksellers, Exchange Place, New Orleans.

The Transactions of the American Medical Association. Vol. XII. Pp. 722. 8vo. Philadelphia, 1859. Printed for the Association. From Messrs. Morgan & Co , booksellers, Exchange Place, New Orleans.

A Practical Treatise on Inflammation of the Uterus, its Cervix and Appendages, and its Connection with Uterine Disease: By James Henry Bennet, M. D., Member of the Royal College of Physicians, etc. etc. etc. Fifth American Edition, from the Third and Revised London Edition; to which is added a Review of the Present State of Uterine Pathology. Pp. 502. 8vo. Philadelphia: Blanchard & Lea, 1860.

A Practical Treatise on Fractures and Dislocations: By Frank Hastings Hamilton, M. D., Professor of Surgery in the University of Buffalo, Surgeon to the Buffalo Hospital of the Sisters of Mercy, etc. Illustrated with 289 wood cuts. Pp. 757. 8vo. Philadelphia: Blanchard & Lea, 1860.

Therapeutics and Materia Medica—a Systematic Treatise on the Action and Uses of Medicinal Agents, including their Description and History: By Alfred Stillé, M. D., late Professor of the Theory and Practice of Medicine in the Medical Department of the Pennsylvania College, etc. etc. etc. In two vols. 8vo. Pp. I, 813; II, 975. Philadelphia: Blanchard & Lea, 1860.

Suggestions on Medical Education: By Joseph Jones, M. D., Professor of Medical Chemistry and Pharmacy in the Medical College of Georgia. Pp. 26. Augusta, Georgia, 1860.

TABLE OF CONTENTS.

ORIGINAL COMMUNICATIONS.

To our Subscribers, Correspondents and Contributors.

All payments should be made, and business letters addressed to Drs. CHAILLÉ and NICHOLS, proprietors; and *not* to the publishers; all literary contributions to Dr. BENNET DOWLER.

Office of the Journal at the University Buildings, on Common street, near Baronne street.

Office hour. from 11 to 12 o'clock.

Copies of the Journal may be purchased, and the Journal subscribed for, at J. C. MORGAN & Co.'s, Exchange Place, at BLOOMFIELD, STEEL & Co's Book Store, No. 60 Camp street, and at T. L. WHITE's, 105 Canal street.

This Journal will be published bi-monthly, each number to contain 152 pages.

The Journal will be sent a second time to those who have not received it one month after the time for its appearance, if the subscriber write that he has not received it.

Those once ordering the Journal to be sent to them, will be considered subscribers until they order its discontinuance, which should be at least two months before they wish it discontinued.

No subscription discontinued unless at the option of the proprietors, until all arrears are paid up.

Numbers of the Journal sent as specimens to gentlemen who are not subscribers will not be continued, unless a written order to continue it is forwarded, with $5 enclosed for the first year.

Payments should be made to those only who bear the written authorization of one of the proprietors. When sent by mail it will be at the proprietor's risk, if registered as a valuable letter.

No personal matters, unless of general interest to the profession, will be published, except as advertisements, and as such must be paid for.

All communications for publication must bear the signature of the writer.

Original articles should be sent two months in advance, should be written on only *one side of the paper*, and those which are short and practical will be preferred.

Postmasters and Booksellers are requested to act as agents both in collecting debts, and procuring new subscribers. To collect debts a written authority will be forwarded upon their application, and they will be allowed to deduct a liberal percentage on any payments passing through their hands.

The contributors to this Journal can have forwarded, to their address, at small expense, 100 copies or more of their articles, in pamphlet form, provided the order to this effect accompany their articles.

TERMS OF THE JOURNAL—Five Dollars per annum, in advance.

TERMS OF ADVERTISEMENTS—always in advance—

> One page, per annum, $50 ; one insertion, $10.
> Half page   "   30:   "   "   5.
> Quarter page, "   15;   "   "   3·

Special arrangements will be made for inserting a few lines, cards, etc.

EDITOR'S OFFICE—NOTICES.

[Managing Editor's Office and Residence, 89 Constance, between Melpomene and Thalia streets; box 106 D, Post Office; box of the Journal at Mr. Morgan's book store, same place, where communications, etc., may be received.]

MAY, 1860.

NEW MEDICAL JOURNALS.

The San Francisco Medical Press—Edited by E. S. Cooper, A. M., M. D., Professor of Anatomy and Surgery in the Medical Department of the University of the Pacific. San Francisco: 1860. No. I, Jan., 1860. Pp. 64. Quarterly.

Hygienic and Literary Magazine—Edited by M. A. Malsbey. No. 1, Jan., 1860: monthly. Atlanta, Ga.

The British American Journal of the Medical and Physical Sciences—Edited by Archibald Hall, M. D., L. R. C. E., Professor of Midwifery, etc., University of McGill College, Montreal. Monthly.

The Kansas City Medical and Surgical Review—G. M. B. Maughs, M. D., and T. S. Case, M. D., Editors. Jan., 1860: Kansas City, Mo.

BOOKS AND PAMPHLETS RECEIVED.

Clinical Lectures and the Principles and Practice of Medicine—By John Hughes Bennett, M. D., F. R. S. E., Professor of the Institutes of Medicine, and Senior Professor of Clinical Medicine, in the University of Edinburgh, etc., etc., etc. From the last London Edition, with 500 Illustrations on Wood. Pp. 952. 8vo. New York: Samuel S. & William Wood. 1860.

The New American Cyclopædia—Edited by George Ripley and Charles A. Dana. Vol. VIII. Pp. 788. Double columns. Royal 8vo. New York: D. Appleton & Co. MDCCCLX. This excellent work appears with great regularity and celerity. Through Mr. Colman, of New Orleans. [B. D.]

A Monograph upon Aconite—Translated from the German of Dr. Reil, Teacher of Medicine, at Halle. By Henry B. Millard, A. M., M. D. Prize Essay. Pp. 168. 8vo. New York: William Radde. 1860.

Brief Expositions of Rational Medicine—By Jacob Bigelow, M. D., etc., etc., etc. 2d edition. Pp. 69. 12mo. New York: Samuel S. & Wm. Wood. 1860.

Nature in Disease: Illustrated in various Discourses and Essays, to which are added Miscellaneous Writings, chiefly on Medical Subjects—By Jacob Bigelow, M. D., etc., etc., etc. 2d edition, enlarged. Pp 410. 12mo. New York: Samuel S. & Wm. Wood. MDCCCLX.

A Treatise on Medical Electricity, Theoretical and Practical, and its use in the Treatment of Paralysis, etc: By J. Althaus, M. D. Pp. 854. 8vo. Philadelphia: Lindsay & Blakiston. 1860.

A Guide to the Practical Study of Diseases of the Eye, with an Outline of their Medical and Operative Treatment—By James Dixon, F. R. C. S., Surgeon to the Royal London Ophthalmic Hospital, etc. From the 2d London edition. Pp. 425. 8vo. Philadelphia: Lindsay & Blakiston. 1860.

Memoir on the Salubrity of the Isle of Pines—By Don José de la Luz Hernandez, Physician and Surgeon of the Royal House of Beneficencia and Foundling Hospital, Member of the Inspection of Studies of the Islands of Cuba and Porto Rico, etc. Pp. 56. Havana. 1857.

Address to the Anatomical Class of the Philadelphia School of Anatomy—By D. Hayes Agnew, M. D., Lecturer on Anatomy, Surgeon to the Philadelphia Hospital, etc. Pp. 20.

On the Difficulties and Advantages of Catheterism of the Air-Passages in Diseases of the Chest—By Horace Green, M. D., LL. D., etc. Pp. 24. New York: 1860.

Monograph on the Pathology of the Pituitary Body—By Middleton Michel, M. D. Pp. 31. Charleston, S. C.: 1860.

An Epitome of Braithwaite's Retrospect. In five parts. Part I. By Walter S. Wells, M. D. Pp. 304. 8vo. C. T. Evans. New York: 1860.

On the Coagulation of the Blood in the Venous System During Life. By George

TABLE OF CONTENTS.

ORIGINAL COMMUNICATIONS.

PROGRESS OF MEDICINE.

BOZEMAN'S HOSPITAL.

90 BARONNE ST., NEW ORLEANS.

This Institution, but recently established, is designed to be a SURGICAL AND WOMAN'S HOSPITAL, and is not, therefore, open to all classes of disease. In the Male department only such cases as require Surgical treatment or operation, will be admitted. The Female department is open, mainly, to cases of Chronic Disease; and, as regards the privacy, convenience, and comfort, of this class of patients, the arrangements are admirably adapted.

The building is situated in one of the most convenient and pleasant parts of the city. It is large, well ventilated, and has been thoroughly repaired and newly furnished.

Good accommodation for Negroes.

For further information apply to Dr. N. Bozeman (late of Montgomery, Ala.), Attending Physician and Surgeon. May 1y

---

ATLANTA MEDICAL COLLEGE.

THE SIXTH COURSE OF LECTURES in this Institution, will open on the FIRST MONDAY IN MAY NEXT, and continue until the last of the following August.

FACULTY:

ALEXANDER MEANS, M. D., Professor of Chemistry and Pharmacy.
H. W. BROWN, M. D., Professor of Anatomy.
JOHN W. JONES, M. D., Professor of Principles and Practice of Medicine and General Pathology.
W. F. WESTMORELAND, M. D., Professor of Principles and Practice of Surgery.
T. S. POWELL, M. D., Professor of Obstetrics.
J. P. LOGAN, M. D., Professor of Physiology, and Diseases of Women and Children.
J. G. WESTMORELAND, M. D., Professor of Materia Medica and Medical Jurisprudence.

Practical Anatomy under the Direction of the Professor of Anatomy.

J. G. McLIN ....*Janitor.*
N. D'ALVIGNY, M. D.............................*Curator of the Museum.*

Clinical Instruction and Dispensary Prescriptions had regularly, as heretofore, during the course.

The Dissecting Room, furnished with good material, will be open by the 15th of April, for those who wish to dissect before Lectures commence.

FEES:

Matriculation Ticket (taken once only).......................................$ 5
Course of Lectures 105
Dissecting Ticket (required only once)....................................... 10
Diploma 25
Good Board can be had for $3 to $4 per week.
For further information address

J. G. WESTMORELAND, DEAN.

Atlanta, Ga., Feb., 16, 1860. May 2m

TABLE OF CONTENTS.

ORIGINAL COMMUNICATIONS.

PROGRESS OF MEDICINE.

To our Subscribers, Correspondents and Contributors.

All payments should be made, and business letters addressed to Drs. CHAILLÉ and NICHOLS, proprietors; and *not* to the publishers; all literary contributions to Dr. BENNET DOWLER.

Office of the Journal at the University Buildings, on Common street, near Baronne street.

Office hour, from 11 to 12 o'clock.

Copies of the Journal may be purchased, and the Journal subscribed for, at J. C. MORGAN & Co.'s, Exchange Place, at BLOOMFIELD, STEEL & Co's Book Store, No. 60 Camp street, and at T. L. WHITE's, 105 Canal street.

This Journal will be published bi-monthly, each number to contain 152 pages.

The Journal will be sent a second time to those who have not received it one month after the time for its appearance, if the subscriber write that he has not received it.

Those once ordering the Journal to be sent to them, will be considered subscribers until they order its discontinuance, which should be at least two months before they wish it discontinued.

No subscription discontinued unless at the option of the proprietors, until all arrears are paid up.

Numbers of the Journal sent as specimens to gentlemen who are not subscribers will not be continued, unless a written order to continue it is forwarded, with $5 enclosed for the first year.

Payments should be made to those only who bear the written authorization of one of the proprietors. When sent by mail it will be at the proprietor's risk, if registered as a valuable letter.

No personal matters, unless of general interest to the profession, will be published, except as advertisements, and as such must be paid for.

All communications for publication must bear the signature of the writer.

Original articles should be sent two months in advance, should be written on only *one side of the paper*, and those which are short and practical will be preferred.

Postmasters and Booksellers are requested to act as agents both in collecting debts, and procuring new subscribers. To collect debts a written authority will be forwarded upon their application, and they will be allowed to deduct a liberal percentage on any payments passing through their hands.

The contributors to this Journal can have forwarded, to their address, at small expense, 100 copies or more of their articles, in pamphlet form, provided the order to this effect accompany their articles.

TERMS OF THE JOURNAL—Five Dollars per annum, in advance.

TERMS OF ADVERTISEMENTS—always in advance—

        One page, per annum, $50; one insertion, $10.
        Half page   "   30; "   "   5.
        Quarter page, "   15; "   "   3.

Special arrangements will be made for inserting a few lines, cards, etc.

CANSTATT'S JAHRESBERECHT

UBER DIE

Portschritte der Gesammten Medizin in allen Laendern.

"CANSTATT'S YEARLY REPORT ON THE PROGRESS OF MEDICINE IN ALL COUNTRIES."

This Report, founded in the year 1841, is published annually, in seven volumes. The first volume contains the Biological Sciences; the second, the General Pathological Disci,lines; the third, the Diseases of the Different Organs and Systems of the Body; fourth, the Different Diseases, Considered from an Ethiological Point of View; fifth, the Therapeutics and Operative Medicine; sixth, the Veterinary Science; seventh, Forensic Medicine and Statistics.

Annual Subscription Price, $8 in advance.

The Editors of this widely-circulated Journal very much regret that they so seldom receive American medical works, and shall be happy if the American authors will communicate with them. Any works sent to the address of the

STAKELSCHE BACHHANDLUNG,

WUERZBURG, BAVARIA,

will be received with pleasure, and mentioned in their yearly report. [July 1.

EDITOR'S OFFICE—NOTICES.

[Managing Editor's Office and Residence, 96 and 98 Constance, between Melpomenia and Thalia sts. ; box 106 D, Post Office ; box of the Journal at Mr. Morgan's book store, same place, where communications, etc., may be received.]

SEPTEMBER, 1860.

NEW MEDICAL JOURNALS.

The Columbus Review: A Journal of Medicine and Surgery. Bi-Monthly. Edited by W. L. McMillen, M. D. Vol. I, No. 1, August, 1860. Columbus (O). ..

American Medical Times—Being a Weekly Series of the New York Journal of Medicine: Edited by Stephen Smith, M. D.; Associate Editors: Elisha Harris, M. D., and George F. Shrady, M. D. No. 1; Vol. 1. New York, 1860.

BOOKS AND PAMPHLETS RECEIVED.

Annales des Maladies Chroniques (Médecine et Chirurgie) et de l'Hydrologie Médicale—Publiées par le docteur Andrieux, de Brioude. Tome premier. Brioud (Haute-Loire): chez le Rédacteur en Chef: 1860.

The Institutes of Medicine—By Martyn Paine, A.M., M.D. LL.D., Professor of the Institutes of Medicine and Materia Medica in the University of the City of New York; Corresponding Member of the Royal Verein für Heilkunde in Preussen ; Corresponding member of the Gessellschaft für Natur und Heilkunde zu Dresden; Member of the Medical Society of Leipsic; of the Medical Society of Sweden ; of the Montreal Natural History Society ; and of many other Learned Societies. 5th edition. Pp. 1109: 8vo. New York: Harper and Bros., 1859.

Du Laryngoscope et de son emploi en Physiologie et en Médecine—Par le docteur J. N. Czermak, Professeur de Physiologie à l'Université de Pest. Edition Française: publiée avec le concours de l'auteur: accompagnée de 2 planches gravées et de 34 figures intercalées dans le texte. Pp. 102. 8vo. Paris: J.-B. Baillière et Fils: 1860.

The Diseases, Injuries, and Malformations of the Rectum and Anus, with Remarks on Habitual Constipation—By T. J. Ashton, Surgeon to the Blenheim street Dispensary, etc. ; with Illustrations. From the third and enlarged English edition. Pp. 242, in 8vo. Philadelphia: Blanchard & Lea. 1860. From Mr. T. L. White, bookseller, 105 Canal st., N. O.

On Obscure Diseases of the Brain and Disorders of the Mind : their Incipient Symptoms, Pathology, Diagnosis, Treatment, and Prophylaxis—By Forbes Winslow, M. D., D.C.L., etc. Pp. 576, in 8vo. Philadelphia: Blanchard & Lea. 1860. From Mr. T. L. White, bookseller, 105 Canal st., N. O.

A Practical Treatise on Diseases of the Lungs, including the Principles of Physical Diagnosis—By Walter Hayle Walshe, M. D., Professor of the Principles and Practice of Medicine in University Medical College, etc. A new American, from the revised third and much enlarged London edition. Pp. 468, in 8vo. Philadelphia: Blanchard & Lea. 1860. From Mr. T. L. White, bookseller, 105 Canal street, N. O.

Electro-Physiology and Electro-Therapeutics : showing the best Methods for the Medical Uses of Electricity—By Alfred C. Garratt, M. D., Fellow of the Massachusetts Medical Society. Pp. 708, in 8vo. Boston: Ticknor & Fields, 1860. From Mr. T. L. White, bookseller, 105 Canal st. N. O.

Proceedings of the Sixty-Eighth Annual Convention of the Connecticut Medical Society —Held at Hartford, May 23d and 24th, 1860. Pp. 74. 8vo. Hartford: 1860.

The Claims and Position of Physiology—An Anniversary Oration delivered before the So. Ca. Medical Association: February 1, 1860: By J. Dickson Bruns, A. M., M.D., Lecturer on Physiology in the Charleston Preparatory Medical School, etc, etc. Pp. 15. Charleston, S. C.: 1860.

Effects of Disease on the Teeth—By Abr: Robertson, D.D.S., M.D. Wheeling, Va.: 1860.

The Half-Yearly Abstract of the Medical Sciences—Edited by W. H. Ranking, M.D., Cantab., and C. B. Radcliffe, London. Apparatu nobis opus est, et rebus exquisitis undique et collectis, arcessitis, comportatis.—Cicero. Pp. 284 8vo. No. XXXI. January—June, 1860. Philadelphia: Lindsay and Blakiston: 1860.

A Treatise on Fever : its Cause, Phenomena, and Treatment : with an Appendix containing Views on some Female Diseases, some Diseases of Children, etc.—By Rezin Thompson, M. D. Pp. 448, 12mo. Nashville, Tenn. 1860. From the author.

TABLE OF CONTENTS.

ORIGINAL COMMUNICATIONS.

PROGRESS OF MEDICINE.

TABLE OF CONTENTS.

ORIGINAL COMMUNICATIONS.

To our Subscribers, Correspondents and Contributors.

All payments should be made, and business letters addressed to Drs. CHAILLÉ
id NICHOLS, proprietors; and *not* to the publishers; all literary contributions
Dr. BENNET DOWLER.

Office of the Journal at the University Buildings, on Common street, near
ronne street.

Office hour, from 11 to 12 o'clock.

Copies of the Journal may be purchased, and the Journal subscribed for, at
C. MORGAN & Co.'s, Exchange Place, at BLOOMFIELD, STEEL & Co's Book
ore, No. 60 Camp street, and at T. L. WHITE's, 105 Canal street.

This Journal will be published bi-monthly, each number to contain 152 pages.

The Journal will be sent a second time to those who have not received it one
onth after the time for its appearance, if the subscriber write that he has not
eceived it.

Those once ordering the Journal to be sent to them, will be considered sub-
cribers until they order its discontinuance, which should be at least two months
efore they wish it discontinued.

No subscription discontinued unless at the option of the proprietors, until all
rears are paid up.

Numbers of the Journal sent as specimens to gentlemen who are not subscribers
ill not be continued, unless a written order to continue it is forwarded, with $5
closed for the first year.

Payments should be made to those only who bear the   authorization of
no of the proprietors. When sent by mail it will be at   proprietor's risk, if
gistered as a valuable letter.

No personal matters, unless of general interest to the profession, will be pub-
hed, except as advertisements, and as such must be paid for.

All communications for publication must bear the signature of the writer.

Original articles should be sent two months in advance, should be written on
y *one side of the paper*, and those which are short and practical will be preferred.

Postmasters and Booksellers are requested to act as agents both in collecting
ts, and procuring new subscribers. To collect debts a written authority will
forwarded upon their application, and they will be allowed to deduct a liberal
entage on any payments passing through their hands.

e contributors to this Journal can have forwarded, to their address, at small
se, 100 copies or more of their articles, in pamphlet form, provided the order
effect accompany their articles.

MS OF THE JOURNAL—Five Dollars per annum, in advance.

MS OF ADVERTISEMENTS—always in advance—

One page, per annum,	$50;	one insertion,	$10.
Half page	"	30;	"	"	5.
Quarter page,	"	15;	"	"	3.

l arrangements will be made for inserting a few lines, cards, etc.

EDITOR'S OFFICE—NOTICES.

[Managing Editor's Office and Residence, 96 and 98 Constance, between Melpomenia and Thalia st box 106 D, Post Office ; box of the Journal at Mr. Morgan's book store, same place, where communi tions, etc., may be received.]

NOVEMBER, 1860.

On the Theory and Practice of Midwifery : By Fleetwood Churchill, M. D., M. R. I A., Professor of Midwifery, etc., in the King and Queen's College of Physician in Ireland, etc. With Additions, by D. Francis Condie, M. D., author of " ; Practical Treatise on the Diseases of Women and Children," etc. With one hur dred and ninety-four Illustrations. A new American, from the fourth correcté and enlarged English edition. Pp. 655. 8vo. Philadelphia : Blanchard & Le 1860. From Mr. T. L. White, Bookseller, 105 Canal street, New Orleans.

The Principles and Practice af Modern Surgery : By Robert Druitt, Licentiate of tb Royal College c̨ ̄icians, London, etc. A new and revised American, froı the eighth enlä nd improved London edition. With four hundred an thirty-two Illustra . Pp. 695. 8vo. Philadelphia : Blanchard & Lea. 186(From Mr. T. L. Whi.e, Bookseller, 105 Canal street, New Orleans.

Physician's Visiting List, 1861. Philadelphia : Lindsay & Blackiston. From J. C Morgan & Co., Booksellers, Exchange Place, New Orleans.

The Transactions of the Academy of Science of St. Louis : With Plates illustratin Papers. St. Louis, Missouri : 1860. Pp. 527 to 726. From the Academy.

This Fasciculus of two hundred pages is the fourth published by this new an energetic Association, than which, no similar one in this country has in tb̮ incipient stage of existence done more in the same time to win the respect scientific men.

The New York Dental Journal : Edited by Frank H. Norton. July, 1860. ҇ York : W. B. Roberts. 1860.),

Artificial Lactation : By Charles M. Wetherill, PH. D., M. D. Pp. 6. ꜰ

The Anatomy and Physiology of the Placenta. The Connection of the Nervous ḯ of Animal and Organic Life : By John O'Reilly, M. D., Fellow of the . College of Surgeons, Ireland ; Resident Fellow of the New York Acadε Medicine, etc., etc., etc. Pp. 111. 8vo. New York : 1860. From the *ʈ ʳ*

Transactions of the Medical Society of the State of Pennsylvania at its Twelfth Session, held in Philadelphia, June, 1860. New Series : Part V. Pp. 181 lished by the Society. Philadelphia : 1860.

"SILLIMAN'S JOURNAL."

THE AMERICAN
JOURNAL OF SCIENCE AND ARTS.

[TWO VOLUMES ANNUALLY, 450 pp. 8vo.]

Published in numbers *(illustrated)* of 152 pages, every other month, viz: 1st of January, March, May, July, September and November,

AT NEW HAVEN, CONNECTICUT,

BY B. SILLIMAN, JR., AND J. D. DANA,

At Five Dollars per Annum, in Advance.

☞ The Journal is sent *(post paid)* after the annual payment is received.

EDITED BY

Professor B. SILLIMAN, of New Haven,
"   B. SILLIMAN, Jr.,   "
"   JAS. DWIGHT DANA, "

IN CONNECTION WITH

Professor ASA GRAY, of Cambridge,
"   LOUIS AGASSIZ, of Cambridge,
Dr. WOLCOTT GIBBS, of New York.

This work has now been established more than forty years, and is the ONLY JOURNAL of the kind in the United States. It is devoted to the general interests of PHYSICAL and CHEMICAL SCIENCE, GEOLOGY, NATURAL HISTORY, GEOGRAPHY, and kindred departments of knowledge, and contains original papers, as well as abstracts of foreign discoveries, on all these topics.

Seventy-eight Volumes have already been published: FIFTY in the *first* and TWENTY-EIGHT in the *second* Series.

Subscribers receiving their copies direct from the Publishers remit their subscriptions to the Office of SILLIMAN'S JOURNAL, NEW HAVEN, CONNECTICUT.

Most of the back volumes can be obtained of the Publishers.

All communications, remittances, etc., to be addressed to

SILLIMAN & DANA,
OFFICE OF "SILLIMAN'S JOURNAL OF SCIENCE,"
jan. 1y   NEW HAVEN, CONNECTICUT.

To our Subscribers, Correspondents and Contributors.

All payments should be made, and business letters addressed to Drs. CHAILLÉ and NICHOLS, proprietors; and *not* to the publishers; all literary contributions to Dr. BENNET DOWLER.

Office of the Journal at the University Buildings, on Common street, near Baronne street.

Office hour, from 11 to 12 o'clock.

Copies of the Journal may be purchased, and the Journal subscribed for, at J. C. Morgan & Co.'s, Exchange Place, at Bloomfield, Steel & Co's Book Store, No. 60 Camp street, and at T. L. White's, 105 Canal street.

This Journal will be published bi-monthly, each number to contain 152 pages.

The Journal will be sent a second time to those who have not received it one month after the time for its appearance, if the subscriber write that he has not received it.

Those once ordering the Journal to be sent to them, will be considered subscribers until they order its discontinuance, which should be at least two months before they wish it discontinued.

No subscription discontinued unless at the option of the proprietors, until all arrears are paid up.

Numbers of the Journal sent as specimens to gentlemen who are not subscribers, will not be continued, unless a written order to continue it is forwarded, with $5 enclosed for the first year.

Payments should be made to those only who bear the written authorization of one of the proprietors. When sent by mail it will be at the proprietor's risk, if registered as a valuable letter.

No personal matters, unless of general interest to the profession, will be published, except as advertisements, and as such must be paid for.

All communications for publication must bear the signature of the writer.

Original articles should be sent two months in advance, should be written on only *one side of the paper*, and those which are short and practical will be preferred.

Postmasters and Booksellers are requested to act as agents both in collecting debts, and procuring new subscribers. To collect debts a written authority will be forwarded upon their application, and they will be allowed to deduct a liberal percentage on any payments passing through their hands.

The contributors to this Journal can have forwarded, to their address, at small expense, 100 copies or more of their articles, in pamphlet form, provided the order to this effect accompany their articles.

Terms of the Journal—Five Dollars per annum, in advance.

Terms of Advertisements—always in advance—

> One page, per annum, $50 ; one insertion, $10.
> Half page   "   30; "   "   5.
> Quarter page, "   15; "   "   3.

Special arrangements will be made for inserting a few lines, cards, etc.

EDITOR'S OFFICE.—NOTICES.

[Managing Editor's Office and Residence, 89 Constance, between Melpomene and Thalia streets; box 106 D, Post Office; box of the Journal at Mr. Morgan's book store, same place, where communications, etc., may be received.]

JAN., 1860.

Communications have been received from several géntlemen too late for consideration, in reference to the present issue of this Journal.

BOOKS AND PAMPHLETS RECEIVED.

NEW MEDICAL JOURNAL.

The Chicago Medical Examiner. Edited by N. S. Davis, M. D., and E. A. Steele, M. D. Published by William Cravens & Co. Chicago: Monthly: Jan., 1860.

A System of Surgery: Pathological, Diagnostic, Therapeutic and Operative: By Samuel D. Gross, M. D., Professor of Surgery in the Jefferson Medical College of Philadelphia; Member of the American Philosophical Society; Fellow of the College of Physicians of Philadelphia; Corresponding Member of the New York Academy of Medicine, and of the Imperial Royal Medical Society of Vienna; Author of a treatise on the Urinary Organs, etc., etc., etc. Illustrated with 936 engravings; in two volumes. 8vo. Pp. 1162 and 1198. Philadelphia: Blanchard & Lea. 1859. From Prof. T. G. Richardson, M. D.

A Practical Treatise on the Diagnosis, Pathology, and Treatment of Diseases of the Heart; By Austin Flint, M. D., Professor of Clinical Medicine, etc., in the New Orleans School of Medicine; Visiting Physician to the Charity Hospital; Honorary Member of the Medical Society of Virginia, of the Kentucky State Medical Society, of the Medical Society of Rhode Island, of the Pathological Society of Philadelphia, etc. Pp. 473. 8vo. Philadelphia: Blanchard & Lea. 1859. From Mr. T. L. White, bookseller, 105 Canal street, N. O.

[The opinion of one who has not had the necessary leisure to read this volume is doubtlessly valueless. However, the antecedents of this accomplished author as an observer, teacher, thinker and chaste writer, are guarantees that this work is worthy of his well established reputation and of the great subject to which this treatise is devoted.]

The Transactions of the Academy of Science of St. Louis, with numerous illustrated Plates; containing contributions from G. G. Shumard, on Geology of New Mexico; Seyffarth, on Lsed's Mummy Coffin; B. F. Shumard, New Fossils; Sligard, Organitaxis; Engelmann, Diœecious Grasses; Prout, bryozoa; Engelmann, Cuscuta, etc. Vol. I, No. 3. Pp. 305-524. 8vo. 1859. From the Academy.

[This learned society appears to be very energetic and prosperous, being already in active *rapport* with one hundred and eighty-one similar associations in America, Europe, Asia, Africa and Australia, and expending for scientific purposes over $1200 per year without exhausting its treasury.]

Alcohol, its Power and Place: By James Miller, Professor of Surgery in the University of Edinburgh, Surgeon in ordinary to the Queen for Scotland, etc., etc. From the 19th Glasgow edition. Pp. 179. 12mo. Philadelphia: Lindsay & Blakiston. 1859. From J. C. Morgan & Co., booksellers, Exchange Place, N. O.

The Use and Abuse of Tobacco: By John Lizars, late Professor of Surgery to the Royal College of Surgeons, etc. From the 8th Edinburgh edition. Pp. 138. 12mo. Philadelphia: 1859. Lindsay & Blakiston. From J. C. Morgan & Co., booksellers, Exchange Place, N. O.

Description of a Deformed, Fragmentary Human Skull, found in an Ancient Quarry-Cave at Jerusalem; with an attempt to determine, by its configuration alone, the ethnical type to which it belongs: By J. Aitken Meigs, M. D., Professor of the institutes of Medicine in the Medical Department of Pennsylvania College; Physician to the Department of Diseases of the Chest in the Howard Hospital and Infirmary for Incurables]; Corresponding Secretary of the Philadelphia County Medical Society; Member of the Academy of Natural Sciences of Philadelphia; Fellow of the College of Physicians, etc., etc. Pp. 22. Philadelphia: 1859. From the author.

Annual Report of the Smithsonian Institution. Pp. 448. 8vo. Washington: 1859. From the Hon. Mr. Stevens.

Proceedings and Debates of the Third National Quarantine and Sanitary Convention, held in the City of New York, April 27-30, 1859. Pp. 728. 8vo. Document No. 9. New York: 1859. From John H. Griscom, M. D.

[The object of this book is most laudable, namely, to enlighten the public in regard to Quarantine, contagion, sanitary measures, etc. As a City Document, No. 9 is, in its dimensions, worthy the largest city in America. But as an original contribution to science its claims are proportionate neither to its magnitude nor to the reputation of the able and learned members of the National Convention whose opinions and votes it promulgates in so far as the first portion or debates are concerned. The fundamental but inaccessible idea elaborated and diluted by several hundred pages, and sanctioned by an almost unanimous (85 to 6) vote, is sufficiently novel, though not at all probable, namely, that a yellow fever patient cannot, while his clothing (*"fomites!"*) can and does communicate that disease to others. As an *auto da fe*, the burning of rags saturated with blood, excrement and black vomit, is well enough; but costly wardrobes, "purple and fine linen," will, as heretofore, escape cremation. The Appendices are really *the* book. Take from 728 pages, 248 of debates and 39 for banquet toasts, and there will remain 447 for special reports on quarantine, sewerage, and sanitary science which form appendices which are not only creditable to the few gentlemen from whom they emanated, but are, perhaps, the best extant.]

Lectures on Surgical Pathology, Delivered at the Royal College of Surgeons of England: By James Paget, F. R. S., lately Professor of Anatomy and Surgery to the College, Assistant Surgeon and Lecturer on Physiology at St. Bartholomew's Hospital; 2nd American edition. Hypertrophy; Atrophy; Repair; Inflammation; Mortification; Specific Diseases; and Tumors. With numerous illustrations. Pp. 700. 8vo. Philadelphia: Lindsay & Blakiston. 1860. From Messrs. J. C. Morgan & Co., booksellers, Exchange Place, N. O.

[This ingenious work develops not only the general principles of surgery, but also those of medical pathology, and is, at the same time, rich in practical suggestions adapted to special diseases.

An Essay on the Climate and Fevers of the South - Western, Southern Atlantic and Gulf States: By James C. Harris, M. D., of Wetumpka, Ala. Pp. 32 New Orleans: 1858. From the author.

Pathological and Practical Observations on Diseases of the Alimentary Canal, Œsophagus, Stomach, Cæcum and Intestines; By S. O. Habershon, M. D., London; Fellow of the Royal College of Physicians; Assistant Physician to Guy's Hospital, etc. Pp. 312. 8vo. Philadelphia: Blanchard & Lea. 1859. From Mr. T. L. White, bookseller, 106 Canal street, N. O.

Researches on Primary Pathology and Laws of Epidemics: By M. L. Knapp, M. D., Member of the Medical and Chirurgical Faculty of Maryland; late Professor of Materia Medica, and President of the College of Physicians and Surgeons of the University of Iowa; late Professor of Midwifery and Diseases of Women and Children in Rush Medical College; Author of Lectures on the Science of Life Insurance, etc. Two vols. Pp. 312 and 336. 8vo. Philadelphia: Published by the Author. 1858. From the Author.

An Introduction to Pharmacy: Designed as a text book for the Student and as a guide for the Physician and Pharmaceutist: By Edward Parrish, Principal of the School of Practical Pharmacy, etc.: 2nd edition; with 246 illustrations. Pp. 720. 8vo. Philadelphia: Blanchard & Lea. 1859. From Mr. T. L. White, bookseller, 105 Canal street, New Orleans.

[This edition, now much enlarged, is one of the most useful books of the past year.]

A Practical Treatise on Operative Dentistry; By J. Taft, Professor of Operative Dentistry in the Ohio College of Dental Surgery: with illustrations. Pp. 383. 8vo. Philadelphia: Lindsay & Blakiston. 1859. From Mr. T. L. White, bookseller, 105 Canal street, New Orleans.

A System of Dental Surgery: By John Tomes, F. R. S., Dentist to the Dental Hospital of London and to the Middlesex Hospital: With 207 illustrations. Pp. 686. 8vo. Philadelphia: Lindsay & Blakiston. 1859. From Mr. T. L. White, bookseller, 105 Canal street, New Orleans.

[These two dental works, if one may judge of their merits by glancing at their contents, must be excellent; at all events, their typographical execution is greatly superior to the average of those books which are printed for doctors of medicine.]

The New American Cyclopædia: A Dictionary of General Knowledge: Edited by George Ripley and Charles A. Dana. Vol. VII. *Edward-Fueros.* Pp. 786. Double columns. Royal 8vo. New York: D. Appleton & Co., 346 and 348 Broadway. London: 16 Little Britain. 1859. Through Mr. Colman, agent.

[Impartial, lucid, scholarly, compendious, reliable, practical, fresh, and American in aim and execution, this work abounds in knowledge which must interest the physician, in science, art, literature, philosophy, biography, chemistry, medicine, surgery, etc. The names of more than two hundred able contributors to the first five volumes have already transpired, among whom are not a few medical gentlemen: Drs. Brown-Séquard, J. W. Francis, C. R. Gilman, H. Goadby, A. A. Gould, A. A. Hayes, S. Kneeland, E. R. Peaslee, N. P. Rice, J. Wynne, and others.]

Method of Education: By J. H. Watters, M. D., Professor of Physiology and Medical Jurisprudence in the St. Louis Medical College. Pp. 20. St. Louis: 1859.

The Annual Report of the Supervisors and Superintendent of the Mississippi State Lunatic Asylum. Pp. 29. Jackson: 1859.

Fifth Annual Report to the Legislature of South Carolina, relating to the Registry and Returns of Births, Marriages and Deaths, for the year ending December 31, 1858. By Robert W. Gibbes, Jr., M. D., Registrar. Pp. 94. Columbia, S. S. 1859. From the author.

The Subjective and Objective Influences of Medicine: By E. B. Haskins, M. D., Professor of the Principles and Practice of Medicine. Pp. 23. Nashville, Tenn.: 1859.

Records of Daily Practice: A Scientific Visiting List for Physicians and Surgeons. New York: Baillière Brothers, 440 Broadway.

TO OUR SUBSCRIBERS.

Our subscribers are hereby notified that JAS. DEERING, and his assistants, are the only general agents authorized to collect for the New Orleans Medical and Surgical Journal, for the year ending December 31, 1861. His authority to collect is limited to the States of Louisiana, Mississippi, Arkansas, Tennessee, Alabama, Georgia, Florida and South Carolina, and to accounts due for three years or more.

To postmasters and others the bills of those subscribers who may reside in their towns or counties are sometimes entrusted, but in all such cases they have our written authority to collect, specifying the names of our debtors, with the amounts due by each.

Any payments due to us which may be paid to parties not indicated above, will be at the subscriber's risk.

Bank bills current at par in the subscriber's State will be received in payment, and if forwarded by mail in letters registered "valuable," will be at the risk of

DRS. CHAILLÉ & NICHOLS,

Proprietors of the N. O. Medical and Surgical Journal.

TO OUR TEXAS SUBSCRIBERS.

Those of our subscribers in Texas who have receipts for subscription to this Journal, and signed by J. D. Hudgins, will please inform the proprietors, giving the date of such receipt, the amount paid, and to what time credited.

J. D. Hudgins held no authority from us to collect, but was authorized by D. Richardson, of Galveston, who was our agent for the year 1859. His receipts are' therefore, good; but as he has failed to render any account to Mr. Richardson, the latter will, therefore, be unable to render to us a proper account, unless those of our subscribers who hold J. D. Hudgin's receipt report to us the fact.

DRS. CHAILLÉ & NICHOLS,

Proprietors of the N. O. Medical and Surgical Journal.

☞ The obituary notice of Dr. A. B. McWhorter has been crowded out for want of space.

TABLE OF CONTENTS.

ORIGINAL COMMUNICATIONS.

ANNUAL ·CIRCULAR

OF THE

MEDICAL DEPARTMENT

OF THE

UNIVERSITY OF LOUISIANA.

SESSION OF 1860–61.

NEW ORLEANS:
PICAYUNE PRINT, 66 CAMP STREET.
1860.

University of Louisiana.

BOARD OF ADMINISTRATORS.

HIS EXCELLENCY T. O. MOORE,

GOVERNOR OF LOUISIANA.

HON. E. T. MERRICK,

CHIEF JUSTICE OF LOUISIANA.

HON. J. T. MONROE,

MAYOR OF THE CITY OF NEW ORLEANS.

EX-OFFICIO.

HON. T. G. HUNT.

DANIEL EDWARDS.

JOHN PEMBERTON.

J. AD. ROZIER.

WM. R. MILES.

ROBERT J. WARD.

ISAAC J. SEYMOUR.

NEWTON RICHARDS.

MEDICAL FACULTY.

JAMES JONES, M. D.,

PROFESSOR OF THE THEORY AND PRACTICE OF MEDICINE.

WARREN STONE, M. D.,

PROFESSOR OF SURGERY.

J. L. RIDDELL, M. D.,

PROFESSOR OF CHEMISTRY.

A. H. CENAS, M. D.,

PROFESSOR OF OBSTETRICS, AND OF THE DISEASES OF
WOMEN AND CHILDREN.

GUSTAVUS A. NOTT, M. D.,

PROFESSOR OF MATERIA MEDICA AND THERAPEUTICS.

T. G. RICHARDSON, M. D.,

PROFESSOR OF ANATOMY.

L. M. LAWSON, M. D.,

PROFESSOR OF CLINICAL MEDICINE.

THOMAS HUNT. M. D.,

PROFESSOR OF PHYSIOLOGY AND PATHOLOGY.

DEMONSTRATORS OF ANATOMY.

S. E. CHAILLE, M. D.
W. C. NICHOLS. M. D.

University of Louisiana.---Medical Department.

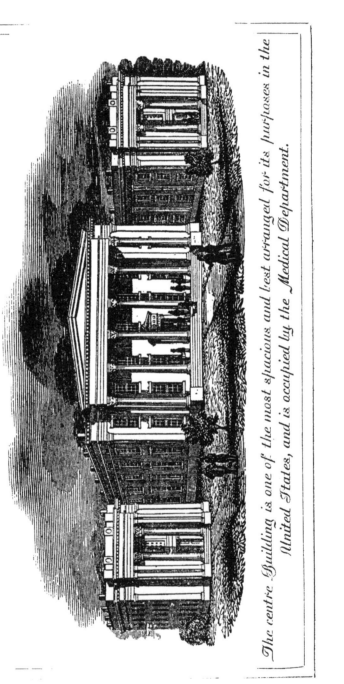

The centre Building is one of the most spacious and best arranged for its purposes in the United States, and is occupied by the Medical Department.

University of Louisiana.

MEDICAL DEPARTMENT.

The Annual Course of Lectures in this Department will commence on Monday, the 12th of November, 1860, and terminate in March, 1861.

Preliminary Lectures will be delivered daily in the Amphitheatre of the Hospital, from the 1st of October, on Clinical Medicine and Surgery and other subjects, without any charge to Students.

In 1859—'60, there were four hundred and two Marticulates, and one hundred and thirteen Graduates in the Department.

The Students of the Class were from Louisiana, Mississippi, Alabama, Texas, Arkansas, Tennessee, Kentucky, Florida, South Carolina, North Carolina, Georgia, Virginia, Missouri, Choctaw Nation, New York and Ohio.

The Faculty announce to the public the continued prosperity of the Medical College of Louisiana.

Three thousand five hundred and sixty names are on the Register of Marticulates.

The College is endowed by the State.

Professor L. M. Lawson has been appointed by the Faculty to deliver a course of Clinical Lectures in this Institution, during the session of 1860—61.

Professor Lawson has already acquired great reputation as a practical teacher of Clinical Medicine.

The Faculty confidently trust, that his labors hereafter will redound to the advantage of this Department, and to the advancement of science.

MUSEUM.

The Museum of Anatomy is extensive. The preparations are chiefly works of Scientific artists in England, France and Italy.

In Human and Comparative Anatomy there are:—

I.—A collection of Muscular preparations, from the Academy of Anatomy at Florence. They represent more than three hundred and fifty separate dissections:

II.—Thibert's Tableaux of the Microscopic Anatomy of the Tissues:

III.—Auzou's Cabinet of Human and Comparative Anatomy:

IV.—A Cabinet of Human Bones, and a collection in Comparative Osteology:

V.—Preparations in Wax, representing the Anatomy of the Viscera; of the Nervous and Vascular Systems; and of every organ in the human body.

The Pathological Department is enriched by models from England and France, which represent diseases of the Eye and diseases of the Skin; and, by a great number of specimens of Urinary and Biliary Calculi, obtained from Dupuytren's Museum, at Paris; from the College of Surgeons, London, and from amongst ourselves.

The models of the diseases of the Skin were made by Mr. Towne, of Guy's Hospital, London. They are perfect, and disease can be studied with their aid almost as well as in nature.

Besides the collections brought from Europe, the Museum contains preparations made by members of the faculty, and others presented by their scientific brethren.

The Pathological collection of Bones is excellent.

The other specimens of Pathological Anatomy are highly interesting and instructive.

CHARITY HOSPITAL.

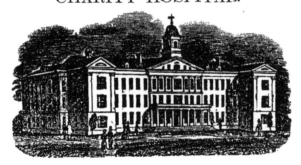

CLINICAL INSTRUCTION.

The number of Admissions into the Hospital in 1859 was 12,775.

The number of Medical cases treated during the last year in the Hospital was about 9,400; the Surgical patients numbered 2,700; and the Obstetrical cases, and those of special diseases of Women and Children, numbered about 675. The number of births was 110.

The College presents opportunities to Students unsurpassed by any institution in the world. The Act which established the University of Louisiana, gives the Professors of the Medical Department the use of the Charity Hospital as a school of practical instruction.

There are about 750 cases usually in the wards of the Charity Hospital. The Professors visit every morning, between 8 and 10 o'clock, the Medical, Surgical and Obstetrical wards, prescribe and make Clinical remarks.

The Students of this Department are taught at the bed-side the nature and treatment of diseases—the modes of examining patients—the practical uses of Auscultation, Percussion, Mensuration, Palpation, and the uses of the Microscope and other instruments, and of Chemical reägents.

The facilities of the Charity Hospital, for professional study, have, after a long series of years of assiduous labor, been improved, and, almost fully developed by the Faculty. So that, in this Hospital, we have in New Orleans a practical School of Medicine and of Surgery, which will bear a favorable comparison with St. Bartholemew's of London, or Hotel Dieu of Paris.

There is no great City of the World which can boast of an institution, where the Student visits every form of disease so unrestrictedly as in the Charity Hospital—where he can so familiarly look disease in the face.

In Rome, Vienna, Paris, London and other justly celebrated Capitals famed for Medical Science and instruction, in Great Britain and in Continental Europe, the Student, at a respectful distance, accompanies the Professor in his visits, listens to his speech, looks at the patients in bed arranged as tableaux, and is favored with glimpses of the picture-like representations of the various forms and phenomena of disease. The Professor informs him of the condition of the pulse, the respiration, the temperature of the body, and of the signs and symptoms which occur during disease, and which the Master observes.

But the pupil cannot place his hand upon the patient—he cannot question him to satisfy his own mind—he is not permitted to speak aloud—and he is excluded from visiting patients except in the presence of his teachers.

In New Orleans the Student can visit patients in the Charity Hospital from morning until night, and devote his talents and industry to the study of every disease in the wards. He can question and examine for himself, that he may the better learn, and resolve his doubts of knowledge.

Members of the Classes of the Medical Department have gratuitous admission to the Hospital, and to all Lectures in the Hospital.

Attendance on cases of Labor in the Obstetrical wards is provided for by the Professor of Obstetrics, from among the candidates for Graduation.

The Professor of Surgery performs operations and dressings in the presence of the Students in the Amphitheatre of the Hospital; and here Lectures are delivered on Wednesday and Saturday of every week, on Clinical Medicine and Surgery, on special Pathological Anatomy, on Physical Diagnosis, and on Auscultation and Percussion.

Post Mortem examinations are also made in presence of the Class.

LECTURES.

I.—The Professor of Anatomy Lectures six days of every week during the session.

II.—The Professor of Physiology and Pathology Lectures five days of every week.

III.—The Professor of the Theory and Practice of Medicine Lectures six days of every week.

IV.—The Professor of Surgery Lectures six days of every week.

V.—The Professor of Obstetrics Lectures four days of every week.

VI.—The Professor of Materia Medica and Therapeutics Lectures four days of every week.

VII.—The Professor of Chemistry Lectures four days of every week.

VIII.—The Professor of Clinical Medicine Lectures six times a week.

The Professors have every thing deemed necessary to aid them in teaching the various branches of Medical Science, viz:

1.—Chemical and Philosophical Apparatus, of modern style.

2.—Specimens of Materia Medica and Chemical products.

3.—Surgical Instruments.

4.—Paintings, Plates, Models, Drawings, Books, and Special Apparatus.

The Medical Department of the University of Louisiana affords the Student ample means of acquiring knowledge of the causes, nature and treatment of diseases peculiar to our climate, and to negroes.

CANDIDATES FOR THE DEGREE OF DOCTOR OF MEDICINE.

I.—The Candidate must be twenty-one years of age, of moral character, and must have studied medicine three years.

II.—He must have attended two full Courses of Lectures, the last of which must have been in this Institution.

III.—He must write a Thesis on a Medical subject, and present it to the Dean one month before the close of the session.

IV.—He must be examined by the Faculty.

The Rooms for Practical Anatomy will be open from the Second Monday in October to the First of April; and from 7 P. M., to 10 P. M., the Demonstrators will be constantly in attendance, for the purpose of instructing the Students.

2

Graduates of respectable schools will be admitted to the course without charge except for Matriculation.

Students who desire further information will address themselves to the Dean.

THOMAS HUNT, M. D., Dean.

NEW ORLEANS, July 1st, 1860.

TERMS:

FOR THE TICKETS OF ALL THE PROFESSORS...$110 00
FOR THE TICKET OF PRACTICAL ANATOMY..... 10 00
MATRICULATION........................... 5 00
DIPLOMA................................. 30 00

☞ FEES FOR TICKETS REQUIRED IN ADVANCE.

Boarding for Students is as cheap in New Orleans as in any other large city in the Union. The Janitor, Mr. P. Borge, will aid the Students in procuring Boarding and Lodging. His residence is in the Medical College of the University buildings, Common street, between Baronne and Philippa streets.

☞ The Administrators of the Charity Hospital elect annually, in April, fourteen Resident Students, who are maintained by the Institution

University of Louisiana.

MEDICAL DEPARTMENT.

SESSION, 1859-60.

STUDENTS.

A

ALSTON, ALFRED A.	Ala.
ANDREWS, CONSTANTINE	La.
ABINGTON, THOMAS W.	La.
ARTHUR, JOHN	La.
AVENT, BENJ. J. A.	Miss.
AUSTIN, RICHMOND P.	Miss.
ALFORD, J. J. (M. D.)	Miss.
ALFORD, S. S.	Miss.
ATMAR, R. M.	Texas.
ABERNETHY, JONES C.	Ala.
ASHTON, WM. H. (M. D.)	Ky.

B

BRADLEY, EDWARD G.	Ark.
BENSON, WALKER S.	Ark.
BRAGG, JUNIUS N.	Ark.
BARBOT, J. C. (M. D.)	La.
BETTES, ALFRED Y.	Ala.
BOURROUM, ANDREW J.	Miss.
BONNEAU, EDWIN A.	Ala.
BELLIN, D. H.	La.
BRIDGES, WALTER L.	Miss.
BALDWIN, JAS. A.	Ark.
BAIN. S. NORVIL	Miss.
BAPTIST, WM. H. (M D.)	Ala.
BUSBY, JOHN J. B.	La.
BONNER, S. L.	Ala.
BLACKSHEAR, JOHN	Texas.
BOOTH, D. W.	Miss.
BUSH, WILLIAMS D.	Ala.
BRACK, J. H.	Miss.
BRUMBY, L. L.	La.
BURKE, SOMERVILLE,	Miss.
BELL, W. T.	Ala.

BLAXOM, J. H. (M. D.)	Miss.
BUCKNER, PRESTON E.	La.
BATCHELOR, T. N.	Miss.
BENSON. BENJ. L.	La.
BRADFIELD, K. G. (M. D.)	Texas.
BAILEY, GEO. H.	Texas.
BATES, C. C.	La.
BADGER, GEO.	N. C.
BRAND, P. S.	La.
BOND, MARSHALL F.	Miss.
BREVARD, E. A.	Fla.
BOND, THOS. J. (M. D.)	Choc. Nation.
BROWN, D. C.	La.
BRYAN, JAMES H. (M. D.)	Ga.
BROWN, BENJ. F.	La.
BROWN, ALEX. PORTER (M. D.)	La.
BROCK, A. G.	Miss.
BANKS, JNO. T. (M. D.)	Ga.
BRITTON, EDW. W.	Texas

C

CHAMBERS, SIDNEY R.	La.
CAMPBELL, J. G.	La.
CURELL, C. M.	La.
CAMERON, JOHN	Texas.
CLOUD, JAS. M.	Miss.
COOK, THOS. B.	Miss.
CAGE, A. H. (M. D.)	Miss.
CARR, ROBERT T.	La.
CUNNINGHAM, WM. H.	Miss.
COLLINS, JOHN W.	Ala.
CROWELL. BENJ. F.	Ala.
CRAIN, PENN	La.
CAULFIELD, WM. J.	Miss.
COOK, JAMES V.	Miss.
CAGE, CHAS. C.	La.

STUDENTS.

CONWAY, CHAUNCEY P. — Miss.
CASTON, SAMUEL N. — Miss.
CLOW, ALBERT B. — La.
CLARK, THOMAS C. — Miss.
COLLINS, O. L. — La.
COOPER, J. C. (M. D.) — La.
COMPTON, JOHN S. — La.
CARROLL, S. D. — Miss.
COWAN, CHAS. G. (M. D.) — Miss.
CUNY, S. E. — La.
CALLOWAY, W. R. (M. D.) — Texas.
CARTER, H. M. (M. D.) — Mo.
CARLEY, J. H. (M. D.) — Ala.
COLE, D. R. (M. D.) — Texas.
CHRISMAN, P. D. (M. D) — La.

D

DAVIS, WILLIAM L. — Miss.
DAVIS, ROBERT — La.
DAVIS, S. R. (M. D) — Miss.
DINKINS, JOE R. — Miss.
DELEE, A. S. — La.
DUFFEL, M. O. E. — La.
DAVIS, JNO. P. — Miss.
DUNN, CHARLES W. — Miss.
DAVIDSON, A. L — La.
DICKEY, EUGENE A. — La.
DEEN, R. M — Miss.
DAVIS, JAMES M. — Ala.
DAILEY, WM. E., Jr., — Texas.
DUGAN, P. B. — Miss.
DALE, W. B. — Ala.
DAVIS, W. G (M. D.) — Miss.
DENMAN, MOSES R. — Texas.
DOUGHARTY, C. M. (M. D.) — Miss.
DAVIS, W. O. (M. D.) — La.
DOWNER, RIALDO J. — La.

E

EGAN, AUGUSTUS W. — La.
EAST, AUGUSTUS L. — La.
EZELL, CHRISTOPHER P. — Ala.
ELLIOTT, JNO. N. — Miss.
ELLIOTT, EBEN — Ohio.
EDDINS, JESSE S. — Texas.

F

FOSTER, JAMES T. — Ark.
FORD, PETER R. — Ark.
FINLEY, WM. P. (M. D.) — Miss.
FAULKNER, SAM H. — La.
FERGUSSON, W. F. — Ga.
FOWLER, VOLNEY D. — Miss.
FLOURNOY, LUCIEN — La.
FLYNT, A. — Texas.
FARR, G. W. — Ala.
FOURNIER, E. H. (M. D.) — Texas.
FRAZER, J. W. — Ark.
FROST, JOHN — Miss.
FORR, ELLY (M. D.) — La.

G

GAUDET, OSCAR — La.
GARRETT, FONTAINE D. — Miss.
GORDON, GILBERT — Miss.
GOLDSBY, MILES W., Jr., — La.
GUERRANT, JOHN WILLIAM — Tenn.
GRIFFIN, ERASMUS F. — Miss.
GILMORE, JOHN W. — Ala.

GIVENS, ALONZO (M. D.) — Miss.
GAVIN, ABSALOM H. — Miss.
GRIFFITH, JAS. E. — Miss.
GODBOLD, WM. L. — Miss.
GINN, JOHN B. — Miss.
GAMBLE, WM. G. — Ala.
GILBERT, F. M. — Miss.
GAHAGAN, O. P. — La.
GREENING, SWEPSON W. — La.
GARDNER, JOHN J. — La.
GIBSON, CHAS. N. — Miss.
GUICE, D. H. — Miss.
GRAHAM CHARLES M. — Texas.
GRACY, J. A. — Tenn.
GATLIN, BINGAMAN F. — Miss.
GUICE, NAPOLEON L. (M. D.) — Miss.
GOODWYN, E. MYDDLETON — S. C.
GILBERT, J. M. — Miss.
GUICE, WM. M. — La.
GASKING, W. A. — La.
GIRGSBY, E. O. (M. D.) — Miss.
GRAVES LEANDER M. — Miss.

H

HOWELL, J. B. — La.
HURD, SETH R. — La.
HILL, CHARLES W. — Miss.
HARALSON, HENRY — Ark.
HIX, JAMES M. — Miss.
HALL, WILLIAM H. — Ala.
HALL, ROBERT A. — Miss.
HOGG, JOHN T. — Texas.
HUNT, LEANDER G. — N. C.
HAYDER, JAMES — Ark.
HARVEY, LEWIS C. — Miss.
HUNT, JAMES M. — Miss.
HOLLIS, HUGH — Tenn.
HICKS, JOHN R., Jr., — Miss.
HARRIS, WILL. V. — Miss.
HOLLONQUIST, R. L. — Ala.
HOLT, THOS. T. — Ala.
HAMILTON, JEFFERSON — La.
HIGDON, DANIEL — La.
HADEN, JAMES E. — Texas.
HOGG, DIXON H. L. — Texas.
HOLDEN, JOHN E. — Miss.
HILLS, THOS. L. — La.
HAYES, WM. H. — Miss.
HARRIS, R. B P. — Miss.
HOLLIDAY, TITUS T. — Miss.
HOWARD, R. G. (M. D.) — La.
HOLCOMBE, JAS. M. — Ark.
HOWE, A. T. (M. D.) — La.
HANNA, WM. S. — Ark.
HEARD, N. A. — Ala.
HICKMAN, C. A. — La.
HERRICK, S. S. — Miss.
HOBSON, O. A. — Miss.
HANNIS, J. — La.
HOOPER, E. M. — La.
HENDERSON, F. B. (M. D.) — Ala.
HILL, D. P. C. — La.
HAWTHORN, WASHINGTON A. — La.
HARRIS, ROBERT L. — Texas.
HOPE, ELAM J. — Miss.
HARWOOD, THOS. B. — Ala.
HEWSON, D. C. (M. D) — Texas.
HAYNES, SAM. B. — La.

STUDENTS.

HAMLIN, CHAS. (M. D.)	La.	McGRAW, A. E.	Ala.
HOLMORN, JNO. T	Miss.	McALPIN, AURELIUS E.	Ark.
		McCLANAHAN, THOS. W.	Texas.
J		MYERS, M. M.	S. C.
JONES, CLEMENT F., Jr.	La.	McCORMICK, HAYFIFLD (M. D.)	La.
JARRATT, ASHBURY L.	Miss.	MERRITT, W. T. (M. D.)	Va.
JONES, JAMES A. (M. D.)	La.	MOSS. WM. A.	La.
JOHNSON. FRANKLIN G.	Miss.	MURPHY, WM. C.	Ala.
JONES, JOHN W.	La.	McDADE, GEO. H.	La.
JACKSON, JAMES W.	La.	MONTGOMERY, JOHN R.	La.
JORDAN. JOHN	Tenn.	MILLS T. L. (M. D.)	La.
JANUARY. DERICK P., Jr.,	La.	MEREDITH, DEMPSEY C.	La.
JONES. VIRGINIUS E.	Miss.	McCREARY, JOHN A.	Ala.
JOHNSON. JAMES T.	Ala.	McKEMLEY, SAMUEL E. (M. D.)	La.
JONES FRANKLIN N.	La.	McGREGOR. THOS.	La.
JENKINS, J. PURVIS	La.	MORGAN, WM. H.	Miss.
		McCLOUD, H. C.	Miss.
K		MEANS, JAMES T.	La.
KNIGHT, J. W.	Texas.		
KENNEDY, NATHAN B.	Ala.	**N**	
KIDD, EUGENE M.	La.	NEAL, VANDY M.	Ala.
KIOLIN, A. C.	Ga.	NUCKOLLS, JOHN M.	Ala.
KENNEDY, J. T.	La.	NEILY, ROBERT M.	Miss.
KIDD. W. J.	La.	NAUL, JESSE W.	La.
KIRKLAND, THOS. J.	Texas.	NAILER. FRANK	Miss.
KENNEDY, WM. H. (M. D.)	Ala.	NIX, REUBEN FITZGERALD	Ala.
KING, WM. B.	Miss.	NOEL, SAMUEL S.	Miss.
KEARNES, CHAS. W.	La.		
KENNON, CHAS. E.	La.	**O**	
KNOWLES, JAS. B. (M. D.)	Ga.	OSWALD, JAS. W. (M. D.)	La.
KIDD ALGERNON G.	Ala.	OFFUT, WM. (M. D.)	La.
L		**P**	
LASCH, JOHN J.	La.	PELAIS, CHAS.	La.
LAROONA, R. T. X. M.	La.	PURVIANCE, JAS. Jr.,	La.
LUCKETT, R. L.	La.	PROFILET, L. E.	Miss.
LAWERY, AUSTIN G.	Miss.	PERDUE, JAMES YANCY	Ark.
LAMBERT, NUMA (M. D.)	La.	PORTWOOD. WM. A.	Miss.
LEWIS, SAMUEL PETE	Miss.	PHILLIPS, JACK	Ala.
LUCKETT, SHERROD G.	Miss.	PARKER, SAMUEL	Ala.
LUTHER, JOHN G. M.	Miss.	PARKER, DANIEL	Ala.
LIVINGSTON, W. P.	Ark.	POSEY, GEORGE W.	Ala.
LEWIS ERNEST S.	La.	PITT, J. S.	Ala.
LITTLE, JEFF. J.	Miss.	PROSSEY, LAWRENCE H.	Miss.
LANDRY, FLORIAN T.	La.	PERRY, O. H.	La.
LETCHER, F. MARION	Ala.	PARKER, LEWIS A.	La.
LEE, ROBERT A.	Ala.	PASSMORE, B. F.	Miss.
LEE, WM. J.	Ala.	PRUITT, SAMUEL	Ala.
LANEUVILLE, JOS. ALEXIS		POST, C. C.	Miss.
LEA, WILLIAM J.	Miss.	PARMLY. SAMUEL P.	Ohio.
LYONS, RAPHAEL	La.	PICKERING, GEO. W. (M. D.)	La.
LEWIS, WALTER	Texas.	PACKWOOD, R. T.	N. Y.
LANE, ROBERT G.	Texas.	PURNELL, HORTENSIUS H.	Miss.
LYON, AUGUSTINE A.	Miss.	PERCY, J. ROWAN (M. D.)	Miss.
LUCAS, JOHN H.	Miss.		
		Q	
M		QUINNEY, R. (M. D.)	Texas.
MORGAN, HENRY W. (M. D.)	La.		
MORRISON, CHARLES M.	Miss.	**R**	
McLEOD, ALEX. G.	Fla.	RIDDELL, SANFORD S.	La.
MARTIN, JAMES	Miss.	RICHARDSON, W. H.	La.
McFARLAND, DUNCAN	Miss.	RUSSELL, JOHN, P.	Ark.
MADDOX, WILLIAM E.	Texas.	ROBERTS, JNO. P. (M. D.)	Ark.
McCUSEL, WM. HARRISON	Tenn.	ROBY, JAMES R.	Miss.
MARSHALL, NAPOLEON B.	Ark.	RICHARDSON, LEMUEL	Miss.
MOODY. ROBERT F.	Ala.	RAINEY, FRANK	Texas.
MARKS, THOS. M.	La.	ROBERTSON, WM. ALLEN	La.
MANERING, THOMAS	La.	ROGERS, WM. J.	Ark.
MURPHY, RUFUS J.	Miss.	RUSHING, F. M.	Ala.
		RHODES, LEMUEL	La.

STUDENTS.

ROBINSON. DICK M. — La.
RAND. J. T. — La.
ROBERTSON. W. F., Jr., — Fla.
RUMPH, WM. P. — Miss.
REAGEN, G. P. — Texas.
RILEY, WM. H. — La.
ROBERTS, J. J. (M. D.) — Texas.
RAGLAND, WM. J. (M. D.) — Texas.

S

SPRAGUE, WH. H. — La.
STICKNEY, JOHN C. — Ala.
SHIFF, HENRY — La.
SMITH, LEOPOLD J. — La.
SLACK, HENRY R. — La.
SMITH, AMBROSE H. F. — La.
SHARMAN, JOHN T. — Miss.
SCOTT, WILLIAM A. — Texas.
SPENCE, ORANGE — La.
STEGER, W. C. — Texas.
STEWART, J. A. — La.
STATHAM, WM. H. — Miss.
STROUD, JONATHAN HENKEL — La.
SMITH, J. DUDLEY (M. D.) — Ark.
SWIFT, THOS. B. — Miss.
STANCELL, RENELL M. — Miss.
SMITH, H. N. — Miss.
SMITH, JOHN PETERS — Ala.
SPINILL, THOS. W. — Ala.
STEVENS, RUFUS K. — Miss.
SAMPLE, JAMES E. — Miss.
SHIVELY, CORNELIUS — La.
SPARKMAN, ACHILLES P. — Miss.
STRINGFIELD, DAVID H. — La.
SHOLARS, AUGUSTUS B. — La.
SARPY, EMILE — La.
STROOPE, S. F. — Ark.
SHERRER, F. L. — Ark.
SHIELDS. BISHLAND — Miss.
SAUNDERS, J. WALKER (M. D.) — La.
SHAW, D. (M. D.) — Texas.
SMITH, MARTIN LUTHER — La.
SAWYER, WM. TEMPLEMAN — Ala.
STROTHER, R. C. (M. D.) — La.
STEWART, J. A. — Ala.
SCHWING, SEBE D. — La.

T

TODD, CHARLES H. — La.
TEBAULT, C. H. — La.

THORPE, HENRY R. (M. D.) — Ala.
TUGGLE, ROBERT — Texas.
THORNTON, VIRGINIUS C. B. — Miss.
TREADWELL, JOEL C. — Ark.
TUBNER, RICHARD G. — Texas.
THOMPSON, H. H. — Miss.
TURPIN, STEVENSON W. — Miss.
TATE. U. O. — Miss.
TILLINGHASTE, E. L. — S. C.
THOMPSON, J. W. — Ala.
TRABUE. WM. C. — La.
THOMPSON K. (M. D.) — La.
TIRRELL, EDWARD T. — Texas.

U

UNDERWOOD, L. M. (M. D.) — Ala.
UPSHAW, W. T. (M. D.) — Ala.

V

VARNER, ALONZO H. — Ark.
VINING, P. W. — Texas.
VINSON, JNO. A. — Texas.

W

WHITE. MARCIUS B. — Ga.
WEATHERLY, ROBERT T. — Miss.
WINSTON, WM. B. — Miss.
WEATHERSBY, WILLIAM — Miss.
WELLS. JOHN R. — Ark.
WRIGHT, JOSEPH M. — Tenn.
WADE, HENRY F. (M. D.) — La.
WILLIAMS, JOHN — Miss.
WILSON, NAPOLEON B. — Miss.
WRIGHT, JAMES W. — Miss.
WALKER, SANDY A. — Miss.
WILLIS, O. R. — La.
WILLIAMS, MELVIN E. — La.
WITHERINGTON, GEORGE — Ala.
WRIGHT, P. H. — Ala.
WAGLAY, JNO. L. — La.
WILLIAMS, W. S. — Miss.
WATT, WM. (M. D.) — Texas.
WALL, EDWARD A. — Miss.
WAILL, J. G. (M. D.) — La.
WYCHE, GEORGE — Texas.
WHITE, ALFRED P. — Miss.

Y

YOUNGBLOOD, S. J. (M. D.) — La.
YERGER, WM. P. — Miss.

SUMMARY OF STUDENTS.

SESSION 1859—1860.

Louisiana	132	Florida	3
Mississippi	127	Ohio	2
Alabama	55	North Carolina	2
Texas	38	Missouri	1
Arkansas	24	Virginia	1
Georgia	6	New York	1
Tennessee	5	Choctaw District	1
South Carolina	3	Kentucky	1

402 Students.

GRADUATES—1860.

EDWARD W. BRITTON.................................Texas.
ROBERT L. LUCKETT.................................Louisiana.
JAMES HARPER......................................Arkansas.
BISLAND SHIELDS...................................Mississippi.
FRED'K L. SHERRER.................................Arkansas.
JAMES T. JOHNSON..................................Alabama.
SIDNEY R. CHAMBERS................................Louisiana.
JONATHAN H. STROUD................................Louisiana.
THOS. M. MARKS....................................Louisiana.
PRESTON E. BUCKNER................................Louisiana.
WILLIAM C. MURPHY.................................Alabama.
WILLIAM A. ROBERTSON..............................Louisiana.
JOHN W. COLLINS...................................Alabama.
ROBT. F. MOODY....................................Alabama.
ROBT. A. LEE......................................Alabama.
CHARLES W. HILL...................................Mississippi.
SAMUEL PARKER.....................................Alabama.
DANIEL PARKER.....................................Alabama.
JOHN R. MONTGOMERY................................Louisiana.
CHARLES M. CURELL.................................Louisiana.
PETER R. FORD.....................................Arkansas.
JOHN B. GINN......................................Mississippi.
JOHN P. DAVIS.....................................Mississippi.
FONTAIN DE G. GARRETT.............................Mississippi.
AUGUSTUS L EAST...................................Louisiana.
WILLIAM A. PORTWOOD...............................Mississippi.
JOHN L. WAGLEY....................................Louisiana.
VANDY M. NEAL.....................................Alabama.
RICHMOND P. AUSTIN................................Mississippi.
JOHN A. McCREARY..................................Alabama.
WILLIAM G. GAMBLE.................................Alabama.
WILLIAM H. CUNNINGHAM.............................Mississippi.
RICHARD G. TURNER.................................Texas.
MILES W. GOLDSBY..................................Louisiana.
JONES C. ABERNETHY................................Alabama.
PEYTON W. VINING..................................Texas.
JAMES W. WRIGHT...................................Mississippi.
STEPHEN E. CUNY...................................Louisiana.
JOHN W. GUERRANT..................................Tennessee.
JOHN CAMERON......................................Texas.
DERRICK P. JANUARY, JR............................Louisiana.
NATHAN B. KENNEDY.................................Alabama.
PATRICK H. WRIGHT.................................Alabama.
MOSES R. DENMAN...................................Texas.
WILLIAM E. MADDOX.................................Texas.
JOHN JORDAN.......................................Tennessee.
JAMES V. COOK.....................................Mississippi.
AUGUSTUS W. EGAN..................................Louisiana.
WILLIAM H. STATHAM................................Mississippi.
WILLIAM C. TRABUE.................................Louisiana.
ERASMUS F. GRIFFIN................................Mississippi.
LEANDER G HUNT....................................North Carolina.
JAMES M HOLCOMBE..................................Arkansas.
LEMUEL RHODES.....................................Louisiana.
RUFUS K. STEVENS..................................Mississippi.
BENJAMIN F. PASSMORE..............................Mississippi.

GRADUATES.

FRANK RAINEY..Texas.
JOHN M NUCKOLLS..Alabama.
JACK PHILLIPS..Alabama.
URIAH O. TATE...Mississippi.
JOHN FROST..Mississippi.
WILLIAM B. KING...Mississippi.
WILLIAM WEATHERSBY..Mississippi.
JOHN A. STEWART...Louisiana.
FRANK NAILER...Mississippi.
CICERO C. BATES..Louisiana.
SHERROD G. LUCKETT...Mississippi.
FRANKLIN M. GILBERT..Mississippi.
JACKSON M. GILBERT...Mississippi.
LEMUEL RICHARDSON..Mississippi.
JAMES W. JACKSON...Louisiana.
JAMES W. FRAZER..Arkansas.
GEORGE BADGER..North Carolina.
SAMUEL L. BONNER...Alabama.
GEORGE WYCHE...Texas.
JOHN P. SMITH..Alabama.
ORLANDO A. HOBSON..Mississippi.
JOHN N. ELLIOTT..Mississippi.
JEFFERSON J. LITTLE..Mississippi.
THOMAS B. HARWOOD..Alabama.
SAMUEL N. CASTON...Mississippi.
WILLIAM F. ROBERTSON Jr....................................Florida.
WALTER LEWIS...Texas.
EPHRIAM A. BREVARD...Florida.
ELAM J. HOPE...Mississippi.
WILLIAM T. SAWYER..Alabama.
FRANKLIN G. JOHNSON..Mississippi.
GEORGE W. POSEY..Alabama.
SAMUEL P. LEWIS..Mississippi.
JOHN H. BRACK..Mississippi.
RICHARD T. PACKWOOD..New York.
BENJAMIN F. BROWN..Louisiana.
WILLIAM M. GUICE...Louisiana.
MARTIN L. SMITH..Louisiana.
EUGENE M. KIDD...Louisiana.
JOHN B. HOWELL...Louisiana.
JOHN W. JONES..Louisiana.
TITUS T. HOLLIDAY..Mississippi.
ALEX. S. De LEE..Louisiana.
JOSEPH A. La NEUVILLE (in Pharmacy)........................Louisiana.
ALFRED A. ALSTON...Alabama.
EDWIN A. BONNEAU...Alabama.
JAMES PURVIANCE..Louisiana.
WILLIAM H. McCORD..Tennessee.
JOSEPH W. THOMPSON...Alabama.
SAMUEL S. NOEL...Mississippi.
THOMAS B. COOK...Mississippi.
WILLIAM H. SPRAGUE...Louisiana.
JOHN J. GARDNER..Louisiana.
SANFORD S. RIDDELL...Louisiana.
CHARLES W GIBSON...Mississippi.
WILLIAM J. LEE...Alabama.
BENJAMIN J. A. AVENT.......................................Mississippi.-113

Lightning Source UK Ltd.
Milton Keynes UK
UKHW012130180219
337529UK00012B/1410/P